F. J. Stucker • C. de Souza • G. S. Kenyon • T. S. Lian • W. Draf • B. Schick (Eds.)

Rhinology and Facial Plastic Surgery

F. J. Stucker • C. de Souza • G. S. Kenyon
T. S. Lian • W. Draf • B. Schick (Eds.)

Rhinology and Facial Plastic Surgery

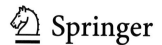 Springer

Fred J. Stucker, MD, FACS
Professor and Chair
Department of Otolaryngology
Louisiana State University
Health Science Center
1501 Kings Highway
Shreveport, LA 71130
USA
E-mail: fstuck@lsuhsc.edu

Chris de Souza, MS, DORL, DNB, FACS
Visiting Assistant Professor in Otolaryngology
State University of New York
Brooklyn
USA
Visiting Assistant Professor in Otolaryngology
Louisiana State University
Health Sciences Center
Shreveport
USA
ENT and Skull base Surgeon
The Tata Memorial Hospital, Lilavati Hospital,
Holy Family Hospital
Mumbai
India
E-mail: christ@mtnl.net.in, Christ@vsnl.com

Guy S. Kenyon, MD, FRCS
Whipps Cross Hospital
Department of Otolaryngology
Whipps Cross Road
Leytonstone, E11 1NR
UK
E-mail: GuyKenyon@aol.com

Timothy S. Lian, MD, FACS
Louisiana State University
Health Science Center
Dept. of Otolaryngology
1501 Kings Highway
Shreveport, LA 71130
USA
E-mail: TLian@lsuhsc.edu

Wolfgang Draf, MD, FRCS
Professor, Director of the Department of Ear,
Nose and Throat Diseases, Head and Neck Surgery
International Neuroscience Institute
at the University of Magdeburg(INI)
Rudolf-Pichlmayr-Str. 4
30625 Hannover
Germany
E-mail: wdraf@aol.com

Bernhard Schick, MD
Professor, Department of Otolaryngology
University Homburg/Saar
Kirrberger Straße
66421 Homburg/Saar
Germany
E-mail: bernhard.schick@uniklinikum-saarland.de

ISBN 978-3-540-74379-8   e-ISBN 978-3-540-74380-4

DOI 10.1007/978-3-540-74380-4

Springer Dordrecht Heidelberg London New York

Library of Congress Control Number: 2008929504

© Springer-Verlag Berlin Heidelberg 2009

Cover design: Frido Steinen-Broo, eStudioCalamar, Figueres/Berlin

Typesetting and Production: le-tex publishing services oHG, Leipzig, Germany

Printed on acid-free paper

Springer is part of Springer Science + Business Media (www.springer.com)

Dedication

To our persistently supportive families and our bright younger colleagues.

Preface

Georg von Bekesey was awarded the Nobel Prize for his seminal work on hearing. It was, however, 43 years later in 2004 that Linda Buck and Richard Axel were awarded the Nobel Prize for their work on olfaction. This is indicative of how the science of rhinology is only now coming into its own. For quite some time, rhinology was thought to be limited in scope. It is now appreciated that the nose is not only an organ of aesthetic appeal, but one that carries out several important, complex functions. The tremendous surge in medical literature in recent times bears witness to this.

The emerging scientific literature involves not only basic sciences, well-planned clinical trials, analyses, and meta-analyses, but also involves astute clinical observation. This is all directed toward good clinical medicine as it should be practiced. Sifting through the vast lists of trials and publications is a daunting task for most practicing rhinologists. The editors thought that a comprehensive book addressing aesthetics, trauma, and the recent rhinological issues would be valuable and helpful for students and practitioners to understand how the nose, paranasal sinuses, and the upper respiratory function in health and how disease affects it. It was with this purpose in mind that this book was written. Most work in rhinology is directed at bringing about uniformity and universality. Uniformity, so as to bring about a commonality in all terms, and staging systems for everyone all over the world. In other words it is directed toward evolving a common scientific language that is spoken uniformly and consistently all over the world. Universality, so that norms, staging systems, etc., can be applied anywhere in the world with equal validity. This can only be achieved through consensus. This book contains not only the genesis and pathogenesis of rhinologic disease, but also what all surgeons want and that is operative steps to bring about successful resolution of disease, with the return of normal function.

All the editors would like to thank the authors for graciously co-operating and contributing to this book. We would also like to thank their families for allowing the authors the time to participate. We thank our families for their help, encouragement, and support.

I would also like to thank Ms. Amy Ray for her help. She has put the extra into the ordinary giving real meaning to the word extraordinary. Amy Ray has been pivotal in this book and has helped resolve many tasks successfully. Amy has been proactive, encouraging, always helpful and continually gracious and generous with her time and help. I don't think we would have been able to complete this book without Amy's assistance. We would like to thank our publishers, Marion Phillip and Irmela Bohn of Springer Verlag, for their kind encouragement, courteousness, and efficient help.

The Editors
January 2009

Contents

Clinical Assessment, Management, Surgery of the Internal Nose

Tumors of the Nose, Paranasal Sinuses, Jaws, Skull Base and Related Problems

Section II
Endonasal Endoscopic Surgery
Bernhard Schick (Editor) and
Wolfgang Draf (Senior Editor)

Anatomy and Imaging

Instrumentation

Endoscopic Surgery of the Nose,
Paranasal Sinuses, and Orbit

Contributors

Bryan T. Ambro
Division of Facial Plastic and Reconstructive Surgery
Department of Otorhinolaryngology – Head and Neck Surgery
University of Maryland Medical Center
16 South Eutaw Street, Suite 500
Baltimore, MD 21201
USA
E-mail: bryanambro@yahoo.com

Vijay K. Anand
Department of Otolaryngology – Head and Neck Surgery
New York Presbyterian Hospital – Weill Medical College
of Cornell University
New York, NY
USA
E-mail: vijayanandmd@aol.com

Peter Andrew
Royal National Throat, Nose and Ear Hospital
London
UK

Marcelo B. Antunes
Department of Otorhinolaryngology – Head and Neck Surgery
University of Pennsylvania
Philadelphia, PA
USA

Farhad Ardeshirpour
Department of Otolaryngology – Head and Neck Surgery
University of North Carolina School of Medicine
Chapel Hill, NC 27599-7070
USA
E-mail: Farhad_ardeshirpour@med.unc.edu

Claus Bachert
Upper Airways Research Laboratory
Department of Otorhinolaryngology
Ghent University
De Pintelaan 185
9000 Ghent
Belgium
E-mail: claus.bachert@ugent.be

Rami K. Batniji
Batniji Facial Plastic Surgery
361 Hospital Road, Suite 329
Newport Beach, CA 92663
USA

Pete S. Batra
Section of Nasal and Sinus Disorders, Head and Neck Institute
Cleveland Clinic Foundation
9500 Euclid Avenue, A71
Cleveland, OH 44195
USA
E-mail: Batrap@ccf.org

Manuel Bernal-Sprekelsen
Servicio de Otorrinolaringología
Hospital Clínic
Barcelona
Spain
E-mail: mbernal@clinic.ub.es

Maurizio Bignami
ENT Department
University of Insubria
Ospedale di Circolo Fondazione Macchi
Viale Borri 57
21100 Varese
Italy
E-mail: m.bigno@virgilio.it

William Binder
University of California–Los Angeles
120 S. Spalding Dr, Suite 340
Beverly Hills, CA 90212-1800
USA
E-mail: info@doctorbinder.com

Andrew Blitzer
Director, NY Center for Voice and Swallowing Disorders
Columbia University
425 W. 59th Street, 10th floor
New York, NY 10019
USA
E-mail: Ab1136@aol.com

Ulrike Bockmühl
Head of the Department of Otorhinolaryngology
Head and Neck Surgery
Klinikum Kassel GmbH
Teaching Hospital of the Philipps-University Marburg
Möncheberstr. 41–43
34125 Kassel
Germany
Email: bockmuehl@klinikum-kassel.de

Aaron I. Brescia
Resident in Otolaryngology, Department of Otolaryngology –
Head and Neck Surgery
University of Cincinnati College of Medicine
Cincinnati, OH
USA

Itzhak Brook
Georgetown University School of Medicine
4431 Albemarle Street, NW
Washington, DC 20016
USA
E-mail: ib6@georgetown.edu, dribrook@yahoo.com

Dominik Brors
Department of Otorhinolaryngology – Head and Neck Surgery
Ruhr University Bochum
St. Elisabeth Hospital
44787 Bochum
Germany
E-mail: dominik.brors@rub.de

Seth M. Brown
Clinical Assistant Professor
University of Connecticut School of Medicine
and
The Connecticut Sinus Institute
12 North Main St., Suite 30
West Hartford, CT 06107
USA
E-mail: sethmbrown@msn.com

Alan R. Burningham
Department of Otolaryngology – Head and Neck Surgery
Louisiana State University Health Sciences Center–Shreveport
1501 Kings Highway
Shreveport, LA 71130
USA
E-mail: alanburningham@hotmail.com,
ABurningham@tpcllp.com

Gabriel G. Calzada
The Bobby R. Alford Department of Otolaryngology –
Head and Neck Surgery
Baylor College of Medicine
Houston, TX
USA

Cecilia Canto-Alarcon
Geisinger Medical Center
Danville, PA
USA

Randolph B. Capone
The Baltimore Center for Facial Plastic Surgery
Johns Hopkins Medical Institutions
6535 North Charles Street #250
Baltimore, MD 21204
USA
E-mail: rcapone@jhmi.edu

Johnny Cappiello
Department of Otorhinolaryngology – Head and Neck Surgery
University of Brescia
25123 Brescia
Italy
E-mail: cappiell@aliceposta.it

Paolo Castelnuovo
II Department of Otorhinolaryngology
Ospedale di Circolo
Fondazione Macchi
University of Insubria
21100 Varese
Italy
E-mail: paologc@tin.it

Javier Cervera-Escario
Servicio de Otorrinolaringología
Hospital Universitario Niño Jesús
Madrid
Spain
E-mail: javiercerver@seorl.net

Anders Cervin
Department of Otorhinolaryngology
Helsingborg Hospital
Department of Clinical Sciences
Lund University
Lund
Sweden
E-mail: anders.cervin@skane.se

Rakesh K. Chandra
Assistant Professor
Northwestern Sinus and Allergy Center
Department of Otolaryngology – Head and Neck Surgery
Northwestern University Feinberg School of Medicine
675 North St Clair, Galter Pavilion 15-200
Chicago, IL 60611
USA
E-mail: RickChandra@hotmail.com

Jon B. Chadwell
Chadwell Facial Plastic Surgery
621 Memorial Drive, Suite 403
South Bend, IN 46601
USA
E-mail: chadwejb@hotmail.com

Martin J. Citardi
Section of Nasal and Sinus Disorders, Head and Neck Institute
Cleveland Clinic Foundation
9500 Euclid Avenue, A71
Cleveland, OH 44195
USA

Sofie Claeys
Upper Airways Research Laboratory
Department of Otorhinolaryngology
Ghent University
De Pintelaan 185
9000 Ghent
Belgium
E-mail: sem.claeys@ugent.be

Noam A. Cohen
Division of Rhinology, Department of Otorhinolaryngology – Head and Neck Surgery
University of Pennsylvania Medical Center
5th Floor Ravdin Building
3400 Spruce Street
Philadelphia, PA 19104
USA
E-mail: Noam.cohen@uphs.upenn.edu

Jannis Constantinidis
Associate Professor, Department of Otorhinolaryngology – Head and Neck Surgery
Aristotle University of Thessaloniki
AHEPA-Hospital, 54 006
Thessaloniki
Greece
E-mail: janconst@otenet.gr

Edwin A. Cortez
14241 Metcalf
Overland Park, KS 66223
USA
E-mail: cortezfps@aol.com

Dary Costa
St. Louis University Department of Otolaryngology – Head and Neck Surgery
6th floor Deslodge Towers
3635 Vista Ave
St. Louis, MO 63110
USA
E-mail: costadj@slu.edu

A. Daudia
Specialist Registrar in Otorhinolaryngology
Queens Medical Centre
University of Nottingham
Nottingham
UK

Francesca De Bernardi
ENT Department
University of Insubria
Ospedale di Circolo Fondazione Macchi
Viale Borri 57
21100 Varese
Italy
E-mail: francescadebernardi@hotmail.com

Louis M. DeJoseph
4553 N. Shallowford Road, Suite 20B
Atlanta, GA 30338-6408
USA

Giovanni Delù
ENT Department
University of Insubria
Ospedale di Circolo Fondazione Macchi
Viale Borri 57
21100 Varese
Italy
E-mail: giovannidelu@tin.it

Joshua C. Demke
Department of Otolaryngology – Head and Neck Surgery
University of North Carolina School of Medicine
Chapel Hill
North Carolina 27599-7070
USA
E-mail: jdemke@unch.unc.edu

Chris de Souza
Visiting Assistant Professor in Otolaryngology
State University of New York
Brooklyn
USA
Visiting Assistant Professor in Otolaryngology
Louisiana State University
Health Sciences Center
Shreveport
USA
ENT and Skull base Surgeon
The Tata Memorial Hospital, Lilavati Hospital,
Holy Family Hospital
Mumbai
India
E-mail: christ@mtnl.net.in, Christ@vsnl.com

Rosemarie A. de Souza
Associate Professor, Department of Internal Medicine
Sion Hospital and LTMG Medical College
Mumbai
India

Anand K. Devaiah
Department of Otolaryngology – Head and Neck Surgery
Boston University School of Medicine
Boston, MA
USA

Matthew J. Dickson
4553 N. Shallowford Road, Suite 20B
Atlanta, GA 30338-6408
USA

Julia Dlugaiczyk
Department of Otolaryngology – Head and Neck Surgery
Friedrich-Alexander University Erlangen-Nuremberg
91054 Erlangen
Germany

Wolfgang Draf
Director of the Department of Ear, Nose and Throat Diseases,
Head and Neck Surgery
International Neuroscience Institute at the University
of Magdeburg (INI)
Rudolf-Pichlmayr-Str. 4
30625 Hannover
Germany
E-mail: wdraf@aol.com

David A. F. Ellis
University of Toronto, About Face Surgical Center
167 Sheppard Avenue West
Toronto, ON M2N 1M9
Canada
E-mail: ellis2106@gmail.com

Ravindhra G. Elluru
Cincinnati Children's Hospital Medical Center
3333 Burnett Avenue, MLC 2018
Cincinnati, OH 45229
USA
E-mail: ravi.elluru@cchmc.org

Fred G. Fedok
Department of Otolaryngology/HNS
Penn State Milton S. Hershey Medical Center
500 University Drive, MC H091
Hershey, PA 17033
USA
E-mail: ffedok@psu.edu

Dan M. Fliss
Department of Otolaryngology – Head and Neck Surgery
Tel-Aviv Sourasky Medical Center
6 Weizmann St.
Tel-Aviv 64239
Israel
E-mail: danf@tasmc.health.gov.il

Philippe Gevaert
Department of Otorhinolaryngology
Upper Airways Research Laboratory
Ghent University
De Pintelaan 185
9000 Ghent
Belgium
E-mail: philippe.gevaert@ugent.be

Ziv Gil
Department of Otolaryngology – Head and Neck Surgery
Tel-Aviv Sourasky Medical Center
6 Weizmann St.
Tel-Aviv 64239
Israel
E-mail: ziv@baseofskull.org

David Goldenberg
Department of Otolaryngology – Head and Neck Surgery
Penn State Milton S. Hershey Medical Center
500 University Drive, MC H091
Hershey, PA 17033
USA
E-mail: dgoldenberg@hmc.psu.edu

Richard L. Goode
Stanford University School of Medicine
300 Pasteur Drive, R135
Stanford, CA 94305
USA
E-mail: goode@stanford.edu

Parul Goyal
Division of Rhinology
Department of Otolaryngology
SUNY Upstate Medical University
Syracuse, NY
USA

Leslie C. Grammer
Division of Allergy and Immunology, Department of Medicine
676 N St Clair, Searle Building 12-561
Chicago, IL 60611
USA

Lisa D. Grunebaum
Division of Facial Plastic and Reconstructive Surgery
Department of Otolaryngology – Head and Neck Surgery
University of Miami
Miami, FL 33124
USA

José-María Guilemany-Toste
Servicio de Otorrinolaringología
Hospital Clínic
Barcelona
Spain
E-mail: 33785jgt@comb.es

C. William Hanson
Department of Otorhinolaryngology – Head and Neck Surgery
University of Pennsylvania
Philadelphia, PA 19104
USA

Gady Har-El
Chairman, Department of Otolaryngology –
Head and Neck Surgery, Lenox Hill Hospital
Professor of Otolaryngology and Neurosurgery
SUNY-Downstate Medical Center
186 East 76th Street, 2nd Floor
New York, NY 10021
USA
E-mail: gadyh@aol.com

Erich Hofmann
Klinik für Diagnostische und Interventionelle Neuroradiologie
Klinikum Fulda gAG
Pacelliallee 4
36043 Fulda
Germany
E-mail: ehofmann.raz@klinikum-fulda.de

Eric H. Holbrook
Massachusetts Eye and Ear Infirmary
Harvard Medical School
243 Charles Street
Boston, MA 02114
USA
E-mail: Eric_Holbrook@meei.harvard.edu

Peter H. Hwang
Stanford Sinus Center
Department of Otolaryngology
Stanford University School of Medicine
Stanford, CA
USA

Bhavin Jankharia
Jankharia Imaging
Bhaveshwar Vihar, 383, Sardar V.P. Road
Mumbai 400004, Maharashtra
India
E-mail: bhavin@jankharia.com

Gert Jeunen
Department of Otolaryngology
Gasthuisberg University Hospital
Catholic University of Leuven
3000 Leuven
Belgium
E-mail: gert.jeunen@gmail.com

Nicholas S. Jones
Professor of Otorhinolaryngology
Queens Medical Centre
University of Nottingham
Nottingham
UK

Mark Jorissen
Ear, Nose, and Throat Department
University Hospital Leuven
Gasthuisberg
Herestraat 49
3000 Leuven
Belgium
E-mail: mark.jorissen@uz.kuleuven.ac.be

Seth J. Kanowitz
Section of Nasal and Sinus Disorders
Head and Neck Institute
Cleveland Clinic Foundation
9500 Euclid Avenue, A71
Cleveland, OH 44195
USA

Guy S. Kenyon
Whipps Cross Hospital
Department of Otolaryngology
Whipps Cross Road
Leytonstone, E11 1NR
UK
E-mail: GuyKenyon@aol.com

Bounmany Kyle Keojampa
Department of Neurological Surgery
Boston University School of Medicine
USA

Robert C. Kern
Department of Otolaryngology – Head and Neck Surgery
Northwestern University Feinberg School of Medicine
Searle Building 12-561
303 E. Chicago Avenue
Chicago, IL 60611
USA
E-mail: r-kern@northwestern.edu

Karen A. Kölln
Department of Otolaryngology – Head and Neck Surgery
UNC-CH School of Medicine
1115 Bioinformatics Bldg. CB# 7070
Chapel Hill, NC 27599-7070
USA
E-mail: KKolln@unch.unc.edu

Mimi S. Kokoska
Otolaryngology – Head and Neck Surgery
Surgical Services (112)
Indianapolis VAMC
1481 W. 10th Street
Indianapolis, IN 46202
USA
E-mail: mimi.kokoska2@va.gov

Iordanis Konstantinidis
First Otorhinolaryngology Department
Aristotle University
Thessaloniki
Greece
E-mail: jokons57@hotmail.com

Stilianos E. Kountakis
Professor of Otolaryngology
Medical College of Georgia
1120 15th Street
Augusta, GA 30907
USA
E-mail: skountakis@mcg.edu

Russell W.H. Kridel
Facial Plastic Surgery Association
6655 Travis Street, Suite 900
Houston, TX 77030-1336
USA
E-mail: rkridel@todaysface.com

John H. Krouse
Department of Otolaryngology – Head and Neck Surgery
Wayne State University
Detroit, MI
USA
E-mail: jkrouse@med.wayne.edu

Jeffrey B. LaCour
Department of Otolaryngology – Head and Neck Surgery
UNC-CH School of Medicine
1115 Bioinformatics Bldg. CB# 7070
Chapel Hill, NC 27599-7070
USA
E-mail: jlacou1@yahoo.com

Wayne F. Larrabee, Jr.
University of Washington
600 Broadway, Suite 280
Seattle, WA 98122-5395
USA
E-mail: larrabee@u.washington.edu

Samson Lee
Lake Washington Facial Plastic Surgery
Bellevue, WA 98008
USA

Donald A. Leopold
Department of Otolaryngology – Head and Neck Surgery
University of Nebraska Medical Center
USA
E-mail: dleopold@unmc.edu

Davide Locatelli
Department of Neurosurgery
University of Pavia
IRCCS Policlinico San Matteo
27100 Pavia
Italy
E-mail: dlocatelli@smatteo.pv.it

Anthony E. Magit
Rady Children's Hospital of San Diego
University of California at San Diego School of Medicine
3030 Children's Way, Suite 402
San Diego, CA 92123
USA
E-mail: amagit@aol.com

Devinder S. Mangat
8044 Montgomery Road, Suite 230
Cinncinati, OH 45236-2919
USA
E-mail: mangat@renewyourlooks.com

Evelyn Linda Maxwell
University of Toronto, About Face Surgical Center
167 Sheppard Avenue West
Toronto, ON M2N 1M9
Canada
E-mail: lindamaxwell22@gmail.com

Susanne Mayr
Department of Otolaryngology – Head and Neck Surgery
Friedrich-Alexander University Erlangen-Nuremberg
91054 Erlangen
Germany
E-mail: susanne.mayr@hno.imed.uni-erlangen.de

Kevin Christopher McMains
Assistant Professor of Otolaryngology
University of Texas Health Science Center at San Antonio
7703 Floyd Curl Drive MC-7777
San Antonio, TX 78229
USA
E-mail: mcmains@uthscsa.edu

Pushkar Mehra
Director, Department of Oral and Maxillofacial Surgery
Boston University Medical Center and Boston Medical Center
Associate Professor and Vice-Chairman
Department of Oral and Maxillofacial Surgery
Boston University School of Dental Medicine
Boston, MA 02118
USA
E-mail: pushkar.mehra@bmc.org

Ralph B. Metson
Department of Otolaryngology
Massachusetts Eye and Ear Infirmary
Zero Emerson Place
Boston, MA 02114
USA
E-mail: Ralph_metson@meei.harvard.edu

Olaf Michel
Poliklinik für Hals-Nasen-Ohrenheilkunde der Universität
zu Köln
Joseph-Stelzmann-Str. 9
50924 Köln-Lindenthal
Germany
E-mail: michel@unikoeln.de.

Giorgio Minonzio
Service of Neuroradiology
Ospedale di Circolo Fondazione Macchi
Viale Borri 57
21100 Varese
Italy
E-mail: giorgiomnnz@alice.it

Amir Minovi
Ruhr University Bochum
Department of Otorhinolaryngology – Head and Neck Surgery
St. Elisabeth Hospital
44787 Bochum
Germany
E-mail: minovi@web.de

Cristina Molina-Martínez
Servicio de Otorrinolaringología
Hospital Clínic
Barcelona
Spain
E-mail: crismol2000@hotmail.com

Robert G. Mynatt
Department of Otolaryngology – Head and Neck Surgery
St. Louis University School of Medicine
3635 Vista Avenue, 6 FDT
St. Louis, MO 63110
USA
E-mail: mynattrg@slu.edu

Piero Nicolai
Department of Otorhinolaryngology – Head and Neck Surgery
University of Brescia
25123 Brescia
Italy
E-mail: pieronicolai@virgilio.it

Erin K. O'Brien
Department of Otolaryngology – Head and Neck Surgery
University of Iowa Hospitals and Clinics
Iowa City, IA
USA

Michael P. Ondik
Department of Otolaryngology – Head and Neck Surgery
Penn State Milton S. Hershey Medical Center
500 University Drive, MC H091
Hershey, PA 17033
USA
E-mail: mondik@hmc.psu.edu

James N. Palmer
Department of Otorhinolaryngology – Head and Neck Surgery
University of Pennsylvania Health System
5 Ravdin, 3400 Spruce Street
Philadelphia, PA 19104
USA
E-mail: James.Palmer@uphs.upenn.edu

Ira D. Papel
The Facial Plastic Surgicenter, Ltd.
Johns Hopkins University
1838 Greene Tree Road
Baltimore, MD 21208-6391
USA
E-mail: idpmd@aol.com

Sunny S. Park
Department of Otolaryngology – Head and Neck Surgery
Penn State Milton S. Hershey Medical Center
500 University Drive, MC H091
Hershey, PA 17033
USA
E-mail: spark@psu.edu

Stephen W. Perkins
170 W. 106th Street
Perkins FPC, P.C.
Indianapolis, IN 46290-1004
USA
E-mail: sperkins@perkinsvannatta.com

Cesare Piazza
Department of Otorhinolaryngology – Head and Neck Surgery
University of Brescia
25123 Brescia
Italy
E-mail: ceceplaza@libero.it

John Pickett
Department of Medical Physics
Barts and the London NHS Trust
London E1 1BB
UK

Andrea Pistochini
Department of Otorhinolaryngology
University of Insubria
Azienda Ospedaliera-Universitaria
Ospedale di Circolo e Fondazione Macchi
Varese
Italy
E-mail: andrea.pistochini@virgilio.it

Jack W. Pou
Louisiana State University Health Sciences Center
1501 Kings Highway
Shreveport, LA 71130
USA

Andreas Prescher
Institut für Neuroanatomie
Universitätsklinikum der RWTH Aachen
Wendlingweg 2
52074 Aachen
Germany
E-mail: aprescher@ukaachen.de

Paul Presti
Lenox Hill Hospital
135 E. 74th Street
New York, NY 10021-3272
USA

Todd W. Preston
Department of Otolaryngology – Head and Neck Surgery
Penn State Milton S. Hershey Medical Center
500 University Drive, MC H091
Hershey, PA 17033
USA
E-mail: subglottis@hotmail.com

Edmund A. Pribitkin
Professor, Academic Vice Chairman
Department of Otolaryngology – Head & Neck Surgery
Thomas Jefferson University
925 Chestnut Street
Sixth Floor
Philadelphia, PA 19107
USA
E-mail: edmund.pribitkin@jefferson.edu

Christopher N. Prichard
The Bobby R. Alford Department of Otolaryngology –
Head and Neck Surgery
Baylor College of Medicine
Houston, TX
USA

Abhijit A. Raut
Lecturer, Radiology Department
Seth G S Medical College and KEM Hospital, Parel
Mumbai
India
E-mail: abhijitaraut@gmail.com

Douglas D. Reh
Department of Otolaryngology, Massachusetts Eye and Ear
Infirmary
Zero Emerson Place
Boston, MA 02114
USA
E-mail: Douglas_reh@meei.harvard.edu

J. Peter Rodrigues
Honorary Head, Department of Otolaryngology
St. Georges Hospital
Mumbai
India

Thomas Romo
Lenox Hill Hospital
135 E. 74th Street
New York, NY 10021-3272
USA
E-mail: docromo@aol.com

Scott B. Roofe
Division of Facial Plastic and Reconstructive Surgery
Department of Otolaryngology – Head and Neck Surgery
Madigan Army Medical Center
9040 Fitzsimmons Drive
Tacoma, WA 98431
USA
E-mail: scottroofe@hotmail.com

Thomas Sanford
Department of Otolaryngology – Head and Neck Surgery
St. Louis University
3635 Vista Ave, 6th Floor Deslodge Towers
St. Louis, MO 63110
USA
E-mail: tsanfor@slu.edu

Bernhard Schick
Professor, Department of Otolaryngology
University Homburg/Saar
Kirrberger Straße
66421 Homburg/Saar
Germany
E-mail: bernhard.schick@uniklinikum-saarland.de

Jerome S. Schwartz
St. Luke's–Roosevelt Hospital Center
NY Center for Voice and Swallowing Disorders
425 W. 59th Street, 10th floor
New York, NY 10019
USA
E-mail: jeromeschwartz@hotmail.com

Kristin A. Seiberling
Department of Otolaryngology – Head and Neck Surgery
Northwestern University, Feinberg School of Medicine
303 E. Chicago Avenue
Chicago, IL 60611
USA

Allen M. Seiden
Professor of Otolaryngology, Department of Otolaryngology –
Head and Neck Surgery
University of Cincinnati College of Medicine
231 Albert Sabin Way #6413MSB
Cincinnati, OH 45267-0528
USA
E-mail: seidenam@ucmail.uc.edu

Brent A. Senior
Department of Otolaryngology – Head and Neck Surgery
University of North Carolina School of Medicine
Chapel Hill, NC 27599-7070
USA
E-mail: brent_senior@med.unc.edu

Gary Y. Shaw
Kansas City University of Medicine and Biomedical Sciences
296 NE Tudor Road
Lee's Summit, MO 54086
USA
E-mail: gshawmd@kc.rr.com

James R. Shire
6151 Shallowford Road, Suite 101
Chattanooga, TN 37421-1616
USA
E-mail: drshire@comcast.net

William E. Silver
4553 N. Shallowford Road, Suite 20B
Atlanta, GA 30338-6408
USA
E-mail: wesilver@PICosmeticSurgery.com

Robert L. Simons
16800 NW 2nd Street, Suite 607
North Miami Beach, FL 33169-5549
USA
E-mail: drsimons@miami-institute.com

Raj Sindwani
Associate Professor of Otolaryngology
Chief of Rhinology & Sinus Surgery
Saint Louis University School of Medicine
Saint Louis University Hospital
3635 Vista Ave, 6 FDT,
Saint Louis, MO 63110
USA
E-mail: sindwani@slu.edu

Peyman Soliemanzadeh
Director of Facial Plastic Surgery
Profiles Beverly Hills
Division of Otolaryngology – Head and Neck Surgery
Cedars Sinai Hospital
Beverly Hills, CA 90211
USA

Phillip C. Song
St. Luke's–Roosevelt Hospital Center
NY Center for Voice and Swallowing Disorders
425 W. 59th Street, 10th floor
New York, NY 10019
USA
E-mail: songphillip@yahoo.com

Melissa Statham
Resident in Otolaryngology, Department of Otolaryngology –
Head and Neck Surgery
University of Cincinnati College of Medicine
Cincinnati, OH
USA

Natalie P. Steele
Department of Otolaryngology – Head and Neck Surgery
University of Illinois at Chicago
1855 West Taylor Street, M/C 648
Chicago, IL 60612
USA

Fred J. Stucker
Professor and Chair
Department of Otolaryngology
Louisiana State University
Health Science Center
1501 Kings Highway
Shreveport, LA 71130
USA
e-mail: fstuck@lsuhsc.edu

Matthew R. Stumpe
Chief Resident, Department of Otolaryngology – Head and Neck Surgery
University of Tennessee Health Science Center
956 Court Avenue, Coleman Building, Suite B224
Memphis, TN 38128
USA
E-mail: mstumpe@utmem.edu

Andrew C. Swift
University Hospital Aintree
Lower lane
Liverpool L9 7AL
United Kingdom
E-mail: andrew_swift@yahoo.com

Jonathan Sykes
2521 Stockton Blvd., Suite 7200
Sacramento, CA 95817-2207
USA
E-mail: jonathan.sykes@ucdmc.ucdavis.edu

Abtin Tabaee
Department of Otolaryngology – Head and Neck Surgery
Beth Israel Medical Center – Albert Einstein College of Medicine
New York, New York
USA
E-mail: atabaee@hotmail.com

Erica R. Thaler
Department of Otorhinolaryngology – Head and Neck Surgery
University of Pennsylvania
Philadelphia, PA 19104
USA
E-mail: Erica.Thaler@uphs.upenn.edu

J. Regan Thomas
Department of Otolaryngology – Head and Neck Surgery
University of Illinois at Chicago
1855 West Taylor Street, M/C 648
Chicago, IL 60612
USA
E-mail: thomasrj@uic.edu

Davide Tomenzoli
Department of Otorhinolaryngology – Head and Neck Surgery
University of Brescia
25123 Brescia
Italy
E-mail: davidetomenzoli@virgilio.it

Alessandro Varini
Department of Otorhinolaryngology
Casa di Cura Salus
Via Bonaparte 4
34123 Trieste
Italy
E-mail: alevarin@tin.it

Shyan Vijayasekaran
Otolaryngology/Head and Neck Surgery
Princess Margaret Hospital for Children
Subiaco
Australia

Trang Vo-Nguyen
Louisiana State University Health Sciences Center
1501 Kings Highway
Shreveport, LA 71130
USA

Emre A. Vural
Otolaryngology – Head and Neck Surgery
John McClellan VA Hospital
Little Rock, AR
USA
and
Department of Otolaryngology – Head and Neck Surgery
University of Arkansas for Medical Sciences
Little Rock, AR
USA
E-mail: vuralemrea@uams.edu

Ben Wallwork
Department of Otorhinolaryngology
Princess Alexandra Hospital
School of Biomolecular and Biomedical Science
Griffith University
Brisbane
Australia

Jeremy Paul Watkins
Department of Otolaryngology
University of Tennessee
956 Court Avenue
Memphis, TN 38163
USA

Rainer Weber
Division of Paranasal Sinus and Skull Base Surgery, Traumatology
Department of ENT
Hospital Karlsruhe
Moltkestrasse 90
76133 Karlsruhe
Germany
E-mail: rainer.weber@klinikum-karlsruhe.com

Randal S. Weber
Professor and Chairman, Department of Head and Neck Surgery
University of Texas MD Anderson Cancer Center
1515 Holcombe Blvd
Houston, TX 77030
USA
E-mail: rsweber@mdanderson.org

Glenn B. Williams
Department of Otolaryngology – Head and Neck Surgery
University of Tennessee
956 Court Avenue
Memphis, TN 38163
USA

Bradford A. Woodworth
Department of Otorhinolaryngology – Head and Neck Surgery
University of Pennsylvania Health System
Philadelphia, PA
USA

Philip A. Young
701 Pike Street
Seattle, WA 98101
USA
E-mail: payoung1@yahoo.com

Daniel M. Zeitler
Resident, Department of Otolaryngology –
Head and Neck Surgery
New York University School of Medicine
New Bellevue Hospital 5E 5
550 First Avenue
New York, NY 10016
E-mail: dmz206@med.nyu.edu

Section I

Advanced Rhinology

Chris de Souza and Guy S. Kenyon (Editors)

Anatomy and Imaging

Chapter 1

Surgical Anatomy of the Nose

Natalie P. Steele and J. Regan Thomas

1

Core Messages

- Expert knowledge of nasal anatomy and function is the key to success in rhinoplasty surgery.
- Facial analysis and facial aesthetic principles must always be a part of the initial patient evaluation.
- Surgical manipulations of the nasal anatomy have functional and aesthetic impact.
- A skilled rhinoplasty surgeon understands the interaction between anatomical units and takes care to preserve these functional relationships to avoid future complications.

Contents

Introduction

Rhinoplasty alone or in combination with septoplasty is one of the most commonly performed surgical procedures in the field of plastic surgery. The nose is a vital part of a person's cosmetic appearance, and any preexisting or postoperative appearance that is unattractive may result in unwanted attention or focus. Although a rhinoplasty or septoplasty is theoretically a relatively straightforward procedure, performing a good rhinoplasty with both a successful cosmetic and functional outcome is challenging. Comprehensive knowledge of facial aesthetics and nasal anatomy is paramount for any surgeon undertaking septoplasty or rhinoplasty procedures. This chapter will discuss both the external and internal anatomy of the nose and septum, particularly with regard to septoplasty and/or rhinoplasty.

Facial Aesthetics

Prior to discussion of rhinoplasty goals, the face must be objectively evaluated in order to determine the patient's existing aesthetics and anatomy, and their goal aesthetics and anatomy. Throughout the history of plastic surgery, the concept of beauty has been objectively analyzed, resulting in specific nasal–facial relationships that comply with these perceptions of beauty. According to facial aesthetic principles, the vertical height of the face can be divided into thirds: from the trichion to the glabella, the glabella to the subnasale, and from the subnasale to the menton. Therefore, the length of the nose should constitute approximately one-third of the vertical height of the face. The lower third of the face is typically subdivided, with the distance from the subnasale to oral commissure being one-third, and the distance from the oral commissure to the menton being two-thirds. Horizontally, the face is divided into fifths – approximating the distance from the helical rim to the lateral canthus, the lateral canthus to the medial canthus, from the medial canthus to the contralateral medial canthus, from the medial canthus to the lateral canthus, and then back to the helical rim. The intercanthal distance should be equal to the distance from alar crease to alar crease at the base of the nose. These fundamental principles should be used to assess the width and length of the nose.

1

Patients presenting for rhinoplasty often need changes in these dimensions in order to create a harmonious facial balance.

Once the basic width and length of the nose have been assessed, the surgeon should next consider other nasal dimensions and the facial angles. The order of analysis of the facial proportions is not necessarily important, but it is essential to adhere to a consistent, reproducible pattern of analysis. For our purposes, a stepwise analysis will begin from the upper third to the lower third of the nose.

The profile view is often the greatest area of concern for the patient. Initially, the nasofrontal angle is evaluated. This is the angle between lines drawn from the nasion or radix to the glabella, and from the nasion to the tip, and typically measures 115–130°. The nasion or radix should be the most depressed area of the nose in profile. In Caucasian patients, the nasion should lie on a horizontal plane with the supratarsal crease. In Asian patients, the nasion is more poorly defined, and is usually located at the pupillary line, making the nasofrontal angle more obtuse. The second important nasofacial angle is the nasolabial angle, which determines the rotation of the nose. This angle lies between a line running from the subnasale to the tip and an intersecting vertical line approximating the upper lip vermilion. In women, this angle should lie between 95 and 110°, and 90 and 95° in men.

Nasal Aesthetics

Projection is another important consideration in preoperative assessment, and can be measured in multiple ways. In a method described by Goode, a line is drawn through the alar crease perpendicular to the Frankfort horizontal plane. A second line is drawn from this line to the nasal tip. A third line is then drawn from the nasion to the nasal tip. For ideal nasal tip projection, the length of the alar–nasal tip line divided by the length of the nasion–nasal tip line should be 0.55 to 0.6. A nose whose ratio is greater than 0.6 is considered to be over-projected [1]. Crumley and Lancer described a 3-4-5 triangle in which nasal projection (the distance from the alar–facial crease to the tip) is approximately 60% of the nasal length (the distance from the nasion to the subnasale) [2]. Yet another alternative is to measure the distance from the subnasale to the nasal tip, and compare it with the distance from the subnasale to the upper lip vermilion border. If the distance from the subnasale to the tip is greater than the distance from the subnasale to the upper lip vermilion border, then the nose is over-projected [3].

Lastly, the relationship of the dorsum to the tip should be analyzed. The dorsum of the nose should be a straight line in profile, just 1–2 mm posterior to the nasal tip. If the nasal dorsum is significantly lower or higher than the nasal tip in profile, it may need augmentation or reduction respectively. Just superior to the tip's defining points should be a slightly more depressed area, corresponding to the supratip. If there is no supratip break, then a 1- to 2-mm depression just above the tip should be fashioned to create an aesthetically optimal result.

Frontal views of the patient also need to be analyzed with regard to aesthetic relationships. Most important to consider is whether or not the nose is straight. This is determined by drawing a vertical line from the glabella to the menton. This preoperative assessment can affect patient expectation, predict intraoperative anatomy, and help formulate a surgical plan. Additionally, the brow-tip aesthetic line, which immediately draws the eyes' attention, must be considered. This line, originating from the brow curvature, follows inferiorly along the nasal sidewall to end at the nasal tip. Any break in the flow of this line will draw the eyes' attention.

Once this overview is completed, a more focused, systematic analysis should take place. For the upper third of the nose from a frontal view width is most important. The width of the upper third, or bony vault, should approximate 70–80% of the interalar distance or the intercanthal distance [4]. This width of the upper third should continue and be consistent inferiorly along the nasal sidewalls through the middle vault. Around the inferior portion of the middle vault, the nose gradually becomes wider until the full width of the interalar distance is reached.

In between the alar creases lies the nasal tip, which is often the most complicated part of the nose to evaluate and surgically correct. The nasal tip has two tip-defining points, which are light reflections seen on a photograph. They are defined as the most projected area on each side of the tip, and correspond to the anterior-most portion, or domes, of the lower lateral cartilages. These reflective points should lie on the same horizontal plane. Bulbosity, bossae, asymmetry, valve collapse, pinching, etc., can all be evaluated from the frontal view. As with the profile view, the relationships of the columella should also be evaluated from the frontal view when the tip is under consideration. In Caucasian patients, the inferior-most point of the columella usually lies on the same horizontal plane as the inferior extent of the ala. Many Asian patients have a retracted columella, which is apparent from the frontal view as a short columella that terminates superior to the ala.

Finally, after the profile and frontal views of the nose have been analyzed, the base view should be evaluated. The base view may provide important information about the nasal anatomy that will be helpful in the operating room. According to aesthetic principles, the soft tissue of the infratip lobule should comprise one-third of the height from the base view, while the columella comprises two-thirds. Postoperatively pinched tips may unevenly increase the height of the infratip lobule. The width of the columella may also be assessed from a base view – this corresponds to the anatomy of the medial crural footplates and/or septum. The contour of the alar rim is the last portion of the nose to be evaluated. Any concavity or collapse seen at rest or on inspiration should prompt the rhinoplasty surgeon to consider cartilage grafting for added support of the external valve.

The unique anatomy of the nose complicates rhinoplasty and septoplasty surgery, and makes them two of the most challenging operations to undertake. It is for this reason that it is imperative to take preoperative photographs, analyze the patient's aesthetics, and realistically alter their photographs to create improvements. Once the aesthetics have been analyzed, the surgeon should have an accurate conception of the underlying anatomy, and the surgical plan.

Nasal anatomy can be subdivided into several categories including the skin-soft tissue envelope (S-STE), septum, lateral nasal walls, bony pyramid, cartilaginous vault, and nasal tip.

The external areas of the nose can be further broken down into aesthetic subunits: the dorsum, side-walls, columella, soft tissue triangle, ala, and tip. Each of these areas will be addressed.

Skin Envelope

To begin, one must evaluate the skin-soft tissue envelope. Thin skin can be very challenging as it exposes every contour irregularity of the osseocartilaginous structures. Furthermore, skin will thin over time, leaving the constant potential of unmasking even the slightest irregularities or asymmetries. Thin skin does have the one advantage of faster postoperative healing due to less tissue edema [5]. Thick skin, on the contrary, complicates rhinoplasty by masking refinements. Even if the underlying bony and/or cartilaginous structures are dramatically changed, the patient's thick skin may mute these results. It may redrape ineffectively, leaving a dead space to be filled in by scar tissue. This can result in bulbous tips and suboptimal supratip contours, or a "pollybeak" deformity. Patients of Asian and African heritage in particular need to be wary of this. In general, skin is thickest near the glabella, thins out toward the middle vault, becomes thinnest in the area of the rhinion (corresponding to the nasal bone/upper lateral cartilage junction), and thickens again at the nasal tip. Lessard and Daniel reported the thickness at the nasofrontal groove to be 1.25 mm, and only 0.6 mm at the rhinion [6]. This differential in skin thickness should be considered during dorsal hump removal. Since the skin is thinner at the rhinion, a slight protrusion of the underlying bony/cartilaginous framework should be maintained at the rhinion in order to create a straight external dorsal profile. Toward the tip, the skin becomes thicker again, due to the increased density of sebaceous glands. Extremely thick skin with large numbers of sebaceous glands can limit skin redraping and good tip definition [7]. Skin thickness is often overlooked in both evaluation and patient expectations, but should not be forgotten.

Subcutaneous Tissue

Subcutaneous tissue is another important consideration in rhinoplasty. This layer lies between the skin and the osseocartilaginous framework. Schlesinger et al. further divided this area into four discrete layers: the superficial panniculus, the fibromuscular layer or nasal superficial musculoaponeurotic system (SMAS), the deep fatty layer, and the periosteum or perichondrium [8]. Ideally, surgical dissection during open rhinoplasty is performed deep to all of these layers. Since the blood supply to the skin-soft tissue envelope flap raised during open rhinoplasty runs into the deep fatty layer, this results in elevation in a relatively avascular plane. Elevating in this plane also prevents disruption of the subcutaneous tissues, decreasing scar formation.

The muscles associated with the nose are covered in a nasal equivalent of the SMAS, and are raised in this S-STE flap during open rhinoplasty. These muscles include elevators, depressors, compressors, and minor dilators [9, 10]. The procerus, levator labii superioris alaeque nasi, and anomalous nasi are elevator muscles, the alar nasalis and depressor septi nasi are depressor muscles, the transverse nasalis and compressor narium minor are compressor muscles, and the dilator naris anterior is a minor dilator [7]. Elevator muscles shorten the nose and dilate the nostrils while the depressor muscles lengthen the nose and dilate the nostrils. Overly active depressor septi nasi muscles can result in tip ptosis during laughing or smiling, which may be bothersome to the patient. The compressor muscles lengthen the nose and narrow the nostrils. Elevating in the proper plane deep to these muscles and the perichondrium/periosteum not only results in an avascular plane with preservation of the soft tissue envelope, but also preserves blood supply to these muscles, which lie within the flap, thus reducing intraoperative bleeding, and postoperative edema and scarring.

Blood Supply

Blood supply to both the skin and the lining of the nose is also worth mentioning, as it is important to consider during preoperative injection for hemostasis, flap design, and nasal incisions. The blood supply to the nose is derived from branches of both the internal and external carotid arteries. Branches of these major arteries form a subdermal plexus, which is most dense in the nasal tip. Superiorly, the anterior and posterior ethmoid arteries branching off of the internal carotid artery supply both the lining of the nose, as well as some of the skin via the external nasal or dorsal nasal arteries. Inferiorly, the labial and angular arteries come off of the facial artery to supply the tip area. The lateral nasal arteries typically branch over the alar groove, while the superior labial arteries continue superiorly through the columella [5, 11]. These arteries are important considerations in open septorhinoplasty. The columellar incision typically bisects the columellar arteries, so the tip of the flap is largely dependent on supply from the lateral nasal arteries coming in over the ala. This anatomy has important implications if alar base reductions are undertaken during open rhinoplasty – in order to preserve an adequate blood supply to the tip, alar base incisions should be no more than 2 mm above the alar groove [5]. Defatting the nasal tip, which is occasionally done in thicker skinned patients, may also endanger nasal tip supply by interrupting the arcade between these two arterial supplies. Branches of the infra-orbital, supra-orbital, and supratrochlear arteries also contribute to the nasal blood supply. Venous drainage is through the facial and angular veins.

Nerve Supply

Nerve supply to the nose is externally derived from branches of the trigeminal nerve. The skin of the nose superiorly at the radix and rhinion is supplied from branches of the supratrochlear termination of the ophthalmic nerve. The anterior ethmoidal nerve, another branch of the ophthalmic, may traverse the dorsum of the nose to supply the tip [12]. In endonasal or in open rhinoplasty, this nerve bundle may be damaged by over-aggressive endonasal incisions violating the fibromuscular layer, or elevation of the S-STE in the wrong plane, resulting in a numb nasal tip. The infraorbital nerve may also contribute branches to the lateral nasal walls, columella, and vestibule. Knowledge of this external nerve supply is necessary to perform adequate nerve blocks for closed reductions, or for rhinoplasty under local anesthesia with sedation.

Intranasal anesthesia is also a prerequisite for these procedures. This may be performed with intranasal cocaine pledgets or other strategically placed topical anesthetics. Perhaps the most important target is the sphenopalatine ganglion located in the posterior portion of the nose just posterior to the middle turbinate. Internal branches of the anterior ethmoid must also be anesthetized in the superior portion of the nose to complete a total nasal block.

Bony Septum

Internally, the nose can be divided into the septum and the lateral wall. The septum can be further divided into a bony and a cartilaginous portion. Unlike the paired nasal bones, the bony septum is a singular, midline structure comprising the perpendicular plate of the ethmoid superiorly, and the vomer inferiorly (Fig. 1.1). The perpendicular plate of the ethmoid is continuous superiorly with the cribriform plate. Any unintended or traumatic manipulation of the superior bony septum, therefore, has the potential to cause a CSF leak and/or anosmia. If this superior portion of the septum is contributing to an obstruction, it must be resected sharply rather than pulled or twisted during a septoplasty procedure. Inferoposteriorly, the vomer forms the midline bony nasal septum. It is typically described as a keel-shaped bone that extends anteriorly from the sphenoid, and superiorly from the nasal crests of the maxilla and the palatine bone. Inferior to the vomer, the nasal crest of the maxilla is positioned anteriorly, and the nasal crest of the palatine bone is positioned posteriorly. These are both thin pieces of bone, but may be deviated or dislocated to form inferior septal spurs that should be resected during septoplasty. The anterior nasal spine and, more posteriorly, the palatine process of the maxilla, are located inferiorly to the nasal crests of the maxilla and palatine bones. The anteroinferior edge of the caudal septum is attached to the anterior nasal spine. In patients with a retruded or underdeveloped maxilla, the anterior nasal spine, and, therefore, the anterior edge of the caudal septum, will be more posteriorly located.

Cartilaginous Septum

The septal cartilage is typically described as being quadrangular in shape. It lays in the midline of the nasal septum nestled between the nasal bones, the perpendicular plate of the ethmoid superiorly, and the vomer and palate inferiorly. The septal cartilage is a major support mechanism of the nose and projects anteriorly to form part of the dorsal profile. The anterior and posterior septal angles are important landmarks during septoplasty and rhinoplasty (Fig. 1.1) The anterior septal angle is the area at the junction of the dorsal and caudal septum. The posterior septal angle is the area where the septum articulates with the nasal spine anteroinferiorly.

Lateral Nasal Wall

Along the lateral nasal wall are bony projections called turbinates. These are paired scroll-shaped bones covered in nasal mucosa, which protrude into the nasal cavity. The inferior, middle, and superior turbinates function to direct airflow through the nose. They also serve as important landmarks for sinus surgery. In rhinoplasty, contact with the turbinates is largely avoided in order to prevent bleeding. The inferior turbinate is useful in osteotomies – mucosal incisions for osteotomies are placed just superior to the inferior turbinate to allow access to the pyriform aperture. Also, the middle turbinate serves as a landmark for the sphenopalatine ganglion, which is an important consideration in nerve blocks for complete intranasal anesthesia.

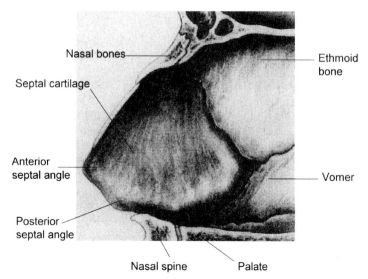

Fig. 1.1 Nasal septal anatomy

Bony Vault

Perhaps the simplest portion of the external nose to discuss anatomically is the bony vault. The bony vault comprises the upper or cephalic third of the nose. The paired nasal bones articulate with the nasal processes of the frontal bones superiorly and the nasal or ascending process of the maxilla laterally. Nasal bones exhibit great variability in their length and width. Generally, though, they assume a pyramidal configuration – wide at the nasofrontal suture, narrowing at the level of the medial canthus, then flaring out laterally as they proceed caudally [13]. The nasal bones are thickest at the nasofrontal junction in the cephalomedial portion of the bones and thin as they broaden inferolaterally [7]. This is the reason why most traumatic nasal fractures occur through the middle or inferior portion of the nasal bones rather than superiorly through the nasofrontal suture [14]. As mentioned previously, from a lateral view, the nasal bones have a natural depression at the radix or nasion area at the level of the supratarsal crease in Caucasian patients. Patients of Asian and African heritage tend to have a more inferiorly located radix approximating the pupillary line. Augmentation or reductions in this area can significantly reduce or deepen the nasofrontal angle, and change the relationship of the nose to the forehead.

Nasal bones average approximately 25 mm in length in Caucasians, but tend to be shorter and lower in profile in patients of Asian and African heritage [15]. It is important to consider the length of the nasal bones prior to surgery, particularly since short nasal bones can be challenging during surgery. Shorter nasal bones can make osteotomies more difficult because of the increased risk of fragmentation. Short nasal bones are also often associated with long upper lateral cartilages that predispose the middle vault to collapse. During any open or closed septorhinoplasty that includes manipulation of the bony vault, the periosteum over the nasal bones should be elevated carefully to avoid tearing. This preserves a pocket lined with periosteum to stabilize the nasal bones after osteotomies [7]. The subperiosteal dissection should continue superiorly, almost to the level of the nasofrontal suture, but at least to the level of the radix.

Typical manipulation of the nasal bones during rhinoplasty involves narrowing of the paired bones via medial and lateral osteotomies. Medial osteotomies are performed in a plane through the midline of the paired nasal bones, and fade out laterally, essentially bisecting the nasal bones in the area of the radix. It is important not to continue the osteotomy superiorly to the level of the nasofrontal suture since this may result in a "rocker deformity" in which the nasal bones are left mobile. Lateral osteotomies are performed through the ascending or nasal processes of the maxilla – not through the nasomaxillary suture. Performing osteotomies through the nasomaxillary suture will result in a palpable step-off, a contour deformity, and an undesirable cosmetic result. Lateral osteotomies should continue medially more superiorly in order to join the lateral extent of the medial osteotomy in the area of the radix.

Another important consideration during osteotomies or any manipulation in the area of the nasal bones is the location of surrounding structures. Posterior to the cephalic portion of the nasal bones are the lacrimal bones – part of the medial orbit. The lacrimal system is situated within a depression in the middle of the lacrimal bone. If surgical osteotomies are too posterior, this area can be easily violated and fractured, with significant sequelae. Just under or posterior to the nasal bones are the nasal septum and perpendicular plate of the ethmoid. Converse first referred to this area where the septum, perpendicular plate of the ethmoid, upper lateral cartilages, and nasal bones meet as the keystone area [16, 17]. In this area, the perpendicular plate of the ethmoid and the septal cartilage provide support for the dorsum. This relationship is important during dorsal hump removal and osteotomies, when the foundation of the nasal dorsum is disrupted.

Cartilaginous Vault

Upper Lateral Cartilages

Inferiorly, the nasal bones are attached to and overlap the cephalic borders of the upper lateral cartilages by 7–10 mm [7]. The upper lateral cartilages comprise the middle third of the nose, or middle vault. These cartilages are extremely important both functionally and cosmetically, and represent a transition zone from the rigid nasal bones to the flexible lower lateral cartilages. They are trapezoidal in shape from a lateral view, flaring out laterally as they proceed inferiorly, smoothing the transition from the more narrow nasal bones to the wider nasal tip. Fibrous connections superior to the nasal bones, medial to the cartilaginous septum, and lateral to the pyriform aperture support the upper lateral cartilages.

Superiorly, the upper lateral cartilages are tucked under the inferior portion of the nasal bones (Fig. 1.2). During rhinoplasty with dorsal hump reduction, removal of significant amounts of dorsal cartilage and bone may alter the relationship of the upper laterals to the septum and nasal bones. Inverted-V deformities and open roof deformities may be the consequence if corrective maneuvers, such as osteotomies, are not performed. Similarly, during rasping of the nasal bones or dorsal hump, the upper lateral cartilage attachments to the nasal bones are at risk of becoming avulsed. Remembering this important anatomic relationship and rasping in an oblique direction should prevent avulsion, and its postoperative sequelae of an inverted-V deformity [7].

Endonasally, the junction of the upper lateral cartilages with the nasal septum forms the internal nasal valve. This valve angle should be between 10 and 15° for adequate nasal airflow, and must be preserved or recreated during rhinoplasty. Even in an unoperated nose, collapse of the internal nasal valve is a concern. Over time, with continued inspiratory negative pressure, the upper lateral cartilages may gradually collapse, resulting in narrowing of the middle vault. This potential is compounded in patients with short nasal bones and poorly supported, long upper lateral cartilages. During rhinoplasty, dorsal hump removal often results in an open roof deformity, which leaves a wider, non-anatomic space between the septum and upper lateral cartilages. If the internal nasal valve is not recreated, inward collapse of the upper lateral cartilages against the septum will narrow the valve, causing functional airway obstruction. Interruption of the mucoperichondrial attachments of the upper lateral car-

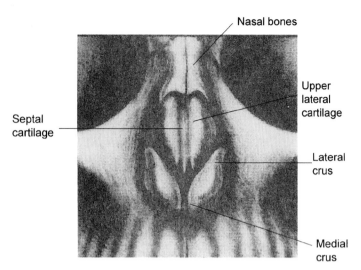

Nasal bones

Upper lateral cartilage

Septal cartilage

Lateral crus

Medial crus

Fig. 1.2 Nasal cartilage anatomy – frontal view

tilages to the septum may also cause nasal valve inadequacy due to problematic scarring. Preservation of this mucosa minimizes collapse and/or posterior displacement of the upper lateral cartilages [18]. In order to prevent this problem of internal valve collapse, a significant percentage of rhinoplasties will require reconstruction of the internal valve with placement of bilateral spreader grafts [19]. These rectangular shaped grafts typically measure 6–18 mm in length, 3–5 mm in height, and 2–4 mm in thickness, and are placed between the cartilaginous septum and remaining upper lateral cartilages [20]. It is important to tuck these grafts under the nasal bones superiorly in order to prevent inverted-V deformities. These grafts are then sutured into place, and act as mechanical bolsters to prevent inward collapse of the upper lateral cartilages.

Lower Third

The tip and ala are largely supported by the lower lateral crura, or alar cartilages. These are C-shaped cartilages typically divided into medial, middle, and lateral crura (Fig. 1.3) [14, 19]. These lower lateral cartilages typically overlap the upper lateral cartilages superiorly in the scroll region, but may underlay or approximate the upper lateral cartilages. This relationship in the scroll region is a major tip support mechanism [7]. Loose areolar tissue and fibrous attachments connect the upper and lower lateral cartilages. With aging, these attachments weaken, contributing to senile ptosis, in which the tip loses its cephalic rotation. In rhinoplasty, transection of these attachments occurs with transcartilaginous or intercartilaginous incisions. These incisions violate this major tip support mechanism, and must be considered and accounted for during tip refinement.

In addition to fibrous attachments to the upper lateral cartilages, the lower lateral cartilage complex is also supported by fibrous attachments to the caudal end of the septum and to the pyriform aperture. The attachments of the medial crura to the membranous septum are important contributors to tip projection. Partial transfixion incisions preserve this support,

but complete transfixion incisions, which separate the medial crural footplates from the membranous septum, sever these attachments and deproject the tip. Similarly, the attachments of the lower lateral cartilages to the pyriform aperture maintain tip rotation and must be preserved. These lateral attachments are most at risk during osteotomies. Therefore, lateral osteotomies are performed in a high-low-high fashion. The initial "high" portion of the osteotomy refers to starting the osteotomy high on the nasal process of the maxilla in order to preserve the fibrous attachments of the lower lateral cartilages, and also the insertions of the nasofacial muscles.

The medial crus of the lower lateral cartilage begins inferiorly at the footplate, and extends into the columella. The middle crus begins inferiorly at the columellar lobule junction, and ends superiorly at the medial extent of the lateral crus. The middle crus may also be referred to as the intermediate crus [7, 21]. The lateral crus starts medially at the lateral end of the middle crus, and ends with a free edge laterally [19]. The transition point from the middle crus to the lateral crus contains the most projected portion of the cartilage, and is referred to as the tip-defining point, or dome. This tip-defining point always lies on the medial aspect of the lateral crus [8].

The medial crura form the cartilaginous support for the columella. They are further divided into a footplate segment and a columellar segment. From a lateral view, the angle of cephalic rotation of the medial crus between these two subdivisions corresponds to the double break portion of the columella. The soft tissue structure of the columella reflects the anatomy of the underlying footplates of the medial crura and their interaction with the caudal septum. Aesthetically, only 2–4 mm of columellar show should be present below the alar margins from a profile view [7]. Anything more than this reflects a "hanging columella" or alar retraction, while any smaller distance represents columellar retraction. Both of these discrepancies are aesthetically displeasing. During an open rhinoplasty approach, it is important to remember that the medial crura have convexities in the area of the columella. Dissection must proceed immediately deep to the skin in order to prevent transecting this convex portion of the cartilages. Occasionally, however, the inferior convexities of the medial crural footplates are intentionally resected to correct a hanging columellar deformity. The membranous septum and caudal edge of the cartilaginous septum also contribute to the columellar shape from this view. All of these relationships must be considered when determining how much of the caudal septum or medial crura to resect or reposition during rhinoplasty. Overaggressive resection of the caudal septum can lead to over-rotation and an unnatural, operated look, while inadequate resection leaves a long caudal septum that pushes the tip down. If no change in tip projection is desired, a transfixion incision should be avoided unless the relationships among the medial crura, membranous septum, and caudal septum are restored. Transfixion incisions are indicated if a significant amount of complex tip work is needed or if deprojection is desired.

From a base view, the divergence of the medial crural footplates determine the width of the columella [8]. These medial crura can be asymmetric, but parallel, flared, or straight. Soft tissue coverage in this area can also change its appearance. If the medial crura are flared, and there is minimal soft tissue coverage, a bifid appearance can result. However, if there is adequate tissue, then the columella just appears wide. Sutures between the medial crural footplates can narrow this area and correct bifidity.

Similar to the medial crura, the middle crura can also be further divided into two segments: the domal and lobular segments. The lobular segment is the more inferior portion of this subdivision, and typically follows the pattern of the columellar segment of the medial crus. That is, if the columellar segment of the medial crus is divergent, then the lobular segment of the middle crus usually is too [22]. The lobular segment does not contribute much to the tip's appearance since it is covered by a thick soft tissue envelope. The domal segment, however, can contribute significantly to the appearance of the tip. It is located between the lobular segment of the middle crus, and the medial portion of the lateral crus. Wide divergence of the middle crura may result in a bifid appearance of the tip, which can be corrected by interdomal sutures during rhinoplasty. Other variations in angulations and convexities of this domal segment of the middle crus can make a tip boxy, narrow or pinched [6, 19].

During rhinoplasty, a variety of suture techniques in this area can significantly change the shape of the tip, increase projection, and improve definition.

Lateral crura also make a large contribution to tip definition and shape, and, therefore, can be manipulated or sculpted in various ways to change its appearance. At their medial extent, the lateral crura begin at the superior edge of the domal segment of the middle crus. This medial segment of the lateral crus contains the tip-defining point – the most anteriorly projected portion of the tip. The lower lateral crura should then take on an outwardly convex configuration laterally over the ala, then curve slightly internally again at their lateral end. This lateral convexity results in a nice arch in the nasal tip and ala. Occasionally, excessive internal recurvature at the lateral aspect of the lateral crura is present, and can cause nasal obstruction. This can be corrected with lateral crural strut grafts during rhinoplasty to reverse the curvature [23].

Typically, as they arch laterally, the lower lateral cartilages also move cephalically. This is an important point to remember during marginal incisions for rhinoplasty – the incision should proceed more cephalically in the lateral portion of the incision to parallel the inferior border of the lateral crura. During tip refinement, however, the caudal margin of the lateral crura should be repositioned to approximate the same plane as the cephalic margin in order to maximize alar support and create a smooth transition from the tip to the supra-alar creases. Alterations in this relationship can give the nasal tip a pinched look, and should be avoided. Interdomal sutures can occasionally change the orientation to a more favorable relationship, but lateral crural strut grafts may be necessary to reposition the lateral crura [23].

Width, length, thickness, and curvature of the lateral crura vary greatly between patients. These cartilages can be cephalically oriented, laterally oriented, thin, thick, extremely wide, deformed, buckled, or concave. Ideally, the lateral crura should deviate from the midline at approximately a 45° angle [23]. More cephalically oriented lateral cartilages cause fullness in the lower third of the nose and a ptotic tip. Fullness is due to excessive width of the cartilages tenting up the skin superior to the alar crease. Typically, only 4–8 mm of lateral crural width

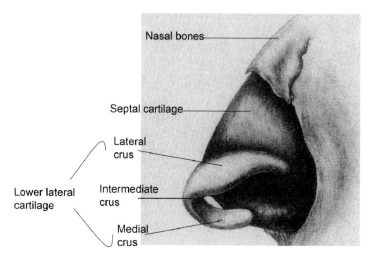

Fig. 1.3 Nasal cartilage anatomy – lateral view

at the medial edge of the lower lateral is required for adequate alar support. More aggressive resection can lead to a pinched tip and/or alar collapse. Cephalically oriented cartilages can also cause derotation of the tip by resisting upward rotation. Excessively long lateral crura may have a similar effect. Trimming the lateral crura (i.e., lateral crural overlay or cephalic trim) and repositioning the lower lateral cartilages in a more horizontal direction (with interdomal sutures or lateral crural strut grafts) may help decrease fullness and increase tip rotation to create a more aesthetic tip.

Soft Tissue of the Nasal Tip

The alar rim is an area of soft tissue adjacent to the caudal edge of the lower lateral cartilages. This area is composed of soft tissue, with no underlying cartilaginous support. Historically in rhinoplasty, the base view was sculpted to become more concave as the alar rims moved toward the nasal tip. This type of sculpting has been proven to contribute to a pinched tip look, long-term alar and/or external valve collapse, and nasal obstruction. The convex structure of the alar rim should be preserved at the nasal tip, not only for functional reasons, but for cosmetic reasons. Leaving this convexity intact creates a smooth transition from ala to tip on the base view. Occasionally, alar rim grafts, which are cartilage grafts measuring 1–2 mm wide and 10 mm long, need to be placed in a pocket immediately adjacent to the alar rim (caudal to the marginal incision) to recreate this contour [23].

The area sandwiched among the alar rim, nostril, infratip lobule, and columella is referred to as the soft tissue triangle. There is no underlying cartilaginous support in this area. During rhinoplasty, any violation of the soft tissue in this area can cause scarring, and may result in notching of the ala. This is an undesirable result, and is a tell-tale sign of rhinoplasty.

At the base of the nose is the nostril sill – a horizontal soft tissue portion at the junction of the nose and upper lip. Just posterior to this is the nasal vestibule, which is the entry to the internal portion of the nose. During rhinoplasty, it is occasionally necessary to perform nasal sill excision or alar base reductions. Internal alar base reductions can reduce flaring, which is a side effect of deprojection of the nose during rhinoplasty.

Conclusion

Although nasal and septal anatomy seems straightforward, there are many intricate anatomic relationships that occur in the nose, particularly in the lower third. A comprehensive understanding of nasal anatomy and the relationships among its individual structures are essential to performing a successful septoplasty or rhinoplasty. Patients must see a visible cosmetic improvement, without compromised function. Furthermore, both the cosmetic result and the functional result must be durable. This is a truly challenging part of rhinoplasty, but it can be accomplished with a solid understanding of the nasal anatomy and relationships.

References

1. Ridley MB. Aesthetic facial proportions. In: Papel ID, Nachlas NE, eds. *Facial plastic and reconstructive surgery*. Philadelphia: Mosby Year Book, 1002:99–109.
2. Crumley RL, Lancer R. Quantitative analysis of nasal tip projection. *Laryngoscope* 1988;98:202–208.
3. Simons RL. Nasal tip projection, ptosis, and supratip thickening. *ENT J* 1982;61(8):452–455.
4. Papel ID. Facial Plastic and Reconstructive Surgery. 2nd Edition. Thieme. New York, NY 2002.
5. Toriumi DM, Mueller RA, Grosch T, Bhattacharyya TK, Larrabee WF Jr. Vascular anatomy of the nose and the external rhinoplasty approach. *Arch Otolaryngol Head Neck Surg* 1996;122(1):24–34.
6. Lessard M, Daniel RK: Surgical anatomy of septorhinoplasty. *Arch Otolaryngol Head Neck Surg* 1985;111(1):25–29.
7. Tardy ME, Surgical Anatomy of the Nose, 1990, Raven Press, New York, NY.
8. Oneal RM, Beil RJ, Schlesinger J. Surgical Anatomy of the Nose. *Otolaryngol Clin North Am*, 32:1, 1999.
9. Griesman BL. The tip of the nose. *Arch Otolaryngol Head Neck Surg* 1952;31(10):551–553.
10. Letourneau A, Daniel RK. Superficial musculoaponeurotic system of the nose. *Plast Reconstr Surg* 1988;82(1):48–57.
11. Rohrich RJ, Gunter JP: Vascular basis for external approach to rhinoplasty. *Surgical Forum* 1990;13:240.
12. Zide BM: Nasal anatomy: The muscles and tip sensation. *Aesthetic Plast Surg* 1985;9(3):193–196.
13. Enlow DH: The Human Face: An Account of Post-Nasal Growth and Development of the Craniofacial Skeleton. New York, Hober, 1968.
14. Rees TD. Aesthetic Plastic Surgery, 1980 WB Saunders, Philadelphia PA.
15. Zingaro EA, Falces E: Aesthetic anatomy of the non-caucasian nose. *Clin Plast Surg*. 1987;14(4):749–765.
16. Converse JM: The cartilaginous structures of the nose. Ann Otol Rhinol Laryngol 1955;64(1):220–229.
17. Converse JM: Corrective surgery of nasal deviations. Arch Otolaryngol Head Neck Surg 1950;52(5):671–708.
18. Toriumi DM, Johnson CM. Open structure rhinoplasty: featured technical points and long-term follow-up. *Facial Plast Clin North Am* 1993; 1:1–22.
19. Sheen JH, Sheen AP. Aesthetic rhinoplasty. St Louis: CV Mosby, 1987.
20. Toriumi DM. Structure approach in rhinoplasty. *Facial Plast Surg Clin North Am*. 2002 Feb;13(1):93–113.
21. Tebbets J. Personal approach to the nasal tip. Presented at the Seventh Annual Texas Rhinoplasty Symposium, Dallas, March 1990.
22. Natvig P, Sether LA, Gingrass RP, Gardner WD. Anatomical details of the osseous cartilaginous framework of the nose. *Plast Reconstr Surg* 1971;48(6):528–532.
23. Toriumi DM. New concepts in nasal tip contouring. *Arch Facial Plast Surg*. 2006;8(3):156–185.

Surgical Anatomy of the Paranasal Sinuses

Robert G. Mynatt and Raj Sindwani

Core Messages

- The paranasal sinuses, orbits, and intracranial cavity are contiguous structures separated by thin bone, and a thorough appreciation of anatomy is essential for safe and efficacious surgery in this region.
- Key major landmarks used for orientation include the middle and superior turbinates, skull base, lamina papyracea of the orbit, and the choana.
- Each sinus cavity has a specific drainage point or ostium through which normal mucociliary clearance is channeled. The outflow tract for mucus can be extremely complicated, as with the frontal drainage pathway, and obstruction may occur at several levels due to the presence of cells that may be pneumatized to varying extents.
- In the clinical setting, the three-dimensional relationships between sinonasal structures and their outflow tracts may be better appreciated through the application of image guidance technology.

Contents

Introduction

Classical anatomy of the nasal cavity and paranasal sinuses was elucidated originally by elegant gross dissection, and more recently with even greater resolution facilitated by modern imaging. Advances in rhinology, including the advent of the rigid nasal endoscope with superior fiber optics and precise localization techniques using surgical navigation systems, have allowed newer perspectives and a better understanding of functional anatomy. Most surgeons today are very familiar with the video display of surgical navigation systems and this technology is now used routinely in the operating room. Image guidance technology utilizing high-resolution CT imaging of the sinuses affords extremely detailed three-dimensional views of the sinonasal anatomy, which, when coupled with the endoscopic image, provides a more complete understanding of complex anatomical relationships. Thorough knowledge of this anatomy is necessary for the sinus surgeon to effectively and safely treat pathology in and around the sinonasal tract. In this chapter we present the sinus anatomy and review key functional regions from the

2

surgical perspective, utilizing an image guidance system (Vectorvision; BrainLAB AG, Munich, Germany) to reinforce three-dimensional relationships.

Embryology

A brief review of embryological development helps to elucidate the intricate anatomy and relationships of the paranasal sinuses and their outflow patterns. A series of bony prominences occurs in the lateral nasal wall between weeks 7 and 9 of fetal development. Generally, six bony ridges from the ethmoid, or ethmoturbinals, are present at week 8, three to four of which will persist. Each ethmoturbinal has an anterior ascending and posterior descending aspect [1, 2]. The ascending and descending portions of the first ethmoturbinal will form the agger nasi and uncinate process respectively. The second lamella gives rise to the bulla ethmoidalis, or ethmoidal "bleb." The third ethmoturbinal becomes the middle turbinate, and the fourth develops into the related superior turbinate. The fifth and sixth ethmoturbinals fuse to become the supreme turbinate. The inferior turbinate arises from a separate entity, the maxilloturbinal, which is not part of the ethmoid, but instead relates to the maxillary and palatine bones [3]. The lamellae of each of these processes gradually develop and give rise to the mature structures described.

Whereas the ridges of the ethmoturbinals form structures, the spaces between the ethmoturbinals, described as furrows, correspond to spaces and clefts of the mature sinus drainage pathways. These furrows can be subdivided into primary or secondary [1, 4]. The first primary furrow gives rise to the infundibulum, hiatus semilunaris, middle meatus, and frontal recess. The second primary furrow corresponds to the superior meatus, and the third primary furrow, the supreme meatus. Secondary furrows form supra and retrobullar recesses, and the ethmoid air cells proper. The frontal recess, and subsequently the frontal sinus, likely develop as an expansion of the furrow between the first and second ethmoturbinals. Whether the frontal sinus originates from the frontal recess, anterior ethmoid air cells, or infundibulum is debatable [4–6].

There is some discussion as to whether the sinuses develop from cartilaginous condensations and subsequent ossification centers primarily, or from the invagination of mucosa with pneumatization secondarily. Primary pneumatization occurs prenatally, while secondary pneumatization and expansion occur largely postnatally [6, 7]. Early in the process of sinus development, a cartilage capsule surrounds the budding nasal cavity and paranasal sinus areas [8]. At week 6 of fetal development, paranasal condensations form lateral nasal swellings and the condensed mesenchyme forms a continuous capsule around the primary nasal cavity with the exception of the early nasal floor [3, 7]. The cartilage condensations are found laterally and centrally. The ectodermal ethmoid plate is at this point a thin cartilaginous plate that laterally forms the concha nasalis and ala orbitalis, which form the second and third ethmoturbinals. In this model, the smooth ectodermal ethmoid complexifies and around weeks 10–12, mucosal folds develop followed by intraconchal cartilage [3]. Sphenoid development, however, seems to favor the latter argument, with largely postnatal development.

This sinus starts to develop around weeks 10–12 of gestation, but is mature by the age of 9–12 years. It begins as a mucosal invagination surrounded by a cartilaginous "cupolar recess of the nasal cavity," which ossifies later to become the "ossiculum of Bertini." The early sphenoid sinus then attaches to the sphenoid bone, and expands into the bone [4, 9]. As mentioned, the frontal sinus can form from expansion of the frontal recess into the frontal bone, or the anterior ethmoid cells directly, or from the infundibulum [10]. The maxillary sinus is thought to develop from a lateral expansion of the infundibulum [6, 11].

The Paranasal Sinuses

The paranasal sinuses are made up of the anteriorly draining group: the maxillary, anterior ethmoid, and frontal sinuses; and the posteriorly draining group: the posterior ethmoid and the sphenoid sinuses. These mucosa-lined, air-containing spaces in the skull are named for the bones into which they have pneumatized. Through a series of narrow spaces and channels, the mucus produced by the sinuses makes its way into the nasal cavity and nasopharynx at which point it is swallowed. Conventional techniques of functional endoscopic sinus surgery (FESS) for chronic inflammatory disease target this complex drainage system by enlarging the openings of the sinuses and their outflow tracts in a mucosa-sparing manner [7]. Although the exact physiologic role of the sinuses is not known for certain, theories on the functions of the paranasal sinuses include: olfactory, respiratory (humidification, buffer pressure changes, local immunologic defense), phonetic (resonance, reduce bone conduction of our own speech), static (reduce weight of the skull), mechanical (trauma protection), and thermal (provide heat insulation).

Sinonasal Mucosa

Three different mucosal types line the nasal cavity and paranasal sinuses. The primary function of the nose pertains to olfaction and this is reflected in the mucosa associated with fibers from the olfactory nerve traversing the cribriform plate. This mucosa is a ciliated, pseudostratified, columnar epithelium with odor receptors and a high concentration of mucous glands. The olfactory receptor cells are bipolar, with their sensory aspect in the nasal cavity and project directly onto the rhinal cortex. This mucosa is centered on the cribriform plate in the roof of the nasal cavity and can extend variably onto the supreme, superior, and middle turbinates, the superior septum, and even parts of the lateral nasal wall. Drying and inflammation of the olfactory mucosa, as well as nasal obstruction, can result in decreased olfactory sensation.

The predominant mucosal surface of the sinonasal tract is the respiratory epithelium, which lines the walls of the nasal and sinus cavities, the nasopharynx, and the nasal floor. This is also ciliated, pseudostratified, columnar epithelium, with an equally high concentration of glands, and greater innervation by the trigeminal nerve (via V2 and some of V1). In the healthy state, the mucosa of the sinonasal tract produces over 600 cc of mucus daily. The mucus is propelled along the surface of the respiratory epithelium by the coordinated beating action of the cilia. This mucociliary clearance (or "mucus flow") occurs in a characteristic pattern both within the sinuses and throughout the nasal cavity [12].

Posteriorly, in the nasopharynx, the respiratory epithelium assumes a different character that may reflect the presence of lymphoid tissue associated with Waldeyer's ring. Anteriorly, the respiratory epithelium transitions into keratinizing stratified squamous epithelium, or skin, in the nasal vestibule. This area has associated hair follicles (forming the nasal vibrissae or hairs), and tends to express cutaneous pathology. Developmentally, the schneiderian membrane is made up of ectoderm and is associated with the olfactory constituent. The respiratory epithelium, on the other hand, is considered to be derived from endoderm.

General Sinonasal Blood Supply

The nasal cavity enjoys a rich blood supply from both the internal and external carotid arteries. The ethmoidal arteries are distal branches of the ophthalmic artery off of the internal carotid artery. They supply the ethmoid sinuses, and portions of the lateral nasal wall and anterior septum. The nasal floor obtains vascular supply from the superior labial and greater palatine arteries anteriorly. The sphenopalatine artery gives a major branch to the septum, and a posterior lateral nasal wall branch that provides blood to the lateral wall, sphenoid rostrum, and turbinates. The posterior nasal cavity may also receive blood from ascending pharyngeal and many tonsillar and palatine branches from the external carotid system.

Innervation

The sinonasal system receives innervation from many sources for various functions. Olfactory function is served by cranial nerve I – the olfactory nerve. The olfactory bulb runs from the temporal lobe through the olfactory groove and sends 50–200 nervelets through the cribriform foramina to innervate the olfactory mucosa in the superior nasal cavity. The maxillary division (V2) of the trigeminal nerve is the major source of sensation from the nasal cavity and sinus system. The nerve branches from the main trigeminal trunk, traverses the cavernous sinus, and exits through the foramen rotundum in the skull base to enter the pterygopalatine fossa. It traverses the inferior orbital fissure and becomes the infraorbital, superior alveolar, palatine, and nasopalatine nerves, and provides branches to the nasal lining. Nasal sensory innervation is also supplied in part by the ophthalmic (V1) branch of the trigeminal nerve, most notably via the nasociliary and anterior and posterior ethmoidal nerves. Parasympathetics from the greater superficial petrosal branch of the facial nerve join with sympathetic nerves from the internal carotid system (lesser superficial petrosal nerve) to form the vidian nerve. The vidian nerve traverses the vidian or pterygoid canal in the region of the lateral sphenoid floor, and supplies secretomotor innervation to the nasal cavity and lacrimal glands.

The Lateral Nasal Wall

The topography of the lateral nasal wall is dominated by the turbinates and the spaces under and between them known as meati. There can be from three to four turbinates in the adult including the inferior, middle, superior, and possibly the supreme turbinate. The key to the relationship between the sinuses and the nasal cavity is the ostiomeatal complex (OMC) anteriorly, and the sphenoethmoid recess posteriorly. As such, obstruction in these areas, most notably at the OMC, has been demonstrated to be responsible for most clinical cases of rhinosinusitis [13]. The OMC is a narrow but high traffic area that captures drainage from the frontal, maxillary, and anterior ethmoid sinuses.

Inferior Turbinate

The inferior turbinate is made up of a bony concha covered with vascularized erectile-type tissue and respiratory mucosa. It is frequently hypertrophic and is commonly a cause of airway obstruction [3]. The anterior insertion of the inferior turbinate is on the lateral wall just posterior to the pyriform aperture, while the posterior insertion is just below that of the middle turbinate, about 1–1.5 cm anterior to the choanae [14]. Its blood supply consists of a branch of the posterior lateral nasal artery from the sphenopalatine artery, and possibly a branch from the descending palatine artery [15]. As shown in Fig. 2.1, this turbinate makes up the inferior boundary of the middle meatus, and lies just inferior to the maxillary ostium. The inferior meatus is the space between the inferior turbinate and the floor of the nasal cavity, and it includes the outflow of the nasal lacrimal duct on the lateral wall just posterior and inferior to the head of the turbinate.

Middle Turbinate

The middle turbinate maintains central importance on the lateral nasal wall and has a complex geometric configuration. It can be divided into anterior, middle, and posterior parts. The most anterior portion is vertically arranged and inserts superiorly at the delicate junction of the ethmoidal fovea and the cribriform plate. Figure 2.2 demonstrates the three-dimensional anatomy of the middle turbinate. The fovea, seen in the coronal view, is quite thin at the middle turbinate insertion (0.2 mm) [1], and represents a common site of cerebrospinal fluid leak during sinus surgery. The middle portion of the middle turbinate is obliquely oriented as it slants toward the lamina papyracea laterally. This area forms a coronally oriented curtain of bone known as the basal lamella (or ground lamella), which separates the anterior ethmoid cells from the posterior cells. This portion of the middle turbinate is well appreciated in Fig. 2.2. The basal lamella, an important surgical landmark, provides the medial and posterior boundary of the anterior ethmoid air cells, and the anterior and inferior boundary of the posterior ethmoid cells [16, 17]. The posterior section of the middle turbinate inserts horizontally onto the lamina papyracea and palatine bone

2

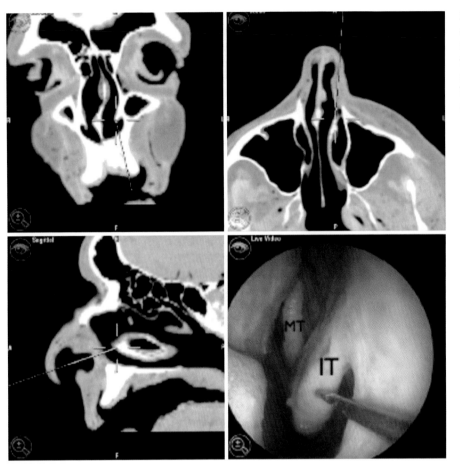

Fig. 2.1 Standard four-quadrant view of an IGS video display (VectorVision; Brainlab, Munich, Germany). The probe tip and corresponding cross-hairs rest upon the anterior aspect of inferior turbinate (*IT*). The middle turbinate (*MT*) and septum can also be seen

laterally. These relationships are best illustrated in the coronal and sagittal CT cuts in Fig. 2.2.

The middle turbinate consists of a bony concha, less vascular erectile tissue than the inferior turbinate, and a layer of respiratory mucosa. It may contain some olfactory mucosa superiorly [3]. This turbinate may be variably pneumatized. If the pneumatization extends into the concha, it is called a concha bullosa [18–20], but if it only extends into the vertical lamellar area, it is strictly called an intralamellar cell [21]. The middle turbinate typically extends inferiorly and posteriorly, with a lower lateral curvature, but may also have a paradoxical lower medial curvature. The presence of a concha bullosa or paradoxical curve may contribute to nasal obstruction, and post-obstructive infection. Figure 2.3 is an excellent demonstration of some common anatomic variants. The blood supply to the middle turbinate is from the anterior and posterior ethmoid arteries, and a branch from the posterolateral nasal artery [15].

Superior and Supreme Turbinates

The superior turbinate, from the 4th and 5th ethmoturbinals, is situated superior and posterior to the middle turbinate [1, 4,

7]. It is much smaller than the previously mentioned turbinates. It is attached to the skull base superiorly and extends inferiorly medial to the middle turbinate, slightly laterally across the sphenoid face (Fig. 2.4). The superior turbinate is the key landmark for identifying the sphenoid ostium (Fig. 5). The lower third of this turbinate is frequently resected to gain better access to the sphenoid ostium during sphenoidotomy. The superior meatus lies between the middle and superior turbinates and contains the drainage pathway of the posterior ethmoid air cells, unless a supreme turbinate is present, in which case the outflow would be into both the superior and supreme meati [16, 17, 22]. The presence of the poorly developed supreme turbinate (Fig. 2.6) is highly variable.

Sphenopalatine Foramen

The sphenopalatine foramen is located on the lateral nasal wall in the vicinity of the lateral middle turbinate attachment. The sphenopalatine artery, a substantial vessel, is the terminal branch of the internal maxillary artery and it enters the posterior nasal cavity from the pterygopalatine fossa via the sphenopalatine foramen. The foramen and pterygopalatine fossa are

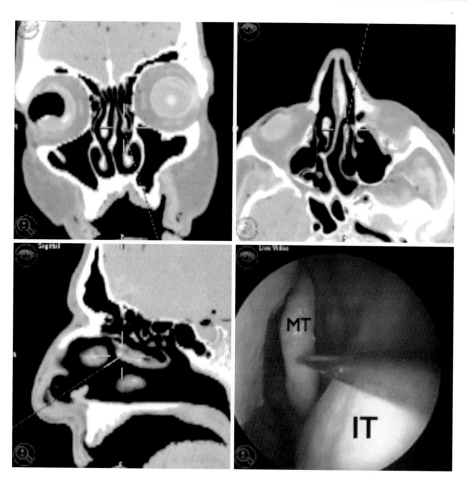

Fig. 2.2 The probe rests upon the anterior aspect of the middle turbinate (*MT*), with the inferior turbinate in the foreground. In the axial view the maxillary line and the uncinate laterally can be seen. The coronal view shows the superior insertion of the MT onto the fovea

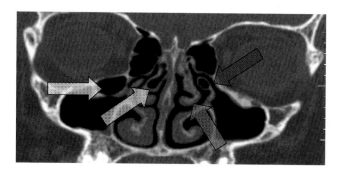

Fig. 2.3 In this coronal CT image, *colored arrows* point out common middle meatal variants including: a paradoxically curved turbinate (*orange arrow*, seen bilaterally), an intralamellar cell (*yellow arrow*), a pneumatized uncinate process (*blue arrow*), and an infraorbital cell (*white arrow*)

epicenters for the development of juvenile nasopharyngeal angiofibroma (JNA) and will be identified during resection of this vascular tumor. In addition, isolation and control of the artery at the foramen are useful for controlling intractable posterior epistaxis. It can be found endoscopically posterior to the posterior fontanel area as it enters the nasal cavity at the level of the posterior maxillary sinus wall, as shown in Fig. 2.7. The crista ethmoidalis, a bony projection of the palatine bone, is a useful landmark for transnasal endoscopic sphenopalatine artery ligation (TESPAL).

Middle Meatus

The middle meatus is contained between the middle and inferior turbinates. This important area houses the OMC (Fig. 2.8). The OMC represents the key anatomic and functional pathway for drainage of the anterior sinuses, including the frontal, maxillary, and anterior ethmoids [13]. It incorporates the hiatus semilunaris, infundibulum, bulla ethmoidalis, maxillary ostium, and the frontal recess [24]. The hiatus semilunaris is not a true space, but a crescent-shaped two-dimensional cleft con-

2

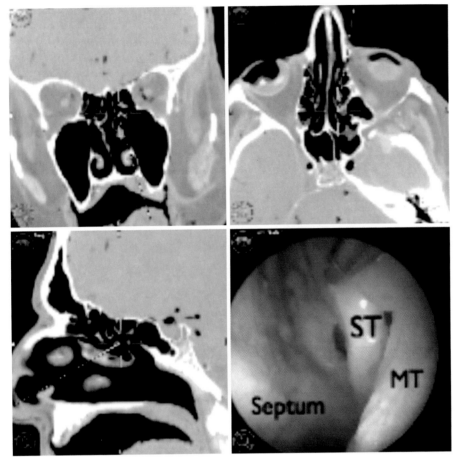

Fig. 2.4 The IGS probe rests upon the anteroinferior aspect of the superior turbinate (*ST*) on the endoscopic view. The middle turbinate (*MT*) is in the foreground and the septum can be seen to the left. In the axial CT panel, the relationship between the ST and the MT and the sphenoid is shown

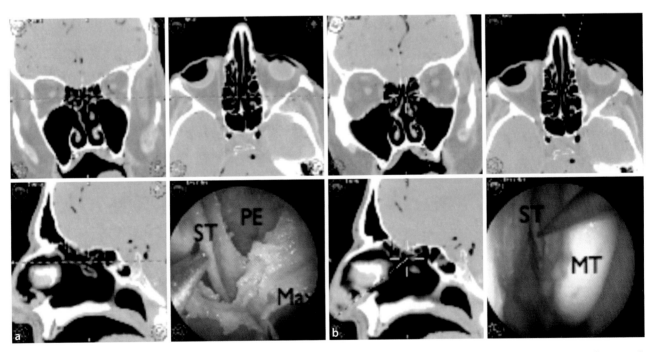

Fig. 2.5 **a** Transethmoid and **b** transnasal approaches to the superior turbinate and sphenoid sinus are demonstrated. In **a**, the IGS probe rests upon the superior turbinate (*ST*), with the posterior ethmoids (*PE*) in the background, and the maxillary antrum in the foreground. **b** shows the IGS probe coursing along the septum to rest on the ST, medial to the middle turbinate (*MT*)

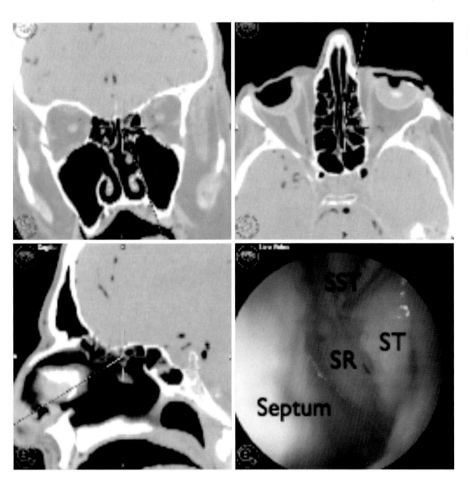

Fig. 2.6 The IGS probe points out the left supreme turbinate (*SST*). In the background lies the sphenoid rostrum (*SR*). The superior turbinate is lateral to this, with the septum medial

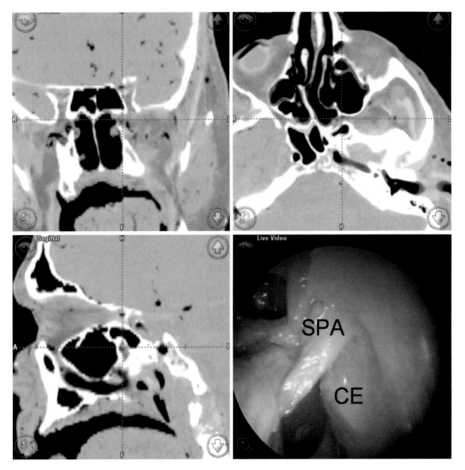

Fig. 2.7 The left sphenopalatine artery (*SPA*) can be seen exiting posterior to the crista ethmoidalis (*CE*) on the endoscopic view. The cross-hairs on the CT panels show the sphenopalatine foramen (best seen on axial CT) in the orthogonal planes. Note its relation to the lateral attachment of the middle turbinate and the posterior wall of the maxillary sinus

necting the middle meatus and nasal cavity to the infundibulum [25]. It is bounded by the anterior face of the ethmoid bulla posteriorly and the posterior free margin of the uncinate process anteriorly. Depending on the insertion of the uncinate, it can be bounded by the frontal recess or lamina superiorly as well [7]. The infundibulum is the actual space that provides common outflow to the maxillary sinus, anterior ethmoids, and possibly the frontal recess. The lateral border of the infundibulum is the lateral nasal wall including the ascending process of the maxilla, lamina papyracea, and palatine bone. The medial boundary is the uncinate and semilunar hiatus. The ethmoid bulla and uncinate process make up the posterior boundary. Superiorly, the infundibulum typically communicates with the frontal recess, depending on the development and location of other structures including the uncinate process, agger nasi cell, and the bulla ethmoidalis (Fig. 2.9) [5, 10].

The Uncinate Process

The uncinate process is a thin curtain of bone oriented in the parasagittal plane. It is attached anteriorly to the ascending process of the maxilla. The uncinate is lined by mucosa on both its medial and lateral aspects. This structure has a variable superior insertion [7], and can insert on the lamina papyracea, the middle turbinate, or the skull base above. This insertion directly influences whether the frontal recess drains into the infundibulum, or more medially into the middle meatus. Laminar insertion dictates more anterior drainage and the creation of a superior recessus terminalis (or terminal recess) within the infundibulum, which is a blind-ended pouch without communication with the frontal recess. Insertion of the uncinate onto the middle turbinate and skull base permit frontal sinus drainage to empty into the infundibulum.

The uncinate runs inferiorly, and then posteriorly forming a hook around the face of the bulla ethmoidalis, thus providing an anterior and inferior boundary for the hiatus semilunaris. In this way, the posterior margin of the uncinate is free and unattached. Inferiorly, this structure inserts onto the inferior turbinate and palatine bone. These relationships are evident in Fig. 2.10. The uncinate may closely approximate the lateral wall in the presence of an atelectatic maxillary sinus, or extend medially at a more obtuse angle in association with maxillary sinus polyposis [26, 27]. It may also occasionally be pneumatized (via the agger nasi or frontal recess cells) as shown in Fig. 2.3. Uncinectomy is the initial step of standard endoscopic sinus surgery, and this

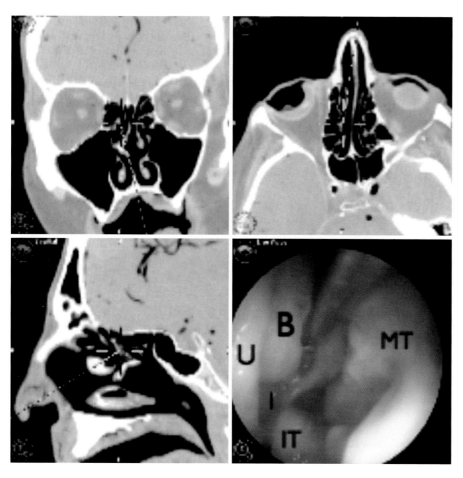

Fig. 2.8 The probe is on the basal lamella of the middle turbinate. The semilunar hiatus can be seen separating the bulla (*B*) and uncinate (*U*). The infundibulum (*I*) is the 3D space entered via the hiatus. *IT* inferior turbinate

structure needs to be removed in order to visualize and access the natural maxillary sinus ostium.

The Maxillary Line

The anterior attachment of the uncinate process to the thick ascending (or frontal) process of the maxilla forms a highly conserved and useful intranasal landmark called the maxillary line. The maxillary line is a curvilinear, mucosal eminence projecting from the anterior middle turbinate attachment superiorly, and inferiorly along the lateral nasal wall to the root of the inferior turbinate (Figs. 2.11, 2.12) [28]. The line is located near the head of the middle turbinate in the anteroposterior dimension. Extranasally, the maxillary line corresponds to the suture line between the lacrimal bone and the maxilla within the lacrimal fossa. In the axial plane, the midpoint of the maxillary line marks the level of the superior aspect of the maxillary sinus ostium, which lies approximately 11 mm posteriorly, and the inferior aspect of the junction of the lacrimal sac and the nasolacrimal duct anteriorly [28]. Noting the location of the maxillary line is useful during uncinectomy (the incision is correctly placed just posterior to the line), and also for identification of the site of the lacrimal fossa (which is approximately bisected by the line) during endoscopic dacryocystorhinostomy (DCR) [29].

The Maxillary Sinus

The maxillary is the first sinus to be addressed utilizing the conventional Messerklinger technique of endoscopic sinus surgery [30]. It has been known as the cheek or dental sinus. Typically well-aerated by the age of 15–18 years, this sinus is the largest and most commonly involved sinus in inflammatory disease. The adult volume can range from 8.5 to 15 ml, but it can also be hypoplastic or atelectatic. A hypoplastic maxillary is often associated with a lateralized uncinate process, which carries a higher risk of inadvertent orbital penetration during uncinectomy [26, 27]. The hard palate and superior alveolar ridge make up the floor of the maxillary sinus. The maxillary and palatine bones comprise the medial wall, and the zygoma provides the lateral wall. Posteriorly, the pyramidal process of the maxilla separates the sinus from the pterygopalatine and infratemporal fossae. The roof is provided by the inferior orbital wall, comprising the lacrimal, sphenoid, and ethmoid bones and the zygomatic process of the maxilla. The maxillary sinus has a posterosupe-

2

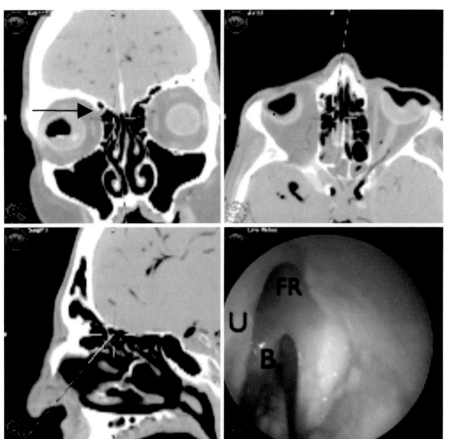

Fig. 2.9 The probe is touching the anterior skull base. The frontal recess (*FR*) drains into the infundibulum medial to the uncinate process (*U*) on the endoscopic view shown. The ethmoid bulla (*B*) can be seen in the background, with the middle turbinate to the right. An *arrow* points to the canal transmitting the anterior ethmoid artery, which is seen crossing the ethmoid air cells on the coronal CT view

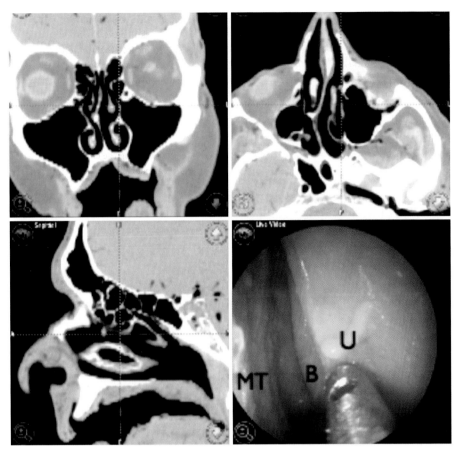

Fig. 2.10 The endoscopic view shows key (*left*) middle meatal structures: uncinate (*U*), the ethmoidal bulla (*B*), and the middle turbinate (*MT*). The coronal CT view demonstrates a laminar insertion pattern of the uncinate and subsequent medial outflow of the frontal recess. The axial view demonstrates both the semilunar hiatus and infundibulum in relation to the uncinate and the cross-hairs

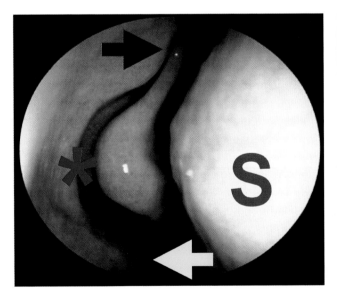

Fig. 2.11 Maxillary line – endoscopic view. This view displays the curvilinear maxillary line (*blue asterisk*) from superior (*black arrow*) to inferior (*yellow arrow*) along the right lateral nasal wall. *S* septum

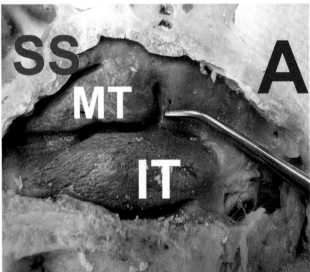

Fig. 2.12 Maxillary line – gross sagittal view. This sagittal cadaveric view of the left lateral nasal wall shows the maxillary line (probe tip) in relation to the inferior (*IT*) and middle turbinate (*MT*). *A* anterior, *SS* sphenoid sinus

2

riorly situated primary or natural ostium located in the lateral nasal wall, within the posterior third of the infundibulum. This "true" maxillary ostium sits in the posteroinferior infundibulum about 72% of the time [16], just inferior to the anterior aspect of the bulla. Secondary openings or accessory ostia can exist, particularly posterior to the primary site in the posterior fontanel (25%), or in the anterior fontanel [16]. The fontanel area is a membranous bony dehiscence in the lateral nasal wall within the infundibulum. A generous maxillary antrostomy can be seen in the endoscopic view in Fig. 2.13, along with other important structures.

Traditional approaches for access to the maxillary sinus interior include the Caldwell-Luc approach and the dependently based inferior meatal antrostomy. These techniques have been outdated by studies demonstrating that physiologic sinus drainage occurs through mucociliary clearance directed exclusively toward the native ostium [31]. Thus, modern sinus surgery addresses a diseased maxillary sinus by widening the OMC and specifically enlarging the natural maxillary ostium. The maxillary sinus can also be used as a portal to approach the orbit, the infratemporal fossa and palate. The sphenopalatine artery and infratemporal nerves (from V2) and vessels can be seen running laterally to medially across the posterior and superior sinus walls. In addition, fontanel and inferior turbinate branches of the posterolateral nasal artery run in close proximity to the ostium [15]. The superior alveolar artery runs in the lateral wall.

Occasionally, tooth roots will erupt through the floor, anteroinferiorly. The canine fossa is the thinnest area of the anterior wall and is a useful location for puncture and diagnostic aspiration. The nasolacrimal duct runs vertically in the anterior portion of the medial wall, in the frontal process of the maxilla. Occasionally, an infraorbital ethmoid cell [32, 34], or Haller cell (Fig. 2.3), may impinge upon the medial and superior wall, possibly compromising drainage. The prevalence of these cells is 8–45% [20, 34].

The Ethmoid Sinuses

The ethmoid sinuses are the most central sinuses in the paranasal sinus system anatomically, and they are also the most central to understanding functional sinus anatomy. These air cells and their variations intimately affect and may potentially obstruct the outflow of all of the other sinuses [35]. The boundaries of the ethmoid labyrinth have been described as an upright matchbox. The lateral wall comprises the lamina papyracea and lacrimal bone and the roof is made up of the fovea ethmoidalis. The middle, superior, and possibly supreme turbinates make up the medial boundary, the sphenoid rostrum is posterior, and the inferior aspect is not bounded by a particular structure, but is open to the nasal cavity, with the exception of the infundibulum, anteriorly [16, 22]. The ethmoid cells are divided into ante-

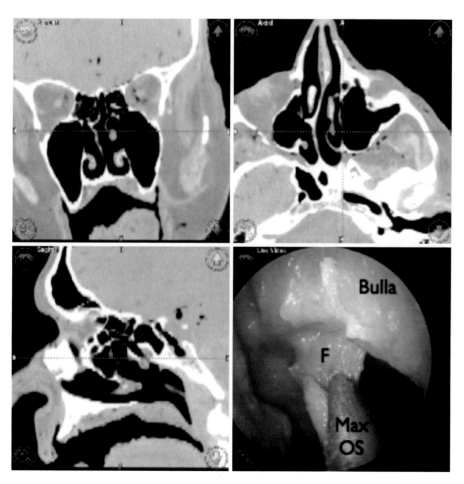

Fig. 2.13 The endoscopic view reveals the posterior fontanel area (*F*), the maxillary ostium (*Max OS*), and the ethmoidal bulla superiorly

rior and posterior groups depending upon their relationship to the basal lamella of the middle turbinate, and also based upon their drainage patterns. Generally, the anterior cells drain into the middle meatus via the ostiomeatal complex (anterior to the basal lamella), and the posterior cells drain into the superior (or supreme) meatus (posterior to the basal lamella) [7, 17]. Anterior cells can number between 2 and 8, and posterior cells between 1 and 5. The total volume is about 15 ml in the adult. The blood supply to this area is from the internal carotid artery via the ophthalmic, and subsequently, the anterior and posterior ethmoidal arteries [15]. Innervation is via the nasocilliary (V1) nerve to the anterior and posterior ethmoid nerves and some V2 inferiorly, with parasympathetics from the vidian nerve and sympathetics running with the arterial supply. Venous drainage is into the cavernous sinus system [3].

The Anterior Ethmoids

The first aspect of the ethmoid system to be addressed during conventional ESS is the bulla ethmoidalis [30]. This reliable air cell is a key feature of the middle meatus. If not aerated, the bulla is known as the torus lateralis. The ethmoid bulla is attached laterally to the lamina papyracea and possibly also to the lacrimal bone. The basal lamella or retrobullar space (when present) lie immediately posterior to it, the skull base and suprabullar recess

(when present) are superior, and the middle turbinate is medial. As mentioned, the anterior face of the bulla forms the posterior border of the hiatus semilunaris. The bulla has a variable superior extent and this structure can greatly influence the character of the frontal recess. Space that develops between the posterior wall of the bulla and the basal lamella is known as the retrobullar space (shown in Fig. 2.14), while space above the bulla (between it and the skull base) forms the suprabullar recess. "Sinus lateralis" is a somewhat dated term that refers to the space lateral to the middle turbinate, but medial to the bulla [2]. This space would be continuous posterior to the bulla with the retrobullar space, and some sources refer to the sinus lateralis and the retrobullar space synonymously. The retrobullar space and the suprabullar recess communicate with the infundibulum posterior and inferior to the bulla. If the bulla pneumatizes completely up to the skull base, a suprabullar space is not present, and frontal sinus drainage occurs more anteriorly and medially. The sagittal CT image of Fig. 2.14 vividly illustrates the relationship of the uncinate process and the ethmoid bulla, highlighting the two-dimensional cleft (hiatus semilunaris) that separates them.

The agger nasi (or "nasal mound") is the most anterior ethmoidal air cell [5]. It appears as a prominence anterior to the superior insertion of the middle turbinate (Fig. 2.15), and it is best delineated radiologically on sagittal CT cuts. Importantly, this air cell forms the anterior boundary of the frontal recess and it may also contribute to the floor of the frontal sinus. Adequate

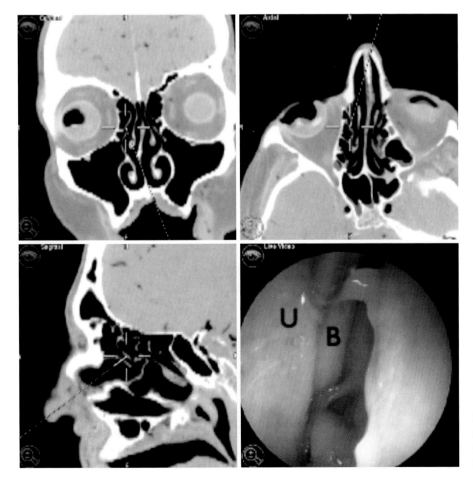

Fig. 2.14 The ethmoid bulla (*B*) can be seen behind the free edge of the uncinate (*U*). It inserts into the lamina laterally (as seen on the coronal CT panel)

2

clearing of the agger nasi and removing the "cap" or superior aspect of this cell is the cornerstone of a complete frontal recess dissection. The anterior ethmoid cells have a unique relationship to the frontal outflow tract. Though air cell development in this area is variable, the drainage pathway intertwines with the bulla, frontoethmoid cells, supraorbital ethmoid cells, and agger nasi cells, and ultimately empties into the middle meatus through the hiatus semilunaris [6, 10]. Frontoethmoid cells have been classified by Kuhn [36] as types I–IV and will be discussed with the frontal recess later in this chapter. The supraorbital cell is possibly a variation of the frontoethmoid cell that pneumatizes into the orbital plate of the frontal bone via the frontal recess or suprabullar recess. Its ostium is usually above the bulla and anterior to the anterior ethmoid artery, and is easily confused with the frontal sinus ostium (which usually lies more medially and anteriorly). A frontal bullar cell occurs when the bulla extends superiorly above the level of the frontal sinus floor. The significance of all of these anterior ethmoid cells is that if well pneumatized and/or diseased, they may compromise the patency of the frontal recess and hamper normal mucociliary clearance from the frontal sinus [5]. They therefore must be systematically identified and addressed, if surgical intervention is to successfully re-establish drainage and ventilation of the frontal sinus.

The anterior ethmoid artery runs posterior to the superior aspect of the bulla and in the posterosuperior aspect of the frontal recess within the anterior ethmoid labyrinth [37]. The anatomy in this location is variably dependent upon the positioning of the bulla and the presence of supraorbital ethmoid

cells. Intraorbitally, the anterior ethmoid artery is located approximately 24 mm posterior to the anterior lacrimal crest; the posterior ethmoid artery is located another 12 mm more posteriorly; and the optic nerve may be found 4–7 mm beyond this [38]. Both arteries can be found along the frontoethmoid suture line. The anterior ethmoid artery crosses the ethmoid roof, from the orbit, and traverses the lateral lamella of the cribriform into the olfactory bulb area, as seen in Fig. 2.9. During its course, this vessel can travel protected through a bony "orbito-cranial canal", or it may be dehiscent and hang exposed from a mesentery below the level of the roof. Its location in the ethmoid roof is not only important for avoidance of hemorrhage, but also because its site of intracranial penetration represents one of the thinnest areas of the ethmoid roof and a potential site of CSF leak. This area has been measured to be 0.05 mm at the artery site, compared with 0.2 mm at the cribriform and 0.5 mm at the fovea [39, 40].

The Posterior Ethmoids

The basal lamella of the middle turbinate represents the anterior boundary of the posterior ethmoid air cells. The cells are bounded laterally by the lamina and palatine bone, and posteriorly by the sphenoid rostrum. The posterior ethmoid artery supplies this area and is usually smaller than its anterior counterpart. The number of posterior ethmoid cells and their arrangement is variable. In addition, aeration of the middle tur-

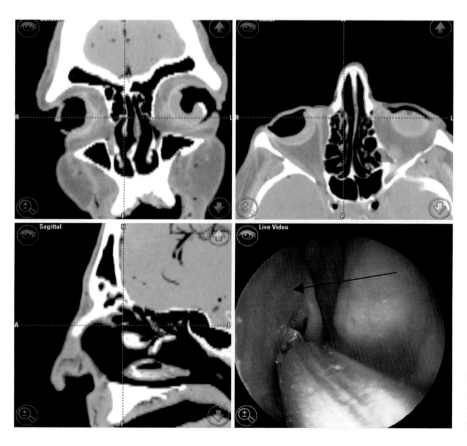

Fig. 2.15 An *arrow* points to the agger nasi, which is located just anterior to the superior insertion of the middle turbinate on the endoscopic view

binate can develop from this area, resulting in a concha bullosa deformity, although this variation may also develop from aberrant pneumatization from the anterior ethmoid cells or even the frontal recess [41]. The sphenoid ostium can be identified at the rostrum posterior to these air cells in an inferomedial position. Occasionally, the posterolateral portion of the ethmoid labyrinth contains an air cell historically described by Onodi [42], which has pneumatized to displace the sphenoid sinus inferiorly and medially. This sphenoethmoid cell (or Onodi cell) is important to recognize because of its proximity to the optic nerve and carotid artery. Frequently, the nerve will be dehiscent in its lateral wall, and is at considerable risk of injury in this location. In fact, approximately 80% of optic nerve injuries are thought to occur in the setting of a sphenoethmoid cell [1]. This air cell is not directly anterior to the sphenoid rostrum as other ethmoid cells are, but instead it extends superior and posterior to it.

Sinonasal Roof

The roof of the nasal cavity and the ethmoid air cells can be described as a linear midline depression between the anterior cranial fossae, from the most anterior aspect at the anterior frontal process in the midline, to the more flattened planum sphenoidale posteriorly. The lateral aspect of this bilateral depression is known as the fovea ethmoidalis, a part of the ethmoid roof. The ethmoid bone forms an intracranial continuation of the septal perpendicular plate called the crista galli, which is flanked by the long aspect of the rectangular cribriform plate on either side. These plates have numerous foramina for tendrils of the olfactory nerves. The fovea ethmoidalis connects the cribriform plate to the superior and laterally arranged thicker orbital plate of the frontal bone. The depth of the olfactory cleft (created by the orientation of the cribriform with the fovea) is thus variable, and has been classified by Keros [33] into three types (see Fig. 2.16). This classification system stratifies risk of injury during ethmoidectomy as directly related to foveal depth. Thus, the skull base is thin in the area of the fovea ethmoidalis (medial and superior), but much thicker and more resilient to injury superolaterally under the area of the frontal bone. The middle

turbinate attaches superiorly at the junction of the cribriform plate (medially) and the fovea ethmoidalis (laterally). This critical area represents a likely site for inadvertent intracranial penetration and CSF leak [39, 40]. The sinonasal roof or skull base slopes downward at an angle of 15° from anterior to posterior [14].

The Sphenoid Sinus

The sphenoid sinus is positioned in the very center of the head, and occupies the most posterior location in the paranasal sinus system (Table 2.1). This partitioned cavity is housed within the sphenoid bone. Anteriorly, the sphenoid is bounded by the posterior ethmoids and nasal cavity and abuts the vomer in the midline. The rostrum is continuous with the clivus posteroinferiorly, while the sella turcica and pituitary gland indent into the posterosuperior aspect of the sinus. The optic chiasm is anterior and superior to this. The superolateral walls are bounded by the cavernous sinus. The petrous apex and clivus meet adjacent to the sinus inferolaterally. Lesions in this area may potentially be approached via a trans-sphenoidal approach. The nasopharynx extends to the sphenoid sinus from below. A bony septum divides the sinus in a midline or paramedian position. Multiple intrasinus septations often exist. Importantly, these bony septations frequently insert onto the carotid canal, which runs in a vertical fashion in the posterolateral wall (Fig. 2.17). Uncontrolled shearing of these septations may cause fractures of the carotid canal and potentially injure the internal carotid artery with resultant catastrophic hemorrhage. The carotid artery may also be dehiscent within the sinus in 8–25% of patients [7, 43]. The optic nerve runs horizontally across the superolateral wall of the sphenoid sinus and may be dehiscent in 4–8%. This number can jump to 50% if associated with a sphenoethmoid cell.

Pneumatization of the sphenoid sinus may extend laterally to incorporate the maxillary nerve (as it traverses the foramen rotundum) or even the pterygoid plates. In an extensively aerated sphenoid, many neighboring structures may be seen indenting the sinus walls. The relationship between the optic nerve and the carotid artery in the lateral sphenoid wall of a well-pneu-

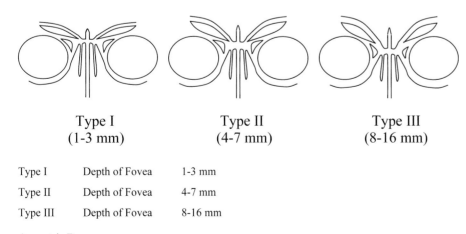

| Type I (1-3 mm) | Type II (4-7 mm) | Type III (8-16 mm) |

Type I	Depth of Fovea	1-3 mm
Type II	Depth of Fovea	4-7 mm
Type III	Depth of Fovea	8-16 mm

Asymetric Fovea

Fig. 2.16 The Keros classification [33]

matized sinus often forms a recess at the level of the anterior clinoid process, known as the opticocarotid recess. This is an important landmark during endoscopic optic nerve decompression surgery [44].

Several neurological structures are in close proximity to the sphenoid sinus. The vidian nerve runs from posterolateral to anteromedial across the floor of this sinus and the maxillary division of the trigeminal nerve (V2) may run adjacent to the lateral wall. Other nearby nerves include the frontal division of the trigeminal nerve (V1), and cranial nerves III, IV, and VI via the cavernous sinus. The sphenoid rostrum, or anterior wall, should be carefully identified on a CT scan prior to surgery, with evaluation for the presence of a sphenoethmoid air cell. These cells can obscure judgment regarding location of the sphenoid ostium. The sphenoid ostium, or opening, is located in the inferomedial aspect of the sphenoid face, between the nasal septum and the superior turbinate (Fig. 2.18). The 2- to 3-mm wide sphenoid ostium is typically situated 1.0–1.5 cm above the choana and 5 mm lateral to the septum, at approximately the level of the maxillary sinus roof (Table 2.2) [14]. The ostium is positioned about 7 cm deep from the nasal sill, at a 30° angle from the nasal floor. It drains into the sphenoethmoid recess.

The sphenoethmoid recess collects sinus drainage from the sphenoid sinus as well as the posterior ethmoid cells. It is bounded by the sphenoid rostrum (containing the sphenoid ostium) posteriorly, by the posterior ethmoid cells anteriorly, and by the superior (and supreme) turbinates laterally. The nasal cavity is inferior, and the nasal septum makes up the medial boundary. As mentioned, the superior turbinate is the major landmark used for identification of the sphenoid ostium and the sphenoethmoid recess during endoscopic surgery. Endoscopic approaches to this region include trans-septal, paraseptal or transnasal, and transethmoidal routes (see Fig. 2.20).

The Frontal Sinus

The frontal sinus is housed within the thick frontal bone. It sits above the orbit, just anterior to the frontal lobe of the brain within the anterior cranial fossa. It is the last sinus to develop. This paired sinus is divided in the midline by a bony septum. The adult volume ranges from 4 to 7 ml. The frontal sinus can be extensively pneumatized, minimally pneumatized or hypoplastic, or even totally absent (unilaterally or bilaterally). Vascular supply occurs largely via the anterior ethmoid artery and venous drainage is provided by the ophthalmic (cavernous sinus) and supraorbital veins (facial vein), and the foramina of Breschet (posterior to the dura). It is innervated by branches of V1. Supraorbital and supratrochlear arteries and nerves (V1) run anterior to the face of the sinus emanating from the orbit.

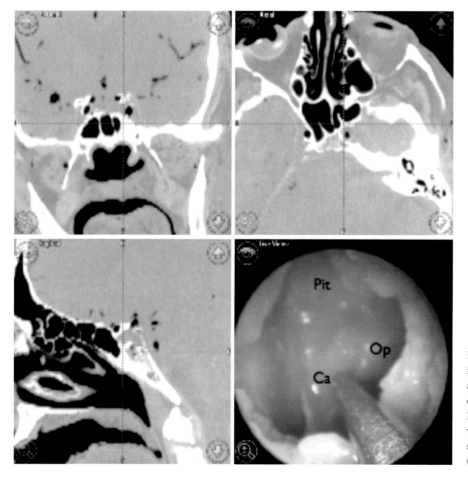

Fig. 2.17 Through a sphenoidotomy, indentations of the internal carotid artery (*Ca*), pituitary gland (*Pit*), and optic nerve (*Op*) can be identified. The IGS probe and cross-hairs point out a vertical septation in the left sphenoid sinus that inserts onto the carotid canal (axial view)

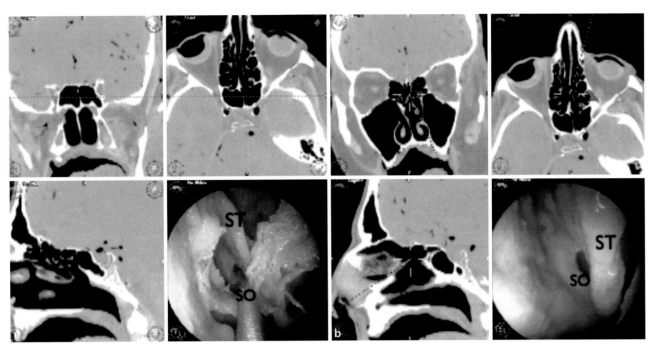

Fig. 2.18 **a** shows the IGS probe traversing a transethmoid route to the left sphenoid ostium (*SO*) through the basal lamella, the posterior ethmoids, medial to the superior turbinate (*ST*), through the spheno- ethmoid recess and into the ostium. **b** shows the transnasal route to the left sphenoid ostium, medial to the middle turbinate and superior turbinate

Table 2.1 Nasal cavity landmark measurements [14]

Nasal floor to roof	46 mm
Anterior nasal spine to choanae	60 mm
Anterior nasal spine to sphenoid ostium	61 mm
Posterior nasal floor to sphenoid ostium	37 mm
Superior aspect of choanae to sphenoid ostium	10 mm

Table 2.2 Classification of frontoethmoid air cells [36]

Type I	Single frontal recess cell above the agger nasi cell
Type II	Tier of cells in frontal recess above the agger nasi cell
Type III	Single massive cell pneumatizing cephalad into the frontal sinus
Type IV	Isolated cell in the frontal sinus
Other cells	
Agger nasi	
Supraorbital ethmoid	
Frontal bulla cells	
Suprabullar cells	
Intrafrontal sinus septal cell	

The frontal sinus has a thin inner and thick outer table of cortical bone. The floor of the sinus also comprises thick bone. The natural ostium lies in the posteromedial aspect of the sinus floor, and it drains into the superoanterior region of the frontal recess below. When viewed endoscopically, the opening into a supraorbital ethmoid cell, part of the anterior ethmoidal cell sys- tem pneumatizing over the orbit posterior to the frontal sinus, may be confused with the frontal sinus ostium, which is gener- ally located more anterior and medial in relation. Use of an im- age guidance system can assist in resolving this confusion. The floor of the frontal sinus may be encroached upon from below by extensively pneumatized cells such as an enlarged ethmoid

2

bulla (frontal bulla), a prominent agger nasi, frontoethmoid cells, suprabullar cells, supraorbital cells, or an interfrontal septal cell [36]. Some of these anterior ethmoid structures may also compromise the outflow tract in the region of the frontal recess. The frontal recess represents the only communication between the sinus and the nasal cavity inferiorly. Any obstruction of this complex area may disrupt normal drainage of the sinus, and result in sinus inflammation. Chronic frontal sinus obstruction and disease is particularly concerning, as it may cause mucocele formation and carries the risk of intracranial or intraorbital spread of infection. Thus, the key to providing a healthy sinus is the maintenance of a patent frontal sinus outflow tract.

The frontal recess constitutes the drainage pathway from the frontal sinus into the nasal cavity [45]. From the recess, mucus empties ultimately into the middle meatus via the hiatus semilunaris; however, the exact route taken depends upon the superior attachment of the uncinate process, the size of the agger nasi and ethmoidal bulla, as well as the specific arrangements of other anterior ethmoid cells. There is no actual "duct" that drains the frontal sinus, but rather an outflow pathway bounded by these variable constituents, which when well-pneumatized, may give the appearance of a duct-like structure. As seen in the

CT views and three-dimensional reconstruction in Fig. 2.19, the frontal sinus and recess create an hourglass shape, with the frontal ostium serving as the isthmus or narrowest point. The ethmoid bulla, suprabullar space, and anterior skull base, along with the anterior ethmoid artery, constitutes varying portions of the posterior boundary of the frontal recess (Table 2.3). The anterior boundary of the frontal recess is the posterior wall of the agger nasi cell. The superoanterior aspect is bounded superiorly by a thick "beak" of frontal bone in the region of the frontal sinus ostium, which strictly represents the floor of the frontal

Table 2.3 Structures of the frontal recess

Anterior:	Agger nasi
Posterior:	Ethmoid bulla and suprabullar space, skull base, supraorbital cell, anterior ethmoid artery
Lateral:	Lamina papyracea
Medial:	Middle turbinate and cribriform plate, uncinate

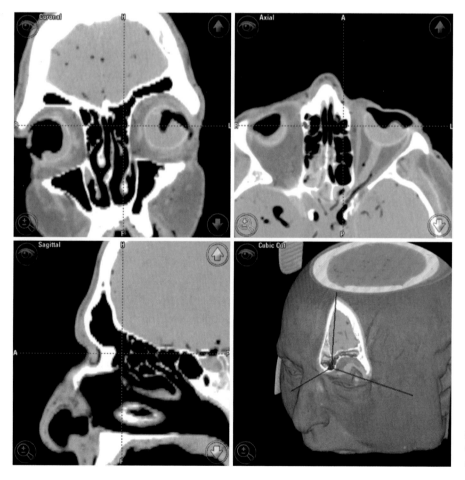

Fig. 2.19 Three-dimensional reconstruction of left frontal recess with orthogonal views. The frontal beak, ethmoid bulla, and agger nasi are shown

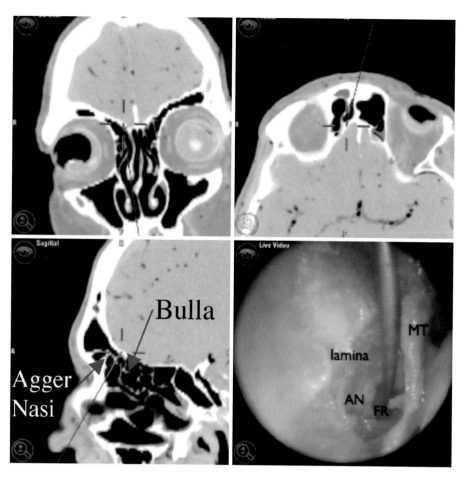

Fig. 2.20 Frontal recess. The IGS probe extends into the right frontal recess (*FR*) onto the skull base as viewed through a 70° endoscope. Note the contributions of the agger nasi (*AN*), lamina, and middle turbinate (*MT*) to the boundaries of the recess. The sagittal CT view best illustrates the relationship between the ethmoid bulla, agger nasi, and skull base in this region

sinus proper. The lamina papyracea makes up the lateral wall of the recess, and the middle turbinate forms the medial boundary, which may also include the uncinate process, depending on its variable superior site of attachment [46].

As demonstrated in Fig. 2.20, conventional approaches to endoscopic frontal recess dissection focus on enlarging the frontal recess in the anteroposterior dimension [47]. This is accomplished primarily by removing the superoposterior walls of the agger nasi and thoroughly removing the ethmoidal bulla [48]. Although dissection of the posterior boundary occurs at the bullar face, it is easy to see why the anterior boundaries provide a safe directionality for more forceful dissection away from the delicate skull base. Further endoscopic exposure of the frontal recess may be achieved by removing the anterior face of the agger nasi (just lateral to the anterior middle turbinate attachment) by performing the agger nasi punch-out procedure, or "POP," which provides a more direct view into the area of the superior frontal recess [49].

The presence of air cells within the frontal sinus or recess can disrupt mucus flow and lead to obstruction. Kuhn and colleagues characterized four major frontoethmoid cell patterns associated with the frontal outflow tract (see Table 2.2) [36]. In addition to providing insight into the pathophysiology of frontal sinus disease, recognition of the types of frontoethmoid cells present also assists in planning a surgical approach aimed at addressing these sites of obstruction. Depending on their exact location, type III or type IV cells may require an above (via trephination) and below (endoscopic) approach to provide the adequate lateral access necessary for their complete resection. As illustrated in Fig. 2.20, frontoethmoid, orbitoethmoid, agger nasi, and ethmoid bulla variations can all significantly impact the anatomy and function of the frontal recess.

It is important to note that every patient presents unique anatomy of the frontal recess (and sinus anatomy in general), and to describe "standard" anatomy of the frontal recess invites complacency that could lead to intraoperative complications. In this area, the risks of violating the skull base, entering the orbit, or lacerating the anterior ethmoid artery are probably the highest. Frontal sinus surgery is technically demanding, due to the inaccessible location of the frontal sinus high in the sinonasal tract, which often requires the use of angled endoscopes and curved instruments. Further, incomplete treatment of the recess invites scarring and stenosis as this narrow inlet is extremely unforgiving during the healing period. Thus, a thorough understanding of the patterns of aeration and frontal sinus outflow in each individual case is mandatory to a successful outcome from

2

surgery. The use of surgical navigation in frontal sinus surgery can decisively confirm safe entrance into the frontal sinus [50] as well as highlighting the intricate nuances of the frontal recess anatomy along the way. Preoperative analysis and planning using particularly the sagittal views from an image guidance system may provide valuable insight in cases involving complex frontal sinus pathology [47].

Conclusion

The surgical anatomy of the paranasal sinuses is complex, and highly variable. The intricate three-dimensional relationships between the sinonasal structures and their outflow tracts may be better appreciated through the application of image guidance technology, which provides accurate localization of specific anatomical references simultaneously in all three orthogonal planes. The paranasal sinuses, orbits, and intracranial cavity are contiguous structures separated by thin bone, and a thorough appreciation of anatomy is essential for safe and efficacious surgery in this complex region.

References

1.   Stammberger, H, Hawke, M, Endoscopic Anatomy of the Lateral Nasal Wall and Ethmoidal Sinuses in Essentials of Endoscopic Surgery. Saint Louis, MO: Mosby: 1993

2   Stammberger HR, Bolger WE, Clement PAR, et al. Anatomic terminology and nomenclature in sinusitis. Ann Otol Rhinol Laryngol 1995;104 (Suppl 167):7–19.

3.   Blitzer, A, Lawson, W, Friedman, W Anatomy and Embryology in Surgery of the Paranasal Sinuses. Philadelphia, PA: W. B. Saunders Company: 1985.

4.   Kennedy, DW, Bolger, WE, Zinreich, SJ. Anatomy of the Paranasal Sinuses in Diseases of the Sinuses: Diagnosis and Management. Hamilton, Ontario, B. C. Decker, Inc.: 2001.

5.   Kuhn FA, Bolger WE, Tisdal RG. The agger nasi cell in frontal recess obstruction: an anatomic, radiologic and clinical correlation. Op Tech Otolaryngol Head Neck Surg 1991;2:226–31.

6.   Schaeffer JP. The genesis, development and adult anatomy of the nasofrontal duct region in man. Am J Anat 1916;20: 125–45.

7.   Levine, HL, Clemente, MP. Surgical Anatomy of the Paranasal Sinus in Sinus Surgery: Endoscopic and Microscopic Approaches. New York, NY: Thieme: 2005.

8.   Wang RG, Jiang SC, Gu R. The cartilaginous nasal capsule and embryonic development of human paranasal sinuses. J Otolaryngol 1994;23:239–43.

9.   Vidic B. The postnatal development of the sphenoidal sinus and its spread into the dorsum sellae and posterior clinoid processes. AJR Am J Roentgenol 1968;104:177–83.

10. Kasper KA. Nasofrontal connections: a study based on one hundred consecutive dissections. Arch Otolaryngol 1936;23:322–44.

11. Schaeffer JP. The sinus maxillaris and its relations in the embryo, child and adult man. Am J Anat 1912;10:313–67.

12. Donald, PJ, Gluckman, JL, Rice, DH, eds. The sinuses. New York: Raven Press, 1995.

13. Stammberger, H. Endoscopic Endonasal Surgery – new concept. Otolaryngol Head Neck Surg 1986; 94: 143–146.

14. Lange, J. Clinical Anatomy of the Nose, Nasal Cavity, and Paranasal Sinuses. New York: Thieme Verlag; 1989:1–50

15. Lee, HY, Kim, HU, Kim, SS, Son, EJ, Kim, JW, Cho, NH, Kim, K-S, Lee, J-G, Chung, IH, Yoon, JH. Surgical Anatomy of the Sphenopalatine Artery in Lateral Nasal Wall. Laryngoscope 2002; 112:1813–1818.

16. Van Alyea OE. Ethmoid labyrinth: anatomic study, with consideration of the clinical significance of its structural characteristics. Arch Otolaryngol 1939;29:881–901.

17. Caldas Navarro, JA. Surgical Anatomy of the Nose, Paranasal Sinuses, and Pterygopalatine Fossa in Micro-endoscopic Surgery of the Paranasal Sinuses and the Skull Base. Berlin, Germany, Springer Verlag: 2000.

18. Zinreich SJ, Mattox DE, Kennedy DW, et al. Concha bullosa: CT evaluation. J Comput Assist Tomogr 1988;12:778–84.

19. Clark ST, Babin RW, Salazar J. The incidence of concha bullosa and its relationship to chronic sinonasal disease. Am J Rhinol 1989;3:11–12.

20. Bolger EW, Butzin CA, Parsons DS. Paranasal sinus bony anatomic variations and mucosal abnormalities – CT analysis for endoscopic sinus surgery. Laryngoscope1991;101:56–64.

21. Grunwald, L. Descriptive und topographische Anatomie der Nase und ihrer Nebenholen. In: Denker, A., Kahler, O., eds. Die Krankenheiten der Luftwege und der Mundhole, Berlin: Springer-Bergman, 1925:1–95.

22. Shambaugh GE. The construction of the ethmoid labyrinth. Ann Otol Rhinol Laryngol 1907;16:771–5.

23. Stammberger, H. Endoscopic Endonasal Surgery – new concept. Otolaryngol Head Neck Surg 1986; 94:143–146.

24. Nauman, H. Pathologische Anatomie der chronischen Rhinitis und Sinusitis. In: Proceedings of the VIII International Congress of Oto-rhino-laryngology. Amsterdam: Exerpta Medical, 1965.

25. Zuckerkandl, E. Normale und pathologische Anatomie der Nasenhole und ihre pneumatischen Anhange. Vienna: Braunmuller, 1882.

26. Bolger WE, Woodruff WW, Morehead J, Parsons DS. Maxillary sinus hypoplasia: classification and description of associated uncinate hypoplasia. Otolaryngol Head Neck Surg 1990;103:759–65.

27. Bolger WE, Kennedy DW. Atelectasis of the maxillary sinus. J Respir Dis 1992;13:1448–50.

28. Chastain J, Cooper M, Sindwani R. The Maxillary Line: Anatomical Characterization and Clinical Utility of an Important Surgical Landmark. Laryngoscope 2005. June; 115(6):990–92.

29. Woog JJ, Sindwani R. Endoscopic Dacryocystorhinostomy and Conjunctivodacryocystorhinostomy. Otolaryngol Clin North Am. 2006;39(5):1001–17.

30. Stammberger H. Functional endoscopic sinus surgery: the Messerklinger technique. Philadelphia, PA: BC Decker; 1991.

31. Donald, PJ, Gluckman, JL, Rice, DH eds. The sinuses. New York: Raven Press, 1995.

32. Von Haller A. First lines of physiology. In: Cullen W, editor, 1st US ed. Edinburgh: Obabran, Penniman and Co; 1803. p. 224.

33. Keros P. Über die praktische Bedeutung der Niveau-Unterschiede der lamina cribrosa des ethmoids. In: Naumann HH, ed. Head and neck surgery. Vol 1. Face and facial skull. Philadelphia, PA: WB Saunders; 1980. p. 392.

34. Kainz J, Braun H, Genser P. Haller's cells: morphologic evaluation and clinico-surgical relevance. Laryngorhinootologie 1993;72: 599–604.

35. Bolger EW, Butzin CA, Parsons DS. Paranasal sinus bony anatomic variations and mucosal abnormalities – CT analysis for endoscopic sinus surgery. Laryngoscope 1991; 101: 56–64.

36. Kuhn, FA (1996). Chronic frontal sinusitis: the endoscopic frontal recess approach. Op Tech Otolaryngol Head Neck Surg vol 7: pp 222–229.

37. Chastain JB, Sindwani R. Anatomy of the Orbit, Lacrimal Apparatus, and Lateral Nasal Wall. Otolaryngol Clin North Am. 2006;39(5):855–64.

38. Kirschner, JA, Yanagisawa, E, Crelin, ES (1961) Surgical anatomy of the ethmoid arteries. Arch Otolaryngol, 74(4):382–386.

39. Kainz J, Stammberger H. The roof of the anterior ethmoid: a place of least resistance in the skull base. Am J Rhinol 1989; vol (3):191–9.

40. Kainz J, Stammberger H. Danger areas of the posterior rhinobasis: an endoscopic and anatomical surgical study. Acta Otolaryngol 1992;112:8

41. Grunwald, L. Deskriptive und topographische Anatomie der Nase und ihrer Nebenholen. In: Denker, A., Kahler, O., eds. Die Krankenheiten der Luftwege und der Mundhole, Berlin: Springer-Bergman, 1925: 1–95.

42. Onodi A. The optic nerve and the accessory sinuses of the nose. London: Bailliere, Tindall and Cox; 1910. 1–26.

43. Bolger, WE, Kennedy, DW Complications in surgery of the paranasal sinuses. In: Eisele DW, editor. Complications in head and neck surgery. Philadelphia, PA: CV Mosby; 1992. 458–70.

44. Pletcher S, Sindwani R, Metson R. Endoscopic Orbital and Optic Nerve Decompression Otolaryngol Clin North Am. 2006;39(5):943–58.

45. Killian, G. Anatomie der Nase menschlicher Embryonen. Arch Laryngol Rhinol. (Berl). 1895; (3):17–47.

46. Metson R, Sindwani R. Frontal Sinusitis: Endoscopic Approaches. Otolaryngol Clin North Am. 2004;37:411–22.

47. Sindwani R, Metson R. Image-Guided Frontal Sinus Surgery. Otolaryngol Clin North Am. 2005;38(3):461–71.

48. Stammberger, H. Uncapping the Egg: The Endoscopic Approach to Frontal Recess and Sinuses. ed. Stammberger, Tuttlingen, Germany, Endo-Press, 2004.

49. Pletcher SD, Sindwani R, Metson R. The Agger Nasi Punch-Out Procedure (POP): Maximizing Exposure of the Frontal Recess. Laryngoscope 2006;116(9):1710–1712.

50. Sindwani R, Metson R. The Impact of Image-Guidance on Osteoplastic Frontal Sinus Obliteration Surgery. Otolaryngol Head Neck Surg 2004; 131:150–5.

Paranasal Sinuses in Health and Disease

Abhijit A. Raut and Bhavin Jankharia

Core Messages

- The CT scan is the modality of choice for evaluation of paranasal sinuses due to its ability to optimally display bone, soft tissue, and air.
- Magnetic resonance imaging (MRI) has the edge over CT with regard to tissue characterization.
- There are a number of variations in nasal anatomy, including middle turbinate, nasal septum, ostiomeatal complex, and uncinate process variations.
- There are five major patterns of inflammatory sinonasal disease: the infundibular, ostiomeatal unit, spheno-ethmoid recess, sinonasal polyposis, and sporadic unclassified patterns.
- The most commonly encountered complication of acute sinusitis is orbital extension.
- Many forms of disease affect the paranasal sinuses.

Contents

Introduction

In the era of endoscopic sinus surgery, the plain radiograph of the paranasal sinuses (PNS) has limited value, in spite of low cost, low radiation dose, and ready availability. Plain radiographs underestimate bony and soft tissue pathology compared with modern imaging techniques like computed tomography (CT) and magnetic resonance imaging (MRI), and these techniques have eclipsed the role of plain radiography in sinus evaluation.

3

Imaging Modalities

CT Scan

The CT scan is the modality of choice for evaluation of PNS due to its ability to optimally display bone, soft tissue, and air [1]. CT can accurately depict the anatomy of the PNS and their normal and abnormal variations, various pathologies, and their extensions. CT of the PNS provides a reliable road map for endoscopic sinus surgery. Limited coronal CT scanning with a low-dose radiation technique can be used for diagnosis of inflammatory sinonasal disease [2]. Additional axial images are useful for evaluation of the anterior and posterior walls of the PNS when there is complete opacification of sinuses and for tumor mapping. Postcontrast evaluation of the PNS is performed in cases of nasal masses and neoplasms for tissue characterization, intracranial and intraorbital extension, and associated cavernous sinus thrombosis.

Prerequisites

All patients should preferably be treated with nasal decongestants prior to the examination and asked to blow the nose just beforehand.

Technique

A prone CT scan of the PNS is performed with hyper-extended chin. Contiguous images with a slice thickness of 3 mm are obtained perpendicular to the hard palate and coverage runs from the anterior wall of the frontal sinus to the posterior wall of the sphenoid sinus.

Axial CT scanning is performed in a supine position so that the hard palate is perpendicular to the table top with 3-mm contiguous images obtained parallel to the inferior orbitomeatal line. The area of coverage should extend from the maxillary teeth to the superior border of the frontal sinuses. In the era of multidetector CT scans, reconstruction can be performed by acquiring axial images in the spiral mode.

Magnetic Resonance Imaging

Magnetic resonance imaging (MRI) has the edge over CT with regard to tissue characterization. It can reliably differentiate between PNS masses and obstructive secretions and inflammatory soft tissue. On T2-weighted images, tumors display intermediate signal intensity, while inflammatory soft tissue is usually hyperintense. Postcontrast MRI is superior in detecting tumors, inflammatory changes, and skull-base invasion. Infected mucosa of the sinonasal cavity shows centrifugal enhancement, while tumors show enhancement toward the center [3]. Tumor extension and perineural spread is best appreciated using the fat saturation postcontrast technique. Contrast-enhanced MRI

improves demonstration of intracranial tumor extension, meningitis, cerebritis, and orbital extension.

However, MRI is not suitable for the routine evaluation of PNS as bones and air within the PNS appear hypointense on all imaging sequences. Ten percent of the patients subjected to MRI may experience claustrophobia. MRI cannot be performed in patients with ocular foreign bodies and cardiac pacemakers. Postcontrast scans demonstrate intense enhancement in tumors and inflammatory pathology, as well as normal mucosa, as a result of which the pathology appears larger than the original size.

Development of Paranasal Sinuses

The face and jaw are derived from three major sources and these include:

1. The ectoderm, which provides surface cover. Ectodermal-mesenchymal interaction forms future developing structures.
2. Neural crest cells form most of the facial mesenchymal structures.
3. The para-axial and prechordal mesoderm develop future myeloblasts of the voluntary craniofacial muscles [4].

The future face is developed from the surface depression, i.e., the stomodeum, which is situated below the developing brain and develops at 4–4.5 weeks' gestation. The stomodeum is surrounded by five mesenchymal prominences.

Paired maxillary prominences lie laterally, while the single frontonasal prominence lies cranial to the stomodeum. Paired mandibular prominences lie caudal to the stomodeum. Bilateral thickening of the ectoderm, i.e., nasal placodes, are formed under the influence of the ventral forebrain at the same time during gestation. At around the fifth week of gestation, the nasal placodes invaginate to form nasal pits.

At around the seventh week of intrauterine gestation the maxillary prominence grows medially, displaying nasal prominences. These nasal prominences fuse at the midline to form the medial upper lip and anterior palate and the maxillary prominences fuse posteriorly to form the posterior palate. The maxillary prominence is separated from the lateral nasal prominence by the nasolacrimal groove, which forms the future nasolacrimal duct. The maxillary prominence forms the cheeks and maxillae. The nasal septum is derived from the frontonasal prominence and grows caudally, fusing with the palate to form the nasal cavities. Bony processes arise from the lateral nasal walls and form turbinates.

During the third fetal month, maxillary sinuses develop, while the sphenoid sinus develops during the fourth fetal month. The ethmoid sinus develops during the fifth fetal month, whereas the frontal sinus does not develop until after birth. At birth, the maxillary and ethmoid sinuses are present, but are usually not aerated. At birth, the sphenoid sinus is usually underdeveloped. At around 6 years of age the frontal sinuses become radiologically visible. The PNS reach their adult configuration after puberty at around 12–15 years of age.

Anatomy

In order to interpret cross-sectional imaging studies of the PNS, the anatomy of the PNS and the nose must be clearly understood. The key to the normal anatomy of the PNS lies in a clear understanding of the structures of the lateral wall of the nose into which most of the paranasal sinuses drain. The anatomy of the lateral wall of the nose is complex compared with the rest of the sinus anatomy.

Lateral Nasal Wall

The PNS drain in the region of the lateral nasal wall. Hence, evaluation of the lateral nasal wall is crucial. Three, or sometimes four, bony lamellae, or conchae, project from the lateral wall of the nose and are named inferior, middle, superior, and sometimes supreme turbinates (Fig. 3.1). The air space beneath the concha is called the meatus. The PNS drain into the nose via the meati. The superior meatus drains the posterior ethmoid air cells and more posteriorly, the sphenoid sinus (via the sphenoethmoid recess). The inferior meatus receives drainage from the nasolacrimal duct. The inferior turbinate is a separate bone, while the superior and middle turbinates are parts of the ethmoid bone [5].

The middle meatus receives drainage from the frontal sinus via the frontal recess, the maxillary sinus via the maxillary ostium, and the anterior ethmoid air cells via the ethmoid cell ostia. The middle meatal attachment is crucial. Superiorly, the middle turbinate is attached to the lateral margin of the cribriform plate. This is called the medial lamella. As it runs posteriorly, the attachment of the middle turbinate curves laterally and is attached to the lamina papyracea. This is called the ground lamella, or basal lamella. This is an important surgical landmark that separates the anterior and posterior ethmoid cells.

Maxillary Sinus

These are paired pyramid-shaped air cavities within the maxillary bones. The roof of the sinus is formed by the orbital floor. The highest portion of the sinus is in the posteromedial portion and lies beneath the orbital apex. The groove and canal for the maxillary nerve are in relation to the roof of the sinus. The floor of the maxillary sinus is formed by the palatine and alveolar process of the maxilla. The medial wall of the sinus forms the lateral wall of the nasal cavity. Posteriorly, the sinus abuts the retromaxillary fat pad and pterygopalatine fossa.

The Ethmoid Sinus

The ethmoid complex consists of four parts, the horizontal lamina called the cribriform plate, the perpendicular plate, and two lateral masses called ethmoid labyrinths. The ethmoid sinus expands within the ethmoid bone or within other sinuses until puberty, forming intramural and extramural ethmoid cells respectively. Extramural expansion of the ethmoid cells can invade frontal, maxillary, and sphenoid sinuses, as well as the ascending processes of the maxilla and lacrimal bones. Lateral extension of the bony basal lamella divides the ethmoid sinus complex into anterior and posterior groups. The anterior ethmoid cells are numerous and smaller in size, whereas the posterior ethmoid cells are larger and fewer. The anterior ethmoid cells are further classified depending upon the drainage pattern into the frontal recess cells, infundibular cells, and basal cells. The posterior ethmoid cells are divided into posterior and postrema cells. The ostia of the ethmoid sinuses are the smallest of all the PNS. There is a higher incidence of mucocele in the anterior ethmoidal cells.

The roof of the ethmoid sinus is in relation to the anterior cranial fossa and is formed by the orbital process of the frontal

Nose and Nasal Cavities

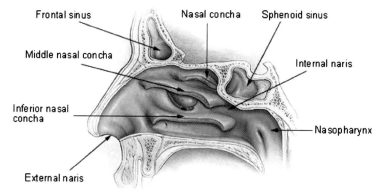

Frontal sinus

Nasal concha

Sphenoid sinus

Middle nasal concha

Internal naris

Inferior nasal concha

External naris

Nasopharynx

Fig. 3.1 Diagram of the sagittal view of the lateral wall of the nose after removal of the turbinates

3

bone and fovea ethmoidalis. The fovea ethmoidalis is 4–7 mm higher than the cribriform plate. An extremely thin bony lamella joins the fovea ethmoidalis and the cribriform plate, and is a common site for surgical injury. The lateral wall of the ethmoid sinus is in relation to the bony orbit.

Frontal Sinus

The frontal sinuses are paired, usually asymmetric, and are located within the frontal bone. They develop independently of the anterior ethmoid cells. The floor of the frontal sinus forms the orbital roof. The posterior wall of the sinus is in relation to the anterior cranial fossa and slopes inferiorly. The primary frontal ostium is located in the midline in the floor of the sinus and is called the frontal recess. This is an hourglass narrowing between the frontal sinus and the anterior middle meatus.

Sphenoid Sinus

This is the posterior-most PNS and shows variable pneumatization. Depending on pneumatization, the sphenoid sinus is classified as nonpneumatized (approximately 1%), presellar (approximately 40%), or sellar (approximately 60%). The roof of the sphenoid sinus is in relation to the anterior cranial fossa, sella turcica, optic chiasm, and juxtasellar space. The lateral wall of the sphenoid sinus is in relation to the orbital apex, optic canal, cavernous sinus, and internal carotid artery. Posteriorly, the sphenoid sinus is in relation to the clivus, the prepontine cistern, and the basilar artery. The sinus floor forms the roof of the nasopharynx. These anatomical relationships of the sphenoid sinus can constitute potential surgical hazards.

Sphenoid sinus septations are usually located in the midline anteriorly and are aligned with the nasal septum. The sphenoid ostium is located medially in the anterosuperior portion of the sinus cavity and communicates with the sphenoethomoidal recess in the posterior aspect of the superior meatus. The sphenoethmoid recess is well displayed in the axial and sagittal planes (Fig. 3.2) [6].

Mucociliary Apparatus

The nose and the PNS are lined by pseudostratified, columnar, ciliated epithelium with interspersed goblet cells. Secretions and mucus from serous and mucus glands opening into the epithelial surface form a mucus blanket that covers the epithelium. Dust from inspired air is deposited on the surface of the mucosa. This mucus blanket is moved by ciliary action toward the pharynx. The cilia beat 250–300 times per minute in a synchronous rhythm. This "mucociliary" system protects the sinuses and the nasal cavity.

Messerklinger demonstrated that the mucociliary clearance of the secretions in the PNS follows genetically predetermined pathways toward the nasal ostia [7]. Normal mucociliary clearance occurs when the drainage channels are patent. When there is contact between two opposing mucosal interfaces, or there is

obstruction of a normal drainage channel, the normal mucociliary action is disturbed, leading to accumulation of mucus and debris with resultant recurrent inflammatory sinonasal disease.

The ostia of the paranasal sinuses are usually not gravity-dependent. It has been proven that in spite of surgically created gravity-dependent nasoantral communication (antrostomy), mucociliary drainage preferentially occurs toward natural sinus ostia. This is the reason for the failure of conventional surgical procedures and is the rationale in favor of functional endoscopic sinus surgery (FESS) [8].

Normal Nasal Variants

Although the nasal anatomy varies from patient to patient, certain anatomical variations are seen more frequently. These variations may narrow normal drainage channels predisposing to chronic sinusitis, while certain variations increase the operative risks. Operating surgeons should be aware of these variations.

Different investigators have reported different prevalence rates; however, often there is a lack of consensus regarding the clinical significance of these variations. Although variations are observed in asymptomatic patients, the prevalence rate of these variations is significantly higher among patients with chronic sinusitis.

Middle Turbinate Variations

The middle turbinate is a thin bony structure that may show varying degrees of pneumatization. Significant pneumatization of the middle turbinate is termed "concha bullosa" (Fig. 3.3). When sufficiently large, this may constrict the middle meatus or encroach upon the infundibulum. Since the air cavity in the concha bullosa is lined with epithelium, it may show inflammatory changes that predispose to mucocele formation. The middle turbinates are usually convex medially. If this convexity is directed toward the lateral nasal wall, it is referred to as a "paradoxical turbinate" (Fig. 3.4) [9].

Nasal Septum Variations

A deviated nasal septum can be congenital or may be post-traumatic and most commonly seen at chondrovomerine articulation. Sometimes there may be associated nasal spurs. The incidence of deviated nasal septum can be up to 20–31% of the population. Significant bowing of the nasal septum results in narrowing of the middle meatus. Associated nasal spurs further compromise the OMU [10].

Variations in Relation to the Ostiomeatal Complex: Haller Cells

Haller cells are extramural ethmoid air cells that project along the medial wall of the floor of the orbit and along the inferior aspect of the lamina papyracea. These cells cause narrowing

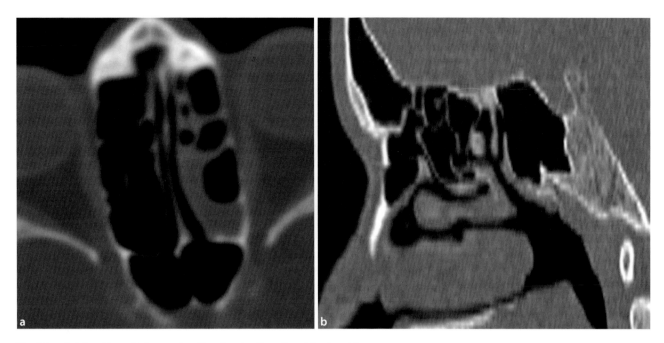

Fig. 3.2 **a** Axial and **b** sagittal reconstruction showing the sphenoid–ethmoid recess

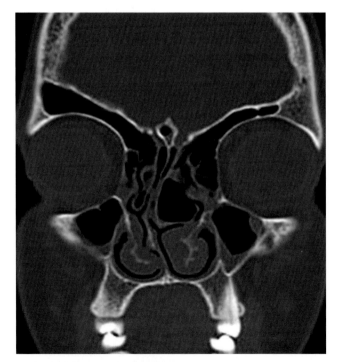

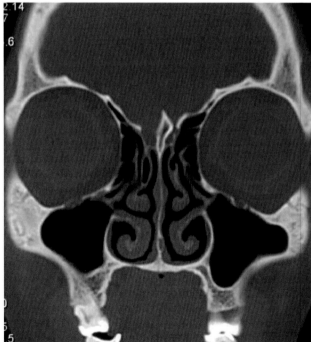

Fig. 3.3 Excessive pneumatization of the left middle turbinate sugges-tive of concha bullosa with mildly deviated nasal septum to the right and compression of left ostiomeatal complex

Fig. 3.4 Bilateral pneumatization of the middle turbinate with lateral convexity suggestive of paradoxical turbinate

of the infundibulum and lead to obstruction of the ostium of the maxillary sinus, thus predisposing to maxillary sinusitis (Fig. 3.5) [11].

Uncinate Process Variations

The uncinate process follows a variable course. The medial deviation of the uncinate process (Fig. 3.6) compromises the middle meatus, while the lateral deviation of the uncinate process (Fig. 3.7) encroaches upon the hiatus semilunaris and infundibulum. Occasionally, the free end of the uncinate process may be pneumatized (Fig. 3.8) and cause narrowing of the maxillary ostium [12]. Sometimes the uncinate process may be attached to the lamina papyracea (Fig. 3.9), lateral surface of the middle turbinate or the fovea ethmoidalis, which may lead to obstruction of the infundibulum. Under such circumstances, care must be taken by the operating endoscopic surgeon not to apply undue force while performing uncinectomy, as this may lead to cerebrospinal fluid rhinorrhea or damage to the anterior cranial fossa and orbital contents.

Onodi Cells

These are the posterior-most ethmoid cells extending into the sphenoid bone situated adjacent to the optic nerve, and they may cause impingement of the latter (Fig. 3.10) [13].

The optic nerve may be surrounded by Onodi cells or may just abut these cells, thereby placing the nerve at surgical risk.

Dehiscence of the Lamina Papyracea

Due to dehiscence of the lamina papyracea, periorbital or orbital content may prolapse into the ethmoid complex and/or infundibulum. This may be a congenital variant or post-traumatic (Fig. 3.11).

Excessive Pneumatization of the Sphenoid Sinus

Pneumatization of the anterior clinoid process secondary to extension of the sphenoid sinus makes the optic nerve vulnerable to surgical complications (Fig. 3.12).

Sometimes the internal carotid artery bulges into the sphenoid sinus. The bone separating the internal carotid artery from the sphenoid sinus is very delicate and measures between 0.5 and 1 mm. Rarely, the internal carotid artery prolapses through the sphenoid sinus and any damage to the artery during sphenoid sinus surgery may lead to catastrophe.

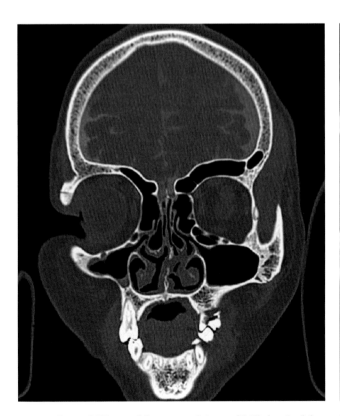

Fig. 3.5 Coronal CT scan of the paranasal sinuses (PNS) showing bilateral concha bullosa with an infraorbital, extramural ethmoid cell suggestive of a Haller cell

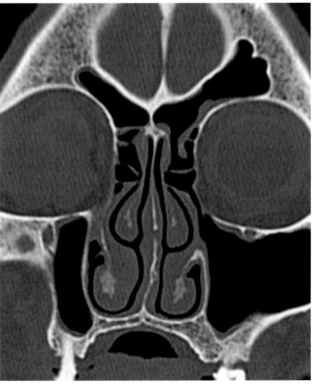

Fig. 3.6 Medial deviation of the uncinate process abutting the middle turbinate

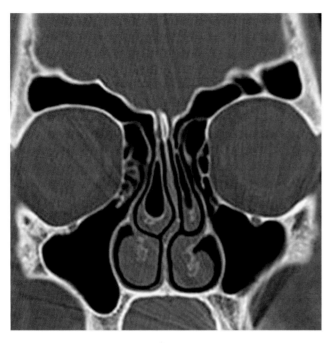

Fig. 3.7 Bilateral concha bullosa. Note lateral deviation of the uncinate process attached to the ethmoid bulla

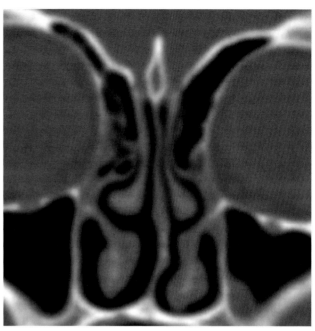

Fig. 3.8 Pneumatization of the right uncinate process

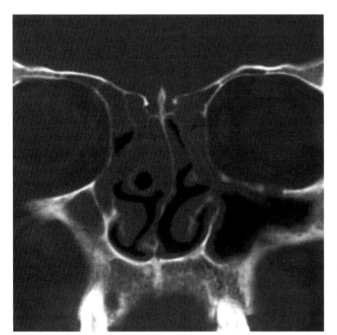

Fig. 3.9 The uncinate process on the left side is attached to the lamina papyracea with bilateral sinusitis. Note the hypoplastic right maxillary sinus

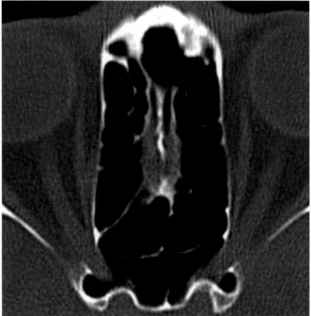

Fig. 3.10 Excessive pneumatization of the bilateral posterior ethmoid sinuses. Note that the optic nerves on both sides show dehiscence

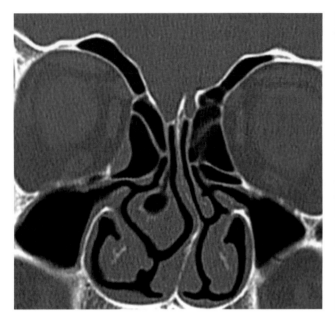

Fig. 3.11 Prolapse of the right orbital fat secondary to the defect in the ipsilateral lamina papyracea

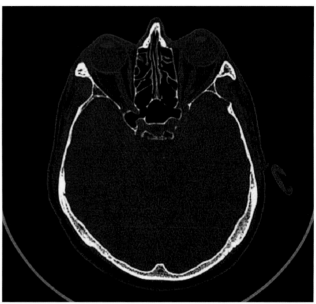

Fig. 3.12 Excessive pneumatization of the sphenoid sinus with resultant asymmetric pneumatization of the anterior clenoid processes

Sinonasal Disease

Anterior Cephalocele

A cephalocele occurs secondary to herniation of the meninges through the cranial defect, i.e., meningocele, or meninges and brain matter, i.e., encephalocele. Anterior cephaloceles may be congenital or post-traumatic and constitute 15% of total cephaloceles. Anterior cephaloceles are classified depending on their craniofacial pathway: frontonasal, nasoethmoidal, and naso-orbital cephaloceles.

Axial and coronal CT can depict the bony defect through which the brain content herniates. However, sagittal and coronal MRI characterize the soft tissue components and help to differentiate between meningoceles and encephaloceles (Fig. 3.13) [14].

Choanal Atresia

The oronasal membrane perforates by the seventh fetal week, the failure of which may result in choanal atresia and may cause

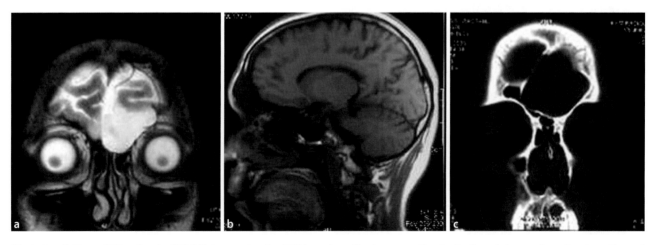

Fig. 3.13 **a,b** Coronal T2 and sagittal T1 MR images showing CSF intensity collection protruding in the frontal sinus and nasal cavity. **c** Coronal bone window of CT showing remodeling of the frontal sinus

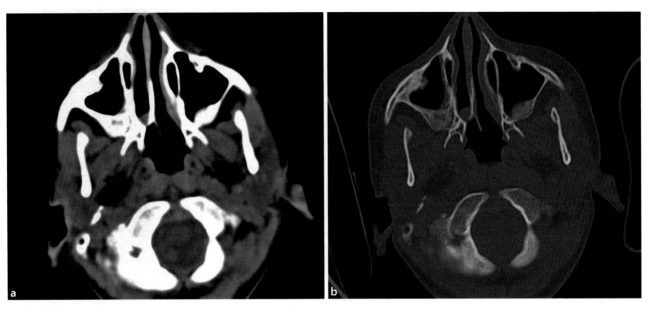

Fig. 3.14 **a,b** Axial soft tissue and bone window showing narrowing and complete occlusion of posterior nasal cavity due to bony choanal atresia

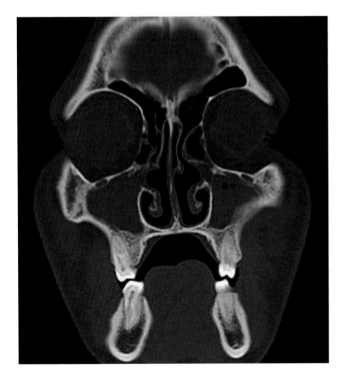

Fig. 3.15 Coronal plain CT scan of the PNS showing a bilateral infundibular pattern of sinusitis secondary to infundibular stenosis

significant respiratory distress in the newborn. It may present as a component of the CHARGE association (C, coloboma; H, heart disease; A, atresia choanae; R, retarded growth and development; G, genital hypoplasia; and E, ear anomalies and/ or deafness). It is often associated with other anomalies [15]. The lesion may be unilateral or bilateral, membranous or bony. CT plays a significant role in the diagnostic and therapeutic approach to congenital choanal atresia. CT evaluation must be performed in neonates with nasal obstruction (Fig. 3.14).

Sinonasal Inflammatory Disease Pattern

Five major patterns of inflammatory sinonasal disease are described. By applying these patterns, we can provide an easy guide to or road map of FESS, allowing tailored endoscopic surgery [16].

Infundibular Pattern

The disease is limited to the maxillary sinus and is due to obstruction of the infundibulum or ostium of the maxillary sinus. The ipsilateral frontal and anterior ethmoid sinuses are unaffected. The common lesions that lead to the infundibular pattern are mucosal swelling at the infundibulum, polyps, and anatomical variants such as Haller cells (Fig. 3.15) and uncinate process variations. Hypoplastic maxillary sinus is usually associated with a long infundibulum that frequently gets blocked.

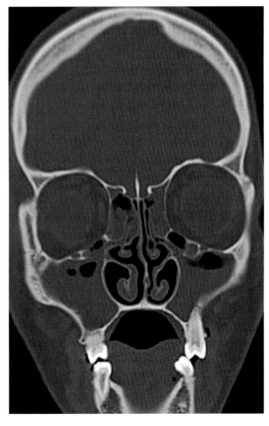

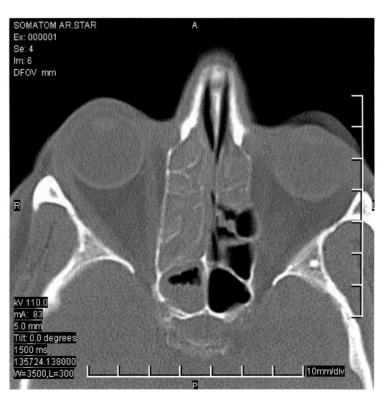

Fig. 3.16 Osteomeatal pattern of sinusitis. Note opacification of bilateral maxillary and ethmoid sinuses

Fig. 3.17 Sphenoethmoid sinusitis secondary to opacification of the sphenoethmoid recess

Ostiomeatal Unit Pattern

The ostiomeatal unit (OMU) pattern is secondary to occlusion of the middle meatus and is the most common pattern of obstructive sinusitis. The ipsilateral frontal, anterior ethmoidal and maxillary sinuses show variable inflammatory involvement. Mucosal swelling, hypertrophied turbinates, polyps, adhesions, nasal tumors, and anatomical variants like concha bullosa, paradoxical turbinate, and deviated nasal septum may be associated with an OMU pattern (Fig. 3.16).

Spheno-ethmoid Recess Pattern

A spheno-ethmoid recess pattern is seen when the ipsilateral posterior ethmoid and the sphenoid sinus are involved. Depending upon mucociliary drainage of the sinuses and location of the obstructive process in the superior meatus, variable involvement of the sphenoid and posterior ethmoid sinus can be seen. Axial (Fig. 3.17) and sagittal images are more helpful for identification of the obstructive pathology.

Sinonasal Polyposis

Sinonasal polyposis is an inflammatory condition associated with characteristic polypoid mucosa of the nose and PNS, with typical radiologic and endoscopic appearance. It is the most troublesome pattern as it may be associated with recurrence and occasionally aggressive behavior. Pathologically edematous hyperplastic mucoperiosteum is heaped up in polypoid fashion. Polysaccharide material present within glands attracts an abnormal amount of water and electrolytes and leads to growth of polyps that appear hypodense on CT scan and are frequently in relation to the middle turbinate. There may be bilateral involvement or sometimes extensive proliferation can be seen. Sinonasal polyposis may be associated with widening of the infundibulum and bony remodeling (Fig. 3.18). Rarely, polyps extrude into the surrounding structures including the orbits and cranial fossa.

Sometimes, polyps can appear hyperdense on plain CT (Fig. 3.19) due to secondary fungal infection, which can be seen in immunocompetent patients. On T2-weighted MRI, polyps appear hyperintense, whereas polyposis associated with fungal involvement shows marked shortening (Fig. 3.20).

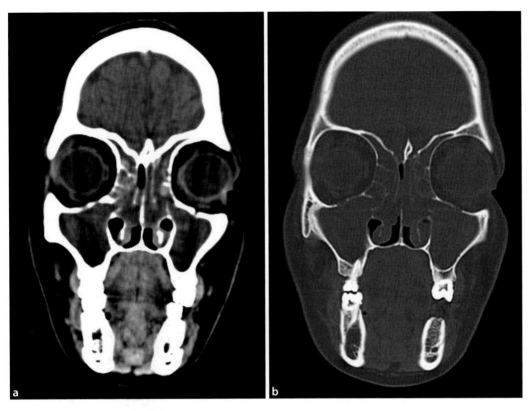

Fig. 3.18 **a,b** Opacification of bilateral maxillary, ethmoidal, and frontal sinus in a known case of polyposis. Hyperdense foci are secondary to super added fungal infection

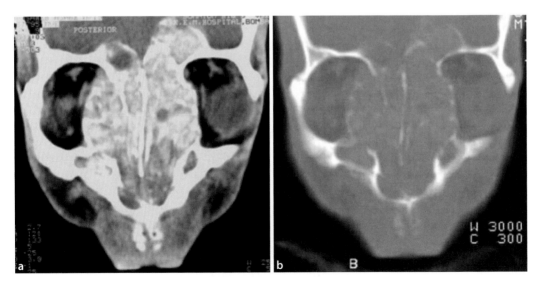

Fig. 3.19 **a,b** Extensive sinonasal polyposis with intra orbital and intracranial extrusion associated with hyperdense concretions due to super added fungal infection in a known case of allergic fungal sinusitis

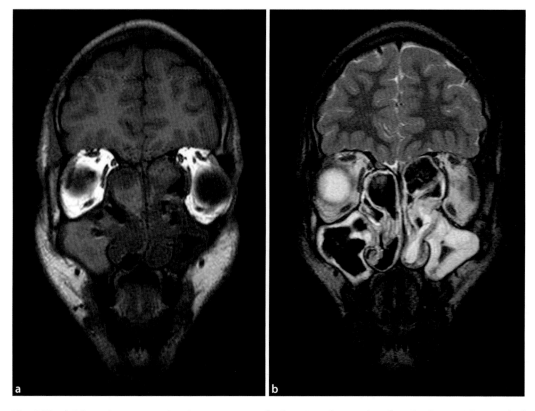

Fig. 3.20 **a,b** Magnetic resonance imaging appearance of polyposis with secondary fungal infection. Note marked shortening on T2-weighted image (**b**)

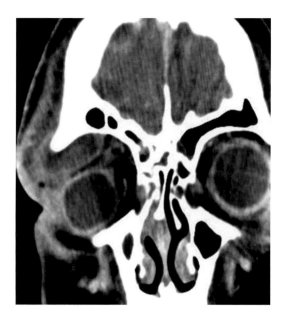

Fig. 3.21 Subperiosteal abscess with mass effect on the right globe secondary to ethmoidal sinusitis

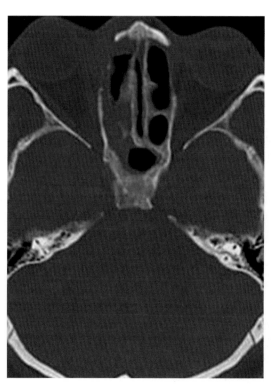

Fig. 3.22 Sclerosis and erosion of the right lamina papyracea with intraorbital extension in a complicated case of ethmoid sinusitis

Sporadic Unclassified Pattern

This includes retention cysts, mucoceles, and mild mucoperiosteal thickening. Postoperative changes after FESS are included in this group.

Complications of Sinusitis

The most commonly encountered complication of acute sinusitis is orbital extension. The ethmoid sinuses are the most common culprits. The infections travel through the thin lamina papyracea, into the valveless veins and may result into orbital cellulitis, subperiosteal abscess, retrobulbar abscess or optic neuritis. On CT images, these inflammatory changes are seen as stranding of the fat planes. The abscesses appear as low-density collections with peripheral enhancement (Fig. 3.21). Bone sclerosis and destruction (Fig. 3.22) may be detected when there is associated osteomyelitis.

Spread of the infection through infected ethmoid cells into the lacrimal apparatus may lead to dacrocystitis and sphenoid sinusitis may lead to optic neuritis.

Intracranial extension may be seen in the form of meningitis, subdural or epidural empyema (Fig. 3.23), brain abscesses, and venous or cavernous sinus thrombosis. The spread of infection is through retrograde thrombophlebitis. Hematogenous and perineural spread have also been described. Postcontrast fat-saturated MRI evaluation of the skull-base is diagnostic for intracranial spread of the disease [17].

Chronic Sinusitis

Repeated or persistent infection leads to chronic sinusitis, which results in atrophy, sclerosis or hypertrophy of the mucosa. These changes are often associated with acute inflammation and the bony sinus wall often shows sclerosis and thickening. These changes are well appreciated in wide soft tissue windows on CT. Hyperdense secretions are seen on the plain CT due to inspissated secretions or due to hemorrhage within or secondary to fungal sinusitis. On MRI, depending upon water and mucus content, the secretions may appear hypo- to hyperintense on T2-weighted images and display variable signal intensity on T1-weighted images.

Cysts and Polyps

Cysts and polyps are common sequelae of inflammation. Obstruction of seromucinous glands leads to formation of mucus retention cysts, while serous retention cysts are formed due to accumulation of fluid in the submucosal layer of the sinus mucosa. These cysts are incidentally seen on imaging and are often asymptomatic. Most commonly they are observed in the maxillary sinus. On CT and MRI, they appear as fluid-filled lesions with smooth convex outer margins (Fig. 3.24). The cyst never fills the sinus completely and air is always present along the superior margin of the cyst. They are commonly seen in the maxillary sinus.

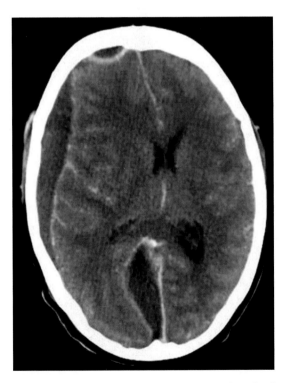

Fig. 3.23 Peripherally enhancing low attenuated subdural collections in the frontal, parietal, and parafalcine regions on the right-hand side due to complicated frontal sinusitis

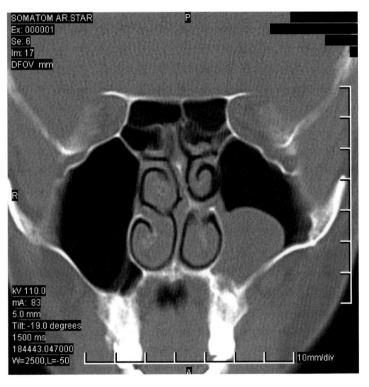

Fig. 3.24 Coronal CT scan showing a solitary water density cyst in the left maxillary sinus

A polyp is heaped-up mucosa elevated by inflammation in a polypoid shape. Polyps are frequently associated with allergic and nonallergic atopic rhinitis, asthma, infection, cystic fibrosis, and Kartagener's syndrome. Polyps may be solitary or extensive. On CT scans they appear as confluent soft tissue masses filling the entire sinonasal cavity. There may be associated demineralization of bony septa, truncation of the middle turbinate tip, infundibular widening or ethmoid sinus wall bulging. When polyposis is severe there may be frank bone destruction. A thin, hypodense mucosal rim usually separates the polyp from the sinus wall. Occasionally, maxillary polyps may expand and prolapse through the sinus ostium and present as a nasal polyp. These are called antrochoanal polyps (Fig. 3.25).

In cases of extensive sinonasal polyposis, there may be associated bony dehiscence and extrusion into the orbit or cranial fossa. Due to fungal infection or inspissated secretions the sinonasal polyposes present as hyperdense soft tissue masses. On CT, *Aspergillus* is the most common culprit and often does not require antifungal agents for treatment [18].

Mucocele

A mucocele is an expansile lesion that has developed within a sinus due to obstruction of a sinus ostium or a compartment of a separated sinus. The sinus cavity is completely filled by mucus material and is airless. The sinus cavity is expanded and there may be associated remodeling of bone. It is most commonly seen in the frontal sinus (60–65% of cases; Fig. 3.26), followed by the ethmoid sinus (20–25% of cases; Fig. 3.27). Only 5–10% of mucoceles occur in the maxillary and sphenoid sinuses [19].

Classically, mucoceles are painless and present with signs and symptoms due to mass effect. Pain is associated with a pyocele or an infected mucocele. On CT, an airless, expanded sinus filled with homogenous mucus is diagnostic of mucocele [20]. There may be associated thinning of the wall of the sinus or sometimes partial erosion. On MRI the signal intensities of mucocele depend upon the protein content of entrapped secretions.

Mucoceles can be differentiated from large retention cysts by absence of air, and associated expansion and remodeling of the sinus wall. Mucoid collection within the antrum and double wall appearance distinguishes odontogenic cysts from mucoceles.

Fungal Sinusitis

A variety of fungal diseases affect the PNS. The common mycotic infections are aspergillosis, mucormycosis, candidiasis, histoplasmosis, and coccidioidomycosis.

There are four distinct patterns of fungal disease, which are described below.

Acute Invasive Disease

Aspergillosis is the commonest causative fungus in immunocompromised patients, while mucormycosis is frequently associated with uncontrolled diabetes. These fungi proliferate in the PNS, causing ischemic necrosis and spread to the adjacent organs. Once tissue invasion is established the fungi further invade the vessel wall, with subsequent thrombosis. The fungi disseminate via perivascular channels and can cross bony par-

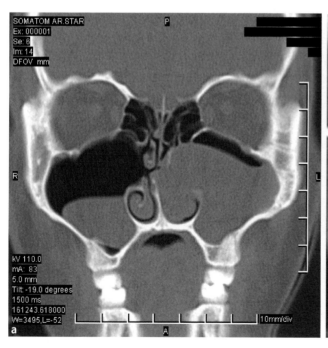
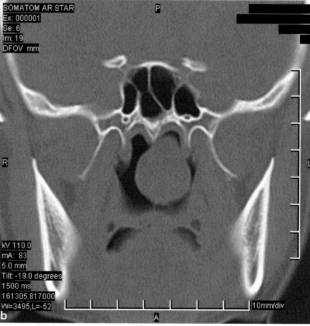

Fig. 3.25 **a,b** Coronal CT scan showing left maxillary polypoid mass prolapsing through the accessory ostium into the oropharynx

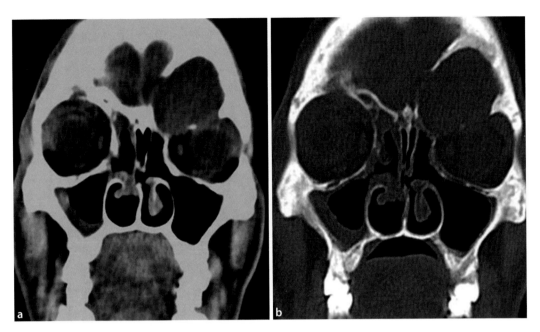

Fig. 3.26 **a,b** Coronal CT scan showing expansile soft tissue attenuated mass in the left frontal sinus displacing the globe inferiorly and laterally in a case of left frontal sinus mucocele

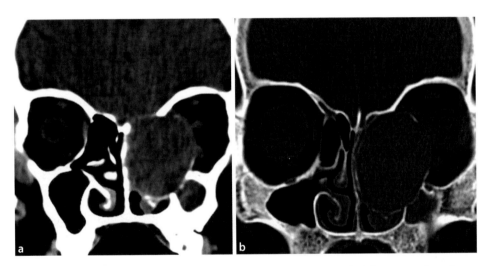

Fig. 3.27 **a,b** Coronal CT scan showing water attenuated expansile mass in the left anterior ethmoid sinus causing remodeling of the lamina papyracea in a diagnosed case of anterior ethmoid mucocele

titions through penetrating blood vessels. Contiguous extension into the orbital apex with involvement of the extraocular muscles may occur. The optic nerve may be enlarged due to direct invasion. The superior ophthalmic vein and ophthalmic artery involvement indicate orbital apex syndrome. Intracranial involvement can be secondary to contiguous spread through the PNS or by hematogenous spread of the disease. Vascular occlusion may be associated with cerebral infarcts (Fig. 3.28). Occasionally, cavernous sinus extension or leptomeningeal enhancement may be seen.

The CT scan shows contiguous PNS involvement associated with mucoperiosteal thickening, and aggressive destruction of bones, which may mimic malignancy (Fig. 3.29). Obliteration of the normal fat planes within any of the periantral components is suggestive of deep tissue extension of the infection (Fig. 3.30). MRI with excellent soft tissue resolution can delineate intracranial and intraorbital extension better than CT scanning. On T2-weighted MRI, the fungal sinusitis shows hypointense soft tissue (Fig. 3.31) [21]. The prognosis for these patients is usually grave.

3

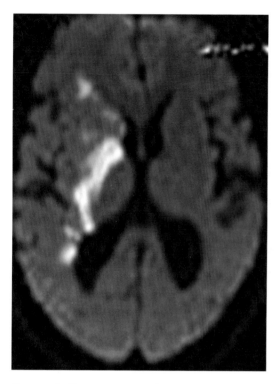

Fig. 3.28 Diffusion MRI image showing restriction of diffusion in the right ganglio capsular region secondary to thrombosis of right MCA in a known case of invasive aspergillosis

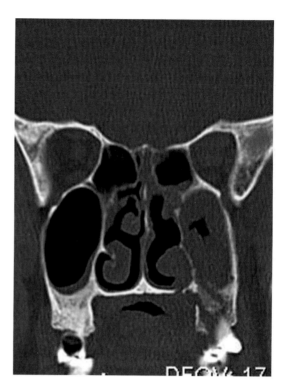

Fig. 3.29 Aggressive destruction of the alveolar margin on the left side. Note oroantral fistula in a known case of mucormycosis

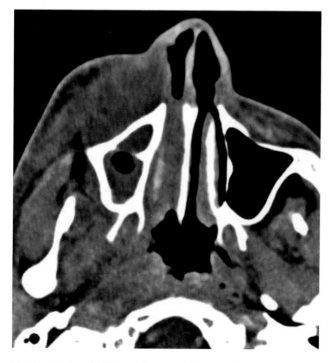

Fig. 3.30 Plain axial CT scan showing soft tissue in the right cheek. Soft tissue is seen in the maxilla. Note obliteration of the posterior periantral fat planes due to aggressive extension of the disease through the intact sinus wall in a diagnosed case of mucormycosis

Chronic Invasive Infection

This may be seen in healthy hosts living in endemic areas as such as Sudan or Saudi Arabia, or in mildly immunocompromised and diabetic patients. These cases respond to antifungal or surgical therapy.

Fungal Ball or Mycetoma

Benign fungal hyphal colonization of the PNS usually develops in response to local changes in the microenvironment, which are commonly seen after surgery, radiotherapy or in marijuana smokers. They respond to conservative management.

Allergic Fungal Sinusitis

Allergic fungal sinusitis (AFS) is usually associated with polyposis, allergic sinusitis or asthma. Aspergillus is the most common causative fungus. These cases show response to conservative and surgical therapy.

Granulomatous Sinusitis

Granulomatous disease involving the sinonasal cavity may be autoimmune or infectious, including rhinoscleroma, leprosy,

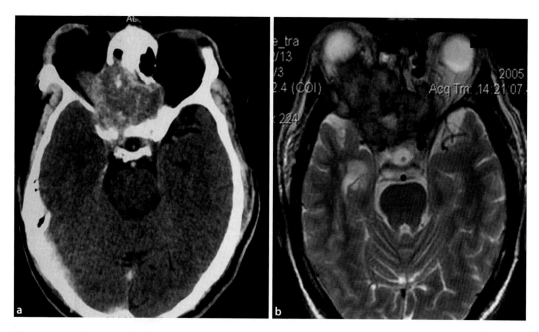

Fig. 3.31 **a** Axial CT postcontrast CT scan demonstrating heterogeneously enhancing soft tissue in the ethmoid complex with aggressive destruction of the lamina papyracea in a known case of invasive aspergillosis. **b** Axial T2-weighted MRI image showing marked T2 shortening of the soft tissue. Note encasement of the ipsilateral internal carotid artery

syphilis, tuberculosis, actinomycosis, lymphoma, idiopathic causes or secondary chronic irritants such as beryllium, chromate salts, and cocaine. Wegener's granulomatosis and sarcoidosis are other examples of granulomatous sinusitis [22].

Destructive granulomatous disease results in variable sinonasal mucosal changes ranging from nonspecific inflammation with mucosal thickening and nasal secretions to localized soft tissue masses. Nasal cavity involvement is preceded by PNS extension. The midline septum may be thickened and bulky and there may be associated extensive erosions. The maxillary and ethmoid sinuses are frequently involved, with sparing of the frontal and sphenoid sinuses. There may be sinomucosal thickening. Thickening of bones and sclerosis are frequently associated chronic inflammatory reactions. Bulky soft tissue masses may be seen in granulomatous sinusitis. These changes are well delineated on CT. On MRI, like any inflammatory disease, granulomatous sinusitis demonstrates hypointense soft tissue on T1-weighted images and hyperintense signal on T2-weighted images. Sometimes, on T2-weighted imaging, reactive sinusitis may display intermediate signal (Fig. 3.32).

Squamous Cell Carcinoma

Squamous cell carcinomas of the nasal and paranasal sinuses are uncommon, but they may be seen among workers who are exposed to nickel, chromium, mustard gas, isopropyl alcohol, and radium. Males aged between 55 and 65 years are usually affected. The most common site is the nasal septum near the mucocutaneous junction and the middle turbinate. The prognosis

of these patients depends upon the extension of the tumor at the time of diagnosis. Local recurrences are seen in 20–50% of patients and around 80% of such recurrences are seen within the first year. The overall 5-year survival rate is up to 62%. Ohngren divided the antrum into posterosuperior and anteroinferior segments by drawing a line on the lateral view of the radiograph (cited in [23]). Tumors limited to the anteroinferior segment have a better prognosis. The most common site of involvement is the maxillary sinus (62%), followed by the nasal cavity (26%), the ethmoid sinus 10%, and the sphenoid sinus (2%). Again, the prognosis of patients with these carcinomas is related to the staging of the tumor at the time of diagnosis.

The American Joint Cancer Commission Modified Staging for carcinoma maxilla is as follows [24]:

TX: The primary tumor cannot be assessed.

To: No evidence of disease.

Tis: Carcinoma in situ.

T1: Tumor limited to the antral mucosa with no erosion or destruction of the bone.

T2: Tumor causes bone erosion or destruction except for the posterior antral wall, including extension into the hard palate and/or middle nasal meatus.

T3: Tumor invasion of any of the following – bone of the posterior wall of the maxillary sinus, subcutaneous tissue, skin of the cheek, pterygoid plates, floor or medial wall of the orbit, infratemporal fossa.

T4: Tumor invasion of the orbital contents beyond the floor of the medial wall including any of the following – the orbital apex, cribriform plate, base of the skull, nasopharynx, sphenoid or frontal sinuses.

3

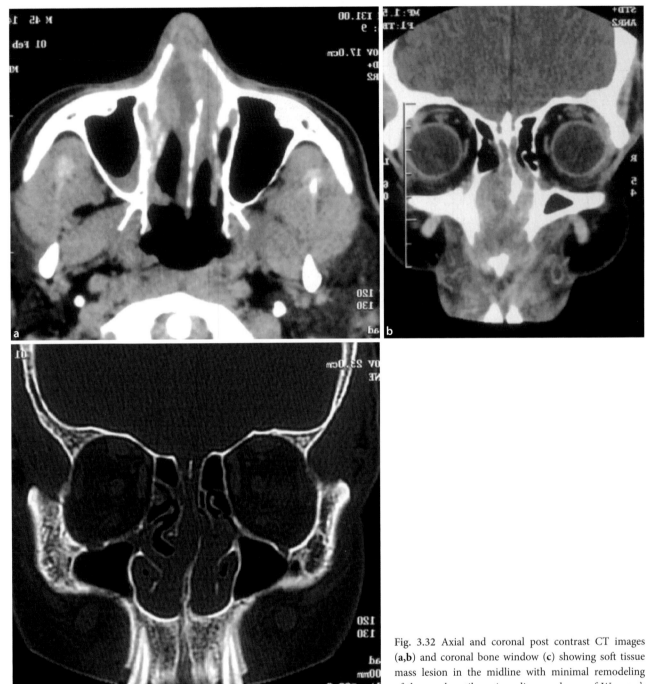

Fig. 3.32 Axial and coronal post contrast CT images (**a,b**) and coronal bone window (**c**) showing soft tissue mass lesion in the midline with minimal remodeling of the nasal cartilages in a diagnosed case of Wegener's granulomatosis

Lymphadenopathy is uncommon in low-grade carcinoma. Once the tumor invades the adjacent structures, the primary drainage is to the retropharyngeal nodes. CT shows a homogenous soft tissue attenuation mass. Large masses are associated with areas of necrosis and hemorrhage. Aggressive destruction of bone is substantial compared with the tumor mass (Fig. 3.33).

On MRI, the mass displays intermediate signal on T1-weighted images and is slightly hyperintense on T2-weighted images. On postcontrast scans, these masses display homogenous enhancement, except when associated with hemorrhage or necrosis (Fig 3.34).

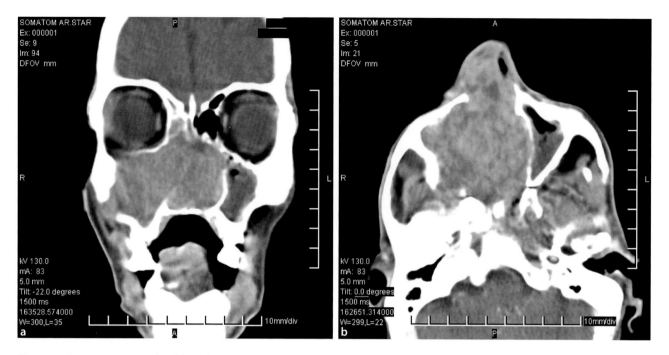

Fig. 3.33 **a** Postcontrast coronal and **b** axial CT scan showing heterogeneous soft tissue mass in the right maxilla causing aggressive destruction of the sinus walls in a diagnosed case of squamous cell carcinoma

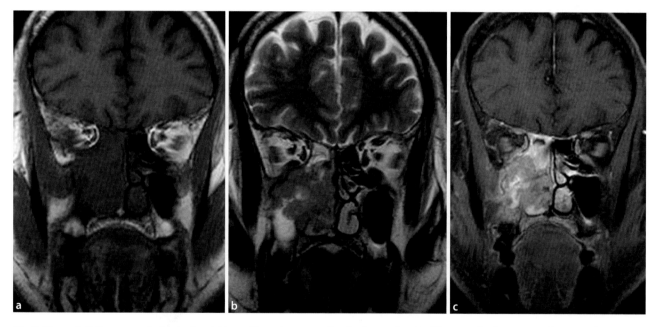

Fig. 3.34 **a–c** Soft tissue mass lesion in the right maxillary sinus extending in the nasal cavity. The mass displays intermediate signal on T2 MR images and shows heterogeneous enhancement on post contrast image

Papilloma

Papillomas are uncommon sinonasal neoplasms and constitute 0.4–4.7% of total sinonasal masses. There are three distinct types of papillomas: fusiform, inverted, and oncocytic.

Fusiform Papillomas

Fusiform papillomas constitute 50% of total papillomas and are seen commonly in men between 20 and 50 years of age. They usually arise from the nasal septum, are solitary, and have very minimal malignancy potential.

Inverted Papillomas

These papillomas make up 47% of the total number of papillomas and are commonly seen in elderly men. The lateral nasal wall near the middle meatus is most commonly affected, from which they extend into the sinus. They cause nasal obstruction, epistaxis, and anosmia [25].

Carcinoma Ex-Inverted Papillomas

This type of papilloma has been described in 3–24% of cases. Squamous cell carcinoma may be associated with inverted papilloma in 2–56% of cases. On cross-sectional imaging they appear as unilateral, soft tissue density, lobulated masses. They are associated with bowing of the midline nasal septum rather than destruction. Calcification is frequently associated with inverted papilloma (Fig. 3.35). A septal, basal polypoid mass strongly suggests fusiform papilloma. When an area of asymmetric destruction is associated with a case of inverted papilloma, the possibility of an underlying carcinoma should be considered.

Adenocarcinoma

These are the second most common neoplasms involving the sinonasal tract and are commonly seen in a middle-aged or elderly population with a high incidence among wood-workers. The ethmoid sinus is more commonly involved than the maxillary sinus. They can be classified as minor salivary gland tumors (e.g., adenoid cystic carcinoma, mucoepidermoid carcinoma, acinic cell carcinoma, and benign and malignant pleomorphic adenoma), an intestinal type of adenocarcinoma, or a sinonasal neuroendocrine type of carcinoma. On imaging they appear to be similar to the squamous cell carcinoma.

Esthesioneuroblastoma

These are also known as olfactory neuroblastomas. They are uncommon malignant tumors and arise from the neuroepithelium of the superior nasal cavity. These tumors have a bimodal age distribution occurring at 10–20 years and 50–60 years and typically grow inferiorly into the nasal cavity with superior extension into the ethmoid sinus. Intracranial extension through the cribriform plate and intraorbital extension through the lamina papyracea are frequent features. On CT, bowing of the walls of the nasal cavity and adjacent PNS is well appreciated. The scan also shows local destruction of the sinus walls, turbinates, and the nasal septum. The tumor may show calcification within. On MRI images, the tumor appears hypointense on T1-weighted images and hyper- to isointense on T2-weighted images. On postcontrast scans, these tumors show heterogeneous enhancement. Peripheral cysts along the intracranial margin of the tumor constitute a specific sign of esthesioneuroblastoma and, when present, are diagnostic (Fig. 3.36) [26].

These tumors are treated by surgical excision and radiotherapy. Local recurrence is seen in up to 5% of the patients.

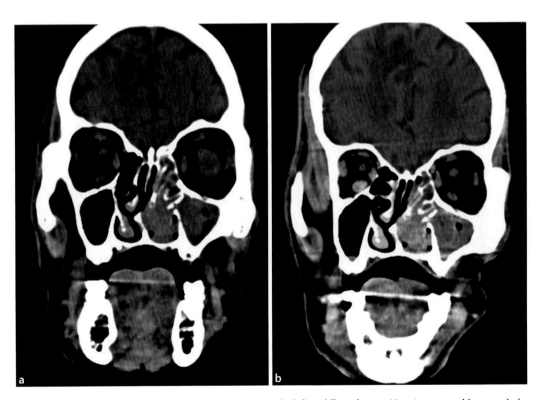

Fig. 3.35 **a,b** Heterogeneous soft tissue mass in relation to the left middle turbinate. Note intact nasal bone and obstructive maxillary sinusitis

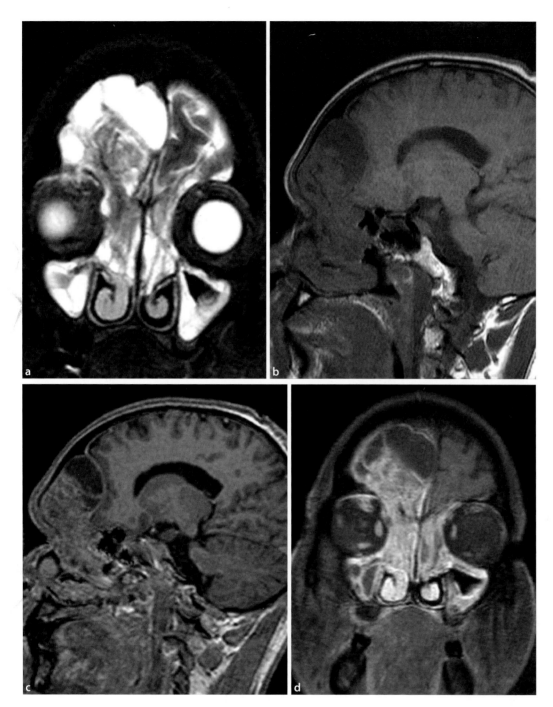

Fig. 3.36 **a–d** T2-weighted coronal, T1-weighted sagittal, and postcontrast images showing intermediate soft tissue mass in the nasal fossa with intracranial extension. Postcontrast images show intense enhancement. The peripherally enhancing cysts are seen at the tumor–cerebral junction. These features are suggestive of esthesioneuroblastoma

Juvenile Nasopharyngeal Angiofibroma

A nasopharyngeal angiofibroma is a benign but locally aggressive tumor arising from the fibrovascular stroma on the posterolateral nasal wall adjacent to the sphenopalatine foramen. The common clinical presentation is of an adolescent male with a nasal mass and history of epistaxis. Extension into the pterygopalatine fossa occurs in 89% of the cases and results in widening of this fossa with resultant anterior bowing of the posterior ipsilateral antral wall. Other directions of tumor spread include posteriorly into the nasopharynx, via the foramen rotundum into the middle cranial fossa, and through the inferior orbital fissure into the orbits. The diagnosis by CT is based upon the site of origin of the lesion in the pterygopalatine fossa. There are two constant features: an enhancing mass in the posterior nasal cavity and pterygopalatine fossa, and erosion of the bone behind the sphenopalatine foramen with extension to the upper medial pterygoid plate (Fig. 3.37). Good bone imaging on CT is essential to show invasion of the cancellous bone of the sphenoid. This is the main predictor of recurrence: the deeper the extension, the larger the potential tumor remnant likely to be left following surgery [27]. The characteristic features on MRI are due to the high vascularity of the tumor, causing signal voids and strong postcontrast enhancement. MRI shows the preoperative soft tissue extent of angiofibroma optimally, but its more important application is to provide postoperative surveillance in order to show any residual or recurrent tumor, record tumor growth or natural involution, and monitor the effects of radiotherapy (Fig. 3.38).

Malignant Melanoma

These are relatively rare sinonasal malignancies and constitute 3–4% of the neoplasms in this region. They are more commonly seen in the nasal cavity than within the PNS. The nasal septum is the most common site. They are common in the elderly population. Up to 65% of patients with melanomas have recurrence or metastasis within the first year after surgery. Metastases are seen in the lung, brain, lymph nodes, and adrenals.

Both hemorrhagic and nonhemorrhagic melanotic melanomas display hyperintense signal on T1-weighted images. Amelanotic melanomas display intermediate signal on T1-weighted images and are difficult to distinguish from other tumors. On T2-weighted images, melanoma shows intermediate signal intensity and shows moderate postcontrast enhancement.

Rhabdomyosarcoma

Rhabdomyosarcoma is one of the most common tumors in children less than 15 years of age. They are seen infrequently in the head and neck region. The maxillary sinus is the most common site.

This tumor appears as a poorly defined, homogenous mass associated with bone remodeling and destruction. On postcontrast scans, they show moderate to generalized enhancement. On MRI examination, they appear isointense to the muscle on T1-weighted images. On T20weighted images they are hypointense to the muscle. Necrosis, hemorrhage, and calcification are not usually associated with these tumors.

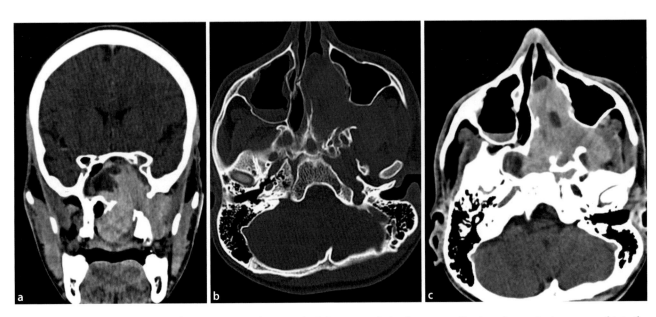

Fig. 3.37 **a–c** Intensely enhancing soft tissue mass in relation to the left pterygopalatine fossa, extending into the masticator space and into the sphenoid sinus, suggestive of juvenile nasopharyngeal angiofibroma. Bone window at the same level demonstrating widening of the pterygopalatine foramina and sphenopalatine fissure

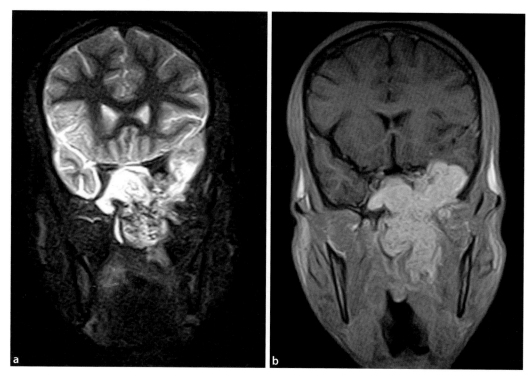

Fig. 3.38 **a** T2-weighted coronal image showing hyperintense mass lesion in relation to the left pterygopalatine fossa. Note flow voids within the lesion, suggestive of rich vascular supply. **b** Intense enhancement is seen on a postcontrast scan in a diagnosed case of juvenile nasopharyngeal angiofibroma

Odontogenic Cysts

Odontogenic and developmental cysts are rare and are derived from cystic expansion of the epithelial remnant of dental apparatus. They are uncommon entities and are classified as follicular, periodontal, odontogenic, nasopalatine, median palatine, and nasolabial cysts.

Follicular cysts, also known as dentigerous cysts, result from accumulation of fluid in relation to the tooth. They are invariably associated with an impacted or unerupted tooth. On imaging they appear as well-circumscribed cysts containing the crown of a tooth. They are usually unilocular. Resorption of the adjacent tooth root may be associated (Fig. 3.39). These cysts may extend into the maxillary sinus and cause expansion of the antra.

Periapical, radicular or dental cysts arise in the erupted, infected tooth. Maxillary teeth are most commonly involved. Remodeling of the maxillary sinus wall is seen, with elevation of the inferior sinus cortex (Fig. 3.40) [28].

Odontogenic keratocysts are aggressively growing lesions and are associated with Marfan's syndrome and basal cell nevus syndrome. They are more common in the mandible than in the maxilla. CT shows a water density, sharply defined, cystic lesion. These cysts may be destructive and invade the adjacent bone (Fig. 3.41).

Odontogenic Tumors

An ameloblastoma is a slowly growing solid and cystic tumor. Twenty percent of ameloblastomas are located in the maxilla. Radiographically, an ameloblastoma may be a unilocular or multilocular radiolucent lesion. On CT, an ameloblastoma appears as a low attenuation cystic lesion intermixed with isodense areas, reflecting the solid component of this lesion (Fig. 3.42). Other odontogenic tumors to involve the PNS are the cementoma, odontoma, and fibromyxoma.

Osteoma

An osteoma is a benign solitary expansile proliferation of mature bone. Multiple osteomas are seen in Gardener's syndrome. They are commonly encountered in membranous bones of the skull and face. The frontal sinus is the most favored site. On imaging, they appear as well circumscribed masses of variable bone density arising from the sinus wall (Fig. 3.43).

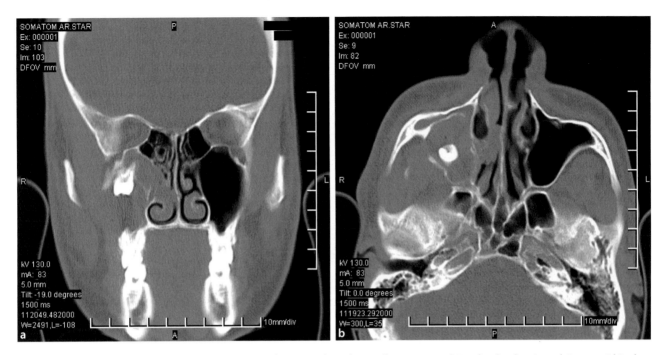

Fig. 3.39 **a** Axial and **b** coronal images showing an expansile mass in the right maxillary sinus involving the alveolus. A tooth is seen within the lesion. These features are seen in dentigerous cysts

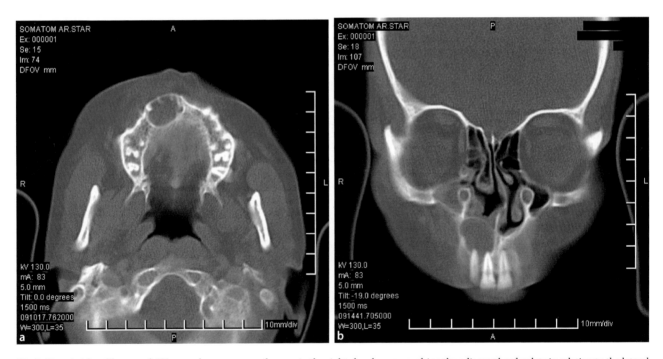

Fig. 3.40 **a** Axial and **b** coronal CT scans show an expansile mass in the right alveolus encroaching the adjacent hard palate in relation to the lateral incisor tooth, suggestive of a dental cyst

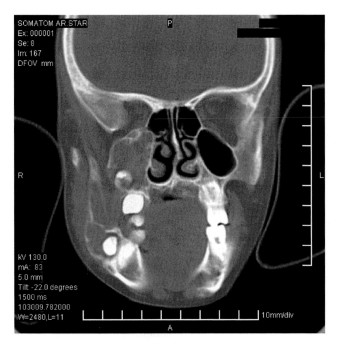

Fig. 3.41 An expansile lytic lesion is seen in the right maxilla in relation to the second molar tooth. Another lytic lesion is seen in relation to the body and ramus of the mandible in a known case of an odontogenic keratocyst

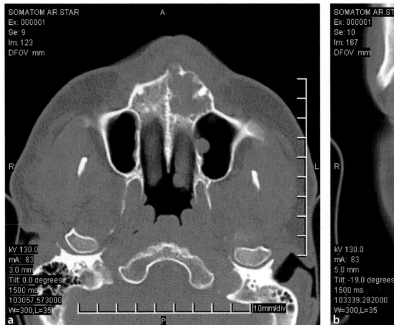

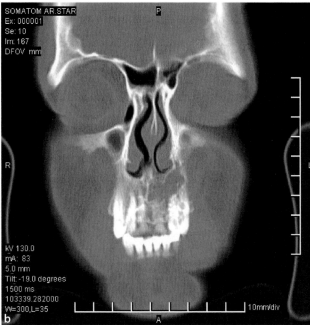

Fig. 3.42 **a–d** Axial and coronal CT scans with soft tissue and bone window showing an expansile lytic lesion in relation to the alveolar margin with an irregular margin associated with isodense soft tissue along the periphery in a proven case of ameloblastoma (**c,d** *see next page*)

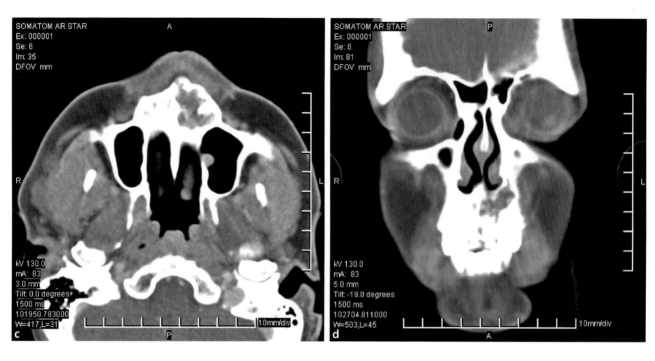

Fig. 3.42 **a–d** (*continued*) Axial and coronal CT scans with soft tissue and bone window showing an expansile lytic lesion in relation to the alveolar margin with an irregular margin associated with isodense soft tissue along the periphery in a proven case of ameloblastoma

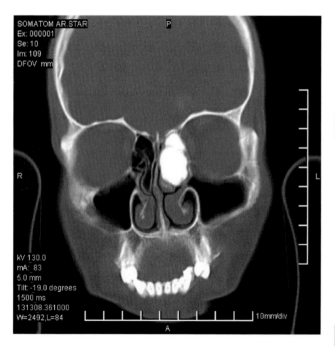

Fig. 3.43 Well-circumscribed sclerotic lesion is seen in the anterior ethmoid cell on the left side, suggestive of osteoma

Fibrous Dysplasia

Fibrous dysplasia is a benign skeletal disorder in which medullary bone is replaced by poorly organized fibro-osseous tissue.

Patients present with obstructive symptoms, due to encroachment of the bony mass into the PNS, nasal fossa or neu-

rovascular channels. On imaging, there is typically ground glass opacity with expansion of the bone and widening of the medullary space. The margin of the tumor is formed by thin, intact cortical bone (Fig. 3.44) [29].

Osteosarcoma

Osteosarcomas account for 0.5–1% of sinonasal tumors. They may occur de novo or may be associated with radiation, Paget's disease or fibrous dysplasia, and are frequently seen in the maxillary sinus. Depending upon the nature of the tumors, aggressive or minimal destruction of the bones may be seen associated with soft tissue. Irregular calcification or aggressive periosteal reaction is well demonstrated on CT. On MRI, these masses are seen as inhomogeneous lesions of intermediate signal intensity with areas of low signal intensity corresponding to ossification.

Chondrosarcoma

Chondrosarcomas rarely involve the nasal cavity and PNS. When present they arise most frequently in the maxilla. Although usually low-grade tumors, local excision is usually associated with a high rate of recurrence; hence, en bloc resection is advisable. Cross-sectional imaging plays an important role in planning definitive surgery. On CT scans they show nodular or plaque-like calcifications. On T1-weighted images these lesions appear heterogeneous and display intermediate signal intensity. On T2-weighted images they demonstrate peripheral hyperintense signal. Postcontrast images show peripheral enhancement.

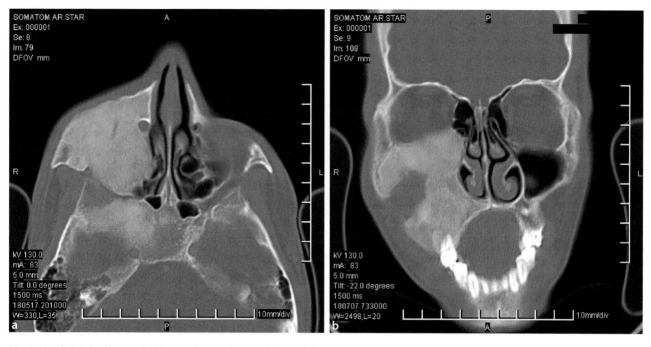

Fig. 3.44 a,b Axial and coronal CT scans show widening of the medullary space secondary to an expansile mass of ground-glass density involving the right maxilla, zygoma, and alveolar process, representing fibrous dysplasia

Metastases to the Paranasal Sinuses

The majority of metastases to the sinonasal tract are through hematologic spread to the bone. Renal, breast, lung, and prostate carcinomas are among the most common malignancies that metastasize to the PNS. The maxillary antrum is frequently involved.

References

1. Zinreich S, Kennedy D, Rosenbaum A, et al. Paranasal sinuses: CT Imaging requirements for endoscopic surgery. Radiology 1987; 163:769–775.

2. Buvoisn B, Landry M, Chapuis L, et al. Low-dose CT and inflammatory disease of the paranasal sinuses. Neuroradiology 1991; 33:403–406.

3. Grossman RI, Youserm DM. Sinonasal disease. In Grossman RI, Yoserm DM (Eds) Neuroradiology. The requisites, 2nd edition. Philadelphia, Mosby.

4. Moore KL, Persaud TVN. The developing human. Clinically oriented embryology, 6th Ed, Philadelphia: Saunders, 1998.

5. Hansberger R. Imaging for the sinus and nose. In Hansberger R, Ed. Head and Neck Imaging Handbook. St. Louis: Mosby – Year Book, 1990; 387–419.

6. Zinreich S, Abidin M, Kennedy D. Cross sectional imaging of the nasal cavity and paranasal sinuses. Operative techniques. Otolaryngol Head Neck Surg 1990; 1:93–99.

7. Messerklinger W. On the drainage of the normal frontal sinus of man. Acta Otolaryngol 1967; 63:176–181.

8. Rice DH. Endoscopic sinus surgery: anterior approach. Otolaryngol Head Neck Surg 1986; 94:143–146.

9. Lloyd GAS. CT of the paranasal sinuses: Study of a control series in relation to Endoscopic sinus surgery. J Laryngol Otol 1990; 104:477–481.

10. Zinreich S. Imaging of inflammatory sinus disease. Otolaryngol Clin. North Am 1993; 26:535–547.

11. Laine F, Smoker W. The Ostiomeatal Unit and endoscopic surgery: anatomy, variations and imaging findings in inflammatory diseases. Am J Roentgenol 1992, 159:849–857.

12. Bolger W, Butzin C, Tarsons D. Paranasal sinus bony anatomic variations and mucosal abnormalities: CT analysis for Endoscopic Surgery. Laryngoscope: 1991; 101:56–64.

13. Stammberger HR, Kennedy DW, Bolger WE et al. Paranasal sinuses anatomic terminology and nomenclature. The Anatomic Terminology Group. Ann Otol Rhinol Laryngol suppl 1995; 167: 7–16.

14. Maidich TP, Ultman NR, Braffman BH, et al. Cephaloceles and related malformations. AJNR Am J Neuroradiol 1992; 13:655–690.

15. Faust RA, Philip CD. Assessment of congenital bony nasal obstruction by 3-dimensional CT volume rendering. Int J Pediatr Otorhinolaryngol 2001 Oct 19; 61(1):71–75. Review.

16. Hansberger HR, Babbel RW, Davis WL. The major obstructive inflammatory patterns of the sinonasal region seen on screening sinus CT. Semin Ultrasound CT MRI 1991; 12:541–560.

17. Larson TL. Sinonasal inflammatory disease: Pathophysiology, imaging and surgery. Semin Ultrasound CT MRI, Volume 20, No. 6, 1999; 379–390.

18. Som PM, Curtin H. Chronic inflammatory sinonasal diseases including fungal infections: The Role of Imaging. Radiol. Clin. North Am 1993; 31:33–44.

19. Zizmor J, Noyek A. Cysts, benign tumours and malignant tumours of PNS. Otolaryngol Clin North Am 1973; 6:487–508.

3

20.	Perugini S, Paraquini V, Menichelli et al. Mucocele in the PNS involving the orbit CT signs in 43 cases. Neuroradiology 1982: 23:133–139.

21.	Fatterpekar G, Mukherji SK, Arbealez A. Fungal disease of the paranasal sinuses. Semin Ultrasound CT MRI: 1999; 20(61) 391–401

22.	Fleming I, Cooper J, Henson D, Som PM, Brandwein M. Inflammatory diseases. In Som PM, Curtin HD (eds): Head and Neck Imaging, 4th edn. St. Louis, Mosby 2003.

23.	Daredes S, Choh, Som M. Total maxillotomy. In: Blitzer A, Lawson W, Fridman W, Eds. Surgery of the Paranasal Sinuses. Philadelphia: Saunders, 1985; 204–216.

24.	American Joint Committee on cancer staging manual. 5th Edition. Philadelphia: Lippincott Raven 1997.

25.	Lund V, Lloyd G. Radiological changes associated with Inverted papillomas of the Nose and Paranasal sinuses. Br J Radiol 1984; 57:455–461.

26.	Som P, Lidov M, Brandwein M et al. Sinonasal esthesioneuroblastoma with intracranial extension. Marginal tumor cyst as a MR finding. Am J Neuroradiol 1994; 15:1259–1262.

27.	Lloyd G, Howard D, Lund VJ, Savy L. Imaging for juvenile angiofibroma. J Laryngol Otol. 2000 Sep; 114(9):727–730. Review.

28.	Stafne E, Gibiliseo J. Oral Roentgenographic diagnosis. 4th ed. Philadelphia: Saunders, 1975; 147–168.

29.	Som P, Lidov M. The benign fibro-osseous lesion: its association with paranasal sinuses mucoceles and its MR appearance. J Comput Assist Tomogr 1993; 17:492–494.

Physiology and Pathophysiology

Chapter 4

Measurement of Nasal Function

Guy S. Kenyon and John Pickett

4

Core Messages

- Of all the techniques available, rhinomanometry is the closest to a "gold standard" for nasal assessment.
- Acoustic rhinometry is also widely used and spirometry has enjoyed some support.
- There is a need for more reliable system of nasal airway measurement.
- Inter- and intra-test variation in measurements of nasal obstruction are too variable for any one means of assessment to be reliable at the present time.
- Utilisation of a combination of measurement techniques together with clinical judgement and the reports of the patients' own sensation of obstruction are the best that can be achieved currently.

Contents

Introduction

It is widely appreciated that the nose acts in order to provide air conditioning and humidification of the inhaled air, as well as a protective function through the mucociliary escalator and through filtration and the secretion of lysozymes and immunoglobulins. When the flow of air is unimpeded the nasal airway also allows odorant to interact with the olfactory epithelium, thus providing the individual with a sense of smell. But it is as a resistor that the nose receives most attention in routine clinical practice, since it is patients with obstructive symptoms who constitute the majority of referrals and who form the bulk of the patients receiving surgery.

Perhaps because of this much effort has been made to try to measure nasal airway performance. Indeed, such measurements are not new. Mirror misting or other assessments of the pattern of exhaled air from the nose as a means of assessing performance was advocated at the end of the 19th and at the beginning of the 20th centuries [1, 2] and Hirschman [3] used a modified cystoscope to examine the sinuses. Unfortunately, as will be shown, in spite of many technical advances our means of accurately assessing patients objectively have not advanced into routine practice at most centres.

This is, perhaps, because efforts to measure nasal airway performance frequently fail to correlate with the pathological processes that are observed within the nose. Empirically, it would seem obvious that the two should be related – but they are not. There appear, in fact, to be four possible states. Thus, a patient may have:
- A normal nose and no complaint.
- A complaint of obstruction that appears to have an obvious cause that can be identified and is corrected medically or surgically with apparent relief, such as rhinitis, a deviated septum or unilateral polyp.
- A highly congested nose with turbinate hypertrophy or septal deviation, but no apparent complaint.
- A complaint of obstruction in the presence of an airway that appears widely patent – the so-called "empty nose syndrome"

This lack of synergy between the patient's symptom and the physical findings is also manifest in a lack of correlation between measurements of resistance and the patient's subjective assessment of their own airway [4]. In the light of this many clinicians in routine practice do no more than ask the patient how readily they believe they can breathe through the nose. Such an assessment is normally accompanied, at least in a research setting, by measurements on a visual analogue scale. But it is a wholly objective analysis that is desirable – especially if surgical and medical intervention is to be properly assessed. To that end much effort has been made to try to devise methods that give a reproducible and objective assessment of nasal airway performance – although many of the papers that have been written on the subject have poor power and are level 4 or 5 evidence at best.

The main methods that have been used for airway assessment will be presented here. The first category makes measurements of the ease with which air passes through the nose, either from the individual's own effort or from an externally generated source. The second measures the dimensions of the nasal cavity and the points at which resistance to flow may be abnormally high. In both of these categories there are a number of different methods that have been developed to accomplish the measurement, each with its own advantages and disadvantages. Finally, there are a miscellany of other methods that have been used and that will be alluded to. In the discussion that follows, each of these processes will be described and the literature surrounding each method outlined.

Techniques

Rhinomanometry

Rhinomanometry provides a direct measurement of nasal resistance. By measuring the pressure gradient across the nasal cavity and the volume flow through the nose, the hydraulic resistance can be calculated, $R = \Delta P / \dot{V}$.

Such measurements can be either active or passive with the pressure measured at either the anterior or posterior nares. Passive methods measure pressure changes while externally generated airflow is directed at a known rate through a mouthpiece. Active anterior rhinomanometry has been found to offer better reproducibility than passive rhinomanometry and the latter measurements do not mimic normal physiological flow. As a result they have been, for all practical purposes, abandoned.

In contrast active methods, where the pressure gradient across the nose is generated while the patient breathes quietly, have been the subject of many reports in the literature. There are two such methods [5]. In posterior active rhinomanometry the pressure is measured in the mouth (Fig. 4.1) and this measurement is presumed to give a recording that is equal to the pressure in the nasopharynx. The pressure gradient across the whole nose can be assessed at a variety of flow rates to give a measure of resistance. In active anterior rhinomanometry, the pressure gradient is assessed by occluding one nostril either by using a nozzle or by applying adhesive tape and measuring the pressure in the anterior nares (Fig. 4.2). No air can, of course, flow into the occluded side, but the pressure measurement made

is assumed to equal the pressure in the nasopharynx and, hence, to represent the pressure gradient on the contra-lateral side. Deriving the pressure in this way is termed anterior rhinomanometry. The total resistance can then be calculated from the unilateral measurements using the formula:

$$1/R_{\text{total}} = 1/R_{\text{right}} + 1/R_{\text{left}}$$

In both posterior and anterior rhinomanometry measurements of flow are usually made using a pneumotachograph connected to a mask covering the nose or nose and mouth. A nozzle can be used to connect this directly to the nostril for anterior rhinomanometry – but this is not commonly done as it is felt to be more likely to distort the nose and disrupt the measurement. A good seal is required, as leaks will cause errors in the flow measurement. A further option is to use a head out body box to derive the flow signal. This eliminates the need to use a mask as, during respiratory movements, air is inspired or expired and air surrounding the body is displaced from the box. If the mouth is closed measurements of air flow therefore reflect the flow through the nose [6].

A graph of the pressure plotted against flow is sigmoid in shape as increasing turbulence at higher flow rates results in higher resistance to flow (Fig. 4.3). Progressively increasing pressures therefore result in progressively smaller increases in flow. There is currently no complete mathematical description of the pressure/flow relationship over the whole breathing cycle and, for this reason, it is necessary to present results in a consistent way to enable meaningful comparisons between centres and operators.

A number of schemes for this have been proposed. As resistance varies at different pressures and flows, and therefore varies across the respiratory cycle, the resistance is often quoted at standard pressure gradients such as 50, 100 and 150, calculated using the formula $R = \Delta P / \dot{V}$ [7]. An alternative method is that outlined by Broms et al. [8]. If the pressure is plotted against flow during the breathing cycle, such that one Pa on the pressure axis is the same length as one cm^3/s on the flow axis, then the equation $V(r) = V_o + c.r$ can be used where:

$V(r) = $ the angle between a line from the intercept of the curve with a circle of radius (r) to the origin and the flow axis

$V_o = $ the angle of the curve to the flow axis at the origin

$C = $ a constant (reflects non-linearity i.e. turbulence)

Taking the radius r as 100 (100 Pa and 100 cm^3/s) and as $r=200$ and $r=300$ is thought to give an adequate description of the whole curve.

O'Neill [9] proposed and validated an improved mathematical model using log transforms of the pressure and flow data. However, this has yet to find routine use and in commercial devices the consensus guidelines of the International Committee for Standardisation of Rhinomanometry (ICSR), published in 1984, are usually followed [7]. These recommended that either the Broms method or the resistance at 150 Pa should be used.

Rhinomanometry has, over the years, become regarded as the 'gold standard' for objective measurement of nasal function – but its validity is in fact still open to question. Even with the adoption of standardised operating procedures as recommended by the ICSR, studies on the accuracy and reproducibility of the technique have reported coefficients of variation for their measurements from less than 5% up to 60% – even when the ICSR protocols are followed [10–12]. It is difficult to believe that such a wide range could not owe something to differences in experimental technique, but in most reports insufficient information as to the protocols used is given to allow meaningful comparisons to be made between different studies. Carney et al. [13] reported coefficients of variation of up to 60% when performing active anterior rhinomanometry according to ICSR guidelines – although this figure was improved to 15% when they used their revised "Nottingham" protocol. The latter involved paying greater attention to removing air leaks and repeating measurements when strict acceptance criteria for the curves were not reached. It seems likely that other investigators adopt similar strategies to achieve lower coefficients of variation, but often such information is omitted when data are reported.

If the reproducibility is operator- and technique-dependent then it is also true that there will be variability due to the mucosal element of resistance over the medium to long term. Decongestion before measurement largely removes this source of variability, but at the cost of limiting the technique to the study of cartilaginous and bony structural abnormalities rather than the mucosal element of resistance.

Relatively few studies in the last 20 years have addressed the accuracy and repeatability of rhinomanometry and, more importantly, the correlation of the results achieved with the patient's perception of obstruction. Clarke et al. [14] found a significant correlation when short-term changes in rhinomanometric variables following decongestion by xylometazoline were related to changes in the sensation of obstruction measured on a visual analogue scale. However, a short-term reduction in resistance, which can be related by the individual to an almost immediate change in sensation of nasal patency, is likely to be different to the long-term view that the patient may have of his or her nasal patency. In the longer term, the variability in both the patient's symptoms and the measurements made during rhinomanometry means that the correlation between the two is likely to be lost. In practice, one might anticipate that rhinomanometry would always be capable of detecting large changes in resistance, such as would be expected after surgery. However, in fact the correlation of rhinomanometric changes with the findings following surgery are often poor. The situation is confused. Thus, among many similar papers, one group of authors found that there was a significant improvement in the measurements made on the narrowed side following septal surgery [15], while others have reported no significant improvement in measurements made in patients having rhinoplasty and functional septoplasty [16]. In the light of this sort of confusion most would therefore conclude that rhinomanometry, as opposed to a subjective impression of patient satisfaction, has limited value in clinical assessment.

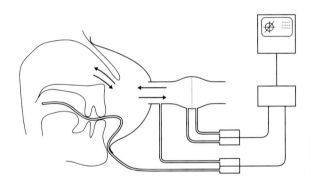

Fig. 4.1 In posterior active rhinomanometry the pressure is measured in the mouth and this measurement is presumed to give a recording that is equal to the pressure in the nasopharynx

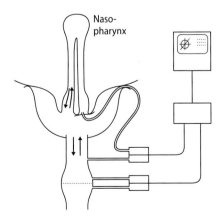

Fig. 4.2 In active anterior rhinomanometry, the pressure gradient is assessed by occluding one nostril either by using a nozzle or by applying adhesive tape and measuring the pressure in the anterior nares

4

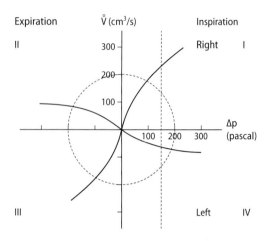

Expiration   V̊ (cm³/s)   Inspiration

II   300   Right   I

200

100

Δp
100 200 300 (pascal)

III   Left   IV

Fig. 4.3 A graph of the pressure plotted against flow is sigmoid in shape as increasing turbulence at higher flow rates results in higher resistance to flow

Acoustic Rhinometry

Acoustic rhinometry is a technique that is able to measure the cross-sectional area of the nasal cavity as a function of the distance from the anterior nares. A sound pulse with a frequency content typically ranging from 100 to 10,000 Hz, or continuous wide band noise of frequencies up to about 25 kHz, is generated by a spark or loudspeaker and is fed into the nose through a probe inserted into the nasal vestibule (Fig. 4.4). The reflected sound waves are detected by a microphone mounted within the probe, which consists of a tube of known dimension with the sound source at one end. The other end is applied, using an adapter, to the nostril. The microphone is mounted in the wall of the sound tube between the sound source and the nose.

Changes in acoustic impedance occur where the cross-sectional area changes. These changes in impedance result in the reflection of the incident sound waves and/with the strength of the reflection being dependent on the magnitude of the impedance changes. By analysing the magnitude and timing of reflected sound pulses the cross-sectional area change and its distance from the microphone detector can be measured (Fig. 4.5). The measured cross-sectional area can be integrated to derive nasal volume.

The method assumes sound is propagated in one direction, that the walls of the nasal cavity are rigid and that there is no loss of sound energy as the sound moves down the nose. It also assumes that the nose is symmetrically bifurcate.

Most recent developments have produced instruments using continuous wide band noise. Comparison of the generated noise and measured noise, which includes the reflected component, allows the reflections to be extracted and from this information an area–distance curve can be plotted. This continuous analysis, as opposed to pulse response analysis, means that the measurement rate can be higher than the 20 per second or so available from the pulse type of acoustic rhinometers.

Acoustic rhinometry is quantitative and quick to perform, although the accuracy of the technique is very dependent on the positioning of both the probe and the patient. Coefficients of variability of 8–12% [17, 18] have been reported for repeated measurements with the probe removed and replaced between measurements. Other errors may be introduced due to nasal airflow and movement during measurement, nasal distortion, an imperfect seal between probe and nostril and the presence of ambient noise. Careful measurement techniques, such as those recommended by the Standardisation Committee on Acoustic Rhinometry, can reduce some of these errors [19]. These techniques include using an acoustic gel to provide a seal between the probe and the nose, ensuring constant room temperature and humidity, training operators and by rejecting poor quality curves. In addition, there must be adequate time for acclimatisation and the patient must be given clear instructions.

Acoustic rhinometry has been validated using physical models (both anatomic and cylindrical tubes), cadavers and by in vivo studies. Model studies have correlated cross-sectional areas and volumes against the known or measured dimensions of the model [20, 21]. In cadavers the dimensions measured by acoustic rhinometry have been compared with CT, water displacement or estimates made from the areas of dissected nasal cavity [21, 22]. In vivo comparisons with CT, MRI and water displacement have also been made [23–29], and comparisons have been made with the result obtained with rhinomanometry, with spirometry and with the patient's subjective symptoms [30–35].

In general the dimensions measured by acoustic rhinometry have tended to agree reasonably with the "true" dimensions in these validation studies – but a number of potential sources of error have been found. These include air leaks between the sound tube and nostril, distortion of the nasal vestibule and valve [36], and, in the posterior part of the nose, both systematic under- and over-estimation of nasal dimensions. Under-estimation beyond a narrow constriction has been attributed to the reflection of the sound impulse at the constriction [37], while the over-estimation has been attributed to sound leakage into the sinuses or the contra-lateral airway [19, 25, 26, 38].

Hamilton et al. [39] found considerable systematic errors in the cross-sectional areas of a plastic tube model measured by acoustic rhinometry, which varied with the area of constriction measured. They concluded that the absolute dimensions measured were unreliable, but that the effects of interventions and dynamic changes could be monitored. Other errors in measurements, especially in children, have been found to be due to a mismatch between the dimensions of the sound tube and the nasal cavity when using adult instruments [20]. Newer instruments with probes designed specifically for infants and children have seemingly addressed this issue [40].

Coefficients of variation of between 2 and 15% have been reported for repeated measurements using acoustic rhinometry [21, 41]. This variability is thought to be due largely to positional variation of the probe within the nares. However averaging repeated measurements only marginally improved day-to-day repeatability in a study on decongested noses [18], which perhaps indicates that the method is prone to other, systematic, errors in measurement and assessment.

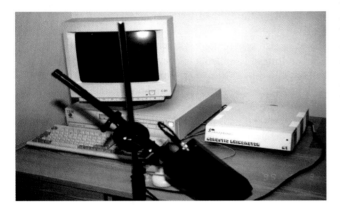

Fig. 4.4 A sound pulse with a frequency content typically ranging from 100 to 10,000 Hz or continuous wide band noise of frequencies up to about 25 kHz is generated by a spark or loudspeaker and is fed into the nose through a probe inserted into the nasal vestibule

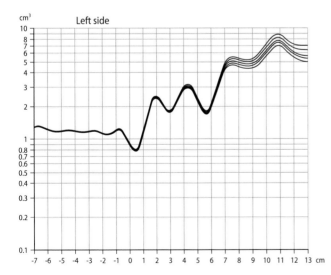

Fig. 4.5 By analysing the magnitude and timing of reflected sound pulses the cross-sectional area change and its distance from the microphone detector can be measured

Spirometric Techniques

The use of spirometry and peak flow measurement in respiratory medicine is well established and such methods of measurement are familiar to most clinicians. Traditionally, spirometers operate by measuring directly the displaced air volume during various breathing manoeuvres. These devices rely on a moving cylinder or bellows arrangement and they are still considered to be the gold standard for such measurements. However newer electronic devices generally use a flow sensor, the output of which is integrated to yield volume: these represent a more flexible and convenient measurement technique and allow inspiratory as well as expiratory measurements.

More popular for nasal assessments have been peak flow rate measurements using a Wright peak flow meter. These small, usually mechanical, meters are frequently used for pulmonary assessment and can be fitted with a nasal mask and used to assess the expiratory phase of respiration. They can also be reversed to give a peak inspiratory measurement. Whilst less accurate than a formal spirometer these devices are inexpensive enough to allow their use for repeated measurements in the consulting room, or even in the patient's home. As such, they have a distinct advantage over other techniques for monitoring relatively slow changes in nasal function.

There has been considerable debate as to which parameters should be routinely measured. The most commonly reported spirometric variables for nasal patency assessment have been nasal peak inspiratory or expiratory flow rates, with other variables, such as forced inspiratory or expiratory volume in 1 s and nasal forced vital capacity, being less favoured. When a number of variables were compared with resistance measured by rhinomanometry, peak inspiratory flow rate correlated better with resistance values (negatively) than other spirometric variables [42]. However coefficients of variability reported for peak nasal inspiratory and expiratory flow rates have ranged from <3% to >9%, with the variability of inspiratory measurements being consistently greater than those for expiration [43]. Despite this greater variability, inspiratory measurements have found greater acceptance – perhaps due to the risk of contamination of the meter with mucus during expiration, and also because there is a proper perception that inspiratory measurements, with a tendency of the lateral wall of the nose to collapse in this respiratory phase, are frequently more relevant to the investigation of the patient's complaint of obstruction.

In fact, opinion is divided on the utility of peak nasal flow measurements in practice. Some authors endorse such measurements in certain circumstances [42, 44–46], while others have found that technical problems such as alar distortion due to the applied pressure needed to seal the mask and alar collapse at high flow rates [43, 47], as well as poor repeatability and diurnal variability [48], make the technique too unreliable for routine use. The effort of forced inspiratory or expiratory manoeuvres has also been shown to act as a mechanical stimulus to the nose in some rhinitic patients, which causes an increase in nasal resistance [49].

As with other methods of measurement, the correlation of peak flow measurements with subjective symptoms is inconsistent. In one study, peak nasal inspiratory flow was found to correlate well with symptom scores in perennial allergic rhinitis sufferers after treatment with corticosteroids or placebo [35]. However, other studies have found either no correlation or a poor correlation between peak nasal inspiratory flow and subjective assessment [43, 50, 51]. Thus, there are doubts not only as to which parameter should be measured, but also as to whether the measurements made represent a realistic insight into the patient's complaint.

Forced Oscillation

The forced oscillation technique involves the superposition of a small-amplitude, low-frequency (usually <100 Hz), oscillating signal onto normal tidal breathing. A loudspeaker is used to generate the signal and the resulting pressure and flow variations are recorded using a pneumotachograph. The resistance derived in this way is of the entire airway. By recording with the nose included in the measurement volume, and then either subtracting the flow recorded at the same pressure with a nasal clip in place and calculating resistance from the resultant nasal-only flow and pressure, or by subtracting the resistance recorded breathing through the mouth only, the nasal resistance can be estimated

$$|Z_{nasal}| = |Z_{total}| - |Z_{oral}|.$$

Relatively few reports on the validity of these measurements are available [52–54]. Potential drawbacks of the technique are that it is complex and time-consuming to perform and the data analysis is not straightforward. The assumption that subtraction of the thoracic and oral components from the total resistance derives nasal resistance may not be entirely valid and dynamic changes in nasal or thoracic resistance could introduce errors, as the total resistance and oral resistance are not recorded simultaneously.

Other Techniques

Many other techniques have attempted to characterise nasal function. Most notably these have included attempts to add objectivity to the Zwaardemaker technique using liquid crystal thermography, but this simple technique has not enjoyed widespread acceptance to date, as it was not found to produce any clinically useful measure of nasal obstruction [55]. More recently, we have also measured the patterns of humidified air exhaled from the nose onto a fixed plate, using a thermal camera (Fig. 4.6) [56].

The plate medium chosen was normal copy paper (Xerox 80 g/m²), as this was found to heat sufficiently quickly to form an image on each consecutive breath. The system was first tested in continuous flow conditions in a temperature-controlled laboratory (23°C±0.5°C), with an air cylinder and control valve, humidifier and rotameter type flowmeter used to supply a controlled flow of humidified and warmed air.

Figure 4.7 shows the typical image obtained and also an isotherm, which was plotted at a value halfway between the peak temperature and ambient temperature (in this case 27.9°C). The area enclosed by this isotherm can be measured and the value obtained normalised by dividing by the area of the whole plate, measured from the same image. An increase in a normalised 50% area is seen with increasing flow and we are currently trying to correlate the measurements made with this technique with the reported sensation of obstruction in normal individuals and patients. We are also currently investigating the use of Schlieren photography to see if we can use the image of the plume of expired air from the nose to make some form of subjective assessment of nasal airflow.

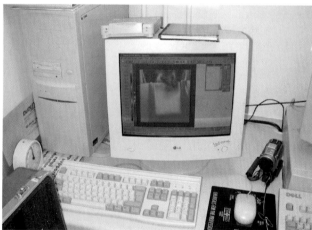

Fig. 4.7 A typical image obtained by the thermal camera and also an isotherm, which was plotted at a value halfway between the peak temperature and ambient temperature (in this case 27.9°C). The area enclosed by this isotherm can be measured and the value obtained normalised by dividing by the area of the whole plate, measured from the same image

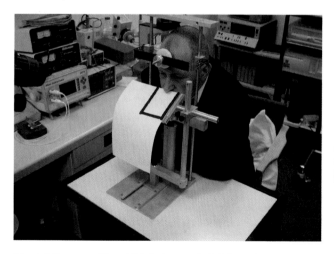

Fig. 4.6 Patterns of humidified air are exhaled from the nose onto a fixed plate and measured using a thermal camera

Conclusions

Of all the techniques available, rhinomanometry is the closest to a "gold standard" for nasal assessment. Acoustic rhinometry is also widely used and spirometry has enjoyed the support of some authors. Other attempts to measure nasal obstruction have also been mentioned in this chapter and those that have not been mentioned in depth include measurements of the proportion of nasal to oral inspired or expired volume [57, 58] and manometric rhinometry – which has been used to measure nasal volume [59]. In addition, endoscopic measurement of the dimensions of the nasal airway using image-processing techniques have been utilised [60]. But, as with the more established methods, all of these techniques have found limited support in practice, principally because no technique has, to date, been found to reliably correlate with the reported symptom of obstruction.

To address this we clearly need a greater understanding of the physiology of normal nasal airflow. In addition, the basic methodologies used may also need altering and refining. We have, for instance, tried to ensure greater validity by utilising mental alerting during measurement, as is done during caloric irrigation, to distract the patient from the task in hand and to try and ensure that individual is unaware of his or her own breathing pattern. We have also favoured non-contact techniques, since the very validity of techniques that require facial contact or the insertion of nozzles or pressure tubes into the nose has to be questioned. This has been the case since it has been known that application of a face mask alters the respiratory breathing patterns of neonates [61] and from this it might be adduced that any form of local stimulation is likely to alter the pattern of respiration and, hence, the performance of the nasal airway. Certainly, the insertion of probes or applications of masks must, at the very least, cause some minor degree of alteration of function and stenting the ala, as is done in acoustic rhinometry, clearly changes the whole dynamic of the external valve. For these reasons, measurements of the pattern of exhaled air are empirically attractive, but whether it will be possible to demonstrate the clinical utility of such "no touch" techniques, and whether they have any advantages over more established methods, remain to be proven.

In a world of evidence-based practice and health care commissioning there is certainly a need to demonstrate objective evidence of outcome from treatment. At present, without a reliable system of nasal airway measurement, there is no such evidence base for much of what is done to the nose by medical and surgical intervention. Frequently, the evidence for or against a particular procedure is contradictory. Where results are available there are often methodological flaws and inconsistencies that invalidate the conclusions drawn and make them difficult to substantiate. Furthermore, most studies on the performance of the various measurement techniques presently available offer level 4 evidence, at best, and do not follow the recently published STARD guidelines for the reporting of studies of diagnostic accuracy [62]. Thus, in a recent systematic review of all the available literature, 942 articles were identified concerning the objective assessment of outcomes from septal surgery. However, only 13 of these papers were found to have any real validity and, in fact, methodological inconsistencies with inadequately specified inclusion criteria ruled out all but three of these for meta-analysis [63].

An ideal technique would quantify the level of obstruction in such a way as to be able to inform the choice of therapy and correlate well with the subjective sensation experienced by the patient. Objective measurements are also necessary to aid comparisons between treatments. However, the reality is that the inter- and intra-test variation in measurements of nasal obstruction are too variable for any one means of assessment to be reliable at the present time and, until we have a better understanding of the basic physiology, the best we can do at present is to utilise a combination of measurement techniques together with clinical judgement and the reports of the patients' own sensation of obstruction.

References

1. Glatzel, P. 1901, "Zur Prüfung der Luftdurchgängigkeit der Nase", *Therapie der Gegenwart*, vol. 42, p. 348.

2. Zwaardemaker, H. 1894, "Atembeschlag als Hilfsmittel zur Diagnose der Nasalen Stenosen", *Archiv für Laryngologie und Rhinologie*, vol. 1, pp. 174–177.

3. Hirschmann, A. 1903, "Über Endoskopie der Nase und deren Nebenhöhlen. Eine neue Untersuchungsmethode", *Archiv für Laryngologie und Rhinologie*, vol. 143, pp. 195–202.

4. Jones, A. S., Willatt, D. J., & Durham, L. M. 1989, "Nasal airflow: resistance and sensation", *Journal of Laryngology & Otology*, vol. 103, no. 10, pp. 909–911.

5. Clement, P. A. 1990, "Different types of rhinomanometers, standardization, pathologic shapes of rhinomanometric recordings, pitfalls, and possible errors", *Facial Plastic Surgery*, vol. 7, no. 4, pp. 230–244.

6. Cole, P. & Havas, T. 1987, "Nasal resistance to respiratory airflow: a plethysmographic alternative to the face mask", *Rhinology*, vol. 25, no. 3, pp. 159–166.

7. Clement, P. A. 1984, "Committee report on standardization of rhinomanometry", *Rhinology*, vol. 22, no. 3, pp. 151–155.

8. Broms, P., Jonson, B., & Lamm, C. J. 1982, "Rhinomanometry. II. A system for numerical description of nasal airway resistance", *Acta Oto-Laryngologica*, vol. 94, no. 1–2, pp. 157–168.

9. O'Neill, G., Tolley, N. S., Hollis, L. J., Hern, J. D., & Almeyda, J. S. 1996, "Analysis of rhinomanometric data based upon a model of nasal airflow and logarithmic transformation of the data", *Clinical Otolaryngology & Allied Sciences*, vol. 21, no. 6, pp. 524–527.

10. Corrado, O. J., Ollier, S., Phillips, M. J., Thomas, J. M., & Davies, R. J. 1987, "Histamine and allergen induced changes in nasal airways resistance measured by anterior rhinomanometry: reproducibility of the technique and the effect of topically administered antihistaminic and anti-allergic drugs", *British Journal of Clinical Pharmacology*, vol. 24, no. 3, pp. 283–292.

11. Schumacher, M. J. 2004, "Nasal dyspnea: the place of rhinomanometry in its objective assessment. [Review] [37 refs]", *American Journal of Rhinology*, vol. 18, no. 1, pp. 41–46.

12. Shelton, D. M. & Eiser, N. M. 1992, "Evaluation of active anterior and posterior rhinomanometry in normal subjects", *Clinical Otolaryngology & Allied Sciences*, vol. 17, no. 2, pp. 178–182.

4

13. Carney, A. S., Bateman, N. D., & Jones, N. S. 2000, "Reliable and reproducible anterior active rhinomanometry for the assessment of unilateral nasal resistance", *Clinical Otolaryngology & Allied Sciences*, vol. 25, no. 6, pp. 499–503.

14. Clarke, R. W., Cook, J. A., & Jones, A. S. 1995, "The effect of nasal mucosal vasoconstriction on nasal airflow sensation", *Clinical Otolaryngology & Allied Sciences.*, vol. 20, no. 1, pp. 72–73.

15. Jalowayski, A. A., Yuh, Y. S., Koziol, J. A., & Davidson, T. M. 1983, "Surgery for nasal obstruction – evaluation by rhinomanometry", *Laryngoscope*, vol. 93, no. 3, pp. 341–345.

16. Courtiss, E. H. & Goldwyn, R. M. 1983, "The effects of nasal surgery on airflow", *Plastic & Reconstructive Surgery*, vol. 72, no. 1, pp. 9–21.

17. Fisher, E. W., Morris, D. P., Biemans, J. M., Palmer, C. R., & Lund, V. J. 1995, "Practical aspects of acoustic rhinometry: problems and solutions", *Rhinology*, vol. 33, no. 4, pp. 219–223.

18. Harar, R. P., Kalan, A., & Kenyon, G. S. 2002, "Improving the reproducibility of acoustic rhinometry in the assessment of nasal function", *Journal of Oto-Rhino-Laryngology & its Related Specialties*, vol. 64, no. 1, pp. 22–25.

19. Hilberg, O. & Pedersen, O. F. 2000, "Acoustic rhinometry: recommendations for technical specifications and standard operating procedures.[erratum appears in Rhinol 2001 Jun;39(2):119]", *Rhinology - Supplement*, vol. 16, pp. 3–17.

20. Buenting, J. E., Dalston, R. M., Smith, T. L., & Drake, A. F. 1994, "Artifacts associated with acoustic rhinometric assessment of infants and young children: a model study", *Journal of Applied Physiology*, vol. 77, no. 6, pp. 2558–2563.

21. Hilberg, O., Jackson, A. C., Swift, D. L., & Pedersen, O. F. 1989, "Acoustic rhinometry: evaluation of nasal cavity geometry by acoustic reflection", *Journal of Applied Physiology*, vol. 66, no. 1, pp. 295–303.

22. Mayhew, T. M. & O'Flynn, P. 1993, "Validation of acoustic rhinometry by using the Cavalieri principle to estimate nasal cavity volume in cadavers", *Clinical Otolaryngology & Allied Sciences*, vol. 18, no. 3, pp. 220–225.

23. Corey, J. P., Gungor, A., Nelson, R., Fredberg, J., & Lai, V. 1997, "A comparison of the nasal cross-sectional areas and volumes obtained with acoustic rhinometry and magnetic resonance imaging", *Otolaryngology – Head & Neck Surgery*, vol. 117, no. 4, pp. 349–354.

24. Gilain, L., Coste, A., Ricolfi, F., Dahan, E., Marliac, D., Peynegre, R., Harf, A., & Louis, B. 1997, "Nasal cavity geometry measured by acoustic rhinometry and computed tomography", *Archives of Otolaryngology – Head & Neck Surgery*, vol. 123, no. 4, pp. 401–405.

25. Hilberg, O., Jensen, F. T., & Pedersen, O. F. 1993, "Nasal airway geometry: comparison between acoustic reflections and magnetic resonance scanning", *Journal of Applied Physiology*, vol. 75, no. 6, pp. 2811–2819.

26. Hilberg, O. & Pedersen, O. F. 1996, "Acoustic rhinometry: influence of paranasal sinuses", *Journal of Applied Physiology*, vol. 80, no. 5, pp. 1589–1594.

27. Mamikoglu, B., Houser, S., Akbar, I., Ng, B., & Corey, J. P. 2000, "Acoustic rhinometry and computed tomography scans for the diagnosis of nasal septal deviation, with clinical correlation", *Otolaryngology – Head & Neck Surgery*, vol. 123, no. 1 Pt 1, pp. 61–68.

28. Min, Y. G. & Jang, Y. J. 1995, "Measurements of cross-sectional area of the nasal cavity by acoustic rhinometry and CT scanning", *Laryngoscope*, vol. 105, no. 7 Pt 1, pp. 757–759.

29. Taverner, D., Bickford, L., & Latte, J. 2002, "Validation by fluid volume of acoustic rhinometry before and after decongestant in normal subjects", *Rhinology*, vol. 40, no. 3, pp. 135–140.

30. Ahmad, R. L. & Gendeh, B. S. 2003, "Evaluation with acoustic rhinometry of patients undergoing sinonasal surgery", *Medical Journal of Malaysia*, vol. 58, no. 5, pp. 723–728.

31. Austin, C. E. & Foreman, J. C. 1994, "Acoustic rhinometry compared with posterior rhinomanometry in the measurement of histamine- and bradykinin-induced changes in nasal airway patency", *British Journal of Clinical Pharmacology*, vol. 37, no. 1, pp. 33–37.

32. Kim, C. S., Moon, B. K., Jung, D. H., & Min, Y. G. 1998, "Correlation between nasal obstruction symptoms and objective parameters of acoustic rhinometry and rhinomanometry", *Auris, Nasus, Larynx*, vol. 25, no. 1, pp. 45–48.

33. Porter, M. J., Williamson, I. G., Kerridge, D. H., & Maw, A. R. 1996, "A comparison of the sensitivity of manometric rhinometry, acoustic rhinometry, rhinomanometry and nasal peak flow to detect the decongestant effect of xylometazoline", *Clinical Otolaryngology & Allied Sciences*, vol. 21, no. 3, pp. 218–221.

34. Roithmann, R., Cole, P., Chapnik, J., Barreto, S. M., Szalai, J. P., & Zamel, N. 1994, "Acoustic rhinometry, rhinomanometry, and the sensation of nasal patency: a correlative study", *Journal of Otolaryngology*, vol. 23, no. 6, pp. 454–458.

35. Wilson, A. M., Sims, E. J., Robb, F., Cockburn, W., & Lipworth, B. J. 2003, "Peak inspiratory flow rate is more sensitive than acoustic rhinometry or rhinomanometry in detecting corticosteroid response with nasal histamine challenge", *Rhinology*, vol. 41, no. 1, pp. 16–20.

36. Hamilton, J. W., McRae, R. D., & Jones, A. S. 1997, "The magnitude of random errors in acoustic rhinometry and re-interpretation of the acoustic profile", *Clinical Otolaryngology & Allied Sciences*, vol. 22, no. 5, pp. 408–413.

37. Cankurtaran, M., Celik, H., Cakmak, O., & Ozluoglu, L. N. 2003, "Effects of the nasal valve on acoustic rhinometry measurements: a model study", *Journal of Applied Physiology*, vol. 94, no. 6, pp. 2166–2172.

38. Djupesland, P. G. & Rotnes, J. S. 2001, "Accuracy of acoustic rhinometry", *Rhinology*, vol. 39, no. 1, pp. 23–27.

39. Hamilton, J. W., Cook, J. A., Phillips, D. E., & Jones, A. S. 1995, "Limitations of acoustic rhinometry determined by a simple model", *Acta Oto-Laryngologica*, vol. 115, no. 6, pp. 811–814.

40. Djupesland, P. G. & Lyholm, B. 1997, "Nasal airway dimensions in term neonates measured by continuous wide-band noise acoustic rhinometry", *Acta Oto-Laryngologica*, vol. 117, no. 3, pp. 424–432.

41. Nurminen, M., Hytonen, M., & Sala, E. 2000, "Modelling the reproducibility of acoustic rhinometry", *Statistics in Medicine*, vol. 19, no. 9, pp. 1179–1189.

42. Jones, A. S., Viani, L., Phillips, D., & Charters, P. 1991, "The objective assessment of nasal patency", *Clinical Otolaryngology & Allied Sciences*, vol. 16, no. 2, pp. 206–211.

43. Enberg, R. N. & Ownby, D. R. 1991, "Peak nasal inspiratory flow and Wright peak flow: a comparison of their reproducibility", *Annals of Allergy*, vol. 67, no. 3, pp. 371–374.

44. Clarke, R. W. & Jones, A. S. 1994, "The limitations of peak nasal flow measurement", *Clinical Otolaryngology & Allied Sciences*, vol. 19, no. 6, pp. 502–504.

45. Frolund, L., Madsen, F., Mygind, N., Nielsen, N. H., Svendsen, U. G., & Weeke, B. 1987, "Comparison between different techniques for measuring nasal patency in a group of unselected patients", *Acta Oto-Laryngologica*, vol. 104, no. 1–2, pp. 175–179.

46. Sims, E. J., Wilson, A. M., White, P. S., Gardiner, Q., & Lipworth, B. J. 2002, "Short-term repeatability and correlates of laboratory measures of nasal function in patients with seasonal allergic rhinitis", *Rhinology*, vol. 40, no. 2, pp. 66–68.

47. Clarke, R. W., Jones, A. S., & Richardson, H. 1995, "Peak nasal inspiratory flow – the plateau effect", *Journal of Laryngology & Otology*, vol. 109, no. 5, pp. 399–402.

48. Blomgren, K., Simola, M., Hytonen, M., & Pitkaranta, A. 2003, "Peak nasal inspiratory and expiratory flow measurements – practical tools in primary care?", *Rhinology*, vol. 41, no. 4, pp. 206–210.

49. Braat, J. P., Fokkens, W. J., Mulder, P. G., Kianmaneshrad, N., Rijntjes, E., & Gerth van, W. R. 2000, "Forced expiration through the nose is a stimulus for NANIPER but not for controls", *Rhinology*, vol. 38, no. 4, pp. 172–176.

50. Gleeson, M. J., Youlten, L. J., Shelton, D. M., Siodlak, M. Z., Eiser, N. M., & Wengraf, C. L. 1986, "Assessment of nasal airway patency: a comparison of four methods", *Clinical Otolaryngology & Allied Sciences*, vol. 11, no. 2, pp. 99–107.

51. Morrissey, M. S., Alun-Jones, T., & Hill, J. 1990, "The relationship of peak inspiratory airflow to subjective airflow in the nose", *Clinical Otolaryngology & Allied Sciences*, vol. 15, no. 5, pp. 447–451.

52. Lemes, L. N. & Melo, P. L. 2003, "Simplified oscillation method for assessing nasal obstruction non-invasively and under spontaneous ventilation: a pilot study", *Medical & Biological Engineering & Computing*, vol. 41, no. 4, pp. 439–444.

53. Shelton, D. M., Pertuze, J., Gleeson, M. J., Thompson, J., Denman, W. T., Goff, J., Eiser, N. M., & Pride, N. B. 1990, "Comparison of oscillation with three other methods for measuring nasal airways resistance", *Respiratory Medicine*, vol. 84, no. 2, pp. 101–106.

54. Tawfik, B., Sullivan, K. J., & Chang, H. K. 1991, "A new method to measure nasal impedance in spontaneously breathing adults", *Journal of Applied Physiology*, vol. 71, no. 1, pp. 9–15.

55. Canter, R. J. 1986, "A non-invasive method of demonstrating the nasal cycle using flexible liquid crystal thermography", *Clinical Otolaryngology & Allied Sciences*, vol. 11, no. 5, pp. 329–336.

56. Pickett, J. A., Levine, M., Birch, M., & Kenyon, G. S. "Thermographic measurement of nasal airway function: a modern approach to an old technique", in *20th Congress of the European Rhinologic Society (ERS) & 23rd International Symposium on Infection and Allergy of the Nose (ISIAN)*, Istanbul, p. 214.

57. Drake, A. F., Keall, H., Vig, P. S., & Krause, C. J. 1988, "Clinical nasal obstruction and objective respiratory mode determination", *Annals of Otology, Rhinology & Laryngology*, vol. 97, no. 4 Pt 1, pp. 397–402.

58. Oluwole, M., Gardiner, Q., & White, P. S. 1997, "The naso-oral index: a more valid measure than peak flow rate?", *Clinical Otolaryngology & Allied Sciences*, vol. 22, no. 4, pp. 346–349.

59. Porter, M. J., Maw, A. R., Kerridge, D. H., & Williamson, I. M. 1997, "Manometric rhinometry: a new method of measuring the volume of the air in the nasal cavity", *Acta Oto-Laryngologica*, vol. 117, no. 2, pp. 298–301.

60. Bellussi, L., Ferrara, G. A., Mezzedimi, C., Passali, G. C., D'Alesio, D., & Passali, D. 2000, "A new method for endoscopic evaluation in rhinology: videocapture", *Rhinology*, vol. 38, no. 1, pp. 13–16.

61. Fleming, P. J., Levine, M. R., & Goncalves, A. 1982, "Changes in respiratory pattern resulting from the use of a facemask to record respiration in newborn infants", *Pediatric Research*, vol. 16, no. 12, pp. 1031–1034.

62. Bossuyt, P. M., Reitsma, J. B., Bruns, D. E., Gatsonis, C. A., Glasziou, P. P., Irwig, L. M., Moher, D., Rennie, D., de Vet, H. C., Lijmer, J. G., & Standards for Reporting of Diagnostic Accuracy. 2003, "The STARD statement for reporting studies of diagnostic accuracy: explanation and elaboration", *Clinical Chemistry*, vol. 49, no. 1, pp. 7–18.

63. Singh, A., Patel, N., Kenyon, G., & Donaldson G. 2005, "Is there objective evidence that septal surgery improves nasal airflow?" *Journal of Laryngology and Otology*, vol. 120, no. 11, pp. 916–920.

Nasal Valve Surgery

Guy S. Kenyon and Peter Andrew

Core Messages

- The interaction of the two nasal valves is not fully understood.
- When routine rhinoplasty surgery is undertaken, violation of the scroll area should be avoided wherever possible and aggressive cartilage resection of the alae should not be undertaken, in order to avoid a delayed complaint of nasal obstruction.
- Medical measures to deal with valve complaints are unlikely to prove satisfactory for many patients and surgery is often necessary.
- Surgery may be difficult, especially in noses where scarring is marked, but the results are often worthwhile.
- Nasal valves should be examined and assessed in all our patients on a routine basis.

Contents

Introduction

The causes of nasal obstruction are often held to be due either to mucosal disease or to anatomical abnormality. In the former group cilial dysfunction and atrophic changes may play a role, but the commonest causes of mucosal dysfunction are undoubtedly a group or disorders that are characterised by the generic term "rhinitis". However, if allergic rhinitis is excluded, it has to be admitted that many of the causes of a hypertrophic and hypersecreting mucosa remain ill-defined.

The exact role of the mucosa in the genesis of a patient with a subjective complaint of obstruction remains obscure as does the manner by which an anatomically deviated nasal septum and hypertrophied nasal turbinates may cause some, but not all, patients to complain. Not only is the size of the nasal airway not immediately correlated with the patient's complaint, but the role of surgical correction of the septum and turbinates remains controversial and unproven [1]. This being so, it is scarcely surprising that a lack of clarity also exists with regard to the role of the nasal valve – although there can be little doubt that abnormality in the structure that is normally referred to in this context can cause nasal obstruction in some cases. In fact, as will be seen, there are two valves that interact one with another in helping to regulate flow in the lower third of the nose and the pathology relating to derangement of the structures in this area, while poorly understood, may be the sole cause of a patient's symptoms. Indeed, some have suggested that valve dysfunction is the cause of symptoms in the majority of patients presenting with nasal blockage [2] – although such a view may well be skewed due to the fact that these surgeons were reporting a cohort of revision patients seen in a plastic surgery practice who had undergone excessive dorsal hump resection and detachment of the upper lateral cartilages. Certainly the notion that such findings are more common than septal or turbinate pathology is unproven, as well as probably being alien to the majority of otolaryngologists.

5

The Internal Nasal Valve

The structure most commonly referred to as "the nasal valve" lies at the isthmus or narrowest part of the nose in the coronal plane at the head of the inferior turbinate. However, to describe this area as a valve is really a misnomer. A valve regulates flow or, in strict anatomical terms, is a "membranous part of a vessel preventing the flow of liquids in one direction and allowing it another" [3]. Such a definition is clearly invalid in the nose where flow is obviously bi-directional and is driven by the phases of the respiratory cycle, which, in turn, are driven by the lungs. Nonetheless, the name has become hallowed by common usage.

The first description of a nasal valve is normally attributed to Mink [4]. He defined the valve as the area of the maximal resistance within the anterior part of the respiratory tract, but there has subsequently been a degree of dispute and contention as to exactly what constitutes this entity anatomically. Van Dishoeck [5] undertook a series of radiological studies that suggested that the narrowest area of the nose was at the junction of the lower and upper lateral cartilages, whereas cadaver impressions have suggested that the narrowest area is the piriform aperture [6]. More dynamic studies with nasal probes have suggested that the area of highest pressure change is in the plane of the head of the inferior turbinate, and the same studies also suggested that this plane actually changes depending on the state of congestion or constriction of the head of the inferior turbinate [7]. The role of the head of the inferior turbinate was also emphasised in studies that have shown that decongestants halve nasal resistance [8]. But, while this may be true, it must also be said that there is a tendency for this area to collapse at high flow rates [9], which implies some variability in flow imposed by the lateral nasal wall at this site.

Misnomer or not, it is now agreed that this area at the nasal isthmus constitutes what has now become known as the internal nasal valve [2, 10]. This area offers the greatest resistance to airflow and can be measured in studies using acoustic rhinometry as the point of minimal cross-sectional area. In strict anatomical terms this valve appears to lie in the coronal plane at the head of the inferior turbinate and the "valve" also consists of the caudal

part of the upper lateral cartilage and the angle between this structure and the dorsal septum just beyond the plane of the piriform aperture (the isthmus nasi). It is shown in diagrammatic form in Fig. 5.1. The shape of the latter structure differs in Caucasian (leptorrhine) and Negroid (platyrrhine) noses [11], but it is generally agreed that the important anatomy at this site is the retention of the angle between the upper lateral and the dorsal septum, which should be between 10 and 15°. If scarring is produced here by trauma or injudicious trimming of the upper lateral cartilages during routine rhinoplasty, nasal obstruction may result.

There is no doubt that the lateral nasal wall at this point also moves in a medial direction with forced inspiration, but this can have little impact on nasal flow – at least in the normal nose. This is because the part of the lower lateral cartilage that can actually exhibit any tendency towards inward movement is limited. In a cephalad direction the upper lateral cartilage is, of course, fixed to and runs slightly under the nasal bones and this must limit movement. In a caudal direction the upper lateral cartilages turn back on themselves in the scroll area and are stented by the lower lateral cartilages, which flare during times of maximal inspiratory flow, and which thus support the lower margins of the upper laterals through the medium of the intercartilaginous ligaments. Movement of the lateral wall in this internal valve area is thus restricted. This argument was supported by experiments in normal individuals that showed that the minimal cross-sectional area of the nose, when measured by acoustic rhinometry, is increased by over 40% when topical vasoconstrictors are applied to the mucosa, whereas external nasal splints have relatively little effect at this site [10].

The External Nasal Valve

The external valve is formed by the external nares and its supporting structures. These consist of the columella medially, which is fixed, and by the lateral crura of the lower lateral cartilages, which are mobile. There is no doubt that these parts of the soft tissue structures of the nose display a tendency to collapse at high rates of inspiratory flow, and this tendency is normally resisted by the function of the overlying dilator nares muscles and by the levator labii alaeque nasi muscle, which is inserted into the lateral crura on each side. Inward collapse is also resisted by the tensile strength of the cartilages, but if these are traumatised or either weakened or over-resected as part of a rhinoplasty operation, then collapse may follow. Equally if there is a high abutment of the lateral crus and a cephalad rotation of this cartilage towards the piriform aperture then the soft tissue triangle at the rim of the nose is unsupported – and the tissues then tend to collapse at high flow rates – particularly in older patients in whom the tissues loose their tensile strength. Finally, because of the importance of the overlying facial muscles in stenting the alae, facial paralysis may also cause an interruption to inspiratory flow and may cause altered flow-pressure relationships as the alae show a tendency to collapse during normal inspiratory efforts [7, 12]. What all this clearly demonstrates is the importance of the integrity of the local anatomy in the maintenance of this outer valve. Physiologically unlike the internal

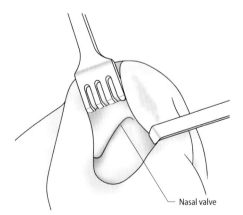

Fig. 5.1 Diagram of internal nasal valve

valve, where flow is primarily influenced by the state of mucosal engorgement, the peak flow is increased substantially by splinting and stenting of this valve and especially by the insertion of a prosthesis such as a Francis alar dilator. By contrast the effects of vasoconstriction on inspiratory flow, while still marked, are less profound [10].

Teleologically, it is impossible to ascertain why these areas exist, although they may be important in allowing a sensation of normal resistance to flow. Moreover, exactly how these two valvular areas interact in response to differing physiological stimuli is also not understood. Clearly in times of maximal inspiratory effort the alae flare and the mucosa decongests with abolition of the nasal cycle, allowing flow rates to increase in response to the body's increased oxygen demand. However, the receptors and reflexes initiating and moderating such a response are not clearly identified – neither at a local level nor more centrally.

Valve Pathology

The causes of obstruction at the internal nasal valve may be primary or secondary. Primary causes are most common due either to high deviations of the septum into the critical area formed by the internal valve angle or to mucosal oedema in the same area. Occasionally a degree of collapse of the upper lateral cartilages in this region may also contribute. Secondary causes following surgery or other trauma include scarring at the apex as well as structural collapse or over-narrowing at the piriform aperture during rhinoplasty surgery. Structural narrowing of the nose in the internal valve area is also more common in noses with short nasal bones and a long narrow middle third, as this leaves the cartilaginous structures relatively unsupported by the short nasal bones. In secondary cases there is a characteristic deformity seen externally that resembles an inverted V (Fig. 5.2).

Causes of obstruction in the external valve area are also best thought of as being either primary or secondary to surgical intervention. In primary cases the lateral crus of the lower lateral cartilage is either weak or malpositioned and the latter category includes patients with a paradoxical inversion or a more cephalid/caudal position of the lateral crus than is normal. As has already been mentioned secondary external valve collapse also follows excessive resection of the lateral crus, with resultant collapse; the latter symptom may present some time distant from the initial surgery and is particularly difficult to correct.

Clinical Assessment

Cottle was the first to highlight the fact that simple septoplasty and turbinate surgery will not cure all patients with nasal blockage and was the first to demarcate and name differing areas within the septum [13]. He divided the septum into five areas: the nostril and vestibule (external valve), the nasal valve angle (internal valve), the attic area, the mid-turbinate area and the posterior turbinate area (Fig. 5.3).

The attic is intimately related to the keystone area of the dorsum where it joins with the caudal part of the nasal bones. This cannot be defiled during normal septal surgery or a saddle deformity may result. The middle and posterior turbinate areas are, however, amenable to septoplasty. In particular, the area of the nasal valve is important and in one series of 500 patients

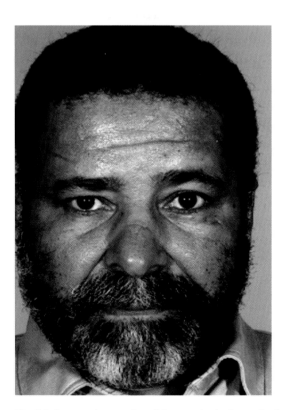

Fig. 5.2 Structural narrowing of the nose in the internal valve area. In secondary cases there is a characteristic deformity seen externally that resembles an inverted V

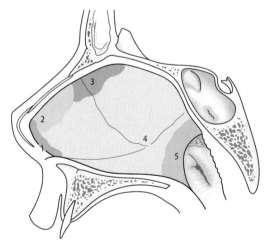

Fig. 5.3 Cottle divided the septum into five areas: the nostril and vestibule (external valve)(1), the nasal valve angle (internal valve)(2), the attic area (3), the mid-turbinate area (4) and the posterior turbinate area (5)

presenting with nasal blockage, 13% had obstruction at the level of the nasal valve [14]. The assessment of the level of septal deviation is thus of paramount importance prior to embarking on a surgical cure for obstructive symptoms.

The clinician must also be aware that pathologies may coexist. Consider the patient with a marked septal deviation and bilateral alar collapse. Prior to surgery angulation of the dorsal septum may mask the co-existent external valve collapse on the narrowed side, as the ala is stented by the septum. On the contralateral side alar collapse also occurs, but passes unnoticed as the cartilage can collapse with impunity into a widely open airway. The patient, who is likely to be complaining of unilateral obstruction, then has successful septal surgery, but no surgery to stiffen or reposition the alae. On the previously narrowed side the stenting of the ala is removed by surgery but the ala can now collapse, with the result that, to the patient, the airway remains obstructed on this side. On the contralateral side, which was previously patent, ala movement is not altered but is now clinically manifest as a complaint of obstruction as the centralisation of the septum causes a relative narrowing of the airway. To everyone's chagrin the patient, who previously enjoyed a nasal airway on one side, now complains of bilateral obstruction.

History and Examination

A full history and examination are obviously mandatory in all patients with symptoms of obstruction. Great detail is clearly redundant in the context of this chapter but a history of previous rhinoplasty or septal surgery is obviously relevant, as are symptoms that suggest that obstruction is not bi-phasic but is, instead, occurring predominantly during the inspiratory phase of respiration. Equally, the clinician should also record whether blockage is unilateral or bilateral, whether it is constant or intermittent and whether it is relieved in whole or in part by nasal steroids or nasal splints. Frequently patients with external valve collapse will have had recourse to Cottle's manoeuvre, in which pulling on the malar skin is routinely employed to open the external valve to avoid obstruction during inspiration (Fig. 5.4) [13]. Sometimes they will have tried external splints, such as the proprietary "Breathe-Right" strips (Fig. 5.5), which are widely available. However, patients may not volunteer such information unless specifically asked.

Clear-cut external deformity may be obvious, but clues as to the true nature of the patient's pathology may nonetheless be ignored. A characteristic inverted V deformity should raise

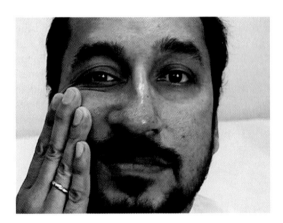

Fig. 5.4 Cottle's manoeuvre, in which pulling on the malar skin is routinely employed to open the external valve to avoid obstruction during inspiration

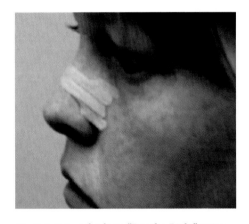

Fig. 5.5 External splints: "Breathe-Right" strips

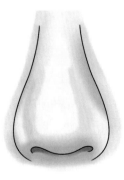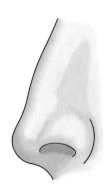

Fig. 5.6 Patients with a high abutment of the ala frequently exhibit what has been called the parenthesis deformity

the suspicion of internal valve pathology. Likewise, the patient with a high abutment of the ala frequently exhibits what has been called the parenthesis deformity (Fig. 5.6) [15]. Simple observation of the nose may also reveal alar or middle third collapse and patients with internal valve deformity often exhibit a pinched look to the middle third during respiration and a loss of the dorsal aesthetic line in repose. If suspicion of pathology is present the Bachman manoeuvre may also be helpful. This latter test assesses the inner valve function by applying a small cotton applicator at the apex of the inner valve. The valve angle is thus enlarged, and a positive result gives further credence to the possibility of inner valve collapse.

Such an examination should also be accompanied by an assessment of the nasal airflow in the resting position during quiet respiration as well as during forced inspiration and expiration. Mirror misting in an out-patient setting is frequently all that is available and is normally sufficient; laboratory confirmation of impaired flow, altered resistance or reduced cross-sectional area, whilst ideal, is not normally necessary.

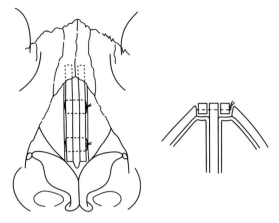

Fig. 5.7 Augmentation of the angle of the internal valve accomplished by the insertion of spreader grafts

Management of Nasal Valve Deficiency

In many cases of nasal valve incompetence, surgical intervention will be required. However, a conservative approach is also possible – especially in minor cases.

Optimising medical treatment with regard to underlying rhinitis, if present, is clearly important and may help to reduce nasal resistance at the internal nasal valve angle and abolish the perception of obstruction. For minor cases of internal valve narrowing external paper splintage may also suffice to alleviate the symptoms, or at least make them tolerable. In patients with major collapse of the external valve a trial of a suitably sized Francis alar dilator is also worthwhile, although these are often rejected due to the discomfort associated with their use.

In the account that follows, surgery for abnormalities of the internal and external valves will be presented. Congenital causes of external valve deficiency, including the cleft palate nose with resultant vestibular stenosis will not be discussed here, although many of the same principles are utilised in their correction.

ring and adhesion, but requires insertion of silastic splints in the postoperative period to reduce the chances of further adhesion formation.

In more complicated cases, and when the angle of the internal valve is severely reduced, the main aim of surgical correction is to augment the angle and this is most readily accomplished by insertion of spreader grafts, as advocated by Sheen (Fig. 5.7 [17]). These are cartilage grafts, normally prepared from autograft cartilage, which are secured with fine sutures so that they lie in an extramucosal pocket on one or both sides of the nose and open the internal valve angle. The original description of spreader grafts was of an endonasal placement and as an adjunct in primary rhinoplasty, for they also have the secondary effect of re-establishing the dorsal aesthetic lines and hence improving the cosmetic appearance of the nose. They may still, of course, be employed as a means of cosmetic enhancement, but they are now more readily used in revision cases where over-resection of the roof of the middle vault has resulted in collapse or pinching of the internal valve. In such patients an external rhinoplasty approach to the dorsum is normally required.

Internal Valve Surgery

Internal valve surgery relies primarily upon reduction of the head of the inferior turbinate, undertaken either alone or in conjunction with manoeuvres designed to enlarge the angle between the upper lateral cartilages and the dorsal septum. Turbinate surgery is widely practised and may be simply accomplished by the use of diathermy, cryotherapy, a laser or – more recently – coblation techniques. Such surgery is not specialised and will not be described further here.

To increase the angle between the septum and upper lateral cartilages two main techniques have been promoted. In minor cases of inner valve deficiency the modified Z-plasty technique is frequently preferred [16]. In this technique a flap of mucosa is rotated into the valve area so as to augment the surface area of the valve. Such a technique is useful in cases of simple scar-

External Nasal Valve Surgery

In patients with external valve collapse it is normally preferable to open the nose using an external rhinoplasty approach as, by so doing, the nature of the pathology can be more readily ascertained and the surgery tailored to the abnormalities revealed. However, there is a role for the internal approach to play in selected cases.

It seems to the authors that in cases in which augmentation is required to strengthen the valve, the general principle should be that, where possible, cartilage is placed as an underlay graft rather than as an overlay. This is clearly more correct empirically, as supporting a collapsing structure is more effective if it is bolstered from below. In addition the graft needs to have some degree of robustness: an onlay graft that has strength may be effective, but if it is also readily palpable it will most probably not be acceptable cosmetically, especially in patients with thin skin. Grafts should therefore be fashioned so that they can be inserted into a mucosal pocket as an underlay to existing structures wherever this is practicable.

Of course a graft may not be necessary in some cases. If the lateral crus is well formed, but is simply placed in too cephalad a position, then such malpositioning can be corrected simply by transposing the crus to a more favourable site. The crus is transected at the junction between the intermediate and lateral crura, rotated 180° and secured in a more caudal position. This straightforward manoeuvre will help to bolster the valve and prevent collapse. Occasionally such transected crura can be swapped from one side to another, and this may improve apposition during suturing.

Two techniques can be used for transection. One technique involves complete dissection of the whole lateral crus and inversion, but this involves dissecting the scroll area and can weaken the attachments between the lower and upper laterals. Therefore, if this technique is used, the free or distal end of the lateral crus needs to be re-attached to the scroll area with PDS or nylon following the transposition. The other technique involves transecting the middle part of the lateral crus only and leaving the free edge attached. In both cases the lateral crura can be further supported by the use of a spanning suture, which will further increase distal flaring and help prevent collapse.

Obviously, in both approaches it is important to dissect and preserve the vestibular mucosa. Moreover, it is also important to appreciate that, especially when operating on the lower lateral cartilages through the external approach, tip projection can be weakened owing to disruption of the inter-domal ligaments. In such circumstances a columella strut placed between the medial crura will help to preserve projection and will help to maintain the airway.

An alternative approach is to bolster the collapsing lateral crus with a batten graft placed deep to the lateral crus (Fig. 5.8) [18]. Such grafts, fashioned either from conchal or from septal cartilage, are ideally placed as caudal as possible to the natural lateral crus and are positioned such that they lie along the supra alar crease and on top of the piriform aperture. These grafts should be slightly concave with the convexity facing the nasal vestibule. They have proved to provide good long-term results in follow-up over an 8-year period [18], and are also effective at dealing with the problem of alar pinching along the supra-alar crease.

When the lateral crus is weak due to previous over-resection, reconstruction is necessary. New cartilages can be fashioned by harvesting the conchal bowl. The two resultant grafts, from the concha cavum and the cymba concha, are almost exactly equal in size and make satisfactory replacement crura. When sutured to the remnant cartilage they are very satisfactory in restoring function and improving the aesthetics in patients with pinched, unnatural looking noses following over-resection.

In more severe cases in which there is also deficiency of the middle vault, restoration of form and function can be achieved using a butterfly graft [19]. These are also harvested from the concha and are rimmed to form a bi-lobed structure, which is then positioned on the dorsum of the middle vault and placed underneath the lateral crura and sutured into position. It is important that the graft springs open the lateral crura for, if this does not happen, function may not be restored. Because of this it may be necessary to reverse the graft with the concavity superiorly, but, while this allows for increased flaring such grafts may produce an adverse cosmetic outcome.

Where facial nerve palsy causes external valve collapse the structure is, of course, likely to be normal. In such patients, a hitching suture placed through an alar crease incision will anchor the ala to the maxillary periosteum. Alternatively, a Gortex sling can be employed, whereby the ala is hitched up and anchored to a titanium screw inserted below the infraorbital ring (Fig. 5.9) [20]. However, this procedure requires three incisions, as sublabial and lower blepharoplasty incisions are required to mobilise subcuticular pockets and insert the screw, and an alar crease incision is also required in order to attach the *Gortex* sling.

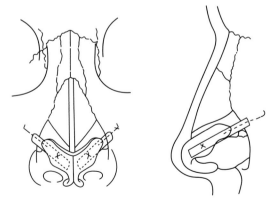

Fig. 5.8 Bolstering of the collapsing lateral crus with a batten graft placed deep to the lateral crus

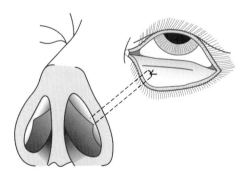

Fig. 5.9 Gortex sling. The ala is hitched up and anchored to a titanium screw inserted below the infraorbital ring (after Paniello,[20])

Conclusions

There is no doubt that disturbance of the function of the nasal valves causes obstruction in some patients. How these two valves interact is not fully understood, but it appears that the paradoxical movements of the alae are essential to support the caudal upper lateral cartilages during inspiration and that, in turn, the supporting structures and muscles play a vital role in maintaining normal nasal patency. When routine rhinoplasty surgery is undertaken, violation of the scroll area should be avoided wherever possible and aggressive cartilage resection of the alae should not be undertaken if a delayed complaint of nasal obstruction is to be avoided.

Medical measures to deal with valve complaints are unlikely to prove satisfactory for many and surgery is, therefore, often necessary. Such surgery may be difficult, especially in noses where scarring is marked, but the results are often highly gratifying and worthwhile. To some extent, what is achieved will depend on the prevailing circumstances. The general principles that result in a successful outcome have been outlined in this chapter, but individual ingenuity is often also required if a reasonable outcome is to be achieved. What is important is that the patient is not dismissed and that we move on, en masse, from the concept of septal and turbinate surgery being the only measures that will suffice in patients presenting to us with symptoms of nasal obstruction. Clearly, there is an emerging consensus to the effect that such an approach is too simplistic and that we should be more aware that the causes of surgically correctable obstruction are more complex than we had previously thought. In that regard it is not too extreme to suggest that the nasal valves should be examined and assessed in all our patients on a routine basis.

References

1. Roblin DG and Eccles R. W*hat, if any, is the value of septal surgery?* Clinical Otolaryngology, 2000. 120(5):580–595.

2. Constantian MB and Clardy RB. *The relative importance of septal and nasal valvular surgery in correcting airway obstruction in primary and secondary rhinoplasty.* Plastic and Reconstructive Surgery, 1996. 98(1): 38–54.

3. Cassell (1999) Cassell's New English Dictionary. Cassell

4. Mink PJ. *Physiologie der oberen Luftwege.* Acta Otolaryngologica, Stock, 1920. supplement 42.

5. Van Dishoeck HA. *Olfactometry in children.* Monatsschrift für Ohrenheilkunde und Laryngo-Rhinologie 1965. 99(10): 460–462.

6. Bachmann W and Legler U. *Studies of the structure and function of the anterior section of the nose by means of luminal impressions.* Acta. Otolaryngologica, 1972. 73: 433–442.

7. Haight J and Cole P. *The site and function of the nasal valve.* Laryngoscope, 1983. 93: 49–55.

8. Jones AS, et al. *The nasal valve: a physiological and clinical study.* Journal of Laryngology and Otology, 1988. 102: 1089–1094.

9. Kasperbauer J and Kern E, *Nasal valve physiology. Implication in nasal surgery.* Otolaryngology Clinics of North America, 1987. 20 (4): 699–719.

10. Shaida AM and Kenyon GS. *The nasal valves: changes in anatomy and physiology in normal subjects.* Rhinology, 2000. 38: 7–12.

11. Ohki M, Naito K, Cole P. *Dimensions and resistances of the human nose: racial differences.* Laryngoscope, 1991. 101 (3): 276–278.

12 Bridger G and Proctor DF. *Maximum nasal inspiratory flow and nasal resistance.* Annals of Otology, Rhinology and Laryngology, 1970. 99: 481–488.

13. Cottle MH. *Rhino-sphygmo-manometry and aid in physical diagnosis.* International Rhinology, 1968. 6: 7.

14. Elwany S and Thabet H. *Obstruction of the nasal valve.* Journal of Laryngology and Otology, 1996. 110: 221–224.

15. Sheen JH and Sheen AP, A*esthetic Rhinoplasty.* 2nd ed. 1987, St Louis: Mosby.

16. Nolste Trenite GJ, R*hinoplasty: A practical guide to functional and aesthetic surgery of the nose.* 3rd edition ed, ed. Nolste Trenite GJ. 2005, The Hague: Kugler.

17. Sheen JH. *Spreader graft: A method of reconstructing the roof of the middle nasal vault following rhinoplasty.* Plastic Reconstructive Surgery, 1984. 73: 230–237.

18. Kalan A, Kenyon G.S, and Seemungal TA. *Treatment of external nasal valve (alar rim) collapse with an alar strut.* Journal of Laryngology and Otology, 2001. 115(10): 788–791.

19. Clark JM and Cook T.A, *The butterfly graft in functional secondary rhinoplasty.* Laryngoscope, 2002. 112(11): 1917–1925.

20. Paniello RC. *Nasal valve suspension. An effective treatment for nasal valve collapse.* Arch. Otolaryngology Head and Neck Surgery, 1996. 122(12): 1342–1346.

Chapter 6

Respiratory Cilia: Principles of Mucociliary Clearance

6

Marcelo B. Antunes and Noam A. Cohen

Core Messages

- Respiratory cilia dynamically respond to environmental and host stimuli to regulate the propulsive force driving mucociliary clearance.
- Phosphorylation and dephosphorylation of ciliary proteins regulate cilia beat frequency.
- Dynamic regulation appears to be blunted in chronic rhinosinusitis in a reversible manner, which may contribute to delayed mucociliary clearance evident in the disease.
- Preservation of mucosa is paramount for restoration of normal mucociliary clearance.

Contents

Introduction

During normal breathing, the airways transport large quantities of environmental air into the lungs. This air is frequently contaminated with a variety of pollutants, particles and bacteria that are deposited in the airways. The nose, paranasal sinuses, trachea, and lower airways are lined with a superficial epithelium consisting primarily of two types of cells: mucus-producing goblet cells (20%) and ciliated cells (80%). This epithelial layer comprises the mucociliary escalator, the primary mode of defense for the entire respiratory system. Mucus produced by goblet cells traps inhaled particulate and infectious debris, while the propulsive force generated by the ciliated cells transports this mucus blanket to the gastrointestinal tract for elimination [1]. Unlike the lower airways or nasal cavity, in which debris-laden mucus can be cleared with a cough or sneeze reflex respectively, the paranasal sinuses are solely dependent on ciliary activity to clear mucus [2]. Mucociliary clearance (MCC) is dynamically regulated by both the inhaled environmental stimuli as well as host factors such as neurotransmitters and cytokines. Although multiple etiologies contribute to the development of chronic rhinosinusitis (CRS), a common pathophysiologic sequela is ineffective sinonasal MCC, leading to stasis of sinonasal secretions, with subsequent infection and/or persistent inflammation. The predominant goal of medical and surgical intervention in the management of CRS is restoration of MCC. Thus, in this chapter we will review respiratory ciliary cell biology and physiology, and the ciliary pathophysiology associated with respiratory diseases.

Ciliary Structure and Function

Respiratory cilia clear mucus and debris from both the upper and lower respiratory passages by beating in a coordinated and rhythmic manner. There are approximately 50–200 cilia per epithelial cell; each measures 5–7 μm in length and has a diameter of about 0.2–0.3 μm [3, 4]. Cilia are organelles located in the apical surface of epithelial cells that are anchored to the basal bodies derived from the centrioles. Each cilium comprises a bundle of interconnected microtubules termed the axoneme and an overlying membrane that is part of the cell plasma membrane. Microtubules comprise protofilaments, which are assembled from α- and β-tubulin dimers. The major β-tubulin in the cilia is the type IV isotype [5], which is much more abundant in the cilia than in the cell and makes for an ideal marker for respiratory cilia in the research setting (Fig. 6.1). The axonemes of motile cilia, which are found in the respiratory system, oviduct, and ventricular ependymal cells, contain two central singlet microtubules surrounded by nine doublet microtubules (Fig. 6.2). The doublet consists of an A-tubule, a complete circle of 13 protofilaments, and a B-tubule, an incomplete circle of 10 protofilaments. The two central microtubules are attached by paired bridges, while the peripheral doublets attach to the central pair via radial spoke heads. Each outer doublet interacts with the adjacent outer doublet via inner dynein arms (IDA), outer dynein arms (ODA), and nexin, each of which have distinct roles in the dynamic motion of cilia bending [6]. Activation of the dynein arms generates a sliding motion of one microtubule doublet against the adjacent doublet. While phosphorylation of the ODA regulates cilia beat frequency, phosphorylation of the IDA regulate the wave form pattern of beating [7, 8]. Although the function of the radial spoke heads is not entirely understood, it seems that they are involved in regionally limiting the sliding between the microtubules during the ciliary stroke, thus converting the sliding motion generated by the dynein arms into the bending motion of the axoneme [9].

Each cilium has a forward effective stroke followed by a recovery stroke. During the effective stroke the cilia is fully extended, and at the apogee of the arc, the distal tip makes contact with the viscous outer mucus layer (see the section "Mucus and Periciliary Fluid"), thereby transmitting directional force to the overlying mucus blanket. During the recovery stroke, the cilia bends 90° and sweeps back to the starting point within the thin periciliary fluid layer. As mentioned above, the mechanism of ciliary motion depends on a series of molecular motors built into the axoneme, which act to produce a vectorial force that causes the outer doublet microtubules to slide relative to one another. The central pair divides the axoneme into opposite halves. As proposed by the "switch point" hypothesis, the dynein motors on one side of the axoneme are predominantly active during the effective stroke, while the motors on the other side are mainly active during the recovery stroke [10]. If the microtubules are numbered in a clockwise fashion from 1 to 9, the effective stroke would involve the ODA on the 9-1-2-3-4 microtubules, and the recovery stroke would involve activity of the dynein in the 5-6-7-8 microtubules [11]. The power generated by the cilium is directly proportional to the number of the dynein–microtubule interactions [12], while under normal circumstances, there is a reserve to increase the power of the stroke [13]. The orientation of the stroke is dictated by the orientation of the basal body of the axoneme [14, 15].

Although it is well established that cilia beat in a coordinated fashion, referred to as a metachronous wave, the mechanism of coordination is not entirely understood. A possible way of explaining the presence of this wave might be the close relationship between the cilia in the cell and the hydrodynamic forces between the cilia, since they beat submerged in a partly liquid environment [16]. Additionally, gap junctions, predominately connexin-43, may generate directional propagation of intracellular calcium waves to adjacent cells driving the metachronous wave [17].

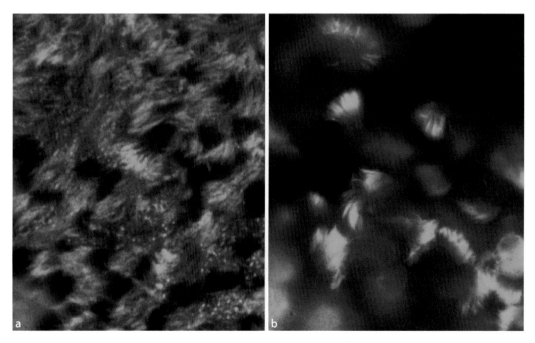

Fig. 6.1a,b Type IV beta-tubulin specifically stains respiratory cilia. **a** Intact and **b** dissociated human paranasal sinus mucosa stained with a monoclonal antibody against type IV beta-tubulin demonstrate intense specific staining of the respiratory cilia

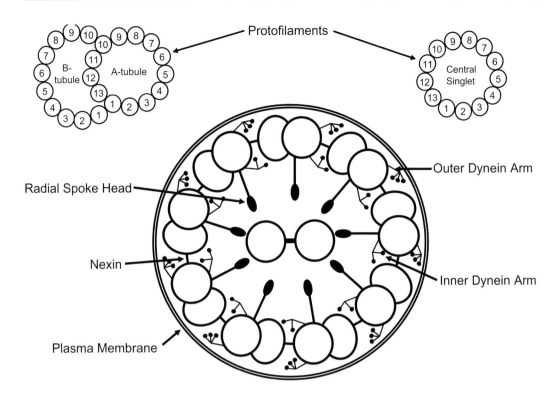

Fig. 6.2 Schematic diagram of axonemal structure. Nine peripheral doublets encircle two central protofilaments. The peripheral doublets are interconnected by nexin and the inner and outer dynein arms, while peripheral and central protofilaments are interconnected by radial spokes. ATPase activity of the dynein arms generates a sliding motion of one microtubule relative to adjacent microtubules, while the semi-rigid structure of nexin and the radial arm spokes translates the sliding motion into bending

Regulation of Ciliary Beat Frequency

Ciliary activity accelerates in response to a variety of mechanical [18], chemical [19, 20], hormonal [21-23], pH [24], and thermal stimuli [25, 26]. Extracellular nucleotides (adenosine and uridine) are especially potent regulators of epithelial functions stimulating MCC through mucus secretion, increasing CBF, and gating ion channels involved in the maintenance of epithelial surface liquid volume [27]. Nucleotides released by the epithelium in response to mechanical and osmotic stimuli work in a paracrine fashion through both metabotropic and ionotropic receptors to potentiate MCC by recruiting adjacent cells to increase CBF [27]. Furthermore, adrenergic [23, 28, 29], cholinergic [30, 31], and peptidergic [32, 33] stimulation have also been demonstrated to stimulate ciliary motility. These environmental and host stimuli are transmitted via surface receptors and channels to trigger activation of second messenger cascades that regulate the phosphorylation status of ciliary proteins, thereby modulating the kinetics of microtubules sliding relative to each other. Inositol triphosphate (IP_3)-mediated calcium transients have been found to correlate with increased CBF [34–36]. Additionally, protein kinase A (PKA)- [31, 37], protein kinase G (PKG)- [38, 39], and nitric oxide (NO)-de-

pendent mechanisms of CBF stimulation have been proposed [20, 40, 41], while activation of protein kinase C (PKC) appears to decrease CBF [33, 42]. To maintain rapid control of ciliary activity, kinase anchoring proteins (AKAPs), kinases, and phosphatases have been demonstrated to be tightly associated with the axoneme [43–45]. Recently, elegant experiments using fluorescence resonance energy transfer (FRET) in primary ciliated cell culture demonstrated direct evidence that activation of protein kinase A (PKA) coincides with an increase in CBF, and that the return to baseline frequency lags behind PKA inactivation, indicating that dephosphorylation by phosphatases is required to terminate CBF stimulation [46].

As mentioned above, environmental stimuli also modulate cilia beat frequency. Small changes in both extracellular and intracellular pH can have a profound impact on CBF. An increase in intracellular pH produces an increase in CBF, while a decrease in pH produces a decrease in CBF [24]. However, it is not known whether this effect is due to modulation of kinase activity, even though an acidic pH has been demonstrated to inhibit PKA function [47], or to direct regulation of the outer dynein arm of the axoneme [48].

Cilia beat has also been shown to be influenced by changes in temperature. Multiple investigations have demonstrated a direct correlation between temperature and ciliary beat frequency [25, 26, 49]. Furthermore, the temperature response appears to be mediated through kinase activity, as activation of protein kinase C shifts the temperature curve to the left [25].

Lastly, cilia beat frequency is also regulated by mechanical factors. Direct mechanical stimulation of the cilia promotes an increase in CBF that coincides with an increase in intracellular Ca^{2+} [18]. Additionally, shear stress applied to the apical surface of mouse tracheal explants has stimulated ciliary beat frequency. The characteristics of this observation include a time-dependent component as well as a directional component, with stimulation resulting from caudally applied shear stress. Furthermore, the response is dependent on purinergic receptor activation as well as intracellular Ca^{2+} and ATP [50].

Inflammatory Mediators

The inflammatory responses found in CRS can be broadly divided into T helper type 1 (T_H1) and T helper type 2 (T_H2) cascades, according to the different cytokines they produce, with a predominance of T_H1 mediators found in CRS without nasal polyposis and T_H2 mediators found in CRS with nasal polyposis [51].

Although no general consensus regarding inflammatory cytokines has been compiled, several molecules are consistently upregulated in diseased mucosa by using various techniques including ELISA, reverse transcriptase coupled to quantitative polymerase chain reaction (RT-PCR), immunohistochemistry, and multiplex technology. The T_H1 cytokines consistently elevated in CRS include TNFα, γIFN, and IL-8 [52, 53], while IL-5, Eotaxin, and RANTES represent consistently elevated T_H2 cytokines [54–57]. Furthermore, several of these factors are reduced following treatment with glucocorticoids [52, 57], a critical component of CRS medical management. Although chemokines and cytokines are primarily responsible for inducing migration, differentiation, activation, and degranulation of subpopulations of leukocytes, several studies have reported cytokine modulation of respiratory cilia function. Recently, IL-8 has been shown to inhibit isoproteranol-stimulated CBF in bovine bronchial epithelial cells [58], while IL-13 has been shown to decrease basal CBF in a dose- and time-dependent manner [59]. Conversely, TNFα and IL-1β increase CBF in bovine bronchial epithelial cells [21]. Therefore, modulation of sinonasal epithelial physiology by CRS-specific inflammatory cytokines/chemokines is a likely mechanism for decreased MCC in the disease state.

Mucus and Periciliary Fluid

Mucus is the second essential component of MCC. Airway mucus possesses a dynamic gel-like composition whose rheologic properties have a tremendous influence on the MCC. Mucus is produced by goblet cells in the mucosa and is approximately 1% NaCl, 0.5–1% free protein, 0.5–1% mucins, which are carbohydrate-rich glycoproteins, with the remaining mass being water, approximately 95% [3]. Additionally, mucus contains in-

nate immune proteins such as lactoferrin, lysozyme, and s-IgA, which aid in the local immune defenses [60]. The two extremes of the rheologic behavior are viscosity (Newtonian) and elasticity (non-Newtonian). An intriguing substance, mucus is viscoelastic, as it is marked by both viscosity (a liquid property) because of its resistance to flow and its capacity to absorb energy when in motion, and by elasticity (a solid property) because of its capacity to store energy that is used to move or deform mass. The physical properties of mucus include spinability, which describes its thread-forming capacity and its internal cohesive force; adhesivity, its ability to bind a solid surface; and wettability, its ability to spread on a surface. All of these rheological and physical properties are influenced by the degree of hydration and the glycoprotein composition, factors that are host-regulated [3, 61].

Over the last decade, with the introduction of perfluorocarbon/osmium fixation [62] detailed transmission electron microscopic examination of airway surface liquid has revealed at least two layers, the outer mucus layer and the inner periciliary layer. As mentioned above, the vast majority of the ciliary stroke occurs in the periciliary fluid with only the distal tip at full extension, making contact with the outer mucus layer comprising high-molecular weight, glycosylated macromolecules that form a network of tangled polymers ideal for trapping inhaled debris [63]. Within the periciliary fluid layer are cell surface-attached mucins forming an apical glycocalyx extending 500–1,500 nm into the airway [64, 65]. The periciliary fluid, both in composition and size, appears to be critical for proper mucociliary transport [66, 67]. If the layer is too short, the glycocalyx of the cell will interact with the mucus and impair mucus clearance.

Mucociliary Clearance and Disease

As discussed above, MCC is dependent on normal ciliary function and mucus composition. Thus, any disease state that compromises any of its components shares the common symptom of recurrent sinopulmonary infections. Primary ciliary dyskinesia (PCD) is a syndrome manifesting as severely impaired MCC due to dysfunctional cilia. PCD patients often present with chronic airway infections and recurrent middle ear infections. Kartagener's syndrome is a subgroup of PCD that includes immotile sperm and situs inversus. The cause of the disturbance is usually a defect in the dynein arms of the axonemal microtubules [68]. Several types of defects have been reported, including complete absence of the dynein arms, outer dynein arms only or inner dynein only [69, 70]. The first of several PCD-associated genes has been cloned that encodes an intermediate chain dynein responsible for coordinating the proper assembly of the heavy chain dyneins [71, 72]. Additionally, subsets of patients with symptoms of PCD demonstrate normal ciliary structure, but have random orientation of the cilia. Thus, even though they have normal motility, the ciliary function is ineffective, resulting in impaired MCC [68]. A number of conditions, such as influenza infection, can disrupt MCC, leading to secondary ciliary dyskinesia (SCD), in which there is no anatomical abnormality of the cilia, but they do not function properly. Traditionally, transmission electron microscopy is considered the gold standard for

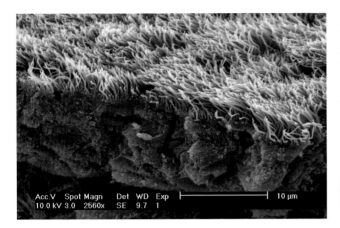

Fig. 6.3 Scanning electron microscopy of rabbit maxillary sinus mucosa. Paranasal sinus mucosa consists of predominantly ciliated cells giving the appearance of a shag carpet

making the diagnosis of PCD (Fig. 6.3). However, sometimes there is no ultrastructural abnormality as previously mentioned, thus limiting this diagnostic modality to only confirming the suspected diagnosis; it does not rule out the diagnosis. Jorissen et al. reported the value of ciliogenesis in cultured cells to establish the diagnosis of PCD [73]. After ciliogenesis, cultures established from patients with PCD will have abnormal ciliary activity, while those established from patients with SCD will regain normal function.

Cystic fibrosis (CF) is a single gene, autosomal recessive disease involving several organ systems that is traditionally considered to be a disease of abnormal mucus production [74]. The genetic defect is found in the cystic fibrosis transmembrane conductance regulator gene product (CFTR), a cAMP-mediated membrane glycoprotein that forms a chloride channel, but also intimately regulates the open probability of the sodium channel, ENaC [75]. Thus, CFTR plays multiple roles in ion flux at epithelial surfaces. Based on these functions, two predominant hypotheses have emerged to explain the pathophysiology of CF: a high salt hypothesis hindering innate immunity function [76] and a low volume hypothesis due to Na^+ hyperabsorption resulting in impeded mucus movement [77]. The controversy between these two hypotheses continues to generate improvement in disease models, as well as analysis of epithelial function.

Chronic rhinosinusitis (CRS), affecting more than 35 million Americans of all ages [78] represents a number of distinct entities that are clinically indistinguishable. While the mortality of the disease is low, the morbidity is high, with CRS patients demonstrating worse "quality of life" scores (for physical pain and social functioning) than those suffering from chronic obstructive pulmonary disease, congestive heart failure or angina [79].

As already mentioned, multiple etiologies contribute to the development of CRS, but a common pathophysiologic complication is ineffective sinonasal MCC, which results in stasis of the sinonasal secretions followed by infection and/or persistent inflammation.

Although the literature is contradictory regarding mucus viscosity [80–82] and basal ciliary beat frequency [81, 83–86] in CRS, recent work has suggested that a subset of patients with CRS have a blunted ciliary response to environmental stimuli [87]. Additionally, air–liquid interface cultures established from patients with CRS have demonstrated increased transepithelial ion transport compared with normal cultures, thereby altering mucus viscosity and potentially contributing to the pathophysiology of the disease [88].

Conclusion

The entire respiratory system is constantly exposed to environmental pollutants, respiratory pathogens and aerosolized toxins. MCC is the primary innate defense mechanism against this constant onslaught. Over the last quarter of a century, techniques to study MCC, and the individual components, cilia and mucus, have evolved. These techniques have advanced our understanding of the interaction of the respiratory epithelium with the airway surface liquid, and have supplied the ability to study pathologic processes involving MCC.

Take-Home Pearls

- Motile cilia are critical for mucociliary clearance.
- Ciliary beat frequency is dynamic and may be pharmacologically manipulated.
- Future work delineating ciliary dysfunction in disease states will generate novel therapeutic modalities in treatment armamentariums.

References

1. Wanner, A., M. Salathe and T.G. O'Riordan, Mucociliary Clearance in the Airways. Am J Respir Crit Care Med, 1996. 154(6 Pt 1): p. 1868–902.

2. Van der Baan, B., Ciliary Function. Acta Otorhinolaryngol Belg, 2000. 54(3): p. 293–8.

3. Houtmeyers, E., R. Gosselink, G. Gayan-Ramirez, et al., Regulation of Mucociliary Clearance in Health and Disease. Eur Respir J, 1999. 13(5): p. 1177–88.

4. Satir, P. and M.A. Sleigh, The Physiology of Cilia and Mucociliary Interactions. Annu Rev Physiol, 1990. 52: p. 137–55.

5. Renthal, R., B.G. Schneider, M.M. Miller, et al., Beta IV Is the Major Beta-Tubulin Isotype in Bovine Cilia. Cell Motil Cytoskeleton, 1993. 25(1): p. 19–29.

6. Hard, R., K. Blaustein and L. Scarcello, Reactivation of Outer-Arm-Depleted Lung Axonemes: Evidence for Functional Differences between Inner and Outer Dynein Arms in Situ. Cell Motil Cytoskeleton, 1992. 21(3): p. 199–209.

6

7. Brokaw, C.J. and R. Kamiya, Bending Patterns of Chlamydomonas Flagella: IV. Mutants with Defects in Inner and Outer Dynein Arms Indicate Differences in Dynein Arm Function. Cell Motil Cytoskeleton, 1987. 8(1): p. 68–75.

8. Brokaw, C.J., Control of Flagellar Bending: A New Agenda Based on Dynein Diversity. Cell Motil Cytoskeleton, 1994. 28(3): p. 199–204.

9. Satir, P. and S.T. Christensen, Overview of Structure and Function of Mammalian Cilia. Annu Rev Physiol, 2007. 69: p. 377–400.

10. Satir, P. and T. Matsuoka, Splitting the Ciliary Axoneme: Implications for A "Switch-Point" Model of Dynein Arm Activity in Ciliary Motion. Cell Motil Cytoskeleton, 1989. 14(3): p. 345–58.

11. Sanderson, M.J. and M.A. Sleigh, Ciliary Activity of Cultured Rabbit Tracheal Epithelium: Beat Pattern and Metachrony. J Cell Sci, 1981. 47: p. 331–47.

12. Holwill, M.E., G.F. Foster, T. Hamasaki, et al., Biophysical Aspects and Modelling of Ciliary Motility. Cell Motil Cytoskeleton, 1995. 32(2): p. 114–20.

13. Johnson, N.T., M. Villalon, F.H. Royce, et al., Autoregulation of Beat Frequency in Respiratory Ciliated Cells. Demonstration by Viscous Loading. Am Rev Respir Dis, 1991. 144(5): p. 1091–4.

14. Satir, P., The Cilium as a Biological Nanomachine. FASEB J, 1999. 13 Suppl 2: p. S235–7.

15. Lee, C.H., S.S. Lee, J.H. Mo, et al., Comparison of Ciliary Wave Disorders Measured by Image Analysis and Electron Microscopy. Acta Otolaryngol, 2005. 125(5): p. 571–6.

16. Gheber, L. and Z. Priel, Synchronization Between Beating Cilia. Biophys J, 1989. 55(1): p. 183–91.

17. Yeh, T.H., M.C. Su, C.J. Hsu, et al., Epithelial Cells of Nasal Mucosa Express Functional Gap Junctions of Connexin 43. Acta Otolaryngol, 2003. 123(2): p. 314–20.

18. Sanderson, M.J. and E.R. Dirksen, Mechanosensitivity of Cultured Ciliated Cells from the Mammalian Respiratory Tract: Implications for the Regulation of Mucociliary Transport. Proc Natl Acad Sci U S A, 1986. 83(19): p. 7302–6.

19. Wong, L.B., I.F. Miller and D.B. Yeates, Stimulation of Tracheal Ciliary Beat Frequency by Capsaicin. J Appl Physiol, 1990. 68(6): p. 2574–80.

20. Jain, B., I. Rubinstein, R.A. Robbins, et al., Modulation of Airway Epithelial Cell Ciliary Beat Frequency by Nitric Oxide. Biochem Biophys Res Commun, 1993. 191(1): p. 83–8.

21. Jain, B., I. Rubinstein, R.A. Robbins, et al., TNF-Alpha and IL-1 Beta Upregulate Nitric Oxide-Dependent Ciliary Motility in Bovine Airway Epithelium. Am J Physiol, 1995. 268(6 Pt 1): p. L911–7.

22. Korngreen, A., W. Ma, Z. Priel, et al., Extracellular ATP Directly Gates a Cation-Selective Channel in Rabbit Airway Ciliated Epithelial Cells. J Physiol, 1998. 508 (Pt 3): p. 703–20.

23. Sanderson, M.J. and E.R. Dirksen, Mechanosensitive and Beta-Adrenergic Control of the Ciliary Beat Frequency of Mammalian Respiratory Tract Cells in Culture. Am Rev Respir Dis, 1989. 139(2): p. 432–40.

24. Sutto, Z., G.E. Conner and M. Salathe, Regulation of Human Airway Ciliary Beat Frequency by Intracellular pH. J Physiol, 2004. 560(Pt 2): p. 519–32.

25. Mwimbi, X.K., R. Muimo, M.W. Green, et al., Making Human Nasal Cilia Beat in the Cold: A Real Time Assay for Cell Signalling. Cell Signal, 2003. 15(4): p. 395–402.

26. Schipor, I., J.N. Palmer, A.S. Cohen, et al., Quantification of Ciliary Beat Frequency in Sinonasal Epithelial Cells Using Differential Interference Contrast Microscopy and High-Speed Digital Video Imaging. Am J Rhinol, 2006. 20(1): p. 124–7.

27. Picher, M. and R.C. Boucher, Human Airway Ecto-Adenylate Kinase. A Mechanism to Propagate ATP Signaling on Airway Surfaces. J Biol Chem, 2003. 278(13): p. 11256–64.

28. Wyatt, T.A. and J.H. Sisson, Chronic Ethanol Downregulates PKA Activation and Ciliary Beating in Bovine Bronchial Epithelial Cells. Am J Physiol Lung Cell Mol Physiol, 2001. 281(3): p. L575–81.

29. Yang, B., R.J. Schlosser and T.V. McCaffrey, Dual Signal Transduction Mechanisms Modulate Ciliary Beat Frequency in Upper Airway Epithelium. Am J Physiol, 1996. 270(5 Pt 1): p. L745–51.

30. Salathe, M., E.J. Lipson, P.I. Ivonnet, et al., Muscarinic Signaling in Ciliated Tracheal Epithelial Cells: Dual Effects on Ca2+ and Ciliary Beating. Am J Physiol, 1997. 272(2 Pt 1): p. L301–10.

31. Zagoory, O., A. Braiman and Z. Priel, The Mechanism of Ciliary Stimulation by Acetylcholine: Roles of Calcium, PKA, and PKG. J Gen Physiol, 2002. 119(4): p. 329–39.

32. Wong, L.B., I.F. Miller and D.B. Yeates, Pathways of Substance P Stimulation of Canine Tracheal Ciliary Beat Frequency. J Appl Physiol, 1991. 70(1): p. 267–73.

33. Wong, L.B., C.L. Park and D.B. Yeates, Neuropeptide Y Inhibits Ciliary Beat Frequency in Human Ciliated Cells Via NPKC, Independently of PKA. Am J Physiol, 1998. 275(2 Pt 1): p. C440–8.

34. Salathe, M. and R.J. Bookman, Coupling of [Ca2+]I and Ciliary Beating in Cultured Tracheal Epithelial Cells. J Cell Sci, 1995. 108 (Pt 2): p. 431–40.

35. Korngreen, A. and Z. Priel, Simultaneous Measurement of Ciliary Beating and Intracellular Calcium. Biophys J, 1994. 67(1): p. 377–80.

36. Lansley, A.B. and M.J. Sanderson, Regulation of Airway Ciliary Activity by Ca2+: Simultaneous Measurement of Beat Frequency and Intracellular Ca2+. Biophys J, 1999. 77(1): p. 629–38.

37. Braiman, A., O. Zagoory and Z. Priel, PKA Induces Ca2+ Release and Enhances Ciliary Beat Frequency in a Ca2+-Dependent and -Independent Manner. Am J Physiol, 1998. 275(3 Pt 1): p. C790–7.

38. Zhang, L. and M.J. Sanderson, The Role of CGMP in the Regulation of Rabbit Airway Ciliary Beat Frequency. J Physiol, 2003. 551(Pt 3): p. 765–76.

39. Wyatt, T.A., J.R. Spurzem, K. May, et al., Regulation of Ciliary Beat Frequency by Both PKA and PKG in Bovine Airway Epithelial Cells. Am J Physiol, 1998. 275(4 Pt 1): p. L827–35.

40. Yang, B., R.J. Schlosser and T.V. McCaffrey, Signal Transduction Pathways in Modulation of Ciliary Beat Frequency by Methacholine. Ann Otol Rhinol Laryngol, 1997. 106(3): p. 230–6.

41. Uzlaner, N. and Z. Priel, Interplay Between the NO Pathway and Elevated [Ca2+]I Enhances Ciliary Activity in Rabbit Trachea. J Physiol, 1999. 516 (Pt 1): p. 179–90.

42. Mwimbi, X.K., R. Muimo, M. Green, et al., Protein Kinase C Regulates the Flow Rate-Dependent Decline in Human Nasal Ciliary Beat Frequency in Vitro. J Aerosol Med, 2000. 13(3): p. 273–9.

43. Porter, M.E. and W.S. Sale, The 9 + 2 Axoneme Anchors Multiple Inner Arm Dyneins and a Network of Kinases and Phosphatases That Control Motility. J Cell Biol, 2000. 151(5): p. F37–42.

44. Kamiya, R., Functional Diversity of Axonemal Dyneins as Studied in Chlamydomonas Mutants. Int Rev Cytol, 2002. 219: p. 115–55.

45. Smith, E.F., Regulation of Flagellar Dynein by the Axonemal Central Apparatus. Cell Motil Cytoskeleton, 2002. 52(1): p. 33–42.

46. Schmid, A., G. Bai, N. Schmid, et al., Real-Time Analysis of Camp-Mediated Regulation of Ciliary Motility in Single Primary Human Airway Epithelial Cells. J Cell Sci, 2006. 119(Pt 20): p. 4176–86.

47. Reddy, M.M., R.R. Kopito and P.M. Quinton, Cytosolic pH Regulates GCL Through Control of Phosphorylation States of CFTR. Am J Physiol, 1998. 275(4 Pt 1): p. C1040–7.

48. Keskes, L., V. Giroux-Widemann, C. Serres, et al., The Reactivation of Demembranated Human Spermatozoa Lacking Outer Dynein Arms Is Independent of pH. Mol Reprod Dev, 1998. 49(4): p. 416–25.

49. Green, A., L.A. Smallman, A.C. Logan, et al., The Effect of Temperature on Nasal Ciliary Beat Frequency. Clin Otolaryngol, 1995. 20(2): p. 178–80.

50. Winters, S.L., C.W. Davis and R.C. Boucher, Mechanosensitivity of Mouse Tracheal Ciliary Beat Frequency: Roles for [Ca2+]O, Purinergic Signaling, Tonicity, and Viscosity. Am J Physiol Lung Cell Mol Physiol, 2007. 292(3): p. L614–24.

51. Hamilos, D.L., Chronic Sinusitis. J Allergy Clin Immunol, 2000. 106(2): p. 213–27.

52. Lennard, C.M., E.A. Mann, L.L. Sun, et al., Interleukin-1 Beta, Interleukin-5, Interleukin-6, Interleukin-8, and Tumor Necrosis Factor-Alpha in Chronic Sinusitis: Response to Systemic Corticosteroids. Am J Rhinol, 2000. 14(6): p. 367–73.

53. Kuehnemund, M., C. Ismail, J. Brieger, et al., Untreated Chronic Rhinosinusitis: A Comparison of Symptoms and Mediator Profiles. Laryngoscope, 2004. 114(3): p. 561–5.

54. Bachert, C., M. Wagenmann, C. Rudack, et al., The Role of Cytokines in Infectious Sinusitis and Nasal Polyposis. Allergy, 1998. 53(1): p. 2–13.

55. Bachert, C., M. Wagenmann, U. Hauser, et al., Il-5 Synthesis Is Upregulated in Human Nasal Polyp Tissue. J Allergy Clin Immunol, 1997. 99(6 Pt 1): p. 837–42.

56. Bachert, C. and P.B. Van Cauwenberge, Inflammatory Mechanisms in Chronic Sinusitis. Acta Otorhinolaryngol Belg, 1997. 51(4): p. 209–17.

57. Woodworth, B.A., K. Joseph, A.P. Kaplan, et al., Alterations in Eotaxin, Monocyte Chemoattractant Protein-4, Interleukin-5, and Interleukin-13 After Systemic Steroid Treatment for Nasal Polyps. Otolaryngol Head Neck Surg, 2004. 131(5): p. 585–9.

58. Allen-Gipson, D.S., D.J. Romberger, M.A. Forget, et al., IL-8 Inhibits Isoproterenol-Stimulated Ciliary Beat Frequency in Bovine Bronchial Epithelial Cells. J Aerosol Med, 2004. 17(2): p. 107–15.

59. Laoukili, J., E. Perret, T. Willems, et al., IL-13 Alters Mucociliary Differentiation and Ciliary Beating of Human Respiratory Epithelial Cells. J Clin Invest, 2001. 108(12): p. 1817–24.

60. Sleigh, M.A., J.R. Blake and N. Liron, The Propulsion of Mucus by Cilia. Am Rev Respir Dis, 1988. 137(3): p. 726–41.

61. Verdugo, P., Goblet Cells Secretion and Mucogenesis. Annu Rev Physiol, 1990. 52: p. 157–76.

62. Sims, D.E., J.A. Westfall, A.L. Kiorpes, et al., Preservation of Tracheal Mucus by Nonaqueous Fixative. Biotech Histochem, 1991. 66(4): p. 173–80.

63. Knowles, M.R. and R.C. Boucher, Mucus Clearance as a Primary Innate Defense Mechanism for Mammalian Airways. J Clin Invest, 2002. 109(5): p. 571–7.

64. Bernacki, S.H., A.L. Nelson, L. Abdullah, et al., Mucin Gene Expression During Differentiation of Human Airway Epithelia In Vitro. Muc4 and Muc5b Are Strongly Induced. Am J Respir Cell Mol Biol, 1999. 20(4): p. 595–604.

65. Lo-Guidice, J.M., M.D. Merten, G. Lamblin, et al., Mucins Secreted by a Transformed Cell Line Derived from Human Tracheal Gland Cells. Biochem J, 1997. 326 (Pt 2): p. 431–7.

66. Tarran, R., B. Button and R.C. Boucher, Regulation of Normal and Cystic Fibrosis Airway Surface Liquid Volume by Phasic Shear Stress. Annu Rev Physiol, 2006. 68: p. 543–61.

67. Tarran, R., L. Trout, S.H. Donaldson, et al., Soluble Mediators, Not Cilia, Determine Airway Surface Liquid Volume in Normal and Cystic Fibrosis Superficial Airway Epithelia. J Gen Physiol, 2006. 127(5): p. 591–604.

68. Rutland, J. and R.U. de Iongh, Random Ciliary Orientation. A Cause of Respiratory Tract Disease. N Engl J Med, 1990. 323(24): p. 1681–4.

69. Sturgess, J.M. and J.A. Turner, Ultrastructural Pathology of Cilia in the Immotile Cilia Syndrome. Perspect Pediatr Pathol, 1984. 8(2): p. 133–61.

70. Afzelius, B.A., Genetics and Pulmonary Medicine. 6. Immotile Cilia Syndrome: Past, Present, and Prospects for the Future. Thorax, 1998. 53(10): p. 894–7.

71. Pennarun, G., E. Escudier, C. Chapelin, et al., Loss-of-Function Mutations in a Human Gene Related to Chlamydomonas Reinhardtii Dynein IC78 Result in Primary Ciliary Dyskinesia. Am J Hum Genet, 1999. 65(6): p. 1508–19.

72. Zariwala, M., P.G. Noone, A. Sannuti, et al., Germline Mutations in an Intermediate Chain Dynein Cause Primary Ciliary Dyskinesia. Am J Respir Cell Mol Biol, 2001. 25(5): p. 577–83.

73. Jorissen, M., T. Willems and B. Van der Schueren, Ciliary Function Analysis for the Diagnosis of Primary Ciliary Dyskinesia: Advantages of Ciliogenesis in Culture. Acta Otolaryngol, 2000. 120(2): p. 291–5.

74. Accurso, F.J., Update in Cystic Fibrosis 2005. Am J Respir Crit Care Med, 2006. 173(9): p. 944–7.

75. Wine, J.J., The Genesis of Cystic Fibrosis Lung Disease. J Clin Invest, 1999. 103(3): p. 309–12.

76. Smith, J.J., S.M. Travis, E.P. Greenberg, et al., Cystic Fibrosis Airway Epithelia Fail to Kill Bacteria Because of Abnormal Airway Surface Fluid. Cell, 1996. 85(2): p. 229–36.

77. Matsui, H., B.R. Grubb, R. Tarran, et al., Evidence for Periciliary Liquid Layer Depletion, Not Abnormal Ion Composition, in the Pathogenesis of Cystic Fibrosis Airways Disease. Cell, 1998. 95(7): p. 1005–15.

78. Murphy, M.P., P. Fishman, S.O. Short, et al., Health Care Utilization and Cost among Adults with Chronic Rhinosinusitis Enrolled in a Health Maintenance Organization. Otolaryngol Head Neck Surg, 2002. 127(5): p. 367–76.

79. Gliklich, R.E. and R. Metson, The Health Impact of Chronic Sinusitis in Patients Seeking Otolaryngologic Care. Otolaryngol Head Neck Surg, 1995. 113(1): p. 104–9.

80. Majima, Y., T. Harada, T. Shimizu, et al., Effect of Biochemical Components on Rheologic Properties of Nasal Mucus in Chronic Sinusitis. Am J Respir Crit Care Med, 1999. 160(2): p. 421–6.

81. Majima, Y., Y. Sakakura, T. Matsubara, et al., Possible Mechanisms of Reduction of Nasal Mucociliary Clearance in Chronic Sinusitis. Clin Otolaryngol, 1986. 11(2): p. 55–60.

82. Atsuta, S. and Y. Majima, Nasal Mucociliary Clearance of Chronic Sinusitis in Relation to Rheological Properties of Nasal Mucus. Ann Otol Rhinol Laryngol, 1998. 107(1): p. 47–51.

83. Majima, Y., Y. Sakakura, T. Matsubara, et al., Mucociliary Clearance in Chronic Sinusitis: Related Human Nasal Clearance and In Vitro Bullfrog Palate Clearance. Biorheology, 1983. 20(2): p. 251–62.

84. Joki, S., E. Toskala, V. Saano, et al., Correlation between Ciliary Beat Frequency and the Structure of Ciliated Epithelia in Pathologic Human Nasal Mucosa. Laryngoscope, 1998. 108(3): p. 426–30.

85. Braverman, I., E.D. Wright, C.G. Wang, et al., Human Nasal Ciliary-Beat Frequency in Normal and Chronic Sinusitis Subjects. J Otolaryngol, 1998. 27(3): p. 145–52.

86. Nuutinen, J., E. Rauch-Toskala, V. Saano, et al., Ciliary Beating Frequency in Chronic Sinusitis. Arch Otolaryngol Head Neck Surg, 1993. 119(6): p. 645–7.

87. Chen, B., J. Shaari, S.E. Claire, et al., Altered Sinonasal Ciliary Dynamics in Chronic Rhinosinusitis. Am J Rhinol, 2006. 20(3): p. 325–9.

88. Dejima, K., S.H. Randell, M.J. Stutts, et al., Potential Role of Abnormal Ion Transport in the Pathogenesis of Chronic Sinusitis. Arch Otolaryngol Head Neck Surg, 2006. 132(12): p. 1352–62.

Chapter 7

The Anatomy and Physiology of Olfaction and Gustation

7

Aaron I. Brescia and Allen M. Seiden

Core Messages

- The olfactory and gustatory systems rely on molecule–receptor-specific binding at specialized receptor sites to transduce afferent stimuli.
- Higher central nervous system centers integrate these combinations of signals to generate perceptions of smell and taste.
- Olfactory receptor bipolar neurons are directly exposed to the external environment, within the nasal vault, making this a unique sensory system.

Contents

Olfaction

The olfactory epithelium is a specialized patch of tissue located in the postero-superior aspect of each nasal vault, on the cribriform plate, upper nasal septum, and upper superior turbinate (Fig. 7.1). It consists of bipolar neurons whose dendritic processes extend directly into the open nasal cavity and are covered by a mucous film, and whose axons stretch back to the primary olfactory bulb in the anterior fossa on the ventral surface of the frontal lobe. Odorant molecules are partitioned into the mucous film overlying this tissue according to their lipid solubility coefficients [1].

The modified respiratory epithelium surrounding these neurons differs from that in the rest of the upper respiratory tract in a number of ways: the supporting cells of the epithelium form tight junctions with each neighboring cell as well as the dendritic processes themselves, helping to ensure strict control of ion and other molecular transport from the overlying mucous film and the underlying sensory neuronal cell bodies; mucous glands within the epithelium secrete not only the critical mucous film in which odorant molecules must partition, but also various odorant binding proteins that help to increase the organic solubility of more hydrophilic odorants, thus enhancing their detection [2, 3].

The olfactory sensory neurons are bipolar neuronal cells whose bodies lie within the middle and deep portions of the olfactory epithelium. Each neuron sends a dendritic process toward the surface of the epithelium and terminates very near the surface in an olfactory knob. The surface of this knob is ciliated, and these ciliated processes extend into the mucous layer in which odorant molecules are partitioned (Fig. 7.2). Odorant receptor molecules are embedded in the cytoplasmic membrane of these 0.1-μm diameter cilia. The axonal processes of these bipolar neurons extend from the neuronal cell bodies to the lamina propria of the olfactory epithelium. Here they are bundled into fascicles of 50–100 axons, and wrapped by a Schwann cell sheath, constituting cranial nerve I. These bundles of unmyelinated axons extend several centimeters, cross the cribriform plate, and synapse with secondary olfactory neurons in the olfactory bulb.

Within the olfactory bulb, synapses between primary and secondary olfactory neurons occur in dense neuronal conglomerates termed glomeruli. It is here that the first processing of peripheral olfactory stimuli occurs. The number of primary olfactory neurons that synapse onto any single secondary olfactory neuron may be as high as 1,000 [4]. The olfactory bulb comprises five layers; namely, the glomerular layer, the external plexiform layer, the mitral layer, the internal plexiform layer, and the granular cell layer. Overall, however, it is simpler to think of the olfactory bulb as having one main input and one main output. The former is represented by cranial nerve I, the latter by the axons of the secondary olfactory neurons, or mitral cells. Mitral cells are second-order neurons that receive both sensory input at their glomerular dendritic processes from primary olfactory neurons, and inhibitory and regulatory input from supportive cells in the other layers of the olfactory bulb, along with other output neurons from regions in the brain such as the amygdala, hippocampus, and substantia nigra.

The axonal processes of the mitral cells, known as the olfactory tract, carry sensory information to the primary olfactory cortex, known as the piriform cortex. This lies within the medial aspect of the temporal lobes. Some fibers from the olfactory tract may cross to the contralateral olfactory cortex via the anterior commissure. Medial tract fibers synapse with interneurons of the anterior olfactory nucleus, whereas lateral tract fibers go on to synapse directly with cortical neurons. Neurons from this primary olfactory cortex project to the dorsomedial nucleus of the thalamus where the conscious sense of smell is aroused. Others project to the amygdala and limbic system where emotional or memory responses to specific odorants are elicited.

Transduction of organic odorant molecules into electrical impulses occurs at receptor sites on the olfactory cilia, after adsorption through the overlying mucous layer. The mucous film itself is an aqueous solution produced mainly by Bowman's glands in response to adrenergic stimulation [5]; the mucous milieu contains various glycosylated sugar molecules and its ion concentration is strictly controlled by sustentacular or supporting cells in the superficial layer of the olfactory epithelium. Sodium, calcium, and chloride concentrations are maintained by complex Ca^{2+}-gated chloride channels and cyclic AMP-gated Ca^{2+}channels to preserve Cl^- efflux-driven neuron depolarization [6, 7].

Volatile odorant molecules will possess intrinsic chemical properties by nature of their unique molecular structures. It has been demonstrated that study participants were able to reliably discriminate between aliphatic alcohols with or without double bonds, and were even able to discriminate based upon the position of the double bond within the overall alcohol structure [8].

Odorant molecules used for receptor characterization have typically been pyrazine-containing, such as the main odorant in bell pepper (2-isobuty-3-[3H]methoxypyrazine) [3], and are found to bind with affinities in the micromolar range. Other common pyrazine-containing odorants include dimethyl pyrazine found in meats, peanut butter, roasted nut, and cocoa. Odorants from the alcohol group include octenol found in plastics, lauryl alcohol in waxes, and α-terpineol from mint. Biochemical properties such as hydrophobicity, functional groups, and aromaticity will influence the concentration and partitioning of odorants across the air–aqueous transition in the mucous film overlying the olfactory receptors. Odorant binding proteins are members of the lipocalin protein family, having most notably β-barrel sequence motifs that form a ligand-binding site. They are expressed by nasal mucosal glands at millimolar levels and dimerize to form binding pockets for more hydrophobic odorant ligands, aiding their transport through the aqueous mucous film. Whether these binding proteins participate in the receptor–ligand binding interaction, or merely act as chaperones, is as yet unresolved [9].

The ciliated ends of the olfactory knobs contain odorant receptor molecules, which in the human, are specific for any one of about 400 active odorant receptor genes. Canines in contrast, express over 1,000 active odorant receptor genes [10]. Currently, it is believed that any single primary olfactory neuron expresses just one receptor phenotype in mammals. However, Duchamp-Viret et al. (1999) showed that the majority of individual rat olfactory receptor neurons tested could respond to five or more different odor stimuli, whereas only about 12% responded to just a single odorant stimulus [11]. Furthermore, it was shown that some olfactory neurons fired in response to certain odorants, but were inhibited by others when compared with basal or spontaneous firing rates. In kind, any one odorant binds to various receptor types with differing affinities, which was shown in mice by isolating single olfactory neurons that respond to a single odorant using Ca^{2+}-based imaging, and reverse cloning the receptor genes of responsive neurons [12]. This lays the basis, therefore, for a higher order discrimination of binding patterns, allowing detection of thousands of different odors. In addition to the hundreds of unique receptor phenotypes and their ability to respond to different odorants, there appears to be at least a rudimentary spatial arrangement of receptor phenotypes within the olfactory epithelium [13]. This organization helps the higher olfactory centers to decode the array of firing patterns from the "front lines" in the nasal vault. These odorant receptors are of the 7-transmembrane domain variety of chemical receptors, and are linked to the G-protein-mediated second messenger system. Adenylate cyclase generates cyclic AMP from ATP, leading ultimately to the opening of membrane-bound Na^+ and Ca^{2+} channels and depolarization of the neuronal cell membrane. Furthermore, Ca^{2+}-mediated Cl^- efflux from high intraneuronal Cl^- stores further depolarizes the cell membrane. Electrical patch clamp studies of olfactory neurons indicate that this subpopulation of primary neurons has relatively high stimulus thresholds compared with other sensory neurons [14]. This action potential is propagated down the long axonal process of these bipolar neurons until glutamate is released at the synapse in the glomerular layer of the olfactory bulb.

Odorant receptor gene probe studies indicate that mammalian primary olfactory neurons of the same phenotype synapse with mitral cells in the olfactory bulb in small and discrete subsets of glomeruli [15]. By segregating the relay of this primary information in this manner, further patterning of information occurs, generating greater complexity for the detection of very subtle differences among a wide array of odors. Binding of glutamate at the apical dendrites of mitral cells leads to their depolarization and subsequent release of glutamate from lateral dendrites onto neighboring granular cells. This interdendritic excitation of granular cells feeds back onto the mitral cell and decreases or prevents that mitral cell's firing rate via GABAergic "lateral inhibition." This constitutes a further level of processing beyond specific odorant–receptor interactions. By varying the action potential firing rate as the result of odorant-evoked potentials based on the concentration and molecular structure of the odorant, mitral and granular cells in the olfactory bulb further contribute to the specificity of odor detection [16].

Action potentials that are propagated along the mitral cell's axon proceed along a collection of mitral cell axons known as the olfactory tract. This white band lies within the olfactory sulcus on the inferior surface of the frontal cortex, eventually dividing into medial and lateral striae. The lateral stria proceeds along the lateral edge of the anterior perforated substance and then turns medially toward the uncus of the hippocampal gyrus. The medial stria turns medially and ends in the subcallosal gyrus.

Detection of the quality of an odorant is a complex combinatorial function of the human brain and involves the stimulation of numerous receptor types by a single odorant molecule. Indeed, it has been shown that different odorants containing the same key functional group known to stimulate mitral cells in the olfactory bulb are often described as having different qualities among different test participants. Furthermore, some odorants are described as having different qualities after simply varying their concentration [17]. Gottfried et al. (2006) showed that differing locations of activity within the olfactory bulb help discriminate quality indeterminate of the odorant's molecular structure [18]. Therefore, there remains much we do not fully understand about the olfactory system. However, it clearly provides for a very rich interaction with our environment.

Gustation

The gustatory system begins with the primary taste organ, the tongue. Special sensory afferent signals from the anterior two-thirds of the tongue are carried by the ipsilateral chorda tympani nerve, whereas those from the posterior third are carried via cranial nerve IX.

The tongue, like the rest of the oropharyngeal cavity, contains nonkeratinized stratified squamous epithelium. It is, however, specialized for chemoreception by way of its unique papillae, which house the primary structures of taste perception, the taste buds.

On the anterior tongue the fungiform papillae are located, typically numbering 200 and housing approximately 1,120 taste buds. The foliate papillae are located on the sides of the tongue, and number five to six per side, housing 1,280 taste buds innervated by the glossopharyngeal nerve. The circumvallate papillae

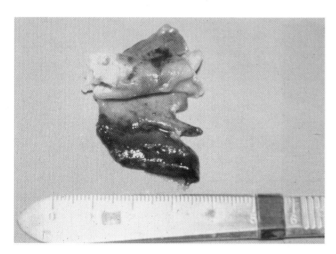

Fig. 7.1 The olfactory cleft, located within the nasal vault, encompasses the cribriform plate, the superior nasal septum, and the upper aspect of the superior turbinate, over which the olfactory epithelium is distributed. This is a cadaver specimen of the middle and superior turbinate, with the septal mucosa flipped superiorly. Notice how narrow is the olfactory cleft

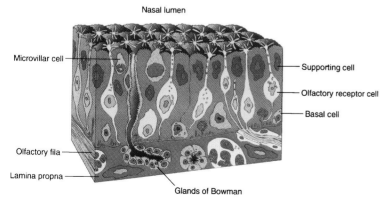

Fig. 7.2 A schematic diagram of the olfactory epithelium, including the bipolar neurons, supporting or sustentacular cells, microvillar cells, and basal cells. Note that each bipolar neuron sends a dendritic process to the surface, terminating in an olfactory knob that is directly exposed to the external environment. Odorant transduction occurs at receptors located on the cilia that line the olfactory knob [Adapted from Gray's Anatomy, 37th edition]

separate the oral tongue from the tongue base, and generally number eight to twelve, housing 2,500 taste buds, also innervated by the glossopharyngeal nerve.

Taste buds are also located on the soft palate, uvula, pharyngeal wall, epiglottis, and larynx, where they are grouped within the epithelium rather than on specialized papillae (Fig. 7.3).

Taste buds are collections of cells adapted for the transduction of chemical signals into electrical impulses. These impulses are projected to the brainstem by cranial nerves VII, IX, or X, depending on their location in the tongue or oropharyngeal mucosa. From the brainstem, these signals are projected to the thalamus, where they are integrated with olfactory signals arising from odorant molecules volatilized during mastication, to produce an overall sense of flavor. Flavor, therefore, more accurately refers to the conscious perception of the end result of chemical transduction from both the gustatory and olfactory systems, whereas taste more accurately describes those sensations arising from the stimulation of the taste bud receptors in the oropharynx and tongue.

Gustatory sensation is initiated when ingested substances are partially solubilized in saliva during mastication. The four basic taste sensations of sweet, sour, bitter, and salt combine to provide the overall signaling pattern that will ultimately contribute to the perceived flavor of the material. Each individual taste bud is composed of specialized receptor cells, termed dark or light cells, depending on the presence or absence of dense granules within them. Any one taste bud contains a combination of light cells, dark cells, and intermediate cells, all of which participate in signal transduction across the taste bud itself. These epithelial cells project microvilli into the apical portion of the taste bud, and these microvilli are arranged to form an apical pore structure that projects through the oral or tongue mucosa into the oropharyngeal cavity. Depending on the taste bud-dependent expression of surface receptors on the microvilli of these dark, light, or intermediate cells, the taste bud will transduce chemical signals of one of the basic taste sensations. As mentioned earlier, each taste bud is innervated at its base by branches of one or more afferent nerves; namely, cranial nerves VII, IX, or X.

The sensations of sour and salt are the result of the manipulation of ion channels at the apical surfaces of taste buds, leading to depolarization of the receptor cells within the taste bud and subsequent depolarization of their respective afferent nerves. More specifically, sour taste arises from acids contained in ingested material. The H+ ions interfere with apical K+ channels of sour-sensing taste bud receptor cells. The resultant blocking of K+ transport leads to depolarization of the cells and the afferent nerve. Salty taste arises when Na+ ions from NaCl in foods are liberated during mastication. Taste buds involved in the

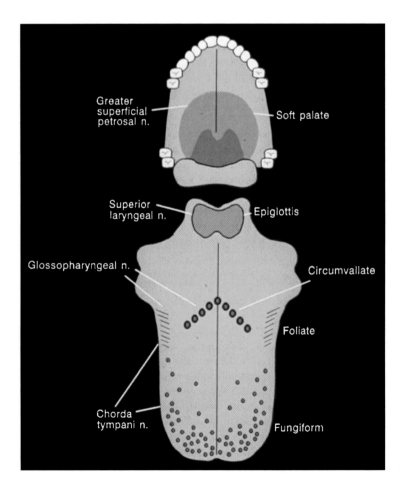

Fig. 7.3 Taste buds located over the tongue and palate

transduction of salty stimuli have simple Na+ ion channels on their surfaces, allowing the passive influx of Na+ across the cell membrane, thereby depolarizing the cell.

The sensations of sweet and bitter stimuli are less well-understood. Bitter-tasting compounds are not easily classified together or predicted from their chemical structures. Caffeine, a methylxanthine molecule, is a bitter tastant that enhances the flavor of coffee, tea, and chocolate. Flavonoids in numerous food sources such as citrus fruits, onions, legumes, and green tea, are of the polyphenol group. These and other bitter tastants enhance the overall taste perception of foods when mixed with other tastant molecules. Conversely, the ammonium cation, denatonium is the most bitter tastant and is added to household items such as nail polish, antifreeze, and paints to discourage human consumption. The ability of taste buds, located primarily in the circumvallate and foliate papillae, to respond to such a diverse array of molecules requires sophisticated second messenger systems such as cAMP and inositol triphosphate (IP_3). A taste-specific G-protein, α-gustducin, has been shown in knock-out murine models to amplify the response to bitter and sweet stimuli, but not salty or sour stimuli [19]. In addition, a family of human bitter-tastant receptor genes has been elucidated, known as the T2R family. These receptors are expressed solely by those taste receptors linked to the α-gustducin G-protein [20].

Sweet tastant receptors are similar to bitter receptors in that they work primarily through second messenger systems. It has been shown in rat circumvallate tissues that saccharin, an amide, and other noncarbohydrate sweeteners, trigger depolarization by eliciting IP_3 to increase intracellular Ca^{2+} concentrations, whereas sucrose and other carbohydrates promote the influx of extracellular Ca^{2+} via cAMP [21].

In addition to the four basic taste qualities with which we are all familiar, a fifth basic taste has been described and is now well accepted by the chemosensory community. First described by Kikunae Ikeda of Japan in 1907, it is a brothy, savory, or meaty taste known as umami (from the Japanese word for savory), and is attributed to amino acids found in protein-rich foods [22]. Ikeda isolated monosodium glutamate as being responsible for the strong taste of seaweed broth, which led to the production and distribution of monosodium glutamate as a flavor enhancer. A receptor for glutamate, mGluR4, was discovered in 1996, and two amino acid receptors, T1R1 and T1R3, were described in 2002 [23].

Conclusion

These special sensory systems utilize simple mechanisms of ion–ion-channel binding as well as the more complex ligand–receptor binding to effect changes within their specialized sensory cells. Despite the enormous progress made over the last 25 years in deciphering these mechanisms, questions remain as to how a relatively small number of receptors can respond to such a vast number of odorants and tastants. Future work will also focus on how the brain decodes all of these signals, and why we humans differ so greatly in our perception of particular scents and foods.

References

1. Seiden, A.M., ed., Taste and smell disorders. 1997, Thieme: New York.

2. Bignetti, E., et al., Purification and characterisation of an odorant-binding protein from cow nasal tissue. Eur J Biochem, 1985. 149(2): p. 227–31.

3. Pevsner, J., et al., Isolation and characterization of an olfactory receptor protein for odorant pyrazines. Proc Natl Acad Sci USA, 1985. 82(9): p. 3050–4.

4. Allison, A.C., The structure of the olfactory bulb and its relationship to the olfactory pathways in the rabbit and the rat. J Comp Neurol, 1953. 98(2): p. 309–53.

5. Chen, Y., et al., Patterns of adrenergic and peptidergic innervation in human olfactory mucosa: age-related trends. J Comp Neurol, 1993. 334(1): p. 104–16.

6. Kaneko, H., et al., Chloride accumulation in mammalian olfactory sensory neurons. J Neurosci, 2004. 24(36): p. 7931–8.

7. Restrepo, D., The ins and outs of intracellular chloride in olfactory receptor neurons. Neuron, 2005. 45(4): p. 481–2.

8. Laska, M., Olfactory discrimination ability for aliphatic c6 alcohols as a function of presence, position, and configuration of a double bond. Chem Senses, 2005. 30(9): p. 755–60.

9. Krieger, M.J. and K.G. Ross, Molecular evolutionary analyses of the odorant-binding protein gene Gp-9 in fire ants and other Solenopsis species. Mol Biol Evol, 2005. 22(10): p. 2090–103.

10. Olender, T., et al., The canine olfactory subgenome. Genomics, 2004. 83(3): p. 361–72.

11. Duchamp-Viret, P., M.A. Chaput, and A. Duchamp, Odor response properties of rat olfactory receptor neurons. Science, 1999. 284(5423): p. 2171–4.

12. Touhara, K., et al., Functional identification and reconstitution of an odorant receptor in single olfactory neurons. Proc Natl Acad Sci U S A, 1999. 96(7): p. 4040–5.

13. Nef, P., et al., Spatial pattern of receptor expression in the olfactory epithelium. Proc Natl Acad Sci U S A, 1992. 89(19): p. 8948–52.

14. Firestein, S. and F. Werblin, Odor-induced membrane currents in vertebrate-olfactory receptor neurons. Science, 1989. 244(4900): p. 79–82.

15. Ressler, K.J., S.L. Sullivan, and L.B. Buck, A zonal organization of odorant receptor gene expression in the olfactory epithelium. Cell, 1993. 73(3): p. 597–609.

16. Margrie, T.W., B. Sakmann, and N.N. Urban, Action potential propagation in mitral cell lateral dendrites is decremental and controls recurrent and lateral inhibition in the mammalian olfactory bulb. Proc Natl Acad Sci U S A, 2001. 98(1): p. 319–24.

17. Laing, D.G., et al., Relationship between molecular structure, concentration and odor qualities of oxygenated aliphatic molecules. Chem Senses, 2003. 28(1): p. 57–69.

18. Gottfried, J.A., J.S. Winston, and R.J. Dolan, Dissociable codes of odor quality and odorant structure in human piriform cortex. Neuron, 2006. 49(3): p. 467–79.

19. Wong, G.T., K.S. Gannon, and R.F. Margolskee, Transduction of bitter and sweet taste by gustducin. Nature, 1996. 381(6585): p. 796–800.

20. Adler, E., et al., A novel family of mammalian taste receptors. Cell, 2000. 100(6): p. 693–702.

21. Bernhardt, S.J., et al., Changes in IP3 and cytosolic Ca2+ in response to sugars and non-sugar sweeteners in transduction of sweet taste in the rat. J Physiol, 1996. 490 (Pt 2): p. 325–36.

22. McCabe, C. and E.T. Rolls, Umami: a delicious flavor formed by convergence of taste and olfactory pathways in the human brain. Eur J Neurosci, 2007. 25(6): p. 1855–64.

23. Palmer, R.K., The pharmacology and signaling of bitter, sweet, and umami taste sensing. Mol Interv, 2007. 7(2): p. 87–98.

7

Olfaction and Gustation: Implications of Viral, Toxic Exposure, Head Injury, Aging, and Drugs

8

Erin K. O'Brien and Donald A. Leopold

Core Messages

- Olfactory disorders are very common in the population with increasing prevalence with advanced age.
- The most common causes of olfactory loss include post-upper respiratory tract infection, post-trauma, nasal and paranasal sinus disease, age and neurodegenerative disease, toxins and medication, and idiopathic.
- Loss of flavor is a loss of retronasal olfaction, whereas loss of taste includes abnormalities in the detection of salty, sweet, bitter or sour flavors.
- Taste disorders can be caused by injury to the tongue mucosa and taste receptors, injury to the cranial nerves relaying taste information, aging, radiation, toxins, and medication.

Contents

Introduction

Chemosensory disorders are common in the population, with a variety of causes of both olfactory and taste dysfunction. The most common causes of olfactory disorders include chronic rhinosinusitis, post-upper respiratory infection (URI) loss, toxic exposure, head injury, aging, and drugs, while among the most common causes of taste disorders are trauma, medication, radiation, and poor oral and dental health, as well as nutritional deficiency. In this chapter, the causes of chemosensory loss will be reviewed and future research into olfactory and taste recovery will be discussed.

Olfactory Disorders

Olfactory receptor neurons (ORNs) are directly exposed to the external environment, leaving them susceptible to injury from inflammatory, infectious, and toxic agents. The prevalence of olfactory dysfunction is underappreciated, as random surveys find a prevalence of self-reported olfactory problems of 1.4% in adults, whereas random samples of adults show a prevalence of olfactory dysfunction of 19–20% (hyposmia 13–16% and anosmia 5–6%), and an increased prevalence with advanced age [2, 16, 25]. The causes of olfactory disorders vary, including most commonly loss after an upper respiratory infection/cold (post-URI) (26%), head trauma (18%), and nasal and paranasal disease (15%), although a large percentage had no identifiable cause (22% idiopathic) [5].

Post-URI Olfactory Loss

Loss of olfaction after viral URI is one of the most commonly reported causes of smell disorders. In studies of olfactory dysfunction, post-URI loss represented 18–42%, with a higher prevalence in women and in the elderly [5, 15, 40, 42]. Olfactory dysfunction during an upper respiratory infection is common, and is usually due to blockage of the airflow to the upper nasal olfactory receptors. Post-URI loss is a sudden neural process that occurs over a few hours or days during the URI. Hyposmia, anosmia or dysosmia may all develop after viral infection, with a higher incidence of hyposmia compared with other causes of olfactory dysfunction [42].

The mechanism of injury resulting in olfactory loss is not known. Biopsies of olfactory epithelium reveal patchy degeneration, suggesting a direct insult to the olfactory neuroepithelium. The olfactory epithelium is markedly disorganized, with few receptors in anosmic patients. In patients with hyposmia, receptors are present, but are reduced in number and distributed in patches [18]. Approximately 30% of patients with olfactory dysfunction after URI recover, but the likelihood of recovery decreases with the duration of olfactory loss, being almost non-existent after 3 years. The likelihood of recovery also decreases with increasing age. This may be due to the decrease in regeneration of olfactory receptor neurons and the decrease in size of the olfactory epithelium with aging [33]. In patients with post-URI olfactory loss, the volume of the olfactory bulb is smaller in patients with anosmia than in those with hyposmia, and is also less in patients with parosmia than in those without. The loss of volume of the olfactory bulb also correlates with the duration of olfactory loss [37].

The loss of olfactory neurons in response to viral exposure may be protective, in that viruses can cause encephalitis if allowed passage to central nervous tissue. While some strains of influenza A can enter the brain via the olfactory route, as demonstrated in mice, other strains of influenza A induce apoptosis in olfactory receptor neurons, and viral components are not detected in the olfactory bulb, as they are enclosed in apoptotic bodies and cleared by the olfactory neuroepithelium. Viral-induced neuronal apoptosis may therefore prevent CNS viral transmission. Herpes simplex virus antigen has been found in postmortem examination of the olfactory tract and cortex and limbic system. HSV causing herpes simplex encephalitis localizes to the frontotemporal region of the brain, supporting the hypothesis that HSV invades the CNS via an olfactory route [29]. While influenza A induces apoptosis in ORNs upon infection, inhibiting viral transmission into the CNS, HSV suppresses olfactory neuronal apoptosis, allowing viral neuroinvasion into the brain [28].

Post-URI olfactory loss may have a seasonal incidence, with a recent report finding peaks in March and May, corresponding to the high incidence of influenza in March and possibly due to other viruses, such as parainfluenza type III, in May [23]. The incidence of acute URIs exhibits a seasonal change, which may be due to the effects of cold temperature on respiratory defense. Cold temperatures lead to a decrease in mucociliary clearance within the nose and paranasal sinuses and a decrease in the phagocytic activity of macrophages, a nonspecific immune defense against viral infections [10].

Toxic Exposure

The prevalence of olfactory dysfunction due to toxic exposure is relatively low (2%), but the number of toxins associated with loss of olfaction is large [5]. The olfactory sensory neurons are directly exposed to the external environment, allow-

ing olfactory transduction, but leaving the neurons vulnerable to environmental toxins. Acute, high levels of toxin exposure may cause immediate olfactory damage, but chronic low-level exposure may also cause gradual olfactory loss. Injury to olfactory epithelium may damage the mature olfactory neurons, but spare the regenerating cells, allowing repopulation of the olfactory neuroepithelium. However, over time, the regeneration decreases with age; the lower rate of regeneration may in part be due to accumulation of toxic injury over a lifetime. The exposure to toxins may be from direct insult from the environment or from systemic toxic exposure. The olfactory epithelium contains high concentrations of xenobiotic enzymes within supporting cells and Bowman's gland cells. More than ten forms of cytochrome P450 mono-oxygenases have been identified in mammalian olfactory epithelium, as have other biotransformation enzymes. The role of these enzymes may be to detoxify inhaled substances, protecting the CNS from toxin exposure as part of the "nose–brain barrier," or may be necessary for processing odorants for receptor activation. In addition to the biotransformation of inhaled substances, enzymes such as P450 may also metabolize systemic compounds, protecting the olfactory tissue from circulating toxins. However, the activity of xenobiotic enzymes may result in the formation of toxic metabolites, resulting in damage to the nasal tissue and olfactory epithelium [6]. The levels of olfactory metabolic enzymes, which can exceed the levels seen in the liver, decrease with age, and this may impact on the effect of toxins on the olfactory epithelium with advancing age [12].

Specific toxins have been associated with olfactory loss in the classes of metals, gases, and solvents. Metal-binding molecules are present in abundance in the olfactory bulb, but gases and solvents, unlike metals, can cross the blood–brain barrier. Metal in the form of dust or fumes can be toxic to the olfactory system. Cadmium, used in the production of batteries, semiconductors, and electroplating, is the most well-known metal linked to olfactory dysfunction [44]. Chromium, like cadmium, is often used with nickel in industrial manufacturing, such as steel production. One study of workers in a chromate-producing factory found that over half had increased olfactory thresholds [46]. Tobacco exposure in current smokers is associated with olfactory dysfunction, and in mice, tobacco exposure led to an increase in apoptosis of olfactory neurons [11, 45].

Head Injury

Like post-URI dysosmia, post-traumatic loss is characterized by a sudden decrease in olfactory ability. Olfactory loss after trauma may result from injury anywhere along the olfactory tract, beginning with stretching or shearing of the olfactory fibers at the cribriform plate, injury to the frontal lobes with or without olfactory bulb damage, or central brain trauma with damage to the temporal cortex. Olfactory deficits secondary to head trauma are more severe than those due to postviral causes and are more likely to include dysosmia [5]. A decrease in both retronasal and orthonasal olfactory function, as well as parosmia, is associated with a reduction in olfactory bulb volume after traumatic head injury. The retronasal olfactory dysfunction is more strongly correlated with a reduction in olfactory bulb volume, and both retronasal dysfunction and parosmia are associated with the presence of cerebral damage [36]. The olfactory epithelium in mice that have undergone removal of the olfactory bulb (bulbectomy) reveals apoptosis of olfactory neurons [21]. As reviewed by Cowan and Roskams, mature olfactory receptor neurons undergo retrograde degeneration after both bulbectomy and olfactory nerve axotomy. Regenerating ORNs have an increased rate of cell death early in development, corresponding to the stage at which they would have reached the bulb, indicating that the bulb likely provides trophic support to maintain the ORN and prevent apoptosis. After axotomy, the rate of ORN degeneration varies, depending on the site of injury, with a delay of degeneration with transection on the dorsal surface of the bulb versus the cribriform plate. After the initial degeneration, the regenerating nerve has the chance to reconnect to the bulb, and therefore does not undergo the same increased rate of apoptosis of new neurons as seen after bulbectomy [4].

Examination of olfactory epithelium in patients with post-traumatic olfactory dysfunction reflects the changes seen in animal models after bulbectomy or axotomy. Histopathology reveals disorganization of the epithelial orientation with thickened epithelium and abnormal dispersement of nuclei, axon proliferation and diminished number of mature olfactory receptors, with those present (the immature neurons) lacking projecting olfactory cilia. This relatively larger number of immature olfactory neurons suggests that their axons are unable to connect to the olfactory bulb, a process required to become mature. This supports the theory of shearing injury or blockage of the olfactory filia at the cribriform plate as the mechanism of injury [18].

Recovery of olfactory function after head trauma is much less likely than recovery after URI, ranging from 10 to 36%, but recovery can occur several years after the trauma [9, 33]. One patient with dysosmia that developed months after head injury had resection of the olfactory bulbs and tracts with findings of an atrophic bulb, a reduced number of intact glomeruli (synapses between axons of olfactory receptor neurons and second-order neurons in the olfactory bulb), and marked gliosis. There was evidence of intact connections between the olfactory mucosa and olfactory bulb, suggesting incomplete regeneration, resulting in dysosmia [19].

Olfactory scores are inversely correlated with the severity of the head injury, although testing of olfactory discrimination is unable to differentiate between central and peripheral damage, such as olfactory nerve shearing [14]. In a study of olfactory function after closed head injuries in children, 3 out of 36 children with hyposmia had lower Glasgow Coma Scale scores and more significant skull/facial fractures and intracranial bleeds [38]. Frontal impact is associated with less dysfunction than back or side impact [9]. Also, patients with facial fractures and olfactory dysfunction were more likely to have sustained severe injuries like nasozygomatic Le Fort fractures, fronto-orbital fractures or pure Le Fort fractures [34].

Magnetic resonance imaging (MRI) can detect injury to the olfactory tract, both acutely and at follow-up. Acute injury may include hyperintensity on T1-weighted images consistent with hemorrhagic contusion and on T2-weighted images consistent with edema of the orbital frontal regions, specifically the gyrus recti and olfactory bulbs and tracts. Later findings may include hyperintensity on T2-weighted images from gliosis and loss of brain substance or atrophy, including the olfactory bulb and tracts [48]. The most common sites of injury in patients with post-traumatic olfactory dysfunction as assessed by MRI are the olfactory bulbs and tracts and inferior frontal lobes. The volume of the olfactory bulbs and tracts is smaller in patients with anosmia than in those with hyposmia, indicating that neural loss occurs at the level of the bulbs or more proximally [51, 52].

Aging

Olfactory impairment can be as high as 70% among elderly people, although self-reporting can be significantly underestimated, with even less accurate self-reporting with increased age [30]. Increased olfactory neuron death with a reduced level of regeneration results in age-related olfactory dysfunction. Medication, cumulative effects of infections, toxic exposure, head trauma or nutritional deficits may all exacerbate olfactory impairment. Examination of the olfactory epithelium (OE) of mice of advanced age reveals an increase in apoptosis of olfactory neurons [21]. Aged OE shows an increase in oxidative stress-related pathways. The OE area decreases with age, which may be caused by an altered response to injury [32]. The OE is replaced with islets of metaplastic respiratory epithelium. Adrenergic innervation within the mucosa decreases with age, as do calcium binding protein elements, making these neurons vulnerable to calcium-mediated cell death. Within the olfactory bulb, the number of mitral cells decreases with age, as does the thickness of the layers of the bulb [24].

Olfactory dysfunction occurs with the onset of Alzheimer's disease (AD), with odor identification altered early and impaired odor detection occurring late in the disease, and impaired olfaction is a marker for cognitive decline [24]. Neurofibrillary tangles and neuritic plaques appear in the olfactory bulb, anterior olfactory nucleus, and prepiriform cortex in patients with AD. Odor threshold scores decline 1 year prior to the diagnosis of AD. Apolipoprotein E type ε4 (APOE4) allele is associated with late onset familial and sporadic AD, and normal, nondemented elderly adults with the APOE4 allele showed a significant decline in performance on odor identification over a 4-year period, but not on odor threshold or dementia rating. Therefore, odor identification may decline prior to other measures of dementia. In addition, individuals with anosmia were at twice the risk of cognitive decline over a 2-year period than those with normosmia. Also, persons with mild cognitive impairment with both poor odor identification and unawareness of smell impairment showed increased incidence of AD [3].

Parkinson's disease (PD) is a neurodegenerative disorder characterized by motor symptoms, but also by damaged odor detection and odor identification. Smell identification tests may be used as an aid in the diagnosis of PD and in differentiating PD from other parkinsonian syndromes. Patients with progressive supranuclear palsy and corticobasal degeneration present with olfaction that is normal or markedly superior to that of patients with PD. Patients with multiple system atrophy do present with odor identification problems, but to a lesser degree than PD patients. Lewy body formation in PD begins first in the olfactory bulb and progresses to other cortical areas [24].

Drugs

Although it is suspected that drugs or drug–drug interactions can have an effect on olfactory ability, it is extremely difficult to prove, because it is usually an uncommon side effect, and multiple other factors (like post-URI losses or aging) are also possible. In one study, patients complaining of dysosmia were more likely to be taking antihypertensives or anxiolytics than control patients [5]. Rarely is a patient's olfactory ability changed with a change in the drugs they are consuming.

One medication that has been implicated in causing anosmia is intranasal zinc gluconate, as used as a treatment for the common cold. Reviewed by Jafek et al. in 2004, zinc application is toxic to olfactory epithelium, as evidenced by resulting anosmia in patients treated with zinc intranasally in failed attempts to prevent polio in the 1930s and in animal experiments. Jafek et al. reported 10 patients with immediate, severe burning of the nose followed by anosmia or severe hyposmia with parosmia after the use of intranasal zinc gluconate [17]. Reports of additional cases also describe the use of intranasal zinc gluconate followed by immediate burning sensation with anosmia developing within a few days, which differs from the typical presentation of post-URI olfactory loss [1].

Future Research

Apoptosis plays a role in the loss of olfactory neurons in response to stressors such as aging, trauma and toxin exposure. Therapeutics aimed at modulation of the apoptotic pathways may be a potential target for pharmacologic intervention for olfactory deficits [21, 45]. Minocycline prevented neuronal apoptosis following olfactory bulbectomy in mice, and is currently undergoing human trials for neurological disorders associated with apoptosis [20].

Retinoic acid is an essential factor in the regeneration of olfactory receptor neurons, and RA administration after olfactory system damage stimulates an immune response and yields a more rapid recovery of olfactory-guided behavior in mice [32]. Preliminary studies in humans, however, have shown no benefit from retinoic acid administration.

Gustatory Disorders

Severe taste losses are far less prevalent than severe olfactory losses. Gustatory disorders include partial loss of taste (hypogeusia), complete loss (ageusia) or altered sensation of taste (dysgeusia). In a large study of patients presenting to a chemosensory center for abnormal smell or taste perception, 20% complained of olfactory dysfunction alone, 58% complained of olfactory and gustatory dysfunction, and 9% complained of taste loss only. On testing, however, in patients who complained of smell and taste dysfunction, only 4% had a demonstrable gustatory deficit. Of patients complaining of only a taste deficit, those with an objective sensory loss were three times more likely to show olfactory dysfunction than gustatory dysfunction [5]. Olfactory dysfunction results in a complaint of loss of taste due to the role of olfaction in appreciating flavor in food and beverages. True gustatory dysfunction reflects a disorder in the ability to detect sweet, sour, bitter, salt or umami (monosodium glutamate).

One difference in the prevalence of taste versus smell disorders may be the anatomic difference in taste function. Although the tongue is the primary receptor area, bilateral innervation by three cranial nerves (VII, IX, and X) provides gustatory sensation with a large number of taste receptors throughout the tongue, palate, larynx, pharynx, and epiglottis. Taste disorders can be divided into interference with access to the primary receptor by stimulant, signal transduction, and central interpretation [31].

Injury Along the Taste Pathway

Patients presenting with a gustatory deficit may have a history of middle ear or oral surgery resulting in damage to the chorda tympani branch of the facial nerve (VII), with the injury occurring from its course through the middle ear, between the medial and lateral pterygoid muscles, or within the lingual nerve. In a large study of patients with olfactory and taste disorders, of the few cases of documented hypogeusia or ageusia, more than 30% were iatrogenic in origin [5].

Aging

Taste dysfunction in the elderly may be due to systemic diseases, their treatment, and medication effects that occur more commonly in elderly people rather than losses secondary to normal aging. Unlike anatomic changes of the olfactory system with advanced age, studies of anatomic changes of taste buds due to aging have been less impressive. Poor oral hygiene, associated with normal aging or disease processes, can affect gustatory function. Dental caries with resultant tooth loss and use of prostheses can interfere with taste function as well as retronasal olfactory function and flavor perception. Xerostomia associated with systemic diseases and treatments more commonly seen in the elderly can also affect gustatory function by decreasing the saliva necessary for molecules to reach taste receptor cells [39].

Irradiation

Taste dysfunction is a common complaint of patients undergoing radiation therapy for head and neck cancer. The causes of taste disorders include disappearance of taste buds and dysfunction of the salivary glands [49]. Hypogeusia, ageusia or dysgeusia often occur in patients receiving external beam radiation for cancers of the head and neck, beginning at a dose of 20 Gy.

In one study on taste thresholds, bitter and salty qualities show the earliest and greatest impairment and sweet quality the least. For doses over 60 Gy, over 90% of patients have a relative taste loss. A partial improvement may begin 1–2 months after treatment ends with recovery at 4 months, although some studies have shown residual impairment more than a year after treatment [35].

Another recent study found a significant decline in the sensitivity of taste for all four basic tastes and umami at 5 weeks after the start of radiation therapy, and significant improvement by week 11. There was no difference in taste sensitivity between those with and without chemotherapy.

In experiments with rats irradiated with 15 Gy in a single fraction, a decline in the number of taste buds and appearance of the papilla was noted on the fourth day after irradiation. By the sixth day, the number of taste-bud cells diminished almost completely, but began to re-emerge and returned to about 80% of the normal level by the 19th day [49].

In a comparison of radiation therapy fields containing the tip of the tongue and the posterior part of the tongue versus only the posterior tongue, only the group with radiation to the tip of the tongue had a significant difference in taste threshold for all four basic tastes, beginning at week 3 of therapy, even with low radiation doses. Recovery of taste was noted 4 months after completing radiation therapy [50].

Treatment of thyroid cancer with radioactive iodine (^{131}I) is associated with taste disturbances as well as xerostomia. Taste alterations can occur immediately after ^{131}I ingestion, and are reported as a side effect of the treatment in 10–26% of patients [22, 27]. One explanation may be radiation-induced sialadenitis of von Ebner glands, located near the circumvallate papilla. Serous saliva from these glands functions to carry food chemicals to taste buds, and loss of this salivary transport may inhibit the ability of chemicals to activate taste buds [26].

Medication

Medication can interfere with taste function on several different levels. Drugs can limit access of tastants to receptors by altering saliva either by reducing the amount of saliva or by changing the ionic content of the saliva, by interacting with the receptor as an agonist or antagonist, disturbing neural propagation by affecting calcium flux, affecting neurotransmitter function, or affecting higher-order neural pathways. Anticholinergics and antidepressants reduce salivary output, causing xerostomia and interfering with the access of molecules to taste receptor cells. The secretion of drugs into the saliva can also affect taste sensation by producing an adverse taste or interfering with normal taste transduction. While hundreds of drugs list taste or smell dysfunction as side effects in a minority of patients, several categories of drugs have documented interference with chemosensory function. Many antimicrobials when taken systemically can be found in salivary secretions and can affect the taste of certain salts. The antifungal terbinafine (Lamisil) can cause deficits in taste in

salty, bitter, sweet, and sour substances, which usually returns after cessation of the drug, but taste difficulties have reportedly persisted long after discontinuance [8]. The elderly and those with a low body mass index were more likely to report taste loss with the use of terbinafine [41]. A number of antivirals also cause taste disorders, either by adversely modifying the taste of other substances or by inducing an unpleasant taste.

Among antihypertensive and antihyperlipidemic medications, over a third list taste and smell dysfunction as a side effect. A majority of angiotensin-converting enzyme (ACE) inhibitors are associated with chemosensory problems, including ageusia, metallic or sweet taste, or taste disturbance or distortion. Taste alterations due to ACE inhibitors may disappear over time while using the drug and usually reverse with discontinuance. Calcium channel blockers have also been associated with taste disturbances by case reports. Diuretics can affect salt taste sensitivity by blocking ion channels on taste buds. Several antihyperlipidemic agents list taste disturbances as a side effect. In patients presenting with dysgeusia, the use of antidepressants or anxiolytics was more common than in patients with no complaints of taste disorder [5].

Chemotherapeutic drugs can affect taste perception by several mechanisms. A bitter taste may be appreciated during intravenous infusion, and a majority of patients on cisplatin reported a metallic taste lasting hours to weeks [47]. As reviewed by Doty and Bromley, the drugs may affect the sensory receptors or pass into the saliva, resulting in a specific taste. In addition to chemotherapeutics, immunosuppressants and corticosteroids can induce candidal overgrowth, altering taste perception. Psychotropic agents, including antidepressants, can affect the intensity of tastants or cause xerostomia [7].

Zinc Deficiency

Heavy metals such as zinc are involved in the physiology of taste function, including the function of alkaline phosphatase in taste buds and the regulation of the pores of the taste buds, which allow entry of stimuli into the taste buds. Patients made experimentally zinc-deficient and in those with diseases causing zinc deficiency had a diminished sense of taste. Hypogeusia in some patients with chronic disease was reversed by the administration of zinc. Zinc sulfate has also improved the symptoms in cancer patients with idiopathic hypogeusia and dysgeusia [35]. In a study of patients with taste impairment, zinc deficiency as measured by serum zinc concentration was found in a minority of patients (7 versus 19). However, zinc nutrition, as measured by the activity of angiotensin-converting enzyme (ACE), a zinc-dependent enzyme, was significantly lower in all patients with taste impairment versus healthy participants, regardless of serum zinc level. As patients with a normal serum zinc level and taste impairment had similar levels of zinc dietary intake to healthy individuals, the cause of the taste impairment was likely malabsorption of dietary zinc [43]. In patients taking ACE inhibitors, serum zinc levels did not decrease, but intracellular levels of zinc in monocytes decreased significantly, further indicating that serum zinc levels do not accurately reflect tissue zinc content. The reduction in the intracellular zinc level may explain the taste disturbances frequently seen as a side effect of ACE inhibitors [13].

Conclusion

When evaluating patients with smell and/or taste complaints, it is very important to listen to their concerns, and gather a thorough history. This, along with an appropriate examination and possibly imaging will give the best determination of the cause of the problem. Unfortunately, except for the conductive losses, there is no proven therapy to reverse most chemosensory losses. Symptoms of distorted smell or taste perception can often be a more disturbing problem for patients than losses. Fortunately, these distortions are usually self-limited in duration.

Continued research into the molecular mechanisms of smell and taste function will likely be the best source to understand how these systems work, and how patients with them can be best helped.

Take-Home Pearls

- Up to 20% of the population may have a diminished (hyposmia) or absent (anosmia) sense of smell, although many patients may not recognize the deficit. The prevalence increases to more than 50% by 65 years of age.
- Olfactory mucosa and olfactory receptor neurons are capable of regeneration, but this decreases with age, and the olfactory epithelium is replaced by respiratory epithelium. This regenerative process may also decrease after viral or toxin exposure.
- Loss of sense of smell is the first presenting sign of Alzheimer's disease and Parkinson's disease, presenting before cognitive deficits or motor symptoms respectively.
- Patients with olfactory disorders must have functioning smoke detectors and natural gas detectors if appropriate, due to safety concerns.

References

1. Alexander TH, Davidson TM (2006) Intranasal zinc and anosmia: The zinc-induced anosmia syndrome. Laryngoscope 116:217–220
2. Bramerson A, Johansson L, Ek L, et al (2004) Prevalence of olfactory dysfunction: The Skovde population-based study. Laryngoscope 114:733–737
3. Calhoun-Haney R, Murphy C (2005) Apolipoprotein epsilon4 is associated with more rapid decline in odor identification than in odor threshold or dementia rating scale scores. Brain Cogn 58:178–182
4. Cowan CM, Roskams AJ (2002) Apoptosis in the mature and developing olfactory neuroepithelium. Microsc Res Tech 58:204–215
5. Deems DA, Doty RL, Settle RG, et al (1991) Smell and taste disorders, a study of 750 patients from the University of Pennsylvania Smell and Taste Center. Arch Otolaryngol Head Neck Surg 117:519–528
6. Doty RL (2003) Handbook of olfaction and gustation. 2nd ed. New York: Marcel Dekker
7. Doty RL, Bromley SM (2004) Effects of drugs on olfaction and taste. Otolaryngol Clin North Am 37:1229–1254
8. Doty RL, Haxel BR (2005) Objective assessment of terbinafine-induced taste loss. Laryngoscope 115:2035–2037
9. Doty RL, Yousem DM, Pham LT, et al (1997) Olfactory dysfunction in patients with head trauma. Arch Neurol 54:1131–1140
10. Eccles R (2002) An explanation for the seasonality of acute upper respiratory tract viral infections. Acta Otolaryngol 122:183–191
11. Frye RE, Schwartz BS, Doty RL (1990) Dose-related effects of cigarette smoking on olfactory function. JAMA 263:1233–1236
12. Genter MB (2004) Update on olfactory mucosal metabolic enzymes: Age-related changes and n-acetyltransferase activities. J Biochem Mol Toxicol 18:239–244
13. Golik A, Zaidenstein R, Dishi V, et al (1998) Effects of captopril and enalapril on zinc metabolism in hypertensive patients. J Am Coll Nutr 17:75–78
14. Green P, Rohling ML, Iverson GL, et al (2003) Relationships between olfactory discrimination and head injury severity. Brain Inj 17:479–496
15. Harris R, Davidson TM, Murphy C, et al (2006) Clinical evaluation and symptoms of chemosensory impairment: One thousand consecutive cases from the nasal dysfunction clinic in San Diego. Am J Rhinol 20:101–108
16. Hoffman HJ, Ishii EK, MacTurk RH (1998) Age-related changes in the prevalence of smell/taste problems among the United States adult population. Results of the 1994 disability supplement to the National Health Interview Survey (NHIS). Ann N Y Acad Sci 855:716–722
17. Jafek BW, Linschoten MR, Murrow BW (2004) Anosmia after intranasal zinc gluconate use. Am J Rhinol 18:137–141
18. Jafek BW, Murrow B, Michaels R, et al (2002) Biopsies of human olfactory epithelium. Chem Senses 27:623–628
19. Kern RC, Quinn B, Rosseau G, et al (2000) Post-traumatic olfactory dysfunction. Laryngoscope 110:2106–2109
20. Kern RC, Conley DB, Haines GK, 3rd, et al (2004) Treatment of olfactory dysfunction, II: Studies with minocycline. Laryngoscope 114:2200–2204
21. Kern RC, Conley DB, Haines GK, 3rd, et al (2004) Pathology of the olfactory mucosa: Implications for the treatment of olfactory dysfunction. Laryngoscope 114:279–285
22. Kita T, Yokoyama K, Higuchi T, et al (2004) Multifactorial analysis on the short-term side effects occurring within 96 hours after radioiodine-131 therapy for differentiated thyroid carcinoma. Ann Nucl Med 18:345–349
23. Konstantinidis I, Haehner A, Frasnelli J, et al (2006) Post-infectious olfactory dysfunction exhibits a seasonal pattern. Rhinology 44:135–139
24. Kovacs T (2004) Mechanisms of olfactory dysfunction in aging and neurodegenerative disorders. Ageing Res Rev 3:215–232
25. Landis BN, Konnerth CG, Hummel T (2004) A study on the frequency of olfactory dysfunction. Laryngoscope 114:1764–1769

26. Mandel SJ, Mandel L (2003) Radioactive iodine and the salivary glands. Thyroid 13:265–271

27. Mendoza A, Shaffer B, Karakla D, et al (2004) Quality of life with well-differentiated thyroid cancer: Treatment toxicities and their reduction. Thyroid 14:133–140

28. Mori I, Nishiyama Y, Yokochi T, et al (2004) Virus-induced neuronal apoptosis as pathological and protective responses of the host. Rev Med Virol 14:209–216

29. Mori I, Nishiyama Y, Yokochi T, et al (2005) Olfactory transmission of neurotropic viruses. J Neurovirol 11:129–137

30. Murphy C, Schubert CR, Cruickshanks KJ, et al (2002) Prevalence of olfactory impairment in older adults. JAMA 288:2307–2312

31. Pribitkin E, Rosenthal MD, Cowart BJ (2003) Prevalence and causes of severe taste loss in a chemosensory clinic population. Ann Otol Rhinol Laryngol 112:971–978

32. Rawson NE, Lamantia AS (2007) A speculative essay on retinoic acid regulation of neural stem cells in the developing and aging olfactory system. Exp Gerontol 42:46–53

33. Reden J, Mueller A, Mueller C, et al (2006) Recovery of olfactory function following closed head injury or infections of the upper respiratory tract. Arch Otolaryngol Head Neck Surg 132:265–269

34. Renzi G, Carboni A, Gasparini G, et al (2002) Taste and olfactory disturbances after upper and middle third facial fractures: A preliminary study. Ann Plast Surg 48:355–358

35. Ripamonti C, Zecca E, Brunelli C, et al (1998) A randomized, controlled clinical trial to evaluate the effects of zinc sulfate on cancer patients with taste alterations caused by head and neck irradiation. Cancer 82:1938–1945

36. Rombaux P, Mouraux A, Bertrand B, et al (2006) Retronasal and orthonasal olfactory function in relation to olfactory bulb volume in patients with posttraumatic loss of smell. Laryngoscope 116:901–905

37. Rombaux P, Mouraux A, Bertrand B, et al (2006) Olfactory function and olfactory bulb volume in patients with postinfectious olfactory loss. Laryngoscope 116:436–439

38. Sandford AA, Davidson TM, Herrera N, et al (2006) Olfactory dysfunction: A sequela of pediatric blunt head trauma. Int J Pediatr Otorhinolaryngol 70:1015–1025

39. Seiberling KA, Conley DB (2004) Aging and olfactory and taste function. Otolaryngol Clin North Am 37:1209–1228, vii

40. Seiden AM (2004) Postviral olfactory loss. Otolaryngol Clin North Am 37:1159–1166

41. Stricker BH, Van Riemsdijk MM, Sturkenboom MC, et al (1996) Taste loss to terbinafine: A case-control study of potential risk factors. Br J Clin Pharmacol 42:313–318

42. Temmel AFP, Quint C, Schickinger-Fischer B, et al (2002) Characteristics of olfactory disorders in relation to major causes of olfactory loss. Arch Otolaryngol Head Neck Surg 128:635–641

43. Ueda C, Takaoka T, Sarukura N, et al (2006) Zinc nutrition in healthy subjects and patients with taste impairment from the view point of zinc ingestion, serum zinc concentration and angiotensin converting enzyme activity. Auris Nasus Larynx 33:283–288

44. Upadhyay UD, Holbrook EH (2004) Olfactory loss as a result of toxic exposure. Otolaryngol Clin North Am 37:1185–1207

45. Vent J, Robinson AM, Gentry-Nielsen MJ, et al (2004) Pathology of the olfactory epithelium: Smoking and ethanol exposure. Laryngoscope 114:1383–1388

46. Watanabe S, Fukuchi Y (1981) Occupational impairment of the olfactory sense of chromate producing workers (author's translation). Sangyo Igaku 23:606–611

47. Wickham RS, Rehwaldt M, Kefer C, et al (1999) Taste changes experienced by patients receiving chemotherapy. Oncol Nurs Forum 26:697–706

48. Wise JB, Moonis G, Mirza N (2006) Magnetic resonance imaging findings in the evaluation of traumatic anosmia. Ann Otol Rhinol Laryngol 115:124–127

49. Yamashita H, Nakagawa K, Tago M, et al (2006) Taste dysfunction in patients receiving radiotherapy. Head Neck 28:508–516

50. Yamashita H, Nakagawa K, Nakamura N, et al (2006) Relation between acute and late irradiation impairment of four basic tastes and irradiated tongue volume in patients with head-and-neck cancer. Int J Radiat Oncol Biol Phys 66(5):1422–1429

51. Yousem DM, Geckle RJ, Bilker WB, et al (1996) Posttraumatic olfactory dysfunction: MR and clinical evaluation. AJNR Am J Neuroradiol 17:1171–1179

52. Yousem DM, Geckle RJ, Bilker WB, et al (1999) Posttraumatic smell loss: Relationship of psychophysical tests and volumes of the olfactory bulbs and tracts and the temporal lobes. Acad Radiol 6:264–272

Chapter 9

The Electronic Nose in Rhinology

Erica R. Thaler and C. William Hanson

9

Core Messages

- The electronic nose (e-nose) is a new technology with many potential applications in rhinology.
- The e-nose is being adapted to provide diagnostic tools for use in rhinology, including cerebrospinal fluid analysis, identification of specific bacteria and bacterial biofilms, and the diagnosis of sinusitis.
- The e-nose is a novel means of breath and secretion analysis that is a potential wave of the future in rhinology.

Contents

Introduction

New technologies abound in 21st century medicine. While there is much to gain from technologic advances in medicine, many advances are costly and target small populations of patients. It is increasingly challenging to find high-impact, low-cost technologies that play have a significant role in the practice of medicine. The electronic nose may be one such technology. This chapter is devoted to the electronic nose and its relevance in medicine, with specific emphasis on research that has involved the field of rhinology.

Over the past decade and a half, chemists have developed a set of technologies widely known as "electronic noses". These technologies are operationally quite similar to the human nose, replicating human olfaction in many facets. The archetypal electronic nose, or e-nose, has an array of nonspecific chemical sensors that may bind to volatile molecules that overlie a substrate. The substrate may be anything that gives off molecules from its surface in vaporized form, such as rotting meat, perfume, or bacteria. The chemical characteristics of the vaporized molecules determine a response pattern by the e-nose: the molecules bind variably to a variety of sensors, and these sensors then react is some measurable way. The measured response is usually represented mathematically as a point in multi-dimensional space, where the number of sensors that respond to the molecules determines the number of dimensions. This point in space is the particular identifier of the vaporized molecules. When samples cluster together in a particular point in space, the e-nose can be trained to recognize the "smell" and identify unknowns having the same odor. Pattern recognition algorithms, such as neural networks and nearest neighbor searches, are trained on "known" samples and then used to identify "unknowns."

While gas chromatographic and mass spectrometric techniques have traditionally been used for the identification of unknown molecular species, for a variety of reasons these devices are not suited for clinical use. E-noses, however, have the advantage of being small, portable, relatively inexpensive and results can be acquired at the time of evaluation by the clinician. These features lend themselves to ease of clinical use. Therefore, it has been widely recognized that medical applications of e-nose technology have the potential to be quite useful. The authors have investigated a wide variety of ways in which the e-nose may have clinical utility. All of these investigations have used the e-nose as a diagnostic tool in areas where current technology or practice leaves gaps in our diagnostic acumen.

In the studies reviewed in this chapter, an e-nose was used consisting of an array of 32 carbon black/polymer composite sensors (Smiths Detection, Pasadena, CA, USA). Carbon black particles are dispersed through a polymer "grid," creating potential conducting pathways [1]. As the polymer interacts with the headspace, molecular odorants diffuse into the polymer causing it to swell, and disrupting the carbon black conducting pathways to a variable degree thereby altering the resistance of the sensor. The specificity of a sensor relates to the specific polymer used in the sensor and the characteristics of the chemicals with which it interacts (for example, polar versus nonpolar, or particular functional groups). The e-nose has a sensitivity down to 0.1% of saturated vapor pressure.

A number of other technologies are used in various electronic noses, including conducting polymer sensors (i.e., polymers that are intrinsically conducting), acoustic sensors, metal oxide sensors and colorimetric sensors. Each technology has its own idiosyncrasies. The conducting polymers, for example, are very sensitive to water vapor, the acoustic wave sensors are not portable, etc. [2].

The data that were garnered by the e-nose in the studies discussed below were subjected to a variety of mathematical models. Standard statistical analysis is not applicable because of the multi-dimensionality of the data. One common methodology is the use of Principle Components Analysis (PCA). PCA uses vectors to evaluate multidimensional data and is a technique for reducing dimensionality while preserving important data. The vectors are calculated to capture meaningful variance among sensor output data. Results can be plotted in one, two or three dimensions to identify differences among odors studied.

Identification of CSF Rhinorrhea

When originally conceptualizing the role of an e-nose in medicine, the authors were faced with several questions. First, would an e-nose be able to react with molecules vaporized from secretions or other samples obtained from the human body? Second, if an e-nose could distinguish such molecules, what exactly were they and why were they characteristic of the disease state? Finally, would the e-nose's ability to distinguish these molecules give it relevance in clinical medicine? As will be evident, these questions have been answered only in part to date.

An initial, compelling question, which was relatively easy to investigate, was to see whether an e-nose could distinguish between various secretions that came from the human nose [3]. It is of clinical interest to be able to determine the character of secretions from the nose, specifically when there is concern about the potential for cerebrospinal fluid (CSF) rhinorrhea. Current practice involves the testing of suspect rhinorrhea for beta-2 transferrin. This test takes up to 24 h to perform, is unavailable in many institutions, and requires at least 0.5 cc for accuracy. For the patient, it is often desirable to have an immediate answer to the question of identification of the fluid.

The following experiments were undertaken. CSF and serum samples were tested in matched sets from a number of patients using between 0.1 and 0.5 cc of fluid. The specimens were measured by micropipette, placed and sealed in headspace-generating vials, and incubated for 30 min on a dry heater block. Controls of saline were used. Alternatively, the specimens were

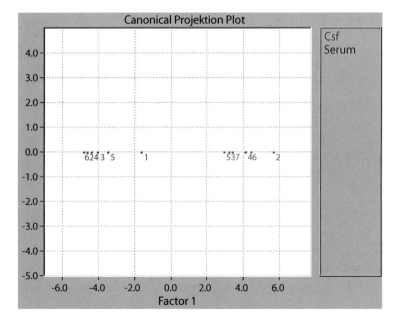

Fig. 9.1 Canonical projection plot of CSF (*red*) and serum (*blue*) samples showing discrimination using 0.5 cc of fluid. The x-axis is the factor or principal component vector demonstrating the greatest variance in data. There is one dimension because only two classes of data are analyzed. Mahalanobis distance = 7.9 (Reprinted with permission from [5], publisher Lippincott Williams and Wilkins)

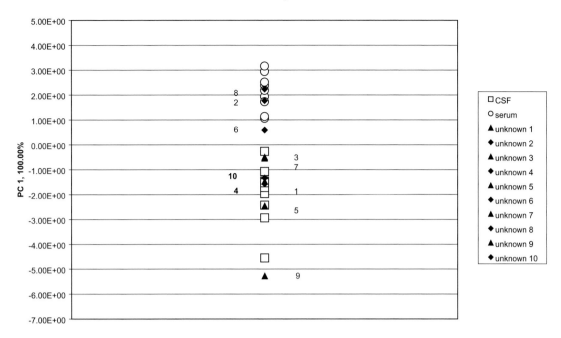

Score Plot in Canonical Space with Mean Center

Fig. 9.2 Canonical projection plot of cerebrospinal fluid pooled samples (*squares*), serum pooled samples (*circles*), and ten unknown samples (*rhombs*/even samples – serum unknowns and *triangles*/odd samples – CSF unknowns). The plot shows discrimination between CSF and serum with a Mahalanobis distance of 4.0183. Unknown CSF samples (odd samples) are placed in the appropriate class of CSF; however, 3 out of 5 serum samples (even samples) are grouped correctly with serum. The y-axis is the factor or principal component vector demonstrating the greatest variance in data (Reprinted with permission from [3], publisher Mosby, Inc.)

collected and placed on cottonoid pledgets. This was done to determine whether or not the nose would be usable for unknown specimens collected intranasally. In each case, the e-nose was able to distinguish readily between CSF and serum. A representative result is shown in Fig. 9.1.

The next set of experiments involved testing the e-nose to see whether it could correctly identify unknown samples as either CSF or serum. This time, samples were collected in matched sets of CSF and serum, and prepared as unknowns. A quantity of 0.3 cc of each specimen was measured with a micropipette, placed in a headspace-generating vial, and incubated for 30 min. A combined probability (Cprob) was calculated for each unknown sample. This is a statistical measure that looks at both the probability of a sample belonging to a class and the distance of that sample from a class (samples with a number close to 1 are more likely to be part of the class). Through a series of experiments, it appeared that the e-nose was able to correctly identify all CSF specimens, with a Cprob range of 0.762 to 1.0. It was able to identify correctly most of the serum samples, with a Cprob range of 0.8744 to 0.9998. Figure 9.2 shows representative data.

These experiments demonstrated that the e-nose did have the ability to distinguish between different bodily secretions with high reproducibility. Because the results of the test were available in about an hour, this testing could be used for the identification of a CSF leak in a clinical setting.

Identification of Bacterial Species

With the success of the above set of experiments, the authors were interested in determining whether or not an e-nose would be able to identify upper and lower respiratory tract bacteria and infections. A series of experiments were designed to determine this.

First, the e-nose was tested for its ability to distinguish between swabs containing bacteria ("positive") and control swabs without bacterial cells ("negative"), using known plated bacteria. Samples were prepared using a sterile nasopharyngeal calcium alginate-tipped applicator (Pur-Wraps Calgiswab Type 1, Hardwood Products, Guilford, ME, USA) to sample a colony of bacterial growth from a variety of bacterial isolates. The swab was then placed in a closed vial with 0.3 cc of normal saline. This system allowed us to generate a humid headspace for sampling. The vials were incubated, and then sampled. The e-nose was able to reproducibly distinguish between controls and bacteria [4].

Second, using the same collection methodology, the e-nose was tested for its ability to distinguish among bacterial pathogens. Again, the e-nose was able to distinguish amongst all specimens tested [5]. Figure 9.3 shows a representative experiment, where individual species of bacteria clustered in individual groups, separate from each other and from saline controls. The analytic approach used in this experiment was cluster analy-

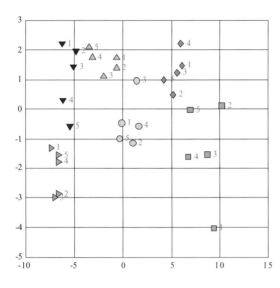

Fig. 9.3 Mean centered canonical projection plot demonstrating clustering of bacterial species, each distinct from the other (*yellow circle* = Pseudomonas aeruginosa, *green square* = Haemophillus influenza, *blue diamond* = Streptococcus pneumonia, *yellow triangle* = Staphylococcus aureus, *purple triangle* = Proteus mirabilis, *turquoise triangle* = Stenotrophomonas maltophilia) (Reprinted with permission from [4], publisher Lippincott Williams and Wilkins)

9

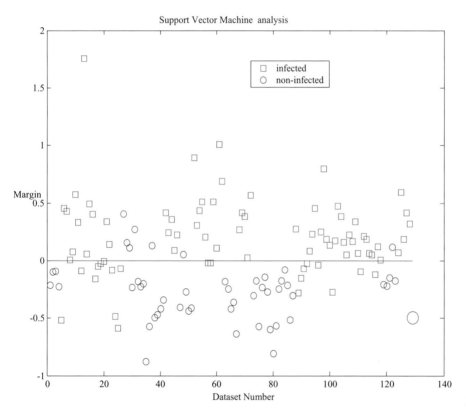

Fig. 9.4 Two-dimensional representation of the support vector machine (SVM) analysis for the second set of samples. *Squares* are infected and *circles* are uninfected. The x-axis is the number of the sample and the y-axis is the margin from the hyperplane created by the SVM analysis (see the methods sections) (Reprinted with permission from [14], publisher Oceanside)

sis, which uses the Mahalanobis distance (MD) to determine whether samples cluster distinguishably. An MD of greater than 5.0 suggests that the e-nose is able to identify an unknown specimen, by correctly placing it in its class. In this experiment, 11 out of 15 comparisons between one bacterial species and another had an MD greater than 5.0.

This kind of experiment has been reproduced elsewhere, using other e-noses, with varying protocols looking at bacterial identification [6–12]. There has been a growing body of work published on the ability of e-noses to identify and distinguish amongst different bacterial species in vitro. The electronic nose has also been shown to be useful in the diagnosis of ventilator-associated pneumonia [13].

Identification of Patients with Bacterial Rhinosinusitis

The authors next turned to in vivo testing, to investigate whether or not the e-nose had the capacity to identify patients with bacterial rhinosinusitis [14]. In this set of experiments, samples were taken from patients presenting with complaints suggestive of bacterial rhinosinusitis. For the most part, these were patients with symptoms suggestive of acute exacerbation of known chronic rhinosinusitis. Healthy volunteers were used as controls. Each participant underwent culture of nasal secretions, which was then analyzed for its microbiologic content. Then, exhaled breath samples were obtained from each participant using a modified nasal CPAP mask connected to the sampling port of the e-nose. The breath samples were then compared with the microbiologic data, which allowed categorization of participants as infected (positive culture) or non-infected (negative culture).

As shown in a representative data set in Fig. 9.4, the e-nose was able to predict with approximately 76% accuracy whether or not the patient was infected. Data analysis for this set of experiments was done using a leave-one-out technique with support vector machine (SVM) analysis. SVM analysis is a linear classification method that minimizes classification error at the same time as maximizing the geometric margin between two sample sets in high-dimensional space, and is well-suited to determining whether there is a difference between two e-nose sample groups. Figure 9.4 shows the results for 25 patients, 15 of whom were considered infected.

These results are significantly better than chance, and the e-nose was able to detect something about the infected patients that was different than the controls. Determination of what exactly the e-nose was distinguishing that made the infected patients different is an as yet unanswered question. It is not clear whether the e-nose is actually detecting the bacteria themselves, fermentation products they produce, or perhaps some aspect of the inflammatory host response to bacteria.

Detection of Biofilms

To better answer the question of what the e-nose may be identifying as a marker of bacterial infection, the authors next investigated biofilm production in bacterial species known to cause sinusitis [15]. Bacterial biofilms are produced by some subtypes of bacterial species such as *Pseudomonas aeruginosa* and *Staphylococcus aureus*, common pathogens in the development of sinusitis. They are created by bacteria that attach to a substrate such as mucosa and form microcolonies. When sufficiently dense, these colonies extrude an exopolysaccharide matrix, a sort of scaffolding on which bacteria proliferate, and survive, despite species-specific anti-microbial therapy. Biofilms have been implicated in many infectious processes.

The experimental design involved the comparison of biofilm-producing bacteria versus non-biofilm-producing bacteria, testing the e-nose's ability to distinguish between organisms. Two strains of *Pseudomonas aeruginosa*, PA01 (Tn7-gfp2-ΩGm) – a biofilm producer, and *Sad36* (flgK)::Tn5B30(Tc) – a non-biofilm

Table 9.1 Real testing result for PA01 versus *Sad36*

	Training	Testing
PA01	100%	100%
Sad36	100%	80.6%

Table 9.2 Real testing result for Staph AB- versus Staph WT

	Training	Testing
Staph AB-	87.7%	72.2%
Staph WT	86.4%	91.7%

producer, and two strains of *Staphylococcus aureus*, WT (Newman) –a biofilm producer, and A/B- (SKM14/Srt A-/Srt B-) – a non-biofilm producer, were utilized for the experiments [16].

The e-nose was then exposed to the different bacterial species a number of times, first to establish the training accuracy of the e-nose, and then to establish its testing accuracy. Logistic regression analysis was used for these studies. This analysis determined that, for 198 samples tested, there was 100% training accuracy for both PA01 and *Sad36*, and 91.4% and 88.4% testing accuracy for PA01 and Sad36 respectively.

In addition, there was 87.1% and 88.2% training accuracy and 75.3% and 76.8% testing accuracy for Staph AB- and Staph WT respectively.

The samples were then tested over a period of 22 days, separating the first 18 days from the last 4 days. Logistic regression analysis was again used to determine the accuracy of the e-nose, are described below.

For PA01 versus *Sad36*, and for Staph AB- versus Staph WT, data collected over 22 days were divided into two data sets. The first 18 days (162 samples) were used as a training set and the remaining 4 days (36 samples) were used as a testing set. The training and testing accuracy for each comparison is summarized in Tables 9.1 and 9.2.

In summary, the e-nose was able to correctly identify biofilm-producing bacteria with an accuracy ranging from 72.2% to 100%. These results suggest that biofilms may be an in vivo marker for certain pathogens in chronic sinusitis.

Future Directions

Electronic nose technology is relatively new and holds great promise as a diagnostic tool in medicine because it is portable, rapid and has potential applicability in a wide range of medical conditions. In addition to the work described above, we and others have demonstrated that the e-nose can be used to identify patients with lung cancer, urinary tract infections, diabetes and bacterial vaginosis [6, 17–24]. Most of the work done to date was performed with first-generation technology both in terms of sensors and analysis.

The field of electronic sensing extends well beyond medicine. Biological and chemical detection has progressed considerably since the 9/11 attacks and sensor arrays (using sensors identical to those in e-noses) have been deployed over major cities as early warning devices. Electronic tongues have been developed for fluid analysis. Nanoscale sensors combining carbon nanotubes with antibodies have shown promise in medicine as well. New statistical methods have evolved in parallel for the evaluation of sensor data from electronic noses, which are inherently high dimensional. Recently developed computer algorithms are particularly suited to the rapid analysis and depiction of this data.

There are three general levels of utility for an electronic nose as a medical device. The first is as a *screening* tool. In this approach the e-nose could be used as a fast, inexpensive method by which patients (i.e., breath) or patient samples (i.e., urine, sputum) in which disease probability is low, could be tested to determine the need for more expensive or invasive tests. This approach uses a Bayesian approach to pre- and post-test probability, and leverages the fact that the test is inexpensive and non-invasive. The e-nose might, for example, be used to test routine urine samples passing through a lab for urinalysis to screen for infection or malignancy. Similarly, an e-nose might be used to guide the physician's prescription of empiric antibiotics.

A second, and greater, level of utility would be the use of an e-nose for *diagnosis*. A sufficiently accurate e-nose might specifically identify the presence of specific infections or malignancies. The e-nose has been shown to accurately distinguish between bacteria and tumor cell lines in laboratory conditions, and might be able to do so in the clinical environment as well.

Finally, the e-nose might be used to identify the onset of a disease (i.e., ventilator-associated pneumonia) and then track its course during treatment, thereby indicating response to treatment or the lack thereof. An e-nose designed for this application could conceivably be integrated into a device (i.e., ventilator, urinary drainage bag) and act as a silent watchdog, much as biodefense sensors are currently used.

In order for the e-nose to be accepted by the medical community as a trusted diagnostic method, further work will need to be done to analyze the molecular odorants in each of the clinical conditions, determine the relationship between those odorants and disease, and develop consistent and transparent statistical approaches.

References

1. Lewis NS, Schauer CL, Sotzing GA, Stitzel SE, Vaid TP, Walt DR: Cross-Reactive Chemical Sensor Arrays. Chemical Reviews 2000; 100: 2595–626

2. Thaler ER, Kennedy DW, Hanson CW: Medical applications of electronic nose technology: review of current status. [Review] [28 refs]. American Journal of Rhinology 2001; 15: 291–5

3. Aronzon A, Hanson CW, Thaler ER: Differentiation between cerebrospinal fluid and serum with electronic nose. Otolaryngology – Head & Neck Surgery 2005; 133: 16–9

4. Lai SY, Deffenderfer OF, Hanson W, Phillips MP, Thaler ER: Identification of upper respiratory bacterial pathogens with the electronic nose. Laryngoscope 2002; 112: 975–9

5. Thaler ER: Candidate's thesis: the diagnostic utility of an electronic nose: rhinologic applications. Laryngoscope 2002; 112: 1533–42

6. Boilot P, Hines EL, Gardnerr JW, Pitt R, John S, Mitchell J, Morgan DW: Classification of bacteria responsible for ENT and eye infections using the Cyranose system. IEEE Sensors J 2002; 2: 247–53

7. Dutta R, Hines EL, Gardner JW, Boilot P: Bacteria classification using Cyranose 320 electronic nose. Biomed Eng Online 2002; 1: 4

8. Gardner JW, Craven M, Dow CS, Hines EL: The prediction of bacteria type and culture growth phase by an electronic nose with a multi-layer perception network. Meas Sci Technol 1998; 9: 120–7

9. Guernion N, Ratcliffe NM, Spencer-Phillips PTN, Howe RA: Identifying bacteria in human urine: Current practice and the potential for rapid, near-patient diagnosis by sensing volatile organic compounds. Clin Chem Lab Med 2001; 39: 893–906

10. Pavlou AK, Turner AP, Magan N: Recognition of anaerobic bacterial isolates in vitro using electronic nose technology. Lett Appl Microbiol 2002; 35: 366–9

11. Searle GE, Gardner JW, Chappell MJ, Godfrey KR, Chapman MJ: System identification of electronic nose data from Cyanobacteria experiments. IEEE Sensors J 2002; 2: 218–29

12. Shin HW, Llobet E, Gardner JW, Hines EL, Dow CS: Classification of the strain and growth phase of cyanobacteria in potable water using an electronic nose system. IEE Proc Sci Meas Technol 2000; 147: 158–64

13. Hanson CW, Steinberger HA: The use of a novel electronic nose to determine the etiology of intrapulmonary infection. Anesthesiology 1997; 87: A269

14. Thaler ER, Hanson CW: Use of an electronic nose to diagnose bacterial sinusitis. American Journal of Rhinology 2006; 20: 170–2

15. Thaler ER, Huang D, Giebeig L, Palmer J, Lee D, Hanson CW, Cohen N: Use of an electronic nose for detection of biofilms. American Journal of Rhinology 2008; 22: 29–33

16. Musk DJ, Jr., Hergenrother PJ, Musk DJJ, Hergenrother PJ: Chemical countermeasures for the control of bacterial biofilms: effective compounds and promising targets. [Review] [136 refs]. Current Medicinal Chemistry 2006; 13: 2163–77

17. Chandiok S, Crawley BA, Oppenheim BA, Chadwick PR, Higgins S, Persaud KC: Screening for bacterial vaginosis: a novel application of artificial nose technology. J Clin Pathol 1997; 50: 790–1

18. Gardner JW, Shin HW, Hines EL: An electronic nose system to diagnose illness. Sensors Actuators B-Chemical 2000; 70: 19–24

19. Thaler ER, Hanson CW: Medical applications of electronic nose technology. [Review] [51 refs]. Expert Review of Medical Devices 2005; 2: 559–66

20.　Wang P, Tan Y, Xie H, Shen F: A novel method for diabetes diagnosis based on electronic nose. Biosensors & Bioelectronics 1997; 12: 1031–6

21.　Di Natale C, Macagnano A, Martinelli E, Paolesse R, D'Arcangelo G, Roscioni C, Finazzi-Agro A, D'Amico A: Lung cancer identification by the analysis of breath by means of an array of non-selective gas sensors. Biosens Bioelectron 2003; 18: 1209–18

22.　Machado RF, Laskowski D, Deffenderfer O, Burch T, Zheng S, Mazzone PJ, Mekhail T, Jennings C, Stoller JK, Pyle J, Duncan J, Dweik RA, Erzurum SC: Detection of lung cancer by sensor array analyses of exhaled breath. American Journal of Respiratory & Critical Care Medicine 2005; 171: 1286–91

23.　Phillips M, Cataneo RN, Cummin AR, Gagliardi AJ, Gleeson K, Greenberg J, Maxfield RA, Rom WN: Detection of lung cancer with volatile markers in the breath [see comment]. Chest 2003; 123: 2115–23

24.　Phillips M, Gleeson K, Hughes JM, Greenberg J, Cataneo RN, Baker L, McVay WP: Volatile organic compounds in breath as markers of lung cancer: a cross-sectional study.[see comment]. Lancet 1999; 353: 1930–3

Clinical Assessment, Management, Surgery of the Internal Nose

Chapter 10

Clinical Assessment and Management of Olfactory Disorders

10

Eric H. Holbrook

Core Messages

- A thorough history provides a diagnosis in most cases of smell disorders.
- A complete head and neck examination helps to confirm the diagnosis.
- Olfactory testing can be performed by all physicians and provides assessment of the degree of smell loss.
- Decisions on obtaining imaging will depend on the history and physical examination.
- Treatment options for smell disorders are limited, but all patients require counseling and education in olfactory loss.

Contents

Introduction

The evaluation of a patient presenting with a chemosensory disorder can be a significant source of frustration for otolaryngologists. Often, these patients present months or years after the onset of symptoms and have been seen previously by multiple care providers. Although they are hopeful for a cure, realization of the permanency of their condition has usually already occurred and they are mostly seeking answers to a multitude of questions. It is the physician's responsibility to diagnose the problem correctly, rule out a potential malignant process, and provide therapy if available. Frustration stems from an incomplete knowledge of the olfactory system and its associated pathology, along with the lack of therapy available for treating the majority of olfactory disorders. Confusion over coding for evaluation of patients with smell disorders (ICD 781.1: disturbances of sensation of smell and taste) and proper procedural coding for smell testing leads to further discouragement from proper evaluation of these patients. Other chapters in this textbook provide information on the physiology of the olfactory system and the common pathology encountered in disorders of the sense of smell. The goal of this chapter is to provide a framework for physicians in which to logically approach a patient who presents with an olfactory disorder and to provide appropriate management options for certain conditions.

Assessment

History

The most important process in the evaluation of a patient complaining of a chemosensory disorder is obtaining the history. A detailed history will provide a diagnosis in the vast majority of cases and therefore most of a physician's time should be spent in discussion with the patient. Although there are hundreds of proposed causes of olfactory disorders, the most common result from upper respiratory infections (URI), head trauma, and rhinosinusitis [1–5]; therefore, significant inquiry should be directed toward these entities. Initially, let the patient describe the symptoms and then gradually ask more directed questions. It is not unusual for them to describe a loss of taste when actually this function is normal and what they are experiencing is a lack of flavor perception due to the absence of smell. Simply confirming that they can detect salty or sweet foods allows you to focus the remainder of the visit on the sense of smell and also gives you the opportunity to educate them on the differences between smell, taste, and flavor. This clarification sometimes puts the patient at ease, knowing it is likely that only one system is affected. Ask them to comment on the severity of the smell loss and how it affects their everyday life. Descriptions of hazardous events including inability to detect cooking fires or natural gas leaks are often relayed by the patient and present an opportunity to counsel the patient on the risks of smell loss. How complete is their loss of the sense of smell and is the flavor of food unchanged? What is the quality of their sense of smell, i.e., is their sense of smell distorted in that things don't smell the way they used to, or do they experience a background odor no one else can smell?

Timing of the onset of the disorder can be very helpful. Sudden onset of smell loss is usually related to an upper respiratory infection (URI) or trauma, whereas gradual smell loss is usually associated with causes such as aging, neurodegenerative disease, and long-term chronic rhinosinusitis (CRS). Fluctuation in the ability to smell is associated frequently with CRS and polyps. Any indication of a gradual improvement in the sense of smell since the initial onset indicates a better prognosis for the return of function. Having no memory of the ability to smell implies a congenital smell loss. In this case, further questions relating to a delay in sexual maturity and family history of the same should be asked to check for Kallmann's syndrome and then an endocrine referral should be considered if the age of presentation is prior to the onset of puberty in order to correct any hormonal deficiency [6].

Answers to questions pertaining to events surrounding the initial onset should be obtained, including the presence of URI symptoms, head trauma (regardless of severity), changes in medications, and use of over-the-counter medications. Physicians should specifically inquire about the use of topical nasal zinc preparations. These medications, designed to prevent or shorten URIs, have been implicated in causing sudden smell loss in some patients [7, 8]. Typically, the smell loss occurs immediately or within hours of the use of the medication, and usually an intense burning sensation to the nasal cavity is experienced after application of the product. However, given that the medication is used commonly during an URI, it may be difficult to distinguish direct causation from the URI itself.

It is important to inquire about concurrent symptoms and other medical problems. Nasal obstruction, drainage, facial pressure/pain, ear complaints, and fatigue suggest rhinosinusitis and/or allergic rhinitis. Unilateral symptoms of obstruction and epistaxis raise concerns for a nasal mass. Questions about memory loss, confusion, and cognitive dysfunction that may suggest a neurodegenerative disorder such as Alzheimer's disease should be asked. Vision changes, headaches, and sensory or motor changes may suggest an intracranial mass or CNS disorder. Past medical and surgical history should be reviewed to uncover possible sources such as nasal trauma, previous nasal surgery, stroke, and thyroid disorders.

Patients disturbed particularly by the presence of abnormal odors such as with parosmia (abnormal perception of a presented odor) or phantosmia (perception of an odor when no odor is present) need special consideration and should be asked for a history of migraines or seizure disorders in addition to questions regarding rhinosinusitis. Patients with phantosmia thought to be related to abnormal olfactory signal processing will often confirm a unilateral presentation to the distorted smell when asked. They often experience relief after periods of sleep and may notice a decrease during episodes of crying or bending over. The abnormal odor is described usually as having a rotten, moldy, swampy, or burning quality, and it is often associated with a decreased sense of smell [9]. This information can help distinguish a causal relationship with a disorder of the olfactory nerves from more central disorders and functional causes such as olfactory reference syndrome [10].

Physical Examination

When conducting an examination of a patient with an olfactory disorder, a routine otolaryngological evaluation should be performed. Cranial nerve function should be assessed to rule out any localizing intracranial lesion. Of course special attention should be given to the examination of the nose; however, excessive manipulation with rhinoscopy or administration of local anesthetic or decongestant sprays should be delayed until after olfactory testing has been performed. The physician should listen for hyponasality of the voice to suggest nasal obstruction and assess nasal patency by gently obstructing the airflow to each naris individually. With anterior rhinoscopy evidence of rhinosinusitis, allergic rhinitis, anatomic obstruction, and polyps, or an obvious mass, especially at the opening to the olfactory clefts, should be looked for.

Anterior rhinoscopy alone has been shown to fail in the diagnosis of a conductive/obstructive olfactory loss in 51% of cases compared with 9% with the use of nasal endoscopy [2]. Nasal endoscopy should be performed in all patients presenting with smell disorders and absence of findings on anterior rhinoscopy. Close attention should be given to the olfactory cleft anteriorly and the area of the superior turbinate posteriorly (Fig. 10.1). In addition to the identification of polyps or masses, assessment for patency of the olfactory cleft region and evidence of CRS with turbinate edema and thickened mucus accumulation should be made.

In cases of patients complaining of phantosmia, unilateral finger occlusion of the nostril will usually result in temporary relief of symptoms if the disorder is related to airflow on the blocked side. This will also help localize the problem to the right or left side. In addition, unilateral topical nasal application of 1 cm^3 of 4% cocaine solution with the body in a supine position and the head extended will anesthetize the olfactory neurons and provide relief of phantosmia if it is related to a disorder of olfactory signal transduction. This procedure will not help with more centrally related causes [9].

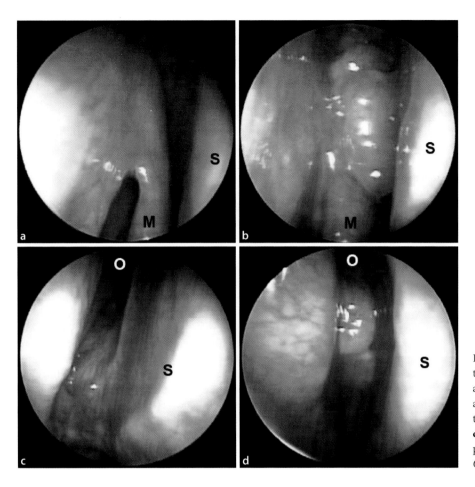

Fig. 10.1a–d Endoscopic examination of the right nasal cavity. **a** Normal anterior olfactory cleft. **b** Comparative anterior region with polyp obstruction. **c** Normal posterior olfactory cleft. **d** Comparative posterior region with polyp obstruction. *M* middle turbinate, *O* olfactory cleft, *S* septum

Olfactory Testing

As part of the work-up in the evaluation of olfactory disorders, testing of olfactory function allows for an objective assessment of the degree of impairment. When olfactory loss is present patients are fairly good at recognizing improving or deteriorating ability [11], but overall olfactory ability compared with that in the general population is impossible with subjective measures alone. Olfactory testing also provides a baseline for a comparison of repeat testing to determine the efficacy of therapy or changes in olfactory ability that may impact upon prognosis. It can also be used as a tool for the detection of malingering in cases of workers' compensation or lawsuits, although many of the tests commonly used can be manipulated by the individual to give the appearance of anosmia with just a little knowledge of the testing paradigm.

Measurements of olfactory ability can be divided into psychophysical and electrophysiologic testing. Psychophysical tests are used most commonly in clinical testing and are based on odor detection, odor identification, and/or odor discrimination. All can be administered unilaterally, which can identify localized lesions and help identify a causative side for phantosmia. Most commonly, odor detection is assessed through forced choice testing of gradually increased concentrations of an odorant, such as butyl alcohol, presented along with a blank sample

[1]. The concentration at which the odor is detected consistently and correctly against the blank is the threshold of detection and is compared with a normal average. Forms of these tests are commercially available, but they can be time consuming and require a knowledgeable test administrator. Tests of identification involve presentation of a battery of stimuli to the individual and asking the patient to choose the smell from a list of possibilities. Samples of olfactory as well as trigeminal stimuli are included, and a composite score, including results of threshold testing is compared with normal values. The Sniffin' Sticks test uses odorant-impregnated felt-tipped pens to test detection threshold, identification, and discrimination [12–14]. A composite score is again derived and compared with normative data. The test can be reused and is easy to perform, but it also requires time commitment from a test administrator.

The most widely used olfactory test in the United States is the University of Pennsylvania Smell Identification Test (UPSIT), commercially marketed as the Smell Identification Test (SIT, Sensonics, Haddon Heights, NJ, USA). This is a self-administered forced-choice smell identification test using microencapsulated beads to present an odor in a scratch-and-sniff manner. Forty items are presented sequentially and the patient is asked to match each smell with a choice of four possible odors. Results are compared with normal data stratified among age and sex. This test of identification has been studied extensively demonstrating reproducibility and good correlation with the degree of odor detection [15]. Test scores can be categorized into grades of hyposmia or anosmia and can reveal probable malingering. A significant advantage for practicing physicians is in the self-administration of the test, allowing the care-provider to see other patients and to free up ancillary office personnel. Potentially, in cases of significant dysosmia, this odorant identification test may exaggerate the degree of smell loss. In addition, some patients may have difficulty with reading and fine motor skills, or they may not speak English well, which results in decreased reliability of the test. It may also become less reliable in the pediatric age groups. In these cases formal threshold testing may be indicated and/or referral to a smell and taste center. For cultural differences in the ability to recognize various odors, the Cross-Cultural Smell Identification Test has been developed, based on the UPSIT, that uses odors consistently identified by individuals across multiple countries and cultures [16].

Electrophysiologic tests are used mostly for research purposes only, but can aid in the detection of malingering if available. Electro-olfactograms (EOG) use electrodes placed on the neuroepithelium to record field potentials during stimulation. However, the placement is uncomfortable since local anesthetic cannot be used and the recoding of potentials can be very difficult [17].

Given the success of auditory brainstem responses in localizing the pathology of hearing loss, odor event-related potentials (OERPs) have been measured in attempt to achieve the same success. An odorant stimulus is presented to the individual in a controlled fashion to avoid confounding stimulation related to airflow and temperature changes while EEG recordings are made. The technique is vulnerable to artifacts, and responses are often difficult to extract from the noisy EEG background. At this point, localization of damage to the olfactory system through OERP recordings is not possible. It may help to identify malingering when OERPs are present; however, the lack of identifiable OERPs does not necessarily predict anosmia [18].

In the absence of formal olfactory function tests, measuring olfactory ability can and should still be a part of the evaluation. A simple screening test developed by Davidson and Murphy [19] uses a standard 70% isopropyl alcohol pad, available in any clinical setting, as a stimulant. The opened pad is first presented to the participant to allow for identification of the odor. The participant is then asked to keep their eyes closed and the pad is then advanced slowly from the level of the umbilicus to the nose with each normal inhalation. The distance from the alcohol pad at the time of first detection to the nose correlates with the degree of olfactory loss. A distance of less than 20 cm indicates hyposmia. It is worth noting that detection of the alcohol pad at the opening of the nares does not rule out anosmia, since the trigeminal nerve can be stimulated with high concentrations of most odorants.

Intentional stimulation of the trigeminal nerve can also be used in cases of potential malingering. An ammonia stick placed quickly in front of the nose will produce burning and lacrimal stimulation regardless of olfactory ability. Often, individuals feigning anosmia who are unfamiliar with innervation of the nose will deny the presence of the stimulus even with obvious trigeminal activation.

With commercially available testing products such as the SIT (www.sensonics.com) that allow for self-administration, physicians have the ability to assess the degree of olfactory loss without committing extensive clinic time. Objective olfactory testing can confirm a suspected smell loss and provide the patient with a number that can be compared with that of the normal population. It may help with prognosis and give the patient a better sense of their condition. If testing is unavailable or inconclusive, patients may be referred to a smell and taste center for further evaluation.

Imaging

In the vast majority of patients who present with olfactory disorders the history will provide the most valuable clues in making a diagnosis, and imaging will not give any useful information. In cases associated with head trauma, imaging has often already been performed, with documentation of contusions to the olfactory bulbs and tracts, inferior frontal lobes, temporal lobes, or the hippocampus known to be related to smell disorders [20]. However, traumatic sheering of olfactory neurons passing through the cribriform plate may be another reason for smell loss after injury and cannot be evaluated through imaging. Therefore, unless the patient presents in the acute setting after trauma, imaging is not needed. A patient with a clear history of causation such as URI-related anosmia and a collaborating normal physical examination needs no further radiographic workup [17]. MRIs are obtained frequently when a patient presents with an olfactory disturbance to avoid missing an intracranial mass. In the setting of an identifiable cause based on history and the absence of abnormal findings on complete examination, MRI is not indicated as part of the evaluation [21]. On the other hand, MRIs may be useful at times when there is an atypical history, when there are neurological findings on physical examination, in evaluation for the absence of olfactory bulbs

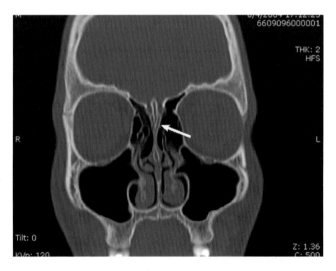

Fig. 10.2 Coronal CT scan of the sinuses in a patient with anosmia. The olfactory clefts are narrowed and obstructed (*arrow*) resulting from large air-filled middle turbinates

in congenital anosmia, when neurodegenerative disorders are suspected, and in evaluation of soft tissue masses identified on endoscopy [17, 22, 23].

Patients with smell disorders related to chronic rhinosinusitis based on history and physical examination will benefit from CT scanning to evaluate for the extent of the disease and for the anticipated endoscopic sinus surgery. Direct nasal/facial trauma is best evaluated with CT scans to inspect the bony detail. Occasionally, non-traumatic obstruction of the olfactory clefts by intranasal anatomy is suspected with endoscopic evaluation even in the absence of subjective nasal obstruction. CT scanning can confirm the presence of medialized or enlarged middle and superior turbinates with severe narrowing of the olfactory cleft and obstruction (Fig. 10.2) [24].

Laboratory Data

Given the variability and multitude of causes of smell disorders, no single battery of laboratory tests is recommended. Specific cases of suspected metabolic disorders or nutritional deficiency suggested by the history and physical examination may warrant specific tests. Smell loss caused by URI is suspected to be related to virus-mediated damage. Serum immunology has been performed in conjunction with epidemiologic studies to suggest parainfluenza type 3 virus as the cause of URI-related smell loss [25, 26]; however, proof of this relationship and blood tests to identify virus-related olfactory loss do not currently exist.

Management

The lack of available therapy for sense of smell disorders is a major source of frustration for physicians evaluating these patients. Zinc supplements were once accepted as a form of therapy for all chemosensory disorders and are still frequently used today; however, a well designed and controlled study has shown no benefit [27]. Various other agents including topical corticosteroids, B vitamins, alpha-lipoic-acid, and theophylline have been suggested for use in olfactory disorders, but are without supportive data. A fraction of most types of olfactory disorders resolve or improve over time with documentation of change occurring years after initial onset [28].

Conductive/Obstructive Causes

The classic description of a conductive form of smell loss is chronic rhinosinusitis (CRS) with polyps with anatomical obstruction of airflow to the olfactory clefts. Although now accepted as also causing potentially a more permanent sensory–neural effect with evidence of apoptosis occurring in the olfactory epithelium of CRS sufferers [29, 30], it is still the most treatable cause of smell loss. These patients often do well with a burst of oral corticosteroids, which can also be a useful diagnostic tool for this type of olfactory dysfunction [2]. Unfortunately, the improvement does not usually last even with the addition of topical nasal steroids. Surgical removal of polyps and ventila-

tion of the sinuses via endoscopic sinus surgery has been shown in many studies to improve smell function (see Raviv and Kern for review [31]), but again incomplete or transient improvement is common. Given the chronic inflammatory state and evidence of sensory–neural damage with CRS, an aggressive combination of medical and surgical therapy seems warranted to prevent permanent damage. It is the author's experience that nasal saline irrigation mixed with corticosteroids in addition to surgery may help improve the duration and quality of olfactory function in these patients by providing better distribution of medication to the olfactory cleft and sinus cavities than conventional corticosteroid sprays.

In cases of anatomical obstruction of the olfactory clefts due to enlarged or medialized turbinates documented with nasal endoscopy and CT scanning, systemic steroids are without benefit [24]. Surgical opening of the olfactory cleft also does not appear to improve function [32]. This may be due to chronic sensory deprivation to the olfactory neurons over an extended period of time and is supported by animal studies [33, 34]. This effect of sensory deprivation on olfactory function may also play a role in CRS with long-standing obstructive polyps and lends further support in favor of aggressive management.

Sensory–Neural Causes

Effective therapies in the treatment of sensory–neural causes of smell loss including URI-related disorders and head trauma are significantly lacking. Part of the dilemma in the assessment of potential therapies and conducting meaningful research in this area is related to the delay in patient presentation when the acute onset and pathologic process has already passed. In the treatment of URI-related smell loss, anti-viral therapy would seem to be a promising area if administered quickly, but without identifying the causative agent, pharmaceutical development is unlikely. Administration of systemic corticosteroids for anosmia/hyposmia has been reported with mixed results in the past. Recently, two separate studies showed long-lasting improvement in olfactory function with a tapering dose of oral steroids in a significant percentage of patients presenting with olfactory loss unrelated to CRS [35, 36]. With these results and the relative safety of short-term systemic steroids, the use of a tapering dose of oral steroids over a 2-week period appears indicated and may provide improvement in function for a number of these patients.

Parosmia/Phantosmia

Distorted sense of smell commonly occurs with an underlying smell loss. This has been suggested to occur at times of the onset of the loss or with improvement of olfactory ability [37]; however, recent studies have shown that the presence of parosmia has no correlation with prognosis [5]. Normally, the parosmia or phantosmia either disappears or decreases to tolerable levels over time. With phantosmia related to patent nasal airflow, temporary improvement can be achieved with the use of saline nose drops in the head down position to occlude the olfactory cleft, or through deliberate induction of rhinitis medicamentosa in the offending naris. In extreme cases the abnormal and usually offending odor may slowly intensify and persist for longer periods of time, greatly affecting quality of life. This can lead to loss of appetite with documented weight loss, severe depression, and social isolation [9]. It is in these rare, severe cases that more aggressive intervention is needed with the use of anti-seizure medication and/or surgery. In the past, surgical procedures were limited to resection of the olfactory bulbs through a craniotomy with the result of complete anosmia [38, 39]. Though technically demanding, use of an alternative approach via endoscopic resection of the olfactory epithelium has shown benefits, with decreased morbidity and frequently with the return of olfactory function [9].

Counseling

Patients with olfactory disorders are notably discouraged by their affliction, with documented decreases in measurements of quality of life [3]. Breakthroughs in research providing us with a better understanding of olfactory physiology have progressed rapidly, but without the transition to human disorders that would allow for therapeutic trials. Although our ability to improve the sense of smell is limited, we as physicians play an important role in educating these patients that in turn will help ease their concerns and frustration. We are obligated to warn them of possible hazards associated with their disability including the inability to smell smoke and the importance of fire detectors, the inability to smell natural gas and the availability of natural gas detectors, and the increased risk of ingestion of spoiled food (patients can be directed to www.nidcd.nih.gov/health/smelltaste for more information). Until research equips us with an effective therapy, we as physicians need to do our best to understand these disorders. Our understanding will then help ease our frustration, allow us to perform complete and logically directed evaluations, and suggest useful treatments with the overall goal of providing optimal care and support for patients afflicted with sense of smell disorders.

> ### Take-Home Pearls
>
> - A thorough history including timing of onset with associated events provides the most information for making a diagnosis.
> - Nasal endoscopy is often necessary to identify obstructive polyps or a mass not identified with anterior rhinoscopy.
> - Smell tests can be performed by all physicians providing an assessment of the degree of olfactory loss and a baseline value for evaluating treatment efficacy.
> - Although treatments are often not available, physicians are obligated to provide care for patients with olfactory disorders in the form of counseling and education.

References

1. Cain WS, Gent JF, Goodspeed RB, Leonard G. Evaluation of olfactory dysfunction in the Connecticut Chemosensory Clinical Research Center. *Laryngoscope* 1988;98:83–88
2. Seiden AM, Duncan HJ. The diagnosis of a conductive olfactory loss. *Laryngoscope* 2001;111:9–14
3. Miwa T, Furukawa M, Tsukatani T, Costanzo RM, DiNardo LJ, Reiter ER. Impact of olfactory impairment on quality of life and disability. *Arch Otolaryngol Head Neck Surg* 2001;127:497–503
4. Temmel AF, Quint C, Schickinger-Fischer B, Klimek L, Stoller E, Hummel T. Characteristics of olfactory disorders in relation to major causes of olfactory loss. *Arch Otolaryngol Head Neck Surg* 2002;128:635–641
5. Reden J, Maroldt H, Fritz A, Zahnert T, Hummel T. A study on the prognostic significance of qualitative olfactory dysfunction. *Eur Arch Otorhinolaryngol* 2007;264:139–144
6. Murphy C, Doty RL, Duncan HJ. Clinical disorders of olfaction. In: Doty RL, ed. *Handbook of Olfaction and Gustation, Second Edition*. New York: Marcel Dekker, Inc., 2003;461–478
7. Jafek BW, Linschoten MR, Murrow BW. Anosmia after intranasal zinc gluconate use. *Am J Rhinol* 2004;18:137–141
8. Alexander TH, Davidson TM. Intranasal zinc and anosmia: the zinc-induced anosmia syndrome. *Laryngoscope* 2006;116:217–220
9. Leopold DA, Loehrl TA, Schwob JE. Long-term follow-up of surgically treated phantosmia. *Arch Otolaryngol Head Neck Surg* 2002;128:642–647
10. Stein DJ, Le Roux L, Bouwer C, Van Heerden B. Is olfactory reference syndrome an obsessive-compulsive spectrum disorder?: two cases and a discussion. *J Neuropsychiatry Clin Neurosci* 1998;10:96–99
11. Gudziol V, Lotsch J, Hahner A, Zahnert T, Hummel T. Clinical significance of results from olfactory testing. *Laryngoscope* 2006;116:1858–1863
12. Kobal G, Hummel T, Sekinger B, Barz S, Roscher S, Wolf S. "Sniffin' sticks": screening of olfactory performance. *Rhinology* 1996;34:222–226
13. Hummel T, Sekinger B, Wolf SR, Pauli E, Kobal G. 'Sniffin' sticks': olfactory performance assessed by the combined testing of odor identification, odor discrimination and olfactory threshold. *Chem Senses* 1997;22:39–52
14. Hummel T, Konnerth CG, Rosenheim K, Kobal G. Screening of olfactory function with a four-minute odor identification test: reliability, normative data, and investigations in patients with olfactory loss. *Ann Otol Rhinol Laryngol* 2001;110:976–981
15. Doty RL, Shaman P, Kimmelman CP, Dann MS. University of Pennsylvania Smell Identification Test: a rapid quantitative olfactory function test for the clinic. *Laryngoscope* 1984;94:176–178
16. Doty RL, Marcus A, Lee WW. Development of the 12-item Cross-Cultural Smell Identification Test (CC-SIT). *Laryngoscope* 1996;106:353–356
17. Wrobel BB, Leopold DA. Clinical assessment of patients with smell and taste disorders. *Otolaryngol Clin North Am* 2004;37:1127–1142
18. Lotsch J, Hummel T. The clinical significance of electrophysiological measures of olfactory function. *Behav Brain Res* 2006;170:78–83

19. Davidson TM, Murphy C. Rapid clinical evaluation of anosmia. The alcohol sniff test. *Arch Otolaryngol Head Neck Surg* 1997;123:591–594

20. Hamilton BE, Weissman JL. Imaging of chemosensory loss. *Otolaryngol Clin North Am* 2004;37:1255–1280, vii.

21. Busaba NY. Is imaging necessary in the evaluation of the patient with an isolated complaint of anosmia? *Ear Nose Throat J* 2001;80:892–896

22. Seiberling KA, Conley DB. Aging and olfactory and taste function. *Otolaryngol Clin North Am* 2004;37:1209–1228, vii.

23. Yousem DM, Geckle RJ, Bilker W, McKeown DA, Doty RL. MR evaluation of patients with congenital hyposmia or anosmia. *AJR Am J Roentgenol* 1996;166:439–443

24. Biacabe B, Faulcon P, Amanou L, Bonfils P. Olfactory cleft disease: an analysis of 13 cases. *Otolaryngol Head Neck Surg* 2004;130:202–208

25. Sugiura M, Aiba T, Mori J, Nakai Y. An epidemiological study of postviral olfactory disorder. *Acta Otolaryngol Suppl* 1998;538:191–196

26. Konstantinidis I, Haehner A, Frasnelli J et al. Post-infectious olfactory dysfunction exhibits a seasonal pattern. *Rhinology* 2006;44:135–139

27. Henkin RI, Schecter PJ, Friedewald WT, Demets DL, Raff M. A double blind study of the effects of zinc sulfate on taste and smell dysfunction. *Am J Med Sci* 1976;272:285–299

28. Duncan HJ, Seiden AM. Long-term follow-up of olfactory loss secondary to head trauma and upper respiratory tract infection. *Arch Otolaryngol Head Neck Surg* 1995;121:1183–1187

29. Kern RC, Conley DB, Haines GK, 3rd, Robinson AM. Pathology of the olfactory mucosa: implications for the treatment of olfactory dysfunction. *Laryngoscope* 2004;114:279–285

30. Holbrook EH, Leopold DA, Schwob JE. Abnormalities of axon growth in human olfactory mucosa. *Laryngoscope* 2005;115(12):2144–2154

31. Raviv JR, Kern RC. Chronic sinusitis and olfactory dysfunction. *Otolaryngol Clin North Am* 2004;37:1143–1157, v–vi.

32. Holbrook EH, Leopold DA. An updated review of clinical olfaction. *Curr Opin Otolaryngol Head Neck Surg* 2006;14:23–28

33. Brunjes PC. Unilateral naris closure and olfactory system development. *Brain Res Brain Res Rev* 1994;19:146–160

34. Holbrook EH, Schwob JE. Naris closure reduces P2 neuron numbers within the normal and lesioned-recovered olfactory epithelium (poster abstract). *Annual Meeting of the Society for Neuroscience*. Atlanta, Georgia, 2006

35. Blomqvist EH, Lundblad L, Bergstedt H, Stjarne P. Placebo-controlled, randomized, double-blind study evaluating the efficacy of fluticasone propionate nasal spray for the treatment of patients with hyposmia/anosmia. *Acta Otolaryngol* 2003;123:862–868

36. Heilmann S, Huettenbrink KB, Hummel T. Local and systemic administration of corticosteroids in the treatment of olfactory loss. *Am J Rhinol* 2004;18:29–33

37. Doty RL. A review of olfactory dysfunctions in man. *Am J Otolaryngol* 1979;1:57–79

38. Kaufman MD, Lassiter KR, Shenoy BV. Paroxysmal unilateral dysosmia: a cured patient. *Ann Neurol* 1988;24:450–451

39. Markert JM, Hartshorn DO, Farhat SM. Paroxysmal bilateral dysosmia treated by resection of the olfactory bulbs. *Surg Neurol* 1993;40:160–163

Chapter 11

Congenital Malformations of the Nose and Paranasal Sinuses

Ravindhra G. Elluru and Shyan Vijayasekaran

Core Messages

■ Congenital malformations of the nose and paranasal sinuses arise from aberrations in the normal developmental pathways of the craniofacial skeleton.

■ Understanding the embryology of the craniofacial skeleton will aide in designing appropriate surgical treatment options for congenital malformations.

■ Radiological evaluation is an important initial step in the diagnosis and management of congenital malformations of the nose and paranasal sinuses.

■ A multidisciplinary approach is often required for treating children with congenital malformations of the nose and paranasal sinuses.

Contents

Introduction

Congenital malformations of the nose and paranasal sinuses are rare. Their presentation ranges form subtle cosmetic deformities to severe deformities that may cause life-threatening acute upper airway obstruction in neonates. This chapter will focus on the most commonly seen congenital lesions in the nose and paranasal sinuses. To facilitate a better understanding of these anomalies, we will briefly review the embryogenesis of this anatomic region.

Embryology of the Nose, Paranasal Sinuses, and Anterior Skull Base

Normal nasal development occurs between the 4th and 12th week of life. During this time, neural crest cells migrate from their origin in the dorsal neural folds around the eye and traverse the frontonasal process. These pluripotent cells undergo rapid proliferation and differentiation into muscle, cartilage, and bone, thus creating the facial structure. During this process, facial prominences develop surrounding the stomodeum, which is formed as an invagination of the ectoderm. The stomodeum is surrounded by the frontonasal prominence superiorly, the maxillary processes laterally, and the mandibular processes inferiorly. The nasal placodes, which are two small thickenings in the frontonasal process, begin to burrow, forming nasal pits. The lateral and medial prominences interact with the developing maxillary process, creating multiple paramedian structures (nasal aperture, nasolacrimal ducts, and upper lip). Eruption of the nasal pits into the choana, fusion of the palatal shelves, and growth of the nasal septum and soft palate coincide with the development of the lateral nasal wall and primitive sinus anatomy. For normal nasal and paranasal growth to occur, all of these rapid changes must occur with complete precision (Fig. 11.1, Table 11.1) [1].

The anterior skull base develops from the frontal, ethmoidal, and nasal bones. The foramen cecum forms a defect in the anterior skull base. This structure is closed by its fusion with the fonticulus frontalis, which represents a space between the developing nasal and frontal bones. It is normal for a projection of dura to extend through the foramen cecum, the prenasal space, and down to the nasal tip. As the foramen closes, the diverticulum of dura detaches from the overlying ectoderm. Faulty closure may enable persistence of neural tissue in the nasal cavity. If the fonticulus also closes abnormally, there may be persistence of an extranasal path such as seen in encephaloceles and gliomas (Fig. 11.2) [1].

Encephaloceles

Encephaloceles are extracranial herniations of cranial contents through a defect in the skull. An encephalocele may include meninges only (termed a *meningocele*), or may include both brain and meninges (termed a *meningoencephalocele*). Estimates of the incidence of these lesions vary considerably, ranging from

1 in 3,000 to 1 in 30,000 births in the western world. The incidence in Asian populations is much higher, with a reported incidence of 1 in 6,000 live births. Encephaloceles have no gender predilection and no familial tendency. Approximately 40% of patients have other associated anomalies [2–4].

Encephaloceles are divided into occipital, sincipital, and basal types (Tables 11.2, 11.3). Although the majority (75%) of lesions in North America and Europe are occipital, their anatomic location excludes them from the scope of the present discussion. Sincipital encephaloceles herniate through a bony defect between the frontal and ethmoid bones anterior to the crista galli, presenting as an external mass over the nose, glabella, or forehead (Fig. 11.3). These lesions are further classified according to their location. Nasofrontal sincipital encephaloceles present as a glabellar mass, causing telecanthus and inferior displacement of the nasal bones. Naso-ethmoidal lesions present as a dorsal nasal mass, causing superior displacement of the nasal bones and inferior displacement of the alar cartilage. Naso-orbital lesions present as an orbital mass, causing proptosis and visual changes [5]. The anatomic course of each of these sincipital encephalocele types is presented in Table 11.2. Basal encephaloceles are less common. They herniate through a bony defect between the cribriform plate and the superior orbital or posterior clinoid fissure, presenting as an intranasal mass (Fig. 11.4). This mass may not be discovered until later in childhood when it causes nasal obstruction and drainage.

Sincipital and basal encephaloceles appear as soft, bluish, compressible lesions that may transilluminate and pulsate. The classic clinical finding is a positive Furstenberg test. Owing to the

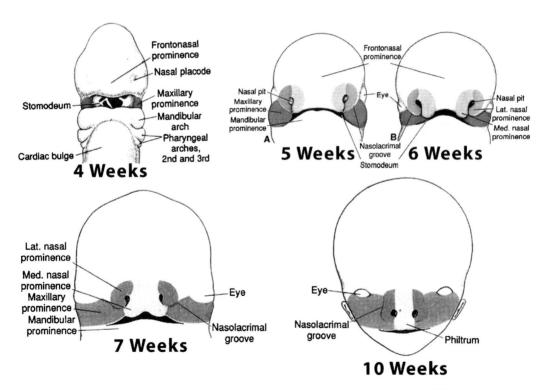

Fig. 11.1 Embryo at 4th, 5th, 6th, 7th and 10th week showing the developing nasal structures [50]

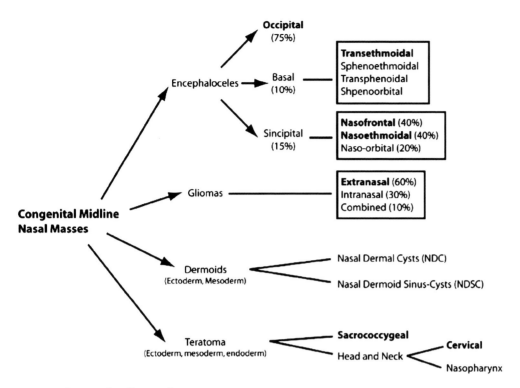

Fig. 11.2 Congenital midline nasal masses

intracranial connection, there is pulsation and expansion of the mass with crying, straining or compression of the jugular veins.

Pathologically, there is a glial component with astrocytes surrounded by collagen, submucosal glands, and sometimes nasal septal cartilage. Some lesions exhibit areas of calcification. It is sometimes difficult to differentiate between gliomas and encephaloceles; however, the presence of ependymal tissue is consistent with an encephalocele [6].

The diagnosis is radiologically confirmed by computed tomography (CT) and/or magnetic resonance imaging (MRI; Fig. 11.5). The CT evaluation should include high-resolution, thin-section, and contrast-enhanced axial and coronal images, which help delineate the infant's cartilaginous skull base. MRI provides complementary information regarding the fluid and soft tissue characteristics of the mass and is valuable in identifying an intracranial connection. It is also useful in helping to differentiate a meningocele from a meningoencephalocele. Imaging additionally helps to exclude associated anomalies such as agenesis of the corpus callosum and hydrocephalus [6].

Encephaloceles are managed surgically. Optimally, there is multidisciplinary involvement that includes both a neurosurgeon and an otolaryngologist. Most authors advocate intervention in the first few months of life [2] to minimize the risk of meningitis and cosmetic deformities. Additionally, early intervention makes the identification of the intracranial connection technically easier and allows more complete repair of the dural defect [2]. The aim of surgery is complete resection of lesions and meticulous closure of the dural defect to prevent cerebral spinal fluid (CSF) leakage. Small lesions with minimal skull base defects may be managed endoscopically. Larger lesions require a combined approach with a craniotomy to resect the lesion and subsequent endoscopic removal of the residual nasal tumor. The skull base defect can then be reconstructed using a pericranial flap or split thickness calvarial bone graft [6]. Neurological function is normal in most patients following surgery. The most commonly encountered postoperative complications are CSF leak, meningitis, and hydrocephalus. Recurrence rates of 4–10% have been reported [7].

Gliomas

Whereas encephaloceles maintain CSF communication with the subarachnoid space, nasal gliomas lack direct central nervous system attachment. Approximately 5–20% of lesions do, however, maintain a fibrous stalk connecting to the subarachnoid space. Gliomas may arise from heterotopic olfactory tissue, neurological tissue within the nasal mucosa, or displaced cells destined to differentiate into neural tissue [6]. It is also possible that these lesions were encephaloceles that were isolated from the CNS as the foramen cecum closed (Fig. 11.6).

These benign masses are extradural collections of glial tissue that present as extranasal (60%), intranasal (30%), or combined (10%) lesions [8]. Extranasal gliomas are smooth, firm, non-compressible masses that occur along the side of the nose, glabella or nasomaxillary suture line [2]. Intranasal gliomas manifest as a pale mass within the nasal cavity, with protrusion from the nostril. The nasal fossa on the involved side may be obstructed. The base of the intranasal gliomas most often arises from the lateral nasal wall near the middle turbinate and occa-

Table 11.1 Structure of the face and the embryological origin

Prominence	Structures
Frontonasal	Nasal dorsum, medial and lateral nasal prominence
Maxillary	Cheeks, lateral portion of upper lip
Medial nasal	Philtrum, columella, nasal tip
Lateral nasal	Nasal alae
Mandibular	Lower lip

Table 11.2 Sincipital encephaloceles

Type	Course	Clinical features
Nasofrontal	Through bone defect between orbits and forward between nasal and frontal bones to the area superficial to the nasal bones	Glabellar mass Telecanthus Inferior displacement of nasal bones
Naso-ethmoidal	Through foramen cecum deep to the nasal bones turning superficially at the cephalic end of the upper lateral cartilage to expand superficial to the upper lateral cartilage	Mass on the nasal dorsum Superior displacement of nasal bones Inferior displacement of the alar cartilages
Naso-orbital	Through the foramen cecum deep to the nasal and frontal bones through a lateral defect in the medial orbital wall	Orbital mass Proptosis Visual changes

Table 11.3 Basal encephaloceles

Type	Course	Clinical features
Transethmoidal	Through the cribriform plate into the superior meatus medial to the middle turbinate	Most common type Nasal obstruction Hypertelorism Broad nasal vault Unilateral nasal mass
Spheno-ethmoidal	Passes through a bony defect between the posterior ethmoid cells and sphenoid	Nasal obstruction Hypertelorism Broad nasal vault Unilateral nasal mass
Trans-sphenoidal	Through a patent craniopharyngeal canal into the nasopharynx	Nasopharyngeal mass Nasal obstruction Associated with cleft palate
Spheno-orbital	Through the superior orbital fissure and out the inferior orbital fissure into the sphenopalatine fossa	Unilateral exophthalmos Visual changes Diplopia

11

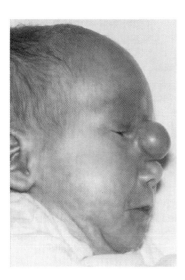

Fig. 11.3 Sincipital encephalocele. A soft bluish compressible mass protruding from the glabellar region

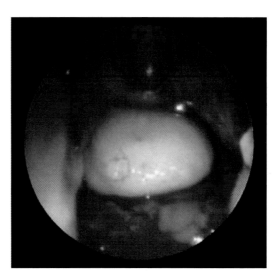

Fig. 11.4 Basal encephalocele seen in nasopharynx with 120° telescope

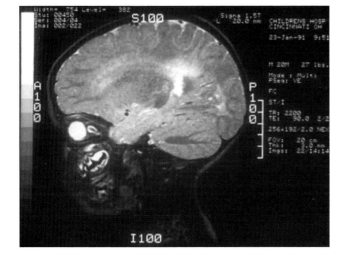

Fig. 11.5 Sagittal MRI of a basal meningoencephalocele protruding into the nasopharynx

sionally from the nasal septum [8]. Although rare, nasal gliomas sometimes extend into the orbit, frontal sinus, oral cavity or nasopharynx. Unlike encephaloceles, gliomas do not change in size with crying or straining and do not transilluminate. They are not familial, but they do have a gender predilection for males (3:2).

The diagnostic evaluation should include a CT scan to assess the bony anatomy of the skull base, MRI to accurately image soft tissue connections to the CNS, and nasal endoscopy to assess the location, origin, and extent of the nasal mass.

Proper management of gliomas requires a multidisciplinary approach that includes professionals from otolaryngology, neuroradiology, and neurosurgery. Surgical extirpation is required, and delaying this intervention may lead to distortion of the sep-

tum or nasal bone, or infection. The surgical approach should allow for excellent exposure and possible exploration of the skull base, and should provide a good cosmetic outcome. The presence of a neurosurgeon at the time of surgery is crucial, should there be an unexpected finding of an intracranial extension. Extranasal gliomas usually require an external incision. Options include lateral rhinotomy, external rhinoplasty, bicoronal incision, and midline nasal incision. The external rhinoplasty approach provides adequate surgical exposure while minimizing facial incisions, and ultimately optimizes the cosmetic outcome. When a fibrous stalk is present that extends deep to the nasal bones toward the base of the skull, a nasal osteotomy is recommended to improve exposure. Following the stalk in its entirety is crucial in determining the possible presence of an intracranial extension. If the nasal mass is large or located in the nasoglabellar region and cannot be safely excised using an external rhinoplasty approach, either a midline nasal incision or a bicoronal approach is required [6]. Due to advancements in surgical instrumentation, image guidance, and surgical techniques, most intranasal gliomas can be treated endoscopically [9, 10]. Recurrence rates are between 4 and 10% [11].

Nasal Dermoids

Nasal dermoids are the most common congenital nasal abnormality. They comprise 1–3% of all dermoids and approximately 10–12% of head and neck dermoids. Unlike teratomas, which contain all three embryonal germ layers, congenital dermoids contain only ectodermal and mesodermal embryonic elements. Mesodermal elements, which include hair follicles, sebaceous glands, and sweat glands are found in the wall of the cyst and thus differentiate these masses from simple epidermoid cysts. Most dermoid cysts occur sporadically, although familial associations have been reported. Associated abnormalities are seen in 5–41% of cases. These include aural atresia, pinna deformity, mental retardation, hydrocephalus, branchial arch sinus, cleft lip and palate, hypertelorism and hemifacial microsomia [12]. Nasal dermoids occur in a sporadic fashion with a slight male preponderance [12, 13].

The etiology of these lesions is controversial and several theories [12, 13] have been proposed to explain nasal dermoid development. The most widely accepted theory, known as the prenasal space theory, is based on the abnormal development of the fonticulus frontalis. This membrane separates the nasal and frontal bones and ossifies to separate the dura and herniating neuroectoderm from the surface epithelium. Normally, the dura separates from the surface epithelium and retracts through the foramen cecum. The retracting dura may drag the surface epithelium inward, causing formation of a sinus tract. In some patients, the sinus tract extends into the intracranial cavity or prenasal space; hence, the dermal sinus or cyst may persist anywhere from the foramen cecum to the nasal tip [14].

Nasal dermoids manifest as a simple cyst, a cyst with a sinus tract, or a sinus tract alone. Lesions usually present as a firm, lobulated, noncompressible midline mass over the nasal dorsum and may be associated with a sinus opening (Fig. 11.7). They show a negative Furstenberg test and do not transilluminate. There may be intermittent discharge or infection. A lesion within the nasal septum will cause nasal obstruction. Although a protruding hair is seen only in a minority of patients, it is pathognomic for a nasal dermoid. Intracranial extension is reportedly involved in 4–45% of cases [12].

Computed tomography and MRI provide complementary information. Fine-cut (1–3 mm) CT in the axial and coronal planes is best for visualizing bony anatomy (Fig. 11.8), whereas MRI is best for assessing soft tissue characteristics. CT scans with intravenous contrast are recommended to differentiate the dermoid from the surrounding nasal mucosa. Common findings include a bifid crista galli and an enlarged foramen cecum. Although these findings do not always indicate the presence of existing intracranial extension, a normal crista galli and fora-

men cecum may be used to exclude intracranial extension [15]. Multi-planar, thin-section, contrast-enhanced MRI is used to depict the anatomy of the anterior skull base. Contrast is used to differentiate the non-enhancing dermoid from enhancing lesions such as hemangiomas and teratomas. The neonatal crista galli does not contain marrow fat and hence a high intensity signal on T1-weighted images is suggestive of an intracranial dermoid (Fig. 11.9).

Because aspiration, incision and drainage, curettage, and subtotal excision are associated with high recurrence rates, these management approaches are generally not advocated. Assessing the degree of intracranial extension is crucial. In patients in whom the likelihood of intracranial extension is low based on clinical and radiological evaluation, an extracranial operative approach may be planned. In patients with features suggestive of intracranial extension, a combined approach should be prepared for in the event of such extension being confirmed at the time of surgery.

Pollock [16] recommended that any approach to a nasal dermoid should fulfill four criteria:
1. Provide excellent access to the midline
2. Allow access to the base of the skull
3. Provide adequate exposure for reconstruction of the nasal dorsum
4. Result in an acceptable scar

Several different extracranial approaches have been described. They include lateral rhinotomy, external rhinoplasty, midline vertical incisions, and medial para-canthal incisions. The external rhinoplasty incision generally has the best cosmetic result and is thus the most widely used approach. Also, this approach gives access to the skull base and allows for exposure of the nasal dorsum; nevertheless, it provides limited access to lesions in the glabellar region. Alternative approaches include lateral rhinotomy or midline vertical incisions, both of which provide excellent access, though with poorer cosmetic outcomes [12]. For lesions in the glabellar area without a sinus opening, a para-canthal incision or a bicoronal approach is recommended. Glabellar lesions with a sinus opening require an elliptical incision to excise the ostium, despite the possibility of a widening scar.

For lesions that extend into the cranial cavity, a craniotomy is sometimes performed; however, controversy exists as to whether this is necessary. Sessions [17] suggested that craniotomy may be avoided and the tract suture ligated if it is devoid of epidermal and adnexal structures at the skull base. This information may be obtained by intraoperative frozen-section biopsy. A number of authors [12, 15] agree with this approach. Posnick [18], however, suggests that epidermal elements may be staggered along the tract and thus postulates that a single biopsy site may provide false-negative information regarding the presence of intracranial extension of the dermoid tract.

If intracranial extension is seen, a multidisciplinary effort is required to perform a frontal craniotomy. This is usually carried out via a coronal incision using a combined intra- and extracranial approach. The overall recurrence rate following adequate excision is low. Lesions may, however, recur years after the initial surgery. As such, long-term follow-up is essential.

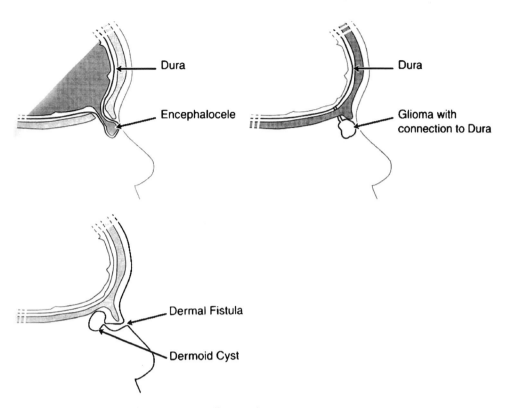

Fig. 11.6 Schematic view of the common midline nasal masses

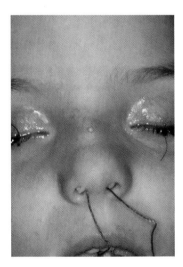

Fig. 11.7 Nasal dermoid presenting as a firm midline nasal swelling associated with a sinus opening

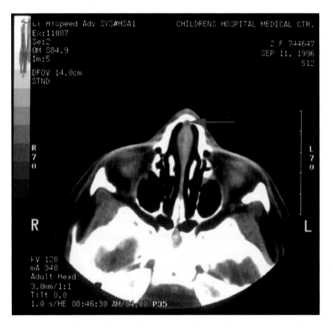

Fig. 11.8 Axial CT of nasal dermoid, evident in the anterior nasal septum as a hypodense lesion

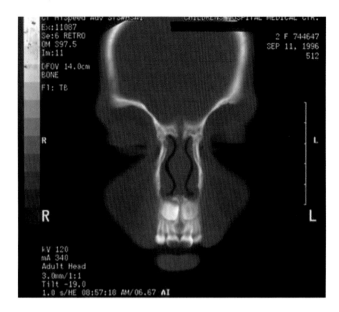

Fig. 11.9 Coronal CT showing a bifid crista galli and an enlarged foramen cecum

Complete Agenesis of the Nose

Congenital absence of the nose, referred to as arhinia, is extremely rare, with only 29 cases described in the literature (Fig. 11.10). This abnormality is part of the spectrum of holoprosencephaly, the most severe form of which is cyclopia with a single median eye and a single-chambered prosencephalon. Arhinia includes absence of the external nose and nasal airways, hypoplasia of the maxilla, a small high-arched plate, and hypertelorism. It is generally sporadic and may occur either as an isolated defect or in association with other facial and cerebral abnormalities [19]. There have also been reports of associations with genetic disorders such as trisomy 10, trisomy 13, and trisomy 21, as well as chromosome 9 inversion and translocation of chromosomes 3 and 12 [3, 19, 20].

Four theories regarding the embryogenesis of arhinia have been proposed. These theories respectively involve:
1. Failure of fusion of the medial and lateral nasal processes
2. Overgrowth and premature fusion of the nasal medial processes
3. Lack of resorption of the nasal epithelial plugs
4. Abnormal migration of neural crest cells [21].

Infants with arhinia display respiratory distress and cyanosis associated with feeding. Older children may gulp food between breaths, which is referred to as "canine eating." Speech is characteristically hypernasal and there are complaints of hyposmia. On physical examination there is an absence of the external nose, nasal septum, and sinuses. There may also be associated abnormalities of the eye, including anophthalmia or hypoplasia of the orbits.

Early management is with a cleft palate feeder or a gastrostomy tube. A prosthetic nose may be used until the child is older and can undergo definitive surgical repair. Surgery requires removing incisor teeth, creating an airway through the maxilla, and releasing the high-arched palate. The nasal passage is then lined with split thickness skin grafts and maintained with long-term stenting. Restenosis is common and serial dilatations are thus required. Reconstruction of the external nose is a multi-staged procedure that requires the use of tissue expanders, bone, cartilage or prosthetic grafts, and local or regional skin flaps. A dacryocystorhinostomy may be required to prevent recurrent conjunctivitis resulting from the absence of nasolacrimal ducts [22].

Craniofacial Clefts

Craniofacial clefts are exceedingly rare and generally not seen in routine clinical practice. The hallmarks of this disorder are: ocular hypertelorism, a broad nasal root, lack of formation of the nasal tip, widow's peak scalp bone anomaly, anterior cranium bifidum occultum, median clefting of the nose, lip, and palate, and unilateral orbital clefting or notching of the nasal ala [1, 23]. DeMyer and colleagues [24] noted an association between hypertelorism, cephalic anomalies, and mental deficiency. These authors also noted that the degree of hypertelorism and extent of extra-cephalic anomalies were associated with the increased likelihood of mental deficiency.

The term "holoprosencephaly" was coined by DeMyer et al. to describe median facial anomalies and the brain morphology associated with these anomalies [25]. Holoprosencephaly is a failure of the embryonic forebrain to cleave sagittally into cerebral hemispheres, transversely into a diencephalon, and horizontally into olfactory and optic bulbs. This failure results in a spectrum of facial anomalies that includes:

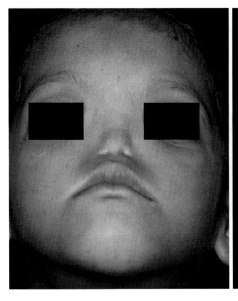
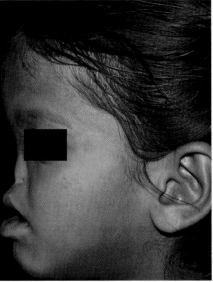

Fig. 11.10 Congenital arhinia

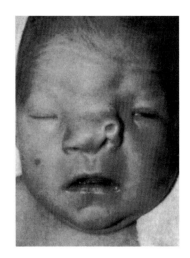

Fig. 11.11 Proboscis lateralis [1]

1. Cyclopia (single eye and single orbit with arhinia and proboscis)
2. Ethmocephaly (extreme hypertelorism, separate orbit arhinia)
3. Cebocephaly (hypertelorism, proboscis-like nose without cleft lip)
4. Median cleft lip (orbital hypertelorism and flat nose)
5. Median philtrum-premaxilla anlage (hypertelorism, bilateral cleft lip, and a median process representing the philtrum maxilla anlage)

The first gene to be associated with holoprosencephaly in humans was the Sonic Hedgehog (SHh) gene. Testing for this gene allows identification of familial forms of holoprosencephaly and evaluation of malformations considered minor variants of the disorder [23].

The Tessier classification of cranial clefts [26] is the most widely used. This classification is based on specific axes (0–14) along the face and cranium. Since the orbit is common to the face and cranium, it distinguishes cranial clefts (9–14) from facial clefts (0–8). For example, a patient with a median nasal cleft would be considered a 0/14 on the Tessier classification.

Median Nasal Clefts

There is a large degree of variability in the severity of median nasal clefts. This deformity, which is also known as bifid nose and internasal dysplasia, can range from a simple median scar at the cephalic end of the nasal dorsum to a completely split nose, forming separate halves, with independent medial nasal walls. A median cleft lip is a frequently seen associated anomaly [27]. The airway is usually adequate, despite the cosmetic appearance. Prior to surgical reconstruction, it is important to rule out a possible dermoid cyst or encephalocele within the nasal-septal area. Surgical reconstruction requires the cooperative efforts of a multidisciplinary team.

Lateral Nasal Clefts

Lateral nasal clefts are rare anomalies that involve defects of the lateral nasal wall or ala. They range from scar-like lines in the ala to triangle-like defects extending into the inner canthal fold and affecting the nasal lacrimal duct system. As with median nasal clefts, lateral nasal clefts require surgical reconstruction using a multidisciplinary approach.

Proboscis Lateralis

Proboscis lateralis is an extremely rare disorder that presents as a tubular sleeve of skin attached to the inner canthus of the orbit and complete agenesis of the paranasal sinuses on the affected side (Fig. 11.11). This lesion is commonly associated with other central nervous system abnormalities.

The most commonly accepted embryologic theory of this disorder is that imperfect mesodermal proliferation occurs in the frontonasal and maxillary processes after formation of the olfactory pits. Epidermal breakdown then occurs, leaving the lateral nasal process sequestered as a tube arising in the frontonasal region. Also, because of this breakdown, the nasolacrimal duct is not formed [1].

The diagnosis is made by physical examination, nasal endoscopy, and CT scanning. Treatment is delayed until facial growth is complete, and a prosthetic device is worn until reconstructive efforts begin. Reconstruction involves the use of bone and carti-lage grafts and surrounding skin, including the tube of anomalous lateral nasal skin. Restenosis is common and serial dilatations and stenting are often required [2].

Polyrrhinia and Supernumerary Nostril

Polyrrhinia (double nose) and supernumerary nostril (accessory nostril) are extremely rare anomalies, with only four reported cases of each [28]. These deformities are associated with pseudohypertelorism, but also have been reported as isolated anomalies. Although there are a number of embryologic theories [1, 28, 29], the event thought to be responsible for this anomaly is the incomplete development of the frontonasal process, which results in separation of the developing lateral portions of the nose. The medial nasal processes and the septum are duplicated, thus forming double noses [1, 2, 11, 26].

Patients with polyrrhinia generally present with a clinical picture similar to that seen in patients with bilateral choanal atresia, and they require the same initial management. The primary step in surgical management is the correction of the choanal atresia. The nasal deformity is later corrected by removing the medial portions of each nose and anastomosing the lateral portions in the midline [2]. The result is a broad flat nose with a depression in the midline that can be corrected by medial infracture of the nasal bones. Supernumerary nostril presents with the external appearance of a small accessory nasal orifice with surrounding redundant soft tissue. The orifice may be lateral, medial or superior to the nose. When there is a true fistula, discharge from this orifice may appear. Treatment entails excision of the supernumerary nostril and primary closure of the defect or closure with the assistance of local flaps [28].

Cleft Lip Nasal Deformity

Children with cleft lip and palate usually have a coexistent nasal deformity. The most severe defects are those associated with a bilateral complete cleft. Children with a bilateral deformity have a flattened nasal tip and a shortened columella 1–2 mm in length. They may also have bilateral maxillary hypoplasia and relative prognathism. Less severe deformity is seen in children with unilateral clefts. In these children, the nasal ala on the side of the cleft is more laterally based, giving the appearance of a flat nostril. The caudal septum is also displaced to the cleft side. The maxilla on the cleft side is hypoplastic and the nasal tip has a bifid appearance.

Treatment options include both primary and secondary rhinoplasty. The former approach, performed at the time of cleft repair, is the technique of choice for many surgeons. This option allows for the possibility of future revision should the functional and cosmetic results of primary repair be suboptimal. Both open and closed rhinoplasty techniques have been used. Given the size of the patient's nasal anatomy, the open approach is generally preferred. Secondary rhinoplasty may either be definitive or intermediate. The latter requires two stages of repair. Stage 1, performed between 4 and 6 years of age, is aimed at providing cosmetic improvement. Stage 2, performed between 8 and12 years of age, follows orthodontic correction, thus making available an optimal skeletal framework. More definitive rhinoplasty is delayed until skeletal growth is completed. As such, it is performed at between 16 and18 years of age [30].

Choanal Atresia

Choanal atresia occurs when the posterior nasal cavity fails to communicate with the nasopharynx [5]. The anatomic deformity comprises:

1. A narrow nasal cavity
2. Lateral bony obstruction by the pterygoid plate
3. Medial obstruction caused by thickening of the vomer
4. Membranous obstruction [31–33]

In a study conducted by Brown et al. [31], the incidence of pure bony atresia was found to be 29%, whereas that of mixed bony-membranous atresia was 71%. None of the patients were found to have purely membranous atresia.

Choanal atresia has a reported incidence ranging from 1 in 5,000 to 1 in 8,000 live births [34]. Fifty percent of patients with choanal atresia have other associated congenital anomalies. Up to two-thirds of cases are unilateral, with atresia most commonly occurring on the right side [5]. Up to 75% of patients affected bilaterally have other associated anomalies [2] such as CHARGE syndrome (*c*oloboma, *h*eart defects, *a*tretic choana, *r*etardation of growth and development, *g*enitourinary disorders and *e*ar abnormalities). Other anomalies include polydactyly, nasal, auricular and palatal deformities, Crouzon's syndrome, craniosynostosis, microcephaly, hypoplasia of the orbit and midface, cleft palate, and hypertelorism [35, 36].

There are several theories of embryogenesis. It is generally thought that choanal atresia is related to persistence of the nasobuccal membrane. This membrane forms at the posterior end of the nasal pits, which have burrowed into the midface mesoderm. It usually ruptures between the fifth and sixth week of gestation to produce choanae. Failure of this membrane to rupture is thought to cause choanal atresia [2]. An alternative theory suggests that abnormal migration of neural crest cells results in choanal atresia. This theory is supported by the high incidence of choanal atresia in patients with mandibulofacial dysostosis, which is associated with abnormal neural crest migration.

Patients with unilateral disease present later in life with rhinorrhea and nasal obstruction. On anterior rhinoscopy, the occluded nasal cavity is typically filled with thick, tenacious secretions. Patients with bilateral choanal atresia present as newborns with cyclical cyanosis relieved by crying. The event begins with increasing efforts to breathe, tight mouth closure, and chest retractions followed by cyanosis. The cycle is broken by crying. A variant of bilateral choanal stenosis presents later in life with mouth breathing, recurrent sinusitis, chronic rhinorrhea, otitis media, malnourishment, and speech defects.

The diagnosis of choanal atresia is made clinically by failure to pass a 6-F catheter through the nose into the nasopharynx. This is supported by endoscopic examination. CT is used to confirm the diagnosis and reveal the nature and thickness of the atresia [37]. Suctioning and vasoconstriction prior to imaging improve resolution (Fig. 11.12). A diagnosis of choanal stenosis is made when there is a narrowed, yet patent, choana. Derkay et al. [38] more specifically define this as a choanal space less than 6 mm and the inability to pass a 6-F catheter more than 32 mm. This diagnosis should be confirmed by endoscopic evaluation (Fig. 11.13).

Unilateral atresia is not an emergency. Treatment is delayed, allowing for growth of the nose, which enhances the ease of surgery and reduces the risk of postoperative complications and restenosis. Bilateral atresia requires an initial intervention to establish an oropharyngeal or orotracheal airway and nasogastric feeding prior to definitive surgery. In some cases, a tracheostomy is indicated for other airway or cardiopulmonary issues. In these cases, definitive surgery is often delayed, allowing for facial growth.

The timing of surgery is variable. Because of the small size of the face in preterm infants, it may be preferable to wait until adequate growth has occurred. Though controversial, some surgeons have advocated the "rule of tens" (the child must weigh 10 lb, have hemoglobin of 10 g/dL, and be 10 weeks old prior to repair).

There has been a shift in the surgical philosophy over the last few decades away from transpalatal (Fig. 11.14) and towards transnasal surgery. The rationale for this change has been the lower risk of dental and facial growth abnormalities associated with the latter approach. The most commonly used approach involves a blunt puncture of the central thin area using a urethral sound or suction instrument. This is carried out under endoscopic guidance using a 0° transnasal telescope or a 120° nasopharyngoscope (Fig. 11.15). Subsequently, backbiting forceps, microdebrider cutters, and/or lasers or drills are used to remove choanal soft tissue and bone. The posterior tip of the middle turbinate is a useful anatomic landmark. Remaining inferior to this structure reduces the risk of intracranial injury [39].

There are several controversial issues regarding atresia surgery. These include the use of stenting, the use of fibroblast inhibitors (mitomycin C), and the preservation of mucosal flaps. Most studies [40, 41] report significant recurrence rates requiring revision surgery. The literature indicates greater success with older children (unilateral atresia), nonsyndromic patients, and with surgical procedures that minimize mucosal trauma.

Congenital Nasal Pyriform Aperture Stenosis

Congenital nasal pyriform aperture stenosis (CNPAS) is an anomaly that occurs secondary to bony overgrowth of the nasal process of the maxilla and typically presents in the first few months of life. The pyriform aperture is the narrowest part of the nasal cavity, and small changes in the cross-sectional area significantly affect airflow by increasing nasal airway resistance. CNPAS most commonly occurs as an isolated anomaly, although it may occur in association with holoprosencephaly.

One theory of embryogenesis maintains that deficient development of the primary palate and bony overgrowth of the nasal process of the maxilla [42] are responsible for this anomaly. A developmental deficiency of the os incisivum could explain the occurrence of a triangular plate, the narrow inferior portion of the nasal cavity, and the associated central maxillary mega-incisor, which is seen in 60% of cases (Fig. 11.16) [43].

Newborns present with symptoms similar to those of choanal atresia and failure to pass through a nasopharyngeal catheter may result in a misdiagnosis of choanal atresia. These symptoms

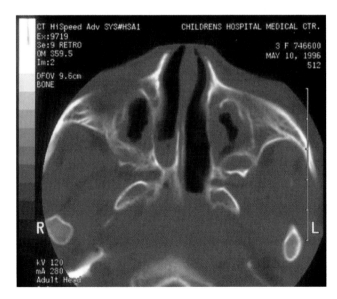

Fig. 11.12 Axial CT scan of unilateral choanal atresia, with a complete bony atretic plate and associated soft tissue

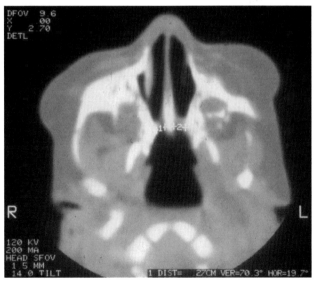

Fig. 11.13 An axial CT scan showing bilateral choanal atresia with soft tissue

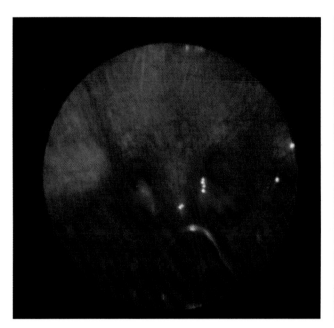

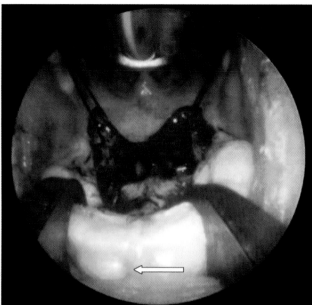

11

Fig. 11.14 A view of bilateral choanal atresia using a 120° nasopharyngoscope

Fig. 11.15 Transpalatal approach to choanal atresia repair. Elevation of a pedicled hard palate mucoperiosteal flap based on the greater palatine artery to expose the choanae

may be triggered by an upper respiratory infection, which further compromises the already narrow airway. The diagnosis of CNPAS is established by physical evaluation and is best confirmed by CT, which shows that the width of the pyriform aperture, the cross-sectional area of the nasal cavity, and the width of the choana are all reduced. In contrast, the height of the nasal cavity and cross-sectional area of the choana are not altered (Figs. 11.17, 11.18). CNPAS is thus an anomaly that results in narrowing of the entire nasal cavity; this narrowing is most severely manifested anteriorly. In a study describing the CT features that facilitate an accurate diagnosis of CNPAS, Belden and colleagues [44] found the most helpful CT measurement to be the width of the pyriform aperture, defined as the distance between the medial aspects of the maxillae at the level of the inferior meatus on images in the axial plane. These authors reported that the width was never >8 mm in their CNPAS group and never <11 mm in their control group. They thus concluded that width is the single most useful measurement for making the radiological diagnosis.

The central maxillary incisor is associated with subtypes of holoprosencephaly. Hypertelorism and a flat nasal bridge are clinical features of the premaxillary dysgenesis associated with holoprosencephaly. Pituitary disorders and dental and facial anomalies are also part of this spectrum, and it is prudent for patients with a central maxillary incisor to undergo a number of investigations, including CT scanning for evaluation of CNS malformations, chromosomal analysis, and pituitary function testing [45].

The prognosis is usually good and surgery is rarely required. Non-operative management with nasal tubes and topical vaso-

constrictive drops may be all that is required until growth results in increased nasal airway size. In patients who require surgery, this is best accomplished through the sublabial approach (Fig. 11.19). A gingival buccal sulcus incision is made through to the periosteum to expose the lateral aspect of the pyriform aperture. The bony lateral margins can then be widened by an otologic drill or curette. Brown et al. [42] recommend the use of nasal stents for up to 4 weeks.

Nasolacrimal Duct Cysts

Nasolacrimal duct cysts are uncommon abnormalities that may lead to nasal obstruction, respiratory distress, and epiphora. Because infants are obligate nasal breathers, the presence of a nasolacrimal duct cyst also makes them susceptible to aspiration and feeding difficulties.

Nasolacrimal duct development begins as a thickening of the ectoderm that becomes buried in the mesoderm between the lateral nasal process and the maxillary process. The duct begins canalization at its lacrimal end and progresses inferiorly. At birth, approximately 30% of all neonates have distal nasolacrimal duct obstruction, although only about 6% have epiphora. When both the superior and inferior aspects of the duct are obstructed, either unilateral or bilateral cyst formation occurs [46].

Symptoms are most marked in patients with bilateral cysts. In most children, however, obstruction spontaneously resolves by 9 months of age. The diagnosis is made by anterior rhinoscopy or nasal endoscopy, which demonstrates a cystic mass in the inferior meatus (Fig. 11.20). This can be confirmed on a CT

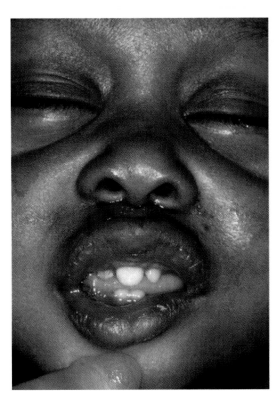

Fig. 11.16 Maxillary mega incisor in association with congenital nasal pyriform aperture stenosis

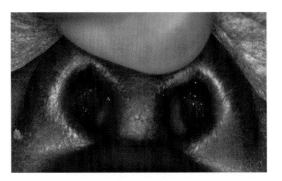

Fig. 11.17 Congenital nasal pyriform aperture stenosis as seen on anterior rhinoscopy

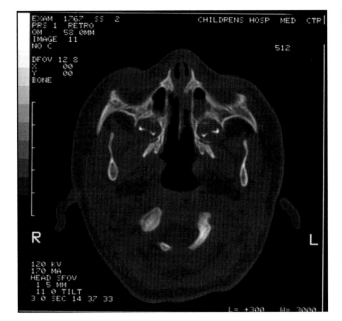

Fig. 11.18 Axial CT scan showing pyriform aperture stenosis secondary to overgrowth of the nasal process of the maxilla, causing reduction in the width of the pyriform aperture

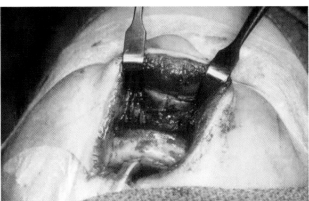

Fig. 11.19 Sub-labial approach to the piriform aperture. A gingivo-buccal sulcus incision is made and a mucoperiosteal flap is raised to expose the piriform aperture

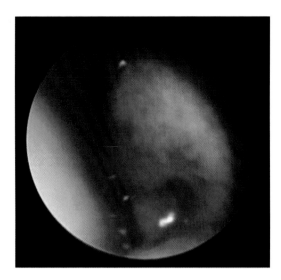

Fig. 11.20 Left nasolacrimal duct cyst in the inferior meatus as seen on anterior rhinoscopy

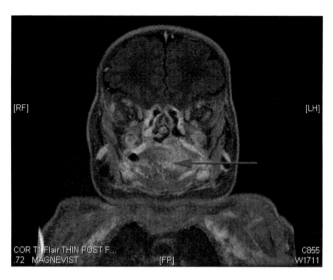

Fig. 11.21 Nasopharyngeal teratoma on coronal MRI with characteristic heterogeneous signal intensity

11

scan. The classic features evident on imaging are a dilated nasal lacrimal duct, an intranasal cyst, and cystic dilatation of the lacrimal sac [46].

Surgery is indicated for infants who have feeding problems, infection, and/or respiratory obstruction. The cyst is marsupialized endoscopically. This is best accomplished by a multidisciplinary team that includes an ophthalmologist who may need to perform nasolacrimal duct probing and possible placement of nasolacrimal duct stents.

Nasopharyngeal Teratomas

Teratomas are the most common germ cell tumors of childhood and are almost always benign. These lesions comprise representative tissues from each of three germ layers of the embryonic disc (ectoderm, endoderm, and mesoderm) and generally contain tissues foreign to the anatomic site of origin. It is thought that teratomas of the head and neck develop from foci of tissue that fail to follow normal embryonic development. These foci may be remnants of normal embryologic structures that break off or do not migrate along well-defined pathways to their normal destination [47].

Teratomas occurring in infancy and early childhood are generally extragonadal, whereas those presenting in older children more commonly occur in the ovary or testis [48]. These neoplasms are most commonly located in the sacrococcygeal region, followed by the ovaries, testes, anterior mediastinum, retroperitoneum, and the head and neck, which accounts for less than 5% of all neonatal teratomas. These rare neoplasms, which reportedly occur in 1 in 20,000 to 40,000 live births, may

be located in the brain, orbit, oropharynx, nasopharynx, or cervical region. The nasopharynx is the second most common site in the head.

Nasopharyngeal teratomas may be sessile or pedunculated and often protrude through the mouth. Anencephaly, hemicrania, and palatal fissures are associated with these lesions. Maternal clinical characteristics may include polyhydramnios due to impaired swallowing and elevated α-fetoprotein levels. Larger lesions are often diagnosed by prenatal ultrasound. This enables planning for an EXIT (ex utero intrapartum treatment) procedure to secure an infant's airway prior to division of the maternal–fetal circulation. The newborn usually presents with severe acute respiratory distress requiring endotracheal intubation or tracheostomy. In patients with smaller lesions, feeding difficulties may be the only presenting symptom [49].

Fine needle aspiration may be used to assist in establishing the diagnosis [49] and imaging can confirm the diagnosis. Lesions present as cystic and solid areas of fat density on CT and MRI (Fig. 11.21). There may be areas of bone and tooth formation. Most nasopharyngeal teratomas usually have no intracranial connections and are well encapsulated. They can be excised through a transoral approach with or without endoscopic assistance. This approach may require splitting of the soft palate or palatal resection. Endoscopic assistance may obviate the need for palatal division or resection [47]. External approaches using a Weber-Ferguson incision or a transcervical incision are also used. If an intracranial component exists, a craniofacial approach is necessary. Outcomes are generally successful and α-fetoprotein levels are periodically measured to monitor recurrence.

References

1. Hengerer AS WR. Congenital Abnormalities of the Nose and Paranasal Sinuses, 4 ed. Philadelphia: Saunders, 2002:4099–4115
2. Brown K RK, Brown OE. Congenital Malformations of the Nose, 4 ed. Philadelphia: Elsevier Mosby, 2005:4099–4109
3. Keeling JW, Hansen BF, Kjaer I. Pattern of malformations in the axial skeleton in human trisomy 21 fetuses. *Am J Med Genet* 1997;68:466–471
4. Sedano HO, Cohen MM, Jr., Jirasek J, Gorlin RJ. Frontonasal dysplasia. *J Pediatr* 1970;76:906–913
5. Silva A SJ. Congenital Malformations of the Nose and Paranasal Sinuses, 1 ed. San Diego: Singular, 1999:381–391
6. Rahbar R, Resto VA, Robson CD, et al. Nasal glioma and encephalocele: diagnosis and management. *Laryngoscope* 2003;113:2069–2077
7. Puppala B, Mangurten HH, McFadden J, Lygizos N, Taxy J, Pellettiere E. Nasal glioma. Presenting as neonatal respiratory distress. Definition of the tumor mass by MRI. *Clin Pediatr (Phila)* 1990;29:49–52
8. Bradley PJ, Singh SD. Nasal glioma. *J Laryngol Otol* 1985;99:247–252
9. Burckhardt W, Tobon D. Endoscopic approach to nasal glioma. *Otolaryngol Head Neck Surg* 1999;120:747–748
10. Yokoyama M, Inouye N, Mizuno F. Endoscopic management of nasal glioma in infancy. *Int J Pediatr Otorhinolaryngol* 1999;51:51–54
11. Van Den Abbeele T, Elmaleh M, Herman P, Francois M, Narcy P. Transnasal endoscopic repair of congenital defects of the skull base in children. *Arch Otolaryngol Head Neck Surg* 1999;125:580–584
12. Rahbar R, Shah P, Mulliken JB, et al. The presentation and management of nasal dermoid: a 30-year experience. *Arch Otolaryngol Head Neck Surg* 2003;129:464–471
13. Pratt LW. Midline Cysts of the Nasal Dorsum: Embryologic Origin and Treatment. *Laryngoscope* 1965;75:968–980
14. Bradley PJ. The complex nasal dermoid. *Head Neck Surg* 1983;5:469–473
15. Pensler JM, Bauer BS, Naidich TP. Craniofacial dermoids. *Plast Reconstr Surg* 1988;82:953–958
16. Pollock RA. Surgical approaches to the nasal dermoid cyst. *Ann Plast Surg* 1983;10:498–501
17. Sessions RB. Nasal dermal sinuses – new concepts and explanations. *Laryngoscope* 1982;92:1–28
18. Posnick JC, Bortoluzzi P, Armstrong DC, Drake JM. Intracranial nasal dermoid sinus cysts: computed tomographic scan findings and surgical results. *Plast Reconstr Surg* 1994;93:745–754; discussion 755–756
19. Shino M, Chikamatsu K, Yasuoka Y, Nagai K, Furuya N. Congenital arhinia: a case report and functional evaluation. *Laryngoscope* 2005;115:1118–1123
20. Kjaer I, Keeling JW, Fischer Hansen B. Pattern of malformations in the axial skeleton in human trisomy 13 fetuses. *Am J Med Genet* 1997;70:421–426
21. Albernaz VS, Castillo M, Mukherji SK, Ihmeidan IH. Congenital arhinia. *AJNR Am J Neuroradiol* 1996;17:1312–1314
22. Ozek C, Gundogan H, Bilkay U, et al. A case of total nasal agenesis accompanied by Tessier no. 30 cleft. *Ann Plast Surg* 2001;46:663–664
23. Ming JE, Muenke M. Holoprosencephaly: from Homer to Hedgehog. *Clin Genet* 1998;53:155–163
24. DeMyer W. The median cleft face syndrome. Differential diagnosis of cranium bifidum occultum, hypertelorism, and median cleft nose, lip, and palate. *Neurology* 1967;17:961–971
25. Demyer W, Zeman W, Palmer CD. Familial Alobar Holoprosencephaly (Arhinencephaly) with Median Cleft Lip and Palate. Report of Patient with 46 Chromosomes. *Neurology* 1963;13:913–918
26. Tessier P. Anatomical classification facial, cranio-facial and latero-facial clefts. *J Maxillofac Surg* 1976;4:69–92
27. Van der Meulen JC, Mazzola R, Vermey-Keers C, Stricker M, Raphael B. A morphogenetic classification of craniofacial malformations. *Plast Reconstr Surg* 1983;71:560–572
28. Williams A, Pizzuto M, Brodsky L, Perry R. Supernumerary nostril: a rare congenital deformity. *Int J Pediatr Otorhinolaryngol* 1998;44:161–167
29. Nakamura K, Onizuka T. A case of supernumerary nostril. *Plast Reconstr Surg* 1987;80:436–441
30. Madorsky SJ, Wang TD. Unilateral cleft rhinoplasty: a review. *Otolaryngol Clin North Am* 1999;32:669–682
31. Brown OE, Pownell P, Manning SC. Choanal atresia: a new anatomic classification and clinical management applications. *Laryngoscope* 1996;106:97–101
32. Harner SG, McDonald TJ, Reese DF. The anatomy of congenital choanal atresia. *Otolaryngol Head Neck Surg* 1981;89:7–9
33. Brown OE, Smith T, Armstrong E, Grundfast K. The evaluation of choanal atresia by computed tomography. *Int J Pediatr Otorhinolaryngol* 1986;12:85–98
34. Pirsig W. Surgery of choanal atresia in infants and children: historical notes and updated review. *Int J Pediatr Otorhinolaryngol* 1986;11:153–170
35. Samadi DS, Shah UK, Handler SD. Choanal atresia: a twenty-year review of medical comorbidities and surgical outcomes. *Laryngoscope* 2003;113:254–258
36. Leclerc JE, Fearon B. Choanal atresia and associated anomalies. *Int J Pediatr Otorhinolaryngol* 1987;13:265–272
37. Crockett DM, Healy GB, McGill TJ, Friedman EM. Computed tomography in the evaluation of choanal atresia in infants and children. *Laryngoscope* 1987;97:174–183
38. Derkay CS, Grundfast KM. Airway compromise from nasal obstruction in neonates and infants. *Int J Pediatr Otorhinolaryngol* 1990;19:241–249
39. Ey EH, Han BK, Towbin RB, Jaun WK. Bony inlet stenosis as a cause of nasal airway obstruction. *Radiology* 1988;168:477–479
40. Manning SC, Bloom DC, Perkins JA, Gruss JS, Inglis A. Diagnostic and surgical challenges in the pediatric skull base. *Otolaryngol Clin North Am* 2005;38:773–794
41. Kubba H, Bennett A, Bailey CM. An update on choanal atresia surgery at Great Ormond Street Hospital for Children: preliminary results with Mitomycin C and the KTP laser. *Int J Pediatr Otorhinolaryngol* 2004;68:939–945
42. Brown OE, Myer CM, 3rd, Manning SC. Congenital nasal pyriform aperture stenosis. *Laryngoscope* 1989;99:86–91

43. Van Den Abbeele T, Triglia JM, Francois M, Narcy P. Congenital nasal pyriform aperture stenosis: diagnosis and management of 20 cases. *Ann Otol Rhinol Laryngol* 2001;110:70–75

44. Belden CJ, Mancuso AA, Schmalfuss IM. CT features of congenital nasal piriform aperture stenosis: initial experience. *Radiology* 1999;213:495–501

45. Arlis H, Ward RF. Congenital nasal pyriform aperture stenosis. Isolated abnormality vs developmental field defect. *Arch Otolaryngol Head Neck Surg* 1992;118:989–991

46. Tabor MH, Desai KR, Respler DS. Symptomatic bilateral nasolacrimal duct cysts in a newborn. *Ear Nose Throat J* 2003;82:90–92

47. Kountakis SE, Minotti AM, Maillard A, Stiernberg CM. Teratomas of the head and neck. *Am J Otolaryngol* 1994;15:292–296

48. Azizkhan RG, Caty MG. Teratomas in childhood. *Curr Opin Pediatr* 1996;8:287–292

49. April MM, Ward RF, Garelick JM. Diagnosis, management, and follow-up of congenital head and neck teratomas. *Laryngoscope* 1998;108:1398–1401

50. Sadler TW. Head and neck embryology. In Langmans's medical. Edn 6, Baltimore,1990, Williams & Wilkins

Chapter 12

Contemporary Management Strategies for Epistaxis

12

Seth J. Kanowitz, Martin J. Citardi, and Pete S. Batra

Core Messages

- Thorough knowledge of the nasal vascular anatomy is paramount for the evaluation and management of epistaxis.
- Multiple factors including local trauma, systemic processes, and medications can contribute to the development of epistaxis.
- Nasal endoscopy is important for accurate diagnosis and effective management of epistaxis of moderate or greater severity.
- Imaging is reserved for special circumstances in patients with maxillofacial trauma and suspected sinonasal neoplasms.
- Mild anterior epistaxis may be controlled with chemical cautery. Moderate to severe anterior epistaxis may require monopolar or bipolar cautery under headlight or endoscopic visualization.
- With the evolution of advanced endoscopic techniques and better appreciation of endoscopic anatomy of the sphenopalatine artery (SPA), transnasal endoscopic SPA ligation (TESPAL) has replaced more traditional surgical approaches such as internal maxillary artery ligation via an extended Caldwell-Luc approach.
- Transarterial embolization of epistaxis remains useful in selected indications (including failed surgical intervention, sinonasal neoplasm, major vascular injury, and vascular malformations).
- External anterior and/or posterior ethmoid artery ligation may be required in special circumstances.

Contents

Introduction

Estimates suggest that 45.2 million people in the United States, or 15.8% of the population, will suffer from 394.6 million incidents of epistaxis annually [3]. Epistaxis accounts for more than 450,000 emergency room visits and 27,000 hospitalizations per year [24]. Epistaxis can span the spectrum ranging from a mere nuisance to a life-threatening emergency. Clearly, most episodes are self-limited and never come to the attention of a physician. However, when more significant bleeding is encountered, the otorhinolaryngologist must implement multiple surgical and nonsurgical maneuvers and integrate these measures into a logical algorithm for the successful treatment of epistaxis.

Nasal Vascular Anatomy

The mucosa of the nasal cavity receives terminal branches from the internal and external carotid arteries with numerous anastomoses between these systems. A thorough understanding of this vascular anatomy is paramount in developing a stepwise approach to the management of epistaxis.

External Carotid Artery System

The external carotid sends two major branches to the nasal cavity: the internal maxillary artery (IMA) and the facial artery.

The IMA travels between the mandibular ramus and the sphenomandibular ligament, either deep or superficial to the lateral pterygoid musculature. It then enters the pterygomaxillary fossa (PMF) and divides into its terminal branches: the sphenopalatine, descending palatine, pharyngeal, pterygoid canal, infraorbital, and posterior superior alveolar arteries. Within this space, the IMA is located within a fat pad and usually more anteroinferior to the vidian and maxillary nerves (Fig. 12.1). The sphenopalatine artery (SPA) gains access to the nasal cavity through the sphenopalatine foramen located along the lateral nasal wall at the junction of the inferior portion of the middle turbinate basal lamella and the medial orbital wall in the region of the crista ethmoidalis. The SPA then divides into the lateral nasal artery, which supplies the lateral nasal wall, and the posterior septal nasal artery, which courses medially over the sphenoid face to supply the corresponding portion of the nasal septum. The descending palatine branch of the IMA supplies the anterior nasal septum and floor of the nose by descending through the greater palatine canal as the greater palatine artery, traveling anteriorly along the lateral hard palate to re-enter the nasal cavity through the midline incisive foramen.

After emerging from the substance of the submandibular gland just deep to the platysma muscle, the facial artery travels obliquely toward the corner of the lip from the lateral aspect of the angle of the mandible. As it reaches the lip, the artery divides into the inferior and superior labial arteries, and then courses superiorly within the nasofacial crease as the angular artery. The superior labial artery sends small branches to supply the nasal vestibule and anterior nasal septum.

Internal Carotid Artery System

The internal carotid artery supplies two terminal branches to the nasal cavity. Both the anterior and posterior ethmoid arteries arise from the ophthalmic artery, the first branch of the internal carotid artery, within the orbit. After exiting the orbit through the suture line of the medial orbital wall, they enter their respective canals and course medially through the ethmoid roof. The anterior ethmoid artery may actually lie 1–3 mm below the roof in a mesentery [24]. The arteries then enter the anterior cranial fossa into the olfactory sulcus at the junction of the eth-

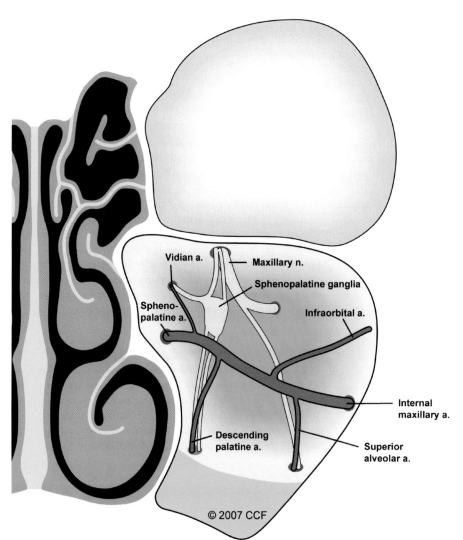

Fig. 12.1 Coronal view of the left pterygomaxillary space demonstrating the internal maxillary artery and its branches. Note the sphenopalatine ganglion and its branches more posteriorly

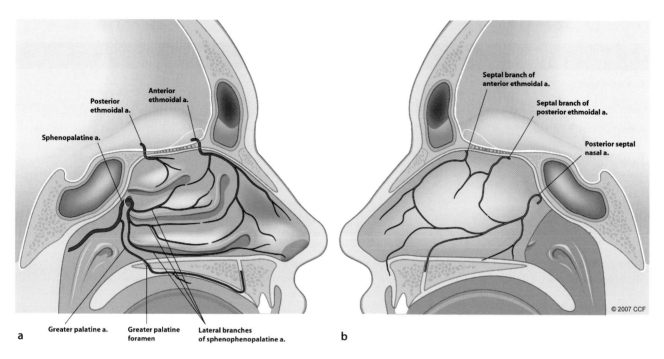

a

Sphenopalatine a.

Posterior
ethmoidal a.

Anterior
ethmoidal a.

Greater palatine a.   Greater palatine
foramen   Lateral branches
of sphenophenopalatine a.

b

Septal branch of
anterior ethmoidal a.

Septal branch of
posterior ethmoidal a.

Posterior septal
nasal a.

© 2007 CCF

Fig. 12.2 **a** Sagittal view of the lateral nasal wall demonstrates the branching pattern of the sphenopalatine, anterior ethmoid, and posterior ethmoid arteries. **b** Sagittal view of the nasal septum demonstrates the branching pattern of the posterior septal, anterior ethmoid, and posterior ethmoid arteries

moid roof and the cribriform plate, only to re-enter the nose via small branches within the cribriform plate. These small terminal branches divide into lateral and septal components. The anterior ethmoid artery is the major blood supply for the lateral and anterior one-third of the nasal cavity, while the posterior ethmoid artery supplies only a small portion of the superior turbinate and adjacent posterior septum (Fig. 12.2).

In up to 31% of cadaver dissections, the posterior ethmoid artery was noted to be absent, while the anterior ethmoid artery was only absent in 10% of cases [17]. The average distance from the anterior lacrimal crest to the anterior ethmoid artery foramen was 18 mm, with the posterior ethmoid foramen located 10 mm more posterior. The posterior ethmoid artery can lie 1–2 mm anterior to the optic nerve.

Little's Area, Kisselbach's Plexus, and Woodruff's Plexus

The confluence of vessels along the anterior nasal septum is known as Kisselbach's plexus, located within Little's area. This area receives vascular supply from the septal branches of the SPA, greater palatine artery, anterior ethmoid artery, and superior labial artery. Consequently, this area represents an anastamotic highway between the internal and external carotid artery systems.

Woodruff's plexus, known as the naso-nasopharyngeal plexus, is located at the posterior 1 cm of the nasal floor, in-

ferior meatus, and middle meatus. This plexus also extends to the vertical strip of mucosa anterior to the eustachian tube cartilage and mucosa lateral and superior to the posterior choana covering the adjacent sphenoid rostrum. Along its inferior extent, it anastomoses with the pharyngeal branches of the IMA [25]

Pathophysiology

Local and Iatrogenic Factors

Injury to or manipulation of the delicate mucosal lining of the nose may induce epistaxis. Simple anterior epistaxis from the septum, in the absence of recent surgery, is usually due to local irritation or dryness leading to mucosal breakdown and vessel wall compromise. If the local irritation is sustained or significant, the perichondrium may become compromised, leading to necrosis of the underlying cartilage and subsequent perforation. If surgery has been performed, or the nasal cavity has been manipulated (i.e., nasal intubation, nasogastric tube, illicit drug use, maxillofacial trauma), more significant bleeding may occur from the arteries in the posterior nasal cavity or lateral nasal wall. A history of persistent or recurrent epistaxis, in the absence of an obvious source, should lead to a work-up for sinonasal neoplasms. A list of common local factors causing epistaxis is provided for reference (Table 12.1).

Table 12.1 Local and systemic factors causing epistaxis

Local factors	Systemic factors
Digital trauma	Medications (acetylsalicylic acid, NSAIDS,
Dry air	warfarin, heparin, vitamin E)
Nasal sprays (decongestants, topical	Supplements (garlic, gingko, ginseng, fish oil,
steroids, topical antihistamines)	cod liver oil, saw palmetto)
Nasal oxygen cannula	Blood dyscrasias (acquired or hereditary)
Nasal CPAP	Hematologic malignancies
Nasal intubation/nasal airway	Platelet dysfunction and thrombocytopenia ($<20,000/mm^3$)
Nasogastric tube	Cardiovascular (increased venous pressure from
Drugs (cocaine, heroin)	congestive heart failure or mitral valve prolapse, hypertension)
Tobacco (cigarette smoke, snuff)	Collagen vascular disorders
Facial trauma (maxillofacial, nasal)	Vitamin A,D,C,E, or K deficiency
Chemical and environmental irritants (pollution)	Malnutrition
Inflammatory disease (rhinitis, sinusitis, pyogenic granuloma)	Alcohol use
Granulomatous disease	Liver failure (chronic or acute)
Structural deformity (septal spurs and perforations	Chronic renal failure and uremia
leading to turbulent nasal airflow)	
Surgery (rhinoplasty, septoplasty, sinus,	
turbinoplasty, midface, skull base)	
Nasal and sinus neoplasms	

Systemic Factors

Interference with the normal coagulation cascade, collagen defects leading to impaired vessel wall integrity, or cardiovascular derangements leading to increased arterial and venous pressure and/or vessel wall damage may manifest as epistaxis in view of the delicate homeostatic balance within the nasal cavity. Hereditary coagulation deficits, such as von Willebrand disease (vWD) and hemophilia, and congenital blood vessel defects, such as hereditary hemorrhagic telangiectasia (HHT; Osler-Weber-Rendu disease), may cause lifelong epistaxis requiring multiple treatment modalities and/or transfusions. Systemic diseases, medications, or nutritional derangements leading to impaired platelet function or coagulopathies may also cause isolated, recurrent, or persistent episodes of epistaxis. Disorders of platelet metabolism and the use of medications that inhibit platelet aggregation may also predispose to epistaxis. A list of common systemic factors causing epistaxis is provided for reference (Table 12.1).

Patient Evaluation

History

A focused history and physical examination is crucial prior to initiating treatment of epistaxis. Basic historical information can be gathered from the patient, family, or the medical chart;

the information outlined in Table 12.1 can serve as a frame of reference. Duration and severity of the current episode, history of previous epistaxis, history of sinonasal and/or skull base surgery, and history of maxillofacial trauma will help determine the severity of the bleeding. Other important historical factors, including nasal obstruction, visual changes, maxillary hypo-/anesthesia, facial asymmetry, or loose teeth should be queried to evaluate for a sinonasal tumor. General medical history, current medications and supplements, and overall medical condition of the patient will also help dictate the management strategy. Family history of bleeding diathesis may be suggestive of an underlying coagulopathy.

Physical Examination

An orderly physical examination ensues after gathering preliminary historical information. Identification of the bleeding source, either with anterior rhinoscopy (see section "Anterior Epistaxis, Mild") or formal nasal endoscopy (see section "Anterior Epistaxis, Moderate to Severe") is paramount in the management of these patients. Indiscriminate nasal packing, especially with nonabsorbable types, should be avoided as this tends to traumatize the nasal mucosa, cause significant patient discomfort, and create new areas of bleeding upon packing removal. Prior to beginning the examination, all necessary equipment should be made available (see Tables 12.2, 12.3). The patient should be positioned upright, preferably in an ENT examination chair if feasible. Universal precautions should be employed and the patient should be draped and provided with an emesis basin.

A complete head and neck examination is necessary to look for diagnostic clues associated with epistaxis (i.e., extraocular muscle restriction, proptosis, or visual disturbance as a result of sinonasal malignancy; petechiae from blood dyscrasias; te-langiectasias from HHT; unilateral middle ear effusion from nasopharyngeal carcinoma). These steps in the physical examination may need to be deferred in patients with active and/or severe epistaxis, and can be performed after the epistaxis is addressed. The oropharynx should be inspected with a tongue blade; the absence of fresh blood within the pharynx indicates that the bleeding source is likely anterior.

Table 12.2 Equipment for epistaxis evaluation and management

Equipment	Medications
Universal protective gear (face shield, mask, gloves, and gown)	0.05% oxymetazoline or 0.5% to 1% phenylephrine
Patient gown and emesis basin	4% lidocaine (xylocaine) for topical application
Headlight and endoscopic light source	1% lidocaine with 1:100,000 epinephrine
Nasal speculums	10-cc sterile water vials
Suction with Frazier tip suctions (8, 10, 12 Fr)	Bacitracin ointment
0 and 30° 4-mm rigid nasal endoscopes	Nasal saline spray
Bipolar cautery	
Supplies	**Absorbable nasal packing**
Silver nitrate sticks	Absorbable hemostatic agents (see Table 12.3)
Cottonoids or cotton	
Tongue blade	
Hemostat or IV tubing clamp	
3- and 10-cc syringes	
18- and 25-gauge needles	
	Non-absorbable nasal packing
	4-, 8- and 10-cm expandable nasal tampon sponges (Merocel® Medtronic Xomed, Jacksonville, FL, USA)
	72×0.5 in petrolatum gauze
	12-Fr Foley catheter with 30-cc balloon
	Telfa® (Kendall, Mansfield, MA, USA)
	Tonsil sponges
	Epistat® (Medtronic Xomed, Jacksonville, FL, USA)
	Rapid Rhino® (ArthroCare ENT, Sunnyvale, CA, USA)

Table 12.3 Absorbable hemostatic agents

Type (comments]	Mode of action	Absorption time	Bactericidal
Porcine gelatin Gelfoam® (Pharmacia & Up-john, Kalamazoo, MI, USA; can expand 200% its initial volume Surgifoam™ (Johnson & Johnson, New Brunswick, NJ, USA; can be mixed with thrombin or saline) Surgiflo™ (Johnson & Johnson Ethicon, New Brunswick, NJ, USA; can be mixed with thrombin or saline)	Mostly mechanical; absorbs many times its weight (×40–45)	4–6 weeks; liquefies 2–5 days in mucosa	No
Oxidized cellulose Oxycel™ (Becton & Dickinson Franklin Lakes, NJ, USA) Surgicel™ (Johnson & Johnson, New Brunswick, NJ, USA) Surgicel Fibrillar™ (Johnson & Johnson Ethicon, New Brunswick, NJ, USA)	Blood bonds with oxidized regenerated cellulose forming an artificial clot; provides surface for fibrin polymerization; effects on clotting cascade largely unknown	1–2 weeks	Yes
Bovine collagen Avitene® (C.R. Bard, Murray Hill, NJ, USA) Collastat™ (Xemax Surgical Products, Napa, CA, USA) Instat™ (Johnson & Johnson Ethicon, New Brunswick, NJ, USA) Helistat® (Integra, Plainsboro, NJ, USA)	Causes platelet aggregation and adhesion	8+ weeks	No
Bovine thrombin and bovine gelatin Floseal™ (Baxter, Deerfield, IL, USA)	Thrombin converts fibrinogen into fibrin monomers, which polymerize to form a reinforced fibrin clot; gelatinous granules restrict blood flow and deliver thrombin to the area; swells 20%	6–8 weeks; grossly within 5–7 days in mucosa	No

12

Laboratory and Radiographic Evaluation

Laboratory work-up is individualized based on the clinical scenario at hand. Laboratory values (complete blood count, coagulation panel, hepatic panel, metabolic panel, bleeding time, blood alcohol level, urine drug panel) may help to identify confounding factors. Radiographic imaging is generally reserved for special circumstances. Computed tomography is indicated in patients with suspected sinonasal neoplasms and maxillofacial trauma. Angiography is warranted in patients with suspected major vascular injury, vascular neoplasms, arteriovascular malformations, and failed surgical interventions.

Management

Anterior Epistaxis, Mild

Anterior epistaxis refers to bleeding that can either be visualized in the anterior aspect of the nasal cavity or controlled with anterior nasal packing. For cases of mild epistaxis, anterior nasal cavity (septum and inferior turbinate head) should be inspected bilaterally with a headlight and nasal speculum. Any clots should be removed as they may obscure any obvious sites of bleeding. Topical decongestion and anesthesia should be applied with an atomizer, on cottonoids, or wisps of cotton. If an obvious bleeding site is identified anteriorly, chemical cautery with silver nitrate can be applied and will generally suffice in cases of mild bleeding. Absorbable gelatin sponge (Gelfoam®; Pharmacia & Upjohn, Kalamazoo, MI, USA) as well as other hemostatic agents (Table 12.2) may be applied over the cauterization site to minimize risk of rebleeding; the application of antibiotic ointment (Bacitracin, Pharmacia & Upjohn; others) helps to promote mucosal healing and to prevent crusting. If an obvious source is not readily identifiable anteriorly, then diagnostic nasal endoscopy is warranted for more detailed nasal evaluation (see section "Anterior Epistaxis, Moderate to Severe"). Even if an apparently obvious source of bleeding is seen during anterior rhinoscopy, formal diagnostic endoscopy may be warranted to confirm the absence of other bleeding sources.

The patient should be instructed to refrain from anticoagulants for 7–10 days (if not medically contraindicated), to avoid strenuous activity, nose blowing or picking, and dry heat, and to utilize nasal saline spray. They should also be counseled regarding the likelihood of expectorating blood clots as the pharynx may collect large quantities of blood during bleeding episodes. This helps to prevent frantic phone calls and unnecessary trips back to the emergency room.

Anterior Epistaxis, Moderate to Severe

For cases of moderate to severe epistaxis, formal diagnostic nasal endoscopy is imperative to successfully identify and control the source of bleeding. Topical decongestion and anesthesia should be applied with an atomizer, on cottonoids, or wisps of cotton. In cases of significant epistaxis that precludes endoscopic visualization, a transoral greater palatine foramen block can be helpful in reducing the bleeding.

Nasal endoscopy is performed in a systematic fashion with a 4.0-mm 30° rigid telescope. The entire nasal cavity is carefully examined for areas of bleeding. The septum, turbinates, middle meatus, and spheno-ethmoid recess should be evaluated for areas of bleeding or potential masses [2]. Particular attention should be given to the sphenopalatine region and Woodruff's plexus in the posterior nasal cavity. Bleeding from the superior nasal cavity without an obvious source may be secondary to anterior ethmoid artery bleeding.

Once the bleeding area is identified, the area should be injected submucosally with 1% lidocaine with 1:100,000 epinephrine. This will help reduce bleeding and will allow for better tolerance of cauterization. Silver nitrate cautery is inadequate for moderate to severe epistaxis and will likely result in recurrent epistaxis and the need for additional procedures. Bipolar electrical cautery, such as Bifrazier™ suction bipolar cautery (Surgical Laser Technologies, Montgomeryville, PA, USA) and Landolt cautery™ (Aesculap, Center Valley, PA, USA), targeted at the site of bleeding, will generally allow for successful control of epistaxis, even in cases of brisk bleeding. Unipolar cautery should be avoided as the transmitted heat to surrounding tissues may cause unnecessary tissue trauma and patient discomfort. This strategy is appropriate for cooperative and stable patients who are able to tolerate office evaluation. In patients unable to tolerate office treatment or deemed medically unstable, the endoscopic examination and cautery can be performed in the operating room under general or monitored care anesthesia.

Often patients presenting with significant epistaxis have undergone previous cautery and packing placement and may be noted to have diffuse local trauma and oozing from the nasal tissues. In these cases, indiscriminate cautery should be avoided and only areas of actual bleeding should be cauterized. In addition, if bipolar electrical cautery is unavailable, placement of nasal packing is appropriate. Both traditional non-absorbable packing (Table 12.2) and absorbable hemostatic agents (Table 12.3) may be used, though absorbable packing is preferred as this will avoid additional iatrogenic trauma from packing removal.

Medically and hemodynamically stable patients can be discharged with the same basic instructions outlined above. Patients with medical comorbidities, especially if deemed to be at high risk of rebleeding, should be monitored in the hospital setting for a minimum of overnight observation.

Posterior Epistaxis

A posterior source may be the culprit in up to 20% of patients with epistaxis [26]. Posterior epistaxis refers to bleeding that occurs in the area of Woodruff's plexus, the SPA, or any bleeding that fails to stop with routine anterior nasal packing. Bleeding in these cases can often stem from an arterial source, such as the sphenopalatine artery or anterior and/or posterior ethmoid artery. Bleeding can be quite severe and may result in significant hemodynamic changes. Aggressive management is imperative in these cases.

Posterior Nasal Packing

Posterior nasal packing refers to an anteroposterior (AP) pack rather than a posterior pack in isolation. The posterior pack is used as a buttress within the nasopharynx for the anterior pack. The AP pack tampanodes the vessels of the anterior and posterior nasal cavity. A 12-Fr Foley catheter with a 30-cc balloon or gauze (2×2s or tonsil balls) is employed for this purpose. Other options include dual balloon epistaxis devices (such as Epistat®; Medtronic Xomed, Jacksonville, FL, USA; Rapid Rhino®; Arthrocare ENT, Sunnyvale, CA, USA). The Foley catheter is placed through the nose, and the balloon is inflated with 5–15 cc of sterile water after adequate visualization. The balloon is tugged back into the nasopharynx, so it ideally abuts the posterior choana. Both nasal cavities are usually packed with petrolatum gauze; alternatively, absorbable packing may be utilized to pack both nasal cavities. The Foley catheter is then secured anteriorly using a G-tube or umbilical clamp. The clamp should never be allowed to rest against the nasal ala to prevent necrosis. Patients are routinely placed on antibiotic therapy to protect against the theoretical risk of toxic shock syndrome from *Staphylococcus aureus* enterotoxins [7]. Patients are then admitted for observation with continuous cardiopulmonary monitoring and supplemental oxygen. Patients with multiple co-morbidities are best managed in the intensive care unit (ICU) setting.

The packs are usually left in place for 3–5 days. When the patient has stabilized, the Foley is deflated and the patient is observed for signs of bleeding. If no bleeding is noted, the Foley can be removed and non-absorbable packing can be removed within 24 h. Alternatively, if absorbable packing is used, this can be left in place and may avoid additional trauma from removal of non-absorbable packing.

Published reviews have demonstrated a 38% failure rate from posterior packing, though rates as high as 52% have been reported [18, 26]. Additionally, posterior nasal packing has its own set of inherent morbidities and potential for mortality, with a complication rate of 20% cited in the literature [30]. Technical issues with insertion, mucosal tearing, failure of the balloon to deflate, alar necrosis, oroantral fistula, otitis media, respiratory obstruction, local infection, poor oral intake leading to malnutrition, aspiration, sleep apnea, significant pain and discomfort, and cardiopulmonary compromise have all been reported [5, 12, 30, 32]. Cardiopulmonary compromise from the presence of an ill-defined nasopulmonary reflex is controversial [11, 14, 16, 20]. More likely, hypoxemia and hypoventilation result from worsening of underlying cardiopulmonary disease due to sedation, aspiration, and possible airway obstruction.

With the advent of endoscopic techniques for the management of epistaxis and the associated risks of posterior packing, this is generally reserved for special circumstances. Patients with profuse bleeding may be temporized with posterior packing until more definitive surgical management can be employed. Patients with multiple co-morbidities may be poor candidates for general anesthesia and thus may be managed with posterior pack placement.

Internal Maxillary Artery Ligation

Originally described by Sieffert in 1928 and then reintroduced by Chandler and Sierens in the 1960s, IMA ligation was popularized by Montgomery in the 1970s. Although IMA ligation has been the workhorse for management of refractory posterior epistaxis for decades, the procedure is now infrequently used. The gingivobuccal approach to the PMF is the preferred method. Prior to performing this approach, a paranasal sinus CT scan should be obtained to verify that the maxillary sinus is aerated and to document the relative position of the orbital floor.

The canine fossa is first identified and the surrounding mucosa is infiltrated with local anesthetic. A standard 3- to 4-cm sublabial incision is made with a healthy cuff of tissue along the gingiva for later closure. The periosteum is incised and superior dissection of the soft tissues ensues off the maxilla until the infraorbital neurovascular bundle is identified. Next, the maxillary sinus is entered just above the canine fossa using a 4-mm osteotome. Kerrison rongeurs are used to enlarge the opening. The remainder of the procedure is then performed under the operating microscope (300-mm lens) or loupes for magnification. The posterior wall of the maxillary sinus is identified and a laterally based mucosal flap is created. The posterior bony wall is

removed in a similar fashion and the fat pad of the PMF is gently explored. The IMA tends to be tortuous and more anteriorly and inferiorly based then the corresponding PMF nerves. After identification and isolation of the vessels with a nerve hook, medium sized vascular clips are applied. The SPA and descending palatine artery should also be clipped to prevent bleeding from collateral vessels. Nasal packing is then removed and the nasal cavity is inspected for any signs of bleeding. If bleeding persists, then the integrity and placement of the vascular clips should be confirmed. If refractory epistaxis persists despite successful IMA ligation, an ipsilateral anterior and posterior ethmoid artery ligation should be performed. The mucosal flap is replaced and the sublabial incision closed with absorbable suture material at the conclusion of the procedure.

Traditionally, IMA ligation has fared well in controlling posterior epistaxis, with re-bleed rates of 10–15% reported in the literature [23, 29]. Most failures are due to technical errors and the inability to adequately identify and clip the IMA [23]. Complications from IMA ligation include facial numbness or hypoesthesia, cranial nerve palsies, epiphora, damage to tooth roots, oroantral fistulae, sinusitis, orbital penetration, and blindness [6]. The advances in the endoscopic techniques and relative availability of angiography, coupled with the associated potential morbidity of the procedure, have limited the use of traditional IMA ligation. Nevertheless, the technique should be part of the surgical armamentarium in instances where endoscopic instrumentation or angiographic facilities are not readily available.

Transnasal Endoscopic Sphenopalatine Artery Ligation

With the evolution of the advanced endoscopic techniques and enhanced knowledge of the nasal vascular anatomy, transnasal endoscopic sphenopalatine artery ligation (TESPAL) is now the preferred method of treatment for intractable, posterior epistaxis. TESPAL combines the advantages of IMA ligation (mainly control of the terminal blood supply) with the advantages of a minimally invasive endoscopic approach. By controlling the SPA as it enters the nose through the sphenopalatine foramen, additional collateral blood flow to the nasal cavity via the SPA is addressed and the multiple branching patterns of the IMA and nerves in the PMF are avoided.

The procedure is performed under general anesthesia. Informed consent should also be obtained for concomitant anterior/posterior ethmoid artery ligation, if clinically dictated. Any nasal packing should be gently removed and the nose should be decongested with topical 0.05% oxymetazoline hydrochloride. The posterolateral insertion of the middle turbinate to the lateral nasal wall is identified and infiltrated with 1% lidocaine with 1:100,000 epinephrine, using a 22G spinal needle. An incision is made in the mucosa just anterior to the crista ethmoidalis of the palatine bone, which can be identified as a small ridge on the lateral nasal wall in this area. Maxillary antrostomy can also be performed to judge the depth of the posterior maxillary wall, but is usually unnecessary. A Cottle elevator or similar instrument is used to raise a medially based mucosal flap off the

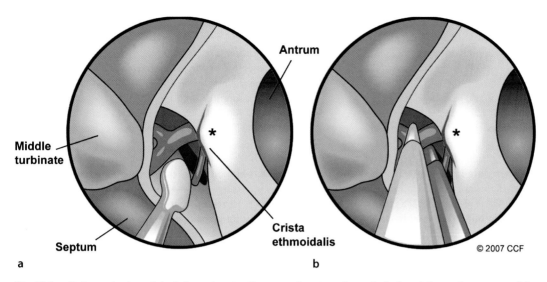

Middle turbinate

Antrum

*

Septum

Crista ethmoidalis

a

*

© 2007 CCF

b

Fig. 12.3 **a** Endoscopic view of the left nasal cavity illustrates elevation of a medially based flap with exposure of the sphenopalatine artery (SPA) and its associated branches. The crista ethmoidalis is an important landmark for identification of the SPA (*asterisk*). **b** Endoscopic view of the left nasal cavity demonstrating bipolar cautery of the SPA

lateral nasal wall (Fig. 12.3a). The SPA is identified as it leaves the sphenopalatine foramen and then carefully isolated with a ball-tipped seeker. The SPA and all associated terminal branches extending across the face of the sphenoid are carefully cauterized with bipolar cautery (Fig. 12.3b). Vascular clips are generally unnecessary, and their stability during future magnetic resonance imaging cannot be ensured. After resolution of the bleeding, the mucosal flap is repositioned and bolstered with small amount of absorbable packing. The patient is usually discharged home the following day, if medically stable.

The complications of TESPAL are similar to those of endoscopic sinus surgery. All patients should be counseled on the possibility of infection and potential intracranial and orbital complications. Crusting and synechiae formation may also be observed. Paresthesia of the palate and nose has also been reported [27].

In a recent review of the literature evaluating the efficacy of TESPAL, pooled data from 11 studies encompassing 127 patients yielded a success rate of 98% [19]. Other, more recent studies have demonstrated similar success [9, 15]. Furthermore, shorter hospital stays and a reduction in the associated medical costs compared with nonsurgical therapy have also been documented [18]. The success of the technique is dependent on the surgical expertise and knowledge of the nasal anatomy, as well as the availability of endoscopic equipment. The procedure is limited by the potential presence of profuse bleeding, which may severely compromise endoscopic visualization.

Anterior and Posterior Ethmoid Artery Ligation

An external anterior and posterior ethmoid artery ligation should be considered when the anterior and/or posterior ethmoid artery is suspected to be the source of bleeding. In addition, these procedures may serve as an important adjunct to

TESPAL and IMA ligation as the anterior ethmoid artery may reconstitute the blood supply to the nose in just a few days and may account for rebleeding episodes. This technique may also be necessary in cases of nasal and maxillofacial trauma where the artery may be lacerated or from arterial injury during endoscopic sinus surgery.

The ethmoid arteries are approached through a standard Lynch incision midway between the medial canthus and midline of the nasal dorsum. The angular vessels should be identified and ligated. After the medial canthal tendon is divided, the lacrimal fossa is identified and the lacrimal sac is gently retracted laterally out of the operative field. The fronto-ethmoid suture line is then visualized. The anterior ethmoid artery arises from the fronto-ethmoid suture line approximately 16 mm (range 14–18 mm) posterior to the anterior lacrimal crest. Two small vascular clips and/or bipolar cautery can be applied prior to division of the vessel. If posterior ethmoid artery ligation is clinically warranted, the artery is found approximately 10 mm posterior to the anterior ethmoid artery. Due to its close proximity to the optic nerve (1–2 mm), clipping or cautery of the posterior ethmoid artery should be carried out with extreme caution. The artery should not be divided given the potential risk of inadvertent injury to the optic nerve. Generally, posterior ethmoid artery ligation is not required, given the high success rates of TESPAL alone or TESPAL combined with anterior ethmoid artery ligation. Complications of external ethmoid artery ligation include scarring, telecanthus, damage to the lacrimal system, hypoesthesia, enophthalmos, orbital hematoma, and blindness.

Transnasal endoscopic ligation of the anterior ethmoid artery has been reported in the literature; however, the feasibility of this technique has recently been called into question [33]. In a cadaver study by Floreani et al., 66% of anterior ethmoid arteries could not be clipped endoscopically. In order for clipping to be effective, the artery had to lie in a bony mesentery, which only occurred in 36% of the cases. A Keros grade 2 or 3 skull base configuration was associated with the anterior ethmoid artery crossing the skull base in a bony mesentery [13].

Arterial Embolization

In 1974, Sokoloff and colleagues first described the technique of arterial embolization for intractable epistaxis in two patients [28]. Since this initial report, multiple studies have further validated this technique. The procedure is usually performed under local anesthesia via transfemoral catheterization. Bilateral external and carotid angiography is performed. If a clear source of bleeding is identified, it is embolized with either polyvinyl alcohol particles, platinum coils, or gelfoam particles. Particle sizes less than 200 μm are avoided, given the risk of migration into intracranial vessels and the potential for stroke [21]. Often a single, clear source of bleeding cannot be identified; bilateral IMA embolization is performed in these cases. Repeat angiography is then performed to assess the extent of embolization and the potential for collateral circulation.

Complications from embolization include groin and/or retroperitoneal hematoma, groin numbness, and femoral artery pseudo-aneurysm. Embolization may result in crusting, sinusitis, facial pain, or paresthesias. The most serious risks are associated with migration of the embolization particles and potential risks of cerebrovascular accident and ophthalmic artery occlusion and blindness. Christensen and colleagues reported 1 case of stroke in 70 patients [4]; Elden et al. reported stroke and central ophthalmic artery occlusion in 1 out of 97 cases [10]. Facial nerve palsy, temporary slough of the nasal tip, and soft tissue necrosis with facial atrophy have also been reported [1, 8, 22, 31].

In a recent review of the literature, Christensen and co-workers identified 23 case series totaling 731 patients [4]. The average success rate for selective embolization was 88% (range 71–100%), with a complication rate of 12% (range 0–50%). Seventy patients (13%) suffered from a major re-bleed within 6 weeks of the procedure. Andersen and colleagues have reported embolization in 22 patients (9 with HHT), with a failure rate of 20% in the HHT group and 13% in the remaining patients [1].

The ability to perform selective arterial embolization under local anesthesia, thus avoiding the risks of general anesthesia, makes this a desirable treatment option. The procedure can also be repeated if hemorrhage recurs. It is especially useful in the medically unstable patient, in vascular malformations, large sinonasal malignancies requiring preoperative or palliative vascular control, and after craniofacial trauma, where normal surgical anatomy may be severely distorted.

References

1. Andersen PJ, Kjeldsen AD, Nepper-Rasmussen J (2005) Selective embolization in the treatment of intractable epistaxis. Acta Oto-Laryngologica 125:293–297
2. Batra PS (2006) The role of endoscopy in the allergist's office. Curr Allergy Asthma Rep 6:228–231.
3. Benninger MS, Marple BF (2004) Minor recurrent epistaxis: prevalence and a new method for management. Otolaryngol Head Neck Surg 131:317–320
4. Christensen NP, Smith DS, Barnwell SL (2005) Arterial embolization in the management of posterior epistaxis. Otolaryngol Head Neck Surg 133:748–753
5. Choy ATK, John DG, van Hasslet CA (1993) Posterior epistaxis and the undeflatable Foley's urinary catheter balloon. J Laryngol Otol 107:142–143
6. Cullen MM, Tami TA (1998) Comparison of internal maxillary artery ligation versus embolization for refractory posterior epistaxis. Otolaryngol Head Neck Surg 118:636–642
7. Derkay CS, Hirsch BE, Johnson JT, et al (1989) Posterior nasal packing: are intravenous antibiotics really necessary? Arch Otolaryngol 115:439–441
8. DeVries N, Verlius RJJ, Snow GB (1986) Facial nerve paralysis following embolization for severe epistaxis. J Laryngol Otol 100:207–210
9. Durr DG (2004) Endoscopic electrosurgical management of posterior epistaxis: shifting paradigm. J Otolaryngol 33:211–216
10. Elden L, Montanera W, Terbrugge K, et al (1994) Angiographic embolization for the treatment of epistaxis: a review of 108 cases. Otolaryngol Head Neck Surg 111:44–50
11. Elwany S, Kamel T, Mekhamer A (1986) Pneumatic nasal catheters: advantages and drawbacks. J Laryngol Otol 100:641–647
12. Fairbanks DNF (1986) Complications of nasal packing. Otolaryngol Head Neck Surg 94:412–415
13. Floreani SR, Nair SB, Switajewski MC, et al (2006) Endoscopic anterior ethmoidal artery ligation: a cadaver study. Laryngoscope 116:1263–1267
14. Hady MRA, Kodeira KA, Nasef AH (1983) The effect of nasal packing on arterial blood gases and acid-base balance and its clinical importance. J Laryngol Otol 97:599–604
15. Holzmann D, Kaufmann T, Pedrini P, et al (2003) Posterior epistaxis: endonasal exposure and occlusion of the branches of the sphenopalatine artery. Eur Arch Otorhinolaryngol 260:425–428
16. Jacobs JR, Levine LA, Davis H, et al (1981) Posterior packs and the nasopulmonary reflex. Laryngoscope 91:279–284
17. Kirchner JA, Yanagisawa E, Crelin ES (1961) Surgical anatomy of the ethmoidal arteries: a laboratory study of 150 orbits. Arch Otolaryngol 74:382–386
18. Klotz DA, Winkle MR, Richmon J, et al (2002) Surgical management of posterior epistaxis: a changing paradigm. Laryngoscope 112:1577–1582
19. Kumar S, Shetty A, Rockey J, et al (2003) Contemporary surgical treatment of epistaxis: what is the evidence for sphenopalatine artery ligation? Clin Otolaryngol 28:360–363
20. Loftus BC, Blitzer A, Cozine K (1994) Epistaxis, medical history, and the nasopulmonary reflex: what is clinically relevant? Otolaryngol Head Neck Surg 110: 363–369
21. Mahadevia AA, Murphy KJ, Obray R, et al (2005) Embolization for intractable epistaxis. Tech Vasc Interv Rad 8:134–138
22. Metson R, Hanson HG (1983) Bilateral facial nerve paralysis following arterial embolization for epistaxis. Otolaryngol Head Neck Surg 91:299–303
23. Metson R, Lane R (1988) Internal maxillary artery ligation for epistaxis: an analysis of failures. Laryngoscope 98:760–764

24. Pallin DJ, Chng Yi-Mei, McKay MP, et al (2005) Epidemiology of epistaxis in US emergency departments 1992 to 2001. Ann Emerg Med 46:77–81

25. Santos PM, Lepore ML. Epistaxis. In Bailey BJ, Calhoun KH, Healy GB, et al (eds) (2001) Head and neck surgery-otolaryngology. Lippincott Williams and Wilkins, Philadelphia, Pennsylvania

26. Schaitkin B, Strauss M, Houck JR, et al (1987) Epistaxis: medical versus surgical therapy: a comparison of efficacy, complications and economic considerations. Laryngoscope 97:1392–1396

27. Snyderman CH, Goldman SA, Carrau RL, et al (1999) Endoscopic sphenopalatine artery ligation is an effective method of treatment for posterior epistaxis. Am J Rhinol 13:137–140

28. Sokoloff J, Waskom T, McDonald D, et al (1974) Therapeutic percutaneous embolization in intractable epistaxis. Radiology 111:285–287

29. Spafford P, Durham JS (1992) Epistaxis: efficacy of arterial ligation and long-term outcome. J Otolaryngol 21:252–256

30. Wang L, Vogel D (1981) Posterior epistaxis: comparison of treatment. Otolaryngol Head Neck Surg 89:1001–1006

31. Wehrli M, Lieberherr U, Valavanis A (1988) Superselective embolization for intractable epistaxis: experiences with 19 patients. Clin Otolaryngol Allied Sci 13:415–420.

32. Wetmore SJ, Scrima L, Hiller FC (1988) Sleep apnea in epistaxis patients treated with nasal packs. Otolarnygol Head Neck Surg 98:596–599

33. Woolford TJ, Jones NS (2000) Endoscopic ligation of anterior ethmoidal artery in treatment of epistaxis. J Laryngol Otol 114:858–860

Chapter 13

Disorders of the Nasal Septum

13

Matthew R. Stumpe and Rakesh K. Chandra

Core Messages

- Nasal septal pathologies may cause significant distress to patients secondary to deviation, perforation, obstruction, epistaxis, and/or cosmetic deformity.
- Numerous infectious, inflammatory, and systemic diseases need to be considered in the differential diagnosis.
- The diagnosis of these entities may require culture, biopsy, specialized laboratory testing, and a high index of suspicion.

Contents

Introduction

Function of the Nasal Septum

The nasal septum is one of the most fully conserved structures in vertebrates. The nasal septum is thought to function in the sensation of smell and perception of pheromones in lower members of the animal kingdom, but such functions in humans have yet to be established. The nasal septum transforms the nasal airway into a parallel circuit. This decreases the total resistance of the nasal airway to less than the smallest resistance of a single nasal cavity alone. Basic physics tells us that the circuit in which resistors are in parallel has less total resistance ($1/R_T = 1/R_1 + 1/R_2 + 1/R_3 + ...$) than a circuit with the same resistors in a series ($R_T = R_1 + R_2 + R_3 + ...$). Thus, the septum reduces the overall resistance of the nasal airway considerably. Septal pathology or perforation consequently has a significant effect on nasal airway. A diverse array of pathology, both local and systemic, can manifest as a disorder of the nasal septum. Patients with nasal septal problems present with a myriad of issues including epistaxis, nasal airway obstruction, pain, crusting, sinusitis, or they can be asymptomatic. A strong foundation in anatomy is also important in the diagnosis and treatment of septal problems. Septal deviation, septal perforation, neoplastic, and inflammatory diseases will be discussed and classified in order to expand the physician's ability to manage this pathology.

Septal Anatomy

The nasal septum is made of multiple layers from lateral to medial as well as differing center support from anterior to posterior. Moving from anterior to posterior the septum is supported by the medial crus of the lower lateral cartilage. Posterior to this is the membranous septum. The quadrangular cartilage is the central component of the cartilaginous septum, receiving its name from the shape this cartilage has in a sagittal plane. The most posterior aspect of the septum is made up of the bony septum with the vomer inferiorly and the perpendicular plate of the ethmoid bone superiorly. The majority of the base of the septum consists of the nasal crest of the maxilla and the posterior part is made up of the nasal crest of the palatine bone. The perpendicular plate of the ethmoid forms approximately the upper third of the nasal septum. This bone articulates with the frontal and nasal bones and the crest of the sphenoid bone outside the nasal septum. The inferior portion of the bony septum, the vomer, articulates superiorly with the body of the sphenoid bone, inferiorly with the nasal crest of the maxilla and palatine bones, and anteriorly with the septal cartilage. The junction of the cartilaginous septum with the bony septum has connective tissue, classifying this junction as a joint, which allows the septal cartilage to deviate without frank dislocation. The anterior aspect of the nasal septum also permits mobility where the membranous septum separates the quadrangular cartilage from the medial crura of the lower lateral cartilage. These nonrigid attachments allow for deformation of the septum without fracture.

Nasal septal blood supply is a rich anastomosis of many contributing vessels. Epistaxis is a common otolaryngologic emergency and the source of bleeding is frequently the anterior nasal septum. The rich arterial area of the anterior nasal septum is routinely described as Little's area or Kiesselbach's plexus. Recent anatomical dissections of the nasal septum have demonstrated a triangular plexus with anastomosis of the anterior ethmoidal artery, superior labial artery, and the "anterior" branch of the sphenopalatine artery [17]. Variable blood supply is found from the posterior septal artery, the posterior ethmoidal artery, and the greater palatine artery. This rich blood supply is susceptible to injury and significant blood loss.

Structural Abnormalities

Septal Deviation

Deviated nasal septum is a very common disorder that may or may not be symptomatic. Symptomatic patients typically present with nasal obstruction, while epistaxis, obstructive sinusitis, pressure, and pain are less common potential complaints. Septal deviation can be divided into congenital or acquired. The traumatic etiology of septal deviation includes traumatic or iatrogenic insult. As described above, the flexibility of the cartilaginous septum and its attachments allows a significant amount of deformation without fracture. The pathophysiology of congenital septal deviation has not been fully elucidated, although it is thought to result from external pressures on the nose during the birthing process. Even the position of the infant during the birthing process can affect the incidence of septal deviation. This has been illustrated by a higher percentage of deformity in children born in a persistent occipitoposterior position [28]. However, this theory is weakened by an incidence of deviation even after cesarean section [28, 58]. Another factor that may be implicated in the origin of congenital deviation is that septal components develop at differing rates leading to deviation from the inner compressive forces of the developing septum. Acquired septal deviation is almost uniformly traumatic (Fig. 13.1) and is occasionally iatrogenic. Chronic pressure from mass effect (e.g., inflammatory polyp or neoplasm) may gradually displace the septum as well.

Deviated nasal symptom may be an incidental finding on physical examination, in which case it does not warrant treatment. However, unilateral nasal obstruction is the most common symptom leading to diagnosis. This may be from direct blockage of the nasal airway, compromise of the cross-sectional area with exacerbation by mucosal inflammation, such as from allergy or contralateral obstruction from a hypertrophied turbinate (Fig. 13.2). The concave side of the septal deviation has been shown to have decreased density of cilia, more inflammation, and a decreased mucociliary transport time [35]. This mucosal pathology on the concave side of the deviation may lead to more symptoms on the nasal side with a larger airway on gross examination. Due to the mucosal effects on the symptoms or the turbinate hypertrophy, medical management should be attempted prior to surgical correction. The treatment goal is to achieve control of mucosal edema and good nasal hygiene with nasal steroids and irrigation. Failure of medical management is an indication for surgery. Septoplasty is often successful as a primary treatment, but may be augmented by nasal turbinate reduction. There are many different approaches to correcting the deformed nasal septum [44]. The main principle is to remove or modify the deviated nasal septum without disrupting uninvolved nasal structures. Elevating a subperichondrial flap on the nasal septal cartilage, the deformed areas are either removed or weakened enough to allow repositioning to the midline. It is mandatory to leave enough suprastructure along the dorsum and the columella to prevent postoperative saddle nose deformity. It should be noted that surgery for nasal septal deviation should be limited to children with severe functional pathology, as the septum is a facial growth center. The mucoperichondrium of the septum is theorized to be the key tissue of the nasal septum regulating facial growth in this region [8]. Septal surgery in children has been shown to have measurable effect on nasal dorsal height [8], and many authors emphasize conservative surgical treatment for childhood septal pathology. However, the effect of septal surgery on *final* nasal height may be minimal [8, 32, 38, 66]. Nonetheless, it appears prudent for

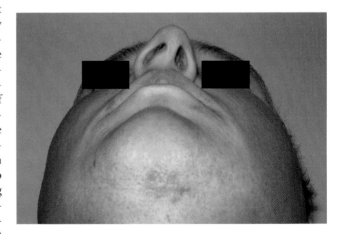

Fig. 13.1 Nasal septal deviation in a patient with a history of nasal trauma

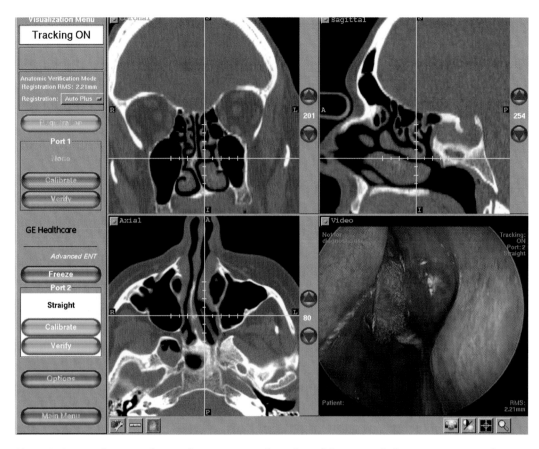

Fig. 13.2 Computed tomography scan demonstrating rightward septal deviation, which is most apparent in the coronal and axial planes (*upper and lower left panels* respectively). These views also demonstrate hypertrophy of the left inferior turbinate in the region of septal concavity

septal surgery in this population to emphasize conservation of the mucoperichondrium and that cosmetic surgery of the nose should be delayed until adult nasal proportions have been accomplished.

Contact Point Headache

Headache may also be a symptom of nasal septal deviation, if associated with a septal spur that impacts a structure of the lateral nasal wall such as the inferior or middle turbinate. Contact point headache is a controversial topic, but has been found to be a valid entity in appropriately diagnosed patients. The diagnosis of contact point headache is supported by relief of the pain with topical vasoconstriction and injection of the contact point with lidocaine. The patient is monitored for resolution of pain. A surgical correction of this point is considered if the pain is terminated with local anesthesia. Studies have shown a decrease in intensity in 91% of headaches following functional endoscopic sinus surgery to correct contact points in a selected group of patients [55]. As is the case with nasal airway obstruction, a full course of medical management including topical nasal steroids is indicated prior to surgical correction. After careful discussion with the patient, septoplasty, turbinate reduction, and/or functional endoscopic sinus surgery may be considered. Symptoms of headache must be discerned from symptoms of facial pain/pressure that may be more indicative of obstructive sinus disease. Patients must be informed of the variable (and sometimes unpredictable) benefit of surgery to headaches thought to be of sinonasal etiology, because the differential diagnosis of headache is broad.

Septal Perforation

Septal perforation (Figs. 13.3, 13.4) is another disorder of the nasal septum that has many differing etiologies. The presence of a perforation in itself may be innocuous. However, it is incumbent upon the otolaryngologist to diagnose the etiology of the perforation and offer treatment if the perforation is symptomatic. Common symptoms of this pathology are whistling, bleeding, rhinorrhea, or crusting [22, 39]. Septal perforation is also a potential symptom of a systemic disorder. Many of these conditions are covered later in the chapter and elsewhere in this book, but etiologies can generally be classified as iatrogenic, traumatic, infectious, or drug-related. However, even after full work-up, the etiology may remain idiopathic in up to half of patients [22].

Most septal perforations are iatrogenic as a result of trauma to the septum during an elective septoplasty or rhinoplasty where opposing mucoperichondrial lacerations heal as a fistula between one side of the nasal cavity and the other. Based on a meta-analysis of the literature, Bateman and Woolford estimated a 2–8% perforation rate from submucous resection and a 1.6–5.4% rate from septoplasty [3].

Management of septal perforation is a complicated issue that should first be focused on identification of the underlying pathology, including infectious and systemic diseases, which are outlined in the remainder of this chapter. Once the underlying pathology has been addressed a sufficient period of stabilization and healing, approximately 6 months, should be allowed to occur prior to surgical correction. Nasal hygiene should be maintained throughout. Formal rhinoplasty should be considered when significant dorsal or tip support structures have been destroyed.

Conservative measures to provide symptomatic relief include nasal saline sprays and lavage. This decreases the incidence of crusting and epistaxis. Conservative management for the sensa-

tion of turbulent airflow or whistling is not effective. Surgical intervention is indicated in these cases. The goals of surgery are both to address symptoms and to regain normal function and physiology with a parallel nasal circuit. Many authors have reported greater than 90% success rates using septal flaps with a connective tissue autograft interposed between to the two mucoperichondrial flaps [23, 39, 54]. Surgical success is dependent on the proportion of nasal septal perforation to the remaining septum and the location. For example, a smaller perforation in a child may be more difficult to repair than a larger one in an adult. Perforations extending to the nasal floor or posterior septum are more technically difficult to access. Both an endonasal approach with or without endoscopic assistance and open techniques have been described [23, 39, 54]. A connective tissue graft between septal flaps is thought to improve success rates. Choices for graft include temporalis fascia, pericranium, acellular dermis, and synthetics such as bioglass [39, 65].

Alternatives to septal mucosal flaps include a pedicled flap from the inferior turbinate [26], silicone septal buttons [57], or surgically enlarging the perforation to reduce surface area for crust accumulation. The latter two techniques are concerned with alleviating the symptoms rather than returning the nose to its physiologically normal state. Septal buttons (Fig. 13.5) are available in standardized sizes, but must be fashioned to the particular dimensions of the pathology. They have a fair rate of success with 59% reporting improvement in crusting, 60% improvement in the nasal airway, and 77% improvement in the occurrence of epistaxis [57].

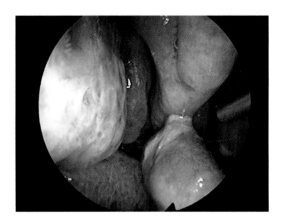

Fig. 13.3 Endoscopy demonstrating a large mature septal perforation. The margins of the perforation are well mucosalized

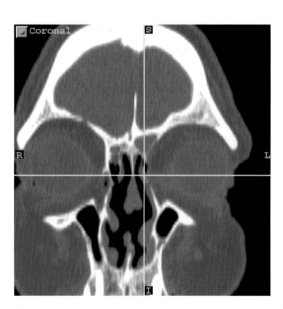

Fig. 13.4 Computed tomography scan demonstrating septal perforation

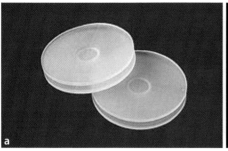
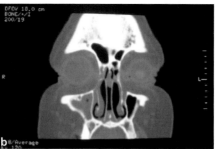

Fig. 13.5 **a** Silastic septal buttons may be fashioned to obturate even septal defects. **b** The coronal CT scan demonstrates septal button closure of a large anterior perforation

Trauma and Hematoma

Direct trauma to the septum with opposing mucoperichondrial disruption can leave a perforation after healing. More commonly, a septal hematoma can develop, separating the mucoperichondrium from the cartilage. Leaving this hematoma in place may deprive the underlying cartilage of its blood supply, which comes exclusively from the overlying perichondrium. Evaluation of the nose in the setting of facial trauma should always include an adequate inspection of the nasal septum for such a hematoma. The treatment of this injury is drainage of the hematoma followed by a bolster of the mucoperichondrium to the cartilage for a short time period with either a nasal tampon or a mattressed suture, subsequently allowing the cartilage to maintain its blood supply. In delayed treatment, the hematoma and necrotic cartilage is an abundant fertilizer for bacterial infection and abscess formation. Incision, drainage, and debridement of necrotic tissues are indicated while attempting to preserve the viable nasal septal tissues. Further infectious complications include cavernous sinus thrombosis, meningitis, or brain abscess [13, 19]. The most commonly implicated organism in these infection complications is *Staphylococcus aureus* [13].

Infections

A variety of infectious agents may cause a septal inflammatory disease, ulceration, perforation, or other septal pathology such as mass effect. Many of these offending agents are unusual, and both fungal and bacterial entities have been implicated. Diagnosis may be difficult and may require culture, biopsy, and/or laboratory testing.

Fungal

Diabetics and patients receiving immunosuppressive chemotherapy make up a majority of these patients. This pathology involves fungal organisms invading through tissue planes resulting in angioinvasion, infarction, and ischemic necrosis (Fig. 13.6). The offending organisms typically include *Aspergillus flavus* or *fumigatus* (septated hyphal forms) or members of the Zygomycetes class/Mucorales order, particularly *Rhizopus oryzae* (nonseptated hyphae). These ubiquitous organisms cause symptoms that can initially mimic a chronic inflammatory condition. However, the disease process is fulminant and quickly proceeds to severe pain, facial anesthesia, cranial neuropathy, proptosis, chemosis, and/or change in visual acuity. Nasal examination reveals necrotic tissues. Management of the underlying condition is essential to return the patient to an immunocompetent state. Treatment requires aggressive debridement of necrotic tissues and intravenous antifungal therapy [33]. The prognosis is nonetheless dismal given the fulminant nature of the process, the proximity of vital structures, and the severity of the predisposing condition.

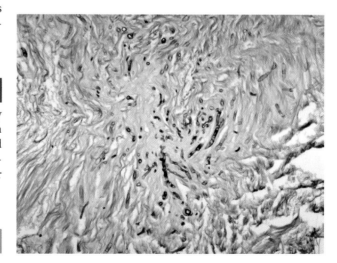

Fig. 13.6 Invasive aspergillosis. Tissue-invasive, branched, septated hyphal forms are demonstrated (Grocott's silver stain, ×200)

13

Syphilis

Syphilis is the sexually transmitted disease caused by infection with *Treponema palladium*. The old saying that, "He who knows all of syphilis, knows all of medicine," Sir William Osler [48], extends to rhinology as well. In the nose, syphilis emerges differently depending on the stage at which it is discovered. Primary syphilis, as in other areas of the body, presents with a chancre at the mucocutaneous border of the septum or nasal vestibule occurring 10–90 days after inoculation [48]. This presentation is very rare in the nose. It is difficult to diagnose because it may appear neoplastic, erosive, scabbed, or have a change in skin pigmentation [48]. The usual history is that these lesions tend to ulcerate and form a minimally painful sore with disproportionate lymphadenopathy in the adjacent nodal basins. Secondary syphilis is often confused with acute rhinitis due to scant thick discharge with stenosis of the nose and irritation to the anterior nares. However, careful examination may reveal discrete mucous patches, erythema, or a solitary plaque on the external nose [48, 67]. It may or may not be associated with syphilitic pharyngitis or laryngitis. Tertiary syphilis presents as a smooth circumscribed swelling covered by inflamed mucosa on the septum. Septal perforation is common and may result in enough cartilage destruction to cause a saddle nose deformity. The diagnosis is made with screening rapid plasma regain (RPR) or Venereal Disease Research Laboratory (VDRL) serology and a fluorescent treponemal antibody absorption (FTA-ABS) test for confirmation or in patients who are at high clinical risk. The treatment is systemic penicillin or other antibiotics.

Tuberculosis

Tuberculosis is thought of as a pulmonary disease caused by *Mycobacterium tuberculosis*. However, this disease can affect the nose either as an extension from the pulmonary infection or, rarely, primarily. In fact, 80–90% of nonpulmonary tuberculosis is found in the head and neck [1]. While cervical lymphadenopathy is the most common head and neck manifestation, the second most frequent otolaryngological presenting complaint is nasal obstruction [1, 50, 53]. Nasal involvement with tuberculosis was first described in 1761 by Giovanni Morgagni (cited in [53]). The diagnosis may be difficult because the organism is not easily cultured and the characteristic caseating granulomas may not be found in a nasal biopsy specimen [4, 18, 53]. Sputum smears may also be negative with primary nasal tuberculosis [53]. The diagnosis may become simplified with the advent of newer technology including polymerase chain reaction. The treatment is a prolonged multi-drug regimen of anti-tuberculous chemotherapy. These drugs need to be specific to geographic regions and guided by drug resistance patterns.

Leprosy

Leprosy is uncommon in North America, but affects 12–15 million people worldwide [40]. It is one of the oldest diseases known to man, originally thought to be a hereditary illness, but now known to be caused by *Mycobacterium leprae*. This acid-fast bacillus has a natural reservoir in the foot pads of mice and the nine-banded armadillo [40]. It cannot be cultured on an artificial medium, but successfully grown only in the cooler tissues of the foot pads of the two aforementioned animals, making it difficult to culture [40]. It is the only bacterium that selectively invades peripheral nerves and causes irreversible cutaneous anesthesia and paralysis of muscles. The estimated incubation time is 3–10 years. Leprosy has a wide spectrum of sequelae, the most severe of which typically presents with intranasal involvement earlier than the systemic symptoms. Nasal symptoms including obstruction, bleeding, crusting and hyposmia are present in up to 94% of people with septal perforation being a relatively late manifestation [40]. Early in the disease, nasal examination reveals isolated nodules or plaques with pale, yellowish thickening of the nasal mucosa. Laboratory testing lacks sensitivity to accurately diagnose this infection, leaving limited culture options and biopsy for diagnosis. Treatment is with anti-leprosy antibiotics such as dapsone, kanamycin, rifampin, or minocycline.

Rhinoscleroma

Rhinoscleroma is a chronic infection of the upper airways. The disease is caused by an infection with *Klebsiella rhinoscleromatis*. Physical findings consistent with rhinoscleroma have been found in Mayan head masks dated between 300 and 600 AD [31]. Females are more frequently affected and increased incidence in areas of crowding, poor hygiene, or poor nutrition [31]. The nose is affected in nearly all of the cases. The first phase is known as the catarrhal atrophic stage or ozaena and is characterized by a foul-smelling purulent nasal discharge that may persist for months. The second or granulomatous stage is when most cases are diagnosed and is associated with nasal deformity. During this time, the nasal lesion has a bluish-red, rubbery granuloma appearance [31]. This eventually subsides into the sclerotic phase where there is growth of granulomas and possible bony destruction [31]. Particularly in the granulomatous phase, multinucleated macrophages with numerous vacuoles containing viable or nonviable bacteria can be seen and are referred to as Mikulicz cells. Russell bodies, which are eosinophilic structures within the cytoplasm of plasma cells, are also seen. These are helpful to guide the diagnosis. Giemsa, Warthin-Starry, or periodic acid-Schiff stains demonstrate the gram-negative rods in the macrophages approximately 50% of the time and are useful for diagnosis [31, 70]. Even though the organism has been shown to be sensitive to a wide variety of antibiotics, treatment is less than definitive. Prolonged treatment with antibiotics and ablation may alter the evolution of the disease.

Rhinosporidiosis

Rhinosporidiosis is a nasal infection that occurs most commonly in India, Sri Lanka, and Southeast Asia, but has been reported rarely in the United States [27]. It is caused by the fungus *Rhinosporidium seeberi*. Nasal involvement is the most common site, presenting with nasal airway obstruction. Physical examination reveals nasal polyps oftentimes arising from the nasal septum. Biopsy demonstrates the fungal agent, which is easily seen on routine light microscopy [6]. However, cultures fail to grow the organism on synthetic medium. The walls of the fungal spores are birefringent under crossed polarized filters and a host granulomatous response with mostly histiocytes and some neutrophils and lymphocytes can be seen [49]. This fungal organism is thought to be transmitted by spores discharged into the nasal secretions, but appears to have a low infectivity [6]. It is believed that the natural reservoir is contaminated water [6]. Surgical excision is the treatment of choice. Dapsone may also be considered for recurrent or disseminated infections [6]. Rhinosporidiosis is considered to be unresponsive to systemic anti-mycotics [49].

Systemic Inflammatory Disease

The nasal septum may be involved in a number of systemic inflammatory disorders. This group includes Wegener's granulomatosis, sarcoidosis, and rheumatic conditions including rheumatoid arthritis and lupus. Giant cell reparative granulomas have also been reported to occur in the nasal cavity [51].

It should also be noted that many of these conditions may be mimicked by drug abuse. Chronic use of vasoconstrictive agents in the nose can lead to septal ulceration or perforation. The classic example of this is cocaine abuse [20, 39, 64, 69]. However, it can occur with over-the-counter sprays such as oxymetazoline, neosynephrine, and others, or secondarily from smoking products containing nicotine [39]. Chronic vasoconstriction leads to ischemic necrosis [61] and perforations from the intranasal abuse of narcotics have also been reported [74]. Aggressive use of thermal or chemical (e.g., silver nitrate) cautery can also cause a septal ulceration and perforation is possible, particularly when apposing places on the septum are cauterized [30]. Septal ulceration or perforation is occasionally associated with use of intranasal steroid sprays. Although contact allergy has been theorized for this phenomenon, the true etiology is unknown [14]. The following discussion will address systemic medical conditions as they may affect the nasal septum.

Wegener's Granulomatosis

Wegener's granulomatosis is an idiopathic, systemic disease characterized by necrotizing, granulomatous inflammation of the upper and lower respiratory tract. This occurs in combination with vasculitis of medium and small arteries and focal or proliferative glomerulonephritis [29]. The incidence ranges from 1–10 cases per million people [29, 68]. The etiology is largely unknown. A common theory is that the disease is immunologically mediated [29]. This initial manifestation of this systemic disease often appears in the head and neck. In fact, rhinologic complaints are the most common presenting symptoms and 30% of patients describe only rhinologic symptoms [29, 52, 68]. It is thus incumbent upon the otolaryngologist to be prepared to diagnose this condition. Prior to the introduction of

cytotoxic pharmacotherapy the prognosis was dismal. With the advent of cyclophosphamide in combination with corticosteroids, the 5-year survival is approximately 72%, increased from 2-year survival of 10% before modern pharmacotherapy [68]. Nasal examination in a patient with active rhinologic disease reveals nasal crusting, erythematous friable mucosa, evidence of sinusitis, or granulation tissue. The nasal crusting and mucosal inflammation can occur anywhere in the nose. However, the septum and turbinates are the most frequently effected. The practitioner should be aware that nasal endoscopy can also be normal in patients with active disease.

Septal perforation is a common finding in Wegener's granulomatosis. However, the actual perforation may not become evident until periods of disease remission. This occurs due to vasculitic involvement of Kiesselbach's plexus resulting in septal cartilage necrosis. Resorption of this necrotic tissue during a time of remission results in a septal perforation. The presence of a perforation does not correlate well with active disease [29] and a high index of suspicion must be maintained in order to make the diagnosis. Cytoplasmic anti-neutrophil antibodies (c-ANCA) are a specific serum marker. However, c-ANCA can be elevated in cocaine abuse [61], leprosy, invasive amebiasis, and infectious endocarditis [29]. Biopsy has been the mainstay of diagnosis for many years prior to the discovery of ANCA testing. It is still very important in the diagnosis of Wegener's granulomatosis as it is very specific, but lacks sensitivity [29]. Biopsy specimens should be generous and include areas of normal tissue for comparison. The location of pathology for biopsy also plays a role in diagnostic accuracy with the paranasal sinus tissue having the highest yield in these cases [29]. In patients in whom Wegener's is highly suspected and the c-ANCA and biopsy are both negative, repeated serology with c-ANCA may reveal the diagnosis over time [37]. The treatment of Wegener's is primarily medical and needs to be approached in coordination with multiple specialties.

Sarcoidosis

Sarcoidosis is a systemic granulomatous disorder characterized by varying degrees of involvement of the skin, viscera, and lymph nodes by noncaseating granulomas. This disease process can involve the nasal septum. Sarcoidosis is characterized by systemic noncaseating granulomas in the absence of any other identifiable cause. The etiology is not fully understood. The incidence is widely variable between geographic locations and between racial groups. The highest incidence is in Sweden and has been reported to be 67 per 100,000 people, with autopsy studies suggesting that the incidence may be much higher [24]. The incidence is higher in African-Americans than in Caucasians in North America and in West Indian populations than Caucasians in London [7, 24]. Head and neck pathology is present in about 10–15% of cases [21, 24], the highest proportion of this being cervical lymphadenopathy [7, 21, 24, 62]. Nasal complaints are rare, with only 1% of patients having nasal complaints in the absence of other symptoms [11]. Otolaryngologic manifestations include nasal obstruction, rhinosinusitis, nasal polyposis, or septal perforation [7, 11, 21, 24, 62]. Otolaryngologists are often the diagnosing physician due to its presenting symptom and the propensity to biopsy a lesion visualized on examination [11]. Diagnosis is that of exclusion and consists of characteristic radiologic findings in the chest, serology, especially elevated angiotensin converting enzyme (ACE) levels, and biopsy demonstrating noncaseating granulomas. Many other disease processes, including tuberculosis, Wegener's, syphilis, leprosy, and Gaucher's disease, must be excluded when making the diagnosis of sarcoidosis [21, 24]. Whenever narrowing the differential diagnosis, stains of nasal biopsies for acid-fast bacilli should be considered. Any cervical lymphadenopathy should also be considered for fine needle aspiration biopsy and may contribute to the diagnosis [25]. Corticosteroids remain the cornerstone of treatment and the drug of choice for exacerbations. The natural history of sarcoidosis is often marked with spontaneous remission and therefore continuous therapy is not always indicated. Central nervous system or ocular involvement constitute medical emergencies and need to be addressed. Topical corticosteroids for nasal symptoms, as are seen in other disease entities, appear to be beneficial [21].

Rheumatoid Arthritis

Rheumatoid arthritis (RA) is a chronic systemic inflammatory disease. The disease primarily affects the peripheral joints symmetrically. The etiology of RA is unknown. Other common manifestations include fatigue, malaise, and morning stiffness. Extra-articular involvement of organs such as the skin, heart, lungs, and eyes can be significant. Nasal septal nodules and perforation have been reported as rare manifestations of this disease [9, 46, 73]. Nasal septal perforations have been attributed to the destructive potential of the vasculitic component of the condition [9]. Raynaud's phenomenon has been described in a subset of these patients and speculation that local vasospasm following inspiration of cold air leading to ischemia in the nose with the similar effect of fingertip ulcers [73]. Treatment of the rhinologic component relies upon control of the underlying pathology.

Systemic Lupus Erythematosus

Systemic lupus erythematosus (SLE) is a chronic, multifaceted inflammatory disease that can affect every organ system of the body. SLE is variable in its manifestations and follows a remitting and relapsing course. This disease involves multisystem microvascular inflammation caused by autoantibodies. Nasal septal pathology is an uncommon feature of SLE, with perforation as the most common septal manifestation [45], and generally occurs during exacerbations and in a context of systemic vasculitis. There are reports of septal perforation being the presenting symptom of SLE [45]. Lesions are typically asymptomatic and patients are many times not aware of their nasal problem. A theory of the pathogenesis of perforation is that the defect begins with ischemia, causing a nasal mucosal ulceration with subsequent chondrolysis [45]. Another theory of vasculitis is as an important etiologic feature in perforation. However, no his-

tological evidence of vasculitis has been documented in the nasal mucosa of SLE patients with nasal septum perforation [45]. Prior to any therapy for the septal pathology, the underlying rheumatologic process needs to be treated.

Crohn's Disease

Crohn's disease is an idiopathic, chronic inflammatory process affecting the bowel. This disease often leads to fibrosis and obstructive symptoms. Crohn's disease usually affects the GI tract anywhere from the mouth to the anus. However, this pathology very rarely involves the nasal structures. The expression of disease in the nasal septum includes intermittent epistaxis, chronic mucosal inflammation, obstruction, and occasionally septal perforation [59]. The condition itself is believed to be the result of an imbalance between proinflammatory and antiinflammatory mediators. The etiology is unknown. Of the 36% of all patients afflicted by Crohn's disease who have extraintestinal involvement, those in whom the nasal septum is affected make up a very small portion [59]. Treatment of the underlying pathology can be effective in treating the nasal manifestations, but does not resolve them in all cases [59].

Systemic Juvenile Idiopathic Arthritis

Systemic juvenile idiopathic arthritis is an inflammatory disease in which the symptoms include chronic arthritis, with common manifestations of fever, evanescent rash, generalized lymphadenopathy, hepatosplenomegaly, and serositis. Patients with systemic juvenile idiopathic arthritis constitute only 10–20% of all cases of idiopathic arthritis, making this disease rare [2]. Septal perforation has been reported in cases of active and inactive disease [2]. The etiology of the perforation is unknown, but potentially related to vascular inflammation leading to ischemic necrosis.

Neoplastic

The nasal septum may be involved in the wide array of benign and malignant neoplasms that affect the sinonasal tract. A full discussion of these entities is beyond the scope of this chapter, but in some of these conditions, the septum is the epicenter of the disease process. These selected disorders are outlined below.

Sinonasal Natural Killer/T-Cell Lymphoma

Sinonasal natural killer (NK)/T-cell lymphoma, occasionally still described as angiocentric T-cell lymphoma, is a malignancy that can be encountered during the work-up of nasal septal disease. In this condition, perforation and rapid fulminant destruction are observed. This pathology may be confused with a more benign granulomatous inflammatory condition (e.g., Wegener's) or cocaine abuse upon initial examination, and his-

13

torically these conditions were indistinguishable by physical examination alone. The previously described disease processes known as *lethal midline granuloma* was a wastebasket term that encompassed both Wegener's granulomatosis and sinonasal NK/T-cell lymphoma [15, 56, 75]. However, with the help of immunohistochemistry and flow cytometry, the distinction was made between this malignant disease and other infectious or inflammatory conditions. Sinonasal NK/T-cell lymphoma shows a predilection for the Asian population, which has an increased prevalence of lymphoma of T-cell origin, in contrast to the western population, which tends to have B-cell lymphoma [15, 41, 75]. Mexicans and South Americans also have an increased prevalence of sinonasal NK/T-cell lymphoma. This disease additionally has a strong association with the Epstein-Barr Virus (EBV) [41]. A biopsy is diagnostic in most cases, where histology reveals pleomorphic tumor cells variably associated with angiocentric infiltration or angiodestructive growth as well as zonal coagulative necrosis [41].

There is interesting evidence demonstrating that the clonal cells may not be T-cells, but rather NK cells or, possibly, a common progenitor [16, 41, 75]. EBV antigens are present in nearly all nasal T-cell lymphomas and may be of use in diagnosis and prognosis, with higher EBV involvement signifying a more aggressive disease [41, 75]. Treatment options continue to evolve and include various protocols of chemotherapy and radiation. As in most malignancies, locoregionally isolated disease has a significantly better 5-year survival, approximately double that observed with systemic disease [41]. For patients with local regional disease at presentation, 5-year survival rates are about 40%, and with those manifesting systemic disease it drops to 7–25% [15, 16, 41, 75]. New strategies including using cisplatinum as a radiation sensitizer or high-dose chemotherapy continue to be explored.

Septal Masses

Any neoplasm with a predilection for the upper respiratory tract can involve all or part of the septum. These include squamous cell carcinoma, minor salivary gland neoplasms, or olfactory neuroblastomas. Metastatic disease from a large number of sources may also involve the nose, affecting the nasal septum. In a 25-year review of cases from the Armed Forces Institute of Pathology, Thompson et al. found that 17% of 115 melanomas of the sinonasal tract involved the nasal septum alone [71]. However, these are exceedingly rare and constitute approximately 0.5% of all sinonasal neoplasms. Other rare tumors include paragangliomas, chordomas [60], chondromas [72], glomus tumors [42], and chondrosarcomas [10, 47].

Sinonasal papillomas are divided into three distinct histologies: exophytic (fungiform), inverted, and cylindrical (oncocytic). It should be noted that the sinonasal membrane and papillomas that occur therein are often named for J.V. Schneider, an early pioneer of the histology of this region. Thus, the alternative terms of Schneiderian membrane and Schneiderian papilloma are occasionally utilized [5, 34].

Inverted papillomas have a predilection for the lateral nasal wall and are characterized by squamous cell architecture with classic papilloma-like features extending into the underlying stroma. Mucinous cysts or cells can be identified either grossly or by special stains [34]. Hyams found a 46% recurrence rate and a 13% malignancy rate in this papilloma subtype [34]. Malignant transformation has also been reported in cylindrical papilloma, but because of its rarity, it is difficult to quantify its malignant potential [34]. Exophytic or fungiform papilloma (Fig. 13.7) is the entity with the highest predisposition for the nasal septum, and the septum is only rarely the site of origin of the other papilloma subtypes. Presenting signs include nasal mass, nasal obstruction, or bleeding. Exophytic papilloma is histologically similar to papilloma found elsewhere on the body, such as the common cutaneous wart. In contrast to the inverting and cylindrical forms, exophytic papilloma does not have any malignant potential [5, 12, 34]. Complete excision is usually curative.

Hereditary Hemorrhagic Telangiectasia

Hereditary hemorrhagic telangiectasia, often referred to as Osler-Weber-Rendu disease, is an autosomal dominant, nonsexlinked condition with multiple telangiectasia throughout the skin and mucous membranes with common hemorrhage. The vascular dysplasia is localized to discrete segments of vessels ranging in caliber from capillaries to large arteries and veins [63]. There is a weakness of the perivascular connective tissues causing a loss of integrity of the vessels [63]. The vessels are unable to vasoconstrict due to the lack of elastic fibers [63]. Recurrent epistaxis is a common symptom of the disease, affecting more than 90% of patients, even though it affects the entire aerodigestive tract, as well as the brain and liver [43]. A common finding is a punctiform spot, or macular telangiectasia. These lesions typically measure 1–3 mm in diameter and are sharply demarcated from the surrounding tissues (Fig. 13.8) [63]. Treatment is directed at protecting these fragile vessels or coagulating them to prevent blood loss. Multiple treatments for hereditary hem-

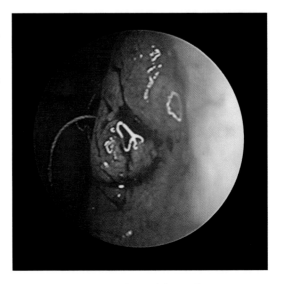

Fig. 13.7 Exophytic papilloma of the nasal septum

orrhagic telangiectasia have been proposed, including cautery, topical and systemic hormone therapy, septodermoplasty, arterial ligation, and laser treatment [43, 63]. Closure of the nasal canal with a modified Young's procedure is indicated for cases of severe epistaxis. Patients should be prepared for dryness of the mouth and throat. Unilateral procedures are indicated in patients with unilateral symptoms and no septal perforation [43]. Laser using KTP and Nd-YAG has been described, with a high rate of success due to the laser absorption by hemoglobin, allowing for specific coagulation of the telangiectasia [63]. In those in whom laser therapy fails, septodermoplasty may be considered. This involves resection of involved mucosa along the septum and skin graft resurfacing. No one treatment will benefit every patient, and each case should be independently evaluated for treatment options.

Reactive Pathology

As indicated above, most variations of nasal polyposis has an affinity for the lateral nasal wall. Although nasal septal polyps are possible, neoplastic changes must be examined and biopsied to rule out malignancy in the evaluation of masses located on the septum. The septal mucosa itself is a columnar epithelium with cilia that is dynamic and constantly plagued with pathogens and irritants. It is susceptible to the development of reactive pathology, as is the entire nasal cavity, including adhesions, the so-called "septal turbinate," and pyogenic granuloma.

Iatrogenic

Adhesions to the lateral nasal wall may appear after the trauma of nasal intubation or surgery. Thus, trauma to the nasal septal mucosa should be minimized or avoided altogether during any nasal surgery. The finding of a "septal turbinate" may be observed in patients who have had resection or partial resection of the middle turbinate. The mucosa of the adjacent septum undergoes focal compensatory hypertrophy in an attempt to fill the void. The resulting septal turbinate may have similar dimensions to the absent portion of the middle turbinate (Fig. 13.9). No specific treatment is necessary for a septal turbinate. This de novo aspect of the septum is rarely a cause of symptomatic nasal or sinus outflow obstruction. However, this variant in nasal anatomy has the potential to lead the unwary surgeon medially and dissection of the nasal cavity in the cribriform area. This has the potential of significant morbidity where the skull base is most inferior and vulnerable to injury.

Pyogenic Granuloma

Pyogenic granuloma (Fig. 13.10) is a reactive lesion that develops secondary to mucosal trauma and hormonal factors, including pregnancy, oral contraceptive, and estrogen replacement. The etiology and exact mechanism is unknown for this pathology. The overall incidence of these lesions in pregnancy is 2–5%. Mucosal lesions more commonly involve the oral cavity rather than the nasal mucosa. However, when they originate in the nasal cavity, the anterior septum is the most common site. A theory for this localization is that the lesion develops during exuberant healing after trauma from nose picking. The most common presenting signs are unilateral epistaxis followed by nasal obstruction. Examination of the pyogenic granuloma reveals a reddish to purple mass located on the septum, most commonly anterior. Pathology reveals numerous vascular channels and chronic inflammation, leading some to term the lesion a lobular capillary hemangioma. It is notable that the lesion does not exhibit either acute bacterial infection or granulomas, making the term "pyogenic granuloma" something of a misnomer. Growth

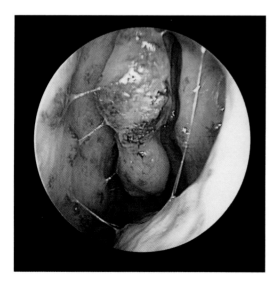

Fig. 13.8 Endoscopy demonstrating hereditary hemorrhagic telangiectasis with lesions involving the septum and turbinates

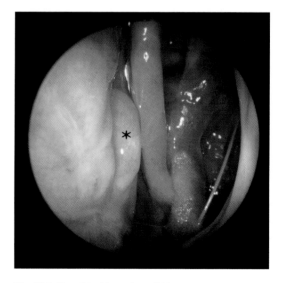

Fig. 13.9 Septal turbinate (*asterisk*)

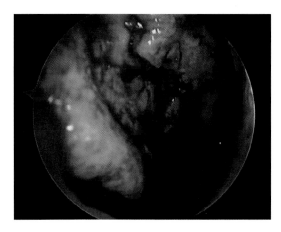

Fig. 13.10 Pyogenic granuloma of the nasal septum

may be rapid, but lesions tend to resolve after pregnancy. For those that do not involve after pregnancy, surgical resection with or without the KTP laser is indicated [36].

Conclusion

The nasal septum is a very important anatomic structure in the normal physiology of the respiratory tract. Nasal septal pathologies may cause significant distress to patients secondary to deviation, perforation, obstruction, epistaxis, and/or cosmetic deformity. Beyond the commonplace deviations and traumatic perforations that are often encountered, numerous infectious, inflammatory, and systemic diseases must be considered in the differential diagnosis. The otolaryngologist must be acutely familiar with these conditions, as many can be life-threatening and thus require prompt medical or surgical intervention. Furthermore, diagnosis of these entities may require culture, biopsy, specialized laboratory testing, and a high index of suspicion.

References

1. Al-Serhani AM (2001) Mycobacterial infection of the head and neck: presentation and diagnosis. *Laryngoscope* 111(11 Pt 1):2012–6.

2. Avčin T, Silverman ED, Forte V, et al (2005) Nasal septal perforation: a novel clinical manifestation of systemic juvenile idiopathic arthritis/adult onset Still's disease. *Journal of Rheumatology* 32(12):2429–31.

3. Bateman ND, Woolford TJ (2003) Informed consent for septal surgery: the evidence-base. *Journal of Laryngology & Otology* 117(3):186–9.

4. Batra K, Chaudhary N, Motwani G, et al (2002) An unusual case of primary nasal tuberculosis with epistaxis and epilepsy. *Ear, Nose, & Throat Journal* 81(12):842–4.

5. Batsakis JG (1981) Pathology consultation. Nasal (Schneiderian) papillomas. *Annals of Otology, Rhinology & Laryngology* 90(2 Pt 1):190–1.

6. Batsakis JG, El-Naggar AK (1992) Rhinoscleroma and rhinosporidiosis. *Annals of Otology, Rhinology & Laryngology* 101(10):879–82.

7. Baum ED, Boudousquie AC, Li S, et al (1998) Sarcoidosis with nasal obstruction and septal perforation. *Ear, Nose, & Throat Journal* 77(11):896–8.

8. Béjar I, Farkas LG, Messner AH, Crysdale WS (1996) Nasal growth after external septoplasty in children. *Archives of Otolaryngology – Head & Neck Surgery* 122(8):816–21.

9. Belloso A, Morar P, Estrach C, et al (2001) Rheumatoid nodule of the nasal septum. *Journal of Laryngology & Otology* 115(10):853–5.

10. Blotta P, Carinci F, Pelucci S, et al (2001) Chondrosarcoma of the nasal septum. *Annals of Otology, Rhinology & Laryngology* 110(2):202–4.

11. Braun JJ, Gentine A, Pauli G (2004) Sinonasal sarcoidosis: review and report of fifteen cases. *Laryngoscope* 114(11):1960–3.

12. Buchwald C, Franzmann MB, Tos M (1995) Sinonasal papillomas: a report of 82 cases in Copenhagen County, including a longitudinal epidemiological and clinical study. *Laryngoscope* 105(1):72–9.

13. Canty PA, Berkowitz RG (1996) Hematoma and abscess of the nasal septum in children. *Archives of Otolaryngology – Head & Neck Surgery* 122(12):1373–6.

14. Cervin A, Hansson C, Greiff L, Andersson M (2003) Nasal septal perforations during treatment with topical nasal glucocorticosteroids are generally not associated with contact allergy to steroids. ORL; Journal for Oto-Rhino-Laryngology and its Related Specialties 65(2):103–5.

15. Chen HL, Cheng PW, Tsai CC (2003) Pathology quiz case. Nasal T/NK-cell lymphoma. *Archives of Otolaryngology – Head & Neck Surgery* 129(10):1135–6.

16. Cheung MM, Chan JK, Lau WH, et al (2002) Early stage nasal NK/T-cell lymphoma: clinical outcome, prognostic factors, and the effect of treatment modality. *International Journal of Radiation Oncology, Biology, Physics* 54(1):182–90.

17. Chiu T, Dunn JS (2006) An anatomical study of the arteries of the anterior nasal septum. *Otolaryngology – Head and Neck Surgery* 134(1):33–36.

18. Choi YC, Park YS, Jeon EJ, et al (2000) The disappeared disease: tuberculosis of the nasal septum. *Rhinology* 38(2):90–2.

19. Chukuezi AB (1992) Nasal septal haematoma in Nigeria. *Journal of Laryngology & Otology* 106(5):396–8.

20. Daggett RB, Haghighi P, Terkeltaub RA (1990) Nasal cocaine abuse causing an aggressive midline intranasal and pharyngeal destructive process mimicking midline reticulosis and limited Wegener's granulomatosis. *Journal of Rheumatology* 17(6):838–40.

21. Dash GI, Kimmelman CP (1988) Head and neck manifestations of sarcoidosis. *Laryngoscope* 98(1):50–3.

22. Diamantopoulos II, Jones NS (2001) The investigation of nasal septal perforations and ulcers. *Journal of Laryngology & Otology* 115(7):541–4.

23. Fairbanks DN (1980) Closure of nasal septal perforations. *Archives of Otolaryngology* 106(8):509–13.

24. Fergie N, Jones NS, Havlat MF (1999) The nasal manifestations of sarcoidosis: a review and report of eight cases. *Journal of Laryngology & Otology* 113(10):893–8.

13

25. Frable MA, Frable WJ (1984) Fine-needle aspiration biopsy: efficacy in the diagnosis of head and neck sarcoidosis. *Laryngoscope* 94(10):1281–3.

26. Friedman M, Ibrahim H, Ramakrishnan V (2003) Inferior turbinate flap for repair of nasal septal perforation. *Laryngoscope* 113(8):1425–8.

27. Gaines JJ, Clay JR, Chandler FW, et al (1996) Rhinosporidiosis: three domestic cases. *Southern Medical Journal* 89(1):65–7.

28. Gray LP (1978) Deviated nasal septum. Incidence and etiology. *Annals of Otology, Rhinology, & Laryngology Supplement* 87(3 Pt 3 Suppl 50):3–20.

29. Gubbels SP, Barkhuizen A, Hwang PH (2003) Head and neck manifestations of Wegener's granulomatosis. *Otolaryngologic Clinics of North America* 36(4):685–705.

30. Hanif, J, Tasca RA, Frosh A, et al (2003) Silver nitrate: histological effects of cautery on epithelial surfaces with varying contact times. *Clinical Otolaryngology & Allied Sciences* 28(4):368–70.

31. Hart CA, Rao SK (2000) Rhinoscleroma. *Journal of Medical Microbiology* 49(5):395–6.

32. Healy GB (1986) An approach to the nasal septum in children. *Laryngoscope* 96(1):1239–42.

33. Hunt SM, Miyamoto RC, Cornelius RS, Tami TA (2000) Invasive fungal sinusitis in the acquired immunodeficiency syndrome. *Otolaryngologic Clinics of North America* 33(2):335–47.

34. Hyams VJ (1971) Papillomas of the nasal cavity and paranasal sinuses. A clinicopathological study of 315 cases. *Annals of Otology, Rhinology & Laryngology* 80(2):192–206.

35. Jang YJ, Myong NH, Park KH, et al (2002) Mucociliary transport and histologic characteristics of the mucosa of deviated nasal septum. *Archives of Otolaryngology – Head & Neck Surgery* 128(4):421–4.

36. Jones JE, Nguyen A, Tabaee A (2000) Pyogenic granuloma (pregnancy tumor) of the nasal cavity. A case report. *J Reprod Med* 45(9):749–53.

37. Jones NS (1999) Nasal manifestations of rheumatic diseases. *Annals of the Rheumatic Diseases* 58(10):589–90.

38. Koltai PJ, Hoehn J, Bailey CM (1992) The external rhinoplasty approach for rhinologic surgery in children. *Otolaryngology – Head and Neck Surgery* 118(4):401–5.

39. Kridel RW (1999) Septal perforation repair. *Otolaryngologic Clinics of North America* 32(4):695–724.

40. Lalwani AK, Tami TA, Gelber RH (1992) Lepromatous leprosy: nasal manifestations and treatment with minocycline. *Annals of Otology, Rhinology & Laryngology* 101(3):261–4.

41. Li CC, Tien HF, Tang JL, et al (2004) Treatment outcome and pattern of failure in 77 patients with sinonasal natural killer/T-cell or T-cell lymphoma. *Cancer* 100(2):366–75.

42. Li XQ, Hisaoka M, Morio T, et al. (2003) Intranasal pericytic tumors (glomus tumor and sinonasal hemangiopericytoma-like tumor): report of two cases with review of the literature. *Pathology International* 53(5):303–8.

43. Lund VJ, Howard DJ (1999) A treatment algorithm for the management of epistaxis in hereditary hemorrhagic telangiectasia. *American Journal of Rhinology* 13(4):319–22

44. Marshall AH, Johnston MN, Jones NS (2004) Principles of septal correction. *Journal of Laryngology & Otology* 118(2):129–34.

45. Mascarenhas R, Tellechea O, Oliveira H, et al (2005) Nasal septum perforation as the presenting sign of lupus erythematosus. *Dermatology Online Journal* 11(2):12.

46. Mathews JL, Ward JR, Samuelson CO, Knibbe WP (1983) Spontaneous nasal septal perforation in patients with rheumatoid arthritis. *Clinical Rheumatology* 2(1):13–18.

47. Matthews B, Whang C, Smith S (2002) Endoscopic resection of a nasal septal chondrosarcoma: first report of a case. *Ear, Nose, & Throat Journal* 81(5):327–9.

48. McNulty JS, Fassett RL (1981) Syphilis: an otolaryngologic perspective. *Laryngoscope* 91(6):889–905.

49. Mears T, Amerasinghe C (1992) Rhinosporidiosis. *Journal of Laryngology & Otology* 106(5):468.

50. Messervy M (1971) Primary tuberculoma of the nose with presenting symptoms and lesions resembling a malignant granuloma. *Journal of Laryngology & Otology* 85(2):177–84.

51. Morris JM, Lane JI, Witte RJ, et al (2004) Giant cell reparative granuloma of the nasal cavity. *American Journal of Neuroradiology* 25(7):1263–5.

52. Nagai H, Takahashi H, Yao K, et al (2002) Clinical review of Wegener's granulomatosis. *Acta Oto-Laryngologica Supplement* (547):50–3.

53. Nayar RC, Al Kaabi J, Ghorpade K (2004) Primary nasal tuberculosis: a case report. *Ear, Nose, & Throat Journal* 83(3):188–91.

54. Newton JR, White PS, Lee MS (2003) Nasal septal perforation repair using open septoplasty and unilateral bipedicled flaps. *Journal of Laryngology & Otology* 117(1):52–5.

55. Parsons DS, Batra PS (1998) Functional endoscopic sinus surgical outcomes for contact point headaches. *Laryngoscope* 108(5):696–702.

56. Pickens JP, Modica L (1989) Current concepts of the lethal midline granuloma syndrome. *Otolaryngology – Head & Neck Surgery* 100(6):623–30.

57. Price DL, Sherris DA, Kern EB (2003) Computed tomography for constructing custom nasal septal buttons. *Archives of Otolaryngology – Head & Neck Surgery* 129(11):1236–9.

58. Roblin DG, Eccles R (2002) What, if any, is the value of septal surgery? *Clinical Otolaryngology & Allied Sciences* 27(2):77–80.

59. Rodriguez-Castro K, Zamora-Barquero H (2006) Nasal septum perforation: rare manifestation of Crohn's disease. *Indian Journal of Gastroenterology* 25(4):214.

60. Scartozzi R, Couch M, Sciubba J (2003) Chondroid chordoma of the nasal septum. *Archives of Otolaryngology – Head & Neck Surgery* 129(2):244–6.

61. Seyer BA, Grist W, Muller S (2002) Aggressive destructive midfacial lesion from cocaine abuse. *Oral Surgery Oral Medicine Oral Pathology Oral Radiology & Endodontics* 94(4):465–70.

62. Shah UK, White JA, Gooey JE, et al (1997) Otolaryngologic manifestations of sarcoidosis: presentation and diagnosis. *Laryngoscope* 107(1):67–75.

63. Siegel MB, Keane WM, Atkins JP, Rosen MR (1991) Control of epistaxis in patients with hereditary hemorrhagic telangiectasia. *Otolaryngology – Head and Neck Surgery* 105(5):675–9.

64. Smith JC, Kacker A, Anand VK (2002) Midline nasal and hard palate destruction in cocaine abusers and cocaine's role in rhinologic practice. *Ear, Nose, & Throat Journal* 81(3):172–7

65. Stoor P, Grenman R (2004) Bioactive glass and turbinate flaps in the repair of nasal septal perforations. *Annals of Otology, Rhinology & Laryngology* 113(8):655–61.

66. Stucker FJ, Bryarly RC, Shockley WW (1984) Management of nasal trauma in children. *Archives of Otolaryngology – Head & Neck Surgery* 110(3):190–2.

67. Sturm HM (1976) Secondary syphilis appearing as a solitary plaque of the nose. *International Journal of Dermatology* 15(9):678–9.

68. Takwoingi YM, Dempster JH (2003) Wegener's granulomatosis: an analysis of 33 patients seen over a 10-year period. *Clinical Otolaryngology & Allied Sciences* 28(3):187–94.

69. Talbott JF, Gorti GK, Koch RJ (2001) Midfacial osteomyelitis in a chronic cocaine abuser: a case report. *Ear, Nose, & Throat Journal* 80(10):738–40.

70. Thompson LD (2002) Rhinoscleroma. *Ear, Nose, & Throat Journal* 81(8):506.

71. Thompson LD, Wieneke JA, Miettinen M (2003) Sinonasal tract and nasopharyngeal melanomas: a clinicopathologic study of 115 cases with a proposed staging system. *American Journal of Surgical Pathology* 27(5):594–611.

72. Unlu HH, Unlu Z, Ayhan S, et al (2002) Osteochondroma of the posterior nasal septum managed by endoscopic transnasal transseptal approach. *Journal of Laryngology & Otology* 116(11):955–7.

73. Willkens RF, Roth GJ, Novak A, Walike JW (1976) Perforation of nasal septum in rheumatic diseases. *Arthritis and Rheumatism* 19(1):119–121

74. Yewell J, Haydon R, Archer S, et al (2002) Complications of intranasal prescription narcotic abuse. *Annals of Otology, Rhinology & Laryngology* 111(2):174–7.

75. Yih WY, Stewart JC, Kratochvil FJ, et al (2002) Angiocentric T-cell lymphoma presenting as midface destructive lesion: case report and literature review. *Oral Surgery Oral Medicine Oral Pathology Oral Radiology & Endodontics* 94(3):353–60.

Chapter 14

The Stuffy Nose

Jeremy Paul Watkins and Rakesh K. Chandra

14

Core Messages

- A thorough history combined with a methodical physical examination including endoscopy is required when evaluating a patient with a stuffy nose.
- Rhinomanometry and acoustic rhinometry are currently most commonly utilized as investigational tools.
- The mainstay of medical therapy for many stuffy nose conditions is topical intranasal steroids.
- Turbinate reduction should be considered in those in whom medical therapy fails.
- If turbinate reduction is contemplated, a technique that preserves the mucociliary surface should be selected.

Contents

Introduction and Background

The obstructed nasal airway is a symptom encountered daily by the otolaryngologist. The etiology of this common complaint is often multi-factorial and can be a source of extreme frustration for both the patient and the physician. Nasal airway obstruction can also result in a significant financial burden. Kimmelman estimated that approximately 5 billion dollars are spent annually to relieve nasal airway obstruction, and an estimated 60 million dollars are spent on surgical procedures intended to relieve nasal airway obstruction [36]. This chapter will focus on anatomical and physiological considerations for the clinician when dealing with "the stuffy nose." This will be followed by a review of diagnostic and therapeutic strategies to assist in the management of this complex problem.

Anatomical Principles

When evaluating the complaint of a "stuffy nose," a clear understanding of nasal anatomy will improve the chances of a satisfactory outcome for both patient and physician. The anatomy of the nose can be divided into external support structures, internal support structures, and internal soft tissue components. When evaluating the nose in this sequential manner, the physician is able to thoroughly evaluate each component separately and determine how much each is contributing to the patient's symptoms.

The bony nasal pyramid provides a foundation of stability for all external support structures of the nose. The nasal bones articulate with the nasal process of the frontal bone superiorly and with the ascending process of the maxilla laterally. They are also important to the shape of the nasal septum as the nasal bones articulate with the superior surfaces of the perpendicular plate of the ethmoid and the cartilaginous nasal septum. The nasal bones overlap the anterior–superior edge of the upper lateral cartilages in the so-called keystone area, providing support to the lateral walls of the middle third of the nose.

The upper and lower lateral cartilages provide critical support to the lower two-thirds of the nose, including the lateral nasal walls and nasal tip. The upper lateral cartilages extend below the cephalic margins of the lower lateral cartilages and are supported laterally by the ascending process of the maxilla. A majority of the upper lateral cartilage is attached medially to the dorsal septum, except for a small cleft that exists caudally in between the septum and the upper lateral cartilages. The upper lateral cartilages are joined inferiorly with the cephalic edges of the lower lateral cartilages, providing one of the major tip supporting structures. Each lower lateral cartilage is composed of a medial and lateral crus. The caudal edge of the lateral crus, along with alar fibro-fatty tissue and the membranous septum, form the external nasal valve [28]. The medial crura are loosely joined to each other and to the nasal septum to contribute to nasal projection and the shape of the columella. The resiliency of the upper and lower lateral cartilages counteract Bernoulli forces during deep inspiration and prevent internal and external nasal valve collapse.

Skin, subcutaneous tissue, and surrounding muscles provide the soft tissue envelope of the nose. The nasal skin and subcutaneous tissue provide minor tip support, while the surrounding musculature plays an important role in the competency of the external nasal valve. The levator labii superioris alaeque nasi is the most important dilator of the external nasal valve, which decreases resistance by widening the nasal ala during inspiration [28].

There are several endonasal structures that play a role in the nasal airway. The nasal septum may be the most important in this regard, as a deviation of the nasal septum often contributes significantly to the symptomatology. The septum is composed of a bony and cartilaginous portion. The bony portion consists of the perpendicular plate of ethmoid, which articulates with the vomer inferiorly. The vomer rests inferiorly on the maxillary and palatine crests [28]. The cartilaginous septum articulates with the perpendicular plate posterior–superior and with the vomer posterior–inferior.

An important endonasal anatomic region is the internal nasal valve (Fig. 14.1), which was first described by Mink in 1903. It is important to differentiate between the nasal valve proper and the "nasal valve area." The components of the nasal valve proper include the dorsal nasal septum medially, the internal caudal edge of the upper lateral cartilage laterally, and the anterior head of the inferior turbinate posteriorly. The "nasal valve area," as described by Kasperbauer and Kern, is the area extending posteriorly from the actual nasal valve to the bony pyriform aperture and extending inferiorly to the floor of the nose [33]. The nasal valve proper is the smallest cross-sectional area of the nasal airway (approximately 40–60 mm^2) and accounts for approximately two-thirds of the total nasal airway resistance. Normally, the angle between the nasal septum and upper lateral cartilage is 10–15° in the leptorrhine nose, and is usually a little wider in the platyrrhine nose.

Patency of the nasal airway is greatly affected by dynamic changes in endonasal soft tissue components, the most important of which is the inferior turbinate. The inferior turbinate extends into the lateral nasal wall as a separate bone, attached to the medial maxilla [28], and is covered by thick mucosal/submucosal tissue (Fig. 14.2). The outermost covering of this layer comprises pseudostratified columnar epithelium with cilia that suspend a bi-layered mucus covering. The thicker outer mucous layer effectively traps particles, while the more serous layer at the base of the cilia promotes the whipping action of the cilia, enhancing mucociliary clearance. The basement membrane lies just under this mucosal layer, which is superficial to the lamina propria [1]. The lamina propria is an important site of several regulators of the nasal airway. This layer is the site where inflammatory cells are released from the microvasculature following stimulation by pro-inflammatory cytokines, and is also the location of the seromucinous glands that generate the outer mucus covering described above. Additionally, the lamina propria contains venous sinusoids located between capillaries and venules in the submucosa. These sinusoids are under sympathetic tone, and some postulate that they are the main contributors of reactive inferior turbinate enlargement [3]. Berger et al. [1] found that patients with bilateral inferior turbinate hypertrophy consistently demonstrated enlargement of the lamina propria area, while the thickness of the epithelial layer remained relatively the same.

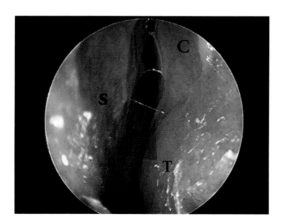

Fig. 14.1 The left nasal valve (*shaded*). The boundaries are the head of the inferior turbinate (*T*), nasal septum (*S*), and internal caudal margin of the upper lateral cartilage (*C*)

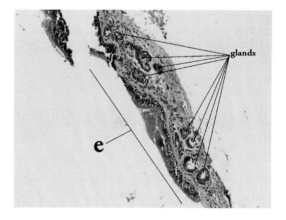

Fig. 14.2 Soft tissue covering of the inferior turbinate. The surface mucosa consists of pseudostratified, columnar, ciliated epithelium (*e*). The submucosa contains seromucinous glands and vascular channels. This specimen exhibits a preponderance of submucous glands, as indicated

Nasal Physiology

Our understanding of nasal physiology has evolved tremendously over the last several thousand years. Aristotle believed that the main function of the nose was sneezing, but it was not until the 20th century that a clearer understanding of nasal function was obtained [36]. The three main functions of the nose are:

1. Modifier of inspired/expired air
2. Olfactory sensory organ
3. Airway resistor

Air that passes through the nose is filtered, moisturized, and warmed to near body temperature before reaching the glottis. When breathing in cold air, nasal resistance increases in order to provide a larger surface area and longer transit time for optimal heat exchange. Upon expiration, the glottis is partially closed, providing turbulence to expired air, allowing for increased mucosal contact in the nose and more efficient resorption of heat and moisture [6]. The filtering mechanism of the nose is at the level of the vibrissae of the nasal vestibule, the mucociliary complex and the side walls of the nasal cavity. The nose is also able to trigger protective reflexes, such as sneezing and coughing, designed to protect the lungs from harmful toxins and allergens.

The temperature of inspired air also plays a role in the perception of nasal airway patency. Cold receptors in the nasal cavity are stimulated as cool air is inspired, resulting in a perceived improvement in nasal airway flow. Substances such as menthol can mimic this phenomenon by altering the sensitivity of cold receptors in the nose; however, nasal resistance is unaffected [57].

Olfactory function in humans is less keen than in other species that rely more heavily on their sense of smell for survival. As humans began to walk upright, they became less reliant on their sense of smell. This evolutionary change resulted in a decrease in size of the olfactory surface area, providing a larger space for nasal breathing [28]. Only an estimated 15% of inspired air actually passes in the olfactory area; however, active sniffing can direct additional airflow superiorly toward the olfactory region [42]. Olfactory sensation is the first means by which we sample the fluid medium in which we live. This sense is important to emotion, perception of flavor, and sensation of danger, and certain professionals such as chefs, wine tasters, and firemen rely heavily on their sense of smell. Our sense of smell acts as a warning of potentially harmful inspired vapors. To complement the olfactory sense, the nose utilizes the trigeminal nerve to detect somatosensory input by chemical and nonchemical stimuli in order to warn us of vapors that may be too hot, too cold, or potentially hazardous [15]. Nasal airway obstruction secondary to severe nasal polyposis (or any obstructive phenomenon) affects our ability to deliver inspired air to the region of the olfactory area. Nasal obstruction may therefore limit important mechanisms of both aesthetic pleasure and survival.

An important role of the nose is to act as an airway resistor. The nasal airway accounts for about 40–50% of total airway resistance, and about 66% of this resistance is provided by the nasal valve. This increased resistance leads to increased pulmonary compliance, providing ample time for gas exchange at the alveolar level [46]. Nasal resistance assists with re-absorption of heat and water, and it also helps prevent alveolar collapse [36].

The nasal cycle is responsible for periodic fluctuations in the resistance of one nasal cavity compared with the other. This phenomenon was first described by Kayser in 1895 and occurs in 80% of the population. Fluctuations in inferior turbinate engorgement last 30 min to 5 h per cycle, resulting in an increase in unilateral nasal airway resistance without affecting total nasal airway resistance. The periodic nasal engorgement of the nasal cycle is under autonomic regulation and can be abolished by topical decongestants. Sympathetic input from the cervical sympathetic chain travels along the deep petrosal nerve to the pterygopalatine ganglion, by way of the vidian nerve, and is responsible for resting vasoconstrictive tone. Parasympathetic input from the greater superficial petrosal nerve travels to the pterygopalatine ganglion, by way of the vidian nerve, and is responsible for vasodilation and engorgement of nasal mucosa.

The phenomenon of the nasal cycle was studied by Lang et al. [39], who measured fluctuations in the nasal cross-sectional area during the nasal cycle using acoustic rhinometry. He was able to show changes in the unilateral nasal cross-sectional area during the nasal cycle; however, little variation was noticed at the nasal valve itself. This may explain why the nasal cycle is often unnoticed unless other pathology exists (septal deviation, allergic rhinitis, etc.).

Nasal resistance is also affected by stimuli such as posture and physical exertion. Nasal resistance is highest when the patient is in the supine position, and decreases as the head is elevated. When the patient is in the lateral decubitus position, the dependent inferior turbinate is engorged and the turbinate in the superior position is constricted. This phenomenon is thought to be related to autonomic shoulder and axillary sensory information linked to nasal reflexes [57]. Physical exertion is thought to decrease nasal resistance either by sympathetic stimulation or by a simple redistribution of blood to the heart, lungs and peripheral muscles [51]. In accordance with Ohm's Law, a decrease in nasal airway resistance requires less work to produce the same amount of flow, which is beneficial during times of physical exertion.

Nasal Airflow

Airflow through the nose is a result of a pressure differential created by negative pressure generated by expanding intra-thoracic volume during inspiration. Nasal airflow takes a parabolic curve (Fig. 14.3) after it enters the nares [6]. Flow is directed above the head of the inferior turbinate and a majority of the airflow passes through the middle meatus. After passing through the middle meatus, airflow curves inferiorly as it passes through the choanae into the nasopharynx. Any disturbance in this pattern (i.e., septal perforation, atrophic rhinitis) can be perceived as nasal airway obstruction.

Nasal airflow can be laminar, turbulent or a combination of the two. Laminar flow occurs through a perfect tube as flow in the center of the tube is more rapid than flow at the periphery. Turbulent flow is characterized by random paths of airflow created by tube irregularities. Because the nose is not a

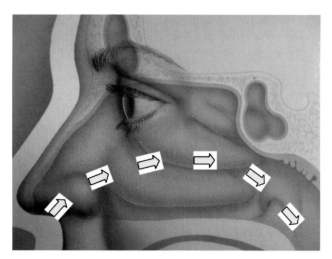

Fig. 14.3 Airflow through the nasal cavity follows a parabolic pattern

perfect tube, flow through the nose is usually more turbulent than laminar. Turbulence is important because it allows for the physiologic mixing of air that improves air modification (warming, humidifying, and filtering) and optimizes olfactory function [36]. Given that nasal airflow is neither purely turbulent nor purely laminar, the sensation of nasal airway obstruction is probably related to the ratio of turbulent to laminar airflow. This ratio depends on the velocity of nasal airflow, as turbulence increases with increasing flow velocity. The most dramatic change in flow velocity occurs at the level of the nasal valve, as air enters a smaller cross-sectional area, causing an increase in airflow velocity. As flow exits the nasal valve and the cross-sectional area of the nose increases, flow is dramatically slowed. Turbulence is greatly increased as the fast moving air immediately exiting the nasal valve area collides with this slow moving air.

History and Physical Examination

As with any clinical disorder, a thorough history is vital to appropriately addressing the problem of nasal airway obstruction. The physician should first begin by localizing the obstructed area, which can be unilateral or bilateral. Important information concerning timing would include onset, duration, and frequency of symptoms. If symptoms of rhinitis are present, the physician should inquire whether a seasonal or perennial pattern is present. Exacerbating and alleviating factors should be elicited, which may reveal certain environmental exposures such as cigarette smoke or toxic fumes. An assessment of associated symptoms should be obtained, such as allergy symptoms (itchy and watery eyes, scratchy throat and sneezing), epistaxis or clear rhinorrhea. It is also important to illicit any history of trauma that may be associated with nasal airway obstruction. Extensive past medical history should be obtained along with an in-depth allergy history. Patients should be questioned on any food allergies, as well as exposure to toxic/allergic substances at

home and at work (including second-hand smoke, old carpet, and house pets). A travel history can also be very useful if fungal infection is a suspected etiology [36].

Once extensive history has been obtained, a complete head and neck examination is performed with particular attention to pertinent non-nasal findings that may point to a diagnosis. Patients with allergic rhinitis may exhibit the classic "allergic shiners" or "allergic salute." Facial nerve function should be assessed, as paralysis of the splinting muscles of the nasal ala may result in a functional nasal airway obstruction. Middle ear effusions may be a manifestation of chronic nasopharyngeal inflammation, adenoid hypertrophy, or an obstructing mass near the Eustachian tube. Midface deformities may be the result of chronic mouth breathing secondary to nasal airway obstruction. A high degree of suspicion for hypothyroidism should be present for patients with chronic nasal congestion, rhinorrhea, post-nasal drip, and globus sensation in the presence of a near normal physical examination [22].

The portion of the physical examination focused on the nasal cavity should be performed in a sequential manner. A suggested method is to focus on external support structures, followed by an assessment of internal support structures, and lastly evaluation of the internal soft tissue structures. This sequential method will ensure that all possible etiologies are evaluated.

When focusing on the external support structures of the nose, the physician should first comment on the overall appearance of the nose. The bony nasal vault should be evaluated for any asymmetries or evidence of prior trauma. Previous deflections secondary to trauma can result in a dorsal septal deviation with nasal valve obstruction. If the patient has a prior history of rhinoplasty, it should be noted if the patient's nasal bridge has been overly narrowed by osteotomies, which could be contributing to the obstruction as well. The columella should be examined for any excessive widening or tilting from a caudal septal deviation. Severe tip ptosis can also contribute to nasal airway obstruction because it can redirect nasal airflow to a more superior route. This detour of the nasal airflow away from the middle meatus can be perceived as nasal airway obstruction. If nasal tip ptosis is contributing to symptoms, tilting the tip superiorly will considerably improve the patient's symptoms. Lastly, the patient should be observed during quiet and deep inspiration and the physician should assess upper and lower lateral cartilage competency. Early collapse during inspiration would suggest valve incompetence.

After examining the external units of the nose, attention should be paid to the internal support structures and soft tissues of the nose. The first area of interest is the internal nasal valve, which is the smallest cross-sectional area in the nasal cavity. Care must be taken not to distort the valve with the nasal speculum, and often the valve can be adequately examined by simply lifting the nasal tip superiorly [37]. The Cottle maneuver is a test of nasal valve integrity. It is performed by retracting the cheek laterally, pulling the upper lateral cartilage away from the septum and widening the internal nasal valve angle (Fig. 14.4). If the patient's symptoms are relieved with this maneuver, this suggests that the cause of the nasal airway obstruction is related to the nasal valve area (e.g., dorsal septal deviation, lack of upper lateral cartilage integrity). False-negatives can be seen with synechiae in the nasal valve, which prevents the valve from opening during the maneuver [37]. Aggressive lateral osteotomies can result in over-medialization of the ascending process of the maxilla, resulting in a decrease in the cross-sectional area of the posterior–lateral nasal valve area, also causing a false-negative finding during the Cottle maneuver. In addition, a cotton swab or nasal speculum can also be used to lateralize the upper lateral cartilage from inside the nose, and the patient is again asked if the symptoms are improved. This technique enables direct observation of the nasal valve area as it widened.

As many nasal airway disturbances are caused or exacerbated by septal abnormalities, the septum should be carefully examined in its entirety (which usually requires decongestion). Anterior deviations in the nasal valve region are more likely than posterior deviations to cause symptoms of obstruction, so not every abnormality of the septum requires surgical correction. Areas of the septum that are normally widened, such as at the septal base and just anterior to the middle turbinate, should not be mistaken for a deviation or spur [46]. When examining the nose, one should also comment on the health of the mucosa of the septum and turbinates. Dry-appearing mucosa with extensive crusting suggests atrophic rhinitis, while boggy or erythematous turbinates can suggest rhinitis.

Complete examination of the septum, turbinates, and internal valve is best accomplished with diagnostic nasal endoscopy. This should be performed before and after decongestion to assess the decongestant response (Fig. 14.5) and to rule out posterior septal deviations, inflammatory disease, polyps (Fig. 14.6), foreign bodies, and neoplasms. If the nasal airway obstruction improves with decongestion alone, this suggests a mucosal inflammatory disorder of the inferior turbinates [8]. No response suggests the etiology of the obstruction is of a rigid, structural nature, such as nasal valve obstruction, septal deviation or bony hypertrophy of the inferior turbinate. It should be noted that some mucosal inflammatory disorders may also exhibit lack of decongestive response, including rhinitis medicamentosa or diffuse nasal polyposis.

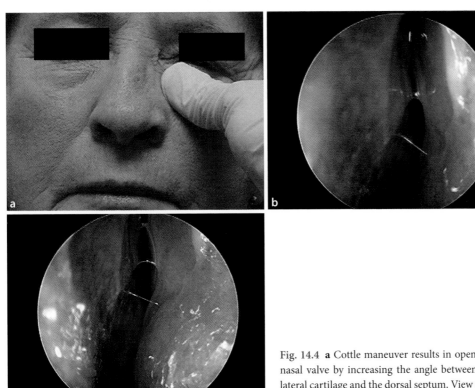

Fig. 14.4 **a** Cottle maneuver results in opening the left nasal valve by increasing the angle between the upper lateral cartilage and the dorsal septum. View of the nasal valve **b** before and **c** during the maneuver

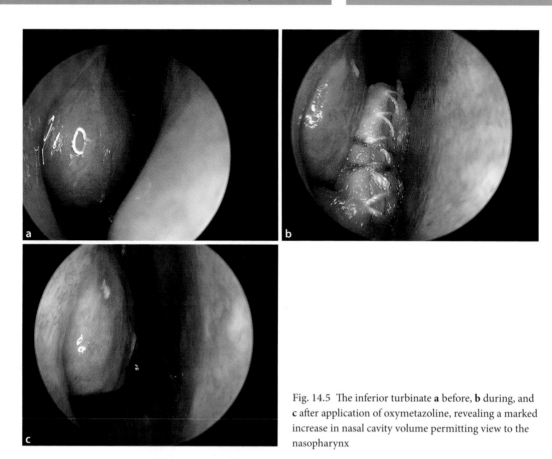

Fig. 14.5 The inferior turbinate **a** before, **b** during, and **c** after application of oxymetazoline, revealing a marked increase in nasal cavity volume permitting view to the nasopharynx

14

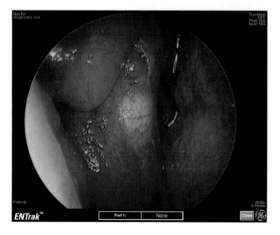

Fig. 14.6 Antrochoanal polyp in a patient whose only complaint was nasal stuffiness

Objective Evaluation and Diagnostic Studies

The rapid technological advances in the field of otolaryngology over the last 50 years have allowed us to obtain a more objective analysis of nasal airway obstruction. Because the source of obstruction is not always evident from patient history and physical examination, radiography may be required to assist with diagnosis. CT may reveal unexpected anatomic findings such as concha bullosa of the inferior turbinate (Fig. 14.7) or a foreign body and can also be used to evaluate structural/bony abnormalities such as a deviated septum, nasal bone fractures, choanal atresia (Fig. 14.8), and sinus disease. MRI, because of its soft tissue detail, is better suited to evaluating the integrity of the dura and to further assessment of certain nasal masses (such as encephalocele or glioma).

Dynamic airway testing is also available as an objective means of evaluating the nasal airway. Hygrometry was one of the first objective measures of the nasal airway. This technique

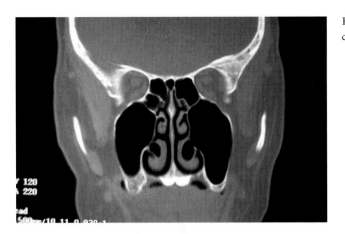

Fig. 14.7 Coronal CT revealing bilateral concha bullosa of the inferior turbinates

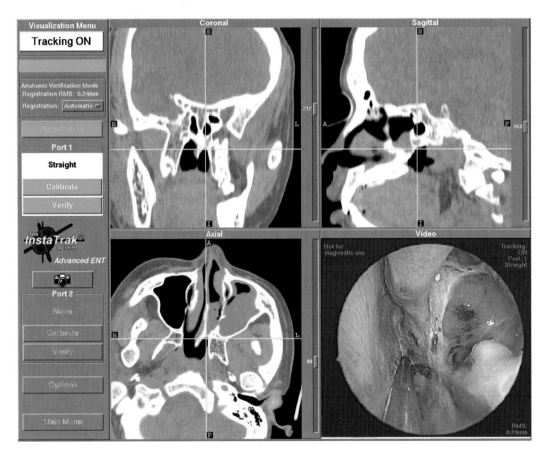

Fig. 14.8 Triplanar CT reconstructions revealing left-sided choanal atresia in an adult who presented with unilateral nasal stuffiness and recurrent sinusitis. This is best visualized in the sagittal (*right upper panel*) and axial (*left lower panel*) views

was described by Zwaardemacher in 1894 and involved having the patient breathe onto a mirror and the diameter of the fog produced by each nostril was compared (cited in [43]). In 1902, Spiess described a technique of nasal airway evaluation that involved having the patient hum while alternating occlusion of each nostril. He used the timbre of sound created during occlusion to assess the nasal airway patency (cited in [26]).

Today, the two most commonly used methods for evaluating nasal obstruction are acoustic rhinometry and rhinomanom-

etry. These objective tests have several uses in both clinical and research settings. They can be used pre- and post-decongestion in an attempt to predict the efficacy of certain medical and surgical therapies. Objective testing is also useful to confirm improved nasal cross-sectional area or resistance after surgery. Lund [42] stresses the importance of objective testing because of the high patient dissatisfaction rate (30%) after surgery to resolve nasal airway obstruction. Acoustic rhinometry and rhinomanometry can also be used for nasal provocational studies in patients with suspected allergic rhinitis and have recently been used for assisting in the diagnosis of obstructive sleep apnea and sleep disordered breathing. Although these objective tests are commonly used in the research setting, clinical use in the US is not as widespread because of issues of expense, availability, and inconsistencies with patient subjective scores [58].

Acoustic Rhinometry

The technology of acoustic rhinometry was originally devised for oil investigation; however, it was not until the 1970s that it was first used in the field of medicine to perform measurements in the distal airway [62]. In 1989, Hilberg was the first to use acoustic rhinometry to measure the cross-sectional area in the nasal airway. The acoustic rhinometer consists of a sound source, wave tube, microphone, filter, amplifier, digital converter, and a computer. A sound wave is transmitted into the nasal cavity, which is then reflected back from the nasal passages and converted into digital impulses that are then constructed on a rhinogram (Fig. 14.9) [38]. This rhinogram provides a two-dimensional anatomic assessment of the nasal airway. The cross-sectional area of the nose differs at different points from the nasal rim, and these variances are detected by changes in acoustic impedance.

Each notch on the rhinogram represents a different anatomic constriction in the nasal cavity [38]. The first notch represents the nasal valve and is usually the MCA (minimal cross-sectional area) in the normal nose. The second notch represents anterior portions of the inferior turbinate or middle turbinate, while the third notch is estimated to be in the area of the middle/posterior end of the middle turbinate [10]. Each notch identifies a site of limitation of nasal airflow and can be used to locate the site of obstruction in the nose.

Acoustic rhinometry has been validated based on other anatomical assessments, and standardized values have been established by several authors [44]. A high correlation of cross-sectional area has been found when comparing acoustic rhinometry with MRI after nasal decongestion [8, 27]. Acoustic rhinometry has also been compared with CT for accuracy of cross-sectional area measurements in the nose. Measurements were found to be very accurate anteriorly, but became less accurate in the posterior portions of the nasal cavity [13, 45].

Rhinomanometry

Rhinomanometry is a functional assessment of airflow and involves measurement of transnasal pressure and airflow. From these measurements one can assess the mean pressure, volume, work (pressure × flow), and resistance (pressure/flow) associated with each breath. Resistance from each side of the nose can be compared with one another and with total nasal resistance, enabling the physician to identify how each nasal passage is contributing to the patient's complaint. The resulting plot, with the x-axis representing the pressure differential and the y-axis representing flow, produces an S-shaped curve (Fig. 14.10). The most common method of reporting results is with inspiratory airflow, as seen on the right side of the graph in Fig. 14.10. The machine consists of a pressure transducer for measuring posterior nasal pressure, a pneumotachometer for measurement of flow, a mask for measurement of anterior nasal pressure and flow, and a computer for converting these measurements into digital signals.

In rhinomanometry, posterior nasal pressure is measured in one of three ways. Anterior rhinomanometry, introduced by Coutade in 1902 (cited in [42]), involves placement of a transducer in the nostril not being tested. Because there is no flow in this nostril, the pressure at the anterior end of this nostril is equal to the pressure in the posterior end of this nostril. This is the most common method used because it is usually well tolerated and it is easier for the patient to cooperate. Limitations of anterior rhinomanometry include its inability to make accurate measurements with septal perforations. Another disadvantage is that a direct measurement of total nasal resistance cannot be made because each nostril is measured separately. Estimations of total nasal resistance can be obtained by calculations; however, these results are not as accurate as those obtained by direct measurement.

Another method of measuring the nasal pressure differential is with posterior (peroral) rhinomanometry, introduced by Spiess in 1899 (cited in [42]). With this method, the pressure detector is in the posterior oropharynx by way of tubing passed through the mouth. It is the only method that can accurately assess the contribution of adenoid hypertrophy to nasal airway obstruction; however, it is not tolerated as well as anterior rhinomanometry. The third method of measuring transnasal pressure is postnasal rhinomanometry. This method involves place-

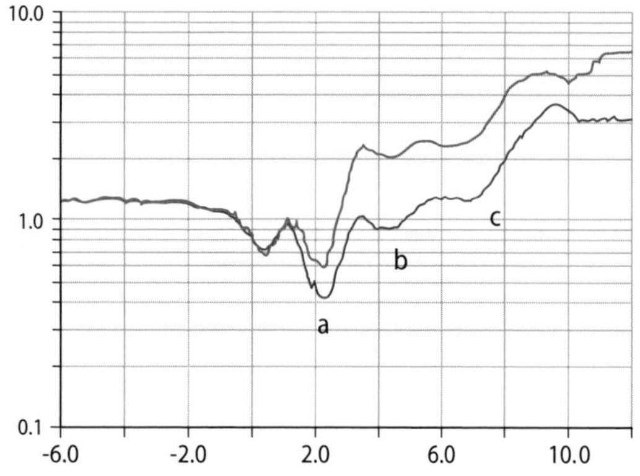

Fig. 14.9 Acoustic rhinometry plot. Before (*red*) and after (*blue*) nasal decongestion. The x-axis represents the distance from the nostril, while the y-axis represents a cross-sectional area of the nasal airway. Notice the increase in the cross-sectional area of the nose after decongestion, more so at the level of *notches b* and *c*. *Notch a* represents the minimal cross-sectional area (MCA or the nasal valve). *Notch b* represents the anterior portions of the inferior turbinate or middle turbinate. *Notch c* represents the area of the middle/posterior end of the middle turbinate. Adapted from [48]

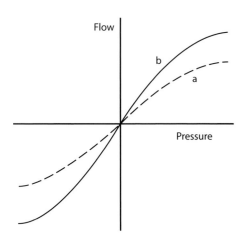

Fig. 14.10 Rhinomanometry plot. *Curve a* represents baseline nasal airway resistance (pressure/flow), while *curve b* represents resistance after decongestion. Notice that as resistance decreases with decongestion, the same pressure differential will produce an increased flow. Adapted from [63]

ment of a posterior nasopharyngeal tube via the test or nontest nostril. Postnasal rhinomanometry is also not commonly used because of issues of poor patient tolerance.

During rhinomanometry airflow can be generated by active or passive means. Active rhinomanometry, the technique most commonly used today, involves using the patient's own respiratory efforts as the source of airflow. Passive rhinomanometry involves pumping air through the nose at a known rate. This method does not imitate true nasal physiology and has been found to reflexively increase mucosal thickness, which could affect the accuracy of its measurements [62].

The measurement of airflow during rhinomanometry can be done by direct or indirect means. With direct methods, airflow is measured at the nasal outlet by way of a nozzle or mask. Masks are most commonly used today because the nozzle can alter the relationship of the nasal ala with the airflow [62]. Indirect methods of airflow measurement are slightly more complicated, using body plethysmography to measure changes in intra-thoracic volume in order to extrapolate air flow.

Odiosoft Rhino

Odiosoft rhino is a new objective technique that converts the frequency of sound generated by nasal airflow into cross-sectional area measurements. The theory behind the technology is that nasal airflow generates a higher frequency sound as turbulence increases [60]. This noninvasive technique, developed by Seren et al. [59], involves a microphone, nasal probe, sound card, and a computer. The nasal probe is connected to a microphone situated 1 cm from the nostril, and the patient is asked to close the other nostril, avoiding any distortion of the test nostril. The sound created during breathing is directly measured with the odiosoft rhino technique, unlike acoustic rhinometry, which measures reflected sounds to calculate nasal cross-sectional area. A recent study published in 2006 [60] shows that this method provides a sensitive and specific assessment of nasal airway patency with better correlation with patient symptom scores than

acoustic rhinometry. Although these findings are encouraging, the search continues for an ideal modality of objective testing.

Variability with Objective Testing

There are several factors that have the ability to cause inconsistencies with objective testing. Hasegawa and Kern noted that the nasal cycle could cause variations in unilateral readings [24]; therefore, most authorities in objective nasal airway testing recommend nasal decongestion before testing to reduce this variability. Several studies have shown a reduction of nasal resistance with exercise [7, 25] and an increase in resistance with a supine position [23], aspirin use [31], and smoking [14]. Ethnicity can also be a source of variability in the nasal airway. Ohki et al. found the greatest nasal resistance in Caucasians, intermediate resistance in Asians, and the lowest nasal resistance in African-Americans [49]. Morgan et al. were able to show similar ethnic trends with nasal cross-sectional areas using acoustic rhinometry [47].

In 1981, to minimize the variability of rhinomanometry, the International Committee on Standardization of Rhinomanometry [35] brought out a set of guidelines. Active, anterior rhinomanometry was labeled the preferred method of testing. Testing should be performed during the same time of day, after the patient has been resting for at least 30 min, and in an environmentally controlled room without any external sunlight. The pressure transducer should be sealed to the nostril with tape without any deformation of the nostril and a transparent face mask should be used to ensure no kinking in the tubing. Recommendations for the standardization of data reporting suggested pressure should be reported in Pascal (Pa), flow reported in cm³/s, and resistance reported in units Pa/cm³/s. The committee also recommended that resistance results be reported at a standard pressure of 150 Pa or "Radius 2" (the intersecting point on the rhinometry graph between 200 cm³/s and 200 Pa).

In 2005, the most recent consensus statement for both rhinomanometry and acoustic rhinometry suggested additional guidelines in an attempt to further standardize objective nasal airway testing [5]. The committee recommended using trained technicians, citing a 3- to 8-fold increase in accuracy. They also made recommendations for standardized decongestion, using two applications that were 5 min apart. For those patients who could not generate pressures of 150 Pa, the committee agreed with reporting resistance at 75, 100, and 150 Pa, as long as the specific pressure was reported. The committee also recommended a standard reference resistance device for rhinomanometry. The European Rhinologic Society has also suggested a similar "standard nose" calibration device for acoustic rhinometry [58].

Comparison of Acoustic Rhinometry with Rhinomanometry

Schumacher [58] suggests that since rhinomanometry is a functional test of the nasal airway, it may be a better screening tool for nasal airway obstruction. A complimentary role for acoustic rhinometry has been suggested as it is better suited to the identification of the site of obstruction [54]. Scadding et al. found comparable results between acoustic rhinometry and rhinomanometry; however, acoustic rhinometry had better patient tolerance and was easier to perform [56]. Passali et al. [50] found that resistance measurements via rhinomanometry were more sensitive and specific in patients with a functional nasal obstruction (such as with rhinitis). Acoustic rhinometry was found to be more sensitive and specific when evaluating nasal airway obstruction secondary to structural abnormalities. It should be noted that in Passali's study, the results of both objective tests had no correlation with either mucociliary transport time or patient symptom scores.

There are several advantages and disadvantages to each method of nasal airway testing. Acoustic rhinometry is rapid (usually takes 10 s for each nostril), minimally invasive, and can identify the exact site of obstruction in the nose. Disadvantages include expense and availability, although the cost of acoustic rhinometry is declining and is currently less expensive than rhinomanometry [9]. Acoustic rhinometry is also unable to accurately measure beyond narrow apertures (i.e., the nasal valve) and is less accurate in the posterior aspect of the nasal cavity [5].

The advantages of rhinomanometry are that it is a more functional test and, in certain circumstances, testing can be done on both nostrils simultaneously. Disadvantages include time (usually takes 20–30 min), and an inability to identify the site of obstruction [9]. Also, rhinomanometry cannot be used in cases of total or near-total nasal obstruction because of the patient's inability to generate sufficient nasal airway pressure and flow.

There are some inherent flaws in both rhinomanometry and acoustic rhinometry. Both tests fail to take tip ptosis or alar collapse into account, as measurements are taken distal to this site. Both testing methodologies also have problems with variability, which is largely operator-dependent. Another concerning flaw of both methods is their poor correlation with patient complaint scores. Tomkinson and Eccles [61] found poor correlation between subjective patient complaints and acoustic rhinometry,

despite significant correlation of acoustic rhinometry with CT, MRI, and rhinoscopy. Gordon et al. [21] found that 22% of patients undergoing septoplasty had persistent subjective obstruction postoperatively despite showing improved rhinomanometric scores. Because of these inconsistencies, objective testing cannot reliably be used to predict successful outcomes after medical or surgical therapy. Although these tests do not provide absolute values to correlate with symptoms, some argue that those patients with high-end resistance/cross-sectional obstruction values are more likely to have subjective improvement after intervention.

Diagnosis and Management

The differential diagnosis of nasal airway obstruction is extensive (see Table 14.1), and detailed description of each etiology is beyond the scope of this chapter. It is important to recognize that multiple etiologies can, and often do, co-exist. The following discussion will address the salient features of some of these underlying conditions and how they may affect management.

Conservative Measures

The treatment of the "stuffy nose" patient will depend on the underlying cause, with surgery usually only being performed after all conservative measures have been exhausted. For patients with nasal airway obstruction secondary to incompetent internal nasal valves, over-the-counter external nasal dilators are sometimes very useful. Portugal et al. [51] was able to show an overall 21% reduction in nasal airway resistance with external nasal dilator use, with better results in the Caucasian nose.

Chronic sinonasal inflammatory disease should be managed as indicated with antibiotics, topical and possibly systemic steroids, and management of co-existing allergy. A complete discussion of medical work-up and management of chronic rhinosinusitis is beyond the scope of this chapter, but it should be noted that conditions such as sinonasal polyposis, allergic fungal sinusitis, aspirin sensitivity triad, cystic fibrosis, and sarcoidosis should also be considered. The history and physical examination must consider salient elements that may cause or contribute to nasal stuffiness, such as use of concomitant medications and underlying endocrine status. Oral contraceptives, estrogen replacement therapy, pregnancy, beta blockers, sildenafil, and hypothyroidism may all be implicated. The patient should also be queried regarding abuse of over-the-counter topical decongestants (rhinitis medicamentosa). These conditions should be managed in conjunction with the primary care physician, and additional symptomatic relief can be achieved with any of the available topical nasal steroids. Oral steroids are occasionally necessary when trying to wean patients who have abused topical decongestants.

Special attention should be paid to endocrine states that can contribute to nasal congestion, such as pregnancy and hypothyroidism. Pregnancy rhinitis is defined as nasal congestion in the last 6 or more weeks of pregnancy, without any other known cause, that resolves within 2 weeks of delivery [16]. It

Table 14.1 Differential diagnosis for nasal airway obstruction

Congenital/Anatomic	Neoplasms
Choanal atresia Adenoid hypertrophy Naso-septal deviation Nasal tip ptosis Internal/external nasal valve incompetence Septal perforation Concha bullosa Cystic fibrosis Ciliary dysmotility	**Benign** – Juvenile nasopharyngeal angiofibroma (JNA) – Hemangioma – Dermoid – Papilloma – Neurofibroma – Nasal osteoma – Benign salivary gland tumor **Malignant** – Esthesioneuroblastoma – Malignant salivary gland neoplasm – Nasopharyngeal carcinoma – Basal cell carcinoma – Adenocarcinoma – Lymphoma – Mucosal melanoma – Squamous cell carcinoma – Sarcoma – Verrucous carcinoma – Metastatic lesion
Inflammatory/Infectious	
Rhinosinusitis Nasal polyposis Inferior turbinate hypertrophy Rhinitis – Allergic rhinitis (seasonal or perennial) – Non-allergic rhinitis (NAR) – Non-allergic rhinitis with eosinophilia (NARES) – Infectious rhinitis (bacterial, viral, fungal) – Vasomotor rhinitis – Atrophic rhinitis – Rhinitis medicamentosa Nasal vestibulitis Syphilis	**Medications**
	Anti-thyroid medications Birth control pills Estrogen replacements Hypertensive medications – Calcium channel blockers – Beta blockers
Trauma	**Neurogenic**
Synechiae Facial nerve paralysis Overaggressive osteotomies Post rhinoplasty nasal valve narrowing Empty nose syndrome (complete turbinate resection) Cocaine abuse Septal perforations	Encephalocele Glioma CSF leak
	Other
Systemic	
Wegener's granulomatosis Sarcoidosis Midline lethal granuloma Rhinoscleroma Histiocytosis X Tuberculosis	Nasal foreign body Hypothyroidism Pregnancy

has been reported to occur as early as 7 weeks' gestation; however, symptoms more commonly occur in the last trimester [16]. The incidence of pregnancy rhinitis has been reported to be as high as 20% and the etiology, although uncertain, is related to hormonal fluctuations during pregnancy that are thought to promote an increase in nasal parasympathetic tone [16]. Treatment involves nasal saline irrigation; external nasal dilators can also be effective. Nasal steroids, although very effective for other forms of rhinitis, have not been shown to provide significant improvement in pregnancy rhinitis [17]. If nasal steroid therapy is contemplated, budesonide should be selected from amongst the available medications of this class because it has been reclassified as pregnancy category B, while the others are class C [20].

Many patients in a hypothyroid state also experience symptoms of chronic rhinitis. In patients who had undergone total thyroidectomy, Chavanne et al. [4] noticed an increase in nasal congestion and secretions, which were relieved with thyroxine injections. The etiology of hypothyroid rhinitis is uncertain and is estimated to occur in approximately 40–60% of patients in a hypothyroid state [22]. The treatment of rhinitis associated with hypothyroidism involves thyroid hormone replacement, in addition to saline irrigation and nasal steroids until the patient is euthyroid.

Management of allergic rhinitis involves several approaches including allergen avoidance, immunotherapy, and management of symptoms with medications. The efficacy of oral decongestants is well known, but use of these medications must be weighed against consideration of central stimulatory and cardiovascular side effects, particularly in patients with hypertension, diabetes, renal insufficiency, and those taking monoamine oxidase inhibitors [19]. Studies have also demonstrated that topical nasal steroids may be equally as effective [63]. Nasal saline is useful in most cases of rhinitis and has been shown to increase mucociliary clearance and minimize crusting [34].

Antihistamines are of potential in the management of allergic rhinitis. First-generation antihistamines (i.e., diphenhydramine) are lipophilic and cause sedation because they easily cross the blood–brain barrier. Second-generation antihistamines (i.e., fexofenadine, cetirizine, loratidine) do not cross the blood–brain barrier as well and are less likely to cause sedation. Studies comparing second-generation oral antihistamines are equally as efficient as one another when compared with placebo [29, 40]; however, there is an increased incidence of drowsiness with cetirizine [29]. Studies have also demonstrated that topical antihistamines (i.e., azalastine) may be superior to cetirizine in the management of congestion [11].

Other options in the management of allergic rhinitis include mast cell stabilizers, anticholinergics, and leukotriene receptor antagonists (i.e., montelukast, zafirlukast). Zafirlukast did show improved subjective nasal obstruction scores when compared with loratadine with or without pseudoephedrine, although no statistically significant differences were seen among the three groups with regard to objective testing [30]. Intra-nasal steroids have been shown to be superior to montelukast when comparing subjective patient scores of nasal congestion [52].

Surgical Management

When conservative measures result in unsuccessful outcomes, surgical intervention is usually offered. Procedures such as endoscopic sinus surgery, rhinoplasty, and septoplasty are covered extensively in other chapters. The focus of this section will be the surgical management of the hypertrophic inferior turbinate.

Hypertrophy of the inferior turbinate is usually associated with an underlying chronic inflammatory process and can cause significant morbidity related to nasal airway obstruction. Berger et al. [1] found that overall turbinate enlargement in the setting of chronic inflammation is usually secondary to an increased proportion of dilated venous sinusoids in the lamina propria of the turbinate. The superficial aspect of this submucosal layer is also associated with increased fibrosis, which explains the decreased responsiveness to medical therapy. Ideally, inferior turbinate reduction would decrease the bulk of the turbinate while preserving the function of the mucociliary surface. Complete turbinate resection should be avoided because it is associated with "empty nose syndrome," characterized by excessive crusting, increased nasal airway turbulence, and a heightened perception of nasal airway obstruction. Berger et al. [1] recommend reducing only the medial and inferior portions of the turbinate because they contain the greatest proportion of venous sinusoids.

Several methods have been described to reduce the hypertrophic inferior turbinate including submucous resection (SMR), radiofrequency ablation (RFA), submucous cautery, and direct electrosurgical reduction. SMR involves resection of the superficial layer of the lamina propria with its glandular and vascular stromal elements (Fig. 14.11) [1], which can be accomplished using a specialized microdebrider blade (Fig. 14.12). RFA involves delivering low-frequency energy to submucosal tissue resulting in internal coagulation of sinusoids and scar contracture with subsequent volumetric reduction, while preserving mucosal integrity [12]. The advantage of this technique is that it can be performed in the office setting with local anesthesia, which may be desirable in cases of isolated turbinate hypertrophy where it may be impractical to proceed with a general anesthetic. Others have utilized electrosurgical reduction using externally applied cautery or argon plasma coagulation. These modalities induce transmucosal destruction of the soft tissue cover of the inferior turbinate. Optimal healing then relies upon regeneration of the ciliated mucosal surface [2]. Submucosal electrocautery, in contrast, causes direct thermal injury to the submucosal tissue, which reduces the turbinate via internal coagulation and scar tissue contracture, without direct insult to the mucosal surface.

The literature abounds with studies demonstrating the efficacy of the various techniques described above, but there is a relative paucity of data comparing the different methodologies of turbinate reduction with one another. In general, it is accepted that the success of the procedure is secondary to reduction of nasal airflow resistance, and augmentation of airflow may even enhance olfaction. It should also be noted that mucociliary clearance is not significantly improved and may be adversely affected after laser procedures [18].

Trials comparing RFA with laser turbinate reduction [53, 55] have demonstrated significant subjective and objective improvement with both techniques. However, patients who underwent RFA had less postoperative crusting with better preservation of mucosal function as measured by saccharin transit time and ciliary beat frequency. Other investigations have also compared submucous cautery to microdebrider-assisted SMR. In this analysis, the latter technique was associated with less crusting, improved endoscopic result, and increased nasal cavity volume as measured by acoustic rhinometry. Furthermore, the improvement with microdebrider-assisted reduction was persistent improvement at 5 years' follow-up [32].

Overall, the preponderance of evidence suggests that primary consideration should be given to techniques such as RFA and SMR with a microdebrider, as these modalities preserve the integrity of the ciliated mucosal surface. One study comparing these two modalities demonstrated that both are associated with significant improvement over baseline at 1 year post-operatively. However, the degree of symptomatic improvement was significantly greater in the microdebrider-treated patients. Objective measurement at 1 year with acoustic rhinometry also revealed a greater increase in the cross-sectional area in this group [41]. Thus, it appears that SMR with a microdebrider is the most efficacious modality and in patients undergoing turbinate reduction in conjunction with another procedure under general anesthetic (i.e., endoscopic sinus surgery), it is our current practice to perform a microdebrider-assisted SMR. In contrast, RFA in the office setting is offered to patients with isolated inferior turbinate hypertrophy in whom medical management has failed.

Conclusions

When evaluating the patient with a stuffy nose, a thorough history combined with a methodical physical exam, including endoscopy, is critical. Several objective techniques are available for assessing nasal congestion. At present, rhinomanometry and acoustic rhinometry are more commonly utilized in the investigational setting, but further study may more fully elucidate the clinical roles of these modalities. Specific underlying causes should be sought and managed. The mainstay of medical therapy for many of these conditions is topical intranasal steroids, and consideration should be given to turbinate reduction in those in whom medical therapy fails. If turbinate reduction is contemplated, a technique that preserves the mucociliary surface should be selected.

Fig. 14.11 Pathology of submucous resection of the inferior turbinate revealing myxoid stroma. This specimen also exhibits multiple islands of glandular epithelium (*asterisk* and *insert*)

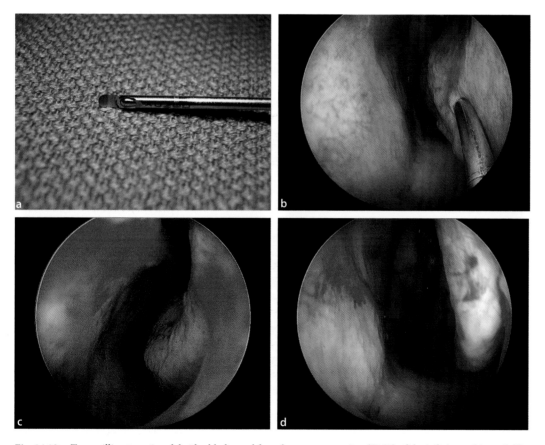

Fig. 14.12 **a** Two-millimeter microdebrider blade used for submucous resection (SMR) of the inferior turbinate. **b** The elevator on the leading edge is used to tunnel submucosally along the medial surface. **c** The hypertrophic turbinate after decongestion is compared with **d** the same turbinate after SMR, revealing marked volumetric reduction with preservation of the mucosal surface

14

References

1. Berger G, Gass S, Ophir D (2006) The histopathology of the hypertrophic inferior turbinate. Arch Otolaryngol Head Neck Surg 132:588–94.

2. Bergler WF, Sadick H, Hammerschmitt N, et al (2001) Long-term results of inferior turbinate reduction with argon plasma coagulation. Laryngoscope 111(9):1593–8.

3. Borum P (1992) Functional anatomy and physiology of the nose. Ear Nose Throat J 71 (1):8–10.

4. Chavanne L (1936) Secretion nasale et glande thyroide. Otorhinolaryngol Int 20:653–64.

5. Clement PA, Gordts F (2005) Standardization Committee on Objective Assessment of the Nasal Airway, IRS, and ERS. Consensus report on acoustic rhinometry and rhinomanometry. Rhinology 43(3):169–79.

6. Cole P (2000) Biophysics of nasal airflow: a review. AJR Am J Roentgenol 14(4):245–9.

7. Cole P, Forsyth R, Haight JS (1983) Effects of cold air and exercise on nasal patency. Ann Otol Rhinol Laryngol 92(2 Pt 1):196–8.

8. Corey JP (1997) A comparison of the nasal cross-sectional areas and volumes obtained with acoustic rhinometry and magnetic resonance imaging. Otolaryngol Head Neck Surg 117:349.

9. Corey JP (2006) Acoustic rhinometry: should we be using it? Curr Opin Otolaryngol Head Neck Surg 14(1):29–34.

10. Corey JP, Gungor A, Nelson R, et al (1998) Normative standards for nasal cross sectional areas by race as measured by acoustic rhinometry. Otolaryngol Head Neck Surg 119(4):389–93.

11. Corren J, Storms W, Bernstein J, et al (2005) Azelastine-Cetirizine Trial No. 1(ACT 1) Study Group. Effectiveness of azelastine nasal spray compared with oral cetirizine in patients with seasonal allergic rhinitis. Clin Ther 27(5):543–53.

12. Coste A, Yona L, Blumen M, et al (2001) Radiofrequency is a safe and effective treatment of turbinate hypertrophy. Laryngoscope 111(5):894–9.

13. Dastidar P, Numminen J, Heinonen T, et al (1999) Nasal airway volumetric measurement using segmented HRCT images and acoustic rhinometry. AJR Am J Roentgenol 13(2):97–103.

14. Dessi P, Sambuc R, Moulin G, et al (1994) Effect of heavy smoking on nasal resistance. Acta Otolaryngol 114(3):305–10.

15. Doty RL, Mishra A (2001) Olfaction and its alteration by nasal obstruction, rhinitis, and rhinosinusitis. Laryngoscope 111(3):409–23.

16. Ellegard EK (2003) The etiology and management of pregnancy rhinitis. Am J Respir Med 2(6):469–75

17. Ellegard EK, Hellgren M, Karlsson NG (2001) Fluticasone propionate aqueous nasal spray in pregnancy rhinitis. Clin Otolaryngol Allied Sci 26(5):394–400.

18. Elwany S, Harrison R (1990) Inferior turbinectomy: comparison of four techniques. J Laryngol Otol 104(3):206–9.

19. Erickson CH, McLeod RL, Mingo GG, et al (2001) Comparative oral and topical decongestant effects of phenylpropanolamine and d-pseudoephedrine. AJR Am J Roentgenol 15(2):83–90.

20. Gani F, Braida A, Lombardi C, et al (2003) Rhinitis in pregnancy. Allerg Immunol 35(8):306–13.

21. Gordon ASD, McCaffrey TV, Kern EB et al (1989) Rhinomanometry for preoperative and postoperative assessment of nasal obstruction. Otolaryngol Head Neck Surg 101:20–26.

22. Gupta OP, Bhatia PL, Agarwal MK, et al (1977) Nasal, pharyngeal, and laryngeal manifestations of hypothyroidism. Ear Nose Throat J 56(9):349–56.

23. Haight JS, Cole P (1986) Unilateral nasal resistance and asymmetrical body pressure. J Otolaryngol 15(Suppl 16):3.

24. Hasegawa M, Kern EB (1978) Variations in nasal resistance in man: a rhinomanometric study of the nasal cycle in 50 human subjects. Rhinology 16(1):19–29.

25. Hasegawa M, Kern EB (1978) The effect of breath holding, hyperventilation, and exercise on nasal resistance. Rhinology 16(4):243–9.

26. Hilberg O, Jackson AC, Swift DL, et al (1989) Acoustic rhinometry: evaluation of nasal cavity geometry by acoustic reflections. J Appl Physiol 66:295.

27. Hilberg, O, Jensen FT, Pederson OF (1993) Nasal airway geometry: comparison between acoustic reflections and magnetic resonance scanning. J Appl Physiol 75:2811.

28. Howard BK, Rohrich RJ (2002) Understanding the nasal airway: principles and practice. Plast Reconstr Surg 109(3):1128–46.

29. Howarth PH, Stern MA, Roi L, et al (1999) Double-blind, placebo-controlled study comparing the efficacy and safety of fexofenadine hydrochloride (120 and 180 mg once daily) and cetirizine in seasonal allergic rhinitis. J Allergy Clin Immunol 104(5):927–33.

30. Jiang RS (2006) Efficacy of a leukotriene receptor antagonist in the treatment of perennial allergic rhinitis. J Otolaryngol 35(2):117–21.

31. Jones AS, Lancer JM, Moir AA, et al (1985) Effect of aspirin on nasal resistance to airflow. Br Med J (Clin Res Ed) 290(6476):1171–3.

32. Joniau S, Wong I, Rajapaksa S (2006) Long-term comparison between submucosal cauterization and powered reduction of the inferior turbinates. Laryngoscope 116(9):1612–6.

33. Kasperbauer JL, Kern EB (1987) Nasal valve physiology: implications in nasal surgery. Otolaryngol Clin North Am 20:699.

34. Keojampa BK, Nguyen MH, Ryan MW (2004) Effects of buffered saline solution on nasal mucociliary clearance and nasal airway patency. Otolaryngol Head Neck Surg 131(5):679–82.

35. Kern EB (1981) Committee report on standardization of rhinomanometry. Rhinology 19(4):231–6.

36. Kimmelman CP (1989) The problem of nasal obstruction. Otolaryngol Clin North Am 22(2):253–64.

37. Kridel RWH, Kelly PE, MacGregor AR, The Nasal Septum. In: Cummings: Otolaryngology (2005) Head and Neck Surgery, 4th ed Mosby: St. Louis, MO.

38. Lal D, Corey JP (2004) Acoustic rhinometry and its uses in rhinology and diagnosis of nasal obstruction. Facial Plast Surg Clin North Am 12(4):397–405.

39. Lang C, Grutzenmacher S, Mlynski B, et al (2003) Investigating the nasal cycle using endoscopy, rhinoresistometry, and acoustic rhinometry. Laryngoscope 113(2):284–9.

40. Lee DK, Gardiner M, Haggart K, et al (2004) Comparative effects of desloratadine, fexofenadine, and levocetirizine on nasal adenosine monophosphate challenge in patients with perennial allergic rhinitis. Clin Exp Allergy 34(4):650–3.

41. Lee JY, Lee JD (2006) Comparative study on the long-term effectiveness between coblation and microdebrider assisted partial turbinoplasty. Laryngoscope 116(5):729–34.

42. Lund VJ (1989) Objective assessment of nasal obstruction. Otolaryngol Clin NA 22(2):279–90.

43. Malm L (1992) Rhinomanometric assessment for rhinologic surgery. Ear Nose Throat J 71:11.

44. Millqvist E, Bende M (1998) Reference values for acoustic rhinometry in subjects without nasal symptoms. AJR Am J Roentgenol 12:341–3.

45. Min YG, Jang YJ, et al (1995) Measurements of cross-sectional area of the nasal cavity by acoustic rhinometry and CT scanning. Laryngoscope 105:757–9.

46. Mirza N, Lanza DC (1999) The nasal airway and obstructed breathing during sleep. Otolaryngol Clin North Am 32(2):243–62.

47. Morgan NJ, MacGregor FB, Birchall MA, et al (1995) Racial differences in nasal fossa dimensions determined by acoustic rhinometry. Rhinology 33(4):224–8.

48. Nigro CEN, Nigro JF, Voegels RL et al (2005) Acoustic rhinometry: anatomic correlation of the first two notches found in the nasal echogram. Rev Bras Otorrinolaringol [online] 71(2):149–154.

49. Ohki M, Naito K, Cole P (1991) Dimensions and resistances of the human nose: racial differences. Laryngoscope 101(3):276–8.

50. Passali D, Mezzedimi C, Passali GC, et al (2000) The role of rhinomanometry, acoustic rhinometry, and mucociliary transport time in the assessment of nasal patency. ENT J 79(5):397–400.

51. Portugal LG, Mehta RH, Smith BE, et al (1997) Objective assessment of the breathe-right device during exercise in adult males. AJR Am J Roentgenol 11(5):393–7.

52. Ratner PH, Howland WC 3rd, Arastu R, et al (2003) Fluticasone propionate aqueous nasal spray provided significantly greater improvement in daytime and nighttime nasal symptoms of seasonal allergic rhinitis compared with montelukast. Ann Allergy Asthma Immunol 90(5):536–42.

53. Rhee CS, Kim DY, Won TB, et al (2001) Changes of nasal function after temperature-controlled radiofrequency tissue volume reduction for the turbinate. Laryngoscope 111(1):153–8.

54. Roithmann R, Cole P, Chapnik J, et al (1994) Acoustic rhinometry, rhinomanometry, and the sensation of nasal patency: a correlative study. J Otolaryngol 23(6):454–8.

55. Sapci T, Sahin B, Karavus A, et al (2003) Comparison of the effects of RF tissue ablation, CO2 laser ablation and partial turbinectomy applications on nasal mucociliary functions. Laryngoscope 113:514–9.

56. Scadding GK, Darby YC, Austin CE (1994) Acoustic rhinometry compared with anterior rhinomanometry in the assessment of the response to nasal allergen challenge. Clin Otolaryngol Allied Sci 19(5):451–4.

57. Schumacher MJ (1989) Rhinomanometry. J Allergy Clin Immunol 83(4):711–718.

58. Schumacher MJ (2002) Nasal congestion and airway obstruction: the validity of available objective and subjective measures. Curr Allergy Asthma Rep 2(3):245–51.

59. Seren F (2005) Frequency spectra of normal expiratory nasal sound. AJR Am J Roentgenol 19:257–61.

60. Tahamiler R, Edizer DT, Canakcioglu S, et al (2006) Nasal sound analysis: a new method for evaluating nasal obstruction in allergic rhinitis. Laryngoscope 116(11):2050–4.

61. Tomkinson A, Eccles R (1996) Comparison of the relative abilities of acoustic rhinometry, rhinomanometry and the visual analog scale in detecting change in the nasal cavity in a healthy adult population. AJR Am J Roentgenol 10:161–5.

62. Zeiders J, Pallanch JF, McCaffrey TV, Evaluation of nasal breathing function with objective airway testing. In: Cummings: Otolaryngology, Head and Neck Surgery, 4th ed. (2005) Mosby: St. Louis, MO.

63. Zieglmayer UP, Horak F, Toth J, et al (2005) Efficacy and safety of an oral formulation of cetirizine and prolonged-release pseudoephedrine versus budesonide nasal spray in the management of nasal congestion in allergic rhinitis. Treat Respir Med 4(4):283–7.

Chapter 15

Surgery of the Nasal Septum

15

Anand K. Devaiah and Bounmany Kyle Keojampa

Core Messages

- The most common indication for septal surgery is to relieve nasal obstruction from septal deviation that hinders airflow through the nose.
- Techniques for septal surgery today emphasize conservative resection and preservation of septal cartilage and bone.
- Morselization is preferred in pediatric patients. With proper preservation of septal cartilage through morselization and repositioning, surgery can be safely undertaken in the pediatric population.
- Septoplasty can provide significant improvement in disease-specific quality of life, high patient satisfaction, and decreased medication use.

Contents

History of Septoplasty

The first documented attempts to correct nasal septal deformities date back to 1757 when Quelmatz recommended daily digital pressure to the septum for gradual correction (cited in [1]). Surgical methods were not attempted until 1875 when Adams described the practice of blunt fracturing and splinting of the nasal septum [2]. Ingals pioneered more radical techniques in 1882 by removing small sections of septal cartilage en bloc with mucosal flap elevation, which was called "window resection" (cited in [1]). Krieg furthered this technique by removing the entire portion of deviated cartilage and Boenninghaus included the resection of the vomer and perpendicular plate of the ethmoid to address more posterior deviations (cited in [1]). In 1899, Asch attempted to alter the tensile curve of septal cartilage instead of resecting it by the use of full-thickness cruciate incisions [1, 3]. Freer and Killian in 1902 developed the foundation of modern septoplasty techniques with the submucous resection. Killian recognized the septum as being an important support structure of the nasal tip and modified his technique to leave a 1- cm dorsal and caudal "L" strut of supporting septal cartilage (cited in [4, 5]).

The era of modern septal surgery began in the 1940s with Cottle, Goldman, and Smith who recognized the disadvantages of submucous resection [6–8]. They favored a more conservative approach to septoplasty with repositioning and removing minimal bone and cartilage. Long-term follow-up studies of patients who had undergone submucous resection frequently showed loss of the support structure of the nose as evidenced by dorsal saddling, retraction of the columella, and alar widening [6–8].

Anatomy

The septum serves several important functions. It provides structural support for the external nose and nasal tip, divides the nose into two cavities, and regulates nasal airflow.

The anterior septum is composed of the quadrilateral cartilage. The bony components of the septum include the nasal crest of the palatine bone, maxilla, and frontal bone, the vomer, the perpendicular plate of the ethmoid, and the spine of the paired nasal bones.

The septum is covered with mucoperichondrial and mucoperiosteal linings. The ophthalmic branch of the internal carotid artery and the maxillary and facial branches of the external carotid artery provide arterial blood supply to the nasal septum. The upper nasal septum is supplied by the anterior and posterior ethmoid arteries, which originate from the ophthalmic branch. The posterior and inferior septum is supplied by the sphenopalatine artery, a branch from the external carotid artery. The septal branch of the superior labial artery provides blood supply to the columella and caudal septum [4, 9].

Preoperative Evaluation

Deviation of the nasal septum is a common cause of unilateral nasal airway obstruction. Iatrogenic trauma to the septum can occur during birth with either forceps placement or during delivery through the pelvic canal. Early septal birth trauma can manifest in nasal obstruction later in life [9].

The most common indication for septal surgery is to relieve nasal obstruction from septal deviation that hinders airflow through the nose. In severe cases, septal deviations can block the ostiomeatal complex, prevent normal sinonasal drainage, and can underlie recurrent episodes of sinusitis.

Septoplasty is also performed in patients with a history of severe epistaxis. Septal deviation can cause turbulent air flow leading to mucosal drying, crusting, and epistaxis. Correction of the deviation can improve this problem by providing normal laminar flow through the nose. Additionally, the septum is an excellent source of donor cartilage for different otolaryngologic procedures, such as rhinoplasty and reconstruction for transsphenoidal approaches to the pituitary [10].

Evaluation of the septum begins with examination of the external appearance of the nose. This examination focuses on the size, shape, symmetry, and alignment of the nose and septum. Observing the patient's nose during normal and effortful nasal breathing is helpful to assess for dynamic obstructions that may be a part of the patient's problem. Anterior rhinoscopy with a nasal speculum allows for internal examination of the septum, the turbinates, and other elements of the nasal valve. The nasal valve is the narrowest area of the airway and its boundaries include the septum, the upper lateral cartilage, and the anterior aspect of the inferior turbinate [9]. These areas may be additional causes of nasal obstruction of which the otolaryngologist should be aware in order to correctly diagnose and treat the patient, as septal deviation may not be the only problem.

Nasal endoscopy with a rigid endoscope can evaluate intranasal structures and assess for polyps or other masses causing nasal obstruction. Additionally, other objective measurements of nasal airway exist, such as rhinomanometry and acoustic rhinometry. However, measurements from these methods do not always correlate with the patient's subjective complaints [4, 11, 12].

Surgical Technique

Today, techniques for septal surgery emphasize conservative resection and preservation of septal cartilage and bone. Derived from a Greek term, *septoplasty* means "to reshape or mold the septum." While there are different variations, what follows is one method employed by the senior author in performing this procedure for conservative resection.

Topical and local anesthesia is necessary for septal surgery, not only for analgesic effects, but also for hemostatic properties. Minimizing bleeding into the operative field allows for adequate exposure and visualization of the nasal septum.

Prior to injection, the nose should be treated with topical agents designed to vasoconstrict the mucosa. Oxymetazoline is the preferred agent of the senior author (AKD), due to the lower risk of cardiac side effects compared with use of topical cocaine, another well-established agent. With a nasal speculum, the septum and nasal cavity are visualized. Cotton pledgets are soaked with oxymetazoline and atraumatically placed in the nasal cavity with bayonet forceps (at least two on each side, one sitting low in the nasal cavity, and one sitting higher).

After decongesting the nasal mucosa, 1% lidocaine with 1:100,000 epinephrine is injected into the submucoperichondrial plane using a 25- or 27-gauge needle. The injection is started at the caudal end of the septum, following a more posterior course until the mucosa is well blanched, or maximum volume based on patient weight is met (Fig. 15.1). Local injection also helps by causing hydrodissection of the mucoperichondrium off the septum. This helps in the development of the mucoperichondrial flap. The contralateral membrane and nasal floor adjacent to the maxillary crest should also be injected.

Several different choices of incisions can be used, each with its advantages and disadvantages. First described by Cottle in 1947, the hemitransfixion incision is made at the caudal-most point of the cartilaginous septum as it adjoins the membranous septum [7, 8]. It is a commonly employed incision as it provides access to both anterior and posterior deviations with only minimal effect on tip support. A no. 15 blade is used to incise the mucosa down to the perichondrium. Identification of the proper subperichondrial layer is essential as it ensures an avascular plane for dissection. Gently scoring the cartilage until one feels its rough surface, after initially lifting the leading edge of the mucoperichondrium, will help reach the proper plane for dissection.

A Killian incision is made more posterior and may be a preferable incision if the anterior septum is straight and the septal deviation is within the posterior third of the nasal cavity [1, 8]. It is created approximately 1–2 cm posterior to the caudal septum and anterior to the septal deviation. Its limitation, however, is that it does not provide access to the caudal septum.

The open rhinoplasty approach can be used to access the septum using marginal and transcolumellar incisions. In the open approach to the septum, the columella is lifted and the medial crura are separated. Tip support can be compromised with this open approach technique and is usually reserved for septal perforation repair or in complex cases in conjunction with an external approach to rhinoplasty [13, 14]. The open rhinoplasty approach is described in further detail elsewhere in this textbook.

15

Whichever incision is chosen, identifying the proper avascular subperichondrial plane is essential. The Cottle elevator is helpful in elevating the mucoperichondrial envelope under direct vision. It has two dissecting surfaces, one sharp and the other more blunt. The sharper spade-like end is used to begin the dissection in the submucoperichondrial plane. After the dissection is started, the flat and blunt end elevates the envelope anteriorly, posteriorly, and inferiorly, while developing a wide mucoperichondrial envelope.

A nasal speculum is then inserted into the mucoperichondrial envelope to allow for visualization and dissection posteriorly. If displacement of the septum off the maxillary crest is encountered, elevation of the mucoperiosteum along the nasal floor will be necessary to realign the septum. An osteotome may be helpful to dissect the septum off the bony nasal crest. After the inferior floor attachments are released, the septum can swing back toward the midline. The mobile septal segment is then realigned to the maxillary crest groove, and the anteriormost aspect is secured to the periosteum of the maxillary crest with a long-lasting absorbable suture.

To prevent cribriform plate injury, the septum should have its segments neither pulled nor twisted without first having had a superior septal incision to disconnect the manipulated segment from the superior connection to the skull base. To decrease the potential for loss of nasal support, the surgeon preserves at least a 1-cm dorsal and 1-cm caudal septal segment, which has been termed the *L-strut* (Fig. 15.2) [5]. After the initial mucoperichondrial flap is elevated, the sharp end of the Cottle or no. 15 blade can be used to incise and penetrate through the cartilage at the point ahead of the offending septal deviation. The surgeon should make sure that there is an adequate strut, as noted above. After the cartilage is incised, this creates a window by which the contralateral mucoperichondrium can be elevated. Once this is done, and the cartilage targeted for resection has had mucoperichondrium elevated from both sides, the swivel knife or Cottle can be used to resect this segment, taking care to preserve the septal strut. Resection of a large central septal segment can be done safely, if required, to address severe septal deviations or if a cartilage graft is needed for rhinoplasty.

After excision of the deviated cartilage or septal spur, the cartilage can be removed or morselized and placed back into the membrane pocket between the mucoperichondrial flaps. Morselization is preferred in pediatric patients. In the pediatric population, it has been shown that septoplasty can be safely performed with proper preservation of septal cartilage through morselization and repositioning; patients were followed for up to 60 months without evidence of deformity or alteration in the growth and development of the nose [15].

The mucoperichondrial envelope with any morselized septal cartilage can then be sutured together with a quilting mattress stitch using 4-0 suture plain gut on a small Keith needle. The quilting mattress suture secures any morselized cartilage, reduces the risk of dead space within the septum where hematoma could form, and brings the mucoperichondrium into contact to nourish the underlying cartilage. Finally, the hemitransfixion or Killian incision is closed with a 5-0 plain chromic suture.

Postoperatively, septal perforations can develop if the mucoperichondrial flaps are both torn at the same level. Having

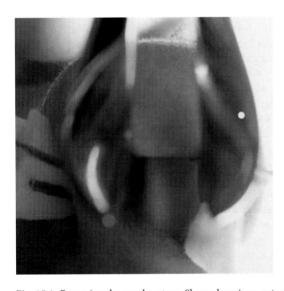

Fig. 15.1 Preparing the nasal septum. Shown here is an anterior rhinoscopic view with pledgets in both nasal cavities. A nasal speculum straddles the nasal septum anteriorly. This helps to identify the septum's caudal edge for injection, and by making the incision for a hemitransfixion approach

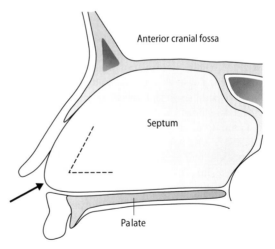

Fig. 15.2 Nasal septum. In this cross-section illustration of the nasal septum, the relationship of the nasal septum to the anterior cranial fossa and palate is shown. Also shown in *dashed lines* is the outline of the nasal septoplasty "L-strut" which is preserved in order to reduce the risk of postoperative nasal deformity. The *large arrow* shows the caudal edge of the nasal septum, which is the starting point in a hemitransfixion incision. A Killian incision is made posterior to the nasal strut, but anterior to the leading edge of a septal deformity

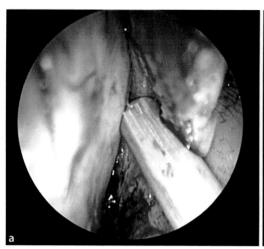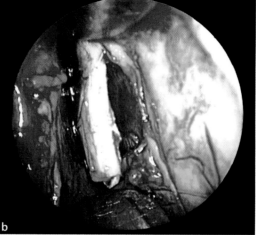

Fig. 15.3a,b Endoscopic septoplasty. **a** Initial dissection of the nasal septum is shown with the mucoperichondrial flap retracted laterally by the suction tip. Note that the instruments are used to not only visualize and dissect, but to simultaneously hold the developed mucoperichondrial pocket open to facilitate the procedure. **b** Visualization of the deeper segments of the septum, including segments prepared for resection, is facilitated by the endoscope

cartilage interposed between flaps that have tears can prevent perforations from forming. Another method for reducing perforation development in the face of a flap tear is the use of silastic splints to keep the edges in a good position and protect them from further trauma; these are cut to size and sutured to the caudal edge of the septum with a 3-0 nylon. Splints can be removed 5–7 days postoperatively, and the patient should be kept on antibiotic coverage while the splints are in place.

Endoscopic approaches to septal surgery are becoming increasingly common, especially when performed concurrently with functional endoscopic sinus surgery. The deviated bone and septum can be resected under direct endoscopic visualization (Fig. 15.3). When compared with standard headlight septoplasty, the endoscopic technique provides several important advantages. Endoscopic visualization allows for improved evaluation of septal deformities in difficult to visualize areas, such as posterior septal deformities. Smaller incisions can be used and a reduced amount of mucoperichondrial dissection can be employed [16, 17]. Furthermore, it is a natural transition between septoplasty and endoscopic sinus surgery when the two procedures are performed at the same time. An endoscopic approach does require more equipment, and special instruments are available to help facilitate this method. However, when extensive deviation is encountered and a wide plane of dissection required, the advantage of the endoscopes is reduced.

Postoperative Care

Nasal packing is usually not necessary for an uncomplicated septoplasty. If splints are used, these are removed between 5–7 days postoperatively. Patients are instructed to use saline nasal irrigation and avoid nose-blowing. Gentle nose blowing is allowed after 2–3 weeks and patients should avoid strenuous activity for a month.

Complications of Septoplasty

Although not common, septal hematoma can be a serious complication in the postoperative period. A hematoma causes separation of the mucoperichondrium from cartilage, causing an interruption in the cartilage's blood supply. Signs and symptoms include intense pain, edema, and complete nasal airway obstruction. The risk of hematoma formation is reduced by the use of septal splints and quilting mattress sutures. Avascular cartilage can be viable for up to 3 days, but without timely evacuation of the hematoma and re-establishment of nutrition to the cartilage, this can be damaging to the septum; this can lead to necrosis, resorption of cartilage, and potential loss of normal nasal form. Management consists of drainage through a mucoperichondrial incision.

Infections after septoplasty are rare, but toxic shock syndrome can occur while nasal packs or septal splints are in place. Patients should be placed on anti-staphylococcal antibiotics prophylaxis until nasal packs and splints are removed. Coating nasal packs with bactroban ointment can help reduce the growth of *Staphylococcus aureus*.

Cerebrospinal fluid leak is rare after septoplasty and usually the result of damage to the cribriform plate during septal manipulation. It is a serious complication when it occurs. Immediate recognition is important, and repair should be done at the time of discovery in surgery. If there is a delay between surgery and discovery of the leak, a CT scan should be obtained to ensure that there is no sign of an intracranial complication such as pneumocephalus. Management involves surgical means to close the leak, and nonsurgical means with bed rest, nasal packing, and oral antibiotics. A lumbar drain may be needed as well. Cerebrospinal fluid leaks usually resolve spontaneously, but it is imperative to watch for signs and symptoms of meningitis, which include headache, photophobia, nuchal rigidity, and fever [18].

A septal perforation can be problematic to patients. It can result in nasal crusting, epistaxis, and whistling during nasal respiration, and can require further intervention in order to reduce the patient's problems.

Failure to maintain an adequate nasal strut through aggressive cartilage resection can lead to nasal deformities. Possible deformities include dorsal saddling, retraction of the columella, and alar widening. Correction of these problems can be difficult and involve extensive reconstructive techniques.

Septoplasty Outcomes

Several studies have been performed recently to evaluate the effectiveness of septoplasty and quality of life outcomes after surgery. Stewart et al. studied the outcomes after nasal septoplasty (NOSE study) and showed that nasal septoplasty resulted in significant improvement in disease-specific quality of life, high patient satisfaction, and decreased medication use. Patients who had a higher degree of symptomatic nasal obstruction had larger improvements after surgery [19].

Tips to Avoid Complications

- The maximum dose for cocaine is 2–3 mg/kg.
- The maximum dose of lidocaine with epinephrine is 7 mg/kg.
- Preserve at least a 1-cm dorsal and 1-cm caudal septal "L" strut.
- When using forceps, completely free the tissue prior to removing it from the nasal cavity. Pulling on tissue can increase the risk of damage to the cribriform plate and cause mucosal tearing.
- A quilting mattress suture can help to re-approximate septal flaps and help prevent postoperative septal hematoma.
- Avoid perforating the mucoperichondrium. Unilateral perforations are common and usually heal spontaneously. Continuous bilateral septal perforations can lead to a persistent perforation that may need to be repaired.

Take-Home Pearls

- Techniques for septal surgery today emphasize conservative resection and preservation of septal cartilage and bone.
- Topical and local anesthesia is necessary for septal surgery for analgesic and hemostatic effects. Minimizing bleeding into the operative field is essential for adequate visualization of the nasal septum.
- Identification of the proper subperichondrial layer is essential as it ensures an avascular plane for dissection.

- Patients should be placed on anti-staphylococcal antibiotics prophylaxis until nasal packs and splints are removed.

References

1. Hinderer KH: History of septoplasty. Fundamentals of anatomy and surgery of the nose, Birmingham, Alabama: Aesculapius Publishing Co.; 1971:1
2. Adams W. The treatment of the broken nose by forcible straightening and mechanical apparatus. *BMJ* 1875; 2:421
3. Asch M. Treatment of nasal stenosis due to deflective septum with and without thickening of the convex side. *Laryngoscope* 1899; 6:340
4. Kridel RW, Kelly PE, MacGregor, AR. The nasal septum. In: Cummings CW, ed. *Otolaryngology-Head and Neck Surgery*. Mosby 2005;948–1001
5. Planas J. The twisted nose. *Clin Plast Surg* 1977; 4:55
6. Bailey BJ. Nasal septal surgery 1896-1899: transition and controversy. *Laryngoscope* 1997 Jan; 107(1):10–6
7. Cottle MH.The 'maxilla-premaxilla' approach to extensive nasal septum surgery. *Arch Otolaryngol Head Neck Surg* 1958; 60:301
8. Cottle MH, Loring RM. Newer concepts of septum surgery: present status. *Eye Ear Nose Throat Monthly* 1948; 27:403
9. Jafek BJ, Dodson BT. Nasal Obstruction In: Bailey BJ et al. 3rd edition *Head and Neck Surgery: Otolaryngology*. Lippincott 2001;293–308
10. Lore JM, Medina, JE. An Atlas of Head and Neck Surgery, 4th edition. Elsevier 2005; 300–6
11. Shemen L, Hamburg R. Preoperative and postoperative nasal septal surgery assessment with acoustic rhinometry. *Otolaryngol Head Neck Surg* 1997; 117:338
12. Wei JL, Remington WJ, Sherris DA. Work-up and evaluation of patients with nasal obstruction. *Facial Plast Surg Clin North Am* 1999; 7:263
13. Rohrich RJ. The deviated nose: optimizing results using a simplified classification and algorithmic approach. *Plast Reconstr Surg* 2002; 110:1509
14. Slavit DH. Reconstruction of caudal end of septum. *Arch Otolaryngol Head Neck Surg* 1995; 121:1091
15. Healy GB. An approach to the nasal septum in children. Laryngoscope. 1986; 96(11):1239–42
16. Giles WC, Gross CW, Abram AC, et al. Endoscopic septoplasty. Laryngoscope 1994; 104(12):1507–9
17. Hwang PH. Endoscopic septoplasty: indications, technique, and results. *Otolaryngol Head Neck Surg* 1999; 120:678
18. Wax MK, Ramadan HH, Ortiz O et al. Contemporary management of cerebrospinal fluid rhinorrhea. *Otolaryngol Head Neck Surg* 1997; 116(4):442–9
19. Stewart MG, Smith TL, Weaver EM. Outcomes after nasal septoplasty: results from the Nasal Obstruction Septoplasty Effectiveness (NOSE) study. *Otolaryngol Head Neck Surg* 2004; 130(3):283–90

Rhinosinusitis – Diagnosis, Differential Diagnosis, Conservative and Surgical Management

Chapter 16

Rhinosinusitis

Chris de Souza and Rosemarie A. de Souza

16

Core Messages

- Inflammation causes changes in the nasal and sinus mucosa.
- Edema occurs and this is followed by a transudate. The effect of edema is that it causes obstruction of the ostia of the sinuses, thereby causing impairment in the drainage of secretions.
- The quality of the mucus changes.
- Inflammation causes the cilia to become paralyzed. This may be temporary or sustained, depending upon the severity of damage.
- The outcome of all these changes is that mucus collects within the sinuses and stasis occurs.
- Initially, the secretions are sterile. They can soon get contaminated with bacteria by nose-blowing, which forces the bacteria into the sinuses from the nasal cavity.
- This results in an acute bacterial infection within the sinuses.
- This can resolve either spontaneously or with the aid of medication. If it does not resolve it can result in chronic disease.
- The criteria for the diagnosis of acute (presumed bacterial) rhinosinusitis include having symptoms that persist for 10 days up to a maximum of 24 days.
- Fever should be present. Symptoms for diagnosis should include anterior and/or posterior nasal discharge, nasal obstruction, and facial pain.
- Objective documentation should include a nasal airway examination for purulent discharge and radiographic evidence of acute rhinosinusitis.
- Both nasal endoscopy and CT are objective measures that can increase the accuracy of the chronic rhinosinusitis (CRS) diagnosis.

- Nasal endoscopic observation of pus, polyps or other disease can help confirm a diagnosis of CRS.
- For areas that cannot be observed with nasal endoscopy, CT can be useful in helping to diagnose disease.
- The use of combining symptoms, findings on nasal endoscopy, and the findings on CT scans can reliably and accurately diagnose and treat CRS.
- Newer instruments and powered tools are now available making mucosal preservation possible.
- Areas in the healing sinus cavity that demonstrate polypoid mucosa are most likely the areas that will demonstrate persistent inflammation. This is likely due to an osteitis reaction.
- Aggressive postoperative debridement of devitalized bone in these areas will result in improved epithelialization of the sinus cavity. Simultaneously, equally aggressive management of infection and inflammation is needed.
- Long-term antibiotics and long-term application of topical steroids are appropriate for the management of these conditions.
- Literature is accumulating in support of the use of topical steroids, which are given preoperatively as well as postoperatively.
- Details of endoscopic sinus surgery are provided elsewhere in this textbook.
- It has been found that a definite relationship exists among allergy, bronchial asthma, and RS.
- The allergic component must be treated appropriately if the management of RS is to be successful.
- Similarly, successful sinus surgery results in a better ability to control bronchial asthma.

Contents

16

What Is Rhinosinusitis?

Rhinosinusitis is a group of disorders characterized by inflammation of the mucosa of the nose and the paranasal sinuses [33].

This was the definition that was accepted by the American Academy of Allergy, Asthma, and Immunology, The American Academy of Otolaryngology – Head and Neck Surgery, The American Rhinologic Society, and the American College of Allergy, Asthma, and Immunology, who had convened a task force of 30 physicians to formulate definitions by consensus.

This consensus group decided to use the term "rhinosinusitis" instead of "sinusitis" because sinusitis is almost always accompanied by concurrent nasal airway inflammation and in many cases sinusitis is always preceded by symptoms of rhinitis.

Furthermore, previously there had been the concept that all cases of chronic rhinosinusitis are caused by ostial obstruction of the sinus. The causes of ostial obstruction are many and diverse. It is now appreciated that rhinosinusitis, especially chronic rhinosinusitis, may be caused by multiple factors such as:

1. Persistent infection caused by biofilms and osteitis
2. Allergy and other disorders of immunity
3. Intrinsic factors of the upper airway
4. Superantigens from *Staphylococcus aureus* in chronic rhinosinusitis (CRS) with nasal polyps
5. Colonizing fungi that induce and sustain eosinophilic inflammation
6. Metabolic disorders including aspirin sensitivity.

Each mechanism may act in concert with other mechanisms or individually for a given patient. This consensus task force also classified rhinosinusitis in the following ways:

1. Acute, presumed bacterial, rhinosinusitis
2. CRS without polyps
3. CRS with polyps
4. Allergic fungal rhinosinusitis (AFRS).

Rhinosinusitis is a clinical diagnosis based largely on history, clinical examination, and imaging modalities. The physical symptoms needed to make a diagnosis of rhinosinusitis are divided into major and minor symptoms.

The major symptoms are:

1. Nasal obstruction/blockage
2. Nasal discharge/purulence/discolored postnasal discharge
3. Hyposmia/anosmia
4. Facial congestion/fullness
5. Facial pain/pressure (facial pain must be accompanied by another major factor to qualify for CRS).

The minor factors are:

1. Fever
2. Halitosis
3. Headache
4. Cough
5. Fatigue
6. Dental pain
7. Ear pain/ear pressure or fullness.

To qualify for a diagnosis of CRS the patient must have at least two major factors or one major factor with two or more minor factors, or nasal purulence on examination [29]. Facial pain is not considered to be a symptom of CRS without other nasal signs and symptoms. The signs and symptoms should persist for at least 12 weeks to qualify as CRS. A separate subcategory for acute exacerbations of CRS was also described. In this category symptoms worsen, but return to baseline following treatment.

Pathophysiology of Rhinosinusitis

Many advances have been made toward the understanding of how rhinosinusitis occurs. Although our understanding has improved, there are still many major gaps in our knowledge. More research and more studies will help improve our knowledge further.

The vicious cycle of rhinosinusitis occurs when a patient is exposed to the numerous upper respiratory viruses. The viral load will result in contamination of the upper respiratory tract. This results in an immune response. The response is a release of inflammatory mediators. These are in the form of the interleukin-8 (Il-8) chemotactic for neutrophils and T lymphocytes, as well as many others.

The inflammatory process will persist and result in edema of the nasal mucosa, an increase in cell membrane permeability, an increase in serous secretions within the mucosa of the nasal cavity and paranasal sinuses, with impairment of normal ciliary clearance. Edema may cause partial or near total obstruction of the paranasal sinus ostia. When obstruction occurs, a relative decrease in barometric pressure within the paranasal sinus is the result. This in turn causes the secretion of a transudate within the sinus cavity. The secretions are free from bacterial contamination. How then does this lead to acute bacterial rhinosinusitis?

Several mechanisms have been postulated. They are:

1. Excessive or abnormally prolonged immune response. The viral inflammation maybe more severe than normal, likely due to a high viral load. Bacteria are then forced into the sinuses by nose blowing. This then leads to secondary bacterial colonization followed by bacterial infection.
2. Immune deficiency of the host. The host's weakened immune system (as a result of diabetes, post-kidney transplant, immune deficiencies, HIV, etc.) predisposes to infections.
3. Impairment in mucociliary clearance (MCC)/stasis of secretions.

In the normal person the respiratory system is kept in a state of equilibrium by mucociliary clearance (MCC). This is to say that all debris, bacteria, etc., are trapped in the mucus and then evacuated by clearance of the beating of the cilia. This can be affected in two ways. The cilia may get paralyzed and not beat or the mucus may not be of the appropriate molecular weight and so cannot be evacuated.

There may be anatomical barriers such as deviated nasal septa, polyps, spurs, etc., that can obstruct drainage. There are three principal disorders of MCC.

1. Primary ciliary dyskinesia is a rare genetic disorder of the ultrastructural apparatus required to propel the cilium in which the nasal nitric oxide is very low due to a deficiency of inducible nitric oxide synthase.
2. Secondary ciliary dyskinesia due principally to microbial or chemical pollutants, toxin-induced dysfunction of the energy pathways required for ciliary clearance.
3. Finally, there are abnormalities in the physicochemical properties of mucus. This will include reduced salt content/osmolality of the mucus, which will prevent it from being cleared.

Dysfunction of the Upper Airway Neurogenic Mechanisms

Stimulation of the nasal sensory nerves during the inflammatory phase of a URT infection results in pain, edema, and a blocked nose. Type C nociceptive nerve endings release neuropeptides including substance P and calcitonin gene-related peptides, which increase plasma extravasation and excess mucus secretions. Recruited parasympathetic nerve fibers cause submucosal gland secretion via acetylcholine and muscarinic receptors. Sneezing, itching, and other reflexes rapidly clear the airway and protect it. However, dysfunction of these nerves may contribute to allergic rhinitis, hyper-responsiveness, and possibly rhinosinusitis. Sympathetic arterial vasoconstriction reduces mucosal blood flow, sinusoidal filling, and vasoconstriction and so restores nasal patency. Loss of sympathetic tone may contribute to chronic non-allergic rhinopathies.

Acute bacterial RS occurs when hypertrophic mucosa develops secondary to a persistent inflammatory process. The acute lymphocytic cellular infiltrate is replaced with monocytes and macrophages. The oxygen content and pH within the sinus cavity reduces, paralyzing the cilia. The bacterial toxins inflict further injury upon the cilia.

In addition, stasis of mucus creates a thick blanket that the cilia cannot clear. The ostia are also obstructed. This then leads to acute bacterial RS.

Interestingly, it has been found that despite this, 50% of bacterial infections resolve spontaneously in healthy individuals without antibiotics, decongestants, NSAIDS, etc.

Those that do not resolve can go on to cause complications or persist as chronic RS (CRS). This will depend upon the severity of the mucosal injury, the presence of anatomical obstructions, and changes in physiology. It should be noted that CRS represents a continuum of acute RS. The difference lies in the progressive severity and irreversible nature of the damage.

Acute (Presumed Bacterial) Rhinosinusitis

Acute rhinosinusitis is caused by the presence of bacteria within the sinus cavity whose ostium is obstructed. Acute rhinosinusitis is usually infectious in nature, while for CRS the causes are varied.

All sinus infections enter the sinus via the nasal cavity. During a cold, nasal fluid containing bacteria, viruses, and inflammatory mediators are blown into the sinuses where they produce inflammation. Mucosal edema, cellular infiltration and mucus thickened by exocytosis of mucin from the numerous goblet cells in the sinus epithelium are the result. It is estimated that of the viral infections only 0.5% to 2% are complicated by secondary bacterial infections [21].

In the immunocompetent person living in the general community acute rhinosinusitis is typically believed to be induced by viruses and usually does not require antibiotics for the first 10–15 days. Beyond this time frame if the symptoms persist, then bacteria are presumed to be present and antibiotics can and should be given [33]. Patients presenting with acute rhinosinusitis usually present with anterior and/or purulent nasal discharge, nasal obstruction, facial pain, and hyposmia.

The duration of acute sinusitis is less than or equal to 4 weeks. The patient's history must include either two or more major factors to be diagnosed as "acute rhinosinusitis".

Most physicians in the field face the following problems:

1. Is an antibiotic necessary? There are proponents for and against when the infection is detected early. Those against prescribing an antibiotic usually cite that most infections are viral and will resolve spontaneously. The medications that can be given are those that provide relief from symptoms. These medications are usually in the form of antipyretic and systemic decongestants. Furthermore, antibiotics given in the presence of a viral infection may result in bacterial resistance and colonization of these bacteria, thus complicating a viral infection. However, if the symptoms are present for more than 2 weeks, then bacteria can be presumed to be present and antibiotics can and should be given. However, all efforts should be made to correctly identify the pathogen causing the acute rhinosinusitis. This will help to choose the appropriate antibiotic.
2. Questions are raised with regard to how to retrieve samples of pus that will accurately reflect the pathogen causing the infection. Most procedures add to costs, are time-consuming and require expertise that may not be available to the primary physician who is invariably the family physician. Thus, in the presence of an acute infection most physicians prefer to use standardized treatment protocols and reserve retrieval of pus samples for special circumstances such as an immunocompromised individual, refractory infections that have not responded to first-line treatment in their treatment protocols and situations where fungal and unusual infections may be suspected. Infections that have been complicated is another situation in which retrieval of the actual bacteria is crucial to effective treatment.
3. Is radiological imaging necessary? Plain X-rays of the nasal cavity and paranasal sinuses have been replaced by CT scanning and MRI. Plain sinus X-ray films might be adequate in situations where acute rhinosinusitis is suspected [33]. Plain X-ray films, although less costly, do have limitations and are much less reliable than CT scans and MRI. In most cases of acute rhinosinusitis most physicians prefer to regard this situation as a clinical diagnosis where the diagnosis is based on history and clinical findings. Imaging modalities such as CT scans and MRI are reserved for situations in which an

acute infection becomes complicated, usually in a situation where the infection has extended beyond the boundaries of the nasal cavity and paranasal sinuses.

4. What is the role of surgery in acute (presumed bacterial) rhinosinusitis? The role of surgery is limited. The role of surgery lies in:

a) Encouraging adequate drainage in a sinus that does not drain, even though adequate and appropriate medication is given.

b) Retrieval of representative samples of pus from the sinus cavity.

c) Surgery is indicated when complications are present. Drainage of the sinus, retrieval of samples of pus, and decompression of the orbit by draining the abscess.

Chronic Rhinosinusitis

Statistics from the Center for Disease Control (CDC) indicate that 32 million adults in the USA (16% of the adult population) suffer from rhinosinusitis [6], with 73 million restricted activity days, 13 million yearly physician visits and a cost of six billion dollars every year. Patients with CRS usually suffer from a significant reduction in the quality of life.

The diagnosis of CRS can be made when the parameters of several criteria are met. Appropriate symptoms of CRS should be present for a period of 12 weeks. Findings on CT scans and nasal endoscopy should be documented and should be indicative of chronic ongoing disease. It should be understood that various forms of CRS exist because the causes of CRS are varied.

Pathological changes of CRS are edema (Fig. 16.1), loss of submucosal glands, ulceration, loss of cilia, fibroplasias, bone remodeling ,and later changes of goblet cell formation.

Physical Findings in CRS

External findings are erythema and swelling over the maxillary, ocular, orbital, and frontal areas.

Anterior rhinoscopy can be used to detect:

- Hyperemia
- Edema
- Crusts
- Pus
- Polyps.

Nasal endoscopy can visualize the following:

- Discoloration of the turbinates
- Pus in the region of the ostiomeatal complex
- Polyp formation.

The specificity of endoscopy is 85%, while that of rhinoscopy is 75% [24]. With the possible exception of deviated nasal septa, anatomic variants do not seem to be significantly associated with CRS [25]. Endoscopic examination by an ENT surgeon is very useful in CRS. There is a high correlation between the findings on endoscopic examination and those on CT scan findings [26]. Prospective endoscopy studies demonstrate a sensitivity of 74% and a specificity of 84% when correlated with CT scans

for CRS. Stankiewicz and Chow [48], in their study, found that nasal endoscopy had a positive predictive value of 74% and a negative predictive value of 64% in CRS.

Radiological Diagnosis

Computed tomography is now the gold standard for imaging of the paranasal sinuses. MRI has better soft tissue detail than CT. MRI is not associated with exposure to ionizing radiation. However, CT scanning is still the preferred imaging method of choice because of the speed of acquisition and the bony detail, which is unavailable with MRI.

However, radiographic findings of CRS are also seen in 27–42% of asymptomatic individuals [16].

Evaluation Scales and Staging Systems

Several evaluation scales exist for patients with chronic rhinosinusitis. For subjective evaluation there are general health status instruments such as the Medical Outcomes Study Short Form 36 (SF 36), as well as disease-specific instruments such as the Chronic Sinusitis Survey (CSS), the Rhinosinusitis Outcome Measure (RSOM 31), Sinonasal Outcome Test (SNOT 20), and the Rhinosinusitis Disability Index (RSDI).

Subjective Outcomes Measures

The SF 36 is a general health status instrument that permits the evaluation of a patient's overall response to treatment. It provides information regarding the functional well-being of the patient. It serves to evaluate not only the response to treatment, but also the need for subsequent intervention through medical or surgical means. The limiting factor of general health status measures is that they do not provide specific evaluation of the disease in question.

Disease-specific health measurement tools are available. The CSS developed at the Massachusetts Eye and Ear Infirmary is duration-based and monitors both symptoms and need for medical therapy over an 8-week period. Studies have demonstrated that the CSS is statistically reliable and is sensitive to clinical change over time.

The RSOM 31 includes components that address health status and quality-of-life measures. It permits evaluation of the magnitude and importance to the patient. The RSOM 31 has undergone several modifications and is now known as the SNOT 20. The SNOT 20 is easier and faster to complete.

The RSDI is unique disease-specific outcome measure in that it evaluates the self-perceived impact of chronic rhinosinusitis in a first-person descriptive format.

The Chronic Sinusitis TyPE (Technology of Patient Experience) specification form is now being used in recent outcomes studies. The TyPE has three forms. It evaluates the patient and previous interventions, if any. The form also includes a post-treatment survey. After statistical and clinical validation in a controlled fashion, these forms appear to provide the best potential for usefulness as management parameters.

16

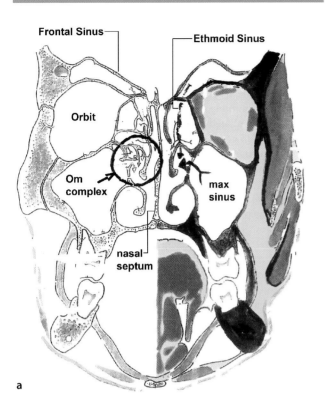

Frontal Sinus

Ethmoid Sinus

Orbit

Om complex

max sinus

nasal septum

a

Fig. 16.1 **a** Edema at the ostium (*circle*) of the maxillary sinus causing obstruction. **b** Continued obstruction of the ostium leads to mucosal hypertrophy and retention of fluid. **c** Edema becomes more pronounced. The fluid has now become purulent. The patient now has fully developed chronic rhinosinusitis

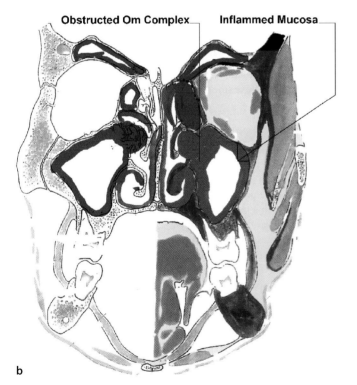

Obstructed Om Complex   Inflammed Mucosa

b

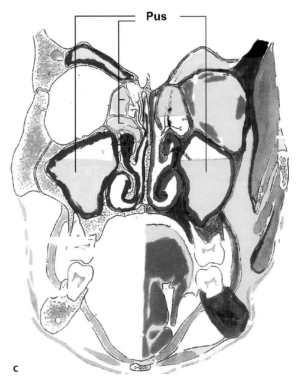

Pus

c

Objective Outcomes Measures

It is becoming evident that objective evaluations incorporating relevant comorbid conditions, extent of radiologic and operative disease, and endoscopic response to therapeutic intervention are objective measurement parameters that have prognostic value. This in turn will likely impact and thereby influence the management of CRS, including the decisions that will involve the surgical and/or medical management of this condition.

CT Scan Staging

Many studies have challenged the guidelines for diagnosing CRS. Studies are being conducted on seeking correlations between objective findings and subjective criteria. In recent years, a discrepancy between the subjective symptoms experienced by patients and their objective endoscopic findings has been demonstrated.

Radiologic staging requires CT scan assessment. Each sinus group (maxillary, anterior ethmoid, posterior ethmoid, sphenoid, and frontal) are graded. Normal (no abnormality) is graded as 0, partial opacification as 1, and total opacification as 2. The ostiomeatal complex is graded as either 0 for normal (no occlusion) or 2 (opacification). Anatomical variants, such as concha bullosa, paradoxical middle turbinate, etc., are noted as being absent (0) or present (1). They do not contribute to the CT scan score.

It is important to remember the time at which a CT scan has been taken. If there is to be a consistent method of staging there must be an agreement on when a CT scan is to be taken. It is best taken after appropriate adequate medical management and when there is no active acute infection present.

Metson et al. [34], at the request of the Rhinology and Paranasal Sinus Committee of the AAO-HNS, attempted to establish a protocol to evaluate CT scan staging systems. Their study found two systems to be favorable toward clinical applications the Glicklich and Metson system and the Lund McKay system.

The Glicklich and Metson system consists of:
- Stage 0: less than 2 mm of mucosal thickening on any sinus wall
- Stage1: unilateral disease and/or anatomical abnormalities
- Stage 2: bilateral disease limited to the ethmoid or maxillary sinuses
- Stage 3: bilateral disease with involvement of at least one sphenoid or frontal sinus
- Stage 4: pansinus disease [20].

The Lund McKay system [31] is based on localization. Points are given for degree of opacification as follows:
- 0 points = normal (no opacification)
- 1 point = partial opacification
- 2 points = total opacification.

This point system is applicable to the maxillary, anterior ethmoid, posterior ethmoid, sphenoid, and frontal sinuses. The ostiomeatal complex was graded as 0 points = normal (no occlusion) or 2 points = opacification.

None of these systems is perfect because they do not take into account conditions like the presence of asthma, Kartagener's syndrome, whether revision surgery is being performed, cystic fibrosis, immune status of the patient, etc. Furthermore, it should be remembered that CT scans are actually a "snapshot" of the disease process. Findings noted at one time may be valid for a short while because the disease process is dynamic, with constant changes occurring all the time.

At an international conference in 1995 [27], patient-perceived data were also used. The patient, using a visual analogue scale (0 [not present] to 10 [present and severe]), addressed system scores. Symptoms included nasal blockage, nasal congestion, nasal pressure, headache, facial pain, olfactory disturbance, and nasal discharge. Patients were asked to rank their three worst symptoms.

Nasal endoscopic examination was quantified by looking for polyps, discharge, edema, adhesions, scarring, and crusting. An absence of polyps was 0, polyps confined to the middle meatus were 1, polyps extending beyond the middle meatus were 2. No nasal discharge was 0, thin serous discharge was 1, and thick purulent discharge was 2.

A staging system for CRS was also devised by Kennedy [26]:
- Stage 1: incorporated anatomic abnormalities, all unilateral sinus disease or bilateral disease limited to the ethmoid sinuses
- Stage 2: bilateral ethmoid disease with involvement of one dependent sinus
- Stage 3: bilateral ethmoid disease with involvement of two or more dependent sinuses on each side
- Stage 4: diffuse sinonasal polyposis.

CT Correlation with CRS

When a patient presents with symptoms of CRS, but there are no findings on a CT scan, alternative diagnoses should be sought. Similarly, if a patient has no symptoms of CRS, but has findings of CRS, such a patient is followed up without intervention.

Several studies have shown that CT scans and symptoms do not necessarily correlate. In the general population there is evidence of findings of disease on CT scans, even though the person is asymptomatic. A prospective study of patients without symptoms of CRS found that 27% had mucosal changes suggestive of CRS on CT scans [16]. A retrospective study demonstrated that symptomatic patients who had CT scans for nonsinus disease were found to have Lund scores as high as 5 [2]. These studies demonstrate that CT alone cannot be used as the only indicator for CRS and that a baseline of mucosal change should be expected in the asymptomatic population. Another retrospective study identified no significant correlation between mucosal abnormalities on CT scans and patients' symptoms [5]. Many authors recommend using CT scans for surgical preparation, but not for the need to determine the need for surgical intervention. Some prospective studies have investigated the discrepancy between symptoms and CT findings. CT scans are not 100% accurate as the sole modality for identifying CRS.

Nasal Endoscopy in Correlation in CRS

Nasal endoscopy can be useful in establishing the diagnosis of CRS. In one report [9] 240 patients who met the criteria of CRS and CT findings were examined using nasal endoscopy. There was a high degree of correlation (75% specificity and 84% sensitivity).

To avoid the problems of a preselected and clearly surgical population, a prospective study examining the findings of nasal endoscopy, CT scans, and CRS symptoms was conducted [48]. In this group, the sensitivity of endoscopy with CT was 46% and the specificity of nasal endoscopy compared with that of CT was 86%. Positive and negative predictive values of nasal endoscopy compared with that of CT was 74% and 64% respectively. This study concluded that nasal endoscopy that was negative for disease correlated well with a negative CT scan.

Pathogenesis of CRS

The Role of Inflammatory Mediators in CRS

Chronic rhinosinusitis is characterized by inflammatory mucosal thickening and polyp formation with a predominantly eosinophilic infiltrate. There is an upregulation (increase) in Th2 cytokines including Il-3, Il-5, and GM-CSF. All these take part in the inflammation, resulting in CRS by increasing the severity and permanence of mucosal damage.

Nitrous oxide (NO) has been discovered in high levels in the respiratory tract. It is thought to contribute to the first line of defense against micro-organisms and aids the upregulation of ciliary activity. Studies on CRS have indicated that in CRS decreased levels of NO are present.

The Role of Altered MCC in CRS

Mucociliary clearance (MCC) aids in transport and clearance that is vital for homeostasis.

Significantly delayed MCC times in patients with CRS have been found. This is influenced by the viscoelasticity of the mucus and depends upon the molecular weight of the mucus secreted. The molecular weight is decided by the release of mediators of inflammation. This results in the slowing down of the metachronous wave of the MCC. Glycoproteins make up the mucus and the molecular weight of the glycoproteins will decide the viscoelasticity of the mucus. Goblet cell activity causes an increase in the mucus. In CRS, the number of goblet cells increases dramatically. This in turn leads to alteration in the quality of mucus. Ciliary disorientation with poor MCC lead to a cycle of chronicity.

Other Factors

Other factors that participate in the pathogenesis of CRS are:
– Osteitis
– Biofilms
– Fungi
– Superantigens
– Allergy.

Chronic rhinosinusitis is due to inflammation, the causes of which are many, while acute rhinosinusitis is usually the result of infection.

Osteitis

Norlander et al. [36] identified a periosteal reaction of fibrosis, bone degradation, and neo-osteogenesis in sinusitis in rabbits. Perloff et al. [39] demonstrated that inflammation could spread to non-involved, non-infected sinus bone in an animal model. Despite the lack of direct infection, inflammation was seen on the bone of the control side that was normal prior to the infection. The infection typically spreads through the haversian canals, resulting in the widening of the spaces through osteoclastic resorption and increased vascularity.

Osteomyelitis Versus Osteitis

The bones of the paranasal sinuses lack the marrow spaces seen in the long bones of the body. Furthermore, in osteomyelitis, bacteria invade the marrow spaces. But in osteitis of the paranasal sinuses no bacteria have been identified. Bolger et al. [7] have found bacteria in the sinus lumen, on the surface of the sinus mucosa, but not in the deep submucosa or in the actual bone.

So how does osteitis occur? While the exact mechanism is not clear at this time, it is postulated that bacteria could cause bony pathology by increasing the inflammatory mediators, prostaglandins, and leukotrienes that stimulate osteoblasts and thus bring about bony remodeling.

Kennedy et al. [28] postulate that frequently, not just debridement of the overlying mucosal disease results in resolution of disease, but also debridement of the underlying bone as well.

How Does Osteitis as a Cause of Chronic Rhinosinusitis Affect Treatment?

Those authors [10] who advocate minimally invasive sinus surgery state that the goal of such surgery is to establish ventilation and drainage. Once this objective has been achieved, they state that rhinosinusitis will resolve and normal drainage will soon be established. However, this is not universally true. Endoscopic sinus surgery should require removal of all bony partitions, especially in the ethmoid sinus. Removal of all the bony partitions serves to remove osteitic bone, bone that might act as a biofilm.

This would not only perpetuate an infection, but it might also impede drainage. Furthermore, such patients will need prolonged antibiotic treatment. Some authors recommend the use of nebulized steroids, topical antifungal agents and oral leukotrienes, and low-dose macrolide therapy [12]. More research is needed to answer many of the questions that surround osteitis as a proposed cause of CRS. Only then would a clear strategy evolve on how such a situation should be treated.

Biofilms

What Is a Biofilm?

A biofilm is a structured community of organisms enclosed in a self-produced polymatrix that is adherent to a living or inert surface. It may be made up of fungi or bacteria that communicate with each other in a co-operative manner. The matrix is slime-like and includes polysaccharides, nucleic acids, and proteins.

Bacterial biofilms are complex organizations of bacteria that are anchored to a living or inert surface. They often originate as a collection of independent, free-floating, planktonic bacteria that attach to a surface and form microcolonies.

Understanding Biofilms

The bacteria accumulate in a community and when a certain amount have accumulated, a "critical point" is reached. At that time, a phenomenon known as "quorum sensing" occurs. This means that a cascade of protein expression occurs that leads to a biofilm phenotype. This phenotype is marked by the formation of towers, layers, and water channels.

Thus, bacteria living in a phenotype can evade host defenses and become less susceptible to systemic or local antibiotics. These biofilms can break off, releasing bacteria in their planktonic form to cause new acute infections and form more biofilms.

How Do Biofilms Resist Antibiotic Therapy?

1. The polysaccharide coat causes slow or incomplete penetration of antibiotics.
2. Once inside a biofilm antibiotics may be deactivated or neutralized when positively charged antibiotics interact with negatively charged polymers of the biofilm.
3. Accumulation of inhibitive waste products or depletion of a needed substrate may put bacteria into a nongrowing (suspended animation) state. This confers relative resistance to antibiotics. Thus, when the antibiotic is stopped the bacteria can start regrowing and cause infections once more.
4. Changing nutrient gradients could also lead to osmotic forces that could cause a stress response, which could result in fewer porins in each bacterial cell wall. This in turn leads to less efficient diffusion of antibiotics into the bacterial cytoplasm.

Five Stages of Biofilm Development

1. Attachment: bacteria attach to a surface. This leads to a cascade of gene expression.
2. Adherence: bacteria adhere tightly to the surface to which they are attached, otherwise biofilm will be impossible.
3. Aggregation: the bacteria aggregate into colonies.
4. Maturation: the biofilm matures and differentiates into complex mushroom-shaped towers
5. Detachment: the bacteria break off from the original biofilm, embolize, and cause acute infections elsewhere and form a new biofilm in a new place.

Superantigens

What are Superantigens?

Superantigens (SAg) are toxins of microbial or viral origin that target the immune system, triggering massive polyclonal T cell proliferation and activation. In genetically susceptible hosts with pre-existing immunopathology and bacterial infections, SAg production may be responsible for the induction of disease and its persistence. SAg are powerful T cell mitogens with concentrations of less than 0.1 pg/mL, sufficient to result in immense uncontrolled systemic release of proinflammatory cytokines. SAg have the unique ability to bypass conventional major histocompatibility complexes (MHC) of the immune systems, activating CD4+ and CD8+ T cells in a major MHC II-dependent but not restricted pattern.

Conventional antigens are typically internalized and processed into smaller peptides by antigen-presenting cells (APC). These are then packaged on the membrane surface in conjunction with MHC molecules for presentation to T cells.

In contrast, unprocessed SAg bind as intact molecules to a region outside the peptide binding groove on the class II MHC molecule, then sequentially bind the T cell receptor (TCR) by means of the variable region of the TCR β-chain. The binding effectively cross-links the TCR and MHC II molecule and results in activation of up to 20–30% of the host T cell population. This is in contrast to the conventional antigen response, which activates only 0.001% to 0.0001% of all T cells. Some pathogens use this mechanism to thwart the immune response. The end result of the SAg leads to corruption of the immune response, which greatly encourages the transmission and virulence of the organism [46].

There is supporting evidence that SAg greatly influence immunomodulatory and proinflammatory cells, and an association exists between SAg and allergic rhinitis and CRS with nasal polyposis (CRS/NP). The SAg hypothesis of CRS with nasal polyposis is supported by the following observations:
1. A high rate of toxin secreting *Staphylococcus* cultured from the nasal cavity of patients who suffer from CRS/NP.
2. A high prevalence of SAg-specific IgE exists in polyp tissue.
3. Variable region of β-chain (VB) skewing is present in polyp lymphocytes.
4. There a correlation between lymphocyte skewing and serum

IgE to SAg in individual patients who have CRS/NP, suggesting a systemic and local response to the same SAg.

5. SAg has been detected in the nasal cavity of patients who suffer from CRS/NP.

Data in support of the SAg hypothesis only account for 50% of patients who suffer from CRS/NP. Since staphylococcal strains are very ubiquitous, this explanation of the observation remains unclear. The complex interaction between SAg and the genetics (MCH II alleles) of the host is one likely explanation. The ability of the SAg to access the host immune system by transcytosis may be highly variable. The genetic susceptibility to mucosal damage may be a major factor in developing CRS with or without nasal polyposis. The most significant area of research would be the demonstration of clinical efficiency of Sag-directed therapy.

The Role of Bacteria in CRS

Potential pathogens can relocate during a viral respiratory tract infection. They can shift from the nasopharynx into the sinus cavity, causing rhinosinusitis. Although bacteria can be found in the sinuses of most patients who have CRS the exact etiology of the inflammation associated with this condition is uncertain. The role of bacteria in CRS associated with nasal polyposis is uncertain. However, many clinicians believe that bacteria play a major role in the causes of CRS and therefore use antimicrobials in the treatment of CRS. The chief difficulty lies in correctly isolating and identifying the causative organism. The difficulties of this are reflected in the available medical literature and are listed below.

1. Various methods are used to sample the sinus cavity. This leads to lack of standardization and unreliability.
2. The area through which the trocar or endoscope is passed is not sterilized.
3. Differences in microbiological culture technique.
4. Failure to evaluate cultures for anaerobes.
5. Lack of assessment of the inflammatory response.
6. Lack of quantification of bacteria.

Studies have described significant differences in the microbial pathogens present in CRS compared with those found in acute rhinosinusitis. *Staphylococcus aureus*, *S. epidermidis*, anaerobes, and Gram-negative bacteria predominate in CRS. The pathophysiology of CRS differs from that of acute rhinosinusitis. The exact events leading to CRS have been difficult to identify or prove. It is postulated [8] that CRS is an extension of unresolved acute rhinosinusitis. It is also postulated that anaerobes play a considerable role in CRS. Adequate and appropriate antibiotics help eradicate disease. Sometimes surgical drainage is needed to make medical treatment effective.

Medical Management of CRS

Recently, there has been increased interest in macrolides in the treatment of CRS. The immunomodulating properties of the macrolides has generated deep interest.

It has been found [11] that there is extensive tissue uptake and intracellular accumulation as far as macrolides are concerned. Macrolides accumulate in inflammatory cells at concentrations several hundred times those found in extracellular fluid. It has been found that cytokines stimulate the accumulation of macrolide antibiotics in macrophages in vitro. This suggests that at sites where inflammation occurs cells may accumulate more macrolides than under normal circumstances. Macrolides are essentially bacteriostatic and bind to the 50S subunit of the ribosome, thus inhibiting protein synthesis. Macrolides are effective against Gram-positive cocci and anaerobes. They have very limited Gram-negative activity. Macrolides reduce the virulence of certain organisms and also alter the architecture and structure of bacterial biofilms. Macrolides decrease interleukin (Il)-8 synthesis. By decreasing Il-8 synthesis neutrophils recruitment is reduced. This blocks the vicious cycle of Il8 production and neutrophils exudation.

Apoptosis (programmed cell death) of inflammatory cells is accompanied by an attenuation of the activity of these cells. Therapeutic induction of apoptosis provides an opportunity by which the inflammatory response can be modulated. Macrolides accelerate apoptosis in human neutrophils. Phagocytic cells can produce toxic reactive oxygen, which destroys bacteria that have been phagocytosed. This oxygen, while it is harmful to bacteria, can also be harmful to the host tissue, especially if it is generated in excess. Macrolides produce a dose-dependent reduction in superoxide that is produced by neutrophils. Recruitment of inflammatory cells to a site of inflammation involves the cells adhering to the vascular endothelium before transmigration. Macrolides down-regulate the expression of cell surface adhesion molecules on neutrophils. Inhibition of molecule expression, therefore, seems to be another possible mechanism by which macrolides exert anti-inflammatory activity. Macrolides have also been found to have beneficial effects on mucus production, as well as to improve mucociliary clearance.

Macrolides are not that effective in situations where the serum IgE is elevated or in situations of allergic fungal CRS. Where macrolides have been found to be effective are cases in which the patient has had persistent purulent rhinorrhea, no allergy is present, and where the patient has not experienced relief with local nasal steroids. Nasal cultures need to be taken and they need to be taken periodically as long as the patient is taking the macrolides. All the macrolides have been found to have a beneficial effect on CRS.

Nasal Polyposis

Nasal polyposis is thought to affect between 1 and 4% of the general population in the USA. However, incidental findings at autopsy may make the figure higher than this. The incidence of allergy is not much higher in patients who have polyps compared with the population as a whole. Patients suffering from nasal polyposis do not have higher rates of positive allergy skin tests. Nasal polyposis is associated with a number of systemic disorders like aspirin intolerance, intrinsic asthma, primary ciliary dyskinesia, and cystic fibrosis. Polyps are frequently observed in chronic rhinosinusitis, allergic CRS, and chronic sinonasal inflammation. Nasal polyposis is now known to have multifactorial causes and these are discussed elsewhere in this book.

How Should CRS Be Treated?

This question is still a matter of debate. Many clinicians have their own protocols, with each claiming success.

The key to successful treatment lies in careful history taking and detailed comprehensive physical examination, which will include nasal endoscopy followed by high-resolution CT scans of the nose and paranasal sinuses. Based on his or her understanding of the cause of CRS and how to bring about a successful resolution of the disease, the clinician can then make a choice with regard to the line of treatment he or she should adopt. The first line of treatment includes the administration of systemic and topical corticosteroids [30]. These may be contraindicated in the presence of fulminant infection or in patients who are immunocompromised, and especially in diabetics.

Appropriate antibiotics can be given. Effectiveness of the macrolides in CRS make them the antibiotics of choice.

Decongestants and sinus drainage procedures did not prove to be superior to saline in the treatment of maxillary rhinosinusitis. The use of bacterial lysates was found to be beneficial, but antihistamines were not found to be beneficial. Randomized control trials found nasal douching to be effective in reducing symptoms, improving the quality of life as well as reversing changes seen on CT and nasal endoscopy.

The role of surgery is effective, but needs to be accompanied by appropriate medication. Endoscopic sinus surgery has evolved significantly, so much so that disease processes that previously needed major surgery accompanied by significantly morbidity and external incisions can now be safely carried out with great expertise with a dramatic improvement in results.

The principles of endoscopic sinus surgery are:
1. Provide adequate drainage by widening the obstructed ostia so that they now drain naturally, freely, and physiologically
2. Provide adequate ventilation of the paranasal sinuses
3. Provide adequate inspection of areas that could not be visualized earlier.

Impact of CRS Versus Nasal Septal Deviations

Bhattacharya [4] notes that traditionally patients with CRS have been treated differently from those with NSD. Patients suffering from CRS reported more symptoms in the nasal symptom domain than patients who only had NSD. Patients with NSD reported higher mean nasal obstruction scores, but lower rhinorrhea and dysosmia symptom severity scores. Bhattacharya notes the higher severity of oropharyngeal symptoms in patients suffering from CRS. Patients suffering from CRS more frequently complain of cough, dental pain, and otalgia than those who have an NSD. Patients suffering from CRS tend to have more extranasal symptoms, which usually result in higher symptom scores. Bhattacharya [4] also notes that patients suffering from

CRS incur a higher economic burden that those who have NSD. Furthermore, the number of work days lost is far more in patients with CRS than in those who have an NSD.

Do Nasal Septal Deviations Cause CRS?

Yasan et al. [50] reported that mild to moderate NSD were not a risk factor for CRS. Only gross NSD present a genuine risk of developing CRS. The greater the septal deviation, the greater the risk of developing CRS. Three pathophysiological hypotheses explain how NSD cause CRS. They are mechanical obstruction, aerodynamic changes, and alterations in sinusal ventilation and antral pressures. NSD, when very significant, can cause dysfunction in these three dynamics, which ultimately affect mucociliary clearance of the sinus and its ostium, which then results in CRS. Unfortunately, there are no further studies that evaluate whether CRS resolves with the surgical straightening of the nasal septum.

The Relationship Between Allergy, Bronchial Asthma, and Rhinosinusitis

There is a well-established relationship between sinusitis and asthma [32]. There is convincing clinical evidence that sinusitis plays a significant part in the pathogenesis of bronchial asthma [47]. Clearing disease from the paranasal sinuses results in significant improvement of asthma.

Allergy and Rhinosinusitis

Rhinosinusitis has been reported to occur in 53–63% of patients who suffer from allergic rhinitis. Allergy has been reported to be present in 20–56% of patients. Savolainen [43] studied 225 patients with documented acute maxillary sinusitis and 103 age-matched controls. A statistically significant increase in definite (25% versus 16.5%) and probable (6.5% versus 3%) allergy was found in individuals suffering from RS compared with the control group.

Several studies [3, 23, 35] have noted a relationship between the severity of RS and the presence of allergy. In these studies correlations were reported between the extent of RS as determined by a CT scan and the presence of specific IgE, as determined by RAST testing.

What Are the Mechanisms That Cause Allergy to Predispose a Person to RS?

Three potential mechanisms are postulated:
1. An IgE-mediated response occurs within the paranasal sinuses.
2. Allergic rhinitis-induced ostial obstructions occur.
3. A constitutional predisposition to sinus mucosal inflammation in allergic patients.

Al Ghamdi et al. [1] and Driscoll et al. [13] have found that both allergic and non-allergic patients manifest increased total CD3 and helper CD4 sinus T cells. Suppressor/cytotoxic CD8 T cells have been reported to be decreased in allergic individuals, but increased in non-allergic patients compared with controls. In addition, only allergic patients have been reported to have increased mast cells, CD20+ B cells and IgE-producing B cell precursors in sinus biopsies. Allergic patients have demonstrated a higher proportion of CD30+ mononuclear cells in sinus mucosa than non-allergic patients. These data suggest that Th2 cytokines and their receptors are important in the eosinophilic inflammation of sinusitis in both allergic and non-allergic patients. However, involvement of different cytokine pathways and effector cells may lead to an increase in inflammation in allergic individuals. The antigen thought to be responsible for stimulating the immunological inflammatory response remains unknown, but is thought likely to be a microbial superantigen [45].

Patients suffering from CRS and bronchial asthma who also have increased total serum IgE along with increased eosinophilia in nasal secretions would likely suggest an allergic component.

Studies indicate that the treatment implications of treating allergic rhinitis occurring concomitantly with CRS need both aspects of this problem to be addressed if successful resolution is to be achieved. Dykewicz and Fineman [14] recommend intranasal steroids, stressing their importance for complete resolution of disease. When combined with antibiotics and other pharmacologic agents, intranasal steroids bring about rapid resolution of disease.

Schlenter and Mann [44] reported improved prognosis when patients suffering from allergic rhinitis and CRS were treated with immunotherapy.

Allergic status may also influence the manner in which a patient responds to surgery for CRS. Kennedy [26] reports that patients who have an extensive thickening of sinus mucosa have poorer outcomes following sinus surgery. In addition, allergic patients who suffer from perennial allergic rhinitis are less likely to benefit from sinus surgery for CRS than those who do not have allergies.

For successful outcomes of CRS in the presence of simultaneously occurring allergy it is also important to treat the allergic component appropriately. Ignoring the allergic component of CRS will likely lead to failure.

Bronchial Asthma and CRS

Fuller et al. [18] and Rossi et al. [42], in their reports, demonstrate that approximately 75% of pediatric patients presenting with status asthmaticus had concomitant RS. TenBrinke et al. [49] reported that a majority of patients suffering from severe bronchial asthma not only had grossly diseased paranasal sinuses, but that the extent of disease was positively linked to airway inflammation. This was seen in increased eosinophils in sputum and peripheral blood as well as levels of nitrous oxide in exhaled air. This indicates an association between sinonasal and lower airway inflammation in patients suffering from severe asthma.

Harlin et al. [22] examined the tissue from patients who had undergone surgery for CRS. Tissue from patients suffering from CRS and bronchial asthma was extensively infiltrated with eosinophils. While the mucosa of patients who were operated for CRS and who did not suffer from asthma had no eosinophils. Immunofluorescent studies demonstrate a significant association between the presence of extracellular deposition of major basic protein and damage to the sinus mucosa. This was similar to that found in asthma. This points to the possibility that sinus disease in patients with asthma may be caused by the same mechanisms that cause damage to bronchial epithelium.

Neural Reflexes

Receptors in the nose, pharynx, and paranasal sinuses give rise to afferent fibers that in turn form part of the trigeminal nerve. This is connected to the vagus in the brain. From the vagus nerve parasympathetic efferent fibers travel to the bronchus. The cholinergic parasympathetic nervous system maintains bronchial muscle tone as well as mediating in acute bronchial responses.

The changes in intrabronchial and extrabronchial reactivity were significantly associated with a marked degree of pharyngitis. It was proposed that the lower airway hyper-responsiveness when RS was present might have been triggered by the seeding of the pharynx. Rolla et al. [41] found a marked thinning of pharyngeal epithelium with a marked increase in pharyngeal nerve fiber density. This would likely encourage increased access of irritants to submucosal nerve endings, thereby inducing the release of sensory neuropeptides via axon reflexes with activation of a neural arc, which would result in reflex airway constriction. This indicates a systemic process rather than a local one.

Rachelefsky et al. [40] reported that children with combined RS and asthma showed significant improvement and resolution of asthma when they were successfully treated for their RS. Similar results were reported by Friedman et al. [17]. Oliveira and Sole [37] reported that in their series of children with asthma and RS, patients improved their bronchial hyper-responsiveness to metacholine and decreased their symptoms when the RS component of their disease was treated successfully.

One study [15] reports that asthma in medically resistant RS resolves following successful surgery for the treatment of RS. Parsons and Phillips [38] also report improvement in asthma following endoscopic sinus surgery. Glicklich and Metson [20] reported that patients in their series who had asthma experienced the greatest improvement in health following endoscopic sinus surgery.

Aspirin-Associated Asthma

This is known as triad asthma or Samter's triad. Aspirin (NSAIDS) sensitivity, nasal polyposis, and asthma occur together. This is due to an abnormality in the arachidonic acid metabolic cycle. Approximately 10% of chronic asthmatics have a response to aspirin or other NSAIDS characterized by the exacerbation of asthma. Aspirin-sensitive asthmatics are characterized by suffering from recurrent nasal polyposis and recurrent RS.

References

1. Al Ghamdi K, Ghaffar O, Small P et al. (1997): IL-4 and IL-13 expression in chronic sinusitis: relationship with cellular infiltrate and effect of topical corticosteroid treatment. *Journal of Otolaryngology* 26:160–166

2. Asraf N, Bhattacharya N (2001): Determination of the "incidental". Lund score for the staging of chronic sinusitis *Otolaryngology Head & Neck Surgery* 125(5):483–486

3. Baroody FM, Suh, SH, Naclerio RM (1997): Total IgE serum levels correlate with sinus mucosal thickness on computerized tomography scans. *Journal of Allergy and clinical Immunology* 100:563–568

4. Bhattacharya N (2005): Symptom and disease severity differences between nasal septal deviation and chronic rhinosinusitis. *Otolaryngology Head & Neck Surgery* 133:173–177

5. Bhattacharya N, Piccirilo Wippold FJ (1997): Relationship between patient based descriptions of sinusitis and paranasal sinus computed tomographic findings. *Archives of Otolaryngology – Head and Neck Surgery* 123;1189–1192

6. Blackwell DL, Collins JG, Coates (2002): Summary health statistics for US adults. *National Health Interview. Vital Health Statistics* 10:205

7. Bolger WE, Leonard D, Dick EJ et al. (1997): Gram negative sinusitis: a bacteriologic and histologic study in rabbits. *American Journal of Rhinology* 11:15–25

8. Brook I (2005): The role of bacteria in chronic rhinosinusitis. *Otolaryngologic Clinics of North America* 38:1171–1192

9. Cassiano R (1997): Correlation of clinical examination with computerized tomography in paranasal sinus disease. *American Journal of Rhinology* 11:193–196

10. Catalano PJ, Setliff RC, Catalano LA (2001): Minimally invasive sinus surgery in the geriatric patient. Operative techniques. *Otolaryngology Head & Neck Surgery* 12(2):85–90

11. Cervin A, Wallwork B (2005): Anti-inflammatory effects of macrolides antibiotics in the treatment of chronic rhinosinusitis. *Otolaryngologic Clinics of North America* 38;1339–1350

12. Chiu AG (2005): Osteitis in chronic rhinosinusitis. *Otolaryngologic Clinics of North America* 38:1237–1242

13. Driscoll PV, Naclerio RM, Baroody FM (1996): CD4+ lymphocytes are increased in the sinus mucosa of children with chronic sinusitis. *Otolaryngology Head & Neck Surgery* 122;1071–1076

14. Dykewicz MS, Fineman S (1998): Diagnosis and management of rhinitis: parameter documents of the joint task force on practice parameters in allergy, asthma and immunology. *Annals of Allergy* 81;463–518

15. English GM (1986): Nasal polypectomy and sinus surgery in patients with asthma and aspirin idiosyncracy. *Laryngoscope* 96:374–380

16. Flinn J, Chapman ME, Wightman AJ, Maran AG (1994): A prospective analysis of incidental paranasal sinus abnormalities on CT head scans. *Clinical Otolaryngology* 19(4) 287–289.

17. Friedman R, Ackerman M, Wald E (1984): Asthma and bacterial sinusitis in children. *Journal of Allergy and Clinical Immunology* 74:185–189

18. Fuller CG, Schoettler JJ, Gilsanz V et al. (1994): Sinusitis in status asthmaticus. *Clinical Pediatrics* 33:712–719

19. Glicklich RE, Metson RA (1994): A comparison of sinus computed tomography (CT) staging systems for outcomes research. *American Journal of Rhinology* 8;291–297

20. Glicklich R, Metson R (1997): Effect of sinus surgery on quality of life. *Otolaryngology Head & Neck Surgery* 117;12–17

21. Gwaltney JM, Wiesinger BA, Patrie JT (2004): Acute community acquired bacterial sinusitis; the value of antimicrobial treatment and the natural history. *Clinical Infectious Diseases* 38;227–233

22. Harlin SI, Ansel DG, Lane SR et al. (1988): A clinical and pathological study of chronic sinusitis: the role of the eosinophil. *Journal of Allergy and Clinical Immunology* 81;867–875

23. Hoover GE, Newman LJ, Platts-Mills TAE et al. (1997): Chronic sinusitis: risk factors for extensive disease. *Journal of Allergy and Clinical Immunology* 100;185–191

24. Hughes R, Jones NS (1998): The role of endoscopy in outpatient management. *Clinical Otolaryngology* 23;224–226

25. Jones NS (2002): CT of the paranasal sinuses: a review of the correlation with clinical, surgical and histopathological findings. *Clinical Otolaryngology* 27;11–17

26. Kennedy DW (1992): Prognostic factors, outcomes and staging in ethmoid sinus surgery. *Laryngoscope* 102;1–18

27. Kennedy DW (1995): Conference on sinus disease: Terminology, staging, therapy. *Annals of Otology, Rhinology and Laryngology* 10410 (supplement pt 2);167

28. Kennedy DW, Senior BA, Gannon FH et al. (1998): Histology and histomorphometry of ethmoid bone in chronic sinusitis. *Laryngoscope* 108;502–507

29. Lanza DC, Kennedy DW (1997): Adult rhinosinusitis defined. *Otolaryngology Head & Neck Surgery* 117;(3) S1–7

30. Lund VJ (2005): Maximal medical therapy for chronic rhinosinusitis. *Otolaryngologic Clinics of North America* 38;1301–1310

31. Lund VJ, McKay IS (1993): Staging in rhinosinusitis. *Rhinology* 31;183–184

32. Marney SR (1996): Pathophysiology of reactive airway disease and sinusitis. *Annals of Otology, Rhinology and Laryngology* 105;98–100

33. Meltzer EO Hamilos DL et al. (2004): Rhinosinusitis: Establishing definitions for clinical research and patient care. *Otolaryngology Head & Neck Surgery* (supplement): 131;(6) 1–62

34. Metson R, Glicklich RE, Stankiewicz JA et al. (1997): comparison of sinus computed tomography staging systems. *Otorhinolaryngology – Head and Neck Surgery* 117;372–379

35. Newman LJ, Platts Mills TAE, Phillips CD et al. (1994): Chronic sinusitis relationship of computed tomographic findings to allergy, asthma and eosinophilia. *JAMA* 271;363–367

36. Norlander T, Westrin KM, Stierna P (1994): The inflammatory response of the sinus and nasal mucosa during sinusitis: Implications for research and therapy. *Acta Otolaryngologica Supplement* 515;38–44

37. Oliveira C, Sole D (1997): Improvement of bronchial hyperresponsiveness in asthmatic children treated for concurrent sinusitis. *Annals of Allergy, Asthma and Immunology* 79:70–74

16

38. Parsons DS, Phillips SE (1993): Functional endoscopic sinus surgery in children: a retrospective analysis of results. *Laryngoscope* 103;899–903

39. Perloff JR, Gannon FH, Bolger WE et al. (2000): Bone involvement in sinusitis; an apparent pathway for the spread of disease. *Laryngoscope* 110;2095–2099

40. Rachelefsky GS, Katz RM, Siegel SC (1984): Chronic sinus disease with associated reactive airway disease in children. *Pediatrics* 73;526–532

41. Rolla G, Colograde P, Scappaticci E, et al. (1997): Damage of the pharyngeal mucosa and hyperresponsiveness of airway in sinusitis. *Journal of Allergy and Clinical Immunology* 100;52–57

42. Rossi OVJ, Pirila T, Laitinen J, et al. (1994): Sinus aspirates and radiographic abnormalities in severe attacks of asthma. *International Archives of Allergy and Immunology* 103;209–216

43. Savolainen S (1989): Allergy in patients with acute maxillary sinusitis. *Allergy* 44;116–122

44. Schlenter WW, Mann WJ (1983): Operative Therapie der chronischen Sinusitis – Erfolge bei allergischen und nichtallergischen Patienten. *Laryngologie, Rhinologie, Otologie* 62;284–288

45. Schubert MS (2001): A superantigen hypothesis for the pathogenesis of chronic hypertrophic rhinosinusitis, allergic fungal sinusitis and related disorders. *Annals of Allergy, Asthma and Immunology* 87;181–188

46. Seiberling KA, Grammer L, Kern RC (2005): Chronic rhinosinusitis and superantigens *Otolaryngologic Clinics of North America* 38;1215–1236

47. Slavin RG (1998): Complications of allergic rhinitis: implications for sinusitis and asthma. *Journal of Allergy and Clinical Immunology* 101;S357–S360

48. Stankiewicz J, Chow J (2002): Nasal endoscopy and the definition and diagnosis of chronic rhinosinusitis. *Otolaryngology Head & Neck Surgery* 126 (6);623–627

49. TenBrinke A, Grootendorst D, Schmidt et al. (2002): Chronic sinusitis in severe asthma is related to sputum eosinophilia. *Journal of Allergy and Clinical Immunology* 109;621–626

50. Yasan H, Dogru H, Baykal B et al. (2005): What is the relationship between chronic sinus disease and isolated nasal septum deviation. *Otolaryngology Head & Neck Surgery* 133;190–193

Chapter 17

Introduction to Evidence-Based Medicine and Pediatric Rhinosinusitis

17

Anthony E. Magit and Cecilia Canto-Alarcon

Core Messages

- Pediatric sinusitis in the otherwise healthy child is primarily a medical disease and surgery should be reserved for patients who are refractory to medical treatment.
- A comprehensive medical history is critical to distinguish between a chronic infection and closely spaced recurrent, uncomplicated upper respiratory infections.
- Adenoidectomy should be considered a primary surgical intervention for chronic sinusitis.
- The presence of infections in multiple anatomic sites leads to consideration of an underlying immunologic disorder.
- Pediatric sinus surgery in a child without an underlying systemic disease is intended to improve aeration of the sinuses and not to remove all diseased tissue.
- Prior to performing sinus surgery consider an allergy and/or immunology evaluation.
- Gastro-esophageal reflux can be responsible for the signs and symptoms of chronic pediatric sinusitis.

Contents

Introduction

Pediatric sinusitis is a multi-factorial disease with significant overlap with several clinical entities. Evaluating the medical literature related to pediatric sinusitis with the intent of creating an evidence-based approach to managing this condition requires an awareness of the clinical ambiguities associated with diagnosing sinusitis in a pediatric patient. This discussion will focus on the pathophysiology, diagnosis, and management of pediatric sinusitis.

The average child is considered to have six to eight upper respiratory infections per year with estimates that between 0.5% and 10% of these episodes will evolve into a bout of sinusitis. Between 3% and 6% of children are thought to have an episode of sinusitis before the age of 3 years [1–3]. The clinician must distinguish between the presence of recurrent, uncomplicated upper respiratory infections and sub-acute or chronic sinusitis.

Pathophysiology

Pathophysiology is directly related to the anatomic considerations of the paranasal sinuses. The interaction of sinus mucosa with conditions resulting in mucosal dysfunction leads to compromised sinus conditions and ultimately sinusitis. Any discussion related to the pathophysiology of sinusitis necessarily involves a great amount of inference, as there are no adequate animal models of pediatric sinusitis.

Maxillary and ethmoid sinuses begin development in the 10th week of gestation and are formed by the 3rd month of gestation. The maxillary and ethmoid sinuses are the only paranasal sinuses that are present at birth, with the ethmoid sinuses being relatively larger than the maxillary [4]. The maxillary and ethmoid sinuses are paired structures and relatively symmetrical in most patients. The maxillary sinuses can consist of a single cavity or have one or several septae, or boney walls dividing the sinus into several components. The ethmoid sinuses consist of anterior and posterior divisions. The ethmoid sinuses are composed of multiple cells created by several intrasinus septae. The sphenoid sinus is typically divided into two or three sections by intrasinus septae and the frontal sinus is commonly asymmetrical, often containing intrasinus septae.

Development of the paranasal sinuses is considered the result of progressive pneumatization of the sinuses. The sphenoid sinus usually begins development at 3 years of age and reaches full size by the age of 7 or 8. The frontal sinus is typically the last to develop and will continue to pneumatize until the child enters late adolescence. The relationship between the degree of pneumatization and sinus disease is thought to be a result of adequate aeration during the period of sinus development.

Cystic fibrosis represents an extreme example of chronically poor aeration of the sinuses resulting in impaired pneumatization and impaired development of the frontal sinuses. Whereas the frontal sinuses are not present at birth and are typically absent or rudimentary in adolescent and adult patients with cystic fibrosis, the explanation is that the presence of diseased mucosa in the area of the future nasofrontal recess impairs pneumatization of the frontal sinus, resulting in minimal or no frontal sinus development. In contrast to the frontal sinus, patients with cystic fibrosis often have enlarged maxillary and ethmoid sinuses as a result of obstruction of the natural openings of these sinuses with soft tissue hypertrophy and thickened secretions, leading to expansion of the bone surrounding the maxillary and ethmoid sinuses.

Acute sinusitis describes inflammation of the lining of the sinuses, the sinus mucosa. The etiology of acute sinus mucosal inflammation is multi-factorial, ranging from an acute viral infection, environmental irritants or allergic reactions. For purposes of this discussion, acute sinusitis will be considered a bacterial or viral infection of the paranasal sinuses. Acute infectious sinusitis is viral in approximately 10% of cases and bacterial in the other 90% [5]. The paranasal sinuses are usually sterile except for transient contamination with bacteria, which are then cleared by normal mucociliary function. Bacteria normally residing within the nasopharynx secondarily infect the paranasal sinuses once the normal aeration of the sinuses is compromised by mucosal obstruction of the natural site of communication between the sinuses and the nasal cavity. The sites of communication with the nasal cavity are the sinus ostia.

Areas of drainage from the paranasal sinuses into the nasal cavity are well defined. The anterior ethmoid, frontal sinus, and maxillary sinuses communicate with the nasal cavity in the area referred to as the ostiomeatal complex. This is located lateral to the middle turbinate and posterior to the uncinate, a prominence of bone located anterior to the natural opening of the maxillary sinus, the maxillary ostia. Mucosal disease in the ostiomeatal complex is considered the single most important factor in the development of sinusitis, leading to obstruction of the natural site of ventilation for the maxillary and anterior ethmoid sinuses. The posterior ethmoid and sphenoid sinuses drain into the nasal cavity via the superior meatus.

Concurrent with obstruction of the sites of communication between the nasal cavity and paranasal sinuses is dysfunction of the cilia located on the surface of the sinus mucosa. In vivo studies have established the patterns of beating of the cilia clearing contaminants from the sinuses. Dysfunction of the cilia, resulting in stasis of material in the sinuses, can result from respiratory viral infections or environmental irritants. Bacteria not readily cleared by the mucocilia will then contribute to an acute bacterial sinus infection.

Definitions

Diagnosing sinusitis is a challenging endeavor with the overlap in clinical symptoms and signs with other disease processes, primarily allergic responses and uncomplicated upper respiratory infections secondary to viral infections. Standard classifications of sinusitis include: acute, sub-acute, recurrent, and chronic [6]. Acute is considered to be of less than 30 days' duration, subacute between 30 and 90 days, and chronic sinusitis implies that signs and symptoms last more than 3 months. Recurrent sinusitis is defined as three episodes of sinusitis within 6 months or four in 1 year, with each episode lasting less than 30 days with at least 10 days between episodes when the patient is asymptomatic.

The primary diagnostic features are based upon history and the physical examination. Unfortunately, the physical findings and history are not specific to sinusitis; these include nasal congestion, rhinorrhea, cough, facial pain, and headache. Pediatric patients may be more likely than adult patients to present with halitosis and "horizontal cough", implying the onset or exacerbation of cough while lying down. Behavioral manifestations of sinusitis in pre-school children can include irritability.

Episodes of acute sinusitis typically begin as uncomplicated upper respiratory infections. By convention, the diagnosis of acute sinusitis depends upon the duration of signs and symptoms. Once signs and symptoms have been present for more than 10 days without evidence of improvement, the patient is considered to have an episode of acute sinusitis. The characteristics of rhinorrhea (i. e., consistency, color) are not specific for differentiating acute sinusitis from an uncomplicated viral upper respiratory infection. The critical feature is the duration of rhinorrhea and symptoms.

Acute Sinusitis

Diagnosis

As discussed previously, acute sinusitis is primarily a clinical diagnosis. The persistence of an upper respiratory infection for more than 10 days with the presence of nasal congestion, rhinorrhea with or without fever, facial pain or cough correlates with the presence of an acute bacterial sinus infection. Acute bacterial sinusitis should be suspected sooner than 10 days of illness if fever is greater than 39°C and purulent nasal discharge is present for 3 or 4 consecutive days.

The role of radiographic evaluation is limited in the diagnosis of acute sinusitis. Plain radiographs have limited utility for paranasal sinus disease. Findings suggestive of sinusitis included opacification of the sinuses, mucosa thickening greater than 4 mm, and the presence of an air–fluid level [7]. Mucosal thickening can be difficult to interpret and is nonspecific with regard to the cause of inflammation. The American Academy of Pediatrics (AAP) Clinical Guideline for Sinusitis recommends against radiographic imaging for the diagnosis of acute sinusitis in children less than 6 years of age; however, the guideline suggests that radiographic imaging may be beneficial for diagnosing severe acute sinusitis in children older than 6 years [8]. A normal plain radiograph is a strong indicator that sinusitis is not present.

Computerized axial tomography (CAT) scans are primarily used if a complication of acute sinusitis is suspected, but are not recommended for the diagnosis of acute, uncomplicated sinusitis. Complications include orbital involvement or intracranial infection. A study by Glasier et al. reported that 100% of young children who experienced an upper respiratory infection in the preceding 2 weeks had soft tissue changes on sinus CAT scans [9].

Transillumination and ultrasound of the paransal sinuses have not been systematically studied in children.

When acute paranasal pain is present and associated with high fever and generalized malaise, obtaining a plain Water's radiograph to aid in establishing the presence of acute maxillary sinusitis may be indicated. The pertinent radiographic finding is an air–fluid level or opacification in a maxillary sinus. For the purposes of obtaining fluid to identify the specific bacteria present, needle aspiration of the sinus transnasally or via a sublabial approach may be appropriate. A trained physician, usually an otolaryngologist, should perform aspiration of the maxillary sinus. Obtaining secretions from the nasal cavity to identify the bacteria in the paranasal sinuses is not helpful as there is relatively no correlation between bacteria in the nasal cavity and that found in the sinuses. Collecting purulent secretions lateral to the middle turbinate may provide meaningful information with regard to the type of bacteria located in the sinuses [10].

Table 17.1   Antimicrobial treatment for acute sinusitis [29]

Severe Symptoms/Daycare/Recent Antimicrobial Treatment
High-dose amoxicillin = 90 mg/kg/day in two divided doses
High-dose amoxicillin-clavulanate acid = 90 mg/kg/day amoxicillin; 6.4 mg/kg/day clavulanate in two divided doses
Mild symptoms
Usual dose amoxicillin = 45 mg/kg/day in two divided doses
High-dose regimen at the discretion of the physician
Penicillin allergic without anaphylaxis
Cefuroxime 30 mg/kg/day in two divided doses
Cefpodoxime 10 mg/kg/day once daily
Cefdinir 14 mg/kg/day once daily
Penicillin allergy with anaphylaxis
Azithromycin 10 mg/kg on day one; 5 mg/kg × 4 days in a single dose
Clarithromycin 15 mg/kg/day in two divided doses
Severe symptoms defined as: temperature of at least 102°F (39°C) and purulent nasal discharge for at least 3 or 4 consecutive days.

Treatment

Antibiotics

A central component to treating acute sinusitis is the knowledge that spontaneous resolution may occur, with rates dependent upon the organism present. Deciding whether or not to treat a patient diagnosed with acute sinusitis is based upon multiple factors, including the presence of any underlying medical conditions, history of previous episodes of sinusitis and confidence that the child will return for re-evaluation if their condition deteriorates.

Antibiotic therapy is the mainstay of medical therapy for acute sinusitis. The AAP evidence-based clinical guidelines for sinusitis suggest a stepwise approach to choice and dosage of antimicrobials (Table 17.1) [8]. Patients treated with antibiotics achieve a more rapid clinical cure. Estimates are that approximately 50–60% of children will improve without antibiotics, with 20–30% with substantially longer recovery times compared with children treated with antibiotics. The primary bacteria associated with acute sinusitis are those found in acute otitis media: *Streptococcus pneumonia*, nontypable *Hemophilus influenzae*, and *Moraxella catharrhalis*. The choice of antibiotic is driven by the spectrum of bacteria found in acute sinusitis and knowledge of the local resistance patterns for antimicrobi-

als. *Streptococcus pneumonia* penicillin and cephalosporin resistance is due to alteration of the penicillin binding protein while beta-lactamase production is responsible for resistance found with nontypable *Hemophilus influenzae* and *Moraxella catarrhalis*. Resistance to amoxicillin is more likely when specific risk factors are present. These risk factors include: attendance in day care, antimicrobial treatment within the past 90 days, and age less than 2 years [11, 12].

The duration of therapy is somewhat controversial. Some authors suggest that the antibiotic should be continued for 1 week beyond the resolution of the signs and symptoms of acute sinusitis with a minimum of 10 days of treatment [13].

Adjuvant Therapy

Clinical trials are limited in support of adjuvant treatment for acute pediatric sinusitis. Given the limited information regarding adjuvant treatment, the clinician should weigh up the potential risks and costs of adjuvant therapy.

Topical steroids in combination with antibiotic therapy have been poorly studied, with results suggesting some reduction in symptoms after 1 week of treatment. Topical and systemic decongestants, antihistamines, and mucolytics have not been extensively studied for acute pediatric sinusitis. Because of cost and side effect concerns, these medications should be used judiciously and with the intent of reducing symptoms and not directly improving the underlying sinus infection [8].

Nasal saline irrigations have the theoretic benefit of reducing intranasal crusting and cleansing the nose with minimal cost or side effects.

Chronic Sinusitis

Creating an evidence-based approach to chronic sinus disease in children is limited by the paucity of prospective studies on pediatric sinusitis. This discussion will focus upon the diagnosis, evaluation, and treatment of sinusitis with an emphasis on the areas where information is lacking to guide the clinician.

Diagnosis

History plays a major role in diagnosing chronic sinusitis. Signs and symptoms associated with chronic sinusitis include: nasal congestion, cough, paranasal facial pain, headache, and malaise. As important as establishing the diagnosis of chronic sinusitis is assessing the patient for evidence of coexisting medical conditions, primarily allergic disease, immune deficiency, and chronic respiratory diseases.

Environmental risk factors for recurrent upper respiratory infections predisposing to chronic sinusitis include attendance in a large daycare institution, presence of siblings in the home, and exposure to environmental smoke.

Evaluation

Physical Examination

Physical findings are nonspecific. The intranasal examination focuses upon the characteristics of the nasal mucosa and evidence of anatomic abnormalities, including severe nasal septal deformities. A significant difference between adult and pediatric patients is the role of the adenoid. Obstructing adenoid tissue may mimic the signs and symptoms of chronic sinusitis for a pediatric patient. A cooperative child may allow flexible or rigid nasal endoscopy in the clinic setting for evaluation of the adenoid. Alternatively, a lateral neck radiograph provides information regarding the degree of nasopharyngeal obstruction secondary to adenoid hypertrophy. The accuracy of nasal endoscopy compared with the lateral neck radiograph in predicting adenoid hypertrophy has not been clearly established.

Radiographic Evaluation

Radiographic evaluation of the paranasal sinuses for a patient with the clinical diagnosis of chronic sinusitis primarily consists of computerized axial tomography (CAT) scans. Plain radiographs are primarily useful for evaluating the presence of a large adenoid pad; magnetic resonance imaging (MRI) is too sensitive for soft tissue inflammation and does not provide adequate information regarding sinus anatomy.

Specific findings on plain radiographs do suggest sinus disease, including mucosal thickening or sinus opacification. A specific situation where plain radiographs can be misleading is the finding of an opacified maxillary sinus where a CAT scan confirms the presence of a hypoplastic maxillary sinus predisposed to chronic sinus disease (Figs. 17.1 and 17.2).

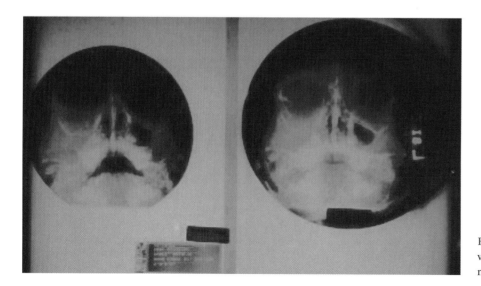

Fig. 17.1 Plain Water's radiographic view interpreted as an opacified right maxillary sinus

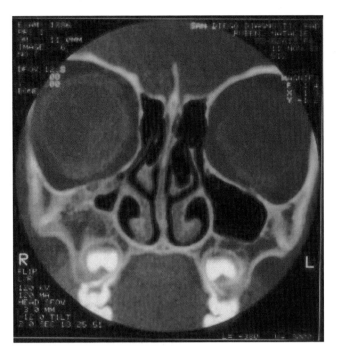

Fig. 17.2 Computerized axial tomography scan confirms hypoplastic right maxillary sinus

Medical Evaluation

Chronic sinus disease in children is primarily a medical disease with surgery indicated in the minority of situations. A thorough evaluation of the patient begins with the history that guides appropriate laboratory testing.

A family history of environmental allergies should prompt an allergy evaluation of the patient. Appropriate allergy evaluation may include skin testing or serologic testing, depending upon the allergy resources available. Allergic rhinitis is present in 15–20% of children with all categories of sinusitis. Approximately 80% of children with chronic sinusitis have a family history of atopy and approximately 50% of children with refractory sinusitis have positive skin tests [14–16].

Immunologic testing is appropriate when an underlying immunologic abnormality is suspected. A child who presents with chronic sinusitis with a history of recurrent infections in other anatomic sites, including recurrent or chronic otitis media, pneumonia or recurrent pharyngitis suggests that an underlying immunologic abnormality might be contributing to chronic sinusitis. The choice of immunologic testing is not well defined. Initial testing may include quantitative immunoglobulins or pneumococcal antibody titers. In locations where universal pneumococcal vaccination is not administered, pre- and postvaccination antibody titers can be a useful assessment of active immunity.

Gastro-esophageal reflux disease is increasingly recognized as a contributing factor to chronic rhinosinusitis. The evaluation for suspected gastro-esophageal reflux ranges from an extensive evaluation by a gastroenterologist to an empiric trial of medical therapy for gastro-esophageal reflux. A descriptive prevalence study of children with chronic sinus disease reported that 19 out of 30 children with chronic sinus disease had gastro-esophageal reflux, as demonstrated by esophageal pH monitoring [17]. In a retrospective review, the symptoms of sinus disease of 30 children considered candidates for endoscopic sinus surgery resolved and surgery was avoided after treatment for gastro-esophageal reflux [18].

Cystic fibrosis is considered when nasal polyps are identified on physical examination, as approximately 25% of patients with cystic fibrosis have nasal polyps [19]. Testing for cystic fibrosis should be considered when the patient presents with recurrent or chronic pulmonary disease or chronic gastrointestinal disease. Initial testing for cystic fibrosis is sweat chloride testing with genetic testing done for confirmation or to delineate the specific genetic deletion.

Intranasal foreign bodies should be considered when a child presents with unilateral nasal discharge without other signs or symptoms of sinusitis.

Treatment

Medical Treatment

Antibiotic therapy has been utilized as primary medical therapy for chronic sinusitis. Empiric use of oral antibiotics has been the mainstay of treatment for chronic sinusitis. The choice of antibiotic and duration of therapy are not well defined. Brook et al., in evaluating the available retrospective studies, suggests that antibiotic therapy should be directed against aerobic and anaerobic beta-lactamase-producing bacteria [20, 21]. It is recommended that therapy be given for at least 21 days and may be continued for 10 weeks.

Intravenous antibiotic therapy has been studied in nonrandomized, retrospective studies. The efficacy of directing antibiotic therapy from culture results from maxillary sinus aspirate has been proposed and may be considered when the patient remains symptomatic after prolonged oral antibiotic therapy and when viable bacteria are recovered from the paranasal sinuses. Several retrospective studies have assessed the efficacy of culture-driven intravenous antibiotic therapy. In these nonrandomized, retrospective studies, between 80 and 100% of patients had initial improvement, with subsequent recurrence of symptoms in approximately 30–55% of the patients. The studies included patients who underwent maxillary sinus aspiration as well as those who had a concurrent adenoidectomy [22–24].

Adjuvant therapy in the form of antifungal agents, decongestants, mucolytics, and antihistamines has not been studied in pediatric sinusitis. Use of these classes of medications should be based upon an understanding of the risks and costs associated with their use. Nasal saline washes have shown efficacy in limited clinical trials and have the benefits of minimal risks and costs.

Surgical Treatment

Surgical treatment for chronic sinusitis should only be considered after a thorough medical evaluation. The three surgical interventions utilized for managing children with chronic sinusitis refractory to medical treatment are adenoidectomy, maxillary sinus aspiration, and endoscopic sinus surgery.

Maxillary sinus aspiration is primarily used to obtain fluid for culture to guide antimicrobial therapy. The specific therapeutic benefit of sinus aspiration has not been well demonstrated.

Adenoidectomy has been used in conjunction with maxillary sinus aspiration as well as endoscopic sinus surgery. The rationale for performing an adenoidectomy for the management of chronic sinusitis has several theoretic benefits. Obstructing adenoid tissue can be responsible for the nasal obstruction associated with chronic sinusitis and contribute to stasis of secretions within the nasal cavity. Any amount of adenoid tissue can harbor bacteria, contributing to paranasal sinus disease in a similar fashion to the relationship between adenoid tissue and otitis media.

Adenoidectomy for chronic sinus disease has not been studied in prospective, randomized trials. Ramadan and Tiu presented retrospective data regarding adenoidectomy and concluded that failures were associated with the presence of asthma and age less than 7 years [25]. In a nonrandomized prospective study, more than 50% of children undergoing adenoidectomy showed improvement in their symptoms, while more than 70% of children undergoing endoscopic sinus surgery with or without adenoidectomy had improved symptoms [26].

In a nonrandomized study by Unkanont of the effect of adenoidectomy on patients with frequent sinusitis and evidence of obstructing adenoid tissue, there was a significant reduction in the frequency of episodes of sinusitis and sleep disturbance following adenoidectomy [27]. In this study, 92% of participants had obstructive sleep disorders and more than 88% had evidence of obstructing adenoid tissue.

Functional endoscopic sinus surgery is intended to improve aeration and drainage of the paranasal sinuses without significant mucosal destruction. This form of endoscopic sinus surgery differs from that performed for patients with extensive nasal and sinus polyps that can be found in cystic fibrosis or allergy-associated polyp disease. Patients with underlying mucociliary dysfunction may benefit from more extensive tissue removal as well.

Endoscopic sinus surgery in children has not been adequately studied with prospective, randomized trials. Stankiewicz provided data for 77 children and adolescents managed with endoscopic sinus surgery [28]. With an average follow-up of 3.5 years, 38% of patients were cured and 55% improved. This cohort of patients included those with cystic fibrosis, allergy, and immunodeficiency. Approximately 50% of patients had closer of at least one maxillary ostium at follow-up examination.

Summary

An evidence-based approach to sinusitis in children is limited by the paucity of prospective, randomized studies evaluating medical and surgical therapies. The available literature provides sufficient information to create reasonable parameters for a rational approach to the various classifications of pediatric sinusitis. Recommendations for the medical and surgical management of acute and chronic sinusitis are presented, with an explanation of the level of evidence.

Acute Sinusitis

Diagnosis

1. Physical examination and history constitute the primary method of diagnosis (strong recommendation based upon literature and opinion).
2. Plain radiographs are not indicated for children under 6 years (strong recommendation).
3. Plain radiographs may be used to confirm diagnosis in children aged over 6 years (equivocal recommendation).
4. CAT scan indicated for suspected complication.

Treatment

1. Antibiotics associated with more rapid resolution of symptoms (moderate recommendation based upon literature and opinion).
2. First-line antibiotic amoxicillin for nonsevere cases with no minimal risk factors for antimicrobial resistance (strong recommendation).
3. High-dose amoxicillin-clavulanate for severe episodes and presence of risk factors (strong recommendation based upon literature and opinion).
4. Adjuvant therapy (decongestants, antihistamines, topical steroids) not indicated (equivocal recommendation based upon side effects and cost).

Chronic Sinusitis

Evaluation

1. Medical evaluation to include allergy and immunologic evaluation (strong recommendation based upon opinion and epidemiology).
2. Plain radiographs to assess adenoids (moderate recommendation based upon overlap in obstructive symptoms between chronic sinusitis and adenoid hypertrophy).

Medical Treatment

1. Antibiotics to cover aerobic and anaerobic beta-lactamase-producing organisms (moderate recommendation based upon literature and opinion).
2. Adjuvant therapy (decongestants, antihistamines) are not indicated (strong recommendation based upon literature).
3. Topical steroids for atopic patients (moderate recommendation based upon opinion).
4. Nasal saline irrigations (strong recommendation based upon opinion).

17

Surgical Treatment

1. Stepwise approach starting with adenoidectomy and endoscopic sinus surgery for failures (strong recommendation based upon opinion).

Tips to Avoid Complications

- Endoscopic sinus surgery in children should be performed with minimal trauma to the middle turbinate to reduce the likelihood of postoperative scar formation.
- A "second-look" procedure to debride sinus cavities is not necessary for the majority of pediatric patients who have had endoscopic sinus surgery.
- Intraoperative image guidance should be considered for revision surgery.
- Irrigation with saline solution is a helpful adjunct for postoperative care to reduce crust formation.
- The presence of nasal polyps should lead to consideration of cystic fibrosis or allergic fungal sinusitis.

Take-Home Pearls

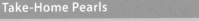

- Manage pediatric sinusitis primarily as a medical condition.
- Adenoidectomy is utilized as the initial surgical intervention in most patients.
- Consider environmental allergies as a contributing factor to pediatric chronic sinusitis.

References

1. Aitken M, Taylor JA. Prevalence of clinical sinusitis in young children followed up by primary care pediatricians. Arch Pediatr Adolesc Med. 1998; 152:244–248.
2. Ueda D, Yoto Y. The ten-day mark as a practical diagnostic approach for acute paranasal sinusitis in children. Pediatr Infect Des J. 1996;15:576–579.
3. Wald ER, Guerra N, Byers C. Upper respiratory tract infections in young children: duration of and frequency of complications. Pediatrics. 1991;87:129–133.
4. Leung A, Kellner J, Acute sinusitis I children: diagnosis and management. J Pediatr Health Care (2004) 21:31–63.
5. Conrad D, Jensen H, Management of acute bacterial rhinosinusitis. Curr Opin Pediatr (2002) 14:86–90.
6. International Rhinosinusitis Advisory Board. Infectious rhinosinusitis in adults: classification, etiology and management. Ear Nose Throat J. 1997;76(suppl):1–22.
7. Wald ER, Chiponis D, Ledesma-Medina J, Comparative effectiveness of amoxicillin and amoxicillin-clavulanate potassium in acute paranasal sinus infections in children: a double-blind, placebo-controlled trial. Pediatrics. 1986;77:795–800.
8. Clinical Practice Guideline: Management of Sinusitis. Pediatrics. 2001;108:798–808.
9. Glasier CM, Mallory GB, Steele RW. Significance of opacification of the maxillary and ethmoid sinuses in infants. J Pediatr. 1989;114:45–50.
10. Gordts F, Abu Nasser I, Clement PA, Pierard D, Kaufman L, Bacteriology of the middle meatus in children. Int J Pediatr Otorhinolaryngol. 1999;48:163–167.
11. Block SL, Harrison CJ, Hedrick JA, et al. Penicillin-resistant Streptococcus pneumoniae in acute otitis media: risk factors, susceptibility patterns and antimicrobial management. Pediatr Infect Dis J. 1995;14:751–759.
12. Levine OS, Farley M, Harrison JH, Lefkowitz L, McGeer A, Schwartz B. Risk factors for invasive pneumococcal disease in children: a population-based case-control study in North America. Pediatrics. 1999;103(3).
13. Wald ER. Sinusitis. Pediatr Ann. 1998;27:811–818.
14. Fireman P, Diagnosis of sinusitis in children: emphasis on the history and physical examination. J Allergy Clin Immunol 1992 90:433–436.
15. Shapiro GG, Rachelevsky GS, Introduction and definition of sinusitis. J Allergy Clin Immunol. 1992 90:417–418.
16. Rachelevsky GS, Goldberg M, Katz RM, Sinus disease in children with respiratory allergy. J Allergy Clin Immunol 1978;61:310–314.
17. Phipps CD, Wood WE, Gibson WS, Cochran WJ. Gastroesophageal reflux contributing to chronic sinus disease in children: a prospective analysis. Arch Otolaryngol Head Neck Surg 2000;126(7);831–6.
18. Bothwell MR, Parson DS, Talbot A, Barbero GJ, Wilder B. Outcome of reflux therapy on pediatric sinusitis. Otolaryngol Head Neck Surg. 1999;121(3):255–62.
19. Orenstein DM, Winnie GB, Altman H. Cystic fibrosis: a 2002 update. J Pediatr. 2002;140:156-–164.
20. Brook I, Thompson DH, Frazier EH. Microbiology and management of chronic maxillary sinusitis. Arch Otolaryngol Head Neck Surg 1994;120:1317–20.
21. Brook I, Yocum P. Management of chronic sinusitis in children. J Laryngol Otol 1995;109:1159–62.
22. Adappa ND, Coticchia JM. Management of refractory chronic rhinosinusitis in children. Am J Otolaryngol 2006;27(6):384–9.
23. Tanner SB, Fowler KC. Intravenous antibiotics for chronic rhinosinusitis: are they effective? Curr Opin Otolaryngol Head Neck Surg 2004;12(1):3–8.
24. Don DM, Yellon RF, Casselbrant ML, Bluestone CD. Efficacy of a stepwise protocol that includes intravenous antibiotic therapy for the management of chronic sinusitis in children andadolescents. Arch Otolaryngol Head Neck Surg. 2001;127(9):1099–1101.
25. Ramadan HH, Tiu J. Failures of adenoidectomy for chronic rhinosinusitis in children: for whom and when do they fail? Laryngoscope 2007;117(6):1080–1083.
26. Ramadan HH. Surgical management of chronic sinusitis in children. Laryngoscope 2004:114(12);2103–9.

27. Ungkanont K, Damrongsak S. Effect of adenoidectomy in children with complex problems of rhinosinusitis and associated diseases. Int J Pediatr Otorhinolgol 2004;68(4):447–51.

28. Stankiewicz JA. Pediatric endoscopic nasal and sinus surgery. Otolaryngol Head Neck Surg. 1995;113(3):204–210.

29. American Academy of Pediatrics. Clinical Practice Guideline: Management of Sinusitis. Pediatrics 2001;108(3):798–808.

17

Chapter 18

Bacteriology of the Paranasal Sinuses and the Nose in Health and Disease

18

Itzhak Brook

Core Messages

- The oral cavity is colonized by aerobic and anaerobic micro-organisms where anaerobic outnumber aerobic bacteria
- Establishment of the correct microbiology of all forms of sinusitis is of primary importance as it can serve as a guide for choosing the adequate antimicrobial therapy.
- Sinus culture should preferably be obtained through sinus puncture or during surgery. Obtaining a culture through sinus endoscopy is an alternative approach.
- Cultures of sinus aspirates should be processed for aerobic and anaerobic bacteria and fungi.

Contents

Introduction

The upper respiratory tract, including the nasopharynx, serves as the reservoir for pathogenic bacteria that can cause respiratory infections including sinusitis [1]. Potential pathogens can relocate during a viral respiratory infection, from the nasopharynx into the sinus cavity, causing sinusitis [2]. Establishment of the correct microbiology of all forms of sinusitis is of primary importance as it can serve as a guide for choosing adequate antimicrobial therapy. This chapter presents the microbiology of all forms of sinusitis and the microbial dynamics of nasopharyngitis.

The Normal Flora of the Oral Cavity

The mucosal and epithelial surfaces of the human body are covered with aerobic and anaerobic micro-organisms [3]. The organisms that reside at these sites are predominantly anaerobic and actively multiply. The trachea, bronchi, esophagus, stomach, and upper urinary tract are not normally colonized by indigenous flora. However, a limited number of transient organisms may be present at these sites from time to time. Microflora also vary at different sites within the body system, as in the oral cavity; the micro-organisms present in the buccal folds vary in their concentration and types of strains from those isolated from the tongue or gingival sulci. However, the organisms that prevail in one body system tend to belong to certain major bacterial species, and their presence in that system is predictable. The relative and total counts of organisms can be affected by various factors, such as age, diet, anatomic variations, illness, hospitalization, and antimicrobial therapy. However, these sets of bacterial flora, with predictable patterns, remain stable throughout life, despite being subject to perturbing factors.

Anaerobes outnumber aerobic bacteria on all mucosal surfaces, and certain organisms predominate at different sites. The number of anaerobes at a site is generally inversely related to oxygen tension [3]. Their predominance in the skin, mouth, nose, and throat, which are exposed to oxygen is explained by the anaerobic micro-environment generated by the facultative bacteria that consume oxygen.

Knowledge of the composition of the flora at certain sites is useful for predicting which organisms may be involved in an infection adjacent to that site and can assist in the selection of a logical antimicrobial therapy, even before the exact microbial etiology of the infection is known.

The normal flora is not just a potential hazard for the host, but also a beneficial partner. Normal body flora also serves as protectors from colonization or subsequent invasion by potentially virulent bacteria. In instances where the host defenses are impaired or a breach occurs in the mucus membranes or skin, however, the members of the normal flora can cause infections.

Microbial Composition

The formation of the normal oral flora is initiated at birth. Certain organisms such as lactobacilli and anaerobic streptococci, which establish themselves at an early date, reach high numbers within a few days. *Actinomyces*, *Fusobacterium*, and *Nocardia* are acquired by the age of 6 months. Following that time, *Prevotella* and *Porphyromonas* spp., *Leptotrichia*, *Propionibacterium*, and *Candida* also become part of the oral flora [3]. *Fusobacterium* populations attain high numbers after dentition and reach maximal numbers at the age of 1 year.

The most predominant group of facultative micro-organisms native to the oropharynx are the alpha-hemolytic streptococci, which include the species *Streptococcus mitis*, *Streptococcus milleri*, *Streptococcus sanguis*, *Streptococcus intermedius*, *Streptococcus salivarius*, and several others [4]. Other groups of organisms native to the oropharynx are *Moraxella catarrhalis* and *Haemophilus influenzae*, which are capable of producing beta-lactamase and may spread to adjacent sites, causing otitis, sinusitis,

or bronchitis. Encapsulated *H. influenzae* also induces serious infections such as meningitis and bacteremia. The oropharynx also contains *Staphylococcus aureus* and *Staphylococcus epidermidis*, which can also produce beta-lactamase and take part in infections.

The normal oropharynx is seldom colonized by Gram-negative Enterobacteriaceae. In contrast, hospitalized patients are generally heavily colonized with these organisms. The reasons for this change in microflora are not known, but may be related to changes in the glycocalyx of the pharyngeal epithelial cells or due to selective processes that occur following the administration of antimicrobial therapy [5]. The shift from predominantly Gram-positive to Gram-negative bacteria is thought to contribute to the high incidence of sinus infection caused by Gram-negative bacteria in patients with chronic illnesses.

Anaerobic bacteria are present in large numbers in the oropharynx, particularly in patients with poor dental hygiene, caries, or periodontal disease. Anaerobic bacteria outnumber their aerobic counterpart at ratios ranging from 10:1 to 100:1 (Fig. 18.1). Anaerobic bacteria can adhere to tooth surfaces and contribute through the elaboration of metabolic by-products to the development of both caries and periodontal disease [4]. The predominant anaerobes are anaerobic streptococci, *Veillonella* spp., *Bacteroides* spp. pigmented *Prevotella* and *Porphyromonas* spp. (previously called *Bacteroides melaninogenicus* group) and *Fusobacterium* spp. [4]. These organisms are a potential source of a variety of chronic infections including otitis and sinusitis, aspiration pneumonia lung abscesses, and abscesses of the oropharynx and teeth.

The microflora of the oral cavity is complex and contains many kinds of obligate anaerobes. The distribution of bacteria within the mouth seems to be a function of their ability to adhere

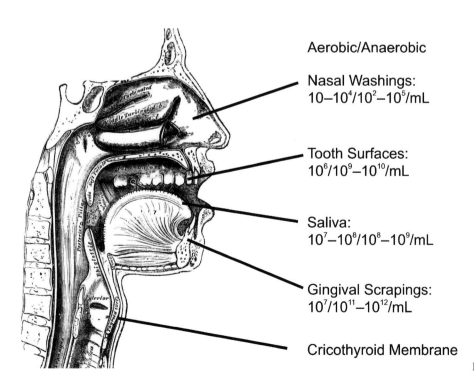

Aerobic/Anaerobic

Nasal Washings:
$10–10^4/10^2–10^5$/mL

Tooth Surfaces:
$10^6/10^9–10^{10}$/mL

Saliva:
$10^7–10^8/10^8–10^9$/mL

Gingival Scrapings:
$10^7/10^{11}–10^{12}$/mL

Cricothyroid Membrane

Fig. 18.1 Oropharyngeal flora

Resistance to β-lactam Antibiotics

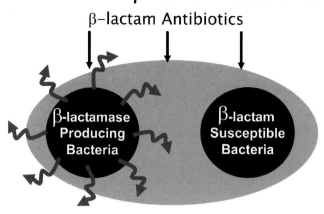

Fig. 18.2 Protection of penicillin-susceptible bacteria from penicillin by beta-lactamase-producing bacteria

to the oral surfaces. The differences in numbers of the anaerobic microflora probably occur because of considerable variations in the oxygen concentration in parts of the oral cavity.

For example, the maxillary and mandibular buccal folds contain 0.4% and 0.3% oxygen respectively, while the anterior and posterior tongue surfaces contain 16.4% and 12.4%. The environment of the gingival sulcus is more anaerobic than that of the buccal folds, and the periodontal pocket is the most anaerobic area in the oral cavity. The ratio of anaerobic bacteria to aerobic bacteria in saliva is approximately 10:1. The total count of anaerobic bacteria is 1.1×10^8/ml (Fig. 18.1). The predominant anaerobic bacteria that colonize the anterior nose are *P. acnes*. *Fusobacterium nucleatum* is the main species of *Fusobacterium* present in the oral cavity. Anaerobic Gram-negative bacilli found in the oral cavity include pigmented *Prevotella* and *Porphyromonas* (previously called black-pigmented *Bacteroides*); *Porphyromonas gingivalis*; *Prevotella oralis*; *Prevotella oris-buccae (ruminicola)*; *Prevotella disiens*; and *Bacteroides ureolyticus*.

Fusobacteria are also a predominant part of the oral flora [6], as are treponemas [7]. Pigmented *Prevotella* and *Porphyromonas* represent less than 1% of the coronal tooth surface, but constitute 4–8% of gingival crevice flora. Veillonellae represent 1–3% of the coronal tooth surface, 5–15% of the gingival crevice flora, and 10–15% of the tongue flora. Microaerophilic streptococci predominate in all areas of the oral cavity, and they reach high numbers in the tongue and cheek [8]. Other anaerobes prevalent in the mouth are *Actinomyces* [9], *Peptostreptococci*, *Leptotrichia buccalis*, *Bifidobacterium*, *Eubacterium*, and *Propionibacterium* [10].

Pigmented *Prevotella*, *Porphyromonas*, and *Fusobacterium* species can produce beta-lactamase [11]. The recovery rate of aerobic and anaerobic beta-lactamase-producing bacteria (BLPB) in the oropharynx has increased in recent years, and these organisms have been isolated in over half of the patients with head and neck infections including sinusitis [11]. BLPB can be involved directly in the infection, protecting not only those species from the activity of penicillins, but also penicillin-

susceptible organisms. This can occur when the enzyme beta-lactamase is secreted into the infected tissue or abscess fluid in sufficient quantities to break the penicillins' beta-lactamase ring before it can kill the susceptible bacteria (Fig. 18.2) [12].

The high incidence of recovery of BLPB in upper respiratory tract infections may be due to the selection of these organisms following antimicrobial therapy with beta-lactamase antibiotics. The emergence of penicillin-resistant flora can occur following only a short course of penicillin [13, 14].

Obtaining Appropriate Sinus Content Cultures While Avoiding the Normal Flora

If a patient with sinusitis develops a severe infection, is immunocompromised or fails to show significant improvement or shows signs of deterioration despite treatment, it is important to obtain a culture, preferably through sinus puncture, as this may reveal the presence of causative bacteria. Obtaining a culture through sinus endoscopy is an alternative approach.

Sinus aspirates for culture must be obtained free of contamination so that saprophytic organisms or normal flora are excluded, and culture results can be interpreted correctly. Because indigenous aerobic and anaerobic bacteria are present on the nasopharyngeal mucous membranes in large numbers, even minimal contamination of a specimen with the normal flora can give misleading results. The use of sinus puncture is the "gold standard" method of obtaining such specimens [15]. There are, however, data that support the use of endoscopically obtained cultures in assessing the microbiology of infected sinuses [16–24].

Sinus Puncture

Obtaining sinus aspirates by puncture is the traditional method of specimens collection. The maxillary sinus is the most accessible of all of the paranasal sinuses. There are two approaches to the maxillary sinus that use puncture: either via the canine fossa or the inferior meatus. The nasal vestibule is often heavily colonized with pathogenic bacteria, mostly *S. aureus*. Therefore, sterilization of the nasal vestibule and the area beneath the inferior nasal turbinate is suggested.

Contamination with nasal flora may, however, occur. To prevent misinterpretation of the culture results, acute infection is defined as the recovery of a high-density bacterial species, i. e., a colony count of at least 10^3–10^4 colony = forming units per milliliter [cfu/mL]. This quantitative definition increases the probability that micro-organisms isolated from the sinus aspirate truly represent in situ infection and not contamination. As most aspirates from infected sinuses contain colony counts above 10^4 cfu/mL. If quantitative cultures cannot be performed, a Gram stain of aspirated specimens enables semiquantitative assessment. If bacteria are readily seen on a Gram stain preparation, the approximate bacterial density is about 10^5 cfu/mL. Out of 12 cases in which an antral puncture showed at least 10^5 cfu/mL pathogens, the Gram stain demonstrated either organisms or white blood cells in all 12 and organisms and white blood cells in 9 out of 12 [16]. A Gram stain is especially useful if organisms are observed on smear and the specimen fails to grow using standard aerobic culture techniques, in which case, anaerobic organisms or other fastidious bacteria or an antibiotic-inhibited flora should be suspected. A Gram stain can also allow an assessment of the local inflammatory response. The presence of many white blood cells in association with a positive high-density bacterial culture makes it probable that a bacterial infection is present. A Gram stain does not, however, differentiate between neutrophils and eosinophils. In contrast, a paucity or absence of white blood cells in association with the presence of a positive low-density culture suggests bacteria contamination.

Endoscopic Cultures

Recently, there has been interest in obtaining cultures of the middle meatus endoscopically, as a substitute or surrogate for cultures of a sinus aspirate. The endoscopically obtained culture is less invasive and associated with less morbidity [16]. Unfortunately, in normal children, the middle meatus has been shown to be colonized with the same bacterial species S. pneumoniae, H. influenzae and M. catarrhalis, as are commonly recovered from children with sinus infection [18]. Accordingly, this technique cannot be recommended for precise bacterial diagnosis in children with sinus infections.

In three recent studies the bacterial species recovered from middle meatal samples obtained from normal adults were coagulase-negative staphylococci (CNS) in 35–50%, Corynebacterium spp. in 16–23%, and Staphylococcus aureus in 8–20% [19–21]. The only overlap between commensals and potential pathogens is S. aureus.

Several studies in adults have shown a good correlation between cultures of the middle meatus and the sinus aspirate in patients with acute sinusitis, especially when purulence is in the middle meatus [16, 21, 22, 25]. However, other studies have not found such a correlation [24, 25].

Concordance on the types and concentrations of organisms recovered by endoscopic aspirates and those isolated during sinus surgery was found in all 6 cases in one study [26]. Sixteen of the 18 anaerobes isolated from sinus aspirates were also found in the concomitant endoscopic sample. Five aerobic isolates were found in both sinus aspirates and endoscopic samples and their concentration was similar. However, contamination by four aerobic Gram-positive bacteria (in numbers of $<10^4$ cfu/sample) were found in the endoscopy samples.

Coagulase-negative staphylococci are usually interpreted as nonpathogens in acute sinusitis. Talbot and colleagues [16] correlated the results of endoscopically obtained cultures and cultures obtained from maxillary sinus aspirates. They reported no situations in which the puncture demonstrated CNS in $>10^5$ cfu/mL; however, a swab of the middle meatus grew CNS in 6 out of 53 patients. Interpretation of the pathogenicity of S. aureus is more difficult. Two out of 53 patients had $>10^5$ cfu/mL, which correlated with the endoscopic swab. However, in an additional 6 patients there was no agreement between sites [16].

In rare instances, neither a sinus aspirate nor a specimen obtained endoscopically is sufficient for the diagnosis of a sinus infection. In this instance, biopsy of the sinus mucosa, and broth culture and appropriate stains, may be required to demonstrate the bacterial etiology.

Discrepancies in the Recovery of Bacteria from Multiple Sinuses in Sinusitis

There are differences in the distribution of organisms in a single patient who suffers from infections in multiple sinuses that emphasize the importance of obtaining cultures from all infected sinuses. A recent study evaluated the discrepancies between infected sinuses by studying the aerobic and anaerobic microbiology of acute and chronic sinusitis in patients with involvement of multiple sinuses [17]. The 155 evaluated patients had sinusitis of either the maxillary, ethmoid or frontal sinuses (any combination) and had organisms recovered from two to four concomitantly infected sinuses. Similar aerobic, facultative, and anaerobic organisms were recovered from all the groups of patients. In patients who had organisms isolated from two sinuses and had acute sinusitis, 31 of the 55 isolates (56%) were found only in a single sinus, and 24 (44%) were recovered concomitantly from two sinuses. In those with chronic infection 31 of the 91 isolates (34%) were recovered only from a single sinus, and 60 (66%) were found concomitantly from two sinuses. Anaerobic bacteria were more often concomitantly isolated from two sinuses (50 out of 70) than aerobic and facultative (10 out of 21, $p < 0.05$). Similar findings were observed in patients who had organisms isolated from three or four sinuses. Beta-lactamase-producing bacteria were more often isolated from patients with chronic infection (58–83%) than from those with acute infections (32–43%). These findings illustrate that there are differences in the distribution of organisms in a single patient who suffers from infections in multiple sinuses and emphasizes the importance of obtaining cultures from all infected sinuses.

Interfering Flora

Competitive interactions between micro-organisms take place in the process of the colonization of mucus membranes, as well as in clinical infections [27]. Bacteria interact with each other when they attempt to establish themselves and dominate their environment [28]. Some of these interactions are synergistic while others are antagonistic, as organisms can interfere with each other's growth and compete for their ecological space. The nasopharynx of healthy individuals is generally colonized by relatively nonpathogenic aerobic and anaerobic organisms [27], some of which possess the ability to interfere with the growth of potential pathogens (Fig. 18.3) [29]. This phenomenon is called "bacterial interference". These organisms include the aerobic alpha-hemolytic streptococci (mostly Streptococcus mitis and Streptococcus sanguis) [30] and anaerobic bacteria (Prevotella melaninogenica and Peptostreptococcus anaerobius) [31]. Many of these organisms produce bacteriocins, which are bactericidal proteins. Nasopharyngeal carriage of upper respiratory tract pathogens, such as S. pneumoniae, H. influenzae, and M. catarrhalis, can, however, occur in healthy individuals and

18

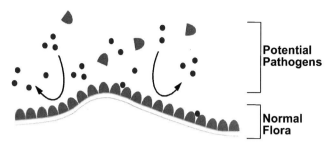

Fig. 18.3 The role of normal flora in preventing colonization and subsequent infection by pathogenic bacteria

increases significantly in the general population of young children during respiratory illness [32]. The number of interfering organisms is also lower in children prone to sinusitis [33]. The absence of these organisms may explain the higher recovery of pathogens in these children. The presence of organisms with interfering potential may play a role in the prevention of colonization by pathogens and the occurrence of upper respiratory infections.

Brook and Gober [34] illustrated that the development of a purulent discharge in nasopharyngitis (NPT) is associated with prior colonization by potential pathogens and the absence of organisms with interfering capabilities in the NP of the patients. However, patients who are not colonized with potential respiratory pathogens, but are colonized with interfering bacteria, or nonpathogens such as *P. acnes* and *Corynebacterium* spp., are not prone to developing purulent NPT.

Administration of antimicrobial agents can influence the composition of nasopharyngeal flora [35]. Members of the oral flora with interfering capability (e. g., aerobic and anaerobic streptococci as well as penicillin-susceptible *P. melaninogenica* strains) can become resistant to amoxicillin, but remain susceptible to amoxicillin-clavulanate. Beta-lactamase-producing *P. melaninogenica* strains are susceptible to amoxicillin-clavulanate. All these organisms are more resistant to second- and third-generation cephalosporin therapy. Therapy with oral second-generation cephalosporins does not eliminate organisms with interfering capabilities, as does amoxicillin [36] or amoxicillin-clavulanate.

Nasal Flora

The origin of organisms that are introduced into the sinuses and may eventually cause sinusitis is the nasal cavity. The normal flora of that site comprises certain bacterial species, which include *S. aureus*, *S. epidermidis*, alpha- and gamma-streptococci, *P. acnes*, and aerobic diphtheroid [37–39]. Potential sinus pathogens have been isolated from healthy nasal cavities, but relatively rarely. These included *S. pneumoniae* (0.5–15%), *H. influenzae* (0–6%), *M. catarrhalis* (0–4%), *Streptococcus pyogenes* (0–1%), and anaerobic bacteria (*Peptostreptococcus* spp. [7–16%] and *Prevotella* spp. [6–8%]) [37–39].

The flora of the nasal cavity of patients with sinusitis is different from healthy flora. While the recovery of *Staphylococcus*

spp. and diphtheroids is reduced, the isolation of pathogens increases: *S. pneumoniae* was found in 36% of patients, *H. influenzae* in over 50%, *S. pyogenes* in 6%, and *M. catarrhalis* in 4% [40–44].

In many studies on the nasal bacterial flora in sinusitis a simultaneous sinus aspirate was not taken [42, 43], while in others the correlation was found to be poor in some [42, 45], but good in others [44, 46]. A good correlation was, however, found in one study [40] in which when the sinus aspirate culture yielded a presumed sinus pathogen, the same organism was found in the nasal cavity sample in 91% of the 185 patients. The predictive value of a pathogen-positive nasal finding was high for *S. pyogenes* (94%), *H. influenzae* (78%), and *S. pneumoniae* (69%), but was low for *M. catarrhalis* (20%). Despite these encouraging data, nasopharyngeal culture is not an acceptable alternative to culture through aspiration.

Normal Sinus Flora

It is known that after sinus surgery, the sinus cavities quickly become colonized with bacteria and are no longer sterile. The question of whether normal bacterial flora exists in the sinuses is controversial. The communication of the sinuses with the nasal cavity through the ostia could enable organisms that reside in the nasopharynx to spread into the sinus. Following closure of the ostium, these bacteria may become involved in the inflammation. Organisms have been recovered from uninflamed sinuses in several studies [47–50]. The bacterial flora of noninflamed sinuses was studied for aerobic and anaerobic bacteria in 12 adults who underwent corrective surgery for septal deviation [47]. Organisms were recovered from all aspirates with an average of four isolates per sinus aspirate. The predominant anaerobic isolates were *Prevotella*, *Porphyromonas*, *Fusobacterium*, and *Peptostreptococcus* spp. The most common aerobic bacteria were *S. pyogenes*, *S. aureus*, *S. pneumoniae*, and *H. influenzae*.

In another study, specimens were processed for aerobic bacteria only, and *Staphylococcus* spp. and alpha-hemolytic streptococci were isolated [48]. Organisms were recovered in 20% of maxillary sinuses in patients who underwent surgical repositioning of the maxilla [49]. In contrast, another report of the aspirates of 12 volunteers with no sinus disease showed no bacterial growth [50].

Jiang et al. evaluated [51] the bacteriology of maxillary sinuses with normal endoscopic findings. Organisms were recovered from 14 out of 30 swab specimens (47%) and 7 out of 17 mucosal specimens (41%).

Gordts et al. [19] reported the microbiology of the middle meatus in normal adults and children. This study noted that in 52 patients 75% had bacterial isolates present, most commonly coagulase-negative staphylococci (CNS) (35%), *Corynebacterium* spp. (23%) and *S. aureus* (8%) in adults. Low numbers of these species were present. In children the most common organisms were *H. influenzae* (40%), *M. catarrhalis* (34%), and *S. pneumoniae* (50%), a marked difference from findings in adults. Nonhemolytic streptococci and *Moraxella* spp. were absent in adults.

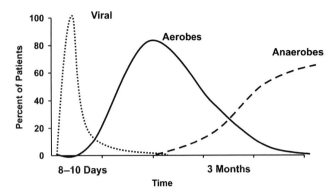

Fig. 18.4 Viral and bacterial causes of otitis and sinusitis

Microbiology of Sinusitis

The pattern of many upper respiratory infections including sinusitis evolves several phases (Fig. 18.4). The early stage is often a viral infection that generally lasts up to 10 days where complete recovery occurs in most individuals [41]. However, in a small number of patients with viral sinusitis (estimated at 0.5%) a secondary acute bacterial infection may develop. This is generally caused by facultative aerobic bacteria (i. e., *S. pneumoniae*, *H. influenzae*, and *M. catarrhalis*). If resolution does not take place anaerobic bacteria of oral flora origin become predominant over time. The dynamic of these bacterial changes were recently demonstrated by performing serial culture in patients with maxillary sinusitis [52].

The Role of Bacterial Superantigens in Sinus Disease

Some micro-organisms (bacteria, viruses, and fungi) can produce exotoxins (sometimes called enterotoxins) that are able to nonspecifically upregulate T lymphocytes by cross-linking the MHC II molecule on antigen = presenting cells with the variable beta (Vβ) region of the T cell receptor (TCR). These exotoxins are called superantigens because they activate in a nonspecific manner subpopulations representing up to 30% of T lymphocytes, in contrast to classical antigens, which activate only <0.01% of T lymphocytes. Furthermore, superantigens can also act as classical antigens, bringing about the concomitant generation of anti-superantigen antibodies, which are often IgE isotypes [53].

Staphylococcus aureus is a common colonizer of the nasal passage of patients with nasal polyps. *S. aureus* superantigens may play a role in nasal polyps as 50% of polyp homogenates contained IgE specific to *S. aureus* exotoxins. Polyps associated with IgE to superantigens had significantly greater eosinophilia and markers of eosinophilic inflammation than controls [54].

Staphylococcal exotoxin-specific serum IgE was present in 5 out of 10 patients with nasal polyposis (50%) and in none of 13 control patients. Patients with IgE to these superantigens have an increase in tissue eosinophilia and a higher incidence of asthma compared with control patients [55].

Staphylococcus aureus was present in 7 out of 13 patients with nasal polyps and all produced exotoxins: staphylococcus enterotoxin A (SEA), toxic shock syndrome toxin-1 (TSS T-1) or staphylococcus enterotoxin B (SEB). A clonal expansion of Vβ specific to the isolated exotoxin was observed in the three patients studied [56].

Viral Infections

Viral illness is the most common predisposing factor for upper respiratory tract infections, including sinusitis [57]. Rhino-, influenzae and para-influenzae viruses are the most common causes of sinusitis [58, 59]. It is not known for certain whether the viral infection precedes or is concurrent with the bacterial infection. The actual mechanisms by which a virus causes sinus disease are unknown. The mechanism whereby viruses predispose to sinusitis may involve microbial synergy, induction of local inflammation that blocks the sinus ostia, increase in bacterial attachment to the epithelial cells, and disruption of the local immune defense (Fig. 18.5).

Epithelial cells are often infected with the common respiratory viruses, which can induce the production of several cytokines [57, 60, 61]. In the case of rhinoviruses, after deposition in the nose the virus is transported to the posterior nasopharynx [60, 62] and attaches to a specific rhinovirus receptor [63]. Following initiation of the infection, several inflammatory pathways are stimulated, as well as the sympathetic nervous system, which generates the classic symptoms of a cold [64]. The common cold not only involves the nasal passages, but also the paranasal sinuses. Sinus computed tomography (CT) scans of 31 young adults with early common colds showed frequent abnormalities in the sinus cavity [65]. Mucosal thickening is observed in radiographs of 87% of patients with colds [66], probably because of excess amounts of mucous discharge from goblet cells. These were observed in the maxillary sinus in 87% of the cases, in the ethmoid sinus in 65%, the frontal in 32%, and the sphenoid in 39%. Similar sinus abnormalities during colds were observed in adults and children [67, 68].

Activation of the inflammatory pathways results in engorgement of the venous erectile tissue in the nasal turbinates, which leads to leakage of plasma into the nose and sinuses, discharge of goblet cells and seromucous glands, sneezing, and sensation of pain.

Computed tomography scans show occlusion of the infundibulum in 77% of patients with viral rhinosinusitis [65]. A malfunction in the ability of cilia to move material deposits toward the ostia, because of the increased amount of viscous material and their induced slowing and paralysis, is also observed [68]. The adverse effect of this dysfunction is compounded by infundibular and ostiomeatal obstruction from mucosal swelling. Some viral infections, such as influenza, can cause destructive epithelial damage that enhances bacterial adherence.

During a cold, nasal fluid containing viruses, bacteria, and inflammatory mediators is suctioned into the sinus cavities where it produces inflammation and/or infection and is thickened by exocytosis of mucin from the numerous goblet cells in the sinus epithelium. The CT abnormalities observed in viral

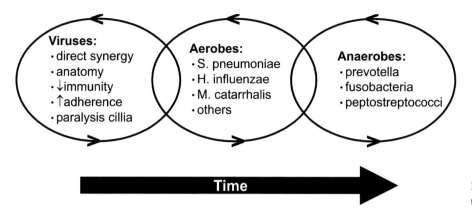

Fig. 18.5 Dynamics of upper respiratory tract infections [90]

sinusitis could, therefore, be due to inflammation alone, or of a viral infection of sinus epithelium cells. In sinus puncture studies in patients with acute community-acquired rhinosinusitis, 15% of the sinus aspirates have yielded rhinovirus, 5% influenza virus, 3% para-influenza virus, and 2% adenovirus [69]. Some of the sinus aspirates yielded both viruses and bacteria.

Bacteria in Acute Sinusitis

Bacteria can be isolated from two-thirds of patients with acute infection of the maxillary, ethmoid, frontal, and sphenoid sinuses [70]. The bacteria recovered from pediatric and adult patients with community-acquired acute purulent sinusitis, using sinus aspiration by puncture or surgery, are the common respiratory pathogens (*S. pneumoniae*, *M. catarrhalis*, *H. influenzae*, and beta-hemolytic streptococci) and those considered to be part of the normal flora of the nose (*S. aureus*; Table 18.1) [71–73]. *S. aureus* is a common pathogen in sphenoid sinusitis [73], while the other organisms are common in other sinuses.

The bacteria that cause the infection in children are generally the same as those found in acute otitis media. *S. pneumoniae* was isolated in 28% of 50 children with acute sinusitis, and *H. influenzae* and *M. catarrhalis* were both isolated in 19% of the aspirates. Beta-lactamase-producing strains of *H. influenzae* and *M. catarrhalis* were found in 20% and 27% of the cases respectively.

The infection is polymicrobial in about a third of the cases. Enteric bacteria are recovered less commonly, and anaerobes were recovered from only a few cases of acute sinusitis. However, appropriate methods for their recovery were rarely employed in most studies of acute sinusitis. Anaerobic bacteria are commonly recovered from acute sinusitis associated with dental disease, mostly as an extension of the infection from the roots of the premolar or molar teeth [74, 75].

Pseudomonas aeruginosa and other Gram-negative rods are common in sinusitis of nosocomial origin (especially in patients who have nasal tubes or catheters), the immunocompromised, patients with Human Immune Deficiency Virus (HIV) infection and patients who suffer from cystic fibrosis [76].

Bacteria in Chronic Sinusitis

Although the exact etiology of the inflammation associated with this chronic sinusitis is uncertain, the presence of bacteria within the sinuses in this patient population has been well documented [77, 78]. Most clinicians believe that bacteria play a major role in the etiology and pathogenesis of most cases of chronic sinusitis, and prescribe antimicrobial therapy for its treatment.

In contrast to the agreement regarding the microbiology of acute sinusitis, there is disagreement regarding the microbiology of chronic sinusitis. Unfortunately, there are several issues that confound the reliability of many of these studies and therefore contribute to the disparity of their results. These issues include: various methods are used to sample the sinus cavity, (i. e., aspiration, irrigation, calcium alginate swab or biopsy); failure to sterilize the area through which the trocar or endoscope is passed; different sinuses or areas that are sampled (i. e., the ethmoid bulla or maxillary antrum, or middle meatus); lack of assessment of the inflammatory response; lack of quantitation of bacteria; previous or current use of antibiotics; variable patient selection, (i. e., age, duration, extent of disease, surgical or non-surgical individuals), presence of nasal polyps, time of culture transport, and method of culture.

Numerous studies have examined the bacterial pathogens associated with chronic sinusitis. However, most of these studies did not employ methods that are adequate for the recovery of anaerobic bacteria. Studies have described significant differences in the microbial pathogens present in chronic sinusitis compared with acute sinusitis. *S. aureus*, *S. epidermidis*, and anaerobic and Gram-negative bacteria predominate in chronic sinusitis. The pathogenicity of some of the low virulence organisms, such *S. epidermidis*, a colonizer of the nasal cavity, is questionable [19, 79]. The absence of quantitation or performance of Gram stains in most studies prevents an assessment of both the density of organisms and the accompaniment of an inflammatory response. The common resistance of *S. epidermidis* to antimicrobials does not prove its pathogenicity. Although *S. epidermidis* is discounted as a pathogen in sinusitis, its role as a pathogen in other body sites has been well documented (i. e. neutropenic sepsis, infections of indwelling catheters, and

Table 18.1 Microbiology of sinusitis (% of patients) [70, 124–126, 177]

Bacteria	Maxillary Acute	Maxillary Chronic N = 66	Ethmoid Acute N = 26	Ethmoid Chronic N = 17	Frontal Acute N = 15	Frontal Chronic N = 13	Splenoid Acute N = 16	Splenoid Chronic N = 7
Aerobic								
S. aureus	4	14	15	24	–	15	56	14
S. pyogenes	2	8	8	6	3	–	6	–
S. pneumoniae	31	6	35	6	33	–	6	–
H. influenzae	21	5	27	6	40	15	12	14
M. catarrhalis	8	6	8	–	20	–	–	
Enterobacteriaceae	7	6	–	47	–	8	–	28
P. aeruginosa	2	3	–	6	–	8	6	14
Anaerobic								
Peptostreptococcus sp.	2	56	15	59	3	38	19	57
P. acnes		29	12	18	3	8	12	29
Fusobacterium sp.	2	17	4	47	3	31	6	54
Prevotella & Porphyromonas sp.	2	47	8	82	3	62	6	86
B. fragilis		6	–	–	–	15	–	–

Gwaltney, 2000
Brook et al., 1989, 2002, 2003

18

in burn patients [80]. Their frequent recovery from swabs obtained from the middle meatus of normal participants marks them as commensals and likely contaminants. In the unusual situation of a large number of white blood cells and organisms being present on the Gram stain and there being heavy growth of S. epidermidis, and proper anaerobic cultures showed no growth of these and other organisms, the possibility of a true infection by S. epidermidis should be entertained [21].

Gram-negative enteric rods were also reported in recent studies [80, 81]. These included P. aeruginosa, Klebsiella pneumoniae, Proteus mirabilis, Enterobacter species, and Escherichia coli. Since these organisms are rarely found in cultures of the middle meatus obtained from normal individuals, their isolation from these symptomatic patients suggests their pathogenic role. These organisms may have been selected following administration of antimicrobial therapy in patients with chronic sinusitis.

The pathophysiology of chronic sinusitis often differs from that of acute sinusitis. The exact events leading to chronic sinusitis have been difficult to identify or prove [82]. It has been proposed that chronic sinusitis is an extension of unresolved acute sinusitis. As mentioned previously, the etiology of acute sinusitis is frequently viral, which can establish an environment that is synergistic with the growth of other organisms, both aerobic and anaerobic. If the infection is not properly treated, the inflammatory process can persist, which, over time, fosters the growth of anaerobic bacteria. Thus, the pathogens in sinusitis appear to evolve over the course of infection – from viruses to aerobic to anaerobic bacterial growth as the symptoms and pathology persist over a period of weeks to months.

The microbiology of chronic sinusitis differs from that of acute sinusitis (Tables 18.1) [83–86]. The transition from acute to chronic sinusitis by repeated aspirations of sinus secretions by endoscopy was illustrated in 5 patients who presented with acute maxillary sinusitis that did not respond to antimicrobial therapy [52]. Most bacteria isolated from the first culture were aerobic or facultative bacteria – S. pneumoniae, H. influenzae, and M. catarrhalis. Failure to respond to therapy was associated with the emergence of resistant aerobic and anaerobic bacteria in subsequent aspirates. These organisms included F. nucleatum, pigmented Prevotella, Porphyromonas spp., and Peptostreptococcus spp. (Fig. 18.6). Eradication of the infection was finally achieved following administration of effective antimicrobial agents and in three cases also by surgical drainage.

This study illustrates that as chronicity develops, the aerobic and facultative species are gradually replaced by anaerobes [52]. This may result from the selective pressure of antimicrobial agents that enables resistant organisms to survive, and from the development of conditions appropriate for anaerobic growth, which include the reduction in oxygen tension and an increase in acidity within the sinus. These are caused by persistent edema and swelling, which reduces blood supply, and by the consumption of oxygen by the aerobic bacteria [87]. Other factors are emergence over time or the selection of anaerobes that possess virulence factors such as a capsule [88].

In chronic infections, when adequate methods are used, anaerobes can be recovered in more than half of all cases; the usual pathogens in acute sinusitis (e. g., *S. pneumoniae*, *H. influenzae*, *M. catarrhalis*) are found with lower frequency [83–86, 89]. Polymicrobial infection is common in chronic sinusitis, which is a synergistic infection [87] and may therefore be more difficult to eradicate with narrow-spectrum antimicrobial agents. Chronic sinusitis caused by anaerobes is a particular concern clinically because many of the complications associated with this condition (e. g., mucocele formation, osteomyelitis, local and intracranial abscess) are caused by these organisms [90].

That anaerobes play a role in chronic sinusitis is supported by the ability to induce chronic sinusitis in a rabbit by intrasinus inoculation of *Bacteroides fragilis* [91, 92] and the rapid production of serum IgG antibodies against this organism in the infected animals [92]. The pathogenic role of these organisms is also supported by the detection of antibodies (IgG) to two anaerobic organisms commonly recovered from sinus aspirates (*F. nucleatum* and *P. intermedia*) [93]. Antibody levels to these organisms declined in the patients who responded to therapy and were cured, but did not decrease in those in whom therapy failed (Fig. 18.7).

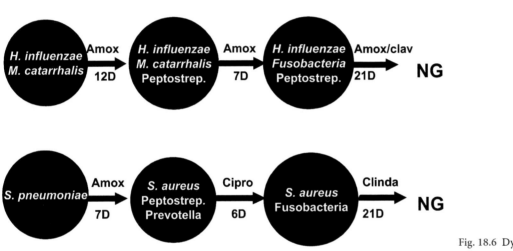

Fig. 18.6 Dynamics of sinusitis [52]

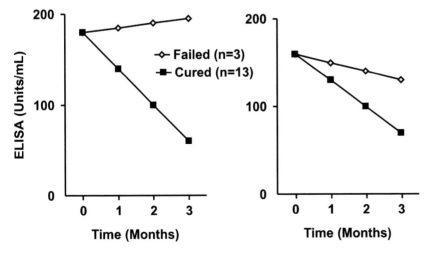

Fig. 18.7 Serum antibodies to *F. nucleatum* and *P. intermedia* in 23 patients with chronic sinusitis [93]

Aside from their role as pathogens the production of beta-lactamase among many Gram-negative anaerobes (e. g., *Prevotella*, *Porphyromonas*, and *Fusobacterium* spp.) can shield or protect other organisms, including aerobic pathogens, from beta-lactamase antibiotics (Fig. 18.2) [12, 94].

Studies in Children

There were 10 studies on the microbiology of chronic rhinosinusitis in children published between 1981 and 2000 [85, 95–103]. Four of these studies were prospective [95, 96, 100, 102] and six were retrospective. In all but two studies, the maxillary sinus was sampled by transnasal aspiration. The most common criteria for evaluation were symptoms that lasted for more than 90 days. An attempt was made to sterilize the nose prior to obtaining the culture in only five studies and bacterial quantitation was rarely done. In two of the studies, normal nasal flora (i. e., *S. epidermidis* and alpha-hemolytic streptococci) were the usual organisms recovered. It is difficult to know what pathologic significance to ascribe to these organisms. In the remaining stud-

ies, the usual sinus pathogens were recovered in about 60% of cases (i. e., *H. influenzae*, *S. pneumoniae*, and *M. catarrhalis*). This was especially true when the criteria for entry included purulent secretions. In the remaining 30–40% of children, contaminants were recovered. Anaerobes were recovered in three studies, the only ones that employed methods for their isolation [85, 95, 102].

Staphylococcus aureus (19%) and alpha-hemolytic streptococci (23%) were the predominant isolates in ethmoid sinusitis in one study [98], and *S. epidermidis* and alpha-hemolytic streptococci were the major ones in another [96]. *M. catarrhalis* was the most common isolate in a study of children with allergies, although 25% of the patients had polymicrobial flora [104]. *S. pneumoniae* and *H. influenzae* predominate in children with acute exacerbations [105].

Brook and Yocum [106] studied 40 children with chronic sinusitis. The sinuses infected were the maxillary (15 cases), ethmoid (13), and frontal (7). Pansinusitis was present in 5 patients. A total of 121 isolates (97 anaerobic and 24 aerobic) were recovered. Anaerobes were recovered from all 37 culture-positive specimens, and in 14 cases (38%) they were mixed with

Table 18.2 Summary of 17 studies that evaluated the role of anaerobes in chronic bacterial sinusitis

Reference	No. of patients	Condition	Patients from whom anaerobic organisms were isolated (%)	Organisms that were anaerobes (%)
[110]	83	Chronic sinusitis	75	52
[111]	66	Acute and chronic sinusitis	39	39
[112]	40 adults	Chronic sinusitis	100	19
[113]	54 adults	Chronic sinusitis	33	42
[114]	15 adults	Chronic sinusitis	38	48
[115]	40	Chronic sinusitis	69	46
[116]	132 adults	Chronic sinusitis	NS	22
[117]	35	Chronic sinusitis	70	39
[85]	40 children	Chronic sinusitis	100	80
[118]	90	Chronic sinusitis	81	29
[119]	10	Chronic maxillary sinusitis	100	60
[102]	93 children	Chronic maxillary sinusitis	93	93
[120]	126 adults	Chronic maxillary sinusitis	90	88
[84]	68 adults	Chronic maxillary sinusitis	100	82
[121]	114 adults	Acute and chronic sinusitis	NS	12
[122]	412	Chronic sinusitis	NS	26
[86]	150 adults	Chronic maxillary sinusitis	54	49

aerobes. The predominant anaerobic organisms were Gram-negative bacilli (36), anaerobic Gram-positive cocci (28), and *Fusobacterium* spp. (13). The predominant aerobic isolates were alpha-hemolytic streptococci (7), *S. aureus* (7), and *Haemophilus* spp. (4).

Brook et al. [95] correlated the microbiology of concurrent chronic otitis media with effusion and chronic maxillary sinusitis in 32 children. Two-thirds of the patients had a bacterial etiology. The most common isolates were *H. influenzae* (9 isolates), *S. pneumoniae* (7), *Prevotella* spp. (8), and *Peptostreptococcus* spp. (6). Microbiological concordance between the ear and sinus was found in 22 of the culture-positive patients (69%).

Erkan et al. [102] studied 93 chronically inflamed maxillary sinuses in children. Anaerobic bacteria were isolated in 81 out of 87 culture-positive specimens (93%), were recovered alone in 61 cases (70%), and mixed with aerobic or facultative bacteria in 20 (23%). Aerobic or facultative bacteria were present alone in 6 cases (7%). A total of 261 isolates, 19 anaerobes, and 69 aerobes or facultatives, were isolated. The predominant anaerobic organisms were *Bacteroides* spp. and anaerobic cocci; the predominant aerobes or facultatives were *Streptococcus* spp. and *S. aureus*.

Studies in Adults

The presence of anaerobic bacteria in chronic sinusitis in adults is clinically significant [107, 108]. Finegold et al. [86], in a study of chronic maxillary sinusitis, found recurrence of signs and symptoms to be twice as frequent when cultures showed anaerobic bacterial counts above 10^3 colony-forming units per milliliter.

Anaerobes were identified in chronic sinusitis whenever techniques for their cultivation were employed. The predominant isolates were pigmented *Prevotella*, *Fusobacterium*, and *Peptostreptococcus* spp. The predominant aerobic bacteria were *S. aureus*, *M. catarrhalis*, and *Haemophilus* spp. Aerobic and anaerobic BLPB were isolated from over one-third of these patients [21, 83, 84, 89, 108, 109]. These BLPB were *S. aureus*, *Haemophilus*, *Prevotella*, *Porphyromonas*, and *Fusobacterium* spp.

A summary of 17 studies of chronic sinusitis performed since 1974, including 1,568 patients (133 were children) is shown in Table 18.2 [84–86, 102, 110–122]. Anaerobes accounted for 12–93% of the isolates were recovered. The variability in recovery may result from differences in the methodologies used for transportation and cultivation, patient population, geography, and use of previous antimicrobial therapy. Brook and Frazier [123] who correlated the microbiology with the history of sinus surgery in 108 patients with chronic maxillary sinusitis found a higher rate of isolation of *P. aeruginosa* and other Gram-negative bacilli in patients with previous sinus surgery. Anaerobes were, however, isolated significantly more frequently in patients who had not had prior surgery.

Brook evaluated the microbiology of 13 chronically infected frontal [124], 7 sphenoid [125], and 17 ethmoid sinuses (Table 18.1) [126]. Anaerobic bacteria were recovered in over two-thirds of the patients. The predominant anaerobes included *Prevotella*, *Peptostreptococcus*, and *Fusobacterium* spp. The main aerobic organisms were Gram-negative bacilli (*H. influenzae*, *K. pneumoniae*, *E. coli*, and *P. aeruginosa*).

Nadel et al. [21] also recovered Gram-negative rods more commonly in previous surgery patients or in those who had had sinus irrigation. *P. aeruginosa* was also more common in patients who received systemic steroids. Other studies have also noted this shift toward Gram-negative organisms in patients who have been extensively and repeatedly treated [80, 81, 127]. The bacterial flora includes *Pseudomonas* spp., *Enterobacter* spp., methicillin-resistant *S. aureus*, *H. influenzae*, and *M. catarrhalis*.

Bacteria in Chronic Maxillary Sinusitis Associated with Nasal Polyposis

Nasal polyps can impair paranasal sinus ventilation and drainage by blockage of the ostiomeatal complex. Several studies have shown that in the majority of cases of chronic sinusitis in which nasal polyps are present, bacterial cultures are negative. Even PCR techniques have failed to demonstrate bacterial infection in most cases [128]. Hamilos et al. [129], who obtained antral culture in 12 individuals with chronic maxillary sinusitis with nasal polyps, isolated organisms in only 3 patients. However, none of these studies employed methods that were adequate for the recovery of anaerobic bacteria.

We evaluated aspirates of 48 chronically inflamed maxillary sinuses from patients who had nasal polyposis that were cultured for aerobic and anaerobic bacteria [130]. Bacterial growth was present in 46 (96%) specimens. Aerobic or facultative bacteria were present in 6 (13%) specimens, anaerobic bacteria alone in 18 (39%), and mixed aerobic and anaerobic bacteria in 22 (48%). There were 110 bacterial isolates (2.4 per specimen). Thirty-nine of the isolates were aerobic or facultative organisms (0.85 per specimen). The predominant aerobic or facultative organisms were: *S. aureus*, microaerophilic streptococci, *H. influenzae*, and *M. catarrhalis*. Seventy-one anaerobes were isolated (1.5 per specimen). The predominant anaerobes were *Peptostreptococcus* spp., *Prevotella* spp., *P. asaccharolytica*, *Fusobacterium* spp., and *P. acnes*. These findings suggest that the microbiology of the maxillary sinus of patients with chronic sinusitis with polyposis is not different from those who develop chronic sinusitis without this condition, as the major isolates are polymicrobial aerobic–anaerobic flora.

Bacteria in Acute Exacerbation of Chronic Sinusitis

Acute exacerbation of chronic sinusitis (AECS) represents a sudden worsening of the baseline chronic sinusitis with either worsening or new symptoms. Typically, the acute (not chronic) symptoms resolve completely between occurrences [131]. We evaluated the microbiology of acute AECS [132] by performing repeated endoscopic sinus aspirations in 7 patients over a period of 125–242 days. Bacteria were recovered from all 22 aspirates and the number of isolates varied between two to four. A total of 54 isolates were isolated, 16 aerobic and facultatives and 38 anaerobic bacteria. The aerobic bacteria were *H. influenzae* (7), *S. pneumoniae* (3), *M. catarrhalis* (3), *S. aureus* (2), and *K. pneumoniae* (1). The anaerobic bacteria included pigmented *Prevotella* and *Porphyromonas* spp. (19), *Peptostreptococcus* spp. (9), *Fusobacterium* spp. (8), and *Propionibacterium acnes* (2). A change in the types of isolates was noted in all consecutive cultures obtained from the same patients, as different organisms emerged, and previously isolated bacteria were no longer recovered. An increase in antimicrobial resistance was noted in six instances. These findings illustrate the microbial dynamics of AECS where anaerobic and aerobic bacteria prevail, and highlight the importance of obtaining cultures from patients with this infection for guidance in the selection of proper antimicrobial therapy.

Brook et al. [133] compared the aerobic and anaerobic microbiology of maxillary AECS with the microbiology of chronic maxillary sinusitis. Included in the study were 32 with chronic sinusitis and 30 with AECS. A total of 81 isolates were recovered from the 32 cases (2.5/specimen) with chronic sinusitis, 33 aerobic, and 48 anaerobic. Aerobes alone were recovered in 8 specimens (25%), anaerobes only were isolated in 11 (34%), and mixed aerobes and anaerobes were recovered in 13 (41%). The predominant aerobic and facultatives were Enterobacteriaceae, and *S. aureus*. The predominant anaerobic bacteria were *Peptostreptococcus* spp., *Fusobacterium* spp., anaerobic Gram-negative bacilli, and *P. acnes*. A total of 89 isolates were recovered from the 30 cases (3.0/specimen) with AECS, 40 aerobic and facultatives, and 49 anaerobic. Aerobes were recovered in 8 instances (27%), anaerobes in only 11 (37%), and mixed aerobes and anaerobes were recovered in 11 (37%). The predominant aerobes were *S. pneumoniae*, Enterobacteriaceae, and *S. aureus*. The predominant anaerobes were *Peptostreptococcus* spp., *Fusobacterium* spp., anaerobic Gram-negative bacilli, and *P. acnes*). This study illustrates that the organisms isolated from patients with AECS were predominantly anaerobic and were similar to those generally recovered in chronic sinusitis. However, aerobic bacteria that are usually found in acute infections (e. g., *S. pneumoniae*, *H. influenzae*, and *M. catarrhalis*) can also emerge in some of the episodes of AECS.

Nosocomial Rhinosinusitis

Patients with nosocomial sinusitis are usually those who require extended periods of intensive care (postoperative patients, burn victims, patients with severe trauma) involving prolonged endotracheal or nasogastric intubation [134]. Nasotracheal intubation places the patient at a substantially higher risk of nosocomial sinusitis than orotracheal intubation [135]. Approximately 25% of patients requiring nasotracheal intubation for more than 5 days develop nosocomial sinusitis [136]. In contrast to community-acquired sinusitis, the usual pathogens are Gram-negative enterics (e. g., *Pseudomonas aeruginosa*, *Klebsiella pneumoniae*, *Enterobacter* spp., *Proteus mirabilis*, *Serratia marcescens*) and Gram-positive cocci (occasionally streptococci and staphylococci) (see elsewhere in this book) [135–139]. Whether these

organisms are actually pathogenic is unclear and they usually represent colonization of an environment with impaired mucociliary transport and foreign body presence in the nasal cavity.

Evaluation of the microbiology of nosocomial sinusitis in 9 children with neurologic impairment revealed anaerobic bacteria, always mixed with aerobic and facultative bacteria, in 6 cases of sinus aspirates and in aerobic bacteria in 3 (33%) [140]. There were 24 bacterial isolates, 12 aerobic or facultative and 12 anaerobic. The predominant aerobic isolates were *K. pneumoniae*, *E. coli*, and *S. aureus* (2 each) and *P. mirabilis*, *P. aeruginosa*, *H. influenzae*, *M. catarrhalis*, and *S. pneumoniae* (1 each). The predominant anaerobes were *Prevotella* spp. (5), *Peptostreptococcus* spp. (4), *F. nucleatum* (2), and *B. fragilis* (1). Organisms similar to those recovered from the sinuses were also isolated from tracheostomy site and gastrostomy wound aspirates in 5 out of 7 instances. This study demonstrates the uniqueness of the microbiologic features of sinusitis in neurologically impaired children, in which in addition to the organisms known to cause infection in normal children, facultative and anaerobic Gram-negative organisms that can colonize other body sites are predominant.

Atypical Organisms

Chlamydia pneumoniae has been isolated from patients with respiratory infection that also included clinical features of sinusitis [141] and serological evidence of its presence in patients, with sinusitis was found in only 2% of 103 patients [142]. However, since it was only isolated in one case of sinus aspirate [143], its exact role in sinusitis is uncertain.

Mycoplasma pneumoniae has been suspected to be a cause of acute sinusitis, but no attempts were made so far to recover it from infected sinuses. However, serological evidence of an increase in antibody titres to suggest a link between sinusitis and *M. pneumoniae* infection [144] in purulent bacterial, and nonpurulent nonbacterial sinusitis.

One study identified *M. pneumoniae*-specific DNA in a small group of participants with sinusitis and/or nasal polyposis [145]. However, a more recent study failed to confirm the presence of bacterial-specific DNA sequences for 16S ribosomal RNA [146].

The Role of Fungi in Sinusitis

Fungal "colonization" of the nose and paranasal sinuses is common in the normal and inflamed sinuses because of the ubiquitous nature of the organisms [147–151]. Under certain conditions, however, clinically significant growth of fungus balls (also called mycetomas) or saprophytic growth of fungus may occur. This can cause the formation and accumulation of fungal mycelia within the nose and paranasal sinuses without significant mucosal inflammation. In such cases extirpation of the offending fungal growth is generally sufficient. However, in other forms the inflammatory response to the fungi may result in clinically significant disease.

18

Fungal sinusitis can be either non-invasive or invasive. Invasive involvement is generally considered to be an acute and fulminant disease. In immunologically deficienct patients, however, the invasive fungal sinusitis is mild or not apparent, and can have a long and chronic course. Diagnosis is confirmed by histological evidence of nasal or sinus invasive fungal involvement lasting longer than 12 weeks.

Management necessitates correction immunologic deficiency, surgical debridement, and long-term systemic and topical antifungal treatment. The disease can progress and recur despite aggressive therapy, and occasionally be fatal.

Fungi can occasionally cause commonly acquired sinusitis [152]. They are especially common in patients with uncontrolled diabetes, HIV disease, and those on prolonged immunosuppression therapy (especially transplant recipients) and those on prolonged courses of antimicrobial therapy. *Aspergillus fumigatus* is the most common fungus associated with sinusitis [153, 154] and can cause disease in the normal as well as the immunocompromised host. The organism is a saprophyte of soil, dust, and decaying organic material. It has an invasive and non-invasive form. The organism's portal of entry is the respiratory tract. Sinusitis due to *Aspergillus* has been associated with the smoking of marijuana, as it contaminates the leaves. The organism can cause non-invasive, invasive, and disseminated forms. The non-invasive form presents as chronic rhinitis and nasal obstruction, and if untreated spreads to the blood stream, seeding numerous sites.

Other *Aspergillus* species have also caused sinusitis in normal hosts and include *Aspergillus flavus* and *Aspergillus niger* [153, 154].

Chronic invasive fungal sinusitis is divided into granulomatous and nongranulomatous subtypes based upon histopathology. Chronic invasive fungal rhinosinusitis has been associated with *Mucor*, *Alternaria*, *Curvularia*, *Bipolaris*, *Candida*, *Sporothrix schenckii*, and *Pseudallescheria boydii* [151]. Other fungi that can cause sinus infection include *Schizophyllum commune* [155], *Emericella nidulans* [156], *Pseudallescheria boydii* [157], *Paecilomyces* spp., *Cryptococcus neoformans*, *Penicillium melinii*, *Scedosporium (monosporium)*, *Apiospermum*, and *Blastomycocis dermatitidis* [158]. Saprophytic fungi causing infections are *Dreschslera* spp., *Alternaria* spp., *Curvularia lunata*, and *Exserohilum* spp. [159]. Mucormycosis is caused by fungi of the Mucurales order. The sinusitis induced occurs in mainly diabetic patients and the immunocompromised.

Allergic sinusitis has been associated with *Alternavia*, *Aspergillus*, *Bipolaris*, *Chrysosporium*, *Dreschlera*, and *Exserohilum* [160]. Allergic fungal sinusitis from *Aspergillus* spp. is similar to allergic bronchopulmonary aspergillosis, with secretions containing eosinophils, Charcot-Leyden crystals, and fungal hyphae [161]. Patients usually have evidence of atopy or asthma. The sinusitis is protracted, and generally involves multiple sinuses. *Myriodontium keratinophilum* also produces allergic-like fungal sinusitis [162]. The patients generally suffer from chronic sinusitis, nasal polyps, and proptosis due to orbital and ethmoid cell invasion. Allergic fungal sinusitis was also described to be associated with Dreschslera [163], Alternaria and Curvularia [164].

Chronic invasive fungal sinusitis is divided into granulomatous and nongranulomatous subtypes based upon histopathology. Chronic invasive fungal rhinosinusitis has been associated with *Mucor*, *Alternaria*, *Curvularia*, *Bipolaris*, *Candida*, *Sporothrix schenckii*, and *Pseudallescheria boydii* [153].

Nasopharyngeal Flora in Health and Disease

Purulent NPT is common in children, especially in the fall, winter, and early spring. This infection is often part of an inflammatory response of the upper respiratory tract that also involves the tonsils, adenoids, uvula, and soft palate.

The nasopharynx (NP) of healthy children is generally colonized by relatively nonpathogenic aerobic and anaerobic organisms [165], some of which possess the ability to interfere with the growth of potential pathogen [30, 166, 167]. Conversely, carriage of potential respiratory aerobic pathogen such as *Streptococcus pneumoniae*, *Haemophilus influenzae*, and *Moraxella catarrhalis*, as well as some anaerobic bacteria (*Peptostreptococcus*, *Fusobacterium*, and *Prevotella* spp.) increases during NPT [37, 168]. The development of purulent NPT in children is associated with the pre-existing colonization by potential pathogens and the absence of interfering organisms in the NP [34].

Microbiological Studies

Most cases of NPT are caused by viral infections. The commonest viral causes of NPT are adeno (types 1 to 7, 7a, 9, 14, and 15) and influenza and para-influenza viruses [169]. Although rhino and respiratory syncytial viral infections are common in children and both always have nasal manifestations (rhinitis), the occurrence of pharyngeal manifestations is uncommon [170].

Staphylococcus pneumoniae, *H. influenzae*, *S. aureus*, and GABHS were recovered in over 75% of patients with purulent nasal discharge and *Corynebacterium diphtheriae* and *Neisseria meningitidis* are rarely recovered [37, 170, 171, 172]. The role of anaerobic bacteria, however, was not investigated in these studies.

Todd et al. [173], who evaluated 144 children with purulent NPT, isolated *S. pneumoniae* in 46%, *H. influenzae* type-b in 21%, and GABHS in 8% of the patients. Nasal crusting was significantly associated with the growth of *S. pneumoniae* or *H. influenzae* type-b. Cisse et al. [174] recovered *S. pneumoniae* (in 60% of the children), streptococci group C (in 41%), *H. influenzae* (in 33%), GABHS (in 20%), and *M. catarrhalis* (in 13%) in the NP of children with NPT in Senegal.

Brook studied the aerobic and anaerobic microbiology of purulent NPT [37] by processing specimens from the inferior nasal meatus of 25 children with purulent NPT and from 25 controls (Table 18.3). A total of 98 isolates (3.9/patient), 45 aerobes (1.8/patient), and 53 anaerobes (2.1/patient) were isolated in patients with purulent NPT. Seventy-three isolates (2.9/patient) were found in the controls, 47 aerobes (1.9/patient) and 26 aerobes (1.0/patient). The organisms recovered in statistically significantly higher numbers in patients with NPT were *S. pneumoniae*, *Haemophilus* spp., *Peptostreptococcus* spp., *Fusobacterium* spp., and *Bacteroides* spp. The organism recovered in

Table 18.3 Bacteria isolated in the nasopharynx of 25 children with nasopharyngitis and 25 controls [37]

Isolates	Nasopharyngitis	Controls
AEROBIC AND FACULTATIVE		
Streptococcus pneumoniae	6[a]	1
Alpha-hemolytic streptococci	6	8
Gamma-hemolytic streptococci	5	6
Group A, beta-hemolytic streptococci	2	–
Group C, beta-hemolytic streptococci	1	–
Group F, beta-hemolytic streptococci	–	1
Staphylococcus aureus	3	8
Staphylococcus epidermidis	1	5
Moraxella catarrhalis	8	7
Haemophilus influenzae	5[b]	1
Haemophilus spp.	2	–
Diphtheroid sp.	4	7
Escherichia coli	1	2
Proteus sp.	1	1
Subtotal	45	47
ANAEROBIC		
Peptostreptococcus spp.	17[b]	4
Microaerophilic streptococci	4	3
Propionibacterium acnes	3	12[c]
Veillonella parvula	2	3
Fusobacterium spp.	3[c]	–
Fusobacterium nucleatum	6[c]	1
Bacteroides spp.	4[c]	1
Pigmented Prevotella and Porphyromonas	11[c]	2
Prevotella oralis	3	–
Subtotal	53	26
Total number of organisms	98	73

Statistically higher number of isolates than other groups: [a]$p < 0.05$, [b]$p < 0.001$, [c]$p < 0.01$

18

significantly higher numbers in controls was *Propionibacterium acnes*.

Current data suggest that the presence of NPT is associated with an increase in the rate of isolation of an aerobic–anaerobic polymicrobial flora. However, the pathogenic role of these organisms in the inflammatory process is unknown.

Microbial Dynamics of Nasopharyngitis

The nasal discharge in children with NPT is generally initially clear and watery; however, in cases that progress, it becomes viscous, opaque, and discolored (white, yellow or green) in a matter of days. Usually the purulent discharge resolves or becomes watery again before disappearing without specific therapy [175].

Cherian et al. [176] evaluated 56 rural Indian children with persistent NPT, and 91 age-matched controls. Chronic ear discharge was noted in 6 of cases (12%), but in none of the controls ($p = 0.007$). *S. pneumoniae* was isolated from NP in 42 out of 49 cases (86%) and 44 out of 80 controls (55%; $p < 0.001$), and *H. influenzae* from 7 cases and 5 controls. *S. pneumoniae* was also isolated in all children with chronic ear discharge and *H. influenzae* was recovered from one child.

A recent study characterizes the aerobic and anaerobic bacterial flora of nasal discharge obtained from children at different stages of uncomplicated NPT [34]. A correlation was made between the bacterial flora and the eventual course of the illness. It also investigated the relationship between colonization of the nasopharynx (NP) with organisms with interfering capability and the subsequent development of purulent NPT.

Serial semi-quantitative NP and quantitative nasal discharge (ND) cultures were taken every 3–5 days from 20 children who eventually developed purulent discharge (Group 1), and a single culture was obtained from a group of 20 who had only clear discharge (Group 2). Aerobic and anaerobic bacteria were isolated from all NP cultures. Bacterial growth was present in 8 patients with ND in Group 2 (40%). Only 7 of the patients with clear ND in Group 1 (35%) showed bacterial growth; the number increased to 14 (70%) at the mucoid stage, and 20 (100%) at the purulent stage. It declined to 6 (30%) at the final clear stage. The number of species and total number of organisms increased in the ND of group 1. Group 1 patients had a higher recovery rate of *S. pneumoniae* and *H. influenzae* in their NP cultures than those in Group 2 ($p < 0.05$). During the purulent stage, *Peptostreptococcus* spp. was isolated in 15 (75%), *Prevotella* spp. in 9 (45%), *Fusobacterium* spp. in 8 (40%), *H. influenzae* in 8 (40%), *S. pneumoniae* in 6 (30%), and beta-hemolytic streptococci in 5 (25%) of ND of Group 1. This was higher than their recovery in the clear stages of both groups and the mucoid stage of Group 1. A total of 8 organisms with interfering capability in the growth of potential pathogens were isolated from the NP of Group 1, compared with 35 from Group 2 ($p < 0.001$).

This study illustrated that the development of purulent NPT is associated with the pre-existing presence in the NP of potential pathogens and the absence of interfering organisms. The potential oropharyngeal pathogens *S. pneumoniae*, *H. influenzae*, and beta-hemolytic streptococci were recovered in the purulent nasal discharge of over three-quarters of the patients. In contrast, these organisms were rarely recovered in patients who did not develop purulent NPT. Children who are not colonized with potential respiratory pathogens, but harbor interfering bacteria, or nonpathogens such as *P. acnes* and *Corynebacterium* spp. may not be prone to developing purulent nasal discharge.

Since no viral cultures were taken, the etiology of NPT in this study was not completely determined. However, the recovery of several aerobic and anaerobic bacteria not generally found as part of the nasal flora, in patients with purulent NPT, may signify their potential pathogenic role. The concomitant presence of these organisms in the inflamed pharynx supports the concept of generalized inflammation that also involves the nasal spaces.

Tips to Avoid Complications

- Preservation of the normal flora, especially that with "interfering" capability, by avoiding unnecessary antimicrobial therapy is of great importance.
- A significant increase occurred in the rate of recovery of methicillin-resistant *Staphylococcus aureus* (MRSA) in patients with acute and chronic maxillary sinusitis.
- *Staphylococcus epidermidis* (coagulase-negative staphylococci) is a common colonizer of the nasal cavity and is therefore a common contaminate of endoscopically obtained cultures.

Take-Home Pearls

- The origin of organisms that are introduced into the sinuses and may eventually cause sinusitis is the nasal cavity.
- The pattern of many upper respiratory infections including sinusitis evolves through several phases: first viral, then aerobic bacteria, and lastly anaerobic bacteria.
- The predominant aerobic bacteria are *S. pneumoniae*, *M. catarrhalis*, and *H. influenzae*.
- Anaerobic bacteria (*Prevotella*, *Porphyromonas*, *Fusobacteria*, and *Peptostreptococcus* spp. predominate in chronic sinusitis.

References

1. Faden H, Stanievich J, Brodsky L, et al. Changes in the nasopharyngeal flora during otitis media of childhood. *Pediatr. Infect. Dis.* 1990;9: 623–6

2. Del Beccaro MA, Mendelman PM, Inglis AF, et al. Bacteriology of acute otitis media: a new perspective. *J. Pediatr.* 1992;120: 856–62

3. Socransky SS, Manganiello SD. The oral microflora of man from birth to senility, *J. Periodontol.* 1971;42:485–96

4. Gibbons, RJ, Socransky SS, Dearaujo WC, et al. Studies of the predominant cultivable microbiota of dental plaque. *Arch. Oral. Biol.* 1964;9:365–70

5. Valenti WM, Trudell RG, Bentley DW. Factors predisposing to oropharyngeal colonization with gram-negative bacilli in the aged. *N Engl J Med* 1978;298:1108–1110

6. Baird-Parker AC. The classification of fusobacteria from the human mouth. *J. Gen. Microbiol.* 1960;22:458–69

7. Smibert RM. Spirochaetales: a review. *CRC Crit. Rev. Microbiol.* 1973;2:491

8. Gibbons RJ. Aspects of the pathogenicity and ecology of the indigenous oral flora of man. In *Anaerobic bacteria, role in disease*, A. Balows et al., editors. Springfield, Ill, 1974, Charles C Thomas

9. Rasmussen EG, Gibbons RJ, Socransky SS. A taxonomic study of fifty Gram-positive anaerobic diphtheroides isolated from the oral cavity of man. *Arch. Oral Biol.* 1966; 11:573–9

10. Gibbons RJ, Socransky SS, Sawyer S, et al. The microbiota of the gingival crevice of man: II. The predominant cultivable organisms. *Arch. Oral Biol.* 1963;8:281–9

11. Brook I. Beta-lactamase producing bacteria in head and neck infection. *Laryngoscope* 1988;98:428–31

12. Brook I. The role of beta-lactamase-producing bacteria in the persistence of streptococcal tonsillar infection. *Rev Infect Dis* 1984;6:601–7

13. Brook I, Gober AE. Emergence of beta-lactamase-producing aerobic and anaerobic bacteria in the oropharynx of children following penicillin chemotherapy. *Clin Pediatr.* 1984;23:338–41

14. Tuner K, Nord CE. Emergence of beta-lactamase-producing microorganisms in the tonsils during penicillin treatment. *Eur J Clin Microbiol.* 1986;5: 399–404

15. American Academy of Pediatrics. Subcommittee on Management of Sinusitis and Committee on Quality Improvement. Clinical practice guideline: management of sinusitis. *Pediatrics* 2001;108:798–808

16. Talbot GH, Kennedy DW, Scheld WM, Granito K. Rigid nasal endoscopy versus sinus puncture and aspiration for microbiologic documentation of acute bacterial maxillary sinusitis. *Clin Infect Dis* 2001;33:1668–75

17. Brook I. Discrepancies in the recovery of bacteria from multiple sinuses in acute and chronic sinusitis. *J Med Microbiol.* 2004;53:879–85

18. Gordts F, Abu Nasser I, Clement PA, Pierad D, Kaufman L. Bacteriology of the middle meatus in children. *Int J Pediatr Otorhinolaryngol* 1999;48:163–7

19. Gordts F, Harlewyck S, Pierard D, Kaufman L, Clement PA. Microbiology of the middle meatus: a comparison between normal adults and children. *J Larynol Otol* 2000;114:184–8

20. Klossek JM, Dubreuil L, Richet H, Richet B, Sedallian A, Beutter P. Bacteriology of the adult middle meatus. *J Laryngol Otol* 1996;110:847–9

21. Nadel DM, Lanza DC, Kennedy DW. Endoscopically guided cultures in chronic sinusitis. *Am J Rhinol* 1998;12:233–41

22. Gold SM, Tami TA. Role of middle meatus aspiration culture in the diagnosis of chronic sinusitis. *Laryngoscope* 1997;107:1586–9

23. Vogen JC, Bolger WE, Keyes AS, Endoscopically Guided Cultures: A Direct Comparison With Maxillary Sinus Aspirate Cultures, *Oto-HNS* 2000;122:370–3

24. Winther B, Vicery CL, Gross CW, Hendley O: Microbiology of the Maxillary Sinus in Adults with Chronic Sinus Disease. *Am J Rhinol* 1996;10:347–50

25. Kountakis SE, Skoulas IG. Middle meatal vs antral lavage cultures in intensive care unit patients. *Otolaryngol Head Neck Surg* 2002;126:377–81

26. Brook I, Frazier EH, Foote PA. Microbiology of chronic maxillary sinusitis: comparison between specimens obtained by sinus endoscopy and by surgical drainage. *J Med Microbiol.* 1997;46:430–2

27. Mackowiak PA. The normal flora. *N Engl J Med.* 1983;307:83–93

28. Brook I. Bacterial interference. *Crit Rev Microbiol.* 1999;25:155–72

29. Sprunt K, Redman W. Evidence suggesting importance of role of interbacterial inhibition in maintaining balance of normal flora. *Ann Intern Med.* 1968;68:579–90

30. Bernstein JM, Sagahtaheri-Altaie S, Dryjd DM, Vactawski-Wende J. Bacterial interference in nasopharyngeal bacterial flora of otitis-prone and non-otitis-prone children. *Acta Otorhinolaryngol Belg.* 1994;48:1–9

31. Murray PR, Rosenblatt JE. Bacterial interference by oropharyngeal and clinical isolates of anaerobic bacteria. *J Infect Dis.* 1976;134:281–5

32. Brook I, Gober A. Bacterial interference in the nasopharynx of otitis media prone and not otitis media prone children. *Arch Otolaryngol Head Neck Surg.* 2000;126:1011–3

33. Brook I, Gober AE. Bacterial interference in the nasopharynx and nasal cavity of sinusitis prone and non-sinusitis prone children. *Acta Otolaryngol.* 1999;119:832–6

34. Brook I, Gober AE. Dynamics of nasopharyngitis in children. *Otolaryngol Head Neck Surg* 2000;122:696–700

35. Foote PA Jr, Brook I. Penicillin and clindamycin therapy in recurrent tonsillitis. Effect of microbial flora. *Arch Otolaryngol. Head Neck Surg.* 1989;15:856–9

36. Brook I, Foote PA. Bacterial interference and beta-lactamase-producing bacteria in the adenoids after antimicrobial therapy. *Clin Inf Dis.* 1997;25:493

37. Brook I. Aerobic and anaerobic bacteriology of purulent nasopharyngitis in children. *J Clin Microbiol.* 1988;26:592–4

38. Savolainen S, Ylikoski J, Jousimies-Somer H. The bacterial flora of the nasal cavity in healthy young men. *Rhinology.* 1986;24:249–55

39. Winther B, Brofeldt S, Gronborg H, Mygind N, Pedersen M, Vejlsgaard R. Study of bacteria in the nasal cavity and nasopharynx during naturally acquired common colds. *Acta Otolaryngol.* 1984;98:315–20

40. Jousimies-Somer HR, Savolainen S. Ylikoski JS. Comparison of the nasal bacterial floras in two groups of healthy subjects and in patients with acute maxillary sinusitis. *J Clin Microbiol.* 1989;27:2736–43

41. Gwaltney JM Jr, Sydnor A, Sande MA. Etiology and antimicrobial treatment of acute sinusitis. *Ann Otol Rhinol Laryngol.* 1981;90(Suppl. 84):68–71

18

42. Lystad A, Berdal P, Lund-Iversen L. The bacterial flora of sinusitis with an in vitro study of the bacterial resistance to antibiotics. *Acta Otolaryngol* Suppl. 1964;188:390–400

43. Nylen O, Jeppsson P-H, Branefors-Helander P. Acute sinusitis. A clinical, bacteriological and serological study with special reference to Haemophilus influenzae. *Scand J Infect Dis.* 1972;4:43–8

44. Björkwall T. Bacteriological examination in maxillary sinusitis: Bacterial flora of the nasal meatus. *Acta Otolaryngol* Suppl. 1950;83:1–32

45. Catlin FI, Cluff LE, Reynolds RC. The bacteriology of acute and chronic sinusitis. *South Med J.* 1965;58:1497–502

46. Savolainen S, Ylikoski J, Jousimies-Somer H. Predictive value of nasal bacterial culture for etiological agents in acute maxillary sinusitis. *Rhinology.* 1987;25:49–55

47. Brook I. Aerobic and anaerobic bacterial flora of normal maxillary sinuses. *Laryngoscopy.* 1981;91:372–6

48. Su WY, Liu CR, Hung SY, Tsai WF. Bacteriological studies in chronic maxillary sinusitis. *Laryngoscope.* 1983;93:931–4

49. Cook HE, Haber J. Bacteriology of the maxillary sinus. *J Oral Maxillofac Surg.* 1987;45:1011–14

50. Sobin J, Engquist S, Nord CE. Bacteriology of the maxillary sinus in healthy volunteers. *Scand J Infect Dis.* 1992;24:633–5

51. Jiang RS, Liang KL, Jang JW, Hsu CY. Bacteriology of endoscopically normal maxillary sinuses. *J Laryngol Otol.* 1999;113:825–8

52. Brook I, Frazier EH, Foote PA. Microbiology of the transition from acute to chronic maxillary sinusitis. *J Med Microbiol* 1996;45:372–5

53. Schubert MS. A superantigen hypothesis for the pathogenesis of chronic hypertrophic rhinosinusitis, allergic fungal sinusitis, and related disorders. *Ann Allergy Asthma Immunol* 2001;87:181–8

54. Bachert C, Gevaert P, Holtappels G, Johansson SG, van Cauwenberge P. Total and specific IgE in nasal polyps is related to local eosinophilic inflammation. J Allergy Clin Immunol 2001;107:607–14

55. Conley DB, Tripathi A, Ditto AM, Grammer LC, Kern RC: Chronic sinusitis with nasal polyps: staphylococcal exotoxin immunoglobulin E and cellular inflammation. *Am J Rhinol.* 2004;18:273–8

56. Bernstein JM, Ballow M, Schlievert PM, Rich G, Allen C, Dryja D. A superantigen hypothesis for the pathogenesis of chronic hyperplastic sinusitis with massive nasal polyposis. *Am J Rhinol* 2003;17: 321–6

57. Subausie MC, Jacoby DB, Richards SM, Proud D. Infection of a human respiratory epithelial cell line with rhinovirus: Induction of cytokine release and modulation of susceptibility to infection by cytokine exposure. *J Clin Invest.* 1995;96:549–57

58. Evans FO Jr, Sydnor JB, Moore WEC, et al. Sinusitis of the maxillary antrum. *N Engl J Med.* 1975;293:735–9

59. Hamory BH, Sande MA, Sydnor A Jr, et al. Etiology and antimicrobial therapy of acute maxillary sinusitis. *J Infect Dis.* 1979;139:197–202

60. Osur SL. Viral respiratory infections in association with asthma and sinusitis: a review. *Ann Allergy Asthma Immunol.* 2002;89:553–60

61. Elias JA, Zheng T, Einarsson O, et al. Epithelial interleukin-11: Regulation by cytokines, respiratory syncytial virus, and retinoic acid. *J Biol Chem.* 1994;269:22261–8

62. Winther B, Gwaltney JM Jr, Mygind N, Turner RB, Hendley JO. Sites of rhinovirus recovery after point inoculation of the upper airway. *JAMA.* 1986;256;1763–7

63. Greve JM, Davis G, Meyer AM, et al. The major human rhinovirus receptor is ICAM-1. *Cell.* 1989;56:839–47

64. Gwaltney JM Jr. Rhinovirus infection of the normal human airway. *Am J Respir Crit Care Med.* 1995;152:S36–9

65. Gwaltney JM Jr, Phillips CD, Miller RD, Riker DK. Computed tomographic study of the common cold. *N Engl J Med.* 1994;330:25–30

66. Puhakka T, Mäkelä MJ, Alanen A, Kallio T, Korsoff L, Arstila P, Leinonen M, Pulkkinen M, Suonpää, Mertsola J, Ruuskanen O. Sinusitis in the common cold. *J Allergy Clin Immunol* 1998;102:403–8

67. Kristo A, Uhari M, Luotonen J, Koivunen P, Ilkko E, Tapiainen T, Alho O-P. Paranasal sinus findings in children during respiratory infection evaluated with magnetic resonance imaging. *Pediatrics* 2003;111:e586–e589

68. Sakakura Y, Sasaki Y, Hornick RB, et al. Mucociliary function during experimentally induced rhinovirus infection in man. *Ann Otol Rhinol Laryngol.* 1973;82:203–11

69. Gwaltney JM Jr. Acute community-acquired sinusitis. *Clin Infect Dis.* 1996;23:1209–25

70. Gwaltney JM Jr, Scheld WM, Sande MA, Sydnor A. The microbial etiology and antimicrobial therapy of adults with acute community-acquired sinusitis: a fifteen-year experience at the University of Virginia and review of other selected studies. *J Allergy Clin Immunol.* 1992;90:457–62

71. Wald ER, Milmore GJ, Bowen AD, Ledema-Medina J, Salamon N, Bluestone CD. Acute maxillary sinusitis in children. *N Engl J Med.* 1981;304:749–54

72. Wald ER, Guerra N, Byers C. Upper respiratory tract infections in young children: Duration of and frequency of complications. *Pediatrics.* 1991;87:129–33

73. Lew D, Southwick FS, Montgomery WW, Weber AL, Baker AS. Sphenoid sinusitis. A review of 30 cases. *N Engl J Med.* 1983;309:1149–54

74. Brook I, Frazier EH, Gher ME Jr. Microbiology of periapical abscesses and associated maxillary sinusitis. *J Periodontal.* 1996;67:608–10

75. Brook I, Friedman EM. Intracranial complications of sinusitis in children. A sequela of periapical abscess. *Ann Otol Rhinol Laryngol.* 1982;91:41–3

76. Shapiro ED, Milmoe GJ, Wald ER, et al. Bacteriology of the maxillary sinuses in patients with cystic fibrosis. *J Infect Dis.* 1982;146:589–93

77. Wald ER, Microbiology of acute and chronic sinusitis in children and adults. *Am J Med Sci* 1998;**316**:13–20

78. Biel MA, Brown CA, Levinson RM et al., Evaluation of the microbiology of chronic maxillary sinusitis. *Ann Otol Laryngol Rhinol* 1998;**107**:942–5

79. Jiang RS, Hsu CY, Jang JW. Bacteriology of the maxillary and ethmoid sinuses in chronic sinusitis. *J Laryngol Otol.* 1998;112:845–8

80. Hsu J, Lanza DC, Kennedy DW. Antimicrobial resistance in bacterial chronic sinusitis. *Am J Rhinol.* 1998;12:243–8

81. Bolger WE. Gram negative sinusitis: emerging clinical entity. *Am J Rhinol* **8** (1994), 279–83

82. Kaliner M, Osguthorpe J, Fireman P, et al. Sinusitis: Bench to Bedside. *Otolaryngol Head Neck Surg.* 1997;116(suppl):S1–S20

83. Nord CE. The role of anaerobic bacteria in recurrent episodes of sinusitis and tonsillitis. *Clin Infect Dis* 1995;20:1512–24

84. Brook I, Thompson D, Frazier E. Microbiology and management of chronic maxillary sinusitis. *Arch Otolaryngol Head Neck Surg.* 1994;120:1317–20

85. Brook I. Bacteriologic features of chronic sinusitis in children. *JAMA.* 1981;246:967–9

86. Finegold SM, Flynn MJ, Rose FV, Jousimies-Somer H, Jakielaszek C, McTeague M, Wexler HM, Berkowitz E, Wynne B. Bacteriologic findings associated with chronic bacterial maxillary sinusitis in adults. *Clin Infect Dis.* 2002;35:428–33

87. Carenfelt C, Lundberg C. Purulent and non-purulent maxillary sinus secretions with respect to Po2, Pco2 and pH. *Acta Otolaryngol.* 1977;84:138–44

88. Brook I. Role of encapsulated anaerobic bacteria in synergistic infections. *Crit Rev Microbiol.* 1987;14:171–93

89. Brook I. Bacteriology of chronic maxillary sinusitis in adults. *Ann Otol Rhinol Laryngol* 1989;98:426–8

90. Brook I. Brain abscess in children: microbiology and management. *Child Neurol.* 1995;10:283–8

91. Westrin KM, Stierna P, Carlsoo B, Hellstrom S. Mucosal fine structure in experimental sinusitis. *Ann Otol Rhinol Laryngol.* 1993;102(8 Pt 1):639–45

92. Jyonouchi H, Sun S, Kennedy CA, Roche AK, Kajander KC, Miller JR, Germaine GR, Rimell FL. Localized sinus inflammation in a rabbit sinusitis model induced by Bacteroides fragilis is accompanied by rigorous immune responses. *Otolaryngol Head Neck Surg.* 1999;120:869–75

93. Brook I, Yocum P. Immune response to *Fusobacterium nucleatum* and *Prevotella intermedia* in patients with chronic maxillary sinusitis. *Ann Otol Rhinol Laryngol* 1999;108:293–5

94. Brook I, Yocum P, Frazier EH. Bacteriology and beta-lactamase activity in acute and chronic maxillary sinusitis. *Arch Otolaryngol Head Neck Surg.* 1996;122:418–22

95. Brook I, Yocum P, Shah K. Aerobic and anaerobic bacteriology of concurrent chronic otitis media with effusion and chronic sinusitis in children. *Arch Otolaryngol Head Neck Surg* 2000;126:174–6

96. Orobello PW, Jr, Park RI, Belcher L et al. Microbiology of chronic sinusitis in children. *Arch Otolaryngol Head Neck Surg* 1991;117:980–3

97. Tinkleman DG, Silk HJ. Clinical and bacteriologic features of chronic sinusitis in children. *Am J Dis Child* 1989;143:938–41

98. Muntz HR, Lusk RP. Bacteriology of the ethmoid bullae in children with chronic sinusitis. *Arch Otolaryngol Head Neck Surg* 1991;117:179–81

99. Otten FWA, Grote JJ. Treatment of chronic maxillary sinusitis in children. *Int J Pediatr Otorhinolaryngol* 1988;15:269–78

100. Otten FWA. Conservative treatment of chronic maxillary sinusitis in children. Long term follow-up. *Acta Otorhinolaryngol Belg* 1997;51:173–5

101. Don D, Yellon RF, Casselbrant M, Bluestone CD. Efficacy of stepwise protocol that includes intravenous antibiotic treatment for the management of chronic sinusitis in children and adolescents. *Otolaryngol Head Neck Surg* 2001;127:1093–8

102. Erkan M, Ozcan M, Arslan S, Soysal V, Bozdemir K, Haghighi N. Bacteriology of antrum in children with chronic maxillary sinusitis. *Scand J Infect Dis.* 1996;28:283–5

103. Slack CL, Dahn KA, Abzug MJ, Chan KH. Antibiotic-resistant bacteria in pediatric chronic sinusitis. *Pediatr Infect Dis J.* 2001;20:247–50

104. Goldenhersh MJ, Rachelefsky GS, Dudley J et al. The microbiology of chronic sinus disease in children with respiratory allergy. *J Allergy Clin Immunol* 1998;**85**:1030–9

105. Wald ER, Byers C, Guerra N *et al.* Subacute sinusitis in children. *J Pediatr* 1989;**115**:28–32

106. Brook I, Yocum P. Antimicrobial management of chronic sinusitis in children. *J Laryngol Otol.* 1995;109:1159–62

107. Finegold SM. Anaerobic bacteria in human disease. Orlando, FL: Academic Press Inc; 1977

108. Brook I. Pediatric Anaerobic Infections. 3rd edition. New York: Marcel Dekker Inc.; 2002

109. Mustafa E, Tahsin A, Mustafa Ö, Nedret K. Bacteriology of antrum in adults with chronic maxillary sinusitis. *Laryngoscope.* 1994;104:321–4

110. Frederick J, Braude AI. Anaerobic infections of the paranasal sinuses. *N Engl J Med.* 1974;290:135–7

111. Van Cauwenberge P, Verschraegen G, Van Renterghem L. Bacteriological findings in sinusitis (1963–1975). *Scand J Infect Dis Suppl.* 1976;(9):72–7

112. Karma P, Jokipii L, Sipila P, Luotonen J, Jokipii AM. Bacteria in chronic maxillary sinusitis. *Arch Otolaryngol.* 1979;105:386–90

113. Berg O, Carenfelt C, Kronvall G. Bacteriology of maxillary sinusitis in relation to character of inflammation and prior treatment. *Scand J Infect Dis.* 1988;20(5):511–6

114. Fiscella RG, Chow JM. Cefixime for the treatment of maxillary sinusitis. *Am J Rhinol.* 1991;5:193–7

115. Sedallian A, Bru JP, Gaillat J. Bacteriologic finding of chronic sinusitis. (Abstract no. P2.71). The 17th International Congress of the Management of Infection. Berlin, 1992

116. Simoncelli C, Ricci G, Molini E, von Garrel C, Capolunghi B, Giommetti S. Bacteriology of chronic maxillary sinusitis. *HNO.* 1992;40:16–8

117. Tabaqchali S. Anaerobic infections in the head and neck region. *Scand J Infect Dis Suppl.* 1988;57:24–34

118. Hartog B, Degener JE, Van Benthem PP, Hordijk GJ. Microbiology of chronic maxillary sinusitis in adults: isolated aerobic and anaerobic bacteria and their susceptibility to twenty antibiotics. *Acta Otolaryngol.* 1995;115:672–7

119. Ito K, Ito Y, Mizuta K, Ogawa H, Suzuki T, Miyata H, Kato N, Watanabe K, Ueno K. Bacteriology of chronic otitis media, chronic sinusitis, and paranasal mucopyocele in Japan. *Clin Infect Dis.* 1995;20 Suppl 2:S214–9

120. Erkan M, Aslan T, Ozcan M, Koc N. Bacteriology of antrum in adults with chronic maxillary sinusitis. *Laryngoscope.* 1994;104(3 Pt 1):321–4

121. Edelstein DR, Avner SE, Chow JM et al. Once-a-day therapy for sinusitis: a comparison study of cefixime and amoxicillin. *Laryngoscope.* 1993;103:33–41

122. Klossek JM, Dubreuil L, Richet H, Richet B, Beutter P. Bacteriology of chronic purulent secretions in chronic rhinosinusitis. *J Laryngol Otol.* 1998;112:1162–6

123. Brook I, Frazier EH. Correlation between microbiology and previous sinus surgery in patients with chronic maxillary sinusitis. *Ann Otol Rhinol Laryngol* 2001;110:148–51

124. Brook I. Bacteriology of acute and chronic frontal sinusitis. *Arch Otolaryngol Head Neck Surg* 2002;128:583–5

125. Brook I. Bacteriology of acute and chronic sphenoid sinusitis. *Ann Otol Rhinol Laryngol* 2002;111:1002–4

126. Brook I. Bacteriology of acute and chronic ethmoid sinusitis. *J Clin Microbiol.* 2005;43:3479–80

127. Bhattacharyya N, Kepnes LJ. The microbiology of recurrent rhinosinusitis after endoscopic sinus surgery. *Arch Otolaryngol Head Neck Surg* 1999;**125**:1117–20

128. Bucholtz GA, Salzman SA, Bersalona FB, Boyle TR, Ejercito VS, Penno L, Peterson DW, Stone GE, Urquhart A, Shukla SK, Burmester JK. PCR analysis of nasal polyps, chronic sinusitis, and hypertrophied turbinates for DNA encoding bacterial 16S rRNA. *Am J Rhinol.* 2002;16:169–73

129. Hamilos DL, Leung DYM, Wood R, Meyers A, Stephens JK, Barkans J, Bean DK, Kay AB, Hamid Q. Association of tissue eosinophilia and cytokine mRNA expression of granulocyte-macrophage colony-stimulating factor and interleukin-3. *J All Clin Immunol* 1993;91:39–48

130. Brook I, Frazier EH, Bacteriology of chronic maxillary sinusitis associated with nasal polyposis. *J Med Microbiol.* 2005;54:595–7

131. Clement PA, Bluestone CD, Gordts F, Lusk RP, Otten FW, Goossens H, Scadding GK, Takahashi H, van Buchem FL, Van Cauwenberge P, Wald ER. Management of rhinosinusitis in children: Consensus meeting, Brussels, Belgium, September 13, 1996. *Arch Otolaryngol Head Neck Surg.* 1998;124:31–4

132. Brook I, Foote PA, Frazier EH. Microbiology of Acute Exacerbation of Chronic Sinusitis. *Laryngoscope.* 2004;114:129–31

133. Brook I. Bacteriology of Chronic Sinusitis and Acute Exacerbation of Chronic Sinusitis. *Arch Otolaryngol Head Neck Surg.* 2006;132:1099–101

134. Bach A, Boehrer H, Schmidt H, Geiss HK. Nosocomial sinusitis in ventilated patients: nasotracheal versus orotracheal intubation. *Anaesthesia* 1992;47:335–9

135. Caplan ES, Hoyt NJ. Nosocomial sinusitis. *JAMA* 1982;247:639–41

136. Kronberg FG, Goodwin WJ. Sinusitis in intensive care unit patients. *Laryngoscope* 1985;95:936–8

137. O'Reilly MJ, Reddick EJ, Black W, et al. Sepsis from sinusitis in nasotracheally intubated patients: a diagnostic dilemma. *Am J Surg* 1984;147:601–4

138. Mevio E, Benazzo M, Quaglieri S, Mencherini S. Sinus infection in intensive care patients. *Rhinology* 1996;34:232–6

139. Arens JF, LeJeune FE Jr., Webre DR. Maxillary sinusitis, a complication of nasotracheal intubation. *Anesthesiology* 1974;40:415–6

140. Brook I, Shah K. Sinusitis in neurologically impaired children. *Otolaryngol Head Neck Surg.* 1998;119:357–60

141. Hahn DL, Dodge RW, Golubjatnikov R. Association of *Chlamydia pneumoniae* (strain TWAR) infection with wheezing, asthmatic bronchitis, and adult-onset asthma. *JAMA.* 1991;266:225–30

142. Thom DH, Grayston JT, Campbell LA, Kuo CC, Diwan VK, Wang SP. Respiratory infection with *Chlamydia pneumoniae* in middle-aged and older adult outpatients. *Eur J Clin Microbiol Infect Dis.* 1994;13:785–92

143. Hashigucci K, Ogawa H, Suzuki T, Kazuyama Y. Isolation of *Chlamydia pneumoniae* from the maxillary sinus of a patient with purulent sinusitis. *Clin Infect Dis.* 1992;15:570–1

144. Savolainen S, Jousimies-Somer H, Kleemola M, Ylikoski J. Serological evidence of viral or *Mycoplasma pneumoniae* infection in acute maxillary sinusitis. *Eur J Clin Microbiol Infect Dis.* 1989;8:131–5

145. Gurr PA, Chakraverty A, Callanan V et al. The detection of *M. pneumoniae* in nasal polyps. *Clin Otolaryngol* 1996;**21**:269–73

146. Bucholtz GA, Salzman SA, Bersalona FB et al. PCR analysis of nasal polyps, chronic sinusitis, and hypertrophied turbinates for DNA encoding bacterial 16S rRNA. *Am J Rhinol* 2002;**16**:169–73

147. Vennewald I, Henker M, Klemm E et al. Fungal colonization of the paranasal sinuses. *Mycosis* 42 Suppl 2:33–6

148. Ponikau JU, Sherris DA, Kern EB et al. The diagnosis and incidence of allergic fungal sinusitis. *Mayo Clin Proc* 1999;**74**:877–84

149. Catten MD, Murr AH, Goldstein JA et al. Detection of fungi in the nasal mucosal using polymerase chain reaction. *Laryngoscope* **111**:399–03

150. Stringer SP, Ryan MW. Chronic invasive fungal rhinosinusitis. *Otolaryngol Clin North Am* 2000;**33**:375–87

151. Ferguson BJ. Definitions of fungal rhinosinusitis. *Otolaryngol Clin North Am* 33:227–35

152. Gwaltney JM Jr. Microbiology of sinusitis. In: Druce HM, ed. Sinusitis: Pathophysiology and treatment. New York: Marcel Dekker. 1994:41–56

153. Morgan MA, Wilson WR, Neil III HB, Roberts GD. Fungal sinusitis in healthy and immunocompromised individuals. *Am J Clin Pathol.* 1984;82:597–601

154. Jahrsdoerfer RA, Ejercito VS, Johns MME, et al. Aspergillosis of the nose and paranasal sinuses. *Am J Otolaryngol.* 1979;1:6–14

155. Kern ME, Uecker FA. Maxillary sinus infection caused by the Homobasidiomycetous fungus Schizophyllum commune. *J Clin Microbiol.* 1986;23:1001–5

156. Mitchell RG, Chaplin AJ, MacKenzie DWR. *Emericella nidulans* in a maxillary sinus fungal mass. *J Med Vet Mycol.* 1987;25:339–41

157. Winn RE, Ramsey PD, McDonald JC, Dunlop KJ. Maxillary sinusitis from Pseudoalles-cheria boydii. Efficacy of surgical therapy. *Arch Otolaryngol.* 1983;109:123–5

158. Adam RD, Paquin ML, Petersen EA, et al. Phaeohyphomycosis caused by the fungal general Bipolaris and Exserohilum. *Medicine.* 1986;65:203–17

159. Zieske LA, Kople RD, Hamill R. Dermataceous fungal sinusitis. *Otolaryngol Head Neck Surg.* 1991;105:567–77

160. Goldstein MF, Dvorin DJ, Dunsky EH, Lesser RW, Heuman PJ, Loose JH. Allergic rhizomucor sinusitis. *J Allergy Immun.* 1992;90:394–404

161. Katzenstein A, Sale SR, Greenberger PA. Pathologic findings in allergic Aspergillus sinusitis. *Am J Surg Pathol.* 1983;7:439–43

162. Maran ACD, Kwong K, Mine LJR, et al. Frontal sinusitis caused by *Myriodontium keratinophilum*. *Br Med J.* 1985;290:207

163. Friedman GC, Hartwick RW, Ro JY, et al. Allergic fungal sinusitis. Report of three cases associated with dermataceous fungi. *Am J Clin Pathol.* 1991;96:368–72

164. Bartynski JM, McCaffrey TV, Frigas E. Allergic fungal sinusitis secondary to dermataceous fungi – *Curvularia lunata* and Alternaria. *Otolaryngol Head Neck Surg.* 1990;103:32–9

165. Mackowiak PA. The normal flora. *N Engl J Med.* 1982;307:83–93

166. Sanders SS, Nelson GE, Sanders WE, Jr. Bacterial interference. IV. Epidemiological determinants of the antagonistic activity of the normal flora against Group A *streptococci. Infect Immun.* 1977;16:599–606

167. Sprunt K, Redman W. Evidence suggesting importance of role of interbacterial inhibition in maintaining a balance of normal flora. *Ann Inter Med.* 1968;68:579–87

168. Faden H, Zaz MJ, Bernstein JM, et al. Nasopharyngeal flora in the first three years of life in normal and otitis-prone children. *Ann Otol Rhin Laryngol.* 1991;100:612–5

169. Engel JP. Viral upper respiratory infections. *Semin Respir Infect.* 1995;10:3–13

170. Heald A, Auckenthaler R, Borst F, et al. Adult bacterial nasopharyngitis: a clinical entity? *J Gen Intern Med.* 1993;8:667–73

171. Hays GC, Mullard JE. Can nasal bacteria flora be predicted from clinical findings? *Pediatrics.* 1972;49:596–9

172. Freijd A, Bygdeman S, Rynnel-Dagoo B. The nasopharyngeal microflora of otitis-prone children, with emphasis on *H. influenzae. Acta Otolaryngol.* 1984;97:117–26

173. Todd JK, Todd N, Damato J, et al. Bacteriology and treatment of purulent nasopharyngitis: a double-blind placebo-controlled evaluation. *Pediatr Infect Dis.* 1984;3:226–32

174. Cisse MF, Sow AI, Thiaw C, et al. Bacteriological study of purulent nasopharyngitis in children in Senegal. *Arch Pediatr.* 1997;4:1192–6

175. Gohd RS. The common cold. *N Engl J Med.* 1954;250:687–91

176. Cherian T, Bhattacharji S, Brahmadathan KN, et al. Persistent rhinorrhoea in rural Indian children: prevalence and consequences. *J Trop Pediatr.* 2000;46:365–7

18

Chapter 19

Chronic Rhinosinusitis and Superantigens

19

Kristin A. Seiberling, Leslie C. Grammer, and Robert C. Kern

Core Messages

- Effects on nasal polyp tissue consistent with local exposure to superantigens are seen in about 50% of patients with chronic rhinosinusitis and nasal polyps.
- It has been hypothesized that polyp formation is potentiated by chronic TH2 stimulation and cytokine release in response to local superantigen production.
- However, superantigens probably do not cause polyps, as a similar phenotypic picture can be demonstrated in their absence.
- Superantigens play no clear role in TH1 polyps such as that seen in cystic fibrosis.
- Superantigens should be considered to be *disease modifiers* rather than causative agents in patients with chronic rhinosinusitis and nasal polyps.
- The presence of superantigens can stimulate polyp formation and growth by accentuating and dysregulating the local mucosal immune response.

Contents

Introduction

Recent expert panels have defined chronic rhinosinusitis (CRS) as a clinical syndrome rather than a discrete disease entity, with emphasis on chronic inflammation rather than infection [1]. In the past CRS was believed to be secondary to anatomic abnormalities leading to ostial obstruction and/or persistent bacterial infection. Symptomatic recurrence of CRS despite adequate surgery, however, resulted in general acceptance of the concept that no one causative factor can fully explain the clinical heterogeneity and pathologic manifestations of the condition. There is growing consensus toward the concept that CRS results from multiple factors that may be working simultaneously or independently in an individual patient. Potential contributing sources can be categorized into: host factors, including anatomic abnormalities, allergy, immune dysfunction, mucociliary defects, metabolic perturbations, such as aspirin intolerance; and environmental factors including micro-organisms, biofilm formation, osteitis, fungal colonization associated with eosinophilia, and bacterial superantigens. The focus of this chapter will be on the hypothesized role of bacterial superantigens (SAg) in CRS with nasal polyps.

Chronic rhinosinusitis is commonly classified into CRS without polyps (CRSsNP) and CRS with polyps (CRSwNP) with SAg playing a proposed role thus far only in the latter. Overall, CRS affects approximately 15% of the American population [1], while CRSwNP occurs in about 20% of those patients with CRS [2]. Patients with polyps represent a distinct group that is clinically more symptomatic and particularly refractory to both medical and surgical therapy. CRSwNP is frequently linked to steroid-dependent asthma and aspirin intolerance. The most common pathology of the sinus mucosa in CRSwNP is similar to that seen in the bronchial mucosa of asthmatics, infiltrates consisting mainly of lymphocytes, plasma cells, and eosinophils. Histologically, nasal polyposis is characterized by a chronic eosinophilic inflammatory pattern in 70–90% of cases [3], tissue edema, and local IgE production. Histologic findings in CRSsNP in general reveal much less tissue eosinophilia and edema with more prominent glandular hyperplasia [4]. The above division of CRS into eosinophilic CRSwNP and relatively non-eosinophilic CRSsNP is somewhat artificial, since polyps with minimal tissue eosinophilia exist in both cystic fibrosis and polyps from Southeast Asia [5, 6]. Nevertheless, despite these exceptions, the triggers for eosinophil recruitment and activation are believed to play a central role in the development of polyps in the vast majority of cases.

Once thought to be an eosinophilic inflammation of allergic origin, evidence has accumulated against allergy in the pathophysiology of nasal polyposis [7]. Furthermore, recent studies have demonstrated that colonization of the nasal cavity with *Staphylococcus aureus* is much more frequent in CRSwNP patients than in those without polyps, suggesting that these bacteria might play a role in the formation of polyps [8]. *S. aureus* is a common microbial agent that is known to release staphylococcal enterotoxins (SE), which act as superantigens (SAg), allergens, and conventional antigens, playing important roles in the development, amplification, and maintenance of the mucosal inflammation in CRSwNP.

What Are Superantigens?

Superantigens are proteins of microbial or viral origin known for their potent lymphocyte-transforming (mitogenic) activity toward human T lymphocytes. Microbial SAg are powerful modifiers of the immune system, which may result in massive T-cell activation, cytokine release, and in some cases systemic shock. SAg are able to trigger excessive and aberrant activation of T cells by bypassing the normal antigen processing step. As depicted in Fig. 19.1, during a conventional response, an antigen is recognized and processed within an antigen processing cell (APC). Peptide fragments of the processed antigen are displayed in the peptide binding groove of the major histocompatibility complex (MHC) class II molecule on the surface of the APC. These fragments are presented to surrounding T lymphocytes. Only those CD4+ T cells that recognize the MHC class II molecule with the bound peptide fragment will be stimulated. This is an extremely specific response that activates only a tiny fragment of the host T cell population (less than 0.01%) [9, 10]. In contrast, SAg bind as intact molecules to a region outside the peptide binding groove of the MHC class II molecule (Fig. 19.1). SAg stimulate both CD4+ and CD8+ T cells in an MHC II-dependent manner; however, T cell receptor (TCR) recognition is not MHC-restricted [11]. Binding to the MHC class II molecule outside the antigen-binding groove prevents the TCR from having cognate recognition of the surface of the MHC molecule, which would be required for usual antigen presentation. SAg bind to the V-beta domain of the TCR and any T cell bearing the appropriate V-beta type will be stimulated by the SAg regardless of the MHC allotype. It is the bridging of the TCR and the MHC class II molecule that leads to massive proliferation and release of cytokines, chemokines, and adhesion molecules, T cell activation, activation-induced apoptosis and anergy [12]. In contrast to the conventional antigen response, which activates less than 0.01% of the host T-cell population, SAg may activate up to 25% [13]. Concentrations of less than 0.1 mg/mL of the bacterial SAg may be enough to stimulate an uncontrolled T cell response, leading to systemic collapse, shock, and death [14].

Staphylococcal Superantigens

To date the most extensively studied SAg are exotoxins produced by the Gram-positive bacteria *S. aureus* and *Streptococcus pyogenes*, organisms commonly found on the skin, in the nose, and in the upper respiratory tract of humans. The number of staphylococcal and streptococcal SAg is evolving as genome sequencing databases grow. As of 2003, 32 staphylococcal and streptococcal SAg have been discovered [15]. The focus of this chapter will be on SE, the SAg that have been linked to CRS, including staphylococcal exotoxins A-Q (SEA-SEQ) and toxic shock syndrome toxin-1 (TSST-1). These are heat-stable proteins ranging from 22.5 to 28 kDa in molecular weight. Overall, these proteins share significant nucleotide and amino acid sequence homology ranging from 32 to 82% and from 21 to 82% respectively [16]. Despite differences in primary amino acid sequencing, the toxins appear as compacted ellipsoidal proteins sharing a common characteristic two-dimensional folding pattern [17, 18]. Despite a highly conserved structural fold, individual bacterial SAg have evolved different mechanisms of binding to MHC class II molecules and TCR. It is likely that staphylococcal and streptococcal SAg have evolved from a single primordial superantigen. The evolution of SAg indicated that for at least some microbes, these toxins confer an advantage and may be an important mechanism for survival.

MHC Class II Binding

As discussed above, SAg bind as intact proteins, directly to the MCH class II molecule outside of the peptide binding groove. SAg have developed three basic mechanisms for binding to the MHC class II molecule [19]. They may bind to a single alpha chain (e. g., SEB), a single beta chain (e. g., SEH) or they may bind and crosslink two MHC class II molecules [20]. Some SAg, like SEH, require a zinc ion to effectively bind the MHC class II molecule [21]. In addition, the affinity of SAg toward different MHC class II isotypes and alleles varies considerably and appears to influence SAg potency [22]. It is thought that SAg recognition by certain T cells is strongly influenced by polymorphic residues of the MHC class II molecule [23]. In humans, the MHC class II molecules can be divided into HLA DR, DQ, and DP isotypes. While in humans, HLA-DR is the predominant MHC class II receptor for most SAg, some appear to have a higher binding affinity for HLA-DQ (Table 19.1) [24]. For example, most staphylococcal exotoxins bind HLA-DR preferentially, whereas many streptococcal pyrogenic exotoxins bind better to HLA-DQ. It has been well established that the MHC polymorphism influences individual SAg activity. Kotb and colleagues showed that certain HLA haplotypes conferred strong protection from severe systemic disease caused by invasive streptococcal infection, whereas other haplotypes increased the risk of severe disease [25]. This may explain why some individuals appear to be relatively protected from the lethal effects of SAg.

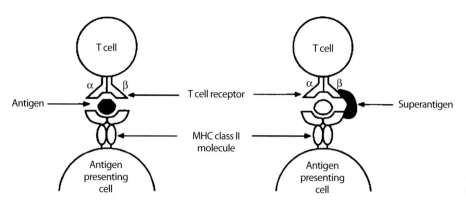

Fig. 19.1 **a, b** Binding mechanism of superantigens [83]

Table 19.1 Binding preference of various superantigens to the different haplotypes of MHC II molecules

Superantigen	MHC II Preference
SEA	HLA DR > DP, DQ
SEB	HLA DR > DP > DQ
SEC1	HLA-DR, DQ
SEC2	HLA-DQ > DR
SED	HLA- DR > DP
SEE	HLA- DR > DP
TSST-1	HLA- DR > DQ > DP

T Cell Interaction with SAg-MHC Class II

While there are TCR consisting of delta and gamma chains, most TCR consist of two chains (alpha and beta), with the beta chain being composed of three segments, variable, joining, and diversity. The alpha chain is composed of a variable and a joining segment. In the conventional antigen response, TCR binding is dependent on the recognition of a combination of each segment. In contrast, the recognition of SAg by the TCR is dependent only on the V-beta chain of the TCR [9]. The number of different V-beta regions of the human T cell repertoire is less than 50 [26], with 24 major types. Most SAg have been found to bind to more than one V-beta domain. This effectively allows each SAg to interact with a large number of T cells (5–30%). Thus, each SAg has a characteristic "V-beta signature" demonstrated by its affinity to various V-beta domains (Table 19.2). The hallmark of SAg activity is noted by clonal expansions of both CD4+ and CD8+ T cells with the appropriate V-beta domain. Using flow cytometry, V-beta clonal expansions have been identified for numerous superantigens.

Superantigen Response

Staphylococcus aureus exotoxins (SE) may act as a conventional antigen, as an allergen, or as a superantigen. As a superantigen, they have an extremely potent stimulatory effect on T lymphocytes (CD4+ and CD8+), B cells, macrophages, antigen-presenting cells (APC), eosinophils, and epithelial cells [27]. SAg modulate the immune response through polyclonal T cell expansion, deletion, and tolerance. As previously mentioned, the conventional antigen response involves processing of the peptide to oligopeptides of 8–20 amino acids in length, binding within the antigen-binding groove of Class I or Class II MHC molecules, presentation to CD8+ or CD4+ T cells respectively and recognition of the TCR in an MHC-restricted manner. This leads to the selective activation of only 0.001–0.0001% of the T cells. Conventional antigens function as T-helper cell epitopes leading to the activation of B-cells and the production of antigen-specific immunoglobulins (i. e., the humoral response). As foreign proteins, SAg will stimulate a humoral response in extremely low concentrations. SAg will be processed as typical antigens by antigen presenting and in the presence of T helper cells will evoke B-cell proliferation and Ig production [28]. Evidence of SAg acting as classical antigens is demonstrated by the presence of anti-superantigen antibodies in the serum.

Acting as a superantigen, these toxins violate the underlying principles of the specific immune response. Although the presentation of SAg is via the MHC II molecule, both CD4+ and CD8+ cells respond. This is in contrast to the conventional peptide antigen that is processed by the APC and presented via MHC II to CD4+ cells or via MHC I to CD8+ cells but not both. SAg efficiently bridge the TCR and MHC class II molecules on APC triggering T cell proliferation/polyclonal expansion (marked by specific V-beta clonal expansion), pro-inflammatory cytokine production, followed by apoptosis, and tolerance (anergy) [29]. In the classic SAg response, APC and T lymphocytes are stimulated, leading to the synthesis and massive release of both TH1 and TH2 cytokines (IL-1, IL-2, IL-4, IL-5, IL-6, IL-8, IL-10, IL-13, TNF-α, GMC-SF) and chemokines, enhanced expression of cell adhesion molecules, T cell proliferation, followed by apoptosis and anergy [30]. SAg may have multiple effects, which are determined by the responding cell, concentration, exposure route, frequency, the nature of the APC

Table 19.2 V-beta associations with various superantigens

SAg	MW (kDa)	Organism	Crystal structure	Zinc binding	MHC II bindin α/β chain	Human TcR Vβ specificity
SEA	27·1	S.aureus	+	+	+/+	1·1, 5·3, 6·3, 6·4, 6·9, 7·3, 7·4, 9·1, 23·
SEB	28·4	S.aureus	+	–	+/–	1·1, 3·2, 6·4, 15·1
SEC1	27·5	S.aureus	–	–	+/–	3·2, 6·4, 6·9, 12, 15·1
SEC2	27·6	S.aureus	+	–	+/–	12, 13, 14, 15, 17, 20
SEC3	27·6	S.aureus	+	–	+/–	5·1, 12
SED	26·9	S.aureus	+	+	+/+	1·1, 5·3, 6·9, 7·4, 8·1, 12·1
SEE	26·8	S.aureus	–	+	+/+	5·1, 6·3, 6·4, 6·9, 8·1
SEG	27·0	S.aureus	–	?	?	3, 12, 13·1, 13·2, 14, 15
SEH	25·2	S.aureus	+	+	–/+	?
SEI	24·9	S.aureus	–	?	?	1·1, 5·1, 5·3, 23
SEJ	28·5	S.aureus	–	?	?	?
SEK	25·3	S.aureus	–	?	?	5·1, 5·2, 6·7
SEL	24·7	S.aureus	–	?	?	?
SEM	24·8	S.aureus	–	?	?	?
SEN	26·1	S.aureus	–	?	?	?
SEO	26·7	S.aureus	–	?	?	?
SEP	26·4	S.aureus	–	?	?	?
SEQ	26·0	S.aureus	–	?	?	2·1, 5·1, 21·3
TSST	21·9	S.aureus	+	–	+/–	2·1

19

and costimulatory ligands, and concurrent or subsequent stimulation with other antigens/toxins [12, 31]. Recent data suggest that chronic stimulation by the SAg may lead to an oligoclonal T cell response rather than the polyclonality seen with acute diseases [32]. Historically, oligoclonality is more consistent with a process driven by a conventional antigen. It is presumed that T cell oligoclonality results from the collaborative effect of the toxin acting both as a superantigen and as a conventional antigen, which in concert enhances/amplifies the antigen-driven response.

Staphylococcal enterotoxins may also act as allergens, promoting a systemic and local IgE response with histamine release on repeated exposure. Studies with TSST-1 have shown that SE may modulate allergic disease by augmenting isotype switching and synthesis of IgE both in vitro [33] and in vivo with a mouse model [34]. TSST-1 may directly and indirectly activate B cells by inducing co-stimulatory molecules CD40 and B7.2 (CD86) respectively [35]. The induced expression on B cells of B7.2 has

been shown to enhance TH2 response and IgE production. IgE-specific to SE have been demonstrated in patients with atopic dermatitis [36] and CRSwNP [37–39]. These toxins likely simultaneously generate both the conventional allergic reaction and a local SAg response. Evidence of this dual functionality is shown in several studies on atopic dermatitis [40, 41] and asthma [42] in which the presence of serum IgE to the SE is associated with higher disease severity.

Effects of Superantigens on Pro-Inflammatory Cells

Proinflammatory cells (eosinophils, macrophages, mast cells, epithelial cells) are known to play an integral part in the pathogenesis of chronic inflammatory states. These cells are known to act as accessory molecules for a T cell activation/proliferation response to SE, in particular the release of cytokines. Direct effects of SE on macrophage activity have been documented, in particular the production of IL-8 [43]. Mast cells may also be directly activated by SE. In heart tissue, SE have been demonstrated to effectively cross-link IgE molecules on mast cells, resulting in an increase in histamine, tryptase, and leukotriene C4 [44]. Studies on eosinophils have primarily described their role as accessory cells, which present SAg to T lymphocytes, by means of MHC class II molecules [45]. SE may also directly and indirectly influence eosinophilia in targeted tissue. Eosinophilia occurs with disease states that demonstrate a bias toward a TH2 cytokine response with release of interleukin (IL)-4 and IL-5. The production of IL-4 and IL-5 is associated with an increase in IgE production and eosinophil proliferation and mast cell activation. In atopic dermatitis, SEB has been shown to stimulate the production of IL-5, which ultimately leads to eosinophilia, a hallmark of severe allergic disease [46]. It is hypothesized that SE may potentiate allergic disease by promoting the production of IL-5, which has been shown to enhance the survival of pro-inflammatory eosinophils via inhibition of apoptosis [47]. Studies using anti-IL-5 antibodies in nasal polyp tissue demonstrated an increase in eosinophil apoptosis and a decrease in tissue eosinophilia [48]. Additionally, IL-5 plays a role in the selective migration of eosinophils from the peripheral circulation into the tissues [49]. Eosinophils are a major source of IL-5, thus creating a possible loop for autocrine activation and survival. Eosinophils are the only human leukocytes with receptors for IL-5, emphasizing the significance of IL-5 in tissue eosinophilia [50]. Eosinophil activation leads to degranulation and deposition of toxic mediators (eosinophilic cationic protein, major basic protein, EDN, eosinophil peroxidase) that play a role in epithelial damage. Recent published reports have demonstrated that SE may activate nasal epithelial cells in vitro, potentially modulating local chemokine and cytokine synthesis and release in disease. Upon exposure to SEB, epithelial cells were shown to release IL-1 and IL-8 [51], cytokines known to activate the immune system. In a similar study, the release of IL-6 from nasal epithelial cells stimulated with SEB has been demonstrated [52]. More recent data confirmed elevated levels of IL-6 in nasal polyp tissue compared with CRSwNP and controls [53]. In addition to chemokine and cytokine release, SE may also adversely affect epithelial ion transport and barrier function [54].

Superantigens in Human Disease

Staphylococcal enterotoxins are most well known for their role in food poisoning and toxic shock syndrome. These SAg are potent gastrointestinal toxins responsible for food poisoning. Classic toxic shock syndrome is caused by *S. aureus* exotoxins, but is also seen with SE produced by some strains of streptococci. Other diseases in which SAg may play a role include: acute rheumatic fever, Kawasaki disease, psoriasis, and certain autoimmune disorders. In addition, bacterial SAg are believed to be involved in the exacerbation and induction of inflammatory skin diseases (e. g., atopic dermatitis) and reactive airway disease. In atopic dermatitis (AD), T cells secrete a T helper (TH2) cytokine profile including IL-4, IL-5, and IL-13, which is known to induce IgE production [55, 56]. Up to 90% of patients with AD are colonized with *S. aureus*, the majority of which are

of the toxin-secreting strain [57, 58, 59]. Studies have shown that the application of SEB to intact normal and atopic skin induces an eczematoid reaction [60]. It is hypothesized that the SE penetrate the skin and induce a TH2 response, which activates cells thought to be important for the initiation of atopic dermatitis lesions. Hofer et al. demonstrated that SAg can augment allergen-specific IgE synthesis and B7.2 expression [35]. Further evidence of SAg activity in atopic dermatitis has been demonstrated by the presence of V-beta skewing (a hallmark of SAg activity) of both CD4+ and CD8+ T cells in the peripheral blood [61].

Similar to AD, there is increasing evidence that SAg may play a role in the pathogenesis and maintenance of upper and lower airway disease, including rhinitis, sinusitis, and asthma. Bronchial asthma is a chronic inflammation of the lower respiratory tract characterized by immune activation of TH2 T cells, which can be detected in bronchial mucosa, bronchoalveolar lavage (BAL), and peripheral blood of patients with asthma [62]. Hauk et al. demonstrated a significant increase in V-beta 8 T cells (both CD4+ and CD8+) of individuals with poorly controlled asthma [63]. This skewing of the V-beta repertoire was greater in BAL T cells than in circulating peripheral blood mononuclear cells (PMBC), suggesting that the respiratory mucosa was the site of SAg exposure. This excess of V-beta 8 T cells was not found in patients with well-controlled asthma or normal controls. It is hypothesized that SAg might cause more potent T cell activation, which maintains the chronic inflammation in severe asthmatics.

Asthma has been linked to CRSwNP and studies on sinus mucosa demonstrated a similar pattern of cellular infiltrates to that seen in asthmatic bronchial mucosa, suggesting an analogous immunopathophysiology [2, 64]. Patients with CRSwNP frequently have asthma, and often develop wheezing and worsening of asthma with untreated sinusitis [65]. This association is clearly demonstrated by patients with Samter's Triad (severe nasal polyposis, aspirin sensitivity, and severe asthma).

Superantigens and CRSwNP

Nasal polyposis most commonly represents a severe T cell-orchestrated eosinophilic inflammation with increased concentrations of IL-5 and local excessive IgE production [66]. Histopathologic findings of polyp tissue reveal epithelial damage, thickening of the basement membrane, edematous stroma with a paucity of glandular structures, and subepithelial eosinophilic inflammation [67]. Eosinophilia is significantly less in CRSsNP. Conclusions made from these observations suggest that eosinophilic inflammation may promote polyp formation and growth in the majority of cases, particularly in Western countries. The eosinophilic inflammation in polyps is orchestrated by activated CD4+ and CD8+ T cells with a mixed TH1and TH2 profile [68] and influenced significantly by IL-5. As discussed above, IL-5 is a key cytokine for the maturation and activation of mature eosinophils and has been found in elevated levels in nasal polyps [69].

Although once thought to represent an eosinophilic allergic process, studies have not clearly shown any differences between polyps from allergic and non-allergic participants [7]. While the etiology of nasal polyps remains unclear, evidence currently points toward the role played by microbial superantigen production within the sinonasal cavity in at least some of the CRSwNP patients, particularly those with very high levels of polyp eosinophilia [37]. The inflammatory reactions and cytokine profile seen in nasal polyposis are strikingly similar to the SAg-induced immune activation described in other chronic inflammatory disorders [70]. It can therefore be hypothesized that in a genetically susceptible host, SAg may induce a sustained TH1/TH2 inflammatory reaction that fosters polyp formation and maintenance; the most likely candidate sources of the SAg are the toxin-producing strains of *S. aureus*. In approximately 25% of the asymptomatic population, the nasal cavity is colonized with *S. aureus* [71]. While this percentage is unchanged in CRSsNP, the colonization rate increases dramatically in CRSwNP, in particular those with extremely high tissue eosinophil counts [8]. Colonization with *S. aureus* was present in 63.6% of patients with nasal polyps and reached as high as 87.5% in patients with coexisting bronchial asthma and aspirin sensitivity. This was significantly higher than the colonization rate in controls and patients with CRSsNP, 33.3% and 27.3% respectively [5]. Although not all strains of *S. aureus* are thought to produce SAg, a recent study using a multiplex polymerase chain reaction (PCR-DNA) enzyme immunoassay against an extended list of staphylococcal enterotoxins (SEA, SEB, SEC, SED, SEE, TSST-1, SEG, SHE, SEI, SEJ), demonstrated an overall rate of toxin gene-positive isolates in 73% of the strains [72]. The difference in colonization rates may be due to disturbances of innate immunity and the mucosal barrier function, which may be major factors in the survival of toxin-secreting staphylococci in the nose. Overall, the differences in staphylococcal colonization rates, as well as the histologic differences mentioned above, suggest that despite some clinical and symptomatic overlap, CRSwNP and CRSsNP are different disease entities with distinct underlying pathologic mechanisms.

Differences in staphylococcal colonization rates provide only indirect support for an SE role in CRSwNP. Identification of IgE antibodies directed against SE in nasal polyp tissue, however, provided the first direct evidence of local superantigen exposure in the nasal cavity of CRSwNP patients. Elevated levels of IgE to SEA/SEB were found in approximately 50% of nasal polyp tissue, as well as increased concentrations of total IgE, IL-5, eotaxin, eosinophil cationic protein (ECP), cys-leukotrienes, and CD23 over controls [37]. In addition, those patients with anti-SEA/SEB IgE had a higher level of total IgE and eosinophils and a higher prevalence of asthma. In another study using a screening assay to detect IgE antibodies SE, elevated levels were found in 27.8% of polyp samples, with rates as high as 53.8% and 80% in subgroups with asthma and aspirin sensitivity, compared with 15% in controls and 6% in patients with CRSsNP [8]. Histologic evidence of local polyclonal IgE formation was later demonstrated by immunohistochemical studies performed on nasal polyp tissue [73]. This study demonstrated the organization of secondary lymphoid tissue, polyclonal IgE associated with the presence of IgE-specific SEA, eosinophilia, and colonization with *S. aureus*. Follicular structures composed of both T and B cells and IgE were found in 25% of nasal polyp

(NP) specimens. Diffuse lymphoid accumulation demonstrating B cell maturation into IgE-producing plasma cells were seen in all NP specimens. Using biotinylated SEA, binding to the follicular structures and lymphoid tissue was demonstrated. This study suggests that microbial colonization with the release of SAg results in the organization of secondary lymphoid tissue with polyclonal B-cell activation as well as IgE isotype switching. This locally generated polyclonal lymphocytic response may aid in the survival of the offending pathogen. A polyclonal response may result in a lack of antibody specificity and T cell response, thus obliterating the specific immune response [74].

Evidence of a systemic IgE response to SE has also been documented; serum IgE directed against at least 1 of 6 superantigenic toxins was detected in 20 out of 23 CRSwNP and in none of the 13 controls [39]. A trend toward increased eosinophilic infiltration was seen in patients positive for IgE to the toxins, which was unrelated to atopic status [38]. It remains unclear, however, whether the systemic anti-SE IgE detected in these studies was related to the CRSwNP, the concomitant asthma, or both.

Superantigens differ in their ability to bind the various V-beta domains of the TCR, some binding with a strong affinity and others binding only weakly. Most SAg bind more than one V-beta domain, leading to a characteristic "clonal signature" that can be demonstrated with flow cytometry. Using this knowledge, Bernstein et al. performed a pilot study on 3 patients with CRSwNP. This study demonstrated clonal expansion of the V-beta domain of the T lymphocytes [75]. A larger study was subsequently performed looking at the pattern of V-beta expression in polyp and peripheral blood T cells (CD4+ and CD8+ cells) in 17 patients with CRSwNP. This study used flow cytometry to evaluate 24 common V-beta motifs for clonal expansion. V-beta skewing was found in all 17 patients, with an average of 11 V-beta domains expanded in polyp tissue versus 2 clonal expansions in blood lymphocytes [38]. The dramatic skewing of V-beta clonal expansions in polyp tissue over peripheral blood suggests a locally occurring process. In addition, samples taken from the blood of normal controls, tissue from the adenoid pad of CRSwNP patients and in patients with antrochoanal polyps did not demonstrate clonal expansions.

Superantigen activation is not classically MHC II-restricted and can involve both CD4+ and CD8+ T cell proliferation. SAg activity should then be marked by clonal expansion in both CD4+ *and* CD8+ T cells, with a high affinity to particular V-beta domains. The human V-beta repertoire consists of approximately 50 types, with 24 of those representing major subtypes. To date, seven of the major subtypes have been associated with a strong affinity toward SAg binding. Using this information, Conley and associates refined their results of the earlier pilot study to look at only those patients who demonstrated V-beta clonal expansions in both CD4+ and CD8+ T-cells with a major SAg association. Out of 20 CRSwNP patients, 35% demonstrated upward skewing in both CD4+ and CD8+ T cells fulfilling the stringent criteria outlined above. In addition, 2 out of 7 patients demonstrated V-beta skewing, representing more than one toxin present [76]. The current data are indicative of a local superantigen reaction in the polyps of these patients with CRSwNP. As was mentioned earlier, SAg also induce a conventional allergic response detected by the presence of toxin-specific IgE in serum and in the polyp tissue itself. Conventional IgE and V-beta clonal proliferation responses to SAg were then concurrently assessed to determine whether the same SAg were eliciting both responses in individual patients. Results demonstrated a strong positive correlation between the IgE response and the T cell response, indicating that the same SE was/were responsible in a given patient [77].

Initial studies provided evidence of the role of SAg in CRSwNP in that a response, characteristic of exposure, was detected in blood and polyp tissue. Direct detection of toxins is more problematic in that they may be present in concentrations of less than 0.1 pg/mL [56]. A recent study, however, using an ELISA kit with a sensitivity of 0.1 ng/mL, was able to directly detect SAg in the nasal cavity of CRSwNP patients [78]. An ELISA immunoassay was used to detect the common staphylococcal exotoxins A, B, C1-3, D, and TSST-1 in both polyp tissue and mucus of patients with CRSwNP. At least one toxin was detected in 14 out of 29 patients with CRSwNP. In addition, 9 of those 14 patients were positive for more than one toxin. Out of the 11 normal controls, none tested positive for toxin and only 1 out of 13 CRSsNP patients had a positive ELISA result.

Historically, the utilization of antibiotics for the treatment of CRSwNP has been minimal, with no clear evidence of polyp shrinkage when used in the absence of corticosteroids. Although the lack of antibiotic efficacy in CRSwNP would appear to constitute an argument against the superantigen hypothesis, two recently observed phenomena have been suggested as explanations. First, staphylococci and other bacteria are capable of forming biofilms in the nose of patients with chronic rhinosinusitis, rendering these organisms resistant to anti-microbial therapy [79]. Second, and perhaps more significant, it has now also been demonstrated that S. aureus is capable of invading human respiratory epithelial cells [80]. In cells of the airway epithelium, S. aureus was found to reside in vacuoles, potentially rendering them resistant to antibiotics [81]. While no direct evidence yet exists, it is hypothetically possible that intracellular bacteria are still capable of secreting toxin with effects on surrounding host tissues. A secondary immune defect, in either the innate or the adaptive system, may be responsible for the invasion, retention, and survival of the microbial agent within the epithelium, possibly explaining why such a ubiquitous organism has an effect on some individuals and not others. Further studies are necessary to validate the clinical significance of either biofilms or intracellular S. aureus in the etiology and pathogenesis of nasal polyps.

Conclusion

In summary, considerable data have been generated by multiple investigators documenting effects on nasal polyp tissue consistent with local exposure to SAg. These effects, including clonal T cell proliferation and IgE formation, are seen in about 50% of CRSwNP patients, typically those with the highest tissue eosinophil counts. Specifically, Bachert and colleagues hypothesize that polyp formation is potentiated by chronic TH2 stimulation and cytokine release in response to local SAg production [69]. It should be emphasized however, that SAg likely do not cause polyps, as a similar phenotypic picture can be demonstrated in

the absence of SAg; specifically, eosinophilic nasal polyps can be present in the absence of any evidence of SAg tissue effects in about half the cases of typical nasal polyps in Western countries. Furthermore, SAg play no clear role in TH1 polyps such as that seen in cystic fibrosis [82]. Consequently, it is probably most accurate at this point to consider SAg to be *disease modifiers* rather than causative agents in CRSwNP. Practically speaking, the presence of SAg in a genetically susceptible host in the proper environmental context likely accentuates and dysregulates the local mucosal immune response, stimulating polyp formation and growth.

References

1. Meltzer, E.O., et al., *Rhinosinusitis: establishing definitions for clinical research and patient care.* J Allergy Clin Immunol, 2004. 114(6 Suppl): p. 155–212
2. Hamilos, D.L., *Chronic sinusitis.* J Allergy Clin Immunol, 2000. 106(2): p. 213–27
3. Mygind, N., R. Dahl, and C. Bachert, *Nasal polyposis, eosinophil dominated inflammation, and allergy.* Thorax, 2000. 55 Suppl 2: p. S79–83
4. Berger, G., et al., *Polypoid mucosa with eosinophilia and glandular hyperplasia in chronic sinusitis: a histopathological and immunohistochemical study.* Laryngoscope, 2002. 112(4): p. 738–45
5. Zhang, N., et al., *An update on the impact of Staphylococcus aureus enterotoxins in chronic sinusitis with nasal polyposis.* Rhinology, 2005. 43(3): p. 162–8
6. Rowe-Jones, J.M., et al., *Polypoidal rhinosinusitis in cystic fibrosis: a clinical and histopathological study.* Clin Otolaryngol Allied Sci, 1997. 22(2): p. 167–71
7. Drake-Lee, A.B. and P. McLaughlan, *Clinical symptoms, free histamine and IgE in patients with nasal polyposis.* Int Arch Allergy Appl Immunol, 1982. 69(3): p. 268–71
8. Van Zele, T., et al., *Staphylococcus aureus colonization and IgE antibody formation to enterotoxins is increased in nasal polyposis.* J Allergy Clin Immunol, 2004. 114(4): p. 981–3
9. Choi, Y.W., et al., *Interaction of Staphylococcus aureus toxin "superantigens" with human T cells.* Proc Natl Acad Sci U S A, 1989. 86(22): p. 8941–5
10. Irwin, M.J. and N.R. Gascoigne, *Interplay between superantigens and the immune system.* J Leukoc Biol, 1993. 54(5): p. 495–503
11. Scherer, M.T., et al., *Superantigens: bacterial and viral proteins that manipulate the immune system.* Annu Rev Cell Biol, 1993. 9: p. 101–28
12. Krakauer, T., *Immune response to staphylococcal superantigens.* Immunol Res, 1999. 20(2): p. 163–73
13. Llewelyn, M. and J. Cohen, *Superantigens: microbial agents that corrupt immunity.* Lancet Infect Dis, 2002. 2(3): p. 156–62
14. Proft, T. and J.D. Fraser, *Bacterial superantigens.* Clin Exp Immunol, 2003. 133(3): p. 299–306
15. Alouf, J.E. and H. Muller-Alouf, *Staphylococcal and streptococcal superantigens: molecular, biological and clinical aspects.* Int J Med Microbiol, 2003. 292(7–8): p. 429–40
16. Munson, S.H., et al., *Identification and characterization of staphylococcal enterotoxin types G and I from Staphylococcus aureus.* Infect Immun, 1998. 66(7): p. 3337–48

17. Papageorgiou, A.C., et al., *Structural basis for the recognition of superantigen streptococcal pyrogenic exotoxin A (SpeA1) by MHC class II molecules and T-cell receptors.* EMBO J, 1999. 18(1): p. 9–21

18. Proft, T., et al., *Immunological and biochemical characterization of streptococcal pyrogenic exotoxins I and J (SPE-I and SPE-J) from Streptococcus pyogenes.* J Immunol, 2001. 166(11): p. 6711–9

19. Petersson, K., G. Forsberg, and B. Walse, *Interplay between superantigens and immunoreceptors.* Scand J Immunol, 2004. 59(4): p. 345–55

20. Petersson, K., et al., *Crystal structure of a superantigen bound to MHC class II displays zinc and peptide dependence.* EMBO J, 2001. 20(13): p. 3306–12

21. Li, Y., et al., *Crystal structure of a superantigen bound to the high-affinity, zinc-dependent site on MHC class II.* Immunity, 2001. 14(1): p. 93–104

22. Mollick, J.A., et al., *Staphylococcal exotoxin activation of T cells. Role of exotoxin-MHC class II binding affinity and class II isotype.* J Immunol, 1991. 146(2): p. 463–8

23. Wen, R., M.A. Blackman, and D.L. Woodland, *Variable influence of MHC polymorphism on the recognition of bacterial superantigens by T cells.* J Immunol, 1995. 155(4): p. 1884–92

24. Herrmann, T., R.S. Accolla, and H.R. MacDonald, *Different staphylococcal enterotoxins bind preferentially to distinct major histocompatibility complex class II isotypes.* Eur J Immunol, 1989. 19(11): p. 2171–4

25. Kotb, M., et al., *An immunogenetic and molecular basis for differences in outcomes of invasive group A streptococcal infections.* Nat Med, 2002. 8(12): p. 1398–404

26. Wei, S. and P. Concannon, *Repertoire and organization of human T-cell receptor alpha region variable genes.* Genomics, 1996. 38(3): p. 442–5

27. Fleischer, B., *Superantigens produced by infectious pathogens: molecular mechanism of action and biological significance.* Int J Clin Lab Res, 1994. 24(4): p. 193–7

28. Ingvarsson, S., et al., *Antigen-specific activation of B cells in vitro after recruitment of T cell help with superantigen.* Immunotechnology, 1995. 1(1): p. 29–39

29. Kappler, J., et al., *V beta-specific stimulation of human T cells by staphylococcal toxins.* Science, 1989. 244(4906): p. 811–3

30. Miethke, T., et al., *Acquired resistance to superantigen-induced T cell shock. V beta selective T cell unresponsiveness unfolds directly from a transient state of hyperreactivity.* J Immunol, 1993. 150(9): p. 3776–84

31. Thibodeau, J., et al., *Molecular characterization and role in T cell activation of staphylococcal enterotoxin A binding to the HLA-DR alpha-chain.* J Immunol, 1997. 158(8): p. 3698–704

32. Kim, K.S., N. Jacob, and W. Stohl, *In vitro and in vivo T cell oligoclonality following chronic stimulation with staphylococcal superantigens.* Clin Immunol, 2003. 108(3): p. 182–9

33. Jabara, H.H. and R.S. Geha, *The superantigen toxic shock syndrome toxin-1 induces CD40 ligand expression and modulates IgE isotype switching.* Int Immunol, 1996. 8(10): p. 1503–10

34. Tumang, J.R., et al., *T helper cell-dependent, microbial superantigen-mediated B cell activation in vivo.* Autoimmunity, 1996. 24(4): p. 247–55

35. Hofer, M.F., et al., *Staphylococcal toxins augment specific IgE responses by atopic patients exposed to allergen.* J Invest Dermatol, 1999. 112(2): p. 171–6

36. Leung, D.Y., et al., *Presence of IgE antibodies to staphylococcal exotoxins on the skin of patients with atopic dermatitis. Evidence for a new group of allergens.* J Clin Invest, 1993. 92(3): p. 1374–80

37. Bachert, C., et al., *Total and specific IgE in nasal polyps is related to local eosinophilic inflammation.* J Allergy Clin Immunol, 2001. 107(4): p. 607–14

38. Conley, D.B., et al., *Chronic sinusitis with nasal polyps: staphylococcal exotoxin immunoglobulin E and cellular inflammation.* Am J Rhinol, 2004. 18(5): p. 273–8

39. Tripathi, A., et al., *Immunoglobulin E to staphylococcal and streptococcal toxins in patients with chronic sinusitis/nasal polyposis.* Laryngoscope, 2004. 114(10): p. 1822–6

40. Breuer, K., et al., *Severe atopic dermatitis is associated with sensitization to staphylococcal enterotoxin B (SEB).* Allergy, 2000. 55(6): p. 551–5

41. Bunikowski, R., et al., *Prevalence and role of serum IgE antibodies to the Staphylococcus aureus-derived superantigens SEA and SEB in children with atopic dermatitis.* J Allergy Clin Immunol, 1999. 103(1 Pt 1): p. 119–24

42. Bachert, C., et al., *IgE to Staphylococcus aureus enterotoxins in serum is related to severity of asthma.* J Allergy Clin Immunol, 2003. 111(5): p. 1131–2

43. Miller, E.J., et al., *Interleukin-8 (IL-8) is a major neutrophil chemotaxin from human alveolar macrophages stimulated with staphylococcal enterotoxin A (SEA).* Inflamm Res, 1996. 45(8): p. 386–92

44. Genovese, A., et al., *Bacterial immunoglobulin superantigen proteins A and L activate human heart mast cells by interacting with immunoglobulin E.* Infect Immun, 2000. 68(10): p. 5517–24

45. Mawhorter, S.D., J.W. Kazura, and W.H. Boom, *Human eosinophils as antigen-presenting cells: relative efficiency for superantigen- and antigen-induced CD4+ T-cell proliferation.* Immunology, 1994. 81(4): p. 584–91

46. Heaton, T., et al., *Staphylococcal enterotoxin induced IL-5 stimulation as a cofactor in the pathogenesis of atopic disease: the hygiene hypothesis in reverse?* Allergy, 2003. 58(3): p. 252–6

47. Yousefi, S., K. Blaser, and H.U. Simon, *Activation of signaling pathways and prevention of apoptosis by cytokines in eosinophils.* Int Arch Allergy Immunol, 1997. 112(1): p. 9–12

48. Ying, S., et al., *T cells are the principal source of interleukin-5 mRNA in allergen-induced rhinitis.* Am J Respir Cell Mol Biol, 1993. 9(4): p. 356–60

49. Bradding, P., et al., *Interleukin-4, -5, and -6 and tumor necrosis factor-alpha in normal and asthmatic airways: evidence for the human mast cell as a source of these cytokines.* Am J Respir Cell Mol Biol, 1994. 10(5): p. 471–80

50. Simon, H.U., et al., *Direct demonstration of delayed eosinophil apoptosis as a mechanism causing tissue eosinophilia.* J Immunol, 1997. 158(8): p. 3902–8

51. Thakur, A., et al., *Modulation of cytokine production from an EpiOcular corneal cell culture model in response to Staphylococcus aureus superantigen.* Aust N Z J Ophthalmol, 1997. 25 Suppl 1: p. S43–5

19

52. Damm, M., et al., *Proinflammatory effects of Staphylococcus aureus exotoxin B on nasal epithelial cells.* Otolaryngol Head Neck Surg, 2006. 134(2): p. 245–9

53. Conley D, T.B., Suh L, Tripathi A, Harris K, Kern R, Schleimer R, Grammer L, *Detection of Immunoreactive IL-6 in Chronic Rhinosinusitis.* Abstract – Triologic Middle Section Meeting, San Diego. Feb 2006, 2006

54. McKay, D.M. and P.K. Singh, *Superantigen activation of immune cells evokes epithelial (T84) transport and barrier abnormalities via IFN-gamma and TNF alpha: inhibition of increased permeability, but not diminished secretory responses by TGF-beta2.* J Immunol, 1997. 159(5): p. 2382–90

55. Hamid, Q., M. Boguniewicz, and D.Y. Leung, *Differential in situ cytokine gene expression in acute versus chronic atopic dermatitis.* J Clin Invest, 1994. 94(2): p. 870–6

56. Marrack, P. and J. Kappler, *The staphylococcal enterotoxins and their relatives.* Science, 1990. 248(4959): p. 1066

57. Leyden, J.J., R.R. Marples, and A.M. Kligman, *Staphylococcus aureus in the lesions of atopic dermatitis.* Br J Dermatol, 1974. 90(5): p. 525–30

58. Hauser, C., et al., *Staphylococcus aureus skin colonization in atopic dermatitis patients.* Dermatologica, 1985. 170(1): p. 35–9

59. Neuber, K. and W. Konig, *Effects of Staphylococcus aureus cell wall products (teichoic acid, peptidoglycan) and enterotoxin B on immunoglobulin (IgE, IgA, IgG) synthesis and CD23 expression in patients with atopic dermatitis.* Immunology, 1992. 75(1): p. 23–8

60. Strange, P., et al., *Staphylococcal enterotoxin B applied on intact normal and intact atopic skin induces dermatitis.* Arch Dermatol, 1996. 132(1): p. 27–33

61. Strickland, I., et al., *Evidence for superantigen involvement in skin homing of T cells in atopic dermatitis.* J Invest Dermatol, 1999. 112(2): p. 249–53

62. Corrigan, C.J. and A.B. Kay, *The roles of inflammatory cells in the pathogenesis of asthma and of chronic obstructive pulmonary disease.* Am Rev Respir Dis, 1991. 143(5 Pt 1): p. 1165–8; discussion 1175–6

63. Hauk, P.J., et al., *Increased T-cell receptor vbeta8+ T cells in bronchoalveolar lavage fluid of subjects with poorly controlled asthma: a potential role for microbial superantigens.* J Allergy Clin Immunol, 1999. 104(1): p. 37–45

64. Schubert, M.S., *A superantigen hypothesis for the pathogenesis of chronic hypertrophic rhinosinusitis, allergic fungal sinusitis, and related disorders.* Ann Allergy Asthma Immunol, 2001. 87(3): p. 181–8

65. Hoover, G.E., et al., *Chronic sinusitis: risk factors for extensive disease.* J Allergy Clin Immunol, 1997. 100(2): p. 185–91

66. Van Cauwenberge, P., et al., *[New insights into the pathology of nasal polyposis: the role of superantigens and IgE].* Verh K Acad Geneeskd Belg, 2005. 67(1): p. 5–28; discussion 29–32

67. Tos, M., et al., *Fireside conference 2. Pathogenesis of nasal polyps.* Rhinol Suppl, 1992. 14: p. 181–5

68. Sanchez-Segura, A., J.A. Brieva, and C. Rodriguez, *T lymphocytes that infiltrate nasal polyps have a specialized phenotype and produce a mixed TH1/TH2 pattern of cytokines.* J Allergy Clin Immunol, 1998. 102(6 Pt 1): p. 953–60

69. Bachert, C., et al., *Superantigens and nasal polyps.* Curr Allergy Asthma Rep, 2003. 3(6): p. 523–31

70. Yarwood, J.M., D.Y. Leung, and P.M. *Schlievert, Evidence for the involvement of bacterial superantigens in psoriasis, atopic dermatitis, and Kawasaki syndrome.* FEMS Microbiol Lett, 2000. 192(1): p. 1–7

71. Farthing MJH, J.D., Anderson J, *Tropical Medicine and Sexually Transmitted Diseases.* 3 ed. Clinical Medicine, ed. C.M. Kumar P. 1994, London: Bailliere Tindall. 1–105

72. Lina, G., et al., *Bacterial competition for human nasal cavity colonization: role of Staphylococcal agr alleles.* Appl Environ Microbiol, 2003. 69(1): p. 18–23

73. Gevaert, P., et al., *Organization of secondary lymphoid tissue and local IgE formation to Staphylococcus aureus enterotoxins in nasal polyp tissue.* Allergy, 2005. 60(1): p. 71–9

74. Reina-San-Martin, B., A. Cosson, and P. Minoprio, *Lymphocyte polyclonal activation: a pitfall for vaccine design against infectious agents.* Parasitol Today, 2000. 16(2): p. 62–7

75. Bernstein, J.M., et al., *A superantigen hypothesis for the pathogenesis of chronic hyperplastic sinusitis with massive nasal polyposis.* Am J Rhinol, 2003. 17(6): p. 321–6

76. Conley D, T.A., Grammer L, Seiberling K, Kern R, *Superantigens and Chronic Sinusitis III: systemic and local response to staphylococcal toxins.* Am J Rhinol, In press.

77. Tripathi, A., et al., *Staphylococcal exotoxins and nasal polyposis: analysis of systemic and local responses.* Am J Rhinol, 2005. 19(4): p. 327–33

78. Seiberling, K.A., et al., *Superantigens and chronic rhinosinusitis: detection of staphylococcal exotoxins in nasal polyps.* Laryngoscope, 2005. 115(9): p. 1580–5

79. Palmer, J.N., *Bacterial biofilms: do they play a role in chronic sinusitis?* Otolaryngol Clin North Am, 2005. 38(6): p. 1193–201, viii.

80. Kintarak, S., et al., *Internalization of Staphylococcus aureus by human keratinocytes.* Infect Immun, 2004. 72(10): p. 5668–75

81. Clement, S., et al., *Evidence of an intracellular reservoir in the nasal mucosa of patients with recurrent Staphylococcus aureus rhinosinusitis.* J Infect Dis, 2005. 192(6): p. 1023–8

82. Claeys, S., et al., *Nasal polyps in patients with and without cystic fibrosis: a differentiation by innate markers and inflammatory mediators.* Clin Exp Allergy, 2005. 35(4): p. 467–72

83. Skov, L., Baadsgaard, O. *Bacterial superantigens and inflammatory skin diseases.* Clin Exp Dermatol 2000. 25: p. 57–61

Chapter 20

Biofilms

Bradford A. Woodworth, Noam A. Cohen, and James N. Palmer

20

Core Messages

- Bacterial biofilms are three-dimensional aggregates of bacteria encased in secreted exopolysaccharides (slime) and lack the susceptibility to antibiotics that planktonic bacteria demonstrate.
- Bacterial biofilms are present in the sinonasal mucosa of some patients with chronic rhinosinusitis.
- The vast majority of bacteria exist in biofilms.
- Bacterial biofilms are a likely contributing factor to medically recalcitrant CRS.
- Strategies developed to treat planktonic bacteria are ineffective against bacteria in a biofilm.
- Understanding how biofilm infections form is fundamental to developing rational strategies for prevention and treatment.

Contents

Introduction

Chronic rhinosinusitis (CRS) affects nearly 16% of the US population each year, resulting in billions of dollars of healthcare expenditure. One of the most common medical complaints, CRS, is responsible for an estimated 13 million physician visits in the United States annually. The disease has a wide-ranging impact on society as well as on quality-of-life issues as assessed by the Short Form-36 quality-of-life survey [1–3]. In fact, patients requiring sinus surgery demonstrated worse scores for physical pain and social functioning than those suffering from chronic obstructive pulmonary disease, congestive heart failure, or angina [4].

The underlying chronic inflammation that seems to be a hallmark of CRS may have various causes. Asthma, allergic rhinitis, Gram-positive and Gram-negative infections, aspirin-sensitive asthma, fungus, osteitis, nasal polyposis, superantigens, and other factors have been implicated in the etiology of CRS. Although multiple etiologies contribute to the development of rhinosinusitis, a common pathophysiologic sequela is ineffective sinonasal mucociliary clearance, resulting in stasis of sinonasal secretions, with subsequent infection and/or persistent inflammation. CRS that is refractory to medical or surgical intervention may involve a particularly resistant form of infection known as a bacterial biofilm.

Bacterial biofilms are three-dimensional aggregates of bacteria encased in secreted exopolysaccharides (slime) and do not have the susceptibility to antibiotics that planktonic bacteria have. They are particularly resistant to antibiotics that attack only dividing cells [5]. However, antibiotic resistance is only one facet of these tenacious infections. Biofilms are strongly resistant to host immunity defense mechanisms and have decreased susceptibility to phagocytic macrophages [5, 6]. The properties of biofilms encourage persistence of bacteria for extensive periods and can result in chronic disease with intermittent acute infections. In addition, these properties allow them to take root in many areas of the body, including the upper respiratory tract where the presence of biofilms has been demonstrated in chronic otitis media, cholesteatoma, and chronic adenoiditis [7]. When CRS develops from acute bacterial sinusitis, the progression into chronic disease parallels these other biofilm-related diseases. For example, patients with Gram-negative bacterial CRS, such as *Pseudomonas*, may become particularly resistant to antibiotic therapy and have the potential to develop chronic disease quite easily.

The senior author was the first to demonstrate bacterial biofilms on the sinus mucosa of patients with CRS (scanning electron microscopy) and in an animal model of *Pseudomonas* sinusitis (Fig. 20.1) [8, 9]. Since then, the presence of bacterial biofilms on the sinonasal mucosa of patients with CRS has been demonstrated by others using a variety of techniques, including scanning and transmission electron microscopy, in situ FISH hybridization, and confocal scanning laser microscopy [10–12]. More recently, Bendouah et al. showed an association between culture-positive *Staphylococcus aureus* and *Pseudomonas aeruginosa* that form biofilms via an in vitro assay and recalcitrant CRS following endoscopic sinus surgery [13]. Furthermore, re-

sults from our laboratory using a similar in vitro assay indicate the presence of biofilm-forming bacteria in approximately 30% of individuals undergoing endoscopic sinus surgery at our institution (Fig. 20.2). Patients evaluated in the outpatient clinic or in the operating room who were found to have sinonasal mucopurulence were cultured in duplicate. While one sample was analyzed by the hospital microbiology lab for culture and sensitivity the duplicate swab was processed for detection of biofilm-forming capacity. In this in vitro assay, cultures are grown in 96-well plates in quadruplicate and compared with positive (wild type PAO1 *Pseudomonas* species) and negative controls (*Sad-31, Sad-36 Pseudomonas*). The *Sad-36* species carries a mutation in the *flagella* gene, which is required for attachment of the *Pseudomonas* to surfaces, thereby making this mutant unable to transition from the planktonic to the adherent phenotype. The *Sad-31* species possesses a mutation in the type IV pili gene, re-

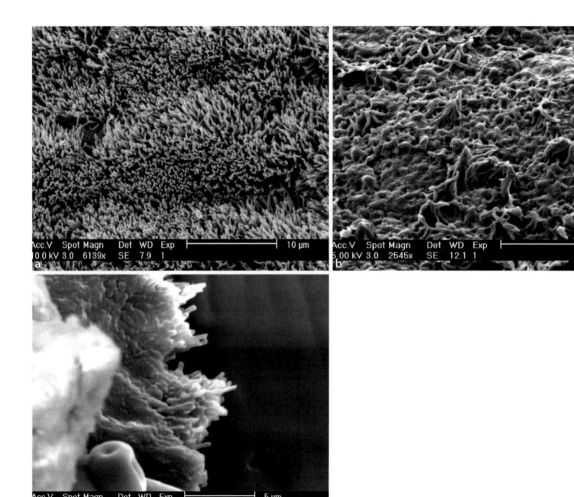

20

Fig. 20.1a–c Bacterial biofilms in sinonasal mucosa from a patient with chronic rhinosinusitis. **a** Scanning electron microscopy (SEM) of normal sinonasal mucosa in which the cilia appear healthy. **b** A thick covering of sinonasal mucosa of a patient with recurrent pan-sensitive *Pseudomonas aeruginosa* chronic rhinosinusitis. There are a number of clumped cilia with the remainder of the "landscape" filled with biofilm towers. **c** At higher power, in the specimen presented in **b** a biofilm tower has been "cracked open" in the preparation process, revealing several rod-like structures representing the pseudomonal rod

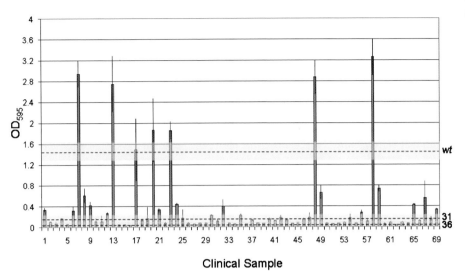

Biofilm Formation in Clinical Isolates

Clinical Sample

Fig. 20.2 Biofilm-forming bacteria demonstrated using endoscopically guided sinonasal cultures (see text for details)

sponsible for auto aggregation, thereby allowing it to adhere to surfaces, but unable to organize into microcolonies and develop into formal biofilms. Biofilm mass is detected by crystal violet staining of inverted pegs incubated in the 96-well plates with bacteria. The crystal violet staining is read at an optical density of 595 nm (OD_{595}). Severe biofilm formation is categorized by OD_{595} greater than PAO-1 (wt), moderate OD_{595} less than wt but greater than *Sad-31*, and minimal as OD_{595} greater than *Sad-31* but greater than *Sad-36*.

Although further investigations into the role of biofilms in CRS are needed, they are a likely contributing factor to medically recalcitrant CRS. A greater understanding of biofilm-induced CRS is required to develop novel therapies directed at prevention and irradiation.

Biofilms and Chronic Disease

The origins of biofilm science were in the engineering and water industries, and only recently have the implications for clinical medicine been noted [14]. Biofilms have now been implicated in many infectious processes, including dental caries, periodontitis, otitis media, musculoskeletal infections, necrotizing fasciitis, biliary tract infection, osteomyelitis, bacterial prostatitis, native valve endocarditis, cystic fibrosis, and pneumonia. Furthermore, there is a long list of nosocomial-type infections in which biofilms are involved. These include ICU pneumonia, sutures, AV shunts, scleral buckles, contact lenses, urinary catheter cystitis, endotracheal tubes, Hickman catheters, central venous catheters, and pressure equalization tubes [7, 15, 16]. In fact, biofilm-forming bacteria are so common that infectious disease researchers at the Centers for Disease Control and Prevention (CDC) estimate that 65% of human bacterial infections involve biofilms [7].

Pathophysiology of Bacterial Biofilms

Bacterial biofilms are a complex association of bacteria anchored to an inert or living surface [14]. Bacterial cells communicate with one another in a cooperative manner and produce a polymeric matrix, which includes mostly polysaccharides, but also nucleic acids and proteins. They begin as a random collection of independent free-floating, planktonic bacteria, which attach to a surface. The bacteria then become densely adherent and begin to form microcolonies. When bacterial density reaches a critical point, inter-bacterial cross-talk triggers a phenomenon known as "quorum sensing." Quorum sensing in turn initiates a cascade of gene and protein expression that ultimately leads to the biofilm phenotype. This phenotype is marked by formation of towers, layers, and water channels (to allow diffusion of nutrients) that comprise individual bacteria demonstrating functional heterogeneity within the community. The mortar for these structures consists of a bacterially extruded exopolysaccharide matrix, which makes up as much as 90% of the biofilm [17]. Single cells or small emboli of cells can produce another biofilm elsewhere when dissociated from the matrix by shear forces and active molecular biofilm processes. A simple analogy for a bacterial biofilm compares free floating plankton in the ocean to planktonic bacteria, and a coral reef to a bacterial biofilm.

It is important to note that biofilms have a heterogeneous morphology, because the biofilm phenotype is highly dependent on the surrounding environment. Bacterial biofilms that have formed on mucosal surfaces have been referred to as *mucosal biofilms* [7], as they are bacterial biofilms that have formed in the special environment of ciliated mucosa, an area expected to have some protection from biofilm formation. Mucosal biofilms will have unique cascades of gene expression and different microenvironments compared with biofilms that form on inert surfaces, because they will be modified by the host inflammatory response and may incorporate some of the host proteins, waste products, and cellular debris. Furthermore, the pathogenicity of biofilm formation may ultimately depend on the causal bacterium.

Staphylococcus aureus and *Pseudomonas aeruginosa* are known pathogens in both upper and lower airway disease. Both organisms are able to produce biofilms. *Staphylococcus aureus* is known to produce exotoxins that act as superantigens to specific immunity. Some believe the superantigens to play a role in the development of CRS in certain individuals [18, 19]. *Pseudomonas aeruginosa* is a Gram-negative bacterium that is frequently associated with long-term upper and lower airway disease. Gram-negative bacterial CRS is particularly recalcitrant in nature. Gram-negative sinusitis, specifically *Pseudomonas*, has been studied extensively in the past, and previous studies have noted an intense transmucosal injury, which is far more intense than experimental sinusitis using other bacteria associated with sinusitis, such as *Streptococcus pneumoniae* [20]. Inflammation and tissue destruction is particularly robust in infectious *pseudomonas*, because secreted enzymes are enhanced by the body's immune defense mechanisms (i. e., neutrophil degradation products) [21]. In these patients, *Pseudomonas aeruginosa* is consistently cultured, yet appropriate antibiotic therapy is often unable to eradicate what appears to be the offending organism. This could be explained by the presence of bacterial biofilms.

Methods of Antibiotic Resistance

As mentioned earlier, biofilms can evade host defenses and demonstrate decreased susceptibility to systemic and local antibiotic therapy [17, 22]. One method of resistance may be the biofilm coat of exopolysaccharide alginate that decreases penetration of antibiotics into the biofilm. However, concentration studies reveal that antibiotics can diffuse efficiently into biofilms, thus contradicting this theory [17]. Water comprises a large portion of the biofilm mass and allows for diffusion of antibiotics down water channels into the core regions of the biofilm. Another proposed method of resistance argues that antibiotics may be deactivated or neutralized when the positively charged antibiotics interact with the negatively charged polymers of the biofilm matrix. A third theory suggests that bacteria might be forced into a nongrowing state in the basal layers of the biofilm due to the accrual of waste products and depletion of needed substrates. This will result in a state of suspended animation that confers relative resistance to antibiotics, because most antibiotics work only on dividing bacteria. Finally, osmotic forces from changing nutrient gradients could create a stress response that results in fewer porins in the bacterial cell wall. This could lead to decreased diffusion of antibiotics into the bacterial cytoplasm. In reality, it is likely that a combination of mechanisms contributes to the hearty antibiotic resistance to biofilms.

Certain antibiotics may potentially induce biofilm formation in some bacteria at subtherapeutic doses. Hoffman et al. demonstrated the induction of biofilm formation in *P. aeruginosa* and *Escherichia coli* secondary to subtherapeutic concentrations

of aminoglycoside antibiotics [23]. Certain *Pseudomonas* may have a gene called the aminoglycoside response regulator (arr) that contributes to this biofilm-specific aminoglycoside resistance. This could be a potential source of bacterial resistance in CRS, especially in those individuals undergoing tobramycin irrigation at subtherapeutic concentrations.

Mucociliary Clearance and Biofilms

Normal airway mucociliary clearance is a critical host defense mechanism that clears the upper airways. This defense mechanism is dependent on the production of mucus and the coordinated beating of ciliated cells. Cilia continually beat at a baseline frequency to sweep debris out the respiratory system for elimination through the GI tract. It is likely that impairment of ciliary motility is important not only in the pathogenesis of CRS, but also asthma and female infertility [24, 25]. Insults such as acute viral and bacterial rhinosinusitis affect mucociliary function and ultimately allow the bacteria to gain a foothold and form a mucosal biofilm, and subsequent CRS.

Treatments for Biofilm-Associated CRS

Various techniques have been evaluated for their capability to manage and control biofilms in environmental science. Materials and coatings to help reduce initial cell adhesion to surfaces and a variety of treatments aimed at decreasing or destroying already formed biofilms, including heat, sonication, chemical treatments, antibiotics, quorum-sensing analogs, cleaning regimens, low-power laser, and lectins [26–31]. Furthermore, new investigations into biological control agents such as protozoa and bacteriophages to reduce biofilms have shown promise [32]. However, the applicability of these treatments to biofilm infections in humans is either questionable or downright prohibitive. Hence, the quest for a reliable means of eliminating biofilm infections in humans is ongoing.

Although CRS may have many independent inciting factors, including bacterial infection (whether planktonic or biofilm-mediated), anatomic abnormality, fungal infection, allergy, genetics, and reactive airways, the mainstays of therapy remain the same: antimicrobial and anti-inflammatory agents combined with surgical ventilation. Surgical ventilation of infected sinuses could be the optimal therapy for combating bacterial biofilms in patients with CRS. Reventilation of the sinuses increases oxygen tension, mechanically disrupts biofilms, and assists with the host's natural defenses to clear infection.

Other treatments for biofilms include novel methods of antibiotic therapy, such as low-dose macrolide therapy. Despite treatment with doses of macrolide that are far below the established minimal inhibitory concentration for *Pseudomonas*, some investigators have demonstrated some success in decreasing biofilm formation [33, 34]. However, the mechanism behind this decrease has yet to be elucidated.

Future directions for biofilm-associated CRS include investigations into the nature of the biofilm at the cellular and molecular levels. Specific molecular targets of the biofilm lifecycle continue to show promise. Interrupting attachment phases by disrupting the type IV pili of *Pseudomonas* is one such potential avenue for therapy [35]. Disrupting quorum sensing could be the most unique and specific target for biofilm therapy. It is possible to interrupt quorum sensing through a variety of novel mechanisms, including the substitution of furanones [36] and the enzymatic cleavage of acyl-homoserine lactones (one of the quorum sensing signals). This shows the promising potential to use quorum-sensing signals as molecular targets to treat biofilms [37].

Bacterial biofilms still evade host defenses and cause disease, despite increasing knowledge and advancements in treatment for these tenacious infections. Biofilms are invariably responsible for at least some recalcitrant CRS. Thus, we should continue to investigate biofilms in CRS and explore potential therapies to develop novel means of therapeutic intervention.

Take-Home Pearls

- Bacterial biofilms are three-dimensional aggregates of bacteria encased in secreted exopolysaccharides that are strongly resistant to host immunity defense and antibiotics.
- Approximately 30% of the bacteria isolated from patients undergoing endoscopic sinus surgery for CRS form biofilms.
- Possible methods of the resistance of bacterial biofilms to antibiotics include:
  - Decreased penetration of antibiotics into the biofilm
  - Deactivation or neutralization of the antibiotic
  - Quiescent bacteria in the biofilm resist antibiotics that only eradicate actively dividing bacteria
  - Decreased porins in the bacterial cell wall that inhibit diffusion of the antibiotic
- Aminoglycosides at subtherapeutic concentrations can induce biofilm formation.
- The mainstays of therapy for biofilm-associated CRS remain antimicrobial and anti-inflammatory agents combined with surgical ventilation.
- Targeting the biofilm life-cycle through interruption of the attachment phase and quorum sensing are likely avenues of future therapy.
- New therapies directed at biofilm prevention and irradication are needed.

References

1. Gliklich, R.E. and R. Metson, *The health impact of chronic sinusitis in patients seeking otolaryngologic care.* Otolaryngol Head Neck Surg, 1995. 113(1): p. 104–9
2. Murphy, M.P., et al., *Health care utilization and cost among adults with chronic rhinosinusitis enrolled in a health maintenance organization.* Otolaryngol Head Neck Surg, 2002. 127(5): p. 367–76
3. Osguthorpe, J.D., *Adult rhinosinusitis: diagnosis and management.* Am Fam Physician, 2001. 63(1): p. 69–76
4. Khalid, A.N., S.A. Quraishi, and D.W. Kennedy, *Long-term quality of life measures after functional endoscopic sinus surgery.* Am J Rhinol, 2004. 18(3): p. 131–6
5. Amorena, B., et al., *Antibiotic susceptibility assay for Staphylococcus aureus in biofilms developed in vitro.* J Antimicrob Chemother, 1999. 44(1): p. 43–55
6. Potera, C., *Forging a link between biofilms and disease.* Science, 1999. 283(5409): p. 1837, 1839
7. Post, J.C., et al., *The role of biofilms in otolaryngologic infections.* Curr Opin Otolaryngol Head Neck Surg, 2004. 12(3): p. 185–90
8. Cryer, J., et al., *Evidence of bacterial biofilms in human chronic sinusitis.* ORL J Otorhinolaryngol Relat Spec, 2004. 66(3): p. 155–8
9. Perloff, J.R. and J.N. Palmer, *Evidence of bacterial biofilms in a rabbit model of sinusitis.* Am J Rhinol, 2005. 19(1): p. 1–6
10. Ferguson, B.J. and D.B. Stolz, *Demonstration of biofilm in human bacterial chronic rhinosinusitis.* Am J Rhinol, 2005. 19(5): p. 452–7
11. Ramadan, H.H., J.A. Sanclement, and J.G. Thomas, *Chronic rhinosinusitis and biofilms.* Otolaryngol Head Neck Surg, 2005. 132(3): p. 414–7
12. Sanderson, A.R., J.G. Leid, and D. Hunsaker, *Bacterial biofilms on the sinus mucosa of human subjects with chronic rhinosinusitis.* Laryngoscope, 2006. 116(7): p. 1121–6
13. Bendouah, Z., et al., *Biofilm formation by Staphylococcus aureus and Pseudomonas aeruginosa is associated with an unfavorable evolution after surgery for chronic sinusitis and nasal polyposis.* Otolaryngol Head Neck Surg, 2006. 134(6): p. 991–6
14. Costerton, J.W., P.S. Stewart, and E.P. Greenberg, *Bacterial biofilms: a common cause of persistent infections.* Science, 1999. 284(5418): p. 1318–22
15. Ehrlich, G.D., et al., *Mucosal biofilm formation on middle-ear mucosa in the chinchilla model of otitis media.* JAMA, 2002. 287(13): p. 1710–5
16. Mah, T.F. and G.A. O'Toole, *Mechanisms of biofilm resistance to antimicrobial agents.* Trends Microbiol, 2001. 9(1): p. 34–9
17. Stewart, P.S. and J.W. Costerton, *Antibiotic resistance of bacteria in biofilms.* Lancet, 2001. 358(9276): p. 135–8
18. Bachert, C., P. Gevaert, and P. van Cauwenberge, *Staphylococcus aureus superantigens and airway disease.* Curr Allergy Asthma Rep, 2002. 2(3): p. 252–8
19. Tripathi, A., et al., *Immunoglobulin E to staphylococcal and streptococcal toxins in patients with chronic sinusitis/nasal polyposis.* Laryngoscope, 2004. 114(10): p. 1822–6
20. Bolger, W.E., et al., *Gram negative sinusitis: a bacteriologic and histologic study in rabbits.* Am J Rhinol, 1997. 11(1): p. 15–25
21. Ratjen, F. and G. Doring, *Cystic fibrosis.* Lancet, 2003. 361(9358): p. 681–9
22. Davies, D.G., et al., *The involvement of cell-to-cell signals in the development of a bacterial biofilm.* Science, 1998. 280(5361): p. 295–8
23. Hoffman, L.R., et al., *Aminoglycoside antibiotics induce bacterial biofilm formation.* Nature, 2005. 436(7054): p. 1171–5
24. Talbot, P., et al., *Identification of cigarette smoke components that alter functioning of hamster (Mesocricetus auratus) oviducts in vitro.* Biol Reprod, 1998. 58(4): p. 1047–53

25. Wyatt, T.A., et al., *Regulation of ciliary beat frequency by both PKA and PKG in bovine airway epithelial cells.* Am J Physiol, 1998. 275(4 Pt 1): p. L827–35

26. Hammer, B.K. and B.L. Bassler, *Quorum sensing controls biofilm formation in Vibrio cholerae.* Mol Microbiol, 2003. **50**(1): p. 101–4

27. Nandakumar, K., et al., *Recolonization of laser-ablated bacterial biofilm.* Biotechnol Bioeng, 2004. 85(2): p. 185–9

28. Oulahal-Lagsir, N., et al., *Ultrasonic methodology coupled to ATP bioluminescence for the non-invasive detection of fouling in food processing equipment – validation and application to a dairy factory.* J Appl Microbiol, 2000. 89(3): p. 433–41

29. Parkar, S.G., S.H. Flint, and J.D. Brooks, *Evaluation of the effect of cleaning regimes on biofilms of thermophilic bacilli on stainless steel.* J Appl Microbiol, 2004. 96(1): p. 110–6

30. Sheehan, E., et al., *Adhesion of Staphylococcus to orthopaedic metals, an in vivo study.* J Orthop Res, 2004. **22**(1): p. 39–43

31. Simoes, M., et al., *Studies on the behaviour of Pseudomonas fluorescens biofilms after Ortho-phthalaldehyde treatment.* Biofouling, 2003. 19(3): p. 151–7

32. Kadouri, D. and G.A. O'Toole, *Susceptibility of biofilms to Bdellovibrio bacteriovorus attack.* Appl Environ Microbiol, 2005. 71(7): p. 4044–51

33. Gillis, R.J. and B.H. Iglewski, *Azithromycin retards Pseudomonas aeruginosa biofilm formation.* J Clin Microbiol, 2004. 42(12): p. 5842–5

34. Wozniak, D.J. and R. Keyser, *Effects of subinhibitory concentrations of macrolide antibiotics on Pseudomonas aeruginosa.* Chest, 2004. 125(2 Suppl): p. 62S–69S; quiz 69S.

35. Gallant, C.V., et al., *Common beta-lactamases inhibit bacterial biofilm formation.* Mol Microbiol, 2005. 58(4): p. 1012–24

36. Koch, B., et al., *The LuxR receptor: the sites of interaction with quorum-sensing signals and inhibitors.* Microbiology, 2005. 151(Pt 11): p. 3589–602

37. Dong, Y.H., et al., *Quenching quorum-sensing-dependent bacterial infection by an N-acyl homoserine lactonase.* Nature, 2001. 411(6839): p. 813–7

Chapter 21

Allergic Rhinitis

John H. Krouse

Core Messages

- Allergic rhinitis is a common upper respiratory illness that is associated with other upper and lower respiratory illnesses, including rhinosinusitis, otitis media, and asthma.
- Allergic rhinitis is present in both children and adults, and is accompanied by impairments in sleep, daytime function, and quality of life.
- Classification systems for allergic rhinitis such as ARIA are useful in modeling the disease and in guiding specific approaches to treatment.
- Treatments for allergic rhinitis fall into three categories: allergen avoidance, pharmacotherapy, and desensitization immunotherapy.
- Pharmacological treatments include: antihistamines, decongestants, mast cell stabilizers, corticosteroids, leukotriene receptor antagonists, and topical anticholinergics.
- Considering allergic rhinitis to be a chronic inflammatory disease that varies in severity and persistence allows rational therapy and appropriate and effective use of treatment options.

Contents

Introduction

Allergic rhinitis is a common clinical condition that affects both children and adults. Patients' complaints of nasal and non-nasal symptoms can range from mildly bothersome to severe, and can significantly impact their quality of life, sleep, and daytime function. The term *rhinitis* implies an inflammatory illness of the nasal mucosa that can be triggered by a variety of stimuli, both allergic and non-allergic. Allergic rhinitis is an atopic disease, representing an expression of IgE-mediated immunity in which patients respond to otherwise innocuous substances to which they have the genetic predisposition to develop hypersensitization. Allergic rhinitis is also strongly associated with other comorbid disorders, such as conjunctivitis, acute and chronic rhinosinusitis, otitis media with effusion, and asthma.

It is essential to realize that allergic rhinitis (AR) is a disease characterized by acute and chronic inflammation. Inflammation can be episodic or intermittent, as in seasonal allergic rhinitis, or can be ongoing and persistent, as in perennial allergic rhinitis. The recognition that persistent inflammation is a hallmark of moderate to severe AR has led to a proposed model of this disease based on the chronicity and temporal course of symptoms rather than the type of triggering stimulus. This model, referred to as ARIA – Allergic Rhinitis and Its Impact on Asthma – will be discussed in detail in this chapter, and represents an international consensus approach to the diagnosis and treatment of the patient with AR.

This chapter will review the traditional and proposed classification systems that are used to frame AR. It will also discuss the pathophysiology of AR, and will present strategies for its diagnosis and treatment.

Classifications of Allergic Rhinitis

Rhinitis is generally classified into one of two broad categories: allergic rhinitis, nasal inflammation due to IgE-mediated, Type I hypersensitivity; and non-allergic rhinitis, which is usually presumed to be irritative or non-immune-mediated. In addition, a third category, *mixed rhinitis,* is often included to describe nasal inflammation that shares characteristics and triggers that are both immune and non-immune. The present chapter will focus on AR, although the reader is referred to other sources for a further discussion of other forms of rhinitis [1].

Allergic Rhinitis

Allergic rhinitis (AR) refers to an inflammatory condition or the nasal mucosa that is triggered by an IgE-mediated Type I immunologic response that occurs in a patient who has the genetic predisposition to develop this type of immune response (atopy), and who has been sensitized to specific substances (antigens) that can provoke a hypersensitivity-type response. The immediate phase of this response is mediated by immunoglobulin E (IgE), and rapid symptomatic expression occurs primarily through the effects of the vasoactive amine, histamine. In addition to this rapid expression of symptoms, a more prolonged and delayed response also occurs in AR that is mediated through the influence of a number of humoral and cellular factors. Traditional schemes for the classification of AR have proposed two relatively discrete categories based upon the time of exposure and development of symptoms, and attributed to separate classes of antigens: seasonal allergic rhinitis (SAR), which occurs with the predictable seasonal increases that are seen with environmental antigens such as pollens and outdoor molds; and perennial allergic rhinitis (PAR), which involves exposure to antigens that are present to some degree throughout the year, such as cat and dog dander, dust mites, cockroaches, and indoor molds [2].

Seasonal Versus Perennial Allergic Rhinitis

Three distinct periods of annual variation in outdoor antigens are generally noted in most temporal climates. These periods correspond to the seasons during which various plant families pollenate, and closely predict the variation in patient symptoms that can be seen in SAR. These seasons are often distinct, with tree pollen commonly present in the spring, grass pollen in the summer, and weed pollen in the fall. In addition, mold spores are often present in the warmer months, and can be present throughout the year in tropical and sub-tropical climates

In contrast, patients with PAR tend to complain of nasal symptoms throughout most of the year, although these symptoms may fluctuate in severity. While perennial antigens are present in the environment on a daily basis, levels of these antigens can vary with weather patterns, use of indoor heating and air-conditioning, ambient humidity, and so forth. In addition, many patients have both seasonal and perennial triggers to their AR, so that seasonal exacerbations of PAR are commonly seen. In addition, non-allergic irritants can also cause fluctuations in allergic symptoms, since many patients have elements of both allergic and non-allergic rhinitis.

ARIA Classification of Allergic Rhinitis

While the system of classifying AR on the basis of type of exposure and presence of seasonal variability has been used effectively for managing patients with AR for many years, there

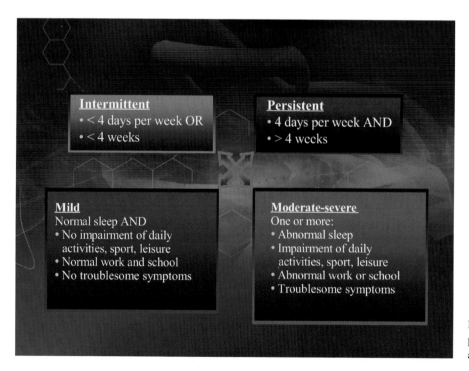

Fig. 21.1 Allergic Rhinitis and Its Impact on Asthma (ARIA) classification of allergic rhinitis [25]

are issues related to this dichotomous classification system that have questioned its utility. For example, in warmer, tropical or sub-tropical climates, pollen seasons can be prolonged and indiscrete. The generalized presence of pollen can cause extended periods of symptoms that appear to be perennial, yet are due to antigens traditionally felt to be "seasonal". This "perennial pollenosis" has led experts to question whether the chronicity of symptoms is of greater importance than the type of antigen trigger.

In 2000, a consensus meeting of physicians from various disciplines met to consider a modified approach to the diagnosis and treatment of AR. This approach, which is based upon the persistence and severity of symptoms of AR, has led to the publication of the ARIA Guidelines (Allergic Rhinitis and Its Impact on Asthma) [3]. These guidelines have been accepted by regulatory agencies in Europe as guidance for the consideration of pharmacotherapeutic treatments for AR. The classification of AR from the ARIA report is similar to that used in various guidelines for the classification and treatment of asthma.

The ARIA guidelines offer four diagnostic categories that are used to diagnose and stage AR:

1. Mild intermittent
2. Moderate-severe intermittent
3. Mild persistent
4. Moderate-severe persistent (Fig. 21.1)

In ARIA, the temporal course of symptoms is divided into two categories: intermittent and persistent. Intermittent AR involves a period of symptoms lasting less than 4 days during any week or less than 4 weeks over the course of a year. Persistent AR, in contrast, involves periods of symptoms lasting more than 4 days a week and occurring for more than 4 weeks a year. In addition, ARIA describes two levels of severity that are based on the physician's assessment of the impact of symptoms on daily function, sleep, and quality of life: mild and moderate-severe. Mild AR involves symptoms that are bothersome to the patient, but are not so severe that they result in significant impact on sleep, daily function, or quality of life. Moderate-severe AR is not only qualitatively different from mild AR, its symptoms adversely impact daytime function, sleep quality, and quality of life. These four categories of temporality and severity will lead to differential treatment recommendations, which will be discussed later in this chapter.

Epidemiology of Allergic Rhinitis

Allergic rhinitis is a common illness that is seen in all parts of the world. Studies suggest that the prevalence of AR is approximately 10–20% of the adult population [4, 5], and may be higher in the pediatric population. While AR can present at any age, most patients first complain of symptoms in childhood, often before the age of 10. The peak symptomatic period appears to be between 10 and 40 years. In addition, it appears that the prevalence of AR is also increasing, with an almost two-fold rise being noted over the past two decades [6]. The economic burden of AR is also significant, with annual direct costs estimated to be in the range of US\$ 2–5 billion [7]. In addition, US\$ 6 billion was spent on prescription medications for the treatment of AR [8]. Worldwide treatment of rhinitis would certainly account for a significant increment of these US figures.

In addition to the financial costs of AR, adverse impact on quality of life and daytime function is severe. Patients with AR complain of cognitive and psychomotor impairment, with impact on daytime alertness, vigilance, concentration, and sleep. These findings are seen in both adults and children [9, 10].

Pathophysiology of Allergic Rhinitis

Allergic rhinitis represents an inflammatory disease of the nasal mucosa. The pathophysiological mechanism in AR involves a type-I immediate hypersensitivity reaction, mediated through T-helper 2 cells (Th2). Individuals with AR must first have the underlying genetic predisposition to develop allergic diseases, a condition that is referred to as *atopy*. In these individuals, there is an upregulated response of the Th2 population that results in sensitization to otherwise innocuous antigens. The recognition of these antigens as foreign stimulates an immune response, whereby exposure to these agents, known as *allergens,* leads to sensitization and memory of immunity in both T and B lymphocytes. In addition, IgE antibodies are produced that are specific to these individual allergens, and are bound to the surface of mast cells in the nasal mucosa, where they maintain surveillance for re-exposure to these antigens.

The acute allergic response in AR is initiated when individuals who have been previously sensitized to an allergen again come into contact with this allergen. Mast cell-bound IgE will then bind these antigens, resulting in cross-linking of adjacent IgE molecules and degranulation of mast cells. This process of degranulation results in the release of preformed pro-inflammatory mediators such as histamine. Histamine release is the major factor responsible for initiating the allergic response, and in stimulating the local and generalized symptoms seen with acute allergen exposure [11]. Histamine then binds to specific histamine (H1) receptors on the surface of target cells, resulting in leakage of plasma in the tissues, edema, and increased mucus production, and other direct inflammatory events [12]. Histamine and other mediators also stimulate nasal sensory fibers, resulting in irritation, sneezing, and itching. Symptoms of AR occur rapidly, within 5–10 min of exposure.

In addition to these immediate effects, delayed symptoms also occur in many patients with AR. This "late-phase response" can lead to symptoms that have their onset at 2–4 h after exposure. Cells such as eosinophils and basophils and soluble mediators such as leukotrienes are important mediators in this delayed response. The allergic response in patients with AR is therefore biphasic, with both immediate and delayed components that are involved in the expression of symptoms.

Diagnosis of the Patient with Allergic Rhinitis

Patients with AR classically present with a cluster of four nasal symptoms, including sneezing, nasal itching, rhinorrhea, and congestion. In addition, they will often complain of other respiratory and ocular symptoms, such as conjunctival redness, tearing, aural blockage, and palatal itching. Patients with AR will often report other allergic diseases such as eczema, asthma, or urticaria. Upper respiratory symptoms such as anosmia and facial pain do occur, but are more commonly seen in combination with acute and chronic rhinosinusitis.

In patients with SAR, symptoms parallel the rise and fall in pollen counts during allergic seasons. Seasonal changes in patients with persistent AR also suggest a seasonal component to the patient's disease. In patients with PAR, symptoms persist throughout most or all of the year. Among these patients, nasal blockage and post-nasal drainage are often more common than sneezing and itching seen among patients with SAR [13]. In addition, the symptoms of chronic rhinosinusitis and non-allergic rhinitis can often overlap symptoms among patients with AR.

The primary component of the patient work-up that will suggest a diagnosis of AR is the patient history. A thorough history is invaluable in guiding the physical examination and testing process among patients with suspected AR, and allows the physician to recommend therapy with confidence. Since AR usually begins in childhood, patients with AR will often report allergic symptoms that began early in life. Young children may not have symptoms of AR, but may have experienced skin allergies, eczema, or food intolerances as infants and toddlers. Respiratory allergy, both AR and asthma, generally present later in childhood, once IgE levels begin to rise at around age 5. This "allergic march" is commonly seen in atopic patients, and its history increases the likelihood that a patient's current symptoms of rhinitis also have an allergic basis. Patients with AR will often be able to identify exposures that incite symptoms; however, not all patients are aware of these triggers. In addition, AR is a disease that has a strong genetic influence. Since patients with AR must have the genetic predisposition and ability to develop an allergic response, it is common for them to have one or both parents with a similar history.

The physical examination of the patient suspected of having AR begins with an inspection of the face for signs of puffiness, edema, asymmetry, or infra-orbital discoloration (allergic shiners). The eyes are examined for conjunctival irritation or erythema. Otoscopy is then used to assess appearance of the tympanic membrane, including mobility, color, thickness, and translucence, as well as the presence of serous or purulent effusion.

The external framework of the nose is then examined for deformity, asymmetry, or other evidence of trauma. A transverse crease in the mid portion of the nasal dorsum is often seen among allergic patients from repeated rubbing of the nose. The internal nose is then examined, with an evaluation of the position and appearance of the nasal septum. The size and appearance of the inferior turbinates is assessed, looking for hypertrophy and mucosal paleness and edema. Among patients with AR, the nasal mucosa is often edematous, resulting in a boggy bluish appearance on examination. In patients with severe AR, the nasal mucosa can have an almost white appearance. The presence and quality of nasal secretions is then assessed. Among patients with AR, secretions may be copious, thin and watery, or thick and tenacious. The presence of nasal polyps is also assessed.

After completion of the nasal examination, an assessment of the oral cavity and oropharynx is undertaken to examine for signs of lymphoid hypertrophy and "cobblestoning" of the posterior pharyngeal wall.

As a complement to the physical examination, allergy testing may be useful in selected patients to assist in achieving a complete diagnosis. It can often be difficult from history and physical examination alone to determine whether rhinitis symptoms are due to allergy. Testing can be performed to assist with the diagnosis, as well as to allow a discussion of avoidance techniques for offending allergens. Antigen-specific allergy testing can be conducted through both skin testing and in vitro techniques. Skin testing can be performed using prick/puncture methods or with intradermal tests [14]. Allergens chosen for testing are selected from common antigens present in the patient's immediate geographic region.

Prick tests are the most commonly used technique for antigen-specific allergy testing. A small volume of each antigen to be tested is introduced through a puncture into the superficial epidermis. Exposure to an antigen on the skin in a sensitized patient results in erythema and induration at the site of testing. The size of the reaction on the skin is used to grade the allergic response. Intradermal testing, in which a small amount of antigen is injected into the superficial dermis, and in vitro tests, often referred to as RAST (radio-allergosorbent test), can also be used to assess allergic sensitivity.

Treatment of the Patient with Allergic Rhinitis

Treatment approaches for the patient with AR are traditionally based on a foundation of three strategies:
1. Allergen avoidance
2. Pharmacotherapy
3. Immunotherapy (Fig. 21.1).

Allergen Avoidance

In patients with AR, avoidance of sensitized antigens can promote better treatment efficacy with fewer symptoms and improved quality of life and function. While environmental control strategies can be useful, they are often difficult for patients to implement effectively. Measures that can reduce exposure to dust mite antigen include the use of allergen-resistant covers for mattresses and pillows and high-efficiency filtration (HEPA filters). Removal of carpeting and curtains has been advocated, although this approach is both costly and of questionable benefit [15].

Several studies have examined the effect of reducing exposure to perennial antigens such as dust mite and cat dander. In a recent study, young children whose family instituted aggressive methods of reducing dust mite antigen were less likely to become sensitized to dust mite antigen over time than were children of families not following these techniques [16].

Another important element of allergen avoidance is the elimination of pets from the environment for patients who are sensitized to them. Cat allergy is among the most potent sensi-

21

tivities, and is associated with both AR and asthma. Families are often reluctant to remove pets from the home, resulting in ongoing exposure to individuals with symptomatic disease. Even when a pet is removed from the home environment, the antigen can persist for months.

While it can be difficult to avoid pollen due to its outdoor location, patients with SAR can perform outdoor activities in the evening during pollen seasons since pollen is released into the environment in the early morning. These patients should also keep their windows closed and use air conditioning and filtration to keep pollen from entering the home and car. Outdoor pets should be washed on entering the home, as they can transport pollen into the home on their fur.

Pharmacotherapy

The use of pharmacotherapy is the mainstay of treatment for the majority of patients with AR. There is a large range of medications and medication classes that are used to treat AR, and these medications vary in their efficacy, mechanisms of action, and safety profiles. It is important to be familiar with the actions and adverse effects of these agents in order to best treat the patient with AR. Table 21.1 offers a comparison of various classes of medications for rhinitis and their relative efficacy.

Antihistamines

Antihistamines are the most frequently used class of medications for the treatment of AR. Antihistamines work at the level of the H_1 receptor in the nasal mucosa. Antihistamines bind to, block, and deactivate these H_1 receptors, which are found on the surface of target cells in the nose. Antihistamines have been in use since the 1940s. Early antihistamines included drugs such as diphenhydramine, and were effective in reducing symptoms of AR. Current antihistamines also have potent antihistaminic effect, yet they suffer performance impairment at recommended doses. These newer antihistamines currently include loratadine, fexofenadine, cetirizine, desloratadine, ebastine, and levocetirizine. In addition, antihistamines can be administered topically for ocular and nasal use, and have little or no sedatory effect when given in this manner. These agents include azelastine, epinastine, and olopatadine.

The primary role of antihistamines in the treatment of the patient with AR is in relieving the acute, histamine-mediated symptoms of allergic rhinitis, including nasal and ocular itching, sneezing, and rhinorrhea. They are therefore often used as first-line therapy in patients with AR. Antihistamines have little effect on nasal congestion and blockage, however; they are not appropriate for single-agent therapy in the AR patient in whom nasal stuffiness is a primary symptom. In this group of patients, antihistamines are frequently used with other classes of medications. Agents such as antihistamine/decongestant combination products are frequently prescribed in this setting, as are intranasal corticosteroids, either with or without antihistamines.

Decongestants

Oral and topical vasoconstrictors are effective medications for the treatment of nasal congestion. Vasoconstrictors are α-adrenergic receptor agonists that decrease venous engorgement in the cavernous sinusoids found primarily in the inferior turbinates. Both oral and topical decongestants are generally well tolerated, although patients may experience adverse sys-

Table 21.1 Medications for allergic rhinitis: effects on symptoms

Agent	Sneezing	Itching	Congestion	Rhinorrhea	Eye Symptoms
Oral antihistamines	+++	+++	+/−	++	+++
Nasal antihistamines	++	++	++	+	−
Intranasal corticosteroids	++	++	+++	++	+
Leukotriene modifiers	+	+	+	+	+
Oral decongestants	−	−	+++	−	−
Nasal decongestants	−	−	+++	−	−
Nasal mast cell stabilizers	+	+	+/−	+	−
Topical anticholinergics	−	−	−	+++	−

+++ = marked benefit; ++ = substantial benefit; + = some benefit; +/− = questionable benefit; − = no benefit

temic effects with decongestants when administered through either route.

Common topical decongestants include naphazoline, phenylephrine, oxymetazoline, and xylometazoline. These medications promote a vigorous vasoconstrictive effect in the nose, which increases airflow and relieves the symptoms of congestion. While topical decongestants show good efficacy, they are associated with tachyphylaxis, even with short-term use. They are therefore recommended for only 3–5 days of use.

In addition to topical medications, oral decongestants are also used for the treatment of nasal obstruction in patients with AR. Commonly used topical decongestants include phenylephrine and pseudo-ephedrine. Oral decongestants are effective in relieving nasal congestion, yet they are associated with significant adverse events, especially in sensitive patients. These adverse effects can include arrhythmias, hypertension, irritability, jitteriness, nervousness, urinary retention, and insomnia. Because of these risks, patients with uncontrolled hypertension and cardiovascular disease should avoid these medications.

Mast Cell Stabilizers

Cromolyn sodium (sodium cromoglycate) is available in a topical form for the treatment of the symptoms of AR. It is administered as a nasal spray, and functions to stabilize mast cell membranes in the nasal mucosa. Through this mechanism, cromolyn sodium inhibits the degranulation of mast cells, and thereby blocks the release of histamine from activated mast cells into the nose. Cromolyn sodium is ineffective once histamine has been released from mast cells, since it does not interfere with histamine's effect on the nasal mucosa. The action of this medication is therefore prophylactic, and it must therefore be used prior to antigen exposure to produce maximum benefit.

Corticosteroids

Corticosteroids are potent anti-inflammatory medications that can be used either systemically or topically for treating patients with AR. Under current guidelines, topical intranasal corticosteroids (INS) are recommended as primary treatment for patients with nasal congestion and with moderate to severe AR [3], in part based on research that shows these agents to be more efficacious than antihistamines [17]. INS are being used with increasing frequency for the treatment of AR. There are a number of preparations that are available for use, including flunisolide, beclomethasone, budesonide, fluticasone propionate, mometasone furoate, triamcinolone acetonide, and two new agents, ciclesonide and fluticasone furoate. Efficacy is similar among all agents of the class, although there is some variability in systemic absorption noted among agents.

Intranasal corticosteroids as a class are generally free of adverse nasal and systemic effects. They are well tolerated among most patients [18]. Agents such as mometasone furoate and fluticasone propionate have been shown in prospective trials to be free of growth suppression and suppression of the hypothalamic–pituitary–adrenal (HPA) axis.

Oral corticosteroids such as prednisone and methylprednisolone are also recommended under the ARIA guidelines in cases of severe and refractory AR. They are appropriate and effective in the treatment of these patients, and can generally be used for short periods of time with little adverse effect. The major risks of corticosteroids are dose-related and cumulative, and involve joint injury, osteoporosis, cataract formation, and other systemic effects. For this reason, when used for the treatment of AR, oral corticosteroids should be used at the lowest effective dose possible and for the shortest time period. Current guidelines recommend against using parenteral depot versions of corticosteroids due to unpredictable absorption, irreversibility once given, and a higher rate of adverse systemic effects.

Leukotriene Receptor Antagonists

Leukotriene receptor antagonists (LTRA) are effective in the treatment of SAR and PAR. LTRA include montelukast, zafirlukast, and pranlukast, although montelukast is the only agent approved for treatment of AR in the United States. Montelukast has been shown to relieve both the nasal and non-nasal symptoms of AR, and has a similar efficacy in the treatment of SAR to loratadine [19]. These agents have demonstrated anti-inflammatory effect in both the lower and upper airways, and can be used in children as young as to 6 months of age. LTRA may also have benefit in AR patients with nasal polyps.

Topical Anticholinergics

Anticholinergic medications block parasympathetic stimulation of the nasal mucosa, resulting in a decrease in the amount of nasal secretions and an increase in their tenacity. These medications have benefit in the treatment of copious, watery rhinorrhea, which is more often present in non-allergic or mixed rhinitis than it is in AR. The agent that is available for topical intranasal use is ipratropium bromide. It has minimal benefit in the treatment of AR, as it has no effect on histamine-mediated symptoms such as sneezing or itching, and no effect on nasal congestion. Its use would generally be limited to supplemental therapy with another agent.

Immunotherapy

The third strategy for treating the patient with AR involves the use of desensitization immunotherapy. Immunotherapy involves the subcutaneous (SC) or sublingual (SL) administration of antigens to which a patient is sensitive, generally in increasing doses. Both SC and SL immunotherapy are designed to decrease the systemic reactivity of the patient to those antigens, and to decrease the symptoms of AR. Immunotherapy has been shown to be an efficacious treatment strategy for patients with AR [20–22], and should be considered when patients have a poor response to pharmacotherapy and avoidance strategies.

With SC immunotherapy, low concentrations of antigen are injected once or twice a week over several years. Antigen

21

concentrations are increased over a period of several months to lessen adverse local and systemic effects, and then held stable over several years. SC immunotherapy is rarely accompanied by serious untoward reactions, and its safety has been well established [23].

With SL immunotherapy, antigen is delivered through the SL rather than the SC route, and European clinical trials have demonstrated its efficacy for the treatment of AR [21, 22]. SL immunotherapy appears to be very safe and is not associated with anaphylaxis, although mild local and systemic reactions have sometimes been seen.

ARIA-Based Treatment of Allergic Rhinitis

A consensus panel sponsored by the World Health Organization (WHO) has offered a rational approach to the diagnosis, classification, and treatment of AR. This panel has developed a model of AR based on the temporal course or chronicity of the symptoms of AR and the severity of the functional impairment of AR, and published this model as the ARIA Guidelines [3]. ARIA is an acronym that represents Allergic Rhinitis and Its Impact on Asthma, and offers treatment guidelines for AR that are similar to those implemented for the diagnosis and treatment of asthma. The ARIA guidelines argue that AR is an inflammatory disease of the upper airway, in the same way that asthma is an inflammatory disease of the lower airway. The ARIA guidelines depart from the traditional model of classifying AR as either SAR or PAR and describe AR through four distinct categories based upon the severity and chronicity of the disease.

The ARIA guidelines suggest a step-care approach to the treatment of the patient with AR (Fig. 21.2). All patients receive education and information regarding allergen avoidance. In mild intermittent AR, treatment can be initiated with an oral or topical nonsedating antihistamine, a topical mast cell stabilizer or an INS. In patients with mild, persistent AR, INS are considered controller medication and are to be used on a daily basis during persistent symptoms; topical antihistamines can be added for acute exacerbations. In moderate-to-severe intermittent AR, and in all patients with persistent AR, INS are recommended as primary treatment, with nonsedating antihistamines added for synergistic effect when necessary. In severe AR oral corticosteroids can be utilized for treatment of severe symptoms or acute exacerbations of persistent AR. Immunotherapy can also be used in patients with significant persistent symptoms to decrease sensitization and improve control. Research has shown that a treatment strategy based on the ARIA guidelines is more effective in controlling symptoms among patients with AR than a strategy that employs routine care [24].

Summary

Allergic rhinitis is a common upper respiratory illness. It is associated with other upper and lower respiratory illnesses, including rhinosinusitis, otitis media, and asthma. AR is present in both children and adults, and is accompanied by impairments in sleep, daytime function, and quality of life. It is important to accurately diagnose AR in patients with nasal symptoms, and to implement appropriate therapy to reduce symptoms and improve quality of life.

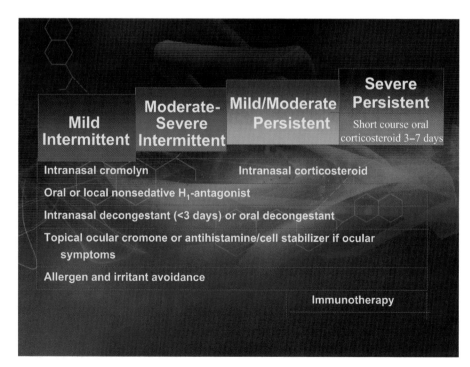

Fig. 21.2 Treatment plan for allergic rhinitis (ARIA) [3]

Classification systems for AR such as ARIA are useful in modeling the disease and in guiding specific approaches to treatment. The use of the ARIA guidelines has been shown to offer an advantage over non-guideline-based treatment approaches. Considering AR to be a chronic inflammatory disease that varies in severity and persistence allows rational therapy and appropriate and effective use of treatment options.

References

1. Krouse JH. Allergic and non-allergic rhinitis. In Bailey BJ, Johnson JT, Newlands SD, et al. (eds.) *Head and Neck Surgery – Otolaryngology*. Philadelphia, Lippincott Williams and Wilkins, 2006

2. Baroody FM. Allergic rhinitis: broader disease effects and implications for management. *Otolaryngol Head Neck Surg* 2003;128:616–631

3. Bousquet J, Van Cauwenberge P, Khaltaev N; ARIA Workshop Group; World Health Organization. Allergic rhinitis and its impact on asthma. *J Allergy Clin Immunol* 2001;108:S147–334

4. Settipane RA. Demographics and epidemiology of allergic and nonallergic rhinitis. *Allergy Asthma Proc* 2001;22:185–189

5. Naclerio R, Solomon W. Rhinitis and inhalant allergens. *JAMA* 1997;278:1842–1848

6. Wright AL. The epidemiology of the atopic child: who is at risk for what? *J Allergy Clin Immunol* 2004;113:S2–7

7. Davies RJ, Rusznak C, Devalia JL. Why is allergy increasing? – environmental factors. *Clin Exp Allergy* 1998;28[Suppl 6]:8–14

8. Reed SD, Lee TA, McCrory DC. The economic burden of allergic rhinitis: a critical evaluation of the literature. *Pharmacoeconomics* 2004;22:345–361

9. Stempel DA, Woolf R. The cost of treating allergic rhinitis. *Curr Allergy Asthma Rep* 2002;2:223–230

10. Juniper EF, Rorhbaugh T, Meltzer EO. A questionnaire to measure quality of life in adults with nocturnal allergic rhinoconjunctivitis. *J Allergy Clin Immunol* 2003;111:484–490

11. Krouse HJ, Davis JE, Krouse JH. Immune mediators in allergic rhinitis and sleep. *Otolaryngol Head Neck Surg* 2002;126:607–613

12. Gomez E, Corrado OH, Baldwin DL, et al. Direct in vivo evidence for mast cell degranulation during allergen-induced reactions in man. *J Allergy Clin Immunol* 1986;78:637–645

13. Krouse JH. Seasonal and perennial rhinitis. In Krouse JH, Chadwick SJ, Gordon BR, et al. (eds), *Allergy and Immunology: An Otolaryngic Approach*. Philadelphia: Lippincott, Williams and Wilkins, 2002

14. Krouse JH, Mabry RL. Skin testing for inhalant allergy 2003: current strategies. *Otolaryngol Head Neck Surg* 2003;129:S33–49

15. Terreehorst I, Hak E, Oosting AJ, et al. Evaluation of impermeable covers for bedding in patients with allergic rhinitis. *N Engl J Med* 2003;17:237–246

16. Arshad SH, Bateman B, Matthews SM. Primary prevention of asthma and atopy during childhood by allergen avoidance in infancy: a randomized controlled study. *Thorax* 2003;58:489–493

17. Stempel DA, Thomas M. Treatment of allergic rhinitis: an evidence-based evaluation of nasal corticosteroids versus nonsedating antihistamines. *Am J Manag Care* 1998;4:89–96

18. Benninger MS, Ahmed N, Marple BF, et al. The safety of intranasal steroids. *Otolaryngol Head Neck Surg* 2003;129:739–750

19. Nayak AS, Philip G, Lu S, et al. Efficacy and tolerability of montelukast alone or in combination with loratadine in seasonal allergic rhinitis: a multicenter, randomized, double-blind, placebo-controlled trial performed in the fall. *Ann Allergy Asthma Immunol* 2002;88:592–600

20. Calderon MA, Alves B, Jacobson M, et al. Allergen injection immunotherapy for seasonal allergic rhinitis. *Cochrane Database Syst Rev* 2007;(1): CD001936

21. Wilson DR, Torres Lima M, Durham SR. Sublingual immunotherapy for allergic rhinitis: systemic review and meta-analysis. *Allergy* 2005;60:4–12

22. Wilson DR, Torres LI, Durham SR. Sublingual immunotherapy for allergic rhinitis. *Cochrane Database Syst Rev* 2003;(2):CD002893

23. Hurst DS, Gordon BR, Fornadley JA, et al. Safety of home-based and office allergy immunotherapy: a multicenter prospective study. *Otolaryngol Head Neck Surg* 1999;121:553–561

24. Bousquet J, Lund VJ, van Cauwenberge P, et al. Implementation of guidelines for seasonal allergic rhinitis: a randomized controlled trial. *Allergy* 2003;58:724–726

25. Bousquet J, van Cauwenberge P, Khaltaev N. Executive Summary of the Workshop Report 7–10 December 1999, Geneva, Switzerland. *Allergy* 2002;841–855

21

Chapter 22

Fungal Rhinosinusitis

22

Chris de Souza and J. Peter Rodrigues

Core Messages

- Target sites for fungal infections include the fungal cell wall and cell membrane, DNA protein synthesis, and alterations in metabolism characteristics.
- Reversal of immunocompromise
- Treatment outcomes of immunocompromised patients suffering from AIDS and invasive aspergillosis infections improve when the infection is diagnosed, identified, and treated as early as possible.
- Those patients who have a fungal ball and are immunocompromised or who will need to be immunosuppressed will need to have surgery to clear out the diseased sinus. This is necessary, for if the fungal ball is allowed to reside in the sinus such patients run the risk of the fungal ball evolving into invasive sinusitis.
- It can be said that the goals of surgery are: removal of all mucin and fungal debris and permanent drainage and ventilation of the affected sinuses, while preserving the integrity of the underlying mucosa.
- Surgery should provide postoperative access to previously diseased areas. This is necessary to facilitate removal of debris and mucin in the clinic and allow inspection of areas of the nasal cavity in the clinic that would not have been possible to visualize under normal circumstances.
- All patients suffering from AFRS appear to need surgical debridement with removal of the fungi and nasal polyps. This is necessary to help initiate mucociliary clearance. At present AFRS is thought to be mucosal hypersensitivity directed at fungal antigens that are deposited on the mucosa of the upper respiratory tract.
- Removing the allergen would reduce the allergic response. This in turn would reduce the subsequent resulting edema. This would then help with the rapid clearance of the fungi by mucociliary clearance, which would be the ultimate goal of treatment of AFRS.
- The use of lipid-based amphotericin B may be a wise alternative for individuals unable to tolerate the nephrotoxicity associated with amphotericin B deoxycholate.

Contents

Introduction

Fungal diseases have emerged as major challenges for physicians, microbiologists and basic scientists. The incidence of mycotic infections and the number and diversity of pathogenic fungi have increased recently. It has now been discovered that immunocompetent as well as immuno-incompetent individuals can be at risk. Prognosis and therapy depend on the proper identification of the fungus causing infection as well as the treatment modalities given taking into account that the patient's immune system can be made competent if it is not. Fungi are ubiquitous organisms. They are commonly found in the respiratory tract including the nose and paranasal sinuses [18]. Microscopic colonization of the nose and paranasal sinuses can be found in the normal and in the diseased state as well. Fungi are eukaryotic organisms and they may exist as yeast or as molds. Yeast is unicellular and reproduces by budding, while molds coalesce as colonies of intertwined hyphae referred to as myceliae.

Of the greater than 50,000 fungal species only about 300 have been documented as playing a role in causing disease in humans. Potential fungal pathogens are confined to three major groups. They are:
1. Zygomycetes
2. *Aspergillus* species
3. Various dematiaceous genera.

There are two basic types of manifestations that comprise the entity "fungal rhinosinusitis." They are invasive and non-invasive manifestations. These maybe divided further into five distinct entities:
1. Acute invasive
2. Chronic invasive (granulomatous and nongranulomatous forms)
3. Fungal balls (mycetomas)
4. Saprophytic colonization
5. Allergic fungal rhinosinusitis.

These manifestations may overlap or progress from a non-invasive form to an invasive form if the immunologic status of the host changes.

The term acute invasive fungal rhinosinusitis is used when vascular invasion is the predominant histopathological feature and the duration of the disease is less than 4 weeks [10]. Usually such patients who present with acute invasive rhinosinusitis are immunologically compromised or immuno-incompetent. Chronic disease exists when the disease progresses gradually over 4 weeks. Some authors [7] have divided the chronic form into granulomatous and nongranulomatous forms.

Diagnosis of Invasive Fungal Rhinosinusitis

Potassium hydroxide (KOH) preps or calcoflour white stains should be obtained from material suspected to contain fungus. Fungal cultures themselves may take weeks to identify. Furthermore, fungal cultures may be positive in patients without invasive fungal infections being present. Necrotic material or biopsy samples should be evaluated through frozen sections. Histologic evidence of fungal invasion is the gold standard for the diagnosis of invasive fungal rhinosinusitis. It is important that a fungal culture be obtained as well to help identify the likely antifungal agents that can be used to treat the fungal infection.

Principles of Treatment of Fungal Infections

1. Reversal of the cause of immunocompromise
2. Administration of systemic antifungal agents
3. Surgical debridement, in which case multiple attempts may be necessary.

How Do Fungi Cause Disease?

To cause an infection the fungus has to first gain access to the host. This necessarily entails a portal of entry, attachment to host cells/host tissues, and the capacity to grow within the host. This implies the ability to replicate at 37°C, obtain nutrients and evade the host's natural defense mechanisms [20]. For dimorphic fungi this also means an initial morphologic conversion to a tissue form of growth.

Some fungi are capable of colonizing surfaces of epithelial tissues without penetrating and invading the surface. Often fungal rhinosinusitis is characterized by colonization rather than invasion. This produces profound inflammatory and immune responses that can be damaging for the host.

On occasion, some fungi can produce potent toxins and mutagens that can cause serious human disease. Less potent irritant and enzymes from fungi attack host cells leading to inflammation or at times immunopathology. Another mechanism is induced when the fungal cell wall antigens stimulate an allergic response in the host [9].

The outcome of inhaling fungal spores depends upon the following factors:
1. The number of spores inhaled
2. The size of the fungal particles
3. The integrity of the nonspecific and specific host defenses
4. The pathobiologic potential or virulence of the particular fungus.

The status of the host's immunity will ultimately determine whether the individual at risk will develop invasive or non-invasive fungal rhinosinusitis. Conditions like diabetic ketoacidosis serve to promote invasion by fungi.

Diagnosing Fungal (Mycotic) Infections

To diagnose accurately the type of fungi present the following are recommended:
1. Microscopic examination of fresh clinical specimens or histopathologic specimens
2. Culture testing of the etiologic agent
3. Serology and skin testing
4. Radiographic imaging
5. Polymerase chain reaction (PCR) methods to detect specific fungal DNA.

Prevention and Prophylaxis in the Immunocompromised Patient

Prevention measures include:
1. Minimizing exposure to fungi most likely to cause rhinosinusitis
2. Using prophylactic antifungal agents to diminish the risk of tissue invasion by infecting organisms.

Risk Factors

Patients with hematologic disease during the neutropenic phase are at risk. The duration of neutropenia is the most important risk factor in leukemic patients. Other factors that increase the risk further are the concomitant use of corticosteroids, broad spectrum antibiotics and the choice of chemotherapeutic agents.

Bone marrow transplant recipients are at greatest risk in the immediate post-transplant period before engraftment and in graft versus host disease (GVHD). Chronic GVHD is associated with increased risk of invasive aspergillosis [14]. Patients suffering from GVHD who are also on corticosteroids usually have a poor outcome.

Prevention

Inhalation of fungal spores sets in motion the train of events that could lead to invasive fungal rhinosinusitis. Thus, prevention seeks to decrease exposure to fungi. Patients, especially those with GVHD, are usually hospitalized for long periods of time and usually develop nosocomial fungal infections. Hospital outbreaks are associated with direct contamination of the ventilation system. Demolition or constructive projects near the hospital can contaminate the ventilation system [1]. Other sources are potted plants, food, fireproofing or insulation materials.

Potted plants and flowers should be avoided and ground pepper should not be used as seasoning. Air ducts should be cleaned regularly. Birds should be discouraged from nesting on sills and on roofs.

Most outbreaks are related to hospital renovations. Dry wall barriers should be used rather than plastic drapes sealing windows. Frequent vacuuming should be carried out.

Prevention with Prophylactic Antifungal Medications

Principles for starting antifungal mediations are:
1. Targeting pathogens most likely to cause infection
2. Identifying subsets of patients at risk of fungal rhinosinusitis
3. Limiting prophylaxis to the period of time when risk is greatest
4. Choosing a safe, well-tolerated drug with minimal side effects
5. Monitoring drug-related side effects and resistance
6. Evaluating the cost of a regimen in relation to its efficacy.

Prophylaxis should be limited to patients likely to develop infection and should be given only during the period of maximum risk.

Aspergillus species is the most common pathogen and medication should be directed at this pathogen [5]. The major target groups based on risk of development of infection should be patients with hematologic malignancies and prolonged neutropenia and those who undergo bone marrow transplantation. The most significant advance against fungal infections has been the use of fluconazole to prevent invasive candidiasis in bone marrow transplant recipients.

Secondary Prophylaxis to Prevent Recurrent Aspergillosis

Secondary prophylaxis against aspergillosis is important in those patients who have suffered a previous attack of aspergillosis in the past and are now undergoing intense chemotherapy or bone marrow transplantation. These patients are at heightened risk of developing a recurrence of an aspergillosis infection [27]. Even with secondary prophylaxis, it has been noted that one-third of patients suffer a relapse of aspergillosis infection.

Recommendations for Preventive Measures

General infection control precautions to ensure that hospital ventilation systems do not transmit filamentous fungi should be routine in all units caring for immunosuppressed patients. HEPA filtration is recommended, but laminar airflow is not.

Diagnosis and Management of Rhinosinusitis Before Scheduled Immunosuppression

It is important to identify, diagnose, and treat pre-existing rhinosinusitis before starting immunosuppressive therapy.

A careful examination with radiological imaging helps to detect patients who may harbor a potentially life-threatening infection, but who are as yet asymptomatic. Other conditions [8] that could lead to rhinosinusitis following immunosuppressive therapy are long-term antibiotic use, indwelling catheters, nasal intubation, steroids, metabolic abnormalities, and chronic rhinosinusitis.

Mucormycosis of the Nose and Paranasal Sinuses

Mucormycosis rarely affects a healthy individual. It commonly affects patients suffering from diabetes. It can, however, occur in any immunocompromised individual.

The mainstay of therapy lies in the following:
1. Reversal of immunocompromise
2. Systemic high dose of amphotericin B
3. Surgical debridement of nonviable tissue

In diabetic patients survivorship ranges from 60 to 90%. When the source of immunocompromise is not quickly reversible survival drops to 20–50%.

Mucormycosis is a term used to refer to any fungal infections of the order Mucorales which belong to the class of Zygomycetes. *Rhizopus oryzae* is the predominant pathogen and accounts for 60% of all forms of mucormycosis. It accounts for 90% of rhinocerebral mucormycosis. All fungi of the order Mucorales reproduce sexually as well as asexually. Members of the family Mucoraceae have characterized sporangia, which envelops numerous asexual spores.

Diabetics presenting with ketoacidosis are disproportionately affected [3]. *Rhizopus* organisms have an active ketone reductase system and thrive in high glucose acidotic conditions. Diabetics also have decreased phagocytic activity because of impaired glutathione pathway. Normal serum inhibits the growth of *Rhizopus* whereas diabetic ketoacidosis stimulates growth [11]. Patients on dialysis treated with deferoxamine B(DFO), an iron and aluminum chelator, are more susceptible to mucormycosis.

Other risk factors are prolonged neutropenia, long-term systemic steroid therapy, protein calorie malnutrition, bone marrow transplantation, immunodeficiency, leukemia and intravenous drug use. The relative infrequency of mucormycosis in AIDS reflects the ability of neutrophils to prevent growth of the fungus. Mucormycosis may have an acute fulminant course or a slower indolent invasive course. When immunocompromise is not easily reversible then the course of the disease is aggressive and rapid.

Signs and Symptoms of Mucormycosis

The leading symptom is fever. This is quickly followed by ulceration in the nose followed by necrosis, periorbital and facial swelling or decreased vision. Ultimately, approximately 80% develop a necrotic lesion on the nasal mucosa. Facial numbness is also present in some patients. The importance of anesthesia of the affected facial areas is an early sign of invasive mucormycosis.

Histopathology

A diagnosis of mucormycosis can be made on histological examination of specimens from a diseased patient. Broad band- or ribbon-like hyphae measuring 10–20 µm branch haphazardly and there is an absence of septations. Mucor stains easily with hematoxylin and eosin. It can also be seen on histopathology that the organism has a distinct predilection for vascular invasion, predominantly arterial invasion.

Treatment

The treatment of mucormycosis includes reversal of immunocompromise, systemic amphotericin B, and surgical debridement. Surgery alone is not curative. Hyperbaric oxygen has also been reported to be a useful adjunct in treatment. It reverses ischemic acidotic conditions that cause fungal infections to perpetuate. Hyperbaric oxygen is usually given at two atmospheres for 1 h on a daily basis for up to 30 sessions. Hyperbaric oxygen does not have a significant impact on mortality. It does, however, limit the area of deformity by decreasing the required area of debridement.

Chronic Invasive Fungal Rhinosinusitis

Chronic invasive fungal rhinosinusitis usually occurs in healthy individuals who are immunologically intact. Usually such patients present with a history of chronic rhinosinusitis symptoms, respiratory tract allergies or nasal polyposis. Some patients who are diabetic even though they are not keto-acidotic present with the granulomatous form of the disease.

Symptoms may take months even years to present. Nasal examination reveals severe nasal congestion and polypoid mucosa. A soft tissue mass can be seen. This is usually covered with debris or thick, inspissated nasal secretions.

Imaging modality of choice is CT in the initial stages. Focal or diffuse areas of hyperattenuation within a sinus are a clue to fungal colonization. Often bone erosion or expansion can be seen. This is usually a sign that an invasive process is about to be initiated (Fig. 22.1).

Magnetic resonance imaging is useful to determine if dural invasion or dural involvement has taken place. Differentiation between a malignant neoplasm and chronic fungal rhinosinusitis may be difficult and is best made on histopathology.

Patients suffering from chronic invasive rhinosinusitis are usually immunocompetent. Some workers performed extensive tests to uncover any hidden immunological abnormality. No specific immunological defects were detected. Instead it was discovered that these immunocompetent individuals were suffering from allergic fungal rhinosinusitis (AFRS). Those patients who had the granulomatous type of disease had a cutaneous type 4 hypersensitivity (delayed skin reaction) to the *Aspergillus* antigen. None of the nongranulomatous patients showed type 4 reactions. De Shazo [6] emphasized in his report that all cases of nongranulomatous, chronic invasive fungal rhinosinusitis occurred in patients with diabetes. The formation of a granuloma requires an indigestible organism and cell-mediated immunity to be directed toward the inciting agent. It is not clear why certain non-immunocompromised individuals develop invasive disease. Some speculate that a hot, dry climate in individuals with nasal obstruction predisposes to *Aspergillus* infections. Others believe that anaerobic conditions in the sinus caused by repeated inflammation predispose the patient to invasive fungal disease. Most authors agree that *Aspergillus* is often a secondary invader of a diseased sinus.

With regard to pathology, periarterial invasion without direct involvement of fungal elements and no true vascular invasion is a typical feature. Three variants are described:
1. Proliferative (granulomatous pseudotubercles in a fibrous stroma)
2. Exudative-necrotizing (with prominent foci of necrosis)
3. A mixed form.

De Shazo [6] described granulomatous chronic invasive fungal rhinosinusitis as granulomas composed of eosinophilic material surrounded by fungus, giant cells, variable lymphocytes and plasma cells. Nongranulomatous chronic invasive fungal rhinosinusitis is characterized by tissue necrosis, dense fungal hyphae and scanty inflammatory infiltrate. The fungi in this form may breach mucosal barriers to invade blood vessels or

22

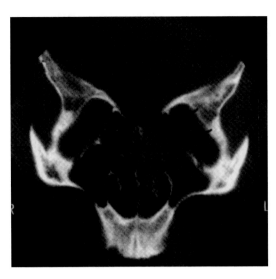

Fig. 22.1 Computed tomography scan showing massive destruction and imminent intracranial invasion by a fungus

just cause arteritis without vascular invasion. Ultimately, both granulomatous and nongranulomatous forms can result in tissue necrosis.

Washburn et al.. [28, 29] feel that the nongranulomatous form should be treated by an aggressive surgical approach, while the granulomatous form responds well to surgery. Current recommendations for both forms are surgery to remove all disease where feasible. This is to be followed by prolonged courses of amphotericin B and itraconazole.

Invasive Fungal Rhinosinusitis in the Acquired Immunodeficiency Syndrome

The increasing prevalence of AIDS has left patients who suffer from this problem at great risk of suffering from fungal infections. Since by definition these patients are immunocompromised the infections that they suffer are usually serious and have poor outcomes. Aspergillosis is the most common pathogen in AIDS patients. It usually causes arterial invasion, thrombosis, and subsequent necrosis of tissue. *Aspergillus fumigatus* is the most common pathogen isolate in the AIDS population.

Infection by HIV causes selective depletion of CD4 (T helper) lymphocytes. Although impaired cellular immunity predisposes to fungal and intracellular bacterial infections, phagocytic polymorphonuclear cells and macrophages are the primary defenses against fungal infections, killing the mycelial and conidial forms of the fungus. AIDS patients demonstrate neutrophil and macrophage dysfunction. Minamoto et al.. [19] cite neutropenia as the single greatest factor predisposing to the development of invasive fungal sinusitis in patients suffering from AIDS. It was also noted that fungal rhinosinusitis was associated with advanced AIDS and low CD4 cell counts.

Fungal Balls (Mycetomas)

Fungal balls of the nose and paranasal sinuses are composed of matted fungal hyphae. Diagnosis is based on the characteristic histopathology of tangled fungal hyphae. Fungal balls are usually found in one sinus. The maxillary sinus is commonly affected followed by the sphenoid sinus. The host is immunocompetent [12] . If immunocompromise occurs then the fungal infection may become invasive and become life-threatening. The clinical symptoms may mimic bacterial sinusitis. The treatment is surgical removal and recurrence is rare. In earlier literature the term "aspergilloma" was used, but the preferred term is "fungal ball".

Older individuals are more commonly affected and no pediatric cases have been reported. There is a female preponderance. The incidence of fungal balls may be geographic and it is felt that this may reflect the infrequency of allergic fungal rhinosinusitis.

Clinical Presentation

Symptoms of fungal balls are identical to those of bacterial rhinosinusitis. They include nasal obstructions, purulent nasal discharge, cacosmia, and facial pain. Other unusual symptoms include epistaxis, fever, and cough. Ten per cent of patients present with nasal polyps.

Radiological Imaging

Computed tomography is the imaging modality of choice. A heterogeneous opacity is commonly seen (Fig. 22.2). Often, radiodensities within the central portion of the soft tissue mass are seen and occasionally, bony destruction, a mucocele, foreign body, or antrochoanal polyp is seen. Air fluid levels that are common in bacterial sinusitis are uncommon in fungal balls. Usually, only a single sinus is involved.

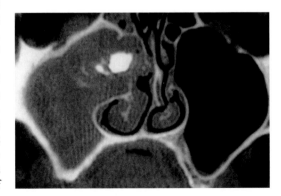

Fig. 22.2 Computed tomography scan of a fungal ball in the maxillary sinus. Note the area of hyperattenuation in the maxillary sinus

Histopathology

Fungal balls are extramucosal manifestations and are non-invasive. Granulomatous reaction is absent, but a tangled mat of fungal hyphae is present (Fig. 22.3). The commonest fungus found is aspergillosis. If immunosuppression develops, then the patient is at risk of developing invasive rhinosinusitis.

The most likely cause of fungal balls is the persistence of fungal spores within the nasal cavity and paranasal sinuses. If the fungal spores do not get cleared out by mucociliary clearance, then they can germinate and cause a fungal ball.

Dental paste as the result of endodontic treatment has been postulated to cause fungal balls. Increased availability of ferritin and zinc can contribute to fungal growth.

Treatment

The treatment for fungal balls is surgical removal. The endoscopic approach is usually sufficient to remove the fungus. Irrigation of the sinus can be done at the same time to ensure total removal. Once removed adequately by surgery, they usually do not recur.

Should an asymptomatic patient undergo surgery for an opacified sinus even though there is no evidence of bony erosion? There are many reports for and against. However, if the patient is asthmatic then surgery can be performed. The rationale for this is the following. There is a possibility that the "opacified" sinus could be contributing to aggravating attacks of asthma. Furthermore, the surgery could provide clues as to why the sinus is opacified and quiescent disease removed before it does further damage. Surgery serves to remove pathology and provide ventilation and drainage. Symptomatic patients need to undergo surgery.

Allergic Fungal Rhinosinusitis

Allergic fungal rhinosinusitis (AFRS) is a term introduced by Robson et al.. [25] to describe a constellation of unusual findings in a unique group of patients suffering from chronic rhinosinusitis.

Allergic fungal rhinosinusitis is believed to be of similar etiology to allergic bronchopulmonary aspergillosis (ABPA) [13]. ABPA is felt to be mediated by both type 1 (IgE) and type III (IgG-antigen immune complexes) Gell and Coombs reactions. The Th2 CD4+ subpopulation of T cells, which are prominent in atopic IgE-mediated disease are felt to cause the escalation of inflammation seen in ABPA. Interleukins 4, 5, 10, and 13 are released by these cells. IL-10 suppresses the alternative Th1 response, IL-4 and IL-13 increase class switching of B cells to produce IgE molecules, and IL-3 and IL-5 function in eosinophil maturation and activation.

Clinical Findings in AFRS

Most patients suffering from AFRS are young, atopic, and immunocompetent [26]. Criteria to determine if the rhinosinusitis is AFRS comprise five typical major characteristics:

1. Gross production of eosinophilic mucin containing non-invasive fungal hyphae
2. Nasal polyposis
3. Characteristic radiographic (CT scan) findings
4. Positive fungal stain or culture
5. Type 1 hypersensitivity.

Six other minor characteristics are:
a) The presence of asthma
b) Unilateral disease
c) Radiographic evidence of bone erosion
d) Fungal culture
e) Charcot-Leyden crystals
f) Serum eosinophilia.

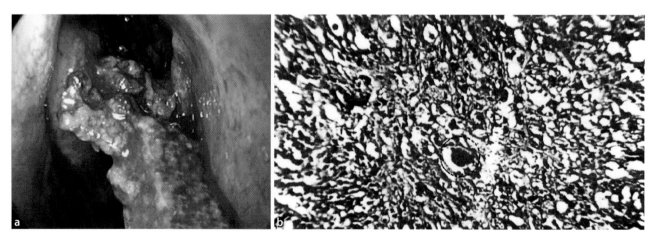

Fig. 22.3 **a** Aspergilloma being removed from the maxillary sinus. **b** Histopathology of blastomycosis of the paranasal sinuses

Allergic fungal rhinosinusitis is initiated when an atopic individual is exposed to inhaled fungi. This provides the initial antigenic stimulus. A Gell and Coombs type 1 (IgE) and 111 (immune complex)-mediated reaction takes place. An intense eosinophilic inflammatory response occurs. This results in mucosal edema, stasis of secretions and inflammatory exudates, which in combination cause obstruction of the sinus ostia. This process may be made worse if other factors like septal deviations and turbinate hypertrophy are also present. The process may then spread to involve adjacent sinuses and produce sinus expansion and erosion. This in turn creates an ideal environment in which fungi proliferate. This further increases antigenic exposure. At some point this cycle becomes self perpetuating. This results in the production of allergic mucin, the accumulation of which causes further obstruction of the involved sinuses, which in turn further propagates the allergic process. Secondary bacterial infection may also occur. Invasion of the underlying mucosa is not a characteristic of AFRS.

The aspergillosis organism itself impairs the host's mucosal defenses. They are capable of altering the host immune response through macrophage and T cell suppression. They reduce the host's defenses by:

1. Reducing ciliary beat frequency
2. Impairing the function of the host fungicidal proteins within the mucus blanket
3. Fungal allergens being able to deactivate the complement system
4. Interfering with phagocytosis
5. Releasing proteolytic enzymes that can destroy the host basement membrane.

Epidemiology

The prevalence of AFRS is between approximately 5 and 10%. AFRS is noted in young age groups from 23 years to 42 years. Pediatric patients present in the same fashion as adults with AFRS. One-third of to one-half of patients suffering from AFRS also suffer from asthma [17]. Cody et al.. [4] described an incidence of 27% of patients who also showed sensitivity to aspirin. Patients with AFRS are by definition atopic.

Signs and Symptoms

The incidence of nasal polyposis is almost 100%. Nasal polyposis is a nonspecific indicator of chronic nasal inflammation.

Allergic fungal rhinitis shows typical findings on CT. The central high attenuation can at times be described as "starry sky", "ground glass", or "serpiginous" pattern. Almost half of patients suffering AFRS have unilateral disease.

Fungal species of the dematiaceous species are most commonly the cause of AFRS. Examination of the mucin retrieved demonstrates eosinophils. Charcot-Leyden crystals and fungal hyphae against a background of eosinophilic material are typical of AFRS. Almost half of AFRS patients have only unilateral disease.

Tests to Confirm a Diagnosis of AFRS

1. Total eosinophil count
2. Total serum IgE
3. Antigen-specific IgE (both fungal and other inhalant allergens either by in vitro testing or by skin testing)
4. Fungal antigen-specific IgG
5. Precipitating antibodies
6. Microscopic evaluation of the mucin that was evacuated during surgery
7. Fungal culture of the material evacuated during surgery

Treatment of AFRS

The traditional treatment for AFRS is surgical clearance of nasal polyposis. Endoscopic clearance is now the widely accepted treatment modality. The gradual accumulation of allergic fungal mucin gives AFRS a predictable characteristic pattern. As the mucus accumulates the involved paranasal sinus begins to resemble a mucocele. The principle of surgery in AFRS is to provide ventilation and drainage while accepting the reality that surgery may not totally eradicate disease. Multiple surgeries may be necessary. Furthermore, the treatment lies in combining surgery with aggressive prolonged medication. Despite all this, recurrences may still occur.

Systemic Steroids

Waxman et al.. [30] suggested the use of systemic steroids in the postoperative period. It should be mentioned that steroids should not be given in the preoperative period as this can cause confusion in the diagnosis. Many studies have provided compelling evidence that the recurrence of AFRS is significantly reduced with the use of systemic steroids. Schubert and Goetz [26] reviewed 67 patients suffering from AFRS and reported that oral corticosteroid therapy significantly delayed the need for revision surgery. Steroids can cause a reduction in or even a total resolution of the eosinophilic mucin that is required to make a diagnosis. It should also be mentioned that steroids are not without their attendant problems.

Immunotherapy

Fungal immunotherapy was proposed as a possible adjuvant therapy to surgical removal of polypoidal tissue and mucin debris. Initial studies addressed the concerns of provoking a Gell and Cooms type 111 reaction caused by immunotherapy. This was extrapolated from warnings regarding the use of immunotherapy in ABPA. A rise in IgE and IgG4 was reported. However, studies [23] revealed that not only was immunotherapy safe, but that it also produced clinical improvements. A longitudinal study of a cohort of patients treated with immunotherapy and followed up for 3 years showed a significant decrease in disease recurrence. Dependence on systemic and topical steroids was less in this study. Furthermore, it was discovered that once surgical removal of mucin and polyps was accompanied by immunotherapy post-surgery, then there was a significant decline in the incidence of revision surgery.

Mabry et al. [16] have made a considerable effort to investigate immunotherapy for AFRS. They injected allergic individuals subcutaneously with small graded doses of allergens against which they are reactive. The effectiveness of therapy and the level of increased IgG obtained was dose-dependent. The initial study by Mabry et al.. did not include a control group for comparison. A more recent follow-up study with a control group showed that immunotherapy reduced reliance on systemic and nasal steroid therapy to control disease compared with patients not receiving immunotherapy after both groups had been treated with surgery followed by systemic steroid therapy. Thus, it may seem that immunotherapy might be a promising new direction in which to develop a supplemental treatment option for surgery and steroid therapy.

A lack of availability of the specific fungal antigens would appear to be a major obstacle to forming a treatment protocol. Precise fungal identification is necessary if the treatment is to work. Thus, crossover from one fungal antigen to another, if proven, may be useful in solving this problem.

Antifungals

Bent and Kuhn [2] studied topical and systemic antifungal therapy for AFRS with mixed results. They demonstrated that ketoconazole and amphotericin B were the most effective agents in vitro.

Topical Antifungals

It has been hypothesized that once fungi were eliminated locally then the disease process could be halted. Ponikau and colleagues [21] treated 51 patients who had CRS that was refractory to all other treatment. These patients were treated with nasal lavages of amphotericin B every alternate day for 3 months. Their findings revealed a decrease in symptoms and improvement in findings on CT scans and endoscopy in 75% of patients. The flaw of Ponikau's study was that it had no control group. This defect was corrected when a follow-up, randomized, placebo-controlled, double-blinded trial [22] found excellent results. There was significant statistical improvement in the CT scan parameters and endoscopic examination in patients treated with amphotericin B nasal lavages compared with the placebo group.

To eliminate the role of nasal lavages (the effect of saline) Weschetta et al.. [31] treated 60 patients who had CRS and nasal polyps refractory to standard medical therapy. This study excluded AFRS. Their study was a double-blinded, randomized controlled trial. Their study showed that amphotericin B nasal lavages was not effective in the treatment of CRS when AFRS was absent.

Richetti et al.. [24] evaluated the effectiveness of amphotericin B nasal lavages that resolved nasal polyposis in 39% of patients.

It can thus be seen that while nasal lavages with amphotericin B appear promising, they need further studying to determine in which situation they will be most effective.

Bent and Kuhn [2] found that the most common pathogens in AFRS were the dematiaceous species (*Curvularia*, *Bipolaris*, *Alternia*) and that these species were sensitive to itraconazole, amphotericin B, nystatin, and ketaconazole. They recommended the topical application of ketaconazole dissolved in an acetic acid solution (0.125% or 1 mg/mL) postoperatively. Alternatively, suspensions of amphotericin B at a dosage of 50 mg in 10 mL of water (not saline or dextrose) irrigated into the nostrils two to four times a day have been used with good results.

In conclusion, it should be said that even the use of the local application of these medications is not conclusively proven. Much work needs to be done before they can be used on a regular basis.

Agents for the Treatment of Invasive Fungal Infections

Antifungal treatment principles include the following:
1. Correct identification of the fungus causing the infection.
2. Correct and appropriate use of standard antifungal regimens.
3. The treating clinician should consider initial therapy as an induction phase with optimization in both dose and duration of antifungal medication. The medication should preferably be fungicidal. Combination therapy may be considered.
4. Reversal or control of immunocompromise
5. Possible drug interactions should be kept in mind
6. Once the patient has stabilized under treatment, the clinician must consider a treatment regimen both in terms of dose as well as choice of medication to complete a defined course of therapy.
7. Follow-up to prevent and control relapses is extremely important.

Amphotericin B Deoxycholate

Amphotericin B deoxycholate is a polyene macrolide. It has a broad spectrum of activity. It is fungicidal and its fungicidal activity is caused by its ability to bind preferably to ergosterol, which is a major component of the fungal cell membrane. Cell membrane permeability is then increased following attachment of this lipophilic structure to the cell wall. This leads to leakage of intracellular components and ultimately results in fungal cell death. Unfortunately amphotericin B also binds to cholesterol in mammalian cell membranes, resulting in toxicity. Amphotericin B interacts with host cell macrophages and has a positive effect on them through an oxidation-dependent process. It is also postulated that amphotericin B may have an immunomodulating effect.

Amphotericin B has an apparent volume distribution of 4 L/kg. Distribution following intravenous administration follows a three-compartment model with high concentrations reaching the liver, spleen, lungs, kidneys, muscle, and skin. Its

22

protein binding capacity is approximately 91–95%. The metabolism of amphotericin B is not clearly understood. Less than half the dose is accounted for by either biliary or renal clearances. Metabolites have not been identified and blood levels are affected by either hepatic or renal failure. Following a biphasic elimination pattern, the initial half-life ranges from 24 to 48 hours with a subsequent terminal half-life of up to 5 days. Only 5% of amphotericin B is absorbed when administered orally.

Intravenous doses ranging from 0.25 to 1.0 mg/kg/day in 5% dextrose are recommended. Doses in adults are 1.2 mg/kg/day while in children the recommended dose is 1.5 mg/kg/day. Some authors recommend a test dose.

Strategies to enhance tolerability to the infusion include the use of hydrocortisone (25 mg added directly to the infusion), which has resulted in a dramatic reduction in febrile reactions. Thrombophlebitis is a common problem associated with the administration of amphotericin B. To avoid this, small amounts of heparin are added to the infusion, using a central line, rotating the infusion site and avoiding highly concentrated preparations. Nephrotoxicity may occur in up to 80% of patients. Azotemia, electrolyte wasting (K+ and Mg+) and a decrease in urine concentrating ability are known to occur. To prevent these attendant problems and minimize the risk of nephrotoxicity, sodium supplementation can be given. Avoidance of concomitant nephrotoxic drugs should also be carried out.

Amphotericin B possesses activity in vitro against most pathogenic fungi found in humans [15]. They are *Blastomycosis dermatidis*, *Cryptococcus neoformans*, *Coccidioides immitis*, *Histoplasma capsulatum*, *Paracoccidioides brasiliensis*, and *Sporothrix schenckii*. Variable in vitro activity is seen against *Aspergillus* and the zygomycetes.

The combination of amphotericin B and flucytosine has demonstrated synergistic fungicidal activity in vitro against the *Candida* species, *C. neoformans*, certain fungi causing chromomycosis, and *Aspergillus* spp. Amphotericin B plus is the drug combination of choice for the treatment of cryptococcal meningitis. Amphotericin B in combination with the triazole compounds, fluconazole and itraconazole, has demonstrated antagonistic effects with itraconazole more consistently exhibiting antagonism than fluconazole. Triple drug therapy in cryptococcal meningitis has been reported to achieve excellent results. Intraperitoneal administration of amphotericin B has been reported to be effective in the management of fungal peritonitis.

Amphotericin B administered empirically has become the gold standard in patients with persistent fever and neutropenia. It remains the treatment of choice for most progressive life-threatening fungal infections, including invasive aspergillosis, zygomycosis, and severe infections of blastomycosis, coccidioidomycosis, sporotrichosis, and histoplasmosis.

Lipid-Based Formulations of Amphotericin B

Amphotericin B lipid complex (ABLC, Abelcet), amphotericin B cholesteryl sulfate complex (ABCD Amphotec) and liposomal amphotericin B (ambisome) use a variety of lipid carriers. The pharmacokinetics of lipid-based formulations of amphotericin B differ significantly from that of amphotericin B deoxycholate.

Lipid-based formulations are preferentially delivered into the reticulo-endothelial tissues such as the liver and spleen. Doses for these preparations are 1–5 mg/kg (liposomal amphotericin B), 5 mg/kg/day (ABLC), and 3–5 mg/kg (ABCD) [15].

Azoles

The azoles offer an alternative to amphotericin B without the attendant problems associated with its use. They include the imidazoles (clotrimazole, ketoconazole, and miconazole) and the triazoles (fluconazole and itraconazole). They have been found to be effective against systemic fungal infections.

The azoles work by primarily inhibiting the cytochrome P450-dependent enzyme lanosterol 14alpha demethylase, which is necessary for the conversion of lanosterol to ergosterol. Ergosterol is a vital component of the cellular membrane of fungi and disruptions in the biosynthesis of ergosterol cause significant damage to the cell membrane by increasing its permeability and ultimately causing cell lysis and cell death.

The triazoles, itraconazole and fluconazole have significant pharmacokinetic differences. Fluconazole is available in the oral and intravenous formulations. It is highly water soluble and in the oral formulation it is absorbed almost completely. A single dose is widely distributed in body fluids. Fluconazole is found in the CSF.

Itraconazole on the other hand is not as well absorbed as fluconazole. The suspension is better absorbed on an empty stomach. Co-administration of acidic beverages such as cranberry juice may enhance absorption. Itraconazole is highly protein bound and achieves relatively low concentrations in the CSF. Metabolism takes place in the liver and is excreted in the urine and the feces.

Daily doses of 200–800 mg of fluconazole have been used. If sera are the concentrations used, then it is recommended that the measured therapeutic concentration be at least equal to or greater than 1 µg/mL.

The metabolism of triazoles takes place in the liver through the cytochrome P450 enzyme system, specifically the 3A4 pathways. There is potential for interactions with other medications that use the same pathway. Fatal interactions have been reported among cisapride, terfenadine, and astemizole. Thus, concomitant use of these medications with the triazoles is contraindicated.

Flucytosine

Flucytosine is a cytosine analog originally formulated for use as an anti-neoplastic agent. It acts directly on the RNA and DNA of yeast cells and is available as an oral medication. Side effects are usually seen when it is given in combination wit amphotericin B. Myelosuppression associated with flucytosine is reversible. The recommended dosage is 10 mg/kg/day in divided doses. Flucytosine has demonstrated antifungal activity in vitro against *Cryptococcus neoformans* and *Candida* species. Resistance to flucytosine occurs because of a single mutation. Thus, flucytosine should not be administered as a single agent. It should be given in combination with Amphotericin B and this combination is the treatment of choice for cryptococcal meningitis.

Terbinafine

Terbinafine is an allylamine compound for oral use. Its fungicidal activity is caused by the inhibition of the enzyme squalene epoxidase, which results in the depletion of ergosterol, which results in cell death. It is now available in the form of topical formulations and tablets. Terbinafine is highly lipophilic and displays a triphasic distribution pattern in humans that consists of a short initial half-life followed by an intermediate half-life of 11–15 h. Terbinafine is indicated for the treatment of various fungal infections of the nails and skin.

New Agents

Voriconazole is a new triazole and is a derivative of fluconazole. Studies evaluating the pharmokinetics of voriconazole demonstrate a bioavailability of 90% and a mean half-life of 6h. Clinical trials indicate that voriconazole is effective against oral and esophageal candidiasis.

Echinocandins are a new class of antifungal agents. They exert antifungal activity by inhibiting 1,3-B glucan synthesis for the fungal cell wall. These agents demonstrate antifungal activity against *Candida* species, *Aspergillus* species, and against *Pneumocystis carinii*. Dual therapy with an azole and even triple therapy in combination with amphotericin B is currently under study.

As our understanding of fungi improves so will the evolution of antifungal agents. The future holds many promising agents and clinical trials are underway.

References

1. Arnow PM, Sadigh M, Costas C et al. 1991): Endemic and epidemic aspergillosis associated with in hospital replication of Aspergillosis organisms. *Journal of Infectious Diseases* 164:998–1000

2. Bent JP and Kuhn FA (1996): Antifungal activity against allergic fungal sinusitis organisms. *Laryngoscope* 106:1331–1334

3. Blitzer A, Lawson W, Meyers BR et al. (1980): Patient survival factors in paranasal sinus mucormycosis. *Laryngoscope* 90:635–648

4. Cody DT, Neel HB, Ferreiro JA et al. (1994): Allergic fungal sinusitis. *Laryngoscope* 104:1074–1079

5. De Carpentier JP, Ramamurthy L, Denning DW et al. (1994): An algorithmic approach to aspergillus sinusitis. *Journal of Laryngology and Otology* 108:314–316

6. De Shazo (1998): Fungal sinusitis. *American Journal of Medical Sciences* 316:39–45

7. De Shazo RD, O'Brien N, Chapin K et al. (1997): A new classification and diagnostic criteria for invasive fungal sinusitis. *Archives of Otolaryngology Head and Neck Surgery* 123:1181–1188

8. Drakos PE, Nagler A, Naparstek E et al. (1993): Invasive fungal sinusitis in patients undergoing bone marrow transplantation. *Bone Marrow Transplant* 12:203–208

9. Ferguson BJ (2000): Definitions of fungal rhinosinusitis. *Otolaryngologic Clinics of North America* 33:227–235

10. Ferguson BJ (1998): What role do systemic corticosteroids, immunotherapy and antifungal drugs play in the therapy of allergic fungal rhinosinusitis? *Archives of Otolaryngology Head and Neck Surgery* 124:1174–1178

11. Gale GR Welch A (1961): Studies of opportunistic fungi. 1. Inhibition of R oryzae by human serum. *American Journal of Medicine* 45:604–612

12. Houser SM and Corey JP (2000): Allergic fungal rhinosinusitis. *Otolaryngologic Clinics of North America* 33:399–408

13. Grosjean P, Weber R (2007): Fungus balls of the paranasal sinuses: a review. *European Archives of Otorhinolaryngology* 264:461–470

14. Janntunen E, Ruutu P, Niskanen L et al. (1997): Incidence and risk factors for invasive fungal infections in allogenic BMT recipients. *Bone Marrow Transplant* 19:801–803

15. Luna B, Drew RH, Perfect JR (2000): Agents for the treatment of invasive fungal infections. *Otolaryngologic Clinics of North America* 33:277–299

16. Mabry RL, Manning SC Mabry CS (1997): Immunotherapy in the treatment of allergic fungal sinusitis. *Otolaryngology Head and Neck Surgery* 116:31–35

17. Manning SC, Holman M (1998): Further evidence for allergic pathophysiology in allergic fungal sinusitis. *Laryngoscope.* 108:1485–1496

18. Menezes RA, de Souza CE, de sa Souza S (1988): Blastomycosis of the paranasal sinuses. *Orbit* 7:3–6

19. Minamoto GY, Barlam TF, Vander Els NJ (1992): Invasive aspergillosis in patients with AIDS. *Clinical Infectious Diseases* 14:66–74

20. Mitchell TG (2000): Overview of basic medical mycology. *Otolaryngologic Clinics of North America* 33:237–249

21. Ponikau JU, Sherris DA, Kern EB (1999): The diagnosis and incidence of allergic fungal sinusitis. *Mayo Clinic Proceedings* 74(9):877–884

22. Ponikau JU, Sherris DA, Weaver A (2005): Treatment of chronic rhinosinusitis with intranasal amphotericin B: a randomized placebo controlled double blind pilot trial. *Journal of Allergy and Clinical Immunology* 115(1):125–131

23. Quinn, J, Wickern G, Whisman B et al. (1995): Immunotherapy in allergic bipolaris sinusitis: a case report. *Journal of Allergy and Clinical Immunology* 95:201–202

24. Robson JMB, Benn RAV, Hogan PG et al. (1989): Allergic fungal sinusitis presenting as a paranasal sinus tumor. *Australia and New Zealand Journal of Medicine* 19:351–353

25. Ricchetti A, Landis BN, Mafoli A (2002): Effect of antifungal nasal lavage with Amphotericin B on nasal polyposis. *Journal of Laryngology and Otology* 116:261–263

26. Schubert MS, Goetz DW (1998): Evaluation and treatment of allergic fungal sinusitis. 1. Demographics and diagnosis. *Journal of Allergy and Clinical Immunology* 102:387–394

27. Viollier AF, Peterson DE, De Jongh CA et al. (1986): Aspergillus sinusitis in cancer patients. *Cancer* 58:366–368

22

28. Washburn RG, Kennedy DW, Begley MG et al. (1988): Chronic fungal sinusitis in apparently normal hosts. *Medicine* 67:231–247

29. Washburn RG (1998): Fungal sinusitis. *Current Clinical Topical Infectious Diseases.* 18:60–74

30. Waxman JE, Spector JG, Sale SR et al. (1987): Allergic aspergillus sinusitis. Concepts in diagnosis and treatment of a new clinical entity. *Laryngoscope* 97:261–266

31. Weschetta M, Rimek D, Formanek M (2004): Topical antifungal treatment of chronic rhinosinusitis with nasal polyps: a randomized double blind clinical trial. *Journal on Allergy and Clinical Immunology* 113:1122–1128

Nasal Polyposis

Melissa Statham and Allen M. Seiden

Core Messages

- Sinonasal polyposis is a common but varied disease process. Nasal polyps are abnormal lesions that emanate from any portion of the nasal mucosa or paranasal sinuses.
- The major histopathologic differences between nasal polyps and normal nasal mucosa include: eosinophilic inflammation, edema, alteration in epithelial growth, and new gland formation.
- Although there is an association between asthma and nasal polyps, the association between polyps and atopic allergy is unclear.
- Polyps in aspirin-sensitive patients are generally more refractory to both medical and surgical therapy.
- In patients with nasal polyps, chronic nasal and paranasal sinus infection is frequently present.
- Complaints typically associated with polyposis are nasal congestion, rhinorrhea, and olfactory dysfunction.
- CT scanning is the imaging method of choice.
- Medical therapy includes corticosteroids, antibiotics, antifungals, antihistamines, and leukatriene modifiers.

Contents

Introduction

Sinonasal polyposis continues to be a common yet varied disease process. Broadly defined, nasal polyps are abnormal lesions that emanate from any portion of the nasal mucosa or paranasal sinuses. Nasal polyps are an end result of varying disease processes within the nasal cavities. Polyps tend to arise from the mucosa of the nasal cavity or from one or more of the paranasal sinuses, often in narrowed spaces such as the outflow tract of the sinuses. Estimated prevalence among symptomatic patients ranges from 1 to 4% of the population [1, 2], with higher rates among patients with asthma and cystic fibrosis [3]. Some autopsy studies that suggest up to 26–42% of patients may develop these during their lifetime [4–7]. However, since most of these cadaveric polyps were small, they were presumptively asymptomatic. When significant intranasal polyposis is present, this can easily be seen by anterior rhinoscopy. Grossly, polyps are generally translucent to pale gray in color, pear-shaped, smooth, soft, and freely mobile.

Polyps may arise from the lateral nasal wall, or in many cases, they are limited to the middle meatus, where they may not be well visualized except on endoscopic examination (Fig. 23.1) [8]. In 200 consecutive patients undergoing endoscopic sinus surgery, Stammberger evaluated the origin of nasal polyps [9] and noted that 80% of polyps originated from the middle meatal mucosa, uncinate process, and infundibulum. In 65% of patients, polyps originated from the ethmoidal bulla and hiatus semilunaris, while 48% originated within the frontal recess (Fig. 23.2). Polyps were found inside the ethmoid bulla in 30% (Fig. 23.3). Inflammatory polyps usually occur bilaterally.

Most sinonasal polyp disease manifests by the age of 40 years, although patients presenting with nasal polyposis before the age of 16 years should be investigated for associated disorders, particularly cystic fibrosis. On gross inspection, the most commonly encountered polyps are benign, semitransparent nasal lesions that are gelatinous in appearance, mobile, and nontender to manipulation (Fig. 23.4). Although multiple etiologies may exist, the end result is an edematous structure that demonstrates a high density of inflammatory cells. Polyps rarely bleed, and bleeding should raise concerns of malignancy.

Medical management of nasal polyps is directed toward minimizing the inciting inflammation, whereas surgical control focuses on removing the mechanical obstruction within the sinus and nasal cavities. Although surgical advances have paralleled improvements in endoscopic sinus surgery, it remains clear that nasal polyposis remains a mucosal disease that often requires medical maintenance. Advances in medical management have hinged on a better understanding of the pathophysiology behind polyp development. Controversy continues with regard to the exact roles of medical and surgical approaches, but a combination of both is often required to adequately treat patients. When polyps are associated with a specific disease entity, such as aspirin sensitivity or autoimmune vasculitis, treatment must also be directed toward the underlying disease process to prevent recurrence.

Nasal polyposis has been found to have a considerable impact on patients' quality of life when measured with a validated questionnaire instrument [10]. Though there were no correlations demonstrated among quality of life, polyp size, computed tomographic scan findings, nasal patency, and allergy, allergic patients had significantly worse scores compared with nonatopic patients.

Histopathology

The major histopathologic differences between nasal polyps and normal nasal mucosa include the following: eosinophilic inflammation, edema, alteration in epithelial growth, and new gland formation (Fig. 23.5). With this in mind, any theory describing the development of nasal polyps must consider the above-mentioned characteristics. Nasal polyposis is not merely edematous change of normal nasal mucosa, but a new inflammatory process that is the result of an array of inflammatory mediators, cytokines, adhesion molecules, and endothelial counter-receptors.

Polyp Formation and Growth

Polyps, by definition, include stromal edema and inflammatory cells, in which activated eosinophils are a prominent feature in about 80% [11]. Albumin and other transudative proteins are deposited within polyps adjacent to the eosinophilic inflammation. Histomorphological characterization of polypoid tissues reveals damaged epithelium, a thickened basement membrane, and a reduced number of vascular and glandular structures with few neural elements [12]. In patients with bilateral polyp disease, polyps appeared to have activated eosinophils present in the luminal compartment of the polyp such that they surround the central cystic portion of the polyp [11]. These findings suggest a central deposition of plasma proteins, regulated by the predominantly eosinophilic subepithelial inflammation, as a principle in the pathogenesis of polyp formation and growth.

Several details regarding polyp development help govern medical management. Polyps tend to occur between narrow areas of mucosal contact, such as the middle meatus [13], especially the narrow clefts in the anterior ethmoid region that create turbulent airflow, and particularly when narrowed by mucosal inflammation. It is theorized that chronic irritation within these narrow areas promotes the release of inflammatory cytokines that attract the migration of other inflammatory cells [14, 15]. During this process, a polyp may form from the mucosa because the heightened inflammatory process from epithelial cells, vascular endothelial cells, and fibroblasts affects the integrity of the sodium channels at the luminal surface of the respiratory epithelial cells in that region of the nasal mucosa. This response increases sodium absorption, leading to water retention and polyp formation.

Polyps, Allergy, and Eosinophilic Inflammation

In patients with a history of rhinologic allergy and physical examination findings of nasal polyps, the inflammatory infiltrate of the nasal mucosa is eosinophilic, and as such, allergy has

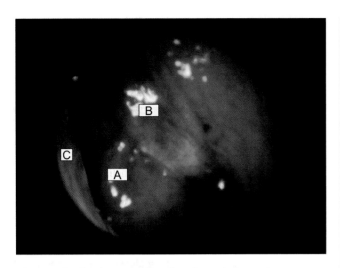

Fig. 23.1 Small polyp protruding from beneath the uncinate process, visualized endoscopically within the left middle meatus. (*A*: polyp, *B*: uncinate process, *C*: middle turbinate)

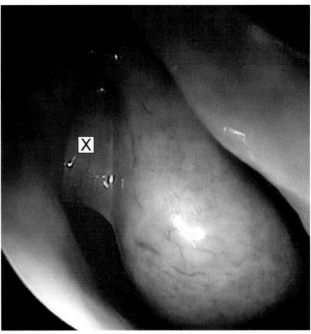

Fig. 23.2 Polyp extending from the right frontal recess (*cross*)

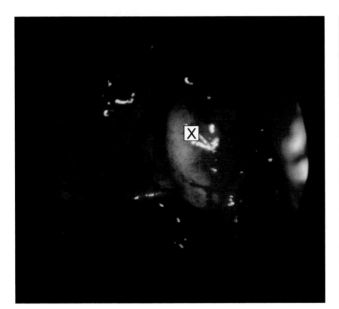

Fig. 23.3 Small polyp found within the right ethmoid bulla at the time of surgery (*cross*)

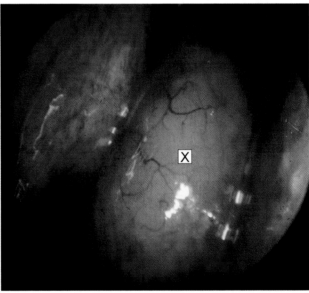

Fig. 23.4 Large polyp filling the right anterior nasal cavity (*cross*)

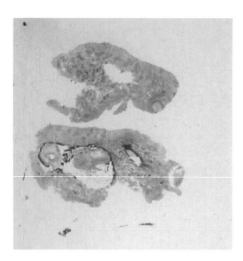

Fig. 23.5 Histologic slide of a nasal polyp. As opposed to normal nasal mucous membrane, nasal polyps demonstrate localized outgrowths of the lamina propria with edema, thickening of the basement membrane, and a variable influx of inflammatory cells

been considered a possibly important etiology for nasal polyps. Although there is an association between asthma and nasal polyps, the association between polyps and atopic allergy is unclear. Kern and Schenck [16] reported nasal polyps in 25.6% of patients with allergy compared with 3.9% of a control group lacking allergy. The prevalence of allergy in patients with nasal polyps varies in the literature from 10 to 64% [17–20]. One study found that patients with nasal polyps have the same prevalence of positive skin prick tests to a series of allergens as that of the normal population [21]. Therefore, many believe that most clinical evidence is against allergy as a causal factor [22].

The mechanisms involved in eosinophilic infiltration of the nasal mucosa and the nasal polyp are not fully elucidated. Epithelial cells from nasal polyps may have a more potent effect on inducing eosinophilic infiltration of the respiratory mucosa than epithelial cells from healthy nasal mucosa [23]. Other studies showed that eosinophil migration into tissues is controlled, in part, by interactions between eosinophil adhesion receptors and counter-structures on the vascular epithelium. Histologic analysis reveals nasal polyps to contain eotaxin, eotaxin-2, and eotaxin-3, suggesting both chemokines are integral in eosinophilia seen in polyposis [24].

Though the number of mast cells within nasal polyps is high [25], the incidence of nasal polyps in patients with allergic rhinitis is again no higher than that found in the non-atopic general population [26–28]. Although mast cell degranulation occurs within polyps, most antihistamines alone have little efficacy in treating patients with nasal polyps [14].

In a study comparing biopsies of nasal polyps versus biopsies of sinonasal mucosa in controls, goblet cells, mast cells, and inflammation with eosinophils were observed in all sinonasal mucosa with no significant difference noted between groups [29]. When comparing atopic and non-atopic patients with nasal polyposis treated with systemic and topical corticosteroids, a significant decrease in mast cells, intra-epithelial eosinophils, squamous metaplasia, and epithelial damage was found in allergic patients after steroid therapy [30]. However, no significant cellular or structural component changes were found in polyp tissues of non-allergic patients after treatment with systemic and topical steroid therapy.

To complicate matters, food allergy may play a role in nasal polyposis. In a population of pre-operative nasal polyposis patients, a significant proportion of patients (70%) had positive skin tests for being allergic to an average of four foods on intradermal allergy testing compared with controls [31]. In this cohort, only 35% of patients also had positive inhalant skin tests, and overall, prevalence of positive inhalant skin tests was similar to controls. These data suggest that IgE- and non-IgE-mediated immunological mechanisms, such as food allergy and delayed food hypersensitivity, may play a role in the etiology of nasal polyps, and dietary manipulation may be indicated, though its role needs further investigation.

Upon stimulus with an offending inspired allergen, preformed and newly generated mediators cause early phase allergic rhinitis symptoms. At the same time, chemotactic factors induce mediator release from eosinophils, basophils, monocytes, and lymphocytes, which eventually cause late-phase allergic rhinitis symptoms. Early-phase mediators include histamine, proteases, cysteinyl leukotrienes (cysLT), prostaglandins, platelet-activating factor, kinins, interleukins, TNF-β, and GM-CSF. Late-phase mediators also include cysLT, which mediate both early- and late-phase symptoms in allergic rhinitis, and other cytokines. Many studies have demonstrated the pro-inflammatory effects of cys-LT in the upper and lower airways as evidenced by their role in allergic rhinitis and chronic hyperplastic rhinitis with nasal polyposis [32, 33].

Cysteinyl leukotrienes (cysLT) exert various effects that contribute to inflammation. The cysLT stimulate mucus secretion by goblet cells and decrease mucociliary clearance. In addition, cysLT can produce or exacerbate nasal congestion by inducing vasodilatation, leading to mucosal edema. They promote inflammatory cell recruitment, eosinophil activation, fibrosis, and airway remodeling acting by means of smooth muscle cell and epithelial cell proliferation in the distal airways.

In patients with polyp disease and concomitant chronic rhinosinusitis and/or allergic fungal sinusitis, the eosinophil is instrumental in the inflammatory process. The eosinophil seems to increase production of cytokines, particularly interleukin (IL)-5, resulting in autocrine stimulation and the chemoattraction of various inflammatory cells [34]. Steroids are effective in reducing the inflammation, resulting in a reduction in polyp size. Even non-eosinophilic polyps, such as those in patients with cystic fibrosis or primary ciliary dyskinesia, are steroid-responsive because of the presence of neutrophils and lymphocytes within polyp tissue [35].

23

Aspirin Sensitivity

Polyps in aspirin-sensitive patients are generally more refractory to both medical and surgical therapy. The abnormal regulation of cyclo-oxygenase pathways characteristic of aspirin sensitivity is critical to the high rate of polyp recurrence among these patients (Fig. 23.6). The formation of prostaglandin E_2 (PGE_2), which has an anti-inflammatory effect on the activation and chemotaxis of eosinophils, seems to be lower in aspirin-sensitive patients, compared with normal controls and aspirin-tolerant patients with polyps [36]. The reduced production of PGE_2 causes enhanced 5-lipoxygenase activity [37]. Hence, the resulting overproduction of cysLT leads to bronchoconstriction and mucosal inflammation among aspirin-sensitive patients. The management of these patients, therefore, must include desensitization to disrupt the inflammatory cascade, resulting in marked improvement of chronic sinus symptoms among these patients [38].

Infectious Etiology

In patients with nasal polyps, chronic nasal and paranasal sinus infection is frequently present. The most common offending pathogens are β-hemolytic streptococci, *Staphylococcus aureus*, *Streptococcus pneumoniae*, and *Haemophilus influenzae*. Neutrophilic, and not eosinophilic, infiltrates predominate in polyps in this setting. In vivo studies of experimental maxillary sinusitis in rabbits demonstrated both granulation-like polyps and edematous-like polyps [39]. In these studies, the sinuses were inoculated with *S. pneumoniae*, *Bacteroides fragilis*, or *S. aureus*, after iatrogenically blocking the maxillary sinus ostium. In this model, granulation-like polyps were noted in regions of deep inflammatory trauma and edematous polyps were found in regions of superficial inflammatory trauma. Polyps were found in all sinusitis groups irrespective of the inducing agent and were not directly related to the presence of a specific microorganism [24]. Viruses also have been proposed as a possible etiology for nasal polyps [40]. However, a viral etiology has not been identified, despite investigations into adenovirus, Epstein-Barr virus, herpes simplex virus, and human papilloma virus [40–42].

Bacterial Superantigens

Recent studies have documented an association of increased IgE levels directed at *Staphylococcus aureus* enterotoxins present within polyp tissue [43]. Staphylococcal and streptococcal toxin-specific IgE antibodies were detected in a significant proportion of patients with chronic rhinosinusitis and nasal polyposis, whereas no controls had IgE to these antigens [44]. In addition, no association was found between severity of sinus disease on CT scan and the presence of staphylococcal and streptococcal toxin-specific IgE antibodies [44]. The impact of bacterial superantigens on medical therapy remains to be seen, but exploring the role of microbial organisms speaks directly to the multi-factorial nature of polyp development.

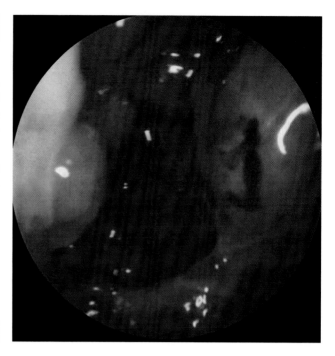

Fig. 23.6 Polyp recurrence within the left ethmoid cavity of an aspirin sensitive patient who has undergone previous surgery

Diagnosis

Complaints typically associated with polyposis are nasal congestion, rhinorrhea, and olfactory dysfunction. A thorough intranasal endoscopic examination is necessary for all patients with polyp disease to assess the gross appearance and sites of origin. When evaluating a patient with nasal polyps, the differential diagnosis of intranasal masses should be entertained, including the possibility of systemic disease. The finding of nasal polyps in children should warrant consideration of cystic fibrosis or a ciliary dysmotility disorder.

As a rule, if the intranasal mass does not have the characteristic appearance of an inflammatory polyp, is unilateral, bleeds easily, or has a stalk that is not clearly identified, imaging studies and possible biopsy are indicated before proceeding with management. Sinonasal neoplasia may display an endoscopic appearance similar to polyps; thus, consideration should be given to the possibility of carcinoma, sarcoma, angiofibroma, meningioma, or esthesioneuroblastoma in certain patients (Fig. 23.7).

Unilateral polyps should raise concern for allergic fungal sinusitis or inverted papilloma. A single, unilateral polyp originating high in the nasal cavity or with a stalk that is not clearly visible may represent an encephalocele or meningocele. Visible pulsations on endoscopy and enlargement of the mass with ipsilateral internal jugular vein compression (Furstenberg's sign) help to confirm this diagnosis. High-resolution CT may reveal bony dehiscences or erosion. Magnetic resonance imaging (MRI) is confirmatory of meningoencephalocele and is advisable when evaluating an area of skull base erosion adjacent to paranasal sinus opacification.

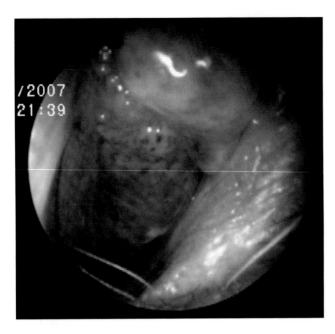

Fig. 23.7 Unilateral left nasal polypoid mass that on biopsy proved to be consistent with melanoma

Role of Imaging

Paranasal sinus CT can be approached in several ways depending on the anticipated disease process. Though plain X-ray radiographs may be used as the initial screening device for evaluating sinusitis or facial trauma, CT scanning is the method of choice for further evaluation of a mass or inflammatory lesion

as this provides superior information on specific sinus involvement by inflammatory processes as well as better delineation of bony sclerosis or destruction (Fig. 23.8). Radiologic studies should be obtained prior to performing a biopsy of any unusual nasal mass.

When endoscopic sinus surgery is anticipated, both coronal and axial non-contrasted CT imaging of the sinuses is necessary for pre-operative evaluation of the extent of sinus disease, to detect anatomic variants, and for planning the surgical approach. This study is done with thin sections ranging from 2 to 3 mm in thickness. A thickness of 5 mm is frequently suboptimal in that it can cause volume-averaging of small structures and obscure the fine details of paranasal sinus anatomy. For an optimal study, both soft-tissue and bone algorithms are used. This differentiates the soft-tissue component, as well as evaluating subtle bony destruction. Coronal imaging may be performed with the neck extended in either the prone or the supine position. An advantage of the prone position is that free fluid in the maxillary sinus layers in a dependent fashion inferiorly. In the supine position, fluid and mucus layer superiorly at the maxillary sinus ostium and may look similar to inflammatory mucosal thickening. Frequently, only the bone algorithm with its edge enhancement properties is needed for evaluating the detailed anatomy of the ostiomeatal complex. The coronal plane is best for evaluating integrity of the cribriform plate. Sinonasal polyps are hypodense on CT scan.

Contrast-enhanced sinus CT is usually unnecessary for routine sinusitis, although when severe nasal polyposis is suspected, contrast may be useful in demonstrating the characteristic "cascading" appearance of the enhancing polyps or to characterize an associated mucocele. A soft-tissue algorithm with soft-tissue windows may be useful when using contrast-enhanced CT for intracranial complications from sinus inflammatory processes.

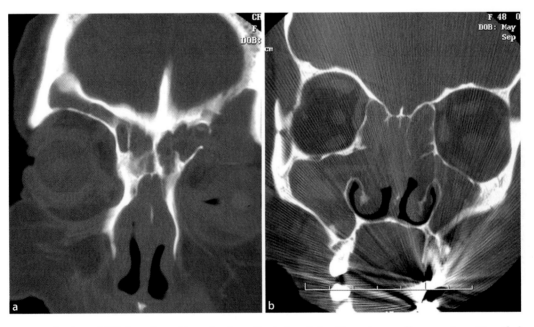

Fig. 23.8a,b Coronal CT of a patient with nasal polyps, allergic fungal sinusitis, and areas of bone erosion. **a** Opacified frontal sinuses with a left frontal mucocele and erosion of the orbital roof. **b** Opacified ethmoid and maxillary sinuses with erosion medially into the nose

A nasal decongestant may be helpful prior to scanning to decrease normal but asymmetric nasal mucosal congestion (normal nasal mucosal cycle) from a mucosa-based mass.

In general, MRI is also useful for identifying the extent of nasal tumors and differentiating tumor from inflammatory mucosal disease and inspissated secretions. Polyps tend to have various signal intensities on magnetic resonance pulse sequences. The MRI characteristics of polyps reflect the various stages of polyps, as well as the various stages of desiccation of the entrapped secretions within crevices between the polyps and on the polyp surfaces [45, 46]. Sinonasal polyps are hypointense on T1-weighted MRI, and hyperintense on T2-weighted MRI.

Mucosal thickening, sinus opacification, or both, are typically more pronounced in chronic rhinosinusitis with nasal polyposis than in those without polyposis. Nasal polyps are seen on CT scans as mucosal protrusions into the nasal cavity. The CT density of polyps cannot be differentiated from hypodense non-polypoid mucosal thickening. When the mucosal thickening appears polypoid in configuration, the CT appearance is suggestive of polypoid disease.

A solitary polyp may not be distinguished from a retention cyst on noncontrasted CT and MRI scans. Unlike cysts, polyps demonstrate moderate-to-marked contrast enhancement [45]. When multiple polyps are present, mucoid secretions become inspissated within the spaces between the polyps, as well as on their surfaces. On CT scans, polyps show soft tissue attenuation values; however, depending on the concentration of the retained secretions, the CT attenuation values increase, and the chronic sinonasal polyposis may show mixed CT attenuation values with areas of increased density, simulating focal or diffuse dystrophic calcifications [45]. These findings suggest that chronic rhinosinusitis with nasal polyposis is complicated further by the presence of allergic fungal rhinosinusitis. In aggres-

sive long-standing polyposis, there may be expansion seen of the paranasal sinuses, as well as focal bone erosion, and these findings are also seen in the setting of allergic fungal rhinosinusitis.

Antral Choanal Polyp

Antral choanal polyps are solitary, unilateral polyps. Although the origin and nature of the antral choanal polyp remains a point of controversy, there is a consensus that the antral choanal polyp originates in the maxillary sinus and passes through the sinus ostium or accessory opening into the nose and toward the choana (Fig. 23.9) [47–49]. The antral choanal polyp is predominantly solitary [50] and represents 3–6% of all nasal polyps [49]; it occurs more commonly in men and possibly children [49, 51, 52]. Chronic inflammatory disease, particularly chronic sinusitis, is widely believed to be the etiology, and recurrence after endoscopic removal in children has been associated with chronic rhinosinusitis [6]. Association with an allergic predisposition is controversial [47, 49, 53]. Nasal obstruction is the main presenting symptom [48, 54]; therefore, the differential diagnosis includes other nasal and paranasal sinus masses, both benign and malignant.

The antral choanal polyp has a distinct appearance on CT, appearing as a hypodense polyp, completely occluding the maxillary sinus and middle meatus, with extension into the nose toward the nasopharynx (Fig. 23.10). On MRI, the polyp most frequently protrudes through the posterior nasal fontanel behind the uncinate process of the lateral nasal wall, where lack of bone provides a path of least resistance for growth [55].

Treatment is surgical because these polyps have few inflammatory cells and therefore do not respond well to corticoster-

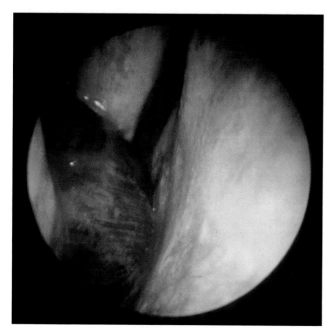

Fig. 23.9 Antrochoanal polyp protruding through an accessory opening of the right maxillary sinus

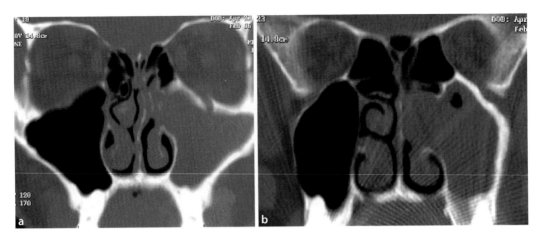

Fig. 23.10a,b Coronal CT of a patient with an antrochoanal polyp involving the left maxillary sinus. **a** Cut through the anterior ethmoid demonstrating an opacified left maxillary sinus with polypoid disease extending into and filling the left middle meatus. **b** Cut through the posterior ethmoid with the polypoid mass extending back toward the posterior choanae

oids [56]. Recurrence rates are reported as high as 28% with limited surgical procedures, such as removal through an antral window [53]. Because antral choanal polyps tend to recur if not excised completely with their underlying mucosa, Caldwell-Luc approaches may be needed in anteriorly based polyps to minimize their recurrence. The Caldwell-Luc maxillary antrotomy with intranasal antrostomy approach may be used for complete removal of the antral portion of the polyp to minimize recurrence [51, 54, 55]. The endoscopic approach has been reported to be effective and is currently the most popular procedure for removal of the antral choanal polyp [48, 49, 51, 54], even in pediatric patients [51]. Endoscopic intranasal resection involves removal of the antral portion of the polyp through the enlarged antrostomy with endoscopic visualization, and the nasopharyngeal portion of the antral choanal polyp is removed transorally if large or transnasally if size permits.

Inverted Papilloma

Inverted papillomas are usually present as polypoid unilateral nasal masses (Fig. 23.11). The histologic findings consist of infolded epithelium that may be squamous, transitional, or respiratory. The incidence of frank malignant transformation approximates 10% [57]. On occasion, they may be found in association with allergic nasal polyps, which accounts for the need to always submit labeled, separate specimens from each side of the nose when performing nasal polypectomy. The frequency of concomitant inverted papilloma in the setting of bilateral nasal polyposis has been shown to be rare, with rates reported between 0.00% and 0.92% [58–61]. In a recent study retrospectively evaluating the frequency of inverted papilloma in patients undergoing surgery for recurrent nasal polyposis, the incidence of inverted papilloma was found to be 0.26% [61].

    Even when not malignant, these lesions must be adequately resected because inadequate excision is likely to result in recur-

rence [62]. The classic approach includes a lateral rhinotomy incision combined with medial maxillectomy to allow adequate margins. However, recent experience with endoscopic sinus surgery has initiated the concept of endoscopic medial maxillectomy to remove inverted papilloma, and the specific procedure may in fact vary depending upon its point of origin. It is now generally accepted that in carefully selected cases, inverting papilloma may be removed endoscopically [63].

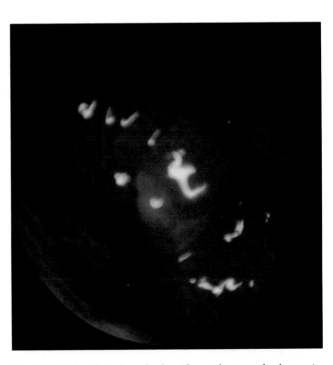

Fig. 23.11 Left unilateral nasal polypoid mass that proved to be consistent with inverted papilloma

Cystic Fibrosis

Cystic fibrosis is an inherited autosomal-recessive disease that gives rise to poor mucus transport. This disease is the most common of the inherited defects causing chronic rhinosinusitis to be identified to date. Cystic fibrosis is defined by abnormal electrolyte and water movement across epithelial cell membranes. The abnormal movement of fluid causes inadequate hydration of the mucus secretions and subsequent thickening, which make the cilia unable to move the mucus in its normal pathways. The mucous plugging that occurs in many sites is thought to give rise to chronic inflammation and subsequent fibrosis. As children rarely develop allergic nasal polyps before the age of 10 years [64], therefore, the presence of nasal polyps in young children requires evaluation for cystic fibrosis.

Nasal polyps have been reported in 1–50% of patients with cystic fibrosis, most frequently in children aged between 4 and 12 years [65–67]. The gross structure of polyps from cystic fibrosis patients does not differ from patients without the disease [68]. In addition, cystic fibrosis may present as nasal polyps in middle age [69]. The diagnosis of cystic fibrosis can be assessed by a sweat chloride test, transepithelial potential difference measurements, or, more accurately, by molecular analysis of the cystic fibrosis transmembrane conductance regulator (CFTR) gene. CFTR gene mutations are frequently detected in adults with various diseases, such as congenital bilateral absence of vas deferens [70, 71], diffuse bronchiectasis [72, 73], or chronic pancreatitis [74], without any other clinical features of cystic fibrosis. Recent studies, conducted in patients with chronic sinusitis or nasal polyposis, have indicated a variable frequency (5–38%) of CFTR gene mutations [75–77]. Among patients with cystic fibrosis and nasal polyposis, nasal polyposis was significantly greater among homozygotes for CFTR mutation ΔF508 [67].

As in aspirin-sensitive patients, nasal polyposis tends to have high recurrence rates in patients with cystic fibrosis [78]. Stammberger [56] has noted that the term recurrence is not really accurate, because the diffuse polypoid inflammatory disease process, polyposis, never really stops. These patients do seem to have marked quality-of-life improvement after sinus surgery, but maintenance therapy with saline rinses and nebulized antibiotics is often needed to decrease the viscosity of secretions. Higher rates of lower respiratory tract colonization with *Pseudomonas* have been associated with the presence of nasal polyps in patients with cystic fibrosis, but this association does not necessarily lead to increased morbidity [79, 80]. Though limited by small numbers, a retrospective review examining post-functional endoscopic sinus surgery (FESS) pulmonary function in patients with cystic fibrosis failed to demonstrate improvement in pulmonary function postoperatively [81]. A review of adult patients with cystic fibrosis, who as children underwent FESS after their first growth spurt but before their second growth spurt, revealed no significant difference in cephalometric analysis to determine facial growth compared with controls [82].

Overall, cystic fibrosis continues to be a challenging chronic disease process, and the nasal polyps in these patients seem to be a result of the underlying mucous stasis and subsequent inflammation rather than causal. A patient with cystic fibrosis can be monitored symptomatically as surgery is generally not performed until these patients are symptomatic, even if nasal polyposis is seen on CT scan or nasal endoscopy. Certainly, each patient is treated on an individual basis.

Primary Ciliary Dyskinesia

Apart from cystic fibrosis, primary ciliary dyskinesia is a disorder affecting airway epithelial cells and is characterized by abnormal ciliary structure and function responsible for impairment of mucociliary clearance and leading to recurrent respiratory tract infections. Inheritance of this disorder is most likely autosomal recessive and can impact almost any point of the cilia. However, the most common defect is in the dynein arms. Immotile cilia and subsequent stasis of secretions gives rise to chronic recurrent sinopulmonary infections. Primary ciliary dyskinesia is usually diagnosed during childhood in the presence of bronchiectasis and chronic purulent sinusitis, associated in about one half of cases with situs inversus (visceral malposition) and infertility [83]. Nasal polyposis occurs in approximately one-third of patients [84]. Primary ciliary dyskinesia has been detected in 6% of children with recurrent upper and lower airway infections [85] and in 13% of adults with diffuse bronchiectasis [86], and primary ciliary dyskinesia has been found in 17% of adult patients with chronic sinusitis and nasal polyposis [87]. Management should include aggressive measures to enhance clearance of secretions and to prevent respiratory infections. As in CF, patients with primary ciliary dyskinesia can be monitored symptomatically because endoscopic sinus surgery and polypectomy are not performed until these patients are symptomatic, even if nasal polyposis is seen on CT scan or nasal endoscopy. Again, each patient is treated on an individual basis.

Churg-Strauss Syndrome

Ear, nose and throat involvement is common in Churg-Strauss syndrome (CSS), usually manifesting as allergic rhinitis and chronic rhinosinusitis with or without nasal polyps. Churg-Strauss syndrome is defined as an eosinophilic, granulomatous inflammation and necrotizing vasculitis of the upper respiratory tract affecting small to medium-sized vessels and is associated with asthma and eosinophilia. In 1990, the American College of Rheumatology established six criteria for the classification of CSS: a history of asthma, eosinophilia (>10% peripheral blood count), mononeuropathy or polyneuropathy, nonfixed pulmonary infiltrates, paranasal sinus abnormalities, and biopsy demonstrating extravascular eosinophils [88]. The disease has been described as occurring in three phases: first, a prodromal phase that may persist for years, consisting of allergic disease, commonly allergic rhinitis and nasal polyposis, and frequently accompanied by asthma; next, progressive peripheral blood and tissue eosinophilia, chronic eosinophilic pneumonia, or eosinophilic gastroenteritis develops; and lastly a life-threatening systemic vasculitis. This syndrome is usually associated with nasal polyps and lacks the diffuse mucosal destruction associated with Wegener's granulomatosis.

Histopathologically, Churg-Strauss syndrome consists of prominent eosinophilic inflammation of vessels and perivascular tissue, with accompanying infiltration of leukocytes, plasma cells, and histiocytes in some patients. All patients are afflicted with vasculitis of the small arteries and veins. The morphologic difference between Wegener's granulomatosis and Churg-Strauss syndrome is that the Wegener's granulomatous inflammation displays more liquefactive necrosis versus the more fibrinoid, necrotizing eosinophilic granulomas seen in Churg-Strauss syndrome. Unlike Wegener's granulomatosis, patients with Churg-Strauss syndrome typically have nasal polyposis rather than crusting and granulation, and the intranasal destructive changes associated with Wegener's granulomatosis are not commonly found in Churg-Strauss syndrome. In addition, serum eosinophilia is not seen in patients with Wegener's granulomatosis. Though both Wegener's granulomatosis and Churg-Strauss syndrome patients have significant pulmonary findings, the infrequency of renal manifestations in Churg-Strauss syndrome also distinguishes it from Wegener's granulomatosis. Churg-Strauss syndrome tends to respond well to systemic corticosteroids and does not respond to cyclophosphamide, as opposed to Wegener's granulomatosis.

No reliable test exists to indisputably confirm or exclude the presence of Churg-Strauss syndrome [89]. It is the specific combination of clinical, radiological, serological, and histological factors, as well as a high index of suspicion, that leads to the final diagnosis.

Peutz-Jeghers Syndrome

Peutz-Jeghers syndrome is an autosomal-dominant hamartomatous polyposis syndrome of the gastrointestinal tract that has been shown to be caused by a germline mutation. Nasal polyposis was described in the original report of the syndrome by Peutz [90]. Recently, a molecular–genetic association between nasal polyposis and Peutz-Jeghers syndrome has been reported, and all patients in a case series from the Netherlands expressed the syndrome's germline mutation [91]. Of note, Peutz-Jeghers syndrome-related nasal polyps revealed significantly less eosinophilia than sporadic nasal polyps.

Medical Therapy

Corticosteroids

Corticosteroids are the mainstay of medical management of nasal polyposis and are by far the best-studied medication in this regard. Systemic steroids are often used as medical polypectomy, reducing inflammation in eosinophilic and noneosinophilically dominated polyps. Their effect has been less well documented than that of intranasal steroids, but several studies have detailed symptomatic improvement in nasal polyposis patients taking systemic steroids, especially for regaining the sense of the smell [92–95]. Systemic (oral, intramuscular, or intravenous) corticosteroids can reduce the size of nasal polyps to an extent that is comparable with surgery [96]. Often a systemic burst is used to shrink large obstructing polyps to provide more area to apply topical steroid therapy. A recent study using this protocol in 152 patients noted 68.5% success after 1-year follow-up, with 31.5% ultimately requiring surgical intervention [97]. Preoperative steroid treatment is also used to minimize polyp size and blood loss, and postoperative steroid pulses can be used for recurrent disease.

A typical taper may be as high as prednisone at 60 mg daily with a taper of 10 mg every several days over a 3-week period. High-risk patients to treat with systemic steroids include diabetics, and patients with glaucoma, gastric ulcers, osteoporosis, hypertension, or psychiatric disorders [98]. These patients, in addition to those requiring repetitive systemic steroid dosing, need to be informed of the risks of systemic steroid use. If sequelae from steroids do arise, the steroid dose can be tapered quickly over 2 to 3 days.

Intranasal steroids have been used extensively as first-line management of nasal polyposis with very few adverse effects. Usually, patients with small polyps and limited involvement on CT scan are good candidates for topical therapy alone. Intranasal steroids have repeatedly been shown to reduce nasal obstruction, drainage, and polyp recurrence [92, 93, 99, 100]. The effect of steroids seems to be nonspecific, improving symptoms in both eosinophilically and non-eosinophilically dominated polyps. Although no studies have confirmed reductions in mucoperiosteal thickening on CT scan [97], intranasal steroids can provide excellent maintenance therapy to help control polyp development [101, 102]. The symptomatic efficacy of intranasal corticosteroid therapy in patients with nasal polyposis is well-documented [103, 104]. During the period of treatment with topical intranasal corticosteroids, symptoms of nasal obstruction, rhinorrhea, and hyposmia are reduced, especially in patients with obstructive polyposis [105]. The improvements in nasal obstruction could be objectively demonstrated via peak nasal inspiratory flow, rhinomanometry, and objective smell testing [106–107]. Specifically, treatment with topical fluticasone nasal drops in patients who had nasal polyposis and chronic rhinosinusitis demonstrated objective improvement in symptom scores, improvement in nasal airflow, decreased polyp volume, and obviated the need for endoscopic sinus surgery in about half of treated patients [109, 110]. Topical corticosteroids reduce polyp recurrence [106, 111] and should be used in the long term, preferably by employing a molecule with low systemic absorption in droplet form and applying it in the head upside-down position [112, 113].

After therapy is initiated, it is recommended that the patient be re-examined in 6–8 weeks to evaluate efficacy [97]. It is generally expected that clinical improvement may take several weeks, but a recent study has noted significant clinical changes within 3 days of treatment [114]. Nasal bleeding is the most common adverse event and can usually be minimized by directing the medication away from the nasal septum. Topical steroid therapy in children with polyps has also been shown to be safe, with no overall effect on attainable height when using clinically recommended doses [115, 116]. Most recently, nasal nebulizers have been used to control refractory rhinosinusitis with antibiotics [117, 118], but no clinical studies have yet documented the benefit of nebulized nasal steroid.

23

Although clinically ill-defined, corticosteroid insensitivity of inflammatory cells may interfere with the efficacy of topical or systemic corticosteroids. Different mechanisms have been proposed to significantly inhibit glucocorticoid signaling, including down-regulation of intranuclear steroid receptors and repression of steroid-responsive transcription [119]. Interestingly, stimulation of normal peripheral mononuclear cells with the *Staphylococcus* superantigen can induce a significant increase in glucocorticoid receptor-β, which is paralleled by corticosteroid insensitivity compared with unstimulated cells [120]. A higher proportion of inflammatory cells expressing this β-isoform has been found in nasal polyps being expressed by T cells, eosinophils, and macrophages [121].

Antibiotic Therapy

Most of the data regarding antibiotic therapy and nasal polyps are based on the efficacy of macrolides. The effectiveness of this group of antibiotics seems to be related to their anti-inflammatory properties rather than their antimicrobial characteristics [122]. Macrolides seem to decrease degranulation of neutrophils and eosinophils and to reduce fibroblast activity in vitro [123].

Recent studies have shown that long-term, low-dose macrolide therapy is effective for treating chronic airway inflammation, and among these are studies suggesting that macrolides play a role in the treatment of chronic rhinosinusitis [124, 125]. Research has helped to clarify the mechanisms by which macrolides suppress inflammation, but their precise action remains unknown. Macrolides inhibit production of proinflammatory cytokines in vitro from various cells [126, 127]. Additionally, they have been shown to decrease airway mucous secretion and inhibit inflammatory cell chemotaxis [128]. Macrolides may also inhibit the migration of inflammatory cells to sites of inflammation as they down-regulate the expression of adhesion molecules in vitro [129]. Recent evidence suggests that macrolides may target the pro-inflammatory nuclear transcription factor-kB (NF-kB), as clarithromycin reduced the DNA-binding activity of NF-kB in human nasal epithelium and fibroblasts [130]. In vitro studies revealed decreased expression of TGF-β and NF-kB in paranasal sinus mucosa [131]. Compared with prednisolone in cultured nasal mucosa from patients with chronic rhinosinusitis, clarithromycin produced an equivalent reduction in IL-5, IL-8, and GM-CSF [127].

Much of the evidence regarding the anti-inflammatory activity of macrolides concerns their effect on neutrophilic inflammation. Though eosinophils have a well-established role in chronic sinus inflammation, macrolide therapy's effect on eosinophilic inflammation is much less clear. Of note, roxithromycin treatment for 3 weeks in a mouse model of asthma was found to inhibit production of IL-5 in lung extracts and decreased bronchial response to systemic methacholine challenge [132]. In a randomized trial of asthmatics treated with clarithromycin or placebo for 8 weeks, those treated with clarithromycin showed significantly decreased peripheral blood and sputum eosinophil counts [133]. Critics have proposed that macrolide therapy in these asthmatic patients actually treated underlying infectious

processes and that their direct anti-inflammatory effects should be regarded critically [134].

Though there are very few in vivo studies investigating the anti-inflammatory effects of macrolides, most of the clinical studies of successful macrolide therapy in nasal polyposis emanate from Japan and have all been uncontrolled studies. Ichimura et al. [135] have noted that roxithromycin, at a dosage of 150 mg/day for 8 weeks, resulted in a reduction of polyps in 52% of the patients with smaller polyps, which are more likely to diminish in size. When cetirizine was added to the treatment group, the success rate for polyp reduction increased to 68%, although this difference was statistically insignificant. In an uncontrolled study treating patients with long-term low-dose macrolide therapy for chronic rhinosinusitis, patients with normal IgE noted significantly higher symptom improvement than patients with elevated IgE and elevated peripheral blood, nasal smear, and nasal mucosal eosinophil counts [136]. This led to the conclusion that macrolides are capable of reducing sinonasal inflammation in chronic rhinosinusitis, but not in patients with IgE or eosinophil-dominated inflammation. This discrepancy between apparent improvement in eosinophilic inflammation in asthmatic patients and no improvement in patients with eosinophilic chronic rhinosinusitis emphasizes the need for placebo-controlled studies to investigate potential symptomatic improvement and changes in inflammatory mediators in vivo. Additionally, some authors have advocated using macrolides in patients when corticosteroid therapy seems to fail [137], but the exact role of macrolides in the paradigm of polyp management remains ill-defined. Randomization of CT staging and consistent definitions of clinical success are needed before the usefulness of macrolide therapy in polyp patients can truly be assessed.

Antifungal Therapy

The exact role fungi play in the development of nasal polyps remains controversial. Because of the high prevalence of fungi noted in some studies [138], some authors believe that fungal antigens may produce chronic inflammation that can lead to nasal polyps. As such, topical intranasal antifungal therapy has been tried as an option to reduce the antigenic load, and, ultimately, the eosinophilic inflammation in chronic rhinosinusitis. The prevalence of fungal infection is also unclear, because fungal exposure differs among countries and within regions of the United States. One disease that is directly related to fungal exposure is allergic fungal rhinosinusitis, in which antifungal immunotherapy may be helpful in reducing mucosal edema and preventing recurrence in patients with fungal allergies [139].

In an open-label study in which patients with chronic rhinosinusitis performed twice daily intranasal irrigations with 20 mL of amphotericin B solution (100 mg/mL) for approximately 1 year, improvements in symptoms and endoscopic staging was noted in 75% of patients [140]. Another uncontrolled study [141] using amphotericin B nasal irrigations in nasal polyp patients noted that 39% of patients experienced endoscopic disappearance of polyps after 4 weeks of irrigations. In another uncontrolled study in which intranasal amphotericin B was applied as a 20-mL suspension per nostril twice daily with a bulb syringe for 4 weeks, Ricchetti et al. reported the disappearance of polyposis on endoscopy in 62% of patients with mild chronic rhinosinusitis and in 42% of patients with moderate chronic rhinosinusitis. However, none of their patients with severe chronic rhinosinusitis and near-obstructing nasal polyps showed improvement [138]. The authors hypothesized that the lack of improvement in the most severe cases could be due to limited access of topical medication to much of the sinus mucosa or the brief duration of therapy. In a double-blind, placebo-controlled trial using a bulb syringe to deliver 20 mL of amphotericin B (250 mg/mL) or placebo to each nostril twice daily for 6 months in patients with chronic rhinosinusitis [142], significantly reduced mucosal thickening was found on CT scans and nasal endoscopy. All patients' nasal mucus contained *Alternaria* proteins pre-treatment, but the changes in *Alternaria* concentrations at 6 months were not statistically different between treatment groups.

An open-label prospective trial in which topical amphotericin B was administered in patients with nasal polyps yielded no improvement in symptoms over 3 months, and for the most part, symptoms in the patients worsened [143]. In a randomized, placebo-controlled trial, patients with nasal polyposis received either topical amphotericin B or placebo four times daily for 8 weeks [144]. No difference in follow-up CT scan scores was observed between groups, and the median post-treatment symptom score was significantly worse in the amphotericin B group than in patients receiving placebo. This study explicitly excluded CRS patients with any suspected fungal etiology, and this choice remains unclear. This patient cohort was further studied to determine the effect of intranasal amphotericin B treatment on nasal eosinophil cationic protein and tryptase levels, which are markers of eosinophilic and mast cell inflammation respectively [145]. Neither topical amphotericin B therapy nor fungal state pre- and post-treatment had a significant influence on activation markers of eosinophilic or mast cell inflammation in chronic rhinosinusitis.

In a prospective, randomized clinical trial [146], patients with nasal polyps and positive mycotic nasal cultures were randomized to either pretreatment with systemic corticosteroids or endoscopic ethmoidectomy and polypectomy and were then treated with either intranasal lysine acetylsalicylate alone or intranasal lysine acetylsalicylate and intranasal amphotericin B. Overall, patients treated surgically had significantly less polypoid recurrence postoperatively than patients pretreated with systemic corticosteroids, and patients treated with both intranasal lysine acetylsalicylate and amphotericin B had significantly less polyp recurrence. These results suggest that long-term topical treatment with lysine acetylsalicylate and amphotericin B may be clinically effective in the treatment of patients with nasal polyposis associated with fungal disease.

Ultimately, the conflicting findings of efficacy of antifungal therapy emphasize the need for further controlled studies to separate out confounding factors of corticosteroid use and different stages of pre-treatment disease among patients before successes can be proven.

Antihistamines

The prevalence of atopy in patients with nasal polyposis reportedly varies from 10 to 64% [147]. Although antihistamines may provide relief of allergic symptoms in patients with nasal polyposis, polyp regression is not significantly seen. In a study examining cetirizine use in nasal polyposis, a reduction in concomitant nasal symptoms of sneezing and rhinorrhea was noted in 45 patients followed for 3 months [148]. Antihistamines are not currently indicated in the primary management of polyp patients unless there is an underlying allergic pathology.

Leukotriene Modifiers

Many studies using the leukotriene receptor antagonist montelukast have demonstrated significant reductions in absolute eosinophil cell counts in peripheral blood and sputum in patients with allergic rhinitis and asthma compared with placebo, confirming the role of leukotrienes in eosinophilic inflammation [149–151]. Patients with chronic hyperplastic rhinosinusitis also had an increase in transcription in leukotriene metabolic precursor proteins. Leukotriene modifiers reduce tissue eosinophilia in asthmatics [152] and will likely provide benefit to patients with chronic sinusitis with nasal polyposis through inhibiting eosinophil recruitment, through decreased activation of sinonasal eosinophils, and through blocking systemic humoral pathways. Although it is clear that zileuton, zafirlukast, and montelukast play an important role in the management of asthma, limited data exist to prove their value in nasal polyposis. Parnes and Chuma confirmed the benefit of zileuton and zafirlukast among nasal polyp patients, with clinical improvement seen in 72% of patients in an open-label trial [153]. A placebo-controlled trial of the 5-lipoxygenase inhibitor, zileuton, was shown to reduce polyp size and improve anosmia [154].

Ulualp et al. studied 18 previously operated sinus patients with aspirin-sensitive polyposis after they had taken zileuton or zafirlukast for longer than 1 month, and found that 60% of patients experienced subjective clinical improvement confirmed by objective endoscopic findings [155]. In an open-label trial of patients with nasal polyposis who were using daily intranasal steroid sprays for a minimum of 6 months, montelukast sodium (10 mg daily) was added for 3 months [156]. Symptom scores significantly improved in 71% of patients and nasal polyp eosinophilia scores significantly improved, with the improvement most noticeable in the patients with perennial allergies.

Therapy of aspirin-exacerbated eosinophilic chronic rhinosinusitis generally includes the combination of systemic and topical steroids, the use of leukotriene modifiers such as the lipoxygenase inhibitor zileuton, and the cysteinyl leukotriene antagonists such as montelukast or zafirlukast.

Aspirin Desensitization

In 1922, the term "aspirin triad" was used by Widal et al. [157] to describe patients with aspirin sensitivity, nasal polyposis, and asthma, and the term was later popularized by Samter and

Beers [158]. Since that time, a much more detailed understanding of the pathophysiology has led clinicians to utilize aspirin desensitization to treat these patients' asthma and nasal polyp disease. Stevenson et al. [38] has developed protocols for inducing aspirin tolerance in these patients through desensitization. The protocol involves progressively increasing oral aspirin in a monitored setting until 450–650 mg of aspirin is tolerated. Once this occurs, daily aspirin is administered with dosages ranging up to 650 mg twice daily for the first month, and then reduced to 325 mg twice daily if the patient's nasal congestion has subsided and sense of smell has returned [159]. If the patient is taking systemic corticosteroids daily or every other day, reducing and discontinuing corticosteroids is recommended before reducing aspirin dose. After reducing the dose of aspirin, if there is a return of nasal congestion, aspirin doses should be increased to previous levels [159]. Nasal responsiveness seems better than bronchial responsiveness, and polyp recurrence in these patients has been shown to be delayed an average of 6 years [38, 159]. These patients also display a significant reduction in the need for both systemic and topical corticosteroids, and there is a concomitant decrease in the frequency of sinus infections annually [38, 159]. If aspirin is discontinued, aspirin sensitivity recurs within 48–96 h, necessitating lifelong therapy. It is recommended that aspirin-sensitive patients undergo endoscopic sinus surgery, followed by desensitization within several weeks, because surgery debulks polypoid disease. Currently aspirin desensitization is recommended for asthmatics unresponsive to medical therapy or requiring high systemic corticosteroid doses and for patients with severe polyps who have required repeated sinus surgery.

Other investigators have also corroborated the beneficial results in chronic polypoid rhinosinusitis. Gosepath et al. [160] have noted that lower doses of aspirin (100 mg) may work as well as higher doses. Typical side effects during desensitization include bronchospasm and nasal-ocular symptoms, both of which are readily controllable [161]. Asthma must be fully controlled before desensitization is started, because bronchospasm is most likely to occur early in the desensitization [38, 159]. Desensitization can thus be considered a critical component of nasal polyp control among these patients.

Topical lysine aspirin seems to have an anti-proliferative effect on fibroblasts from nasal polyps in vitro [162]. A controlled study revealed postoperative treatment with lysine aspirin in both aspirin-tolerant and aspirin-sensitive patients diminished the recurrence rates of polyps [163]. Because both groups benefited equally, lysine aspirin may act as an anti-inflammatory agent rather than through true desensitization. Sousa et al. demonstrated an increase in the cys-leukotriene1 receptor in inflammatory cells, polyps, and epithelium of patients with aspirin-sensitive eosinophilic rhinosinusitis [164]. Moreover, these authors also demonstrated that application of lysine aspirin resulted in significant down-regulation of cysL1-receptor expression compared with placebo.

Although other non-steroidal anti-inflammatory drugs may provoke symptoms in aspirin-sensitive patients, desensitization only can be adequately accomplished with oral aspirin or topical lysine aspirin [165]. For optimal treatment, these authors recommend nasal polypectomy to be performed initially, followed by aspirin desensitization with concomitant leukotriene inhibition.

Intranasal Furosemide

Polyps are well-known to be edematous structures, probably absorbing plasma and water into the lamina propria. Interestingly, intranasal furosemide at a dose of 100 μg to each nostril daily has been shown to significantly minimize postoperative relapse in nasal polyps compared with topical intranasal mometasone [166]. In a randomized prospective trial [167], 7 days of preoperative treatment with oral methylprednisolone (1 mg/kg/day) or inhaled topical furosemide (6.6 mmol/L solution nebulized – maximum dose 20 mg daily), subjective symptoms and endoscopy scores did not differ significantly between the groups post-treatment, and though steroid treatment significantly reduced eosinophil counts, no effect on mast cells or edema was noted. Though furosemide treatment did not affect inflammatory cell counts significantly, it significantly reduced edema in previously unoperated patients. No difference in intraoperative bleeding was observed between the groups. Though its use has not become widespread, topical furosemide may be a useful preoperative adjunct in patients who are unable to tolerate systemic corticosteroid therapy.

Topical Decongestants

To assess whether topical decongestion invalidates the estimation of polyp size in clinical and scientific practice, a double-blind, placebo-controlled randomized study was performed to examine the effect of the decongestants nafazoline and epinephrine on nasal polyp size as assessed by means of endoscopic scoring [168]. No significant effect of decongestion on polyp size could be demonstrated for either treatment.

Intranasal Capsaicin

Capsaicin, the pungent agent in hot pepper, has been used intranasally in nasal polyp patients with subjective and objective success in improving symptoms. Its method of action appears to be blocking neurogenic inflammation in the nose after topical application, resulting in a depletion of neurokinins [169]. This treatment has been used before and after sinus surgery [170], with significant improvement in nasal symptoms and significant reduction in recurrence of nasal polyposis for 9 months post-polypectomy compared with a placebo control group. Capsaicin may provide a low-cost alternative to corticosteroids that could be used in developing countries [171].

Surgical Management

Controversy continues regarding the exact role of surgery in the management of nasal polyp disease. It remains clear that nasal polyposis is a chronic mucosal disease and that surgery is used as an adjunct to control the disease process once it is refractory to medical therapy. The exact timing of this intervention is debatable and may be tailored to individual patients. In those patients with nasal polyp disease and concomitant asthma, surgical intervention may be considered when repeated sinus infections are causing a worsening of the lower airway disease. A position statement has noted that surgery should not be considered before completion of 1 month of medical treatment, as many patients will not require surgical therapy [172]. Given the potential dramatic response that can be seen with a combination of systemic and topical steroids, this strategy seems reasonable when approaching surgical therapy in these patients.

It is well understood that endoscopic sinus surgery has improved the ability to obtain safe and thorough cleansing of paranasal sinus cavities with excellent outcomes, even among polyp patients with extensive disease. Weber et al. [139] have noted that outcomes were successful in 92% of patients even up to 10 years post-sinus surgery. Surgery controls the severity of polypoid obstruction, and the resulting enlargement of paranasal sinus openings facilitates topical application of medications despite many patients continuing to experience radiographic mucoperiosteal thickening. Many studies, however, note that patients with nasal polyposis, especially patients who are aspirin-sensitive, experience high rates of recurrence [56, 173]. Clearly, surgery cannot be evaluated alone, but more appropriately as one of many therapeutic modalities to control nasal polyp disease. Comparative studies of medical versus surgical therapy are often unrealistic, because there are confounding factors and selection bias for both groups and the treatment regimens often rely integrally on one another.

The extent of surgery to be performed remains controversial. Polypectomy alone is incapable of effectively achieving permanent eradication of disease and has largely been abandoned for more complete removal of affected air cells. McFadden et al. [174] were among the first to compare conservative (simple ethmoidectomy) versus radical (Caldwell Luc/trans-sphenoethmoidectomy) surgery in aspirin triad patients and noted that none of the 9 patients undergoing the more radical procedure had recurrence, contrasted against the 6 out of 16 patients undergoing conservative therapy requiring revision. Unfortunately, this retrospective study was not controlled to include disease severity as a confounder.

To some degree, it seems logical that the severity of disease on CT scan should dictate the extent of surgery. Many patients with isolated disease in the ostiomeatal complex require limited surgery, whereas patients with diffuse polypoid mucosa and large obstructive polyps require a more radical surgical approach. Therefore, the operative approach to polyp removal may be based upon the same underlying principles that govern endoscopic sinus surgery in the absence of nasal polyps. The introduction of powered-instrumentation (microdebriders) has also facilitated sinus surgery by preserving normal anatomy and causing less blood loss, and thereby improving visualization during operative cases. Although complete resolution of mucosal abnormalities is rare, continued medical management and vigilant follow-up make revision surgery unnecessary in the vast majority of patients. Successful treatment ultimately depends on a commitment by both the patient and the physician to an intensive postoperative course, which may be quite prolonged and involve multiple debridements.

Although surgical intervention alone does not appear to improve olfaction more than medical treatment alone [175], improved aeration may allow a subset of patients to apply corticosteroids to previously unreachable areas. A postoperative steroid burst may prove helpful in controlling polypoid mucosa along the roof of the ethmoid and cribriform to improve nasal airflow in the olfactory cleft.

Aspirin-sensitive patients are particularly challenging with regard to surgical outcomes. However, among these patients, a number of studies have documented favorable results [174, 176, 177]. When extirpative surgery is combined with aspirin desensitization, patients can experience improved disease-free sinus and asthma intervals. Outcomes have shown that more than 80% of patients will obtain improvement in nasal symptom score and asthma severity [38]. Usually, surgery in aspirin-sensitive polyposis is more extensive in nature than in general polyp patients, and postoperative systemic steroids may be needed to maintain the patient's improvement before desensitization.

In a review of randomized controlled trials, nonrandomized comparative studies, and case series studies that described outcomes associated with endoscopic sinus surgery performed for the excision of nasal polyps, symptomatic improvement ranged from 78 to 88% for FESS compared with 43 to 84% for comparative procedures, which included endoscopic polypectomy, Caldwell-Luc, and intranasal ethmoidectomy [178].

In a prospective, blind, randomized controlled trial, patients were randomized to receive a unilateral transoral infiltration of the pterygopalatine fossa with 2 mL of 2% lidocaine and 1:80,000 adrenalin [179]. Improved intraoperative hemostasis was noted on the injected side, and this could prove useful in sinus surgery for nasal polyposis.

Surgical Complications

In a review of randomized controlled trials, nonrandomized comparative studies, and case series studies that described outcomes associated with endoscopic sinus surgery performed for the excision of nasal polyps [179], major complications ranged from 0 to 1.5% (median, 0%) and minor complications ranged from 1.1 to 20.8% (median, 7.5%). The potentially most serious complications were cerebrospinal fluid leaks, injury to the internal carotid artery, exposure of the dura mater, postoperative meningitis, intraoperative and postoperative bleeding requiring transfusion, periorbital and/or orbital fat exposure, and orbital penetration.

In a large study of patients undergoing sinonasal surgery in England and Wales [181], major complications (orbital or intracranial complications, bleeding requiring vessel ligation or orbital decompression, or return to the operating room) occurred in 0.4% of patients. Minor complications occurred in 6.6% of patients, and these included excessive perioperative bleeding (5.0%) and postoperative hemorrhage requiring intervention (0.8%). These authors found the complication rate to be

23

linked to the extent of disease measured in terms of preoperative symptom severity, the extent of polyposis, extent of opacification on CT scan, and patients having medical co-morbidities based on American Society of Anesthesiologists (ASA) scores, but complication rates were not associated with surgical characteristics (extent of surgery, use of powered instrumentation, and the training level of the surgeon) [180]. In a review of objective and subjective outcomes after revision sinus surgery for chronic rhinosinusitis, the only patients noted to fail after revision surgery were patients with nasal polyposis [181].

References

1. Bateman N, Fahy C, Woolford T. Nasal polyps: still more questions than answers. *J Laryngol* 2003;117:1–9.

2. Hedman J, Kapiro J, Poussa T, *et al*. Prevalence of asthma, aspirin intolerance, nasal polyposis, and chronic obstructive pulmonary disease in a population-based study. *Int J Epidemiol*. 1999; 28 (4): 717–22.

3. Settipane G. Nasal polyps: epidemiology, pathology, immunology and treatment. *Am J Rhinol* 1987;1:119–26.

4. Larsen PL, Tos M. Origin of nasal polyps. *Laryngoscope* 1991; 101: 305–12.

5. Larsen PL, Tos M. Origin of nasal polyps. Transcranially removed nasoethmoidal blocks as a screening method for nasal polyps in an autopsy material. *Rhinology* 1995; 33: 185–8.

6. Larsen PL, Tos M, Baer S. En bloc removal of the ethmoid and ostiomeatal complex in cadavers, with a practical application. *Rhinology* 1994; 32: 62–4.

7. Larsen PL, Tos M. Origin of nasal polyps: an endoscopic autopsy study. *Laryngoscope*. 2004;114 (4): 710–9.

8. Andrews AE, Bryson JM, Rowe-Jones JM. Site of origin of nasal polyps: relevance to pathogenesis and management. *Rhinology*. 2005; 43(3): 180–4.

9. Stammberger H. Functional endoscopic sinus surgery. The Messerklinger technique. Toronto, Philadelphia: BC Decker; 1991.

10. Alobid I, Benitez P, Valero A, *et al*. The impact of atopy, sinus opacification, and nasal patency on quality of life in patients with severe nasal polyposis. *Otolaryngol Head Neck Surg*. 2006; 134(4): 609–12.

11. Bachert C, Wagenmann M, Hauser U, *et al*. Nasal polyposis: from cytokines to growth. *Am J Rhinol* 2000; 105 (4): 782–7.

12. Tos M, Sasaki Y, Ohnishi M, *et al*. Pathogenesis of nasal polyps. *Rhinol Suppl* 1992; 14: 181–5.

13. Stammberger H. Examination and endoscopy of the nose and paranasal sinuses. In: Mygind N, Lindholt T, ed. Nasal polyposis: an inflammatory disease and its treatment. Copenhagen (Denmark): Munksgaard; 1997; 120–36.

14. Mygind N, Dahl R, Bachert C. Nasal polyposis, eosinophil dominated inflammation, and allergy. *Thorax* 2000; 55(2): S79–83.

15. Bernstein JM, Gorfien J, Noble B. Role of allergy in nasal polyposis: a review. *Otolaryngol Head Neck Surg* 1995; 113(6): 724–32.

16. Kern RA, Schenck H-P. Allergy: a constant factor in the etiology of so-called mucous nasal polyps. *J Allergy* 1933; 4: 483.

17. Delaney JC. Aspirin idiosyncrasy in patients admitted for nasal polypectomy. *Clin Otolaryngol* 1976; 1: 27–30.

18. Blumstein GI, Tuft L. Allergy treatment in recurrent nasal polyposis. Its importance and value. *Am J Med Sci* 1957; 234: 269–80.

19. Moloney JR. Nasal polyps, nasal polypectomy, asthma and aspirin sensitivity. Their association in 445 cases of nasal polyps. *J Laryngol Otol* 1977; 91: 837–46.

20. English GM. Nasal polyposis. In: English GM, ed. Otolaryngology, Vol. 2. Philadelphia: Harper and Row. 1985; p.1–30.

21. Pepys J, Duveen GE. Negative skin tests in allergic rhinitis and nasal polyposis. *Int Arch Allergy* 1951; 2: 147–60.

22. Mygind N. Nasal allergy. Oxford: Blackwell; 1978.

23. Xaubet A, Mullol J, Lopez E, *et al*. Comparison of the role of nasal polyp and normal nasal mucosal epithelial cells on *in vitro* eosinophil survival. Mediation by GM-CSF and inhibition by dexamethasone. *Clin Exp Allergy* 1994; 24: 307–17.

24. Olze H, Forster U, Zuberbier T, *et al*. Eosinophilic nasal polyps are a rich source of eotaxin, eotaxin-2 and eotaxin-3. *Rhinology*. 2006; 44: 145–50.

25. Ruhno J, Howie K, Anderson M, *et al*. The increased number of epithelial mast cells in nasal polyps and adjacent turbinates is not allergy-dependent. *Allergy* 1990; 4545: 370–4.

26. Settipane G, Chafee F. Nasal polyps in asthma and rhinitis. A review of 6,037 patients. *J Allergy Clin Immunol* 1977; 59: 17–21.

27. Wong D, Dolovich J. Blood eosinophilia and nasal polyps. *Am J Rhinol*. 1992; 6: 195–8.

28. Jamal A, Marant A. Atopy and nasal polyposis. *J Laryngol Otol*. 1987; 101: 355–8.

29. Kitapci F, Muluk NB, Atasoy P, Koc C. Role of mast and goblet cells in the pathogenesis of nasal polyps. *J Otolaryngol*. 2006; 35(2): 122–32.

30. Alatas N, Baba F, San I, *et al*. Nasal polyp diseases in allergic and nonallergic patients and steroid therapy. *Otolaryngol Head Neck Surg*. 2006; 135: 236–42.

31. Collins MM, Loughran S, Davidson P, *et al*. Nasal polyposis: prevalence of positive food and inhalant skin tests. *Otolaryngol Head Neck Surg*. 2006; 135: 680–3.

32. Haberal I, Corey JP. The role of leukotrienes in nasal allergy. *Otolaryngol Head Neck Surg*. 2003; 129: 274–9.

33. Borish L. The role of leukotrienes in upper and lower airway inflammation and the implications for treatment. *Ann Allergy Asthma Immunol*. 2002; 88S: 16–22.

34. Denburg J. Nasal polyposis: cytokines and inflammatory cells. In: Mygind N, Lildholt T, editors. Nasal polyposis: an inflammatory disease and its treatment. Copenhagen (Denmark): Munksgaard; 1997. p. 78–87.

35. Sorensen H, Mygind N, Tygstrup I, *et al*. Histology of nasal polyps of different etiology. *Rhinology* 1977; 15: 121–8.

36. Mullol J, Fernandez-Morata J, Roca-Ferrer J, *et al*. Cyclooxygenase 1 and cyclooxygenase 2 expression is abnormally regulated in human nasal polyps. *J Allergy Clin Immunol* 2002; 109(5): 824–30.

37. Szczeklik A, Stevenson D. Aspirin-induced asthma: advances in pathogenesis and management. *J Allergy Clin Immunol* 1999; 104(1): 5–13.

38. Stevenson D, Hankammer M, Mathison D, *et al.* Aspirin desensitization treatment of aspirin-sensitive patients with rhinosinusitis-asthma: longterm outcomes. *J Allergy Clin Immunol* 1996; 98(4): 751–8.

39. Norlander T, Fukami M, Westrin KM, *et al.* Formation of mucosal polyps in the nasal and maxillary sinus cavities by infection. *Otolaryngol Head Neck Surg.* 1993;109:522–9.

40. Weille FL, Gohd RS. The virus theory of nasal polyp etiology and its practical applications. *Ann Otol Rhinol Laryngol.* 1957; 65: 443–9.

41. Kozak F, Mahoney J, Chernesky M, *et al.* Nasal polyposis: in search of viral etiology using DNA hybridization. *J Otolaryngol.* 1991; 20: 404–7.

42. Tos M, Larsen PL. Nasal polyps: Origin, Etiology, Pathogenesis, and Structure. In: Diseases of the Sinuses: Diagnosis and Treatment. Kennedy DM, Bolger WE, Zinreich SJ ed. Hamilton: B.C. Decker, 2001; p. 57–65.

43. Bachert C, Gevaert P, Holtappels G, *et al* Total and specific IgE in nasal polyps is related to local eosinophilic inflammation. *J Allergy Clin Immunol* 2001; 107: 607–14.

44. Tripathi A, Conley DB, Grammer LC, *et al.* Immunoglobulin E to staphylococcal and streptococcal toxins in patients with chronic sinusitis/nasal polyposis. *Laryngoscope.* 2004; 114: 1822–6.

45. Mafee MF, Nasal cavity and paranasal sinuses. In: Mafee MF, Valvassori GE, Becker M, Ed. Imaging of the Head and Neck, (Stuttgart), Thieme. 2005; pp. 353–474.

46. Mafee MF. Imaging methods for sinusitis. *JAMA,* 1993; 269: 2808.

47. Min YG, Chung JW, Shin JS, *et al.* Histologic structure of antrochoanal polyps. *Acta Otolaryngol.* 1995; 115: 543–7.

48. Hong SK, Min YG, Kim CN, *et al.* Endoscopic removal of the antral portion of the antrochoanal polyp by powered instrumentation. *Laryngoscope.* 2001;111: 1774–8.

49. Cook PR, Davis WE, McDonald R, *et al.* Antrochoanal polyposis: a review of 33 cases. *Ear Nose Throat J.* 1993; 72: 401–10.

50. Kamel R. Endoscopic transnasal surgery in antrochoanal polyps. *Arch Otolaryngol Head Neck Surg.* 1990; 116: 841–4.

51. Sato K, Nakashima T. Endoscopic sinus surgery for chronic sinusitis with antrochoanal polyp. *Laryngoscope.* 2000; 110: 1581–3.

52. Lee T, Huang S. Endoscopic sinus surgery for antrochoanal polyps in children. *Otolaryngology – Head and Neck Surgery.* 2006; 135: 688–92.

53. Heck WE, Hallberg HE, Williams HL. Antrochoanal polyp. *Arch Otolaryngol.* 1950; 52:538–48.

54. Berg O, Carenfelt C, Silfversward C, *et al.* Origin of the choanal polyp. *Arch Otolaryngol Head Neck Surg.* 1988; 114: 1270–1.

55. Bailey BJ, Calhoun KH, Healy GB, *et al,* eds. *Head and Neck Surgery—Otolaryngology.* Vol 1. 3rd ed. Philadelphia, Pa: Lippincott Williams & Wilkins; 2001: 336–361.

56. Stammberger H. Surgical treatment of nasal polyps: past, present, and future. *Allergy* 1999; 54 (Suppl 53): 7–11.

57. Hyams VJ. Papillomas of the nasal cavity and paranasal sinuses. A clinicopathological study of 315 cases. *Ann Otol Rhinol Laryngol.* 1971; 80(2): 192–206.

58. Alun-Jones T, Hill J, Leighton SE, et al. Is routine histological examination of nasal polyps justified? *Clin Otolaryngol* 1990; 15: 217–19.

59. Diamantopoulos II, Jones NS, Lowe J. All nasal polyps need histological examination: an audit-based appraisal of clinical practice. *J Laryngol Otol* 2000; 114: 755–759.

60. Kale SU, Mohite U, Rowlands D, et al. Clinical and histopathological correlation of nasal polyps: are there any surprises? *Clin Otolaryngol* 2001; 26: 321–3.

61. Romashko AA, Stankiewicz JA. Routine histopathology in uncomplicated sinus surgery: is it necessary? *Otolaryngol Head Neck Surg* 2005; 132: 407–12.

62. Cummings CW, Goodman ML. Inverted papilloma of the nose and paranasal sinuses. *Arch Otolaryngol.* 1970; 92: 445–9.

63. Han JK, Smith TL, Loehrl T, *et al.* An evolution in the management of sinonasal inverting papilloma. *Laryngoscope* 2001; 111: 1395–400.

64. Schramm VL, Myers EN, Kennerdell JS. Orbital complications of acute sinusitis: evaluation, management, and outcome. *Trans Am Acad Ophthalmol Otolaryngol* 1978; 86: 221.

65. Schramm VL, Effron MZ. Nasal polyps in children. *Laryngoscope* 1980; 90: 1488–95.

66. Triglia JM, Belus JF, Dessi P, et al. Rhinosinusal manifestations of cystic fibrosis. *Ann Otolaryngol Chir Cervicofac.* 1993; 110:98–102.

67. Sakano E, Ribeiro AF, Barth L, *et al.* Nasal and paranasal sinus endoscopy, computed tomography and microbiology of upper airways and the correlations with genotype and severity of cystic fibrosis. *Int J Pediatr Otorhinolaryngol.* 2007; 71: 41–50.

68. Tos M. Cystic fibrosis (mucoviscidosis). In: English CM, editor. Otolaryngology, Vol. 2. Philadelphia: Harper and Row; 1985. pp. 1–23.

69. Thaler ER, Smullen SM, Kennedy DW. Adult cystic fibrosis presenting with nasal polyposis and chronic sinusitis. *Am J Rhinol.* 1994; 8: 237–9.

70. Casals T, Bassas L, Ruiz-Romero J, et al. Extensive analysis of 40 infertile patients with congenital absence of the vas deferens: in 50% of cases only one CFTR allele could be detected. *Hum Genet* 1995; 95: 205–11.

71. Costes B, Fanen P, Goossens M, Ghanem N. A rapid, efficient, and sensitive assay for simultaneous detection of multiple cystic fibrosis mutations. *Hum Mutat* 1993; 2: 185–91.

72. Pignatti PF, Bombieri C, Marigo C, et al. Increased incidence of cystic fibrosis gene mutations in adults with disseminated bronchiectasis. *Hum Mol Genet* 1995; 4: 635–9.

73. Girodon E, Cazeneuve C, Lebargy F, et al. CFTR gene mutations in adults with disseminated bronchiectasis. *Eur J Hum Genet* 1997; 5: 149–55.

74. Sharer N, Schwarz M, Malone G, *et al.* Mutations of the cystic fibrosis gene in patients with chronic pancreatitis. *N Engl J Med* 1998; 339: 645–52.

75. Irving RM, McMahon R, Clark R, *et al.* Cystic fibrosis transmembrane conductance regulator gene mutations in severe nasal polyposis. *Clin Otolaryngol* 1997; 22: 519–21.

76. Wang X, Moylan B, Leopold DA, et al. Mutation in the gene responsible for cystic fibrosis and predisposition to chronic rhinosinusitis in the general population. *JAMA* 2000; 284: 1814–9.

77. Coste, A, Girodon E, Louis S, *et al.* Atypical Sinusitis in Adults Must Lead to Looking for Cystic Fibrosis and Primary Ciliary Dyskinesia. *Laryngoscope.* 2004; 114: 837–43.

23

78. Triglia J, Nicollas R. Nasal and sinus polyposis in children. *Laryngoscope* 1997; 107: 963–6.

79. Henriksson G, Westrin KM, Karpati F, *et al*. Nasal polyps in cystic fibrosis: clinical endoscopic study with nasal lavage fluid analysis. *Chest* 2002; 121: 40–7.

80. Kingdom T, Lee K, FitzSimmons S, *et al*. Clinical characteristics and genotype analysis of patients with cystic fibrosis and nasal polyposis requiring surgery. *Arch Otolaryngol Head Neck Surg*. 1996; 122: 1209–13.

81. Madonna D, Isaacson G, Rosenfeld RM, *et al*. Effect of sinus surgery on pulmonary function in patients with cystic fibrosis. *Laryngoscope*. 1997; 107: 328–31.

82. Van Peteghem A, Clement PA. Influence of extensive functional endoscopic sinus surgery (FESS) on facial growth in children with cystic fibrosis. Comparison of 10 cephalometric parameters of the midface for three study groups. *Int J Pediatr Otorhinolaryngol*. 2006; 70: 1407–13.

83. Meeks M, Bush A. Primary ciliary dyskinesia (PCD). *Pediatr Pulmonol*. 2000; 29: 307–16.

84. Leigh LW. Primary ciliary dyskinesia. *Semin Respir Crit Care Med*. 2003; 24: 653–62.

85. Chapelin C, Coste A, Reinert P, *et al*. Incidence of primary ciliary dyskinesia in children with recurrent respiratory diseases. *Ann Otol Rhinol Laryngol*. 1997; 106: 854–58.

86. Verra F, Escudier E, Bignon J, *et al*. Inherited factors in diffuse bronchiectasis in the adult: a prospective study. *Eur Respir J*. 1991; 4: 937–44.

87. Coste, A, Girodon E, Louis S, *et al*. Atypical Sinusitis in Adults Must Lead to Looking for Cystic Fibrosis and Primary Ciliary Dyskinesia. *Laryngoscope*. 2004; 114: 837–43.

88. Masi AT, Hunder GG, Lie JT, *et al*. The American College of Rheumatology 1990 criteria for the classification of Churg-Strauss syndrome (allergic granulomatosis and angiitis). *Arthritis Rheum* 1990; 33: 1094–100.

89. Bacciu A, Bacciu S, Mercante G, *et al*. Ear, nose and throat manifestations of Churg-Strauss syndrome. *Acta Otolaryngol*. 2006; 126: 503–9.

90. Peutz JLA. Combined familial polyposis of the mucous membranes of the intestinal tract and of the nose and throat coupled with peculiar pigmentations of skin and mucous membranes. *Ned Maandschr v Geneesk* 1921; 10: 134–46.

91. De Leng WW, Westerman AM, Weterman M, Jansen M, van Dekken H, Giardiello FM, de Rooij FW, Wilson P, Offerhaus GJ, Keller JJ. Nasal polyposis in Peutz-Jeghers syndrome: a distinct histopathologic and molecular genetic entity. *J Clin Pathol*. 2007; 60: 392–6.

92. Mygind N, Lildholt T. Medical management. In: Settipane G, Lund V, Bernstein J, Tos M, eds. Nasal polyps: epidemiology, pathogenesis, and treatment. Providence, RI: Oceanside Publications; 1997; pp. 147–55.

93. Lildholt T, Dahl R, Mygind N. Effect of corticosteroids. Evidence from controlled trials. In: Mygind N, Lildholt T, eds. Nasal polyposis: an inflammatory disease and its treatment. Copenhagen (Denmark): Munksgaard; 1997; pp. 160–9.

94. Van Camp P, Clement P. Results of oral steroid treatment in nasal polyposis. *Rhinology* 1994; 32: 5–9.

95. Heden Blomqvist E, Lundblad L, Anggard A, *et al*. A randomized controlled study evaluating medical treatment versus surgical treatment in addition to medical treatment of nasal polyposis. *J Allergy Clin Immunol* 2001; 107: 224–8.

96. Lindholdt T, Rundcrantz H, Bende H, *et al*. Glucocorticoid treatment for nasal polyps: the use of topical budesonide powder, intramuscular betamethasone, and surgical treatment. *Arch Otolaryngol Head Neck Surg*. 1997; 123: 595–600.

97. Nores JM, Avan P, Bonfils P. Medical management of nasal polyposis: a study in a series of 152 consecutive patients. *Rhinology* 2003; 41: 97–102.

98. Holmstrom M, Holmberg K, Lundblad L, *et al*. Current perspectives on the treatment of nasal polyposis: a Swedish opinion report. *Acta Otolaryngol*. 2002; 122: 736–44.

99. Bernstein JM. Nasal polyps: finding the cause, determining treatment. *J Respir Dis*. 1997; 18: 847–56.

100. Bonfils P, Nores JM, Halimi P, Avan P. Corticosteroid treatment in nasal polyposis with a three-year follow-up period. *Laryngoscope*. 2003; 113: 683–7.

101. Virolainen E, Puhakka H. The effect of intranasal beclomethasone dipropionate on the recurrence of nasal polyps after ethmoidectomy. *Rhinology*. 1980; 18: 9–18.

102. Karlsson G, Rundcrantz H. A randomized trial of intranasal beclomethasone dipropionate after polypectomy. *Rhinology*. 1982; 20: 144–8.

103. Badia L, Lund V. Topical corticosteroids in nasal polyposis. *Drugs*. 2001; 61: 573–8.

104. Fillaci F, Passali D, Puxeddu R, *et al*. A randomized controlled trial showing efficacy of once daily intranasal budesonide in nasal polyposis. *Rhinology* 2000; 38: 185–90.

105. Tos M, Svenstrup F, Arndal H, *et al*. Efficacy of an aqueous and a powder formulation of nasal budesonide compared in patients with nasal polyps. *Am J Rhinol* 1998; 12: 183–9.

106. Holmberg K, Juliusson S, Balder B, *et al*. Fluticasone propionare aqueous nasal spray in the treatment of nasal polyposis. *Ann Allergy Asthma Immunol*. 1997; 78: 270–6.

107. Keith P, Nieminen J, Hollingsworth K, *et al*. Efficacy and tolerability of fluticasone proprinate nasal drops 400 microgram once daily compared with placebo for the treatment of bilateral polyposis in adults. *Clin Exp Allergy*. 2000; 30: 1460–8.

108. Weber R, Keerl R, Radziwill R, *et al*. Videoendoscopic analysis of nasal steroid distribution. *Rhinology*. 1999; 37: 69–73.

109. Lund V, Flood J, Sykes AP, *et al*. Effect of fluticasone in severe polyposis. Arch *Otolaryngol Head Neck Surg* 1998; 124: 513–8.

110. Aukema AAC, Mulder PGH, Fokkens WJ. Treatment of nasal polyposis and chronic rhinosinusitis with fluticasone propionate nasal drops reduces need for sinus surgery. *J Clin Allergy Clin Immunol*. 2005; 115: 1017–23.

111. Ruhno J, Andersson B, Denburg J, *et al*. A double-blind comparison of intranasal budesonide with placebo for nasal polyposis. *J Allergy Clin Immunol*. 1990; 86: 946–53.

112. Keith P, Nieminen J, Hollingworth K, *et al*. Efficacy and tolerability of fluticasone propionate nasal drops 400mgs once daily compared with placebo for the treatment of bilateral polyposis in adults. *Clin Exp Allergy*. 2000; 30: 1460–8.

113. Pentila M, Poulsen P, Hollingworth K, et al. Dose-related efficacy and tolerability of fluticasone propionate nasal drops 400 mg once daily and twice daily in the treatment of bilateral nasal polyposis: a placebo-controlled, randomised study in adult patients. *Clin Exp Allergy*. 2000; 30: 94–102.

114. Johansson L, Holmberg K, Melen I, et al. Sensitivity of a new grading system for studying nasal polyps with the potential to detect early changes in polyp size after treatment with a topical corticosteroid (budesonide). *Acta Otolaryngol*. 2002; 122: 49–53.

115. Agertoft L, Pedersen S. Short-term lower leg growth rate in children with rhinitis treated with intranasal mometasone furoate and budesonide. *J Allergy Clin Immunol*. 1999; 104: 948–52.

116. Schenkel E, Skoner D, Bronsky E, et al. Absence of growth retardation in children with perennial allergic rhinitis after one year of treatment with mometasone furoate aqueous nasal spray. *Pediatrics*. 2000; 105: E22.

117. Desrosiers M, Salas-Prato M. Treatment of chronic rhinosinusitis refractory to other treatments with topical antibiotic therapy delivered by means of a large-particle nebulizer: results of a controlled trial. *Otolaryngol Head Neck Surg*. 2001; 125: 265–9.

118. Vaughan W, Carvalho G. Use of nebulized antibiotics for acute infections in chronic sinusitis. *Otolaryngol Head Neck Surg*. 2002; 127: 558–68.

119. Schaaf KJ, Cidlowski JA. Molecular mechanisms of glucocorticoid action and resistance. *J Steroid Biochem Mol Biol*. 2002; 83: 37–48.

120. Herz U, Ruckert R, Wollenhaupt K, et al Airway exposure to bacterial superantigen (SEB) induces lymphocyte-dependent airway inflammation associated with increased airway responsiveness: a model for non-allergic asthma. *Eur J Immunol*. 1999; 29: 1021–31.

121. Hamilos DL, Leung DY, Muro S, et al. GR-beta expression in nasal polyp inflammatory cells and its relationship to the anti-inflammatory effects of intranasal fluticasone. *J Allergy Clin Immunol*. 2001; 108: 59–68.

122. Iino Y, Sasaki Y, Kojima C, et al. Effect of macrolides on the expression of HLADR and costimulatory molecules on antigen-presenting cells in nasal polyps. *Ann Otol Rhinol Laryngol*. 2001; 110: 457–63.

123. Nonaka M, Pawankar R, Saji F, et al. Effect of roxithromycin on IL-8 synthesis and proliferation of nasal polyp fibroblasts. *Acta Otolaryngol*. 1998; 539: S71–5.

124. Cervin A, Kalm O, Sandkull P, et al. One-year low-dose erythromycin treatment of persistent chronic sinusitis after sinus surgery: clinical outcome and effects on mucociliary parameters and nasal nitric oxide. *Otolaryngol Head Neck Surg* 2002; 126: 481–9.

125. Hashiba M, Baba S. Efficacy of long-term administration of clarithromycin in the treatment of intractable chronic sinusitis. *Acta Otolaryngol* 1996; 525: S73–8.

126. Kawasaki S, Takizawa H, Ohtoshi T, et al. Roxithromycin inhibits cytokine production by and neutrophil attachment to human bronchial epithelial cells *in vitro*. *Antimicrob Agents Chemother* 1998; 42: 1499–502.

127. Wallwork B, Coman W, Feron F, et al. Clarithromycin and prednisolone inhibit cytokine production in chronic rhinosinusitis. *Laryngoscope* 2002; 112: 1827–30.

128. Tamaoki J. The effects of macrolides on inflammatory cells. *Chest* 2004; 125: S41–50.

129. Lin H, Wang C, Liu C, et al. Erythromycin inhibits beta2-integrins (CD11b/CD18) expression, interleukin-8 release and intracellular oxidative metabolism in neutrophils. *Respir Med* 2000; 94: 654–60.

130. Miyanohara T, Ushikai M, Matsune S, et al. Effects of clarithromycin on cultured human nasal epithelial cells and fibroblasts. *Laryngoscope* 2000; 110: 126–31.

131. Wallwork B, Coman W, Mackay-Sim A, et al. Effect of clarithromycin on nuclear factor-kappa B and transforming growth factor-beta in chronic rhinosinusitis. *Laryngoscope* 2004; 114: 286–90.

132. Konno S, Asano K, Kurokawa M, et al. Antiasthmatic activity of a macrolide antibiotic, roxithromycin: analysis of possible mechanisms *in vitro* and *in vivo*. *Int Arch Allergy Immunol* 1994; 105: 308–16.

133. Amayasu H, Yoshida S, Ebana S, et al. Clarithromycin suppresses bronchial hyper-responsiveness associated with eosinophilic inflammation in patients with asthma. *Ann Allergy Asthma Immunol* 2000; 84: 594–8.

134. Culic O, Erakovic V, Parnham M. Anti-inflammatory effect of macrolide antibiotics. *Eur J Pharmacol* 2001; 428: 209–29.

135. Ichimura K, Shimazaki Y, Ishibashi T, et al. Effect of new macrolide roxithromycin upon nasal polyps associated with chronic sinusitis. *Auris Nasus Larynx*. 1996; 23: 48–56.

136. Cervin A. The anti-inflammatory effect of erythromycin and its derivatives, with special reference to nasal polyposis and chronic sinusitis. *Acta Otolaryngol*. 2001; 121: 83–92.

137. Suzuki H, Ikeda K, Honma R, et al. Prognostic factors of chronic rhinosinusitis under long-term low-dose macrolide therapy. *ORL J Otorhinolaryngol Relat Spec* 2000; 62: 121–7.

138. Ricchetti A, Landis BN, Maffioli A, et al. Effect of anti-fungal nasal lavage with amphotericin B on nasal polyposis. *J Laryngol Otol* 2002; 116: 261–3.

139. Weber R, Draf W, Keerl R, et al. Endonasal microendoscopic pansinus operation in chronic sinusitis. II. Results and complications. *Am J Otolaryngol* 1997; 18: 247–53.

140. Ponikau JU, Sherris DA, Kita H, et al. Intranasal antifungal treatment in 51 patients with chronic rhinosinusitis. *J Allergy Clin Immunol* 2002; 110: 862–6.

141. Ponikau J, Sherris D, Kern E, et al. The diagnosis and incidence of allergic fungal sinusitis. *Mayo Clin Proc* 1999; 74: 877–84.

142. Ponikau JU, Sherris DA, Weaver A, et al. Treatment of chronic rhinosinusitis with intranasal amphotericinB: a randomized, placebo-controlled, double-blind pilot trial. *J Allergy Clin Immunol* 2005; 115: 125–31.

143. Helbling A, Baumann A, Hanni C, et al. Amphotericin B nasal spray has no effect on nasal polyps. *J Laryngol Otol*. 2006; 120: 1023–5.

144. Weschta M, Rimek D, Formanek M, et al. Topical antifungal treatment of chronic rhinosinusitis with nasal polyps: a randomized, double-blind clinical trial. *J Allergy Clin Immunol* 2004; 113: 1122–8.

145. Weschta M, Rimek D, Formanek, M, et al. Effect of Nasal Antifungal Therapy on Nasal Cell Activation Markers in Chronic Rhinosinusitis. *Arch Otolaryngol Head Neck Surg*. 2006; 132: 743–7.

146. Corradini C, Del Ninno M, Buonomo A, *et al.* Amphotericin B and Lysine Acetylsalicylate in the Combined Treatment of Nasal Polyposis Associated With Mycotic Infection. *J Investig Allergol Clin Immunol.* 2006: 16: 188–93.

147. European Academy of Allergology and Clinical Immunology. European position paper on rhinosinusitis and nasal polyps. *Rhinology* 2005; 18: S1–87.

148. Haye R, Aanesen J, Burtin B, *et al.* The effect of cetirizine on symptoms and signs of nasal polyposis. *J Laryngol Otol* 1998; 112: 1042–6.

149. Borish L. The role of leukotrienes in upper and lower airway inflammation and the implications for treatment. *Ann Allergy Asthma Immunol* 2002; 88: 16–22.

150. Braccioni F, Dorman SC, O'Byrne PM, *et al.* The effect of cysteinyl leukotrienes on growth of eosinophil progenitors from peripheral blood and bone marrow of atopic subjects. *J Allergy Clin Immunol* 2002; 110: 96–101.

151. Reiss TF, Chervinsky P, Dockhorn RJ, *et al.* Montelukast, a once-daily leukotriene receptor antagonist, in the treatment of chronic asthma. *Arch Intern Med* 1998; 158: 1213–20.

152. Pizzichini E, Leff JA, Reiss TF, et al. Montelukast reduces airway eosinophilic inflammation in asthma: a randomized, controlled trial. *Eur Respir J* 1999; 14: 12–18.

153. Parnes SM, Chuma AV. Acute effects of antileukotrienes on sinonasal polyposis and sinusitis. *Ear Nose Throat J* 2000; 79: 18–21, 24–5.

154. Dahlen B, Nizankowska E, Szczeklik A, *et al.* Benefits from adding the 5-lipoxygenase inhibitor zileuton to conventional therapy in aspirin-intolerant asthmatics. *Am J Respir Crit Care Med* 1998; 157: 1187–94.

155. Ulualp S, Sterman B, Toohill R. Antileukotriene therapy for the relief of sinus symptoms in aspirin triad disease. *Ear Nose Throat J* 1999; 78(8): 604–6, 608, 613, passim.

156. Kieff DA, Busaba NY. Efficacy of montelukast in the treatment of nasal polyposis. *Ann Otol Rhinol Laryngol.* 2005; 114: 941–5.

157. Widal M, Abrami P, Lenmoyez J. Anaphylaxie et idiosyncrasie. *Presse Med* 1922; 30: 189–92.

158. Samter M, Beers R. Intolerance to aspirin. Clinical studies and consideration of its pathogenesis. *Ann Intern Med* 1968; 68: 975–83.

159. Stevenson DD, Simon RA. Selection of patients for aspirin desensitization treatment. *J Allergy Clin Immunol* 2006; 118: 801–4.

160. Gosepath J, Schaefer D, Amedee RG, *et al.* Individual monitoring of aspirin desensitization. *Arch Otolaryngol Head Neck Surg* 2001; 127: 316–21.

161. Mardiney M, Borish L. Aspirin desensitization for chronic hyperplastic sinusitis, nasal polyposis, and asthma triad. *Arch Otolaryngol Head Neck Surg* 2001; 127: 1287.

162. Bruzzese N, Sica G, Iacopino F, *et al.* Growth inhibition of fibroblasts from nasal polyps and normal skin by lysine acetylsalicylate. *Allergy* 1998; 53: 431–4.

163. Nucera E, Schiavino D, Milani A, *et al.* Effects of lysine-acetylsalicylate (LAS) treatment in nasal polyposis: two controlled long term prospective follow up studies. *Thorax* 2000; 55: S75–8.

164. Sousa AR, Parikh A, Scadding G, *et al.* Leukotriene-receptor expression on nasal mucosal inflammatory cells in aspirin-sensitive rhinosinusitis. *N Engl J Med* 2002; 347: 1493–9.

165. Szczeklik A, Stevenson DD. Aspirin-induced asthma: advances in pathogenesis, diagnosis, and management. *J Allergy Clin Immunol.* 2003; 111: 913–21.

166. Passali D, Bernstein JM, Passali FM, *et al.* Treatment of recurrent chronic hyperplastic sinusitis with nasal polyposis. *Arch Otolaryngol Head Neck Surg.* 2003; 129: 656–9.

167. Kroflic, B, Coer, A, Baudoin, T, *et al.* Topical furosemide versus oral steroid in preoperative management of nasal polyposis. *Eur Arch Otorhinolaryngol* 2006; 263: 767–71.

168. Johansson L, Oberg D, Melen I, *et al.* Do topical nasal decongestants affect polyps? *Acta Otolaryngol* 2006; 126: 288–90.

169. Lacroix J, Buvelot J, Polla B, Lundberg J. Improvement of symptoms of non-allergic chronic rhinitis by local treatment with capsaicin. *Clin Exp Allergy* 1991; 21: 595–600.

170. Zheng C, Wang Z, Lacroix JS. Effect of intranasal treatment with capsaicin on the recurrence of polyps after polypectomy and ethmoidectomy. *Acta Otolaryngol.* 2000; 120: 62–6.

171. Holmstrom M, Holmberg K, Lundblad L, *et al.* Current perspectives on the treatment of nasal polyposis: a Swedish opinion report. *Acta Otolaryngol.* 2002; 122: 736–44.

172. Bikhazi NB. Contemporary management of nasal polyps. *Otolaryngol Clin N Am.* 2004; 37: 327–37.

173. Senior BA, Kennedy DW, Tanabodee J, *et al.* Long-term impact of functional endoscopic sinus surgery on asthma. *Otolaryngol Head Neck Surg* 1999; 121: 66–8.

174. McFadden E, Kany RJ, Fink J, Toohill R. Surgery for sinusitis and aspirin triad. *Laryngoscope* 1990; 100: 1043–6.

175. Heden Blomqvist E, Lundblad L, Anggard A, *et al.* A randomized controlled study evaluating medical treatment versus surgical treatment in addition to medical treatment of nasal polyposis. *J Allergy Clin Immunol* 2001; 107: 224–8.

176. Nakamura H, Kawasaki M, Higuchi Y, *et al.* Effects of sinus surgery on asthma in aspirin triad patients. *Acta Otolaryngol* 1999; 119: 592–8.

177. Uri N, Cohen-Kerem R, Barzilai G, *et al.* Functional endoscopic sinus surgery in the treatment of massive polyposis in asthmatic patients. *J Laryngol Otol* 2002; 116: 185–9.

178. Dalziel K, Stein K, Round A, *et al.* Endoscopic sinus surgery for the excision of nasal polyps: A systematic review of safety and effectiveness. *Am J Rhinol.* 2006; 20: 506–19.

179. Wormald PJ, Athanasiadis T, Rees G, *et al.* An evaluation of effect of pterygopalatine fossa injection with local anesthetic and adrenalin in the control of nasal bleeding during endoscopic sinus surgery. *Am J Rhinol.* 2005; 19: 288–92.

180. Hopkins C, Browne JP, Slack R, *et al.* Complications of surgery for nasal polyposis and chronic rhinosinusitis: the results of a national audit in England and Wales. *Laryngoscope.* 2006; 116: 1494–9.

181. McMains KC, Kountakis SE. Revision functional endoscopic sinus surgery: objective and subjective surgical outcomes. *Am J Rhinol.* 2005; 19: 344–7.

Chapter 24

Complications of Rhinosinusitis

24

Seth M. Brown, Abtin Tabaee, and Vijay K. Anand

Core Messages

■ The spread of infections from the paranasal sinuses to the orbit and intracranial cavity is due to the close proximity of these structures and the presence of valveless veins.

■ The increased incidence of serious complications from acute sinusitis in children mandates early treatment with antibiotics and close observation.

■ In patients with complicated sinusitis, fine-cut CT with contrast remains the imaging method of choice and image-guided protocols can be performed in those patients who may require operative intervention.

■ A team approach is often warranted in the management of these complex patients including otolaryngology, neurosurgery, intensive care, ophthalmology, infectious disease, and pediatrics.

Contents

Orbital Complications

Epidemiology

The most frequent serious complication from sinusitis is infection spreading to the orbit, accounting for approximately 80–90% of cases of complicated sinusitis [23, 25]. This is predominately a disease of childhood, with a peak incidence between the ages of 5 and 10 years [12]. In one recent analysis, nearly 80% of patients with orbital infections from sinusitis were less than 18 years old [37]. As a result, sinus infections are the most common cause of unilateral proptosis in children and the third most common cause in adults following Graves' orbitopathy and pseudotumor [24, 37].

Etiology

Most orbital infections secondary to sinusitis are the result of ethmoid disease [37]. This is due in part to the close proximity of the ethmoid sinus to the orbital cavity. In addition, the two are separated by the thin lamina papyracea of the ethmoid bone which frequently has congenital or traumatic dehiscences within it. Furthermore, erosion of the lamina may occur as a result of the infection or inflammatory sinus disease such as polyposis or allergic fungal sinusitis. Alternative routes of infectious spread include the anterior and posterior ethmoidal neurovascular foramina [24] and the venous system. The ophthalmic venous system, made up of the superior and inferior ophthalmic veins, is valveless, allowing for free-flowing communication of infection from the nose and ethmoid sinus to the orbit.

Clinical Presentation

Patients with an orbital infection from sinusitis normally present with gross swelling of the orbit (Fig. 24.1). The initial manifestation of lid edema may progress rapidly to cause chemosis and visual changes such as diplopia. Orbital infections may be characterized by their location in relation to the orbital septum, with more severe disease located in the postseptal compart-

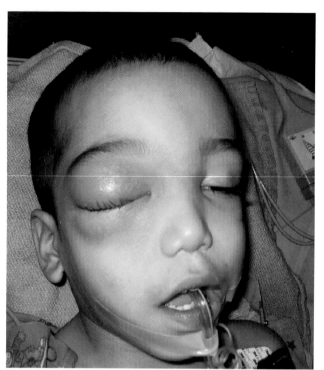

Fig. 24.1 Child with an intraorbital abscess secondary to ethmoid sinusitis

ment. Presentation and examination can help differentiate the location of the infection, as proptosis and ophthalmoplegia are found in a significantly higher number of patients with postseptal disease [30].

Perhaps the most studied infection of the orbit related to sinusitis is subperiosteal abscess. This infection is characterized by a purulent collection between the lamina papyracea and orbital periosteum and most commonly presents as erythema and edema of the eye [1]. The majority of patients with a subperiosteal infection also have chemosis, limitation of extraorbital motion, proptosis, and pain with eye movement [1]. As the infection continues to spread to become an intraorbital abscess, visual changes will continue to evolve. Eventually, visual compromise can occur from several proposed mechanisms: increase in intraocular pressure and pressure ischemia, traction on the optic nerve secondary to proptosis, optic neuritis as a reaction to the infection, or ischemia from thrombophlebitis [1, 27]. If the infection is not adequately treated, symptoms may continue to progress to lethargy, headache, fever, and confusion, as the infection continues to spreads to the cavernous sinus.

Evaluation

The evaluation of a patient with a presumed orbital complication of sinusitis consists of orbital and sinus computed tomography (CT) scans to help characterize the extent of disease in the orbit and the origin of infection in the paranasal sinuses. If orbital swelling is minor and no visual changes or restriction of gaze exist, it can be presumed that the infection is preseptal and treatment can often be initiated without imaging. However, if a brief trial of medical treatment has failed, or signs and symptoms are consistent with a postseptal infection, then imaging becomes necessary.

It is recommended that imaging be performed with the addition of intravenous contrast to better demarcate abscess formation. A non-contrast CT or gadolinium-enhanced magnetic resonance imaging (MRI) scan may be performed in patients with sensitivities to iodine-based contrast. Initially obtaining the scan with an image-guided protocol may minimize the need for a second scan if operative intervention becomes necessary. In addition to imaging, standard blood tests should be obtained including a white blood cell count and blood cultures.

Ophthalmology should be consulted early to help evaluate the condition of the orbit as well as to provide a baseline examination to help determine response to treatment. Ophthalmology examination should consist of tests of visual acuity, ocular range of motion, pupillary reactivity, and a funduscopic evaluation for papilledema and pallor of the optic disc [27, 37].

Staging

The extent of spread of sinusitis to the orbit is most commonly grouped into five different areas increasing in severity. The most accepted scheme was first proposed by Hubers, was modified by Chandler in the 1970s [7], and is as follows:

- Group I: Inflammatory edema (preseptal cellulitis)
- Group II: Orbital cellulitis
- Group III: Subperiosteal abscess
- Group IV: Orbital abscess
- Group V: Cavernous sinus thrombosis.

The classification system is helpful as it demonstrates the potential progression of disease. Patients presenting with early-stage disease can often avoid surgery if recognized early and treated with appropriate medical therapy. Furthermore, as the disease progresses to a more advanced stage, morbidity will significantly increase.

Treatment

Regardless of the ultimate treatment plan, broad-spectrum antibiotics should be initiated immediately after the initial evaluation. If culture and sensitivity data become available, the regimen may be tailored accordingly. However, a broad-spectrum approach should be used even with a positive culture result given the possibility of a multibacterial process and lack of sensitivity of cultures, particularly for anaerobes. The organisms that need to be covered include both the typical pathogens in sinusitis as well as organisms often not encountered in sinus infections. In several larger studies of orbital infections secondary to sinusitis, *Staphylococcus* and *Streptococcus* species were most commonly isolated [1, 25]. Methicillin-resistant *Staphylococcus*

24

aureus needs to be considered in nosocomial infections as well as in patients not responding to standard antibiotic regimens.

For preseptal infections, medical management with close observation may be sufficient. In a study looking at orbital complications of sinusitis, all 27 cases of preseptal or orbital cellulitis responded to medical therapy alone [37]. In another study, 101 patients with preseptal cellulitis responded to a course of intravenous antibiotics without surgery [30]. Medical treatment should consist of broad-spectrum antibiotics and topical nasal decongestion. If there is lack of improvement or progression in symptoms and examination findings within 24–48 h of initiating therapy, additional evaluation and treatment may be necessary to prevent further spread of the infection. Ultimately, the indications for surgical intervention include a combination of factors including clinical history and examination, imaging findings, and response to therapy [27].

It has been suggested that subperiosteal abscess is only a relative indication for surgery and that select patients can be managed medically [13]. This is only appropriate in select patients without changes in visual acuity or ocular mobility. This also relies on a patient that can be accurately examined and thus would not be applicable for most small children. Management of these patients may consist of a brief trial of broad-spectrum intravenous antibiotics with frequent ophthalmologic examinations in an inpatient setting. In one retrospective study of 19 pediatric patients, initially treated with broad-spectrum antibiotics with surgical intervention reserved only for worsening of ophthalmologic examination or lack of improvement in 24–36 h, only proptosis of more than 2 mm was found as a predictor of need for surgical intervention [28].

Brown et al. compared patients with subperiosteal abscess requiring surgical intervention versus those only receiving medical treatment. They found that the patients not requiring surgery were younger (5.1 years versus 11 years), had less restriction of ocular motility (−1.0 mm versus −2.3 mm), and were hospitalized for fewer days (6.5 days versus 9.6 days). They concluded that patients with subperiosteal abscess under the age of 6 years, with minimal restriction of gaze, and without evidence of intracranial infection could be treated medically [6].

The surgical management of orbital complications of sinusitis has evolved from an open to an endoscopic technique. Multiple reports in the literature have supported this approach even in pediatric patients [21, 28, 37]. This is best carried out in experienced hands as endoscopic sinus surgery in the setting of an acute infection is significantly more difficult due to the increase in bleeding and inflammatory distortion of landmarks. Open procedures can be performed when the abscess is in an area poorly accessed through the nose (i. e., superiorly or laterally positioned), in those patients with difficult anatomy including small children, or in the hands of surgeons not skilled in endoscopic techniques. External approaches may involve an external ethmoidectomy via a Lynch incision with placement of a drain either externally or through the nose.

An endoscopic procedure may be an option in patients with orbital complications from sinusitis, but should only be performed by experienced surgeons. The endoscopic technique commences with adequate topical vasoconstriction and injection of lidocaine with epinephrine as hemostasis is essential in order to perform a safe and adequate endoscopic procedure. A sphenopalatine block is helpful to decrease bleeding during the procedure. Topical vasoconstriction should continue throughout the surgery in order to keep the operative field as dry as possible. Involved sinus cells should be opened and a wide exposure of the orbital walls should be performed initially. This typically involves an uncinectomy, maxillary antrostomy, and total ethmoidectomy at a minimum. Following this, the lamina papyracea should be removed to expose and drain the abscess. The lamina papyracea is easily visualized and its removal can be done completely endoscopically in experienced hands. This is similar to the procedure done for orbital decompression in patients with Graves' orbitopathy. Any purulent secretions should be sent for culture and sensitivities. At the completion of the procedure packing should be avoided as much as possible to allow further drainage of purulence.

Image guidance provides an intraoperative, triplanar radiographic road map. This may be important in these cases that typically involve a bloody, infected field in a pediatric patient.

Prognosis

The key to a successful outcome is early recognition of the disease and appropriate treatment. Preseptal disease is associated with minimal to no long-term morbidity when treated early to prevent further spread. However, when infection spreads beyond the orbital septum, morbidity remains high; recent reports have noted an incidence of blindness of up to 10.5% [27]. This is only a 50% reduction from the reported 20% incidence of blindness in the preantibiotic era.

Intracranial Complications

Epidemiology

Although not as common as orbital infections, intracranial complications secondary to sinusitis remain a real entity. In one study looking at all patients admitted with sinusitis over a 13-year period, 3.7% were found to have an intracranial complication [8]. It is well accepted that intracranial complications from sinusitis are more common in adolescent boys. This may be due to a peak in the vascularity of the diploic venous system of this age group [17]. One study looked at admissions for sinusitis and found a strong gender predilection for men and a statistically significant correlation with adolescent boys and intracranial complications secondary to sinusitis [19]. Other studies have also found a predominance of men in patients with intracranial complications of sinusitis [35–37].

Etiology

Similar to orbital infections, intracranial spread may result from direct extension or through the valveless venous system. This is in part due to foramina that exist in the frontal sinus through which the diploic veins of Breschet pass. These passages allow for frontal sinus mucosal capillaries to communicate directly with dural sinuses [22]. In addition to the spread of infection through neurovascular foramen, infection may also spread through congenital or traumatic bony dehiscences. Epidural abscesses specifically are thought to arise from retrograde bacterial spread via the diploic veins. They are also not infrequently associated with skull osteomyelitis and this may be the cause of the epidural collection in many cases [10].

Intracranial spread may result from both acute and chronic sinusitis, with many patients not having a history of sinus disease. In one study only 24% of patients had a history of chronic sinusitis [8]. Different sinuses have been implicated in the disease depending on the origin and site of the intracranial infection. In one study looking at 21 patients with meningitis secondary to sinogenic sources, all patients had affected ethmoid and sphenoid sinuses [36]. Conversely, in patients with epidural abscesses, the most common concurrent sinus disease was unilateral frontal sinusitis present in 85% of patients and unilateral ethmoiditis found in 71% in another study [35]. In patients with frontal lobe abscesses, although usually considered a result of frontal sinusitis, one study found that 54% of patients had concurrent ethmoid disease and 27% had isolated ethmoid disease [8]. In subdural abscesses resulting from a paranasal sinus infection, the frontal and ethmoid sinuses are often implicated [10].

Clinical Presentation

The most common presenting symptoms of patients with intracranial complication of sinusitis are fever and headache [8–10]. Additional symptoms include periorbital or frontal swelling, seizures, and altered mental status [15]. The location of the infection often dictates the presenting signs and symptoms. When the abscess involves the frontal lobe, symptoms tend to be more subtle such as mood and behavioral changes. In contrast, subdural infections tend to have a common flow of events; headache, fever, and lethargy, followed by seizures and coma [36]. This is usually life-threatening as patients often

deteriorate rapidly. Interestingly, another study found that 83% of patients had a preceding upper respiratory infection (URI), however, the mean onset from the URI to the diagnosis of an intracranial infection was 15 days making the clinical utility of this finding minimal [15].

In patients with presumed meningitis, imaging needs to be performed prior to performing a lumbar puncture to rule out increased intracranial pressure, a structural lesion, or a space-occupying collection. Patients who present with headache need to have a good history and physical examination. In those patients with preceding URIs, imaging of the brain should be considered. All patients presenting with orbital swelling and a headache need to have imaging of the brain performed to rule out an intracranial process.

Evaluation

Magnetic resonance imaging as well as CT scanning is necessary in patients with intracranial complications of sinusitis. When evaluating for intracranial complications, a gadolinium-enhanced brain MRI is complementary to CT scanning (Fig. 24.2). In a study looking at CT and MRI for diagnosis of an intracranial abscess from sinusitis, the accuracy rate for CT was 92% versus 100% for MRI [35]. CT scans should be done in all of these cases, and need to include fine-cut images of the paranasal sinuses in both axial and coronal planes. The CT scan will help by demonstrating the inciting sinus disease as well as additional affected sinuses. The CT scan can also be helpful in its superior evaluation of bony structures and can assist in surgical planning by displaying skull base dehiscence. The soft tissue delineation of MRI, in contrast, is superior to CT scans, and is necessary when evaluating intracranial structures. With the addition of gadolinium it can often show meningeal enhancement that may otherwise be missed. The diagnosis of meningitis requires a lumbar puncture which should only be performed after a CT has been done to evaluate for brain swelling.

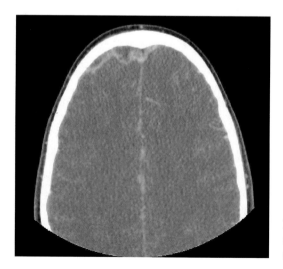

Fig. 24.2 Contrast-enhanced axial MRI scan demonstrating an epidural abscess in an adolescent boy with acute frontal sinusitis

24

Infections

Intracranial infections are usually categorized based on location. This includes meningitis, epidural abscess, subdural abscess, and intracranial abscess. There is disagreement in the literature over which location is most common from the spread of sinusitis. Various authors have identified meningitis [37], epidural abscess [9], subdural abscess [15], and frontal lobe abscess [8] each as the most common intracranial complication of sinusitis. This may be due to the occurrence of multiple simultaneous processes [10]. It is also possible that meningitis is underrepresented as these patients may escape sinus CT [11].

Meningitis involves inflammation and infection of the meninges. It can be the result of a bacterial or viral process. Epidural abscesses are typically found just posterior to the frontal sinus where free venous communication and loose dura predispose to the formation of an abscess [12]. They are found between the bony cranial vault and the dura. Subdural abscesses are found just deep to the dura. Patients usually are ill, appearing with meningismus, fever, and other signs of systemic infection. These abscesses are not uncommonly multiloculated. Brain abscesses are most commonly found at the junction of white and gray matter and clinical diagnosis is often difficult because of lack of focal neurologic signs when the process involves the frontal lobe [12].

Treatment

Treatment is tailored to the site and severity of the infection and incorporates a multidisciplinary team approach including otolaryngology, neurosurgery, neurology, and intensive care specialists. Meningitis originating from a sinus infection may be treated initially with intravenous antibiotics and decongestants, with drainage reserved for failure [10]. For those infections with a collection in the intracranial cavity, simultaneous drainage of the abscess and inciting infection in the sinuses is prudent. This is often from a frontal sinus infection. In an acutely infected sinus image guidance may be useful, particularly in children who have variable anatomy [26].

The methods used to treat the intracranial process include both craniotomy as well as burr holes. The latter may be performed with stereotactic guidance, particularly in intracerebral abscesses, where disruption of the abscess cavity could potentially cause spillage of the infection. However, this may require more than one operation with a subsequent formal craniotomy later should the abscess re-collect. Even following a craniotomy, a secondary intracerebral procedure may be necessary, as evidenced by the need for 20 craniotomies in one study of 13 patients [11].

Drainage of the sinuses is often important even when the intracranial operation is not necessary as it facilitates clearing of the original infection and provides important culture and sensitivity information. In a study looking at the bacteriology of acute frontal sinusitis, the most common organisms were *Haemophilus influenzae*, *Streptococcus pneumoniae*, and *Moraxella catarrhalis* [5]. In another study of intracranial infections from sinusitis in children, 43% of cultured infections were polymicrobial [11]. When looking specifically at the intracranial collection, *Staphylococcus aureus* and *Streptococcus* species were the most frequently cultured. One study found *Staphylococcus aureus* as the most commonly isolated single organism from an intracranial abscess followed by anaerobic streptococci [8]. Other studies have found *Streptococcus* species as the most frequently isolated [10, 11, 15].

Prognosis

Despite the modern development of antimicrobials, neuroimaging, and evidence-based treatment algorithms, the mortality and morbidity of intracranial complications from sinusitis remain high with long-term morbidity rates as high as 20–30% [8, 15, 32]. Neurologic sequela remain the most common source of morbidity with a 17% incidence of hemiparesis or hypoesthesia and a 12% incidence of chronic seizure disorders in one study [8]. In another study of 47 patients with intracranial complications, 15% developed epilepsy, 4 of whom had only an extradural process [15].

It is thought that a subdural abscess may have the highest incidence of permanent neurologic sequelae [10]. Subdural abscesses may also be life-threatening with rapid deterioration [36]. Regardless of the location of the infection intracranially, it can be expected that these patients will have a long inpatient course, with recent studies reporting average length of stays of 29–31 days [10, 15].

Cavernous Sinus Thrombosis

Cavernous sinus thrombosis is a thrombophlebitis of the cavernous sinus. It may result from both septic and aseptic sources, but, when caused by sinusitis, is infectious and thus septic in nature [20]. Although it may originate from any source, it is commonly a result of a central facial infection in the so-called "danger triangle" due to the valveless venous drainage in this area, most frequently in the setting of a sinus infection with either orbital or intracranial spread. In this instance the infection has spread to the cavernous sinus via the venous system, from osteomyelitis or through direct spread through a bony defect [4].

In addition to cavernous sinus thrombosis, superior sagittal sinus thrombosis is reported as a complication from sinusitis and should be treated in a similar fashion [9, 36]. Superior sagittal sinus thrombosis is much less frequently reported and may result from meningitis, ethmoid or maxillary sinusitis, epidural abscess, as well as other non-sinus etiologies [31].

Most patients present with headaches as their predominant symptom, however meningitis is not infrequently coexistent when patients present with cavernous sinus thrombosis [33]. The headaches progress to fevers and periorbital edema after a lag of several days [31]. The usual clinical course of cavernous sinus thrombosis is a picket fence fever pattern in addition to the other features of sepsis. Orbital findings tend to follow as venous congestion occurs in the orbital veins causing chemosis, periorbital edema, and proptosis which in most cases will spread to the opposite eye within 48 h [4]. Concurrent cranial nerve palsies are often found as well, usually involving the optic and abducens nerves [33].

The most common bacteria found in cavernous sinus thrombosis is *Staphylococcus aureus* [33]. This underscores the need for broad antibiotic coverage and adequate coverage for the possibility of methicillin-resistant *Staphylococcus aureus*. There may be a role for operative intervention by the otolaryngologist, with studies reporting that drainage of an offending sinus (often sphenoid) has resulted in a marked improvement [31]. The other part of treatment is the frequently debated issue of adding anticoagulation to the regimen. Studies on anticoagulation are limited secondary to the rarity of this condition today. In theory, anticoagulation may prevent further propagation of the thrombus. The argument against anticoagulation is the concern that its use may trigger septic emboli and increase the risk for intracranial bleeding [4]. To date, however, only two cases exist in the English literature of intracranial hemorrhage secondary to anticoagulation for cavernous sinus thrombosis [4]. In one small study a statistically significant reduction in morbidity was noted in patients treated with antibiotics and anticoagulation versus antibiotics alone, however, there was no difference in mortality [20]. One larger study of 86 patients found a significant reduction in mortality, 14% versus 36%, in patients treated with heparin [31].

Prior to 1960, the mortality of cavernous sinus thrombosis was estimated at 80% in a review of 878 cases from the literature [34]. Even today the mortality is high, with rates approaching 30% in the literature [4, 31]. Despite the improvement in survival, the incidence of cranial neuropathies in survivors remains close to 50%, particularly of the abducens or oculomotor nerves [20]. Patients with cavernous sinus thrombosis need to be treated aggressively with broad-spectrum antibiotics and monitored closely in an intensive care setting.

Mucoceles

Mucoceles are cystic mucus-containing structures usually found in the frontal sinuses (Fig. 24.3). They are the result of long-standing inflammation in the setting of ostial obstruction. This can be secondary to trauma, previous surgical treatment, or chronic sinusitis. They are divided by some into two distinct types of mucocele: a "pressure" mucocele in an obstructed sinus and a "trauma" mucocele resulting from regeneration after infection or blunt trauma to the sinus mucosa [29]. Chronic sinusitis can result in mucocele formation by obstructing the sinus ostia by inflammation or scarring allowing mucus to build up under pressure in a closed sinus cavity [29]. This can occur slowly over the course of many years [12]. Mucoceles are po-

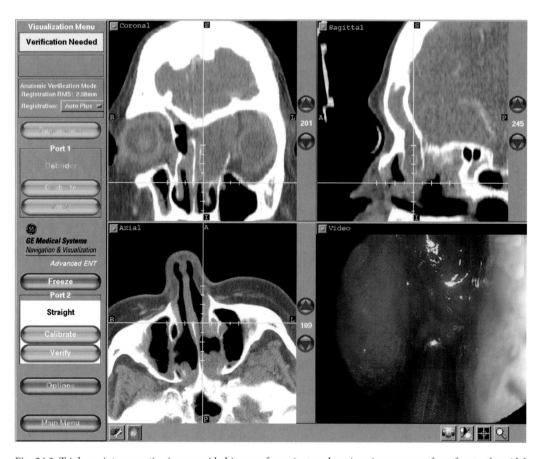

Fig. 24.3 Triplanar intraoperative image-guided image of a patient undergoing sinus surgery for a frontoethmoidal mucocele

tentially dangerous as they may erode into surrounding structures such as the orbit and brain putting pressure on these areas, become secondarily infected and form a mucopyocele, and be associated with osteomyelitis [32].

Treatment of mucoceles has traditionally involved open approaches with obliteration of the involved sinus. Recently reports have shown success with endoscopic approaches with decompression and marsupialization of the mucocele [14].

Bony Complications

Osteomyelitis

Osteomyelitis from sinusitis is almost always a disease of the frontal sinus [12]. The diploic veins of Breschet in addition to connecting to the valveless venous system, also communicate to the marrow cavity of the frontal bone providing a way for osteomyelitis to evolve from frontal sinusitis [22]. Pott's puffy tumor is frontal bone osteomyelitis secondary to acute frontal sinusitis with associated subperiosteal abscess [18]. Although originally described as a complication from trauma, it is more commonly seen resulting from frontal sinusitis [2]. Although rare in the antibiotic era, it is still an entity that needs to be recognized as it appears to be increasing in frequency and is associated with a high risk of meningitis, intracranial abscess, and venous sinus thrombosis. Early diagnosis and treatment are required to prevent long-term complications [18]. Treatment consists of broad-spectrum antibiotics, medical management of sinusitis, and surgical drainage of the abscess with debridement of necrotic and osteomyelitic bone. Cultures taken at the time of surgery may be used to guide therapy.

Hyperostosis

It is well known that sinusitis can cause bone remodeling and infection of the bone within and surrounding the sinus cavity. This entity, known as hyperostotic sinusitis, is often seen on CT scans where bony thickening can be seen at sites of inflammation. Furthermore, it has been observed that patients can often localize signs and symptoms to the site of bony thickening [16]. This bony inflammation and infection is significant in that its treatment often requires surgery to remove the infection from the sinus and 6–12 weeks of intravenous antibiotics to clear the bony infection, similar to osteomyelitis.

Systemic Complications

Pulmonary

Sinusitis and polyposis are well known to aggravate coexisting lung disease. This is particularly true in patients with allergic fungal sinusitis (AFS) and asthma as well as patients with cystic fibrosis and other forms of ciliary dysfunction. For patients with sinusitis and lung disease, it is important to actively follow the patients' pulmonary status by performing spirometry or peak flows on a regular basis. Aggressive medical treatment of the sinuses is essential, as well as strict smoking cessation. There is also a role for allergy workup and treatment and possibly aspirin desensitization in those patients with Samter's triad.

Sepsis

Sinusitis, like most diseases of infectious etiology, can spread systemically and cause septic shock. This is particularly true in the immunocompromised patient. Any patient who is presumed to have sepsis should have a full fever workup including blood cultures. Antibiotics should be culture-directed when possible and there may be a role for sinus cultures in patients presumed to have sepsis from a sinus source. These cultures can usually be obtained bedside by placing a culture stick in the middle meatus under endoscopic visualization. Recent studies have supported this to be at least as efficacious as maxillary sinus punctures [3].

Tips to Avoid Complications

- A full head and neck examination is essential in assessing whether a patient has a complication of sinusitis and the severity of the condition.
- Imaging can help delineate the extent of disease and the need for intervention.
- Assistance in management of these patients, including ophthalmologic and neurosurgical consultations, can help optimize care.
- When surgical intervention is necessary, experience in these procedures is essential and controlling the operating field with adequate hemostasis is of the utmost importance.

Take-Home Pearls

- Despite improvements in treatment and antibiotics, there still remains a real risk of loss of vision and mortality in patients with intraorbital complications of sinusitis.
- The thin-walled lamina papyracea dividing the ethmoid sinuses from the orbit may allow direct spread of disease to the orbit.
- The venous system of the sinuses is a vast network and consists of numerous valveless veins allowing direct spread of infections intracranially.
- Despite advances in endoscopic sinus surgery and image guidance, open approaches may still play a role in the patient with complicated sinusitis.

> • Cultures need to be taken in cases of complicated sinusitis as there is an increasing incidence of antibiotic resistance, specifically methicillin-resistant *Staphylococcus aureus*.

References

1. Arjmand EM, Lusk RP, Muntz HR (1993) Pediatric sinusitis and subperiosteal orbital abscess formation: diagnosis and treatment. Otolaryngol Head Neck Surg 109:886–894

2. Bambakidia NC, Cohen AR (2001) Intracranial complications of frontal sinusitis in children: Pott's puffy tumor revisited. Pediatr Neurosurg 35:82–89

3. Benninger MS, Payne SC, Ferguson BJ, et al. (2006) Endoscopically directed middle meatal cultures versus maxillary sinus taps in acute bacterial maxillary rhinosinusitis: a meta-analysis. Otolaryngol Head Neck Surg 134:3–9

4. Bhatia K, Jones NS (2002) Septic cavernous sinus thrombosis secondary to sinusitis: are anticoagulants indicated? A review of the literature. J Laryngol Otol 116:667–676

5. Brook I (2002) Bacteriology of acute and chronic frontal sinusitis. Arch Otolaryngol Head Neck Surg 128:583–585

6. Brown CL, Graham SM, Griffin MC, et al.(2004) Pediatric medial subperiosteal orbital abscess: medical management where possible. Am J Rhinol 18:321–326

7. Chandler JR, Langenbrunner DJ, Stevens ER (1970) The pathogenesis of orbital complications in acute sinusitis. Laryngoscope 80:1414–1428

8. Clayman GL, Adams GL, Paugh DR, et al.(1991) Intracranial complications of paranasal sinusitis: a combined institutional review. Laryngoscope 101:234–239

9. Gallagher RM, Gross CW, Phillips CD (1998) Suppurative intracranial complications of sinusitis. Laryngoscope 108:1635–1642

10. Giannoni CM, Stewart MG, Alford EL (1997) Intracranial complications of sinusitis. Laryngoscope 107:863–867

11. Glickstein JS, Chandra RK, Thompson JW (2006) Intracranial complications of pediatric sinusitis. Otolaryngol Head Neck Surg 134:733–736

12. Goldberg AN, Oroszlan G, Anderson TD (2001) Complications of frontal sinusitis and their management. Otolaryngol Clin North Am 34:211–225

13. Goodwin WJ (1985) Orbital complications of ethmoiditis. Otolaryngol Clin North Am 18:139–147

14. Har-El G (2001) Transnasal endoscopic management of frontal mucoceles. Otolaryngol Clin North Am 34:243–251

15. Jones NS, Walker JL, Bassi S, et al.(2002) The intracranial complications of rhinosinusitis: can they be prevented? Laryngoscope 112:59–63

16. Kacker A, Huang C, Anand V (2002) Incidence of chronic hyperostotic rhinosinusitis in patients undergoing primary sinus surgery compared to revision surgery. Rhinology 40:80–82

17. Kaplan RJ (1976) Neurological complications of infections of the head and neck. Otolaryngol Clin North Am 9:729–749

18. Kombogiorgas D, Solanki GA (2006) The Pott puffy tumor revisited: neurosurgical implications of this unforgotten entity. J Neurosurg (2 Suppl Pediatrics) 105:143–146

19. Lebovics RS, Moisa II, Ruben RJ (1989) Sex predilection in patients with acute frontal sinusitis. Ear Nose Throat J 68:433–437

20. Levine SR, Twyman RE, Gilman S (1988) The role of anticoagulation in cavernous sinus thrombosis. Neurology 38:517–522

21. Manning SC (1993) Endoscopic management of medial subperiosteal orbital abscess. Arch Otolaryngol Head Neck Surg 119:789–791

22. McLaughlin RB, Rehl RM, Lanza DC (2001) Clinically relevant frontal sinus anatomy and physiology. Otolaryngol Clin North Am 34:1–22

23. Mortimore S, Wormald PJ (1999) Management of acute complicated sinusitis: a 5-year review. Otolaryngol Head Neck Surg 121:639–642

24. Osguthorpe JD, Hochman M (1993) Inflammatory sinus diseases affecting the orbit. Otolaryngol Clin North Am 26:657–671

25. Oxford LE, McClay J (2005) Complications of acute sinusitis in children. Otolaryngol Head Neck Surg 133:32–37

26. Parikh SR, Brown SM (2004) Image-guided frontal sinus surgery in children. Operative Tech Otolaryngol Head Neck Surg 15:37–41

27. Patt BS, Manning SC (1991) Blindness resulting from orbital complications of sinusitis. Otolaryngol Head Neck Surg 104:789–795

28. Rahbar R, Robson CD, Petersen RA, et al.(2001) Management of orbital subperiosteal abscess in children. Arch Otolaryngol Head Neck Surg 127:281–286

29. Schenck NL, Rauchbach E, Ogura JH (1974) Frontal sinus disease. II. Development of the frontal sinus model: occlusion of the nasofrontal duct. Laryngoscope 84:1233–1247

30. Sobol SE, Marchand J, Tewfik TL (2002) Orbital complications of sinusitis in children. J Otolaryngol 31:131–136

31. Southwick FS, Richardson EP Jr, Swartz MN (1986) Septic thrombosis of the dural venous sinuses. Medicine 65:82–106

32. Stankiewicz JA, Newell DJ, Park AH (1993) Complications of inflammatory diseases of the sinuses. Otolaryngol Clin North Am 26:639–655

33. Thatai D, Chandy L, Dhar KL (1992) Septic cavernous sinus thrombophlebitis: a review of 35 cases. J Indian Med Assoc 90:290–292

34. Yarington CT Jr (1961) The prognosis and treatment of cavernous sinus thrombosis: review of 878 cases in the literature. Ann Otol Rhinol Laryngol 70:263–267

35. Younis RT, Anand VK, Davidson B (2002) The role of computed tomography and magnetic resonance imaging in patients with sinusitis with complications. Laryngoscope 112:224–229

36. Younis RT, Lazar RH, Anand VK (2002) Intracranial complications of sinusitis: a 15-year review of 39 cases. Ear Nose Throat J 81:636–642

37. Younis RT, Lazar RH, Bustillo A, et al.(2002) Orbital infection as a complication of sinusitis: are diagnostic and treatment trends changing? Ear Nose Throat J 81:771–775

24

Chapter 25

Macrolides and Their Role in the Treatment of Chronic Rhinosinusitis

25

Anders Cervin and Ben Wallwork

Core Messages

- Long-term, low-dose macrolide antibiotics have immune-modulating effects in inflammatory airway disease.
- The efficacy of long-term, low-dose macrolide antibiotics in CRS has been shown in a placebo-controlled study.
- Long-term, low-dose macrolide antibiotic treatment is more likely to be effective in the non-atopic patient.

Contents

Introduction

The first macrolide antibiotic, erythromycin, was identified in a soil sample from the Philippines and is a metabolic product of *Streptomyces erythreus* [1]. Over the years a number of semi-synthetic derivates have been developed, clarithromycin, azithromycin and roxithromycin being the most used. Macrolides have a special indication in treating intracellular pathogens such as *Chlamydia*, *Mycoplasma* and *Helicobacter pylori*.

They have been used for decades as an important antibiotic, especially in respiratory infections, but in the last decade macrolides have also been of interest in a variety of diseases including secondary prevention of cardiovascular disease and Alzheimer's disease. It is the anti-inflammatory effects of erythromycin and its derivates that have attracted the most attention in recent years.

Endemic in Japan, diffuse panbronchiolitis presents with chronic cough, dyspnoea and mucopurulent expectoration. Almost all patients have chronic rhinosinusitis (CRS). Long-term treatment with erythromycin was tried in the mid 1980s and changed the 10-year survival rate from 25% to over 90% and simultaneously resolved the CRS [2, 3]. Unfortunately, most reports were written and published in Japanese journals and interest from the medical community of the western world was delayed. Kikuchi and colleagues published the first report with an English abstract concerning the use of long-term, low-dose erythromycin treatment of CRS [4]. Since then there has been increasing interest in the role of macrolide antibiotics in the treatment of chronic sinusitis. Of note are the findings that their efficacy is seen at lower doses and with a slow onset compared to the anti-infective effect and in many cases in the absence of an identifiable pathogen. These findings, together with the in vitro research demonstrating the immune-modulating effects of erythromycin and its derivates, have led to the concept of long-term, low-dose macrolide treatment as primarily an immune response modifying treatment and not an antibacterial treatment.

In the present chapter we will explore the evidence for macrolide antibiotics immune-modulating effects and present a treatment algorithm for managing the difficult CRS patient with long-term, low-dose macrolide antibiotics.

In Vitro Studies

Chronic inflammation is central in the pathogenesis of CRS. The inflammatory process therefore represents a target for therapy of this disorder. As evidence has emerged that long-term, low-dose macrolide treatment may have a beneficial effect in disorders of chronic airway inflammation, interest has grown in determining the targets of this apparent anti-inflammatory effect. In this section, we will focus on studies that have investigated the possible anti-inflammatory effect of macrolides in CRS.

Antimicrobial Effect

Macrolides have a well-established antimicrobial activity and have been used in the treatment of a variety of bacterial infections for several decades. They are primarily bacteriostatic and bind to the 50S subunit of the ribosome, thus inhibiting bacterial protein synthesis. Macrolides are active against gram-positive cocci (including anaerobes), with the exception of enterococci, and have limited gram-negative activity. They are currently used as an alternative to the β-lactam antibiotics for the treatment of gram-positive cocci in β-lactam allergic patients. In addition macrolides are the drug of choice for the treatment of respiratory infections caused by *Corynebacterium diphtheriae*, *Bordetella pertussis*, *Legionella pneumophila*, *Mycoplasma pneumoniae* and *Chlamydia pneumoniae* [5].

Some organisms, for example *Pseudomonas aeruginosa*, are resistant to the direct antibacterial effect of macrolides. However, macrolides have been shown to exert an effect on infections produced by these organisms via less direct means. For example, macrolides have been shown to attenuate the effect of various virulence factors produced by *P. aeruginosa*. Hirakata et al. [6] showed that erythromycin inhibits the release of elastase, protease, phospholipase C and eotaxin A by *P. aeruginosa*. Another study showed that erythromycin was able to suppress the production of toxic lectins, protease and haemolysin [7].

Another indirect effect of macrolide treatment on bacterial infection may be on bacterial biofilm formation. Biofilm-producing bacteria such as *Staphylococcus*, *Haemophilus* and *Pseudomonas* benefit from an enhanced ability to adhere to host epithelium, a resistance to phagocytosis and a reduction in the efficacy of antimicrobial agents. Macrolides have been shown to alter the structure and function of biofilm produced by *P. aeruginosa* [8]. Takeoka et al. [9] demonstrated that macrolide treatment of *P. aeruginosa* biofilms resulted in an enhanced ability of neutrophil phagocytosis. Azithromycin has been shown to inhibit interbacterial communication (also referred to as quorum-sensing). Quorum-sensing is important in bacterial virulence factor production and biofilm formation. The same study revealed reduced pseudomonal mobility and an impaired oxidative stress response (resulting in reduced production of toxic oxygen species) following macrolide exposure [10]. In conclusion, these findings therefore suggest that macrolides may be able to reduce tissue damage caused by certain bacteria, without exerting a direct antibacterial effect.

Intracellular Accumulation

Macrolides have been shown to accumulate in inflammatory cells at concentrations several hundredfold higher than concentrations in extracellular fluid. For example, azithromycin concentrates in neutrophils, macrophages and fibroblasts at concentrations 10–100 times higher than serum levels [11]. In addition, inflammatory cytokines have been shown to stimulate the accumulation of macrolides into macrophages [12]. This suggests that, at sites of inflammation, cells may accumulate even more macrolide than under normal physiological conditions. This intracellular accumulation may aid macrolides in treating intracellular pathogens, as well as altering host cell intrinsic functions.

Cytokines

Cytokines constitute a large family of molecules that includes the interleukins, the interferons, the colony-stimulating factors and the tumour necrosis factors. They are key regulators of immune cell growth and differentiation and are thought to regulate or determine the activity of a disease process. The effect of macrolides on cytokines in CRS has been examined in detail.

Interleukin-8 (IL-8) is a potent neutrophil chemoattractant cytokine and has been shown to be one of the principal cytokines involved in chronic sinusitis [13]. IL-8 production by whole sections of CRS mucosa in vitro was shown to be reduced in a dose-dependent fashion by clarithromycin. This reduction was equal to that seen when the mucosa was treated with prednisolone [14]. Neutrophils in the nasal discharge of patients with CRS secrete approximately twice as much IL-8 as those in peripheral blood, indicating that they are activated and hence may induce further neutrophil migration. Erythromycin at concentrations of 10^{-5} and 10^{-6} has been shown to significantly inhibit IL-8 secretion by exudative neutrophils by 54% and 34%, respectively. These drug concentrations are approximately the same as levels found in sinus mucosa and nasal discharge during macrolide therapy [15]. Macrolides therefore seem capable of inhibiting the production of IL-8 by a variety of cell types and may help break the vicious cycle of neutrophil recruitment and further inflammation in chronic airway disease.

Other cytokines shown to be inhibited by macrolide treatment in vitro include IL-5, granulocyte-macrophage colony-stimulating factor and transforming growth factor-β (TGF-β) [14, 16]. TGF-β was shown to have reduced expression following in vitro treatment of cultured CRS mucosa; however, a similar reduction in expression was not seen following in vivo treatment with a long-term, low-dose course of macrolide. This finding highlights the important issue of whether the impressive anti-inflammatory effects of macrolides that have been demonstrated in vitro are seen with the in vivo treatment of patients.

Apoptosis

Therapeutic induction of apoptosis results in an attenuation of the inflammatory response. Both erythromycin and roxithromycin have been shown to accelerate apoptosis in isolated human neutrophils [17]. Aoshiba et al. [18] reported similar findings with erythromycin, roxithromycin and midecamycin.

Oxidative Burst

Phagocytic cells are capable of producing toxic, reactive oxygen species that are used to destroy phagocytosed micro-organisms. These oxygen species are damaging to bacteria and also potentially to host tissues if generated in excess. Macrolides have been reported to produce a dose-dependent reduction in superoxide production by neutrophils [19]. An interesting study by Braga et al. [20] showed that rokitamycin was also capable of inhibiting the oxidative burst of neutrophils and that, after washing the cells to remove the macrolide, the oxidative burst ability was restored.

Adhesion

Macrolides can reduce inflammatory cell adhesion via inhibition of adhesion molecule expression. This effect may result in reduced recruitment of inflammatory cells at sites of inflammation. Erythromycin has been shown to reduce the expression of cell-surface adhesion molecules on neutrophils [21]. Matsuoka et al. [22] reported that clarithromycin markedly inhibited the expression of intercellular adhesion molecule-1 and vascular cell adhesion molecule-1 by synovial (fibroblast-like) cells.

Molecular Mechanism of Activity

Nuclear factor-κB (NF-κB) is a key nuclear transcription factor involved in the upregulation of the inflammatory process. It controls the expression of the genes for multiple cytokines and adhesion molecules [23]. Miyanohara et al. [24] examined the activity of clarithromycin on cultured human nasal epithelial cells and fibroblasts obtained from nasal polyps. They suggested that clarithromycin may decrease the expression of IL-1β mRNA through suppression of activation of NF-κB. Desaki et al. [25] showed that erythromycin inhibited the activation of the transcription factors NF-κB and AP-1 in human bronchial epithelial cells. It is postulated, therefore, that macrolides may produce their wide-ranging anti-inflammatory effect by inhibition of the actions of NF-κB.

Effects on Mucociliary Clearance

In addition to their anti-inflammatory and antibiotic effects, macrolides produce effects on mucus production and mucociliary clearance. In rabbits, roxithromycin treatment increased the rate of tracheal mucociliary transport [26]. A further animal study demonstrated that goblet cell hypersecretion in the guinea pig trachea was reduced by clarithromycin [27]. In patients with CRS treated with clarithromycin, the abnormal viscoelastic properties of their nasal mucus was improved and thus made more suitable for effective mucociliary clearance [28]. These findings support the observations of clinical studies in which mucus secretion was reduced and mucociliary clearance was increased [29, 30].

Conclusion of In Vitro Findings

As outlined above, considerable evidence now exists to show that macrolides have potentially wide-ranging anti-inflammatory and immunomodulatory activities. The authors of this chapter have the impression that the most crucial of these effects is the inhibition of neutrophilic inflammation through the suppression of IL-8 production, which may be secondary to inhibition of NF-κB activation. An additional exciting and potentially powerful mechanism is the inhibition of bacterial virulence and biofilm formation. However, it is important to note that, in many cases, these in vitro effects are yet to be shown to also be present in in vivo studies. The next section will discuss the findings of the clinical studies that have been performed.

Clinical Background

The majority of clinical trials studying the efficacy of long-term, low-dose macrolide treatment in CRS have been small and open. One recent exception, a randomised prospective, placebo-controlled study demonstrating efficacy of macrolides on CRS was published in 2006 [31]. However, to fully understand the in vivo effect of long-term, low-dose macrolide therapy on the respiratory epithelium one has to include studies from the lower airways. It is also here that we find the majority of the placebo-controlled trials.

Effects in Cystic Fibrosis

The remarkable effect on the survival rate in diffuse panbronchiolitis has already been mentioned [3, 32]. In cystic fibrosis (CF) several studies have shown a positive effect, even if the patient is infected with *P. aeruginosa*. In one study, CF patients were treated with 250 mg of clarithromycin every second day resulting in a marked reduction of the cytokine levels, tumour necrosis factor-α (TNF-α), IL-8, IL-4 and interferon-γ, both in sputum and plasma specimens. These changes were associated with a significant improvement in lung function [33]. A placebo-controlled study showed an effect on selected patients in lung function parameters and a reduction in the number of antibiotic treatments but no significant overall effect [34]. Further exploring the possible mechanisms showed no alterations of the adhesion of *Pseudomonas* to the respiratory epithelium [35]. Another placebo-controlled study using azithromycin showed an undisputed effect on respiratory and clinical parameters regardless of pseudomonal infection [36, 37]. This has been reproduced in yet another placebo-controlled trial using azithromycin in adults with CF. Treatment significantly improved quality of life, reduced C-reactive protein levels in serum and the number of respiratory exacerbations, as well as reducing the rate of decline in lung function compared to placebo [38].

Effect in Asthma

A randomised placebo-controlled study using roxithromycin in subjects with asthma and IgG antibodies to *Chlamydia pneumoniae* led to a significant improvement in asthma control after 6 weeks of treatment but the effect was not sustained for more than 3 months [39]. Clarithromycin or placebo treatment in 64 patients for 6 weeks reduced bronchial hyper-responsiveness [40]. In a randomised controlled study, 54 patients with stable asthma and a positive polymerase chain reaction (PCR) for *C. pneumonia* were randomised to placebo or clarithromycin for 6 weeks. Both the PCR-positive and PCR-negative subjects who received clarithromycin demonstrated a reduction in TNF-α, IL-5 and IL-12 mRNA in bronchoalveolar lavage (BAL) and TNF-α mRNA in airway tissue. However, lung function was only improved in the PCR-positive group [41]. Although it is believed that macrolides are more effective in neutrophilic inflammation it has been shown in aspirin-sensitive asthmatics that markers for eosinophilic activity both in blood and sputum is significantly reduced after 8 weeks of roxithromycin therapy [42].

Effects in Chronic Obstructive Pulmonary Disease (COPD)

Sixty-seven patients with stable COPD were treated with clarithromycin or placebo for 3 months. The treatment did not improve health status, sputum bacterial numbers or exacerbation rate [43]. A similar trial from the same authors showed that clarithromycin had no significant effect on neutrophil count or cytokine levels in sputum. However, clarithromycin did cause a small reduction in the neutrophil differentia [44].

Effects in Other Inflammatory Airway Disease

Smaller studies have been made in patients with non-CF bronchiectasis and chronic bronchitis with favourable outcome [45, 46].

Conclusion from the Lower Airways

To sum up the findings from the lower airways, there are some placebo-controlled randomised trials showing a beneficial effect on airway inflammation in CF and asthma. The clinical effect seems to go hand in hand with a reduction in proinflammatory cytokines. This suggests an anti-inflammatory effect in vivo. However, not all studies have used a reduced dose of the macrolide and an antibacterial effect cannot be ruled out. In one study the effect was most notable where intracellular pathogens were present. A few studies showed no or little effect, especially in COPD, suggesting that there is a subset of patients not re-

sponding. The reason for this is unclear and could be attributed to several possible explanations, such as the individual host immunological phenotype (type of inflammation present), the type of microbial infection or colonisation of the airway, and poor absorption or fast metabolism of the macrolide drug.

Studies in Chronic Rhinosinusitis

Eleven non-placebo-controlled studies have been published on the efficacy of long-term (>2 months) macrolide antibiotics in CRS. Another three studies have used macrolides for 1 month or less. Ten of the studies have used a dose lower than the one suggested for an antibacterial effect. Recently the first placebo-controlled study by the present authors has been published confirming results from the open studies [31] (Table 25.1).

What are the conclusions that can be drawn from the different studies in CRS?

Effect on Markers of Inflammation

In a short-term, open study 25 patients with chronic purulent rhinosinusitis were treated with clarithromycin 500 mg twice daily for 2 weeks. A significant reduction was seen in eosinophilic activity, macrophages, IL-6, IL-8, TNF-α and elastase. However, bacterial culture was only performed for *C. pneumoniae*, which was ruled out. The effect of the treatment lasted only for 2 weeks after cessation of medication [47]. In two studies where long-term (>2 months), low-dose roxithromycin or clarithromycin was used, a reduction of IL-8 levels in nasal lavage was seen as well as a reduction in the size of nasal polyps [48, 49]. In our placebo-controlled trial a reduction of nasal IL-8 was observed in nasal lavage in the treatment group [31]. Taken together with the studies from the lower airways it is clear that low-dose macrolide antibiotics reduce the concentration of cytokines and inflammatory cells in the sinonasal mucosa.

Effect on the Rheological Properties of Mucus

Eighteen patients with CRS were treated with clarithromycin 500 mg/day for 4 weeks. The spinnability and elasticity was increased and viscosity decreased suggesting secretions that transport and clear more easily [50]. Similar findings were made by Rubin and colleagues in acute rhinosinusitis where they also found a 30% increase in mucociliary transport [29]. It is also the author's personal experience that the extremely tenacious secretions sometimes seen can be reduced by macrolide treatment and this has a positive impact on the patient's sleep and quality of life.

Effect on Nasal Polyps

Twenty patients with CRS and nasal polyps were treated for at least 3 months with clarithromycin 400 mg/day. In the group whose polyps were reduced in size, the IL-8 levels dramatically

Table 25.1 Studies supporting the use of macrolide antibiotics in rhinosinusitis

Type of study	Dosage 24 h (mg)	Duration (months)	Macrolide	Results	Reference
Prospective, double-blind, placebo-controlled	150	3	RXM	Improvements in SNOT-20 score, nasal endoscopy, saccharine transit time and IL-8 levels in lavage fluid ($p<0.05$)	[31]
Prospective, randomised, $n = 90$	1,000 (2 weeks) 500 (10 weeks)	3	CAM	As effective as surgery in chronic sinusitis	[54]
Prospective, open, $n = 17$	500	12	EM	Twelve responders, mucociliary transport, headache, postnasal drip, all improved, $p < 0.05$	[53]
Prospective, open, $n = 20$	1,000	0.5	CAM	Improvement in CD68, IL-6, IL-8, TNF-α and clinical parameters	[47]
Prospective, open, $n = 20$	400	3	CAM	Reduction of IL-8 in nasal lavage, decreased nasal polyp size	[49]
Prospective, open, $n = 16$	200, 150		CAM, RXM	Patients with normal IgE have higher response rate	[56]
Prospective, open, $n = 20$	1,000	0.5	CAM	Reduction of secretion volume, improvement in mucociliary transport	[29]
Prospective open, $n = 30$	150	3	RXM	Approx. 80% of patients respond. Postnasal drip, headache	[57]
Prospective, open, $n = 12$	150		RXM	Reduction of nasal IL-8, CT better aeration	[48]
Prospective, open? $n = 45$	400	2–3	CAM	Approx. 71% overall improvement	[52]
Prospective, open, $n = 20$ (+20 in combination with azelastine)	150	>2	RXM	Reduction of nasal polyps associated with CRS in at least 52% of patients	[51]
Prospective, open, $n = 32$	400	1	CAM	Reduction of secretion volume, improvement in mucociliary transport	[30]
Retrospective, open, $n = 149$	200–600	3–6	EM	Postoperative treatment with EM improves results compared to no treatment, 88% improvement versus 68%	[55]
Prospective, open, $n = 16$	600	>6	EM	Approx. 85% overall improvement	[58]
Prospective, open	400–600	8	EM	Approx. 60% overall improvement	[4]

Source: Modified from Cervin A, Wallwork B (2005) Anti-inflammatory effects of macrolide antibiotics in the treatment of chronic rhinosinusitis. Otolaryngol Clin North Am 38:1339–1350
EM erythromycin, *CAM* clarithromycin, *RXM* roxithromycin

decreased from 231.2 to 44.0 pg/ml ($p < 0.05$) and were significantly higher before macrolide treatment than those in the group whose polyps showed no change [49]. In another uncontrolled trial 40 patients altogether were treated with either roxithromycin 150 mg alone or in combination with an antihistamine (azelastine) for at least 8 weeks. Smaller polyps were more likely to shrink and this happened in about half of the patients [51]. The use of nasal steroids as the first option is well established and should not be abandoned. However, in nasal polyps with signs of chronic infection adding macrolide treatment may be an alternative.

Duration of Treatment

The rate of improvement is related to the number of weeks the patient is treated. One study showed that response rate varied from 5% at 2 weeks to 71% at 12 weeks [52]. One of our own studies showed that further improvement in responders was seen at 12 months compared to 3 months in mucociliary transport, postnasal drip and headache [53]. Our policy is to treat for 10–12 weeks and then evaluate. One is expecting to see a response rate among 60–80% of the patients at that time interval. Responders may continue with medication whereas one has to seek other alternatives for the non-responding patients.

Presurgical Treatment

Ninety patients with CRS were randomised to either macrolide therapy for 3 months or surgical therapy. Both groups also received a topical steroid and nasal douche with saline. Final assessment was made after 1 year. Both groups showed improvement and there was no significant difference between groups except for nasal volume where surgery was more effective. It was concluded that CRS should be initially targeted with maximal medical therapy before turning to surgery [54]. Unfortunately a placebo group or a group with only topical treatment is lacking.

Postsurgical Treatment

Persisting CRS after adequate surgery is not uncommon. It puts a strain on the relation between the surgeon and the patient and alternative treatments are warranted. Fifty-seven patients with persisting symptoms of CRS 1 year after sinus surgery were treated with erythromycin in doses initially 600 mg/day reduced approximately every second month by 200 mg. Ninety-two patients served as controls. The clinical improvement in the treated group was 88% compared to 69% in the untreated patients [55]. An uncontrolled study from our own research group showed that in our most desperate postsurgical cases, 12 out of 17 responded with significant improvement in headache, nasal congestion and postnasal drip as well as improved mucociliary clearance after 3 months of erythromycin 250 mg twice daily [53].

Randomised Controlled Trials

As opposed to the lower airways, placebo-controlled trials studying the effects of long-term, low-dose macrolide therapy in CRS have been missing until recently. In a study published by Wallwork et al., 64 patients with CRS and without nasal polyps were recruited. Subjects received either 150 mg roxithromycin daily for 3 months or placebo. Outcome measures included the Sinonasal Outcome Test-20 (SNOT-20), measurements of peak nasal inspiratory flow, saccharine transit time, olfactory function, nasal endoscopic scoring and nasal lavage assays for IL-8, fucose and α2-macroglobulin. There were statistically significant improvements in SNOT-20 score, nasal endoscopy, saccharine transit time and IL-8 levels in lavage fluid ($p < 0.05$) in the macrolide group. A correlation was noted between improved outcome measures and low IgE levels. No improvement in any outcome was noted in the placebo-treated patients [31]. The result confirms the findings from previous open studies. Additional placebo-controlled studies are anticipated in the near future.

Macrolides and Their Role in the Treatment of Chronic Rhinosinusitis

Where does macrolide treatment fit in the management of the patient with CRS? Are macrolides most wisely used as a presurgical option to reduce the number of patients going to surgery? Or, considering the risk of evolving resistant bacterial strains, should long-term, low-dose macrolide therapy be withheld until the surgical option has failed? The only true answers to these questions lie in performing placebo-controlled studies targeting specific outcomes, both in presurgical and postsurgical treatment as well as exploring the long-term efficacy of macrolide treatment in CRS. To further complicate matters the possible effect on emerging antibiotic resistance due to increased use of macrolide antibiotics has to be evaluated. One has to bear in mind that, although more placebo-controlled research is warranted, macrolide antibiotics are more extensively investigated than other antibiotics in CRS.

How to Select Patients

The present data support the use of macrolides irrespective of previous surgery or not. The first question to be answered before initiating macrolide treatment is; are there ways to select patients that are more likely to respond? It is the authors' experience, and supported by the Suzuki group, that a high level of serum IgE or marked eosinophilia in nasal smear, sinus mucosa or peripheral blood tells against a favourable outcome [31, 56]. Macrolide therapy has also been found to not be effective in primary ciliary dyskinesia (K. Ichimura, personal communication). From a practical point of view, patients with marked atopy are less likely to respond. The ideal patient is the one with persistent purulent discharge where nasopharyngeal culture is negative, there is no atopy and they experience little or no effect from nasal steroids (Table 25.2).

Table 25.2 How to choose your patient

In favour of macrolide treatment	Against macrolide treatment
Normal serum IgE	High serum IgE
Few allergies, non-atopic	Highly allergic or atopic
Negative culture	(Positive culture)[a]
Steroids not effective	Nasal steroids effective
Symptoms dominated by purulent discharge, post-nasal drip, facial pain and headache	Symptoms dominated by clear runny nose, sneezing
	Primary ciliary dyskinesia
	Allergic fungal sinusitis

Source: Modified from Cervin A, Wallwork B (2005) Anti-inflammatory effects of macrolide antibiotics in the treatment of chronic rhinosinusitis. Otolaryngol Clin North Am 38:1339–1350
[a]Targeted treatment with appropriate antibiotics first

The Work-up

If the patient fits the description above, long-term, low-dose macrolide therapy is likely to be beneficial for the patient. A nasal swab and culture is advised. It can rule out pathogens not susceptible to macrolide antibiotics, for example, the effect on *Haemophilus influenzae* is poor. It is recommended to repeat the nasal culture every 3 months to monitor the possible development of macrolide-resistant bacterial strains. Hepatic side effects are rare and reversible, but it is recommended to check liver enzymes at the start of treatment as well as red and white blood cell counts. Follow-up with new blood tests after 3 months (Fig. 25.1).

Which Macrolide?

Erythromycin, roxithromycin and clarithromycin have all shown an effect in open studies on CRS. Erythromycin is the cheapest but suffers from poor absorption from the gastrointestinal tract with more side effects, especially gastric pain. Roxithromycin and clarithromycin have a better uptake from the gastrointestinal tract. Efficacy in CRS has been shown in open studies for both, but only for roxithromycin in a placebo-controlled study. Azithromycin has not been used in CRS, although its efficacy has been proven in the lower airways. The near future will most likely prove azithromycin to be as effective as the other macrolides. For now clarithromycin or roxithromycin seem to be the drugs with the best evidence supporting efficacy in CRS. Also bear in mind the possible interactions between macrolide antibiotics and, most importantly, dicumarol, antiepileptic drugs, trephenadine, methotrexate and antidepressant drugs.

What Dosage?

Low dose usually means one half the dose used for treating respiratory infections. It is possible to start with the standard dose for treating infections and then reduce the dose after 2–4 weeks. Some authors state that starting with a standard dose will relieve the symptoms quicker than the lower dose [54, 55]. However, it may increase the risk of side effects. From a practical point of view, erythromycin 250 mg twice daily, clarithromycin 250 mg/day or roxithromycin 150 mg/day is adequate.

For How Long?

The patient has to be informed and accept that the effect sets in very slowly. A few patients experience an improvement already after 2 weeks and half of the patients experience improvements after 4–6 weeks. But it may take up to 10 weeks before the patient notices an improvement and the treatment should continue for 12 weeks before a proper evaluation is made. Our recommendation is to see the patient in the office or contact by telephone after 6 weeks in order to check for side effects and to encourage those patients who have yet to experience improvement of symptoms to continue the medication.

If the minimum treatment period is 12 weeks, how long is it advisable to continue? There is no definite answer. Further improvement can be seen up to a year of continuous treatment [53]. If the patient has had a marked improvement there is usually a wish from the patient to continue. It is the authors' experience that this can readily be done for up to a year without risking any side effects. However, the strategy in most cases would be to stop treatment after 3–6 months and wait and see. Some

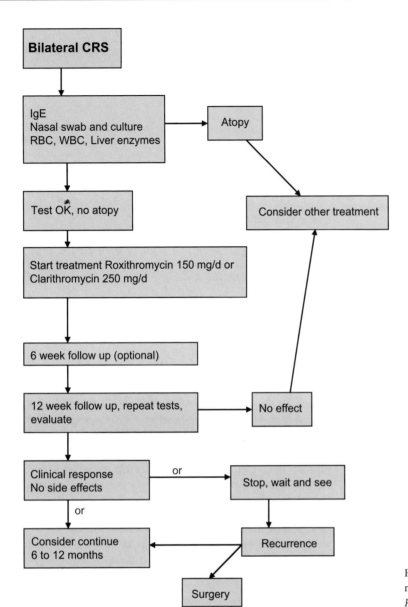

Fig. 25.1 A treatment algorithm for long-term, low-dose macrolide antibiotics in chronic rhinosinusitis (*CRS*). *RBC* red blood cell count, *WBC* white blood cell count

25

patients remain improved, but for others recurrence may come as soon as a month after therapy has stopped. Unfortunately data on recurrence rates are missing. If recurrence occurs, it is possible to start again and if the patient responded the first time it is very likely that it will work in the future as well. Another strategy in the difficult patient is to treat during infection-prone months (winter) and take a break during the summer months.

If Macrolides Do Not Work

It is our experience that with careful selection long-term, low-dose macrolide treatment will work in about 70–80% of your patients. But there is a subset of patients whose symptoms are not relieved. There are some possible explanations that are worthwhile to explore:

1. Is the patient taking the medication?
2. Poor absorption? If the patient is taking erythromycin one could consider switching to a semi-synthetic macrolide (clarithromycin or roxithromycin) with better absorption from the gastrointestinal tract.
3. Is there a simultaneous infection with bacteria not sensitive to macrolides? A nasal swab and culture is recommended. We usually treat simultaneous infection without stopping the macrolide treatment.
4. Is the diagnosis correct? Primary ciliary dyskinesia, cystic fibrosis, immune deficiency and atopy have to be investigated.

However, in some cases, due to our incomplete understanding of the complex immune system, a satisfactory explanation cannot be found and other treatment alternatives have to be found.

Emerging Resistant Bacterial Strains to Macrolides

If during treatment, a bacterial strain resistant to macrolides emerges it is our experience that it is best to stop the medication. A new nasal culture after a couple of weeks will usually show that the resistant bacteria has disappeared. We do occasionally treat the resistant bacterial strain with other antibiotics if the patient's symptoms suggest that this is necessary.

Summary

Long-term, low-dose macrolide administration in CRS is associated with downregulation of the non-specific host inflammatory response as well as clinical improvement. The effect is most likely attributed to the immune-modulating properties of macrolides. The clinical effect is shown in less facial pain, less headache, less postnasal drip, fewer exacerbations of sinusitis and improved quality of life. The treatment is more effective in the non-atopic patient. The treatment should be targeted towards patients with bilateral disease whereas in unilateral disease, surgery is the first option. Macrolide-resistant bacterial strains have to be monitored, but to date they have not been of clinical importance.

Tips to Avoid Complications

- Select patients accordingly (Table 25.2)
- Check for interactions between the macrolide and current medication of the patient
- Follow-up every 3 months
- Use nasal swab and culture to monitor bacterial strains
- Check liver enzymes and red and white blood cells

Take-Home Pearls

- Long-term, low-dose macrolide antibiotic treatment should be targeted at the non-atopic patient with bilateral chronic rhinosinusitis.

References

1. McGuire JM, Bunch R, Anderson RC, Boaz HE, Flynn EH, Powell HM, et al.(1952) 'Ilotycin' an new antibiotic. Antibiot Chemother 2:281–283
2. Nagai H, Shishido H, Yoneda R, Yamaguchi E, Tamura A, Kurashima A (1991) Long-term low-dose administration of erythromycin to patients with diffuse panbronchiolitis. Respiration 58:145–149
3. Kudoh S, Kimura H, Uetake T, et al.(1984) Clinical effect of low-dose, long-term macrolide antibiotic chemotherapy on diffuse panbronchiolitis. Jpn J Thorac Dis 22:254
4. Kikuchi S, Susaki H, Aoki A, Ito O, Nomura Y (1991) Clinical effect of long-term low-dose erythromycin therapy for chronic sinusitis (in Japanese with English abstract). Pract Otlo (Koyoto) 84:41–47
5. Stein GE, Havlichek DH (1992) The new macrolide antibiotics. Azithromycin and clarithromycin. Postgrad Med 92:269–272, 77–82
6. Hirakata Y, Kaku M, Mizukane R, Ishida K, Furuya N, Matsumoto T, et al.(1992) Potential effects of erythromycin on host defense systems and virulence of Pseudomonas aeruginosa. Antimicrob Agents Chemother 36:1922–1927
7. Sofer D, Gilboa-Garber N, Belz A, Garber NC (1999) 'Subinhibitory' erythromycin represses production of Pseudomonas aeruginosa lectins, autoinducer and virulence factors. Chemotherapy 45:335–341
8. Wozniak DJ, Keyser R (2004) Effects of subinhibitory concentrations of macrolide antibiotics on Pseudomonas aeruginosa. Chest 125(2 Suppl):62S–69S; quiz 9S
9. Takeoka K, Ichimiya T, Yamasaki T, Nasu M (1998) The in vitro effect of macrolides on the interaction of human polymorphonuclear leukocytes with Pseudomonas aeruginosa in biofilm. Chemotherapy 44:190–197
10. Nalca Y, Jansch L, Bredenbruch F, Geffers R, Buer J, Haussler S (2006) Quorum-sensing antagonistic activities of azithromycin in Pseudomonas aeruginosa PAO1: a global approach. Antimicrob Agents Chemother 50:1680–1688
11. Stein G, Havlicheck DH (1992) The new macrolide antibiotics: azithromycin and clarithromycin. Postgrad Med 92:269–282
12. Bermudez L, Inderlied C, Young LS (1991) Stimulation with cytokines enhances penetration of azithromycin into human macrophages. Antimicrob Agents Chemother 35:2625–2629
13. Lennard CM, Mann EA, Sun LL, Chang AS, Bolger WE (2000) Interleukin-1 beta, interleukin-5, interleukin-6, interleukin-8, and tumor necrosis factor-alpha in chronic sinusitis: response to systemic corticosteroids. Am J Rhinol 14:367–373
14. Wallwork B, Coman W, Feron F, Mackay-Sim A, Cervin A (2002) Clarithromycin and prednisolone inhibit cytokine production in chronic rhinosinusitis. Laryngoscope 112:1827–1830
15. Suzuki H, Asada Y, Ikeda K, Furukawa M, Oshima T, Takasaka T (1999) Inhibitory effect of erythromycin on interleukin-8 secretion from exudative cells in the nasal discharge of patients with chronic sinusitis. Laryngoscope 109:407–410
16. Wallwork B, Coman W, Mackay-Sim A, Cervin A (2004) Effect of clarithromycin on nuclear factor-kappa B and transforming growth factor-beta in chronic rhinosinusitis. Laryngoscope 114:286–290
17. Inamura K, Ohta N, Fukase S, Kasajima N, Aoyagi M (2000) The effect of erythromycin on human peripheral neutrophil apoptosis. Rhinology 38:124–129
18. Aoshiba K, Nagai A, Konno K (1995) Erythromycin shortens neutrophil survival by accelerating apoptosis. Antimicrob Agents Chemother 39:872–877
19. Hand W, Hand D, King-Thompson N (1990) Antibiotic inhibition of the respiratory burst response in human polymorphonuclear leukocytes. Antimicrob Agents Chemother 34:863–870

20. Braga P, Maci S, Dal Sasso M, Fonti E, Ghessi A (1997) Effects of rokitamycin on phagocytosis and release of oxidant radicals of human polymorphonuclear leukocytes. Chemotherapy 43:190–197

21. Lin H, Wang C, Liu C, Yu C, Kuo H (2000) Erythromycin inhibits beta2-integrins (CD11b/CD18) expression, interleukin-8 release and intracellular oxidative metabolism in neutrophils. Respir Med 94:654–660

22. Matsuoka N, Eguchi K, Kawakami A, Tsuboi M, Kawabe Y, Aoyagi T, Nagataki S (1996) Inhibitory effect of clarithromycin on costimulatory molecule expression and cytokine production by synovial fibroblast-like cells. Clin Exp Immunol 104:501–508

23. Baeuerle P, Henkel T (1994) Function and activation of NF-kappaB in the immune system. Annu Rev Immunol 12:141–179

24. Miyanohara T, Ushikai M, Matsune S, Ueno K, Katahira S, Kurono Y (2000) Effects of clarithromycin on cultured human nasal epithelial cells and fibroblasts. Laryngoscope 110:126–131

25. Desaki M, Takizawa H, Ohtoshi T, Kasama T, Kobayashi K, Sunazuka T, Omura S, Yamamoto K, Ito K (2000) Erythromycin suppresses nuclear factor kappa-B and activator protein-1 activation in human bronchial epithelial cells. Biochem Biophys Res Commun 267:124–128

26. Nakano T, Ohashi Y, Tanaka A, Kakinoki Y, Washio Y, Nakai Y (1998) Roxithromycin reinforces epithelial defence function in rabbit trachea. Acta Otolaryngol Suppl 538:233–238

27. Tamaoki J, Takeyama K, Yamawaki I, Kondo M, Konno K (1997) Lipopolysaccharide-induced goblet cell hypersecretion in the guinea pig trachea: inhibition by macrolides. Am J Physiol 272:15–19

28. Rhee C, Majima Y, Arima S, Jung H, Jinn T, Min Y, Sakakura Y (2000) Effects of clarithromycin on rheological properties of nasal mucous in patients with chronic sinusitis. Ann Otol Rhinol Laryngol 109:484–487

29. Rubin B, Druce H, Ramirez OE, Palmer R (1997) Effect of clarithromycin on nasal mucus properties in healthy subjects and in patients with purulent rhinitis. Am J Respir Crit Care Med 155:2018–2023

30. Nishi K, Mizuguchi M, Tachibana H, et al.(1995) Effect of clarithromycin on symptoms and mucociliary transport in patients with sino-bronchial syndrome. Nippon Shikkan Gakkai Zasshi 33:1392–1400

31. Wallwork B, Coman W, Mackay-Sim A, Greiff L, Cervin A (2006) A double-blind, randomized, placebo-controlled trial of macrolide in the treatment of chronic rhinosinusitis. Laryngoscope 116:189–193

32. Kudoh S, Azuma A, Yamamoto M, Izumi T, Ando M (1998) Improvement of survival in patients with diffuse panbronchiolitis treated with low-dose erythromycin. Am J Respir Crit Care Med 157:1829–1832

33. Pukhalsky AL, Shmarina GV, Kapranov NI, Kokarovtseva SN, Pukhalskaya D, Kashirskaja NJ (2004) Anti-inflammatory and immunomodulating effects of clarithromycin in patients with cystic fibrosis lung disease. Mediators Inflamm 13:111–117

34. Equi A, Balfour-Lynn IM, Bush A, Rosenthal M (2002) Long term azithromycin in children with cystic fibrosis: a randomised, placebo-controlled crossover trial. Lancet 360:978–984

35. Equi AC, Davies JC, Painter H, Hyde S, Bush A, Geddes DM, et al.(2006) Exploring the mechanisms of macrolides in cystic fibrosis. Respir Med 100:687–697

36. Saiman L, Mayer-Hamblett N, Campbell P, Marshall BC (2005) Heterogeneity of treatment response to azithromycin in patients with cystic fibrosis. Am J Respir Crit Care Med 172:1008–1012

37. Saiman L, Marshall BC, Mayer-Hamblett N, Burns JL, Quittner AL, Cibene DA, et al.(2003) Azithromycin in patients with cystic fibrosis chronically infected with Pseudomonas aeruginosa: a randomized controlled trial. JAMA 290:1749–1756

38. Wolter J, Seeney S, Bell S, Bowler S, Masel P, McCormack J (2002) Effect of long term treatment with azithromycin on disease parameters in cystic fibrosis: a randomised trial. Thorax 57:212–216

39. Black PN, Blasi F, Jenkins CR, Scicchitano R, Mills GD, Rubinfeld AR, et al.(2001) Trial of roxithromycin in subjects with asthma and serological evidence of infection with Chlamydia pneumoniae. Am J Respir Crit Care Med 164:536–541

40. Kostadima E, Tsiodras S, Alexopoulos EI, Kaditis AG, Mavrou I, Georgatou N, et al.(2004) Clarithromycin reduces the severity of bronchial hyperresponsiveness in patients with asthma. Eur Respir J 23:714–717

41. Kraft M, Cassell GH, Pak J, Martin RJ (2002) Mycoplasma pneumoniae and Chlamydia pneumoniae in asthma: effect of clarithromycin. Chest 121:1782–1788

42. Shoji T, Yoshida S, Sakamoto H, Hasegawa H, Nakagawa H, Amayasu H (1999) Anti-inflammatory effect of roxithromycin in patients with aspirin-intolerant asthma. Clin Exp Allergy 29:950–956

43. Banerjee D, Khair OA, Honeybourne D (2005) The effect of oral clarithromycin on health status and sputum bacteriology in stable COPD. Respir Med 99:208–215

44. Banerjee D, Honeybourne D, Khair OA (2004) The effect of oral clarithromycin on bronchial airway inflammation in moderate-to-severe stable COPD: a randomized controlled trial. Treat Respir Med 3:59–65

45. Koh YY, Lee MH, Sun YH, Sung KW, Chae JH (1997) Effect of roxithromycin on airway responsiveness in children with bronchiectasis: a double-blind, placebo-controlled study. Eur Respir J 10:994–999

46. Nakamura H, Fujishima S, Inoue T, Ohkubo Y, Soejima K, Waki Y, et al.(1999) Clinical and immunoregulatory effects of roxithromycin therapy for chronic respiratory tract infection. Eur Respir J 13:1371–1379

47. MacLeod CM, Hamid QA, Cameron L, Tremblay C, Brisco W (2001) Anti-inflammatory activity of clarithromycin in adults with chronically inflamed sinus mucosa. Adv Ther 18:75–82

48. Suzuki H, Shimomura A, Ikeda K, Oshima T, Takasaka T (1997) Effects of long-term low-dose macrolide administration on neutrophil recruitment and IL-8 in the nasal discharge of chronic sinusitis patients. Tohoku J Exp Med 182:115–124

49. Yamada T, Fujieda S, Mori S, Yamamoto H, Saito H (2000) Macrolide treatment decreased the size of nasal polyps and IL-8 levels in nasal lavage. Am J Rhinol 14:143–148

50. Rhee CS, Majima Y, Arima S, Jung HW, Jinn TH, Min YG, et al.(2000) Effects of clarithromycin on rheological properties of nasal mucus in patients with chronic sinusitis. Ann Otol Rhinol Laryngol 109:484–487

25

51. Ichimura K, Shimazaki Y, Ishibashi T, Higo R (1996) Effect of new macrolide roxithromycin upon nasal polyps associated with chronic sinusitis. Auris Nasus Larynx 23:48–56

52. Hashiba M, Baba S (1996) Efficacy of long-term administration of clarithromycin in the treatment of intractable chronic sinusitis. Acta Otolaryngol Suppl (Stockh) 525:73–78

53. Cervin A, Kalm O, Sandkull P, Lindberg S (2002) One-year low-dose erythromycin treatment of persistent chronic sinusitis after sinus surgery: clinical outcome and effects on mucociliary parameters and nasal nitric oxide. Otolaryngol Head Neck Surg 126:481–489

54. Ragab SM, Lund VJ, Scadding G (2004) Evaluation of the medical and surgical treatment of chronic rhinosinusitis: a prospective, randomised, controlled trial. Laryngoscope 114:923–930

55. Moriyama H, Yanagi K, Ohtori N, Fukami M (1995) Evaluation of endoscopic sinus surgery for chronic sinusitis: post-operative erythromycin therapy. Rhinology 33:166–170

56. Suzuki H, Ikeda K, Honma R, Gotoh S, Oshima T, Furukawa M, et al.(2000) Prognostic factors of chronic rhinosinusitis under long-term low-dose macrolide therapy. ORL J Otorhinolaryngol Relat Spec 62:121–127

57. Kimura N, Nishioka K, Nishizaki K, Ogawa T, Naitou Y, Masuda Y (1997) Clinical effect of low-dose, long-term roxithromycin chemotherapy in patients with chronic sinusitis. Acta Med Okayama 51:33–37

58. Iino Y, Sugita K, Toriyama M, Kudo K (1993) Erythromycin therapy for otitis media with effusion in sinobronchial syndrome. Arch Otolaryngol Head Neck Surg 119:648–651

Chapter 26

The Frontal Sinus

Parul Goyal and Peter H. Hwang

Core Messages

- Despite many advances in our understanding of frontal sinus anatomy, physiology, and pathology, management of frontal sinus disease remains challenging.
- Endoscopic techniques have enabled surgeons to manage frontal sinus disease with less patient morbidity than ever before.
- Success in treating frontal sinus disease requires a thorough understanding of frontal sinus anatomy and contemporary frontal sinus surgical techniques.
- Radiographic findings indicating the presence of inflammatory frontal sinusitis should not be the sole criteria in selecting patients for frontal sinus surgery. Candidates should be carefully selected by placing the radiographic findings in context with patient symptoms and endoscopic findings.

Contents

Anatomy

Although older texts and literature have referred to the presence of a nasofrontal duct, in actuality no true ductal structure exists at the outflow tract of the frontal sinus. Instead, the frontal sinus narrows to an ostium, and this ostium communicates with a space in the anterosuperior ethmoid sinus termed the frontal recess. The frontal recess serves as an antechamber to the frontal sinus and is bounded by the lamina papyracea laterally, the middle turbinate and cribriform plate medially, the nasofrontal beak anteriorly, and the ethmoid bulla and skull base posteriorly [15].

Development of the frontal recess and frontal sinus starts early in fetal life and continues into the teenage years. Up to four sets of folds and furrows appear in the frontal recess, and development of these regions may ultimately give rise to the frontal sinus and different types of cells in the frontal recess [10]. The multiple cells that can pneumatize the frontal bone all maintain a separate communication with the frontal recess. The frontal sinus itself may develop as an extension of the frontal recess, from extension of an anterior ethmoid cell, or from extension of the ethmoid infundibulum [3]. The pneumatization patterns of the various cells impact the size, location, and shape of the frontal sinus outflow tract. The development is variable, leading to the complexity of the anatomy in this region.

The major cell types found in the frontal recess include agger nasi cells, frontal cells (types I–IV), supraorbital ethmoid cells, suprabullar cells, and intersinus septal cells. The variable presence and configuration of these cells can encroach upon the drainage pathway of the frontal sinus. The agger nasi cell is the most constant of the frontal recess cells, while other cell types have wider variability in their prevalence [13]. The mere presence of agger nasi cells and frontal cells may not increase the likelihood of frontal sinus disease; however, when extensively pneumatized, these cells can make surgical dissection of the frontal recess more difficult [4].

One of the primary determinants of frontal sinus drainage is the insertion of the superiormost aspect of the uncinate process. Most commonly, the superior aspect of the uncinate process attaches laterally onto the orbital wall, in which case the frontal sinus drains medial to the superior attachment of the uncinate

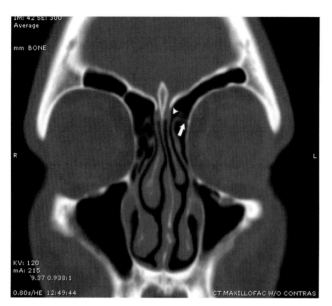

Fig. 26.1 A coronal CT image shows the uncinate process attaching laterally to the lamina papyracea (*arrow*), leading the frontal sinus to drain medial (*arrowhead*) to the superior uncinate attachment. The space in which the arrow is positioned is the recessus terminalis

(Fig. 26.1) [11]. In 10–35% of individuals the uncinate process attaches more medially, to the ethmoid skull base or to the lateral lamella of the cribriform plate [11, 20]. In such cases, the frontal sinus thus drains lateral to the uncinate process, directly into the ethmoid infundibulum. Awareness of the uncinate configuration is critical to successful frontal sinusotomy.

Detailed review of imaging studies is essential to understanding the anatomic variants of the frontal recess that may affect the surgical approach to the frontal sinus. Computerized tomography (CT) is the imaging modality of choice for detailed definition of the bony anatomy. The coronal views are of primary interest and may be acquired in a direct coronal plane with contiguous slices no thicker than 3.0 mm. Alternatively, excellent coronal and sagittal reconstructions can be derived from thin-section axial sections using multidetector CT technology. The sagittal view is particularly helpful for studying the relationship of adjacent frontal recess cells [13]. The CT scan serves as a critical "road map" during surgical dissection and should be referred to frequently during the course of frontal recess surgery. CT images can also be utilized for surgical navigation, which can be a helpful adjunct to endoscopic visualization. However, the use of navigation technology does not negate the need for adequate anatomic knowledge, surgical skill, and surgeon experience.

Imaging is usually not necessary in the evaluation of acute rhinosinusitis because the diagnosis is most commonly based on a history and physical examination. However, in cases of complications of sinusitis, CT and magnetic resonance imaging (MRI) may be indicated. CT provides excellent definition of the bony paranasal sinus anatomy, and contrast-enhanced CT can be useful in defining orbital and intracranial abscesses. MRI provides better definition of soft tissue, which can be especially useful in imaging intracranial processes such as dural venous thrombosis [7]. In patients with severe complications related to frontal sinusitis, both CT and MRI may be indicated because they provide complementary information.

Frontal Sinus Surgical Techniques

The decision regarding when to perform frontal sinus surgery for chronic sinusitis can be a difficult one. In a study of 243 patients with chronic sinusitis, 35% of the frontal sinuses had evidence of inflammatory disease based on CT [20]. However, radiographic evidence of disease should not be the sole criterion used to determine a patient's candidacy for frontal sinus surgery. Instead, the imaging studies should be reviewed in conjunction with a careful assessment of patient symptoms and examination findings before opting for surgical intervention.

Frontal sinus surgery is technically demanding due to the intrinsic narrowness of the frontal recess and the potential for injury to adjacent structures such as the cribriform plate, ethmoid skull base, and orbit. Extreme care must also be taken to avoid iatrogenic complications such as scarring and stenosis. Surgical treatment should be considered only after ascertaining that the frontal sinus disease is refractory to comprehensive medical therapy. Indications for surgical intervention include symptomatic chronic frontal sinusitis, frontal sinus mucoceles, neoplastic processes involving the frontal recess and sinus, skull base defects in the region of the frontal recess, and frontal sinus trauma. In principle, the surgical approach should be tailored to balance surgical aggressiveness against optimizing mucosal preservation. Regardless of the approach taken, the surgeon must ensure a regimen of frequent, meticulous postoperative care and monitoring in order to achieve successful outcomes in frontal sinus surgery.

Endoscopic Frontal Sinusotomy

Endoscopic frontal sinusotomy has supplanted external frontoethmoidectomy and "headlight" intranasal frontoethmoidectomy as the first-line surgical approach for medically refractory chronic frontal sinusitis. The Draf classification categorizes endonasal approaches to the frontal sinus according to the extent of dissection performed. The Draf type I frontal sinusotomy consists of removing ethmoidal cells that may be obstructing the frontal recess without altering the frontal sinus ostium itself. Draf type II techniques have been further categorized into type IIA and type IIB. Draf type IIA frontal sinusotomy involves removal of ethmoidal cells that may be protruding into the frontal sinus. In the type IIB frontal sinusotomy, the ipsilateral frontal sinus floor is removed from the lamina papyracea to the nasal septum [21]. The type III technique involves the creation of a common midline outflow tract for both frontal sinuses after removal of the frontal sinus floor bilaterally as well as a portion of the anterosuperior nasal septum.

The surgical technique for Draf type I and II procedures is similar. The superior attachment of the uncinate process can determine the location of the frontal sinus outflow tract. Most commonly, the superior aspect of the uncinate has a lateral attachment, leading the frontal sinus to drain medially into the frontal recess [11, 20]. As the uncinate process is resected, surgical dissection in these cases is carried out medial to the superiormost aspect of the uncinate process. Angled telescopes (30, 45, or 70 degrees) and curved instruments are used for visualization and dissection. Initially, it is helpful to probe for the frontal sinus outflow tract with a blunt tipped, curved frontal sinus seeker. If agger nasi or frontal cells are present, these can be collapsed with a frontal curette in order to clear obstruction of the outflow tract (Fig. 26.2). These cells are always anterior to the frontal sinus outflow tract. Using a curved curette to collapse these cells anteriorly and inferiorly will allow visualization of the frontal sinus outflow tract (Fig. 26.3). Bone fragments and partitions are meticulously removed using cutting giraffe forceps and through-cutting punches to ensure a patent outflow tract. The curved microdebrider can be useful in clearing polypoid tissue but must be used judiciously, especially when the

tip of the blade is beyond the visual field of the endoscope. In all cases, it is important to preserve mucosa wherever possible, especially along the circumference of the frontal sinus ostium itself. In the Draf type IIB technique, the floor of the frontal sinus is removed from the ipsilateral lamina papyracea to the nasal septum [21]. This can be performed using a drill or frontal sinus punches.

The Draf type III frontal sinusotomy is an extended approach to the frontal sinus by which a single, common nasofrontal communication is created between both frontal sinuses and the nasal cavity. The floor of both frontal sinuses is resected, along with contiguous portions of the superior nasal septum and the frontal intersinus septum (Fig. 26.4). Also termed the modified Lothrop procedure, endoscopic removal of the floor of the frontal sinus is typically performed using curved drills or cutting punches [5]. Meticulous postoperative care, including serial debridement, is necessary to minimize the risk of stenosis, which can be as high as 20% [18].

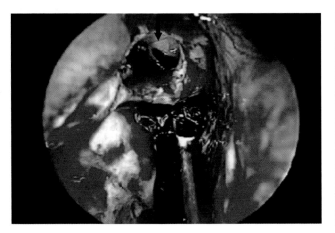

Fig. 26.2 As an endoscopic frontal sinusotomy (Draf type IIA) is being performed, a frontal sinus curette is being used to collapse and remove the agger nasi cell (*arrow*)

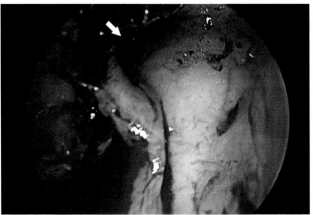

Fig. 26.3 After removal of the agger nasi cell, a patent frontal sinus outflow tract (*arrow*) can be visualized using a 45-degree endoscope

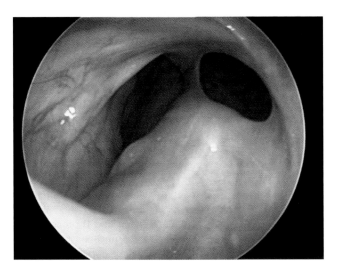

Fig. 26.4 A postoperative view of a Draf type III frontal sinusotomy shows a common outflow tract to both frontal sinuses

Results of Endoscopic Frontal Sinus Surgery

Endoscopic frontal sinus surgery has been reported to have high success rates in improving patient symptoms. Jacobs reviewed his experience of 148 endoscopic frontal sinusotomies [10]. With a mean follow up of 16 months, he found that 84% of the patients had improvement in their symptoms. However, the rate of frontal sinus patency based on endoscopy was found to be 42.6%. Many of the patients did have nasal polyposis, and this may have contributed to difficulty visualizing the outflow tract postoperatively.

Friedman et al. reviewed their long-term results with patients undergoing endoscopic frontal sinusotomy [6]. They reported on a series of 157 patients with a mean follow up of 72 months. These authors found symptomatic improvement in 92% of their patients, with 78% of the patients reporting significant symptom improvement. Fifty-seven patients were available for endoscopic evaluation, and the authors found a 67.6% patency rate after the initial surgical procedure. Of the patients with pathology in the frontal recess on follow up, the most common findings were polyps and scarring [6].

In reviewing their experience with 635 patients undergoing Draf type I frontal sinusotomy and 312 undergoing type II frontal sinusotomy, Weber et al. found significant symptomatic improvement without the need for revision surgery in over 85% of type I patients and 79% of type II patients [21].

Wormald et al. reported the results of their experience with 83 patients undergoing an endoscopic modified Lothrop procedure [23]. The success rate in terms of frontal sinus ostium patency based on endoscopic assessment was 93% with an average follow up period of 21 months. Samaha et al. reviewed their combined experience with Draf type IIB and Draf type III frontal sinusotomy [18]. In 34 patients undergoing type IIB procedures and 66 patients undergoing type III procedures, the authors found an 80% success rate in terms of frontal sinus patency and control of patient symptoms with a mean follow up of 4.1 years.

Frontal Sinus Trephination

Frontal sinus trephination is a technique that can be quite useful in treating a variety of frontal sinus pathology. Trephination has traditionally been performed in the inferomedial aspect of the frontal sinus. After making a skin incision overlying the inferomedial portion of the frontal sinus, a small opening is created through the anterior table of the sinus using a drill. Trephination can be useful as a first-line treatment for acute frontal sinusitis complicated by intracranial or orbital extension. Because inflammation and bleeding can complicate endoscopic frontal recess dissections in an acutely inflamed milieu, it is often preferable to decompress the acute infection via trephination. After the acute inflammation has resolved, a definitive endoscopic frontal sinusotomy can then be performed.

Trephination can also be useful in treating non-acute sinus pathology. The technique can be used to access areas of the frontal sinus that cannot be reached using endoscopic techniques alone. For example, pathology located in the superior and lateral aspects of the sinus can be difficult to visualize and instrument [2]. Examples of pathology that may be difficult to manage entirely endoscopically include frontal sinus neoplasms, fibro-osseous lesions, and frontal sinus skull base defects. Positioning the trephination over the site of the frontal sinus pathology can maximize exposure while minimizing the amount of dissection needed. Computerized navigation can be helpful in guiding the location of the skin incision and the trephination [25].

In selected cases, a transethmoid endoscopic frontal sinusotomy can be performed concurrently with the trephination to provide additional access and exposure. By providing two access points for passing endoscopes and instruments, the "above-and-below" approach offers increased versatility in approaching complex frontal sinus lesions. In addition, the transethmoid frontal sinusotomy provides a portal for long-term endoscopic surveillance of the frontal sinus in the outpatient clinic setting [1]. Combined external and endoscopic approaches to the frontal sinus may obviate the need for more aggressive external approaches such as the frontal osteoplastic flap.

Frontal Sinus Obliteration

Osteoplastic flap techniques were initially described in the late nineteenth century in Europe, and were popularized in the USA by Goodale and Montgomery in the 1950s [10, 19]. These approaches have been used to manage a variety of frontal sinus pathology and were considered the gold standard for treatment of frontal sinus pathology for many years [17]. Although endoscopic techniques are now primarily used for frontal sinus pathology, the osteoplastic flap approach does provide excellent exposure to the entirety of the frontal sinus and may be indicated in selected clinical situations; these may include the management of extensive frontal sinus trauma, frontal sinus neoplasms, and cases of inflammatory disease that have failed endoscopic approaches [19].

Exposure can be obtained by using coronal, forehead, or brow incisions. After exposure of the frontal region, the outlines of the frontal sinus are delineated using transillumination, plain x-ray templates, or, most accurately, computerized navigation [14]. The periosteum is incised, and a saw is used to enter the sinus along its outer margins. This allows the flap to be elevated and downfractured while being left attached along the periosteum in the region of the supraorbital rims. For limited pathology, the mucosa can be left intact if a patent outflow tract is established. If obliteration is planned due to more extensive pathology, care must be taken to remove the mucosa in its entirety. A variety of materials have been used for obliteration, but autologous materials tend to be associated with fewer complications than alloplastic ones [16].

Although frontal sinus obliteration has been shown to be an effective procedure in the management of certain frontal sinus pathologies, patients who have undergone obliteration can present with a variety of postoperative problems, both immediate and delayed. These problems include incomplete obliteration, frontal mucocele, infection of the fat, bone flap osteitis, cosmetic deformity, chronic pain, anesthesia, or paresthesias [8, 12, 22]. Most patients have temporary paresthesias and numbness after surgery, but the likelihood of persistent supraorbital and fore-head numbness has been reported to range from 8% to 35% [8, 22]. The rate of mucocele formation and cosmetic deformity was found to be approximately 10% in a series of 59 patients undergoing obliteration [22]. The time course of mucocele formation was found to be highly variable, ranging from 11 to 130 months after surgery [22]. Mucoceles occurring after frontal sinus obliteration can selectively be managed through conservative endoscopic techniques, avoiding the need for revision obliteration [9, 24].

An additional disadvantage of frontal sinus obliteration is that endoscopic and radiographic evaluation is difficult in patients presenting with recurrent symptoms after obliteration. CT and MRI can provide helpful information, but are often inconclusive in a patient who had undergone previous obliteration. For these reasons, it is best to reserve obliteration procedures for patients that are not able to be managed using less invasive techniques.

Tips to Avoid Complications

- Before embarking on frontal sinus surgery, perform a detailed review of the anatomy of the frontal sinus and frontal recess using the preoperative CT scans.
- When using endoscopic techniques, take extra effort and care to preserve mucosa in the frontal recess.
- Ensure adequate postoperative care, intervening with office debridement and manipulation when necessary, in order to ensure a patent frontal sinus outflow tract as the healing process proceeds.

Take-Home Pearls

- Frontal sinus surgery remains challenging despite recent advances.
- The vast majority of patients with frontal sinus disease can be effectively managed using minimally invasive surgical techniques.
- Due to the greater morbidity of external procedures, it is best to reserve these procedures for patients who cannot be managed effectively using endoscopic techniques.
- Newer technologies such as computerized navigation can be helpful aids for surgeons performing frontal sinus surgery. However, the use of such technology does not negate the need for adequate anatomic knowledge, surgical skill, and surgeon experience.

References

1. Batra PS, Citardi MJ, Lanza DC (2005) Combined endoscopic trephination and endoscopic frontal sinusotomy for management of complex frontal sinus pathology. Am J Rhinol 19:435–441

2. Becker SS, Bomeli SR, Gross CW, Han JK (2006) Limits of endoscopic visualization and instrumentation in the frontal sinus. Otolaryngol Head Neck Surg 135:917–921

3. Bolger WE (2001) Anatomy of the paranasal sinuses. In: Kennedy DW, Bolger WE, Zinreich SJ (eds) Diseases of the sinuses. Decker Hamilton, Ontario

4. DelGaudio JM, Hudgins PA, Venkatraman G, Beningfield A (2005) Multiplanar computed tomographic analysis of frontal recess cells: effect on frontal isthmus size and frontal sinusitis. Arch Otolaryngol Head Neck Surg 131:230–235

5. Dubin MG, Kuhn FA (2005) Endoscopic modified Lothrop (Draf III) with frontal sinus punches. Laryngoscope 115:1702–1703

6. Friedman M, Bliznikas D, Vidyasagar R, Joseph NJ, Landsberg R (2006) Long-term results after endoscopic sinus surgery involving frontal recess dissection. Laryngoscope 116:573–579

7. Germiller JA, Monin DL, Sparano AM, Tom LW (2006) Intracranial complications of sinusitis in children and adolescents and their outcomes. Arch Otolaryngol Head Neck Surg 132:969–976

8. Hardy JM, Montgomery WW (1976) Osteoplastic frontal sinusotomy: an analysis of 250 operations. Ann Otol Rhinol Laryngol 85:523–532

9. Hwang PH, Han JK, Bilstrom EJ, Kingdom TT, Fong KJ (2005) Surgical revision of the failed obliterated frontal sinus. Am J Rhinol 19:425–429

10. Jacobs JB (1997) 100 years of frontal sinus surgery. Laryngoscope 107:1–36

11. Landsberg R, Friedman M (2001) A computer-assisted anatomical study of the nasofrontal region. Laryngoscope 111:2125–2130

12. Lawson W, Reino AJ (1996) Management of embossment following the frontal osteoplastic operation. Laryngoscope 106:1259–1265

13. Lee WT, Kuhn FA, Citardi MJ (2004) 3D computed tomographic analysis of frontal recess anatomy in patients without frontal sinusitis. Otolaryngol Head Neck Surg 131:164–173

14. Melroy CT, Dubin MG, Hardy SM, Senior BA (2006) Analysis of methods to assess frontal sinus extent in osteoplastic flap surgery: transillumination versus 6-ft Caldwell versus image guidance. Am J Rhinol 20:77–83

15. Palmer JN, Kennedy DW (2005) Revision endoscopic sinus surgery. In: Cummings CW (ed) Otolaryngology head and neck surgery. Elsevier Mosby, Philadelphia

16. Petruzzelli GJ, Stankiewicz JA (2002) Frontal sinus obliteration with hydroxyapatite cement. Laryngoscope 112:32–36

17. Salamone FN, Seiden AM (2004) Modern techniques in osteoplastic flap surgery of the frontal sinus. Oper Tech Otolaryngol Head Neck Surg 15:61–66

18. Samaha M, Cosenza MJ, Metson R (2003) Endoscopic frontal sinus drillout in 100 patients. Arch Otolaryngol Head Neck Surg 129:854–858

19. Sillers MJ (2005) Frontal sinus obliteration: an operation for the archives or modern armamentarium. Arch Otolaryngol Head Neck Surg 131:529–531

20. Turgut S, Ercan I, Sayin I, Basak M (2005) The relationship between frontal sinusitis and localization of the frontal sinus outflow tract: a computer-assisted anatomical and clinical study. Arch Otolaryngol Head Neck Surg 131:518–522

21. Weber R, Draf W, Kratzsch B, Hosemann W, Schaefer SD (2001) Modern concepts of frontal sinus surgery. Laryngoscope 111:137–146

22. Weber R, Draf W, Keerl R, Kahle G, Schinzel S, Thomann S, Lawson W (2000) Osteoplastic frontal sinus surgery with fat obliteration: technique and long-term results using magnetic resonance imaging in 82 operations. Laryngoscope 110:1037–1044

23. Wormald PJ (2003) Salvage frontal sinus surgery: the endoscopic modified Lothrop procedure. Laryngoscope 113:276–283

24. Wormald PJ, Ananda A, Nair S (2003) Modified endoscopic Lothrop as a salvage for the failed osteoplastic flap with obliteration. Laryngoscope 113:1988–1992

25. Zacharek MA, Fong KJ, Hwang PH (2006) Image-guided frontal trephination: a minimally invasive approach for hard-to-reach frontal sinus disease. Otolaryngol Head Neck Surg 135:518–522

26

Chapter 27

The Lothrop and Extended Lothrop Procedures

27

Abtin Tabaee, Seth Brown, and Vijay K. Anand

Core Messages

- Advanced endoscopic frontal sinus surgery, including the endoscopic modified Lothrop procedure (EMLP), requires a thorough understanding of the anatomy of the frontal recess and its variations.
- A stepwise algorithm allows for a graded approach for refractory disease of the frontal sinus.
- The EMLP, although technically challenging, is associated with a high rate of efficacy and may help avoid the need for frontal sinus obliteration.
- A maximal recess opening and meticulous postoperative care following the EMLP are required to avoid frontal sinus stenosis.
- Image guidance is a useful adjunct to frontal sinus surgery.

Contents

Introduction

The management of chronic frontal sinusitis remains one of the most challenging aspects of rhinology. Although the majority of patients may be effectively treated with medical therapy or functional endoscopic sinus surgery, a subgroup with refractory stenosis of the frontal recess requires advanced surgical techniques. The variability in pneumatization patterns, proximity of the surgical dissection to the intracranial and orbital cavities, frequent presence of hyperostosis, and propensity for re-stenosis in these patients increase the challenges of surgery. A variety of surgical approaches have been described for management of frontal sinus pathology with the general distinctions of external versus endoscopic and functional versus obliterative. Although frontal sinus obliteration through an osteoplastic approach has traditionally represented the "gold standard" for refractory frontal sinus disease requiring surgery, modern improvements in endoscopic instrumentation and visualization have spurred an interest in advanced endoscopic approaches. The goals of this chapter are to present an algorithm, surgical technique, strategies for complication avoidance, and outcomes associated with surgical management of chronic frontal sinusitis with an emphasis on the endoscopic modified Lothrop procedure (EMLP).

Anatomy of the Frontal Recess

The frontal sinus outflow tract has an hour glass configuration with the potential for significant variability. The ostium represents the narrowest point of the outflow tract. The frontal recess is below this area and is bordered by the middle turbinate medially, lamina papyracea laterally, agger nasi anteriorly, and the bulla ethmoidalis posteriorly. Significant variations may exist in the outflow tract including the presence of a pneumatized ager nasi cell, suprabullar ethmoid cell, and accessory frontal cells [18, 22, 30]. The relation of the recess to the attachment of the uncinate process is also variable. In patients where the uncinate process attaches either to the lamina papyracea or the anterior skull base, the natural pathway of the frontal recess is lateral to the uncinate attachment in the area of the ethmoid infundibulum. Conversely, when the uncinate process attaches to the middle turbinate, the presence of a suprabullar recess is expected with the opening of the frontal recess localized medially to the uncinate process [21, 29]. A thorough understanding of this anatomy and its variations is a critical prerequisite to performing advanced surgical procedures.

Algorithm for Frontal Sinus Surgery

The indications for frontal sinus surgery are based on the patient's clinical history, endoscopy, and CT scan findings. The overall goal of frontal sinus surgery is to either restore the normal sinus physiology or obliterate the sinus. Secondary goals include minimization of morbidity and cosmetic deformity. A graduated approach from least to most invasive is thus advocated for patients with frontal sinusitis. In patients without evidence of frontal sinus disease on preoperative evaluation, the frontal sinus outflow tract should not be explored at the time of surgery. Avoidance of tissue manipulation in this area will minimize the risk of iatrogenic frontal recess stenosis. Additionally, patency of the middle meatus should be optimized. The authors advocate preservation of the middle turbinate in most cases as the stump of an amputated middle turbinate may lateralize and obstruct the frontal recess. Additionally, postoperative debridement and endoscopic management of synechia in the middle meatus may promote postoperative patency.

In patient's with clinical symptoms and radiographic evidence of frontal sinusitis undergoing primary surgery, the frontal recess is explored endoscopically and enlarged. Angled endoscopes, image guidance technology, and frontal sinus instruments (probes, curettes, cutting forceps) are utilized during the dissection. Identification of the natural recess may be challenging given the variability in this area. Following an ethmoidectomy including a complete uncinectomy and opening a pneumatized agger nasi cell, the bony overhang of anterior eth-

moid cells overlying the frontal recess is dissected with either a curved probe or curette ("uncapping the egg") [17]. In patients with frontal sinus disease and a narrow recess, the identified ostium is sequentially enlarged atraumatically to minimize circumferential mucosal and bony scarring.

In patients with recurrent frontal sinusitis following surgery, endoscopic and radiographic examination is critical in determining the nature of the failure. In the majority of patients, a limited frontal sinus exploration addressing the same issues as in primary surgery may be adequate, including maximal opening of the uncinate process, agger nasi cell, and superior ethmoid cells. The role of balloon sinuplasty for this indication is currently unclear as long-term studies are pending [4]. In patients with stenosis of the frontal recess secondary to lateralization of an amputated middle turbinate, the "frontal sinus rescue" procedure is indicated. This involves removal of the middle turbinate bony stump and the lateral aspect of the mucosa followed by draping of the medial aspect of the mucosa over the ethmoid roof [9, 19].

The indications for extended frontal sinus surgery include persistent clinical and radiographic evidence of complete frontal recess stenosis following primary or revision endoscopic frontal sinus surgery (Fig. 27.1). Additional indications include benign neoplastic lesions such as inverted papilloma and osteoma. Finally, in patients with a prior history of frontal sinus obliteration and recurrent symptoms, an obliterated cavity may be reversed with an endoscopic procedure [37]. The technical challenges of surgery in this area require a facile expertise in advanced endoscopic frontal surgery techniques. Multiple names are ascribed to these procedures including the frontal recess drill-out, EMLP, and Draf II, III [10, 12, 16, 20]. The original description by H.A. Lothrop in 1914 involved the enlargement of the frontal recess in continuity with removal of the superior nasal septum and floor and intersinus septum of the frontal sinus through an external frontal-ethmoidectomy approach. In the modern era,

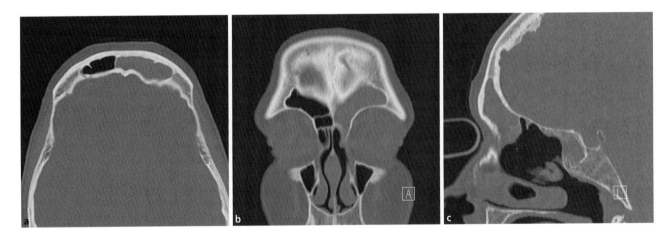

Fig. 27.1a–c Axial (a), coronal (b), and sagittal (c) CT images of a 57-year-old woman with frontal sinusitis following endoscopic sinus surgery and failed frontal sinus rescue procedure for a lateralized middle turbinate. The anterior-posterior distance of the frontal recess is favorable for the endoscopic modified Lothrop procedure

Table 27.1 The Draf classification of surgery for the frontal recess

Name	Surgical goals
Draf type I	Patency of the middle meatus; ethmoidectomy with specific attention to uncinate process and anterior ethmoid cells
Draf type IIA	Removal of the ethmoid cells obstructing the frontal recess from the lamina papyracea to the middle turbinate ("uncapping the egg")
Draf type IIB	Unilateral resection of the entire floor of the frontal sinus between the lamina papyracea and the perpendicular plate of the ethmoid (nasal septum)
Draf type III (endoscopic modified Lothrop)	Resection of the floor of the frontal sinus bilaterally, intersinus septum of the frontal sinus, and adjacent superior nasal septum

W. Draf provided a nomenclature for progressively more invasive approaches to the frontal recess (Table 27.1). Although his description incorporated the use of a microscope, the overall goals of the various procedures are applicable to endoscopic techniques. The EMLP is described in detail in this chapter.

Frontal sinus obliteration through an osteoplastic flap (OPF) approach has been considered the "gold standard" in the management of refractory frontal sinusitis over the past century. A bicoronal or forehead incision is used to expose the anterior table and an OPF is used enter the frontal sinus and recess [16]. Meticulous attention to removal of the sinus mucosa and drilling of the sinus contours with a diamond burr minimizes the risk of delayed mucocele formation. The recess is plugged and the frontal sinus is filled with autologous fat. The osteoplastic bone graft is then replaced. The largest series to date was published in 1976 by Hardy and Montgomery. In a review of 250 patients, they reported no symptoms at follow up (range 3–19 years) in 93% of patients and a complication rate of 18% [17]. Several modern series have similarly reported a greater than 90% success rate following OPF surgery [11, 32, 33]. However, several limitations are identified with the procedure including intraoperative CSF leak, cosmetic deformity, frontal neuralgia, trigeminal hypoesthesia, donor site infections, and long-term potential for recurrent disease including mucocele formation. Additionally, a major limitation of this procedure compared to endonasal procedures is the challenges in following these patients postoperatively. The inability to distinguish postoperative changes from recurrent disease endoscopically or radiographically limits postoperative surveillance of these patients. The collective interest in the EMLP is partly based on these shortcomings. The endonasal approach involved in the EMLP obviates the cosmetic issues associated with the OPF. Additionally, the ability to endoscopically and radiographically survey the postoperative field following EMLP allows for an improved understanding of the patient's symptoms and treatment requirements.

Endoscopic Modified Lothrop Procedure

Preoperative Evaluation

Evaluation of a patient for revision sinus procedures including the EMLP includes a thorough review of the patient's clinical, treatment, and operative history. A variety of underlying diagnoses may result in frontal sinus pathology amenable to EMLP including chronic inflammatory sinusitis with or without polyposis, allergic fungal sinusitis, mucocele, benign neoplasms (inverted papilloma, osteoma), and trauma. Additionally, patients with failed frontal sinus obliteration as evidenced by persistent symptoms or radiographic findings (mucocele) are candidates for the EMLP. An assessment of the patient's symptom complex, response to medical therapy, and comorbidities is performed. A dilemma exists in patients with headaches as the only symptom and radiographic findings suggestive of chronic sinusitis. Primary headache syndromes including migraine should be considered in the differential diagnosis of these patients.

Endoscopic examination of the sinonasal cavity and frontal recess outflow tract is performed with both straight and angled endoscopes. Critical areas of consideration in patients being evaluated for revision surgery include the presence of a residual uncinate process, synechia formation in the middle meatus, identification of inflammatory changes (mucosal edema, polyps) in the expected location of the frontal recess, and the presence and location of the middle turbinate (i. e., lateralized, amputated). Evaluation of the patient's CT scan prior to the first procedure may provide insight into the presurgical level of disease and anatomy. However, the most recent CT scan provides critical radiographic information including the identification of frontal sinus pathology, anatomy of the frontal recess and surrounding structures, presence of hyperostosis, and routine evaluation of the other sinonasal areas (Fig. 27.2). Specifically, the anteroposterior dimension of the frontal recess is evaluated on the sagittal images. Patients with a small anterior-posterior distance of the frontal recess (less than 1 cm) may not be appropriate candidates for the EMLP given the greater likelihood

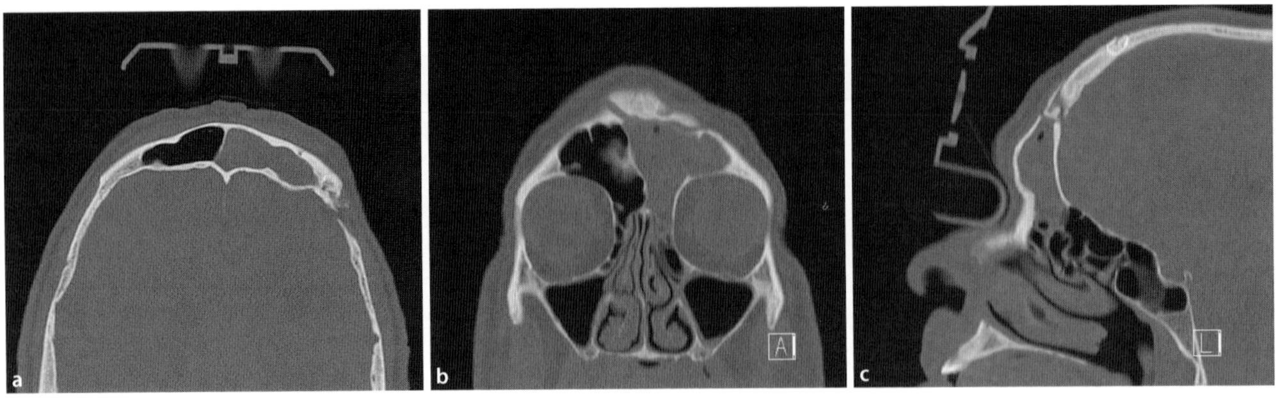

Fig. 27.2a–c Axial (**a**), coronal (**b**), and sagittal (**c**) CT images of a 71-year-old man who developed frontal sinusitis following a craniotomy approach for an orbital apex tumor. A unilateral frontal sinus drill-out procedure was used to successfully restore physiologic frontal sinus outflow

of CSF leak and postoperative stenosis. These issues may also occur more frequently in patients with significant hyperostosis, especially at the area of the frontal sinus "beak".

Surgical Technique

The goal of the EMLP is the creation of a large outflow tract by enlarging the natural recess and removing surrounding bony partitions including the floor of the frontal sinus, superior aspect of the nasal septum, and intersinus septum of the frontal sinus. This may be performed bilaterally (Draf III, EMLP) or unilaterally (Draf IIA, IIB) if the disease process is limited to one side and an adequate opening can be created. The surgical technique has been described previously [10, 12, 16]. The procedure is performed under general anesthesia with the use of image guidance [1]. Maintenance of a low blood pressure and pulse as tolerated decreases the bleeding that would otherwise interfere with visualization during surgery. Neurosurgical pledgets soaked in vasoconstrictive material are placed in the nasal cavity and the region of the middle meatus. The sinonasal cavity is inspected with both straight and angled endoscopes with particular attention to the area of the frontal recess and areas of potential middle meatus obstruction (residual uncinate, synechia, lateralization of the middle turbinate). Local injection into the mucosa and sphenopalatine foramen is performed and allowed to work for a period of 10 min. Following vasoconstriction, a total ethmoidectomy is performed if required. Although these patients typically have had prior sinus surgery, areas of residual ethmoid cells or scar formation may need to be addressed. The performance of a total ethmoidectomy prior to surgery of the frontal recess not only addresses the presence of coexisting disease but also helps delineate critical landmarks including the fovea ethmoidalis, the anterior ethmoid artery, and lamina papyracea.

In patient's undergoing bilateral surgery, surgery is commenced on the easier side. If possible, cannulation of the frontal recess is performed with a curved frontal sinus probe. Frequently, the natural frontal sinus recess may not be identifiable

secondary to scar formation and neo-osteogenesis. The use of image guidance may be useful in these cases to identify the expected area of the recess. Additionally, a small trephination procedure with instillation of colored dye (fluorescein, methylene blue) from above may help aid in identification of the recess endoscopically. The anterior aspect of the bony recess (frontal "beak") is drilled under angled visualization. Care is taken to preserve the posterior mucosa to minimize the risk of circumferential scarring. Additionally, drilling in a posterior to anterior direction helps to avoid intracranial injury and CSF leak. Following identification and enlargement of the frontal recess on one side, the floor of the frontal sinus is entered. This involves a partial septectomy of the perpendicular plate of the ethmoid just anterior to the vertical attachment of the middle turbinate. A segment of the septum measuring approximately 2 × 2 cm is removed early during the procedure. The mucosa and bone are removed in controlled fashion. The frontal sinus floor is entered initially with a probe once the bone has been adequately thinned. The bony floor and intersinus septum are then drilled open. Finally, the contralateral recess is explored in continuity in a similar posterior to anterior manner. A variety of stents are available including Silastic sheeting and non-absorbable packing material.

Postoperative Care

Patients are placed on culture-directed antibiotics and consideration is given to a 3-week course of steroids if there are no medical contraindications. The utility of postoperative stent placement in this area is controversial. Although a stent could theoretically increase the rate of patency, the potential for inciting increased scarring from a foreign body reaction with a negative overall impact on healing has been noted. Additionally, stents may be associated with significant discomfort both while in place and at the time of removal. Finally, the possibility of the presence of bacterial biofilms on stents may act as a nidus for chronic infection [26]. Several papers in the recent literature discuss the use of stents in frontal sinus surgery [3, 13, 34]. The variability in surgeon preference in stent material and duration of stenting supports the need for further study.

Meticulous, long-term postoperative care is required in these patients including routine debridement of crusting, granulation tissue, and scarring. The impact of various adjuncts including topical antibiotics, mitomycin C, and steroids is currently unclear and lacks clear evidence-based support. Our practice is to employ topical medications as we would routinely in postoperative patients with inflammatory sinusitis. Long-term follow up with serial endoscopic examination of the recess is required given the significant potential for complete re-stenosis.

Outcomes of the Endoscopic Modified Lothrop Procedure

Interpretation of the available literature on outcomes following the EMLP is challenging. Direct comparison of surgical results is limited by the variability in surgical indications, underlying disease, surgical technique, and postoperative care strategies. Additionally, long-term follow up describing both patient symptomatology and endoscopic confirmation of patency of the recess is required. Performance of an adequately powered, prospective, randomized study is therefore not feasible. Our understanding of the role of this procedure is based on the collective experience of multiple case series.

In a large, multi-institutional review of 1,286 patients undergoing endonasal frontal sinusotomy, Weber et al. presented a stepwise approach to chronic frontal sinusitis with the extended procedures reserved for patients with persistent disease following initial surgery. They reported a 91.5–95% success rate in 156 patients undergoing the Draf III approach (both endoscopic and microscopic) with a follow up ranging from 12 to 98 months [35]. In a series of 21 patients undergoing EMLP, Casiano and Livingston reported ostial patency of 90% at last follow up (2–24 months) [7]. The authors describe an ideal recess size of greater than 16 mm laterally and 8 mm anterior-posterior at the conclusion of the surgery to minimize the chance for restenosis. Samaha et al. reported the need for additional surgery following a frontal sinus drill-out procedure (Draf type II and III) in 20 of the 100 reported patients [27]. The authors highlighted the importance of long-term follow up especially in patients undergoing unilateral surgery. In a retrospective comparison of outcomes of EMLP versus OPF procedure by Ulualp et al., 2 of the 15 patients required subsequent obliteration within the first 6 months postoperatively [32]. A systematic review performed by Scott et al. in 2003 identified nine studies investigating outcomes following EMLP compared to OPF [28]. The authors noted reporting of higher rates of intraoperative CSF leak (6–11%) but overall a lower incidence of adverse events with the EMLP. Importantly, data on long-term patency rates following EMLP were inadequate to support meaningful conclusions. P.J. Wormald reported his experience with EMLP in 83 consecutive patients [36]. A 93% success rate at initial surgery was noted with a mean follow up of 21.9 months.

Several general conclusions can be made from these and other reported studies. The EMLP has an important and likely evolving role in the surgical management of recalcitrant frontal sinusitis. Postoperative patency is likely dependent on multiple factors including the size of the surgically created recess. However, long-term follow up is critical in these patients given the potential for re-stenosis requiring additional surgery.

Image Guidance

The use of a CT-based image guidance system is indicated in the entire spectrum of surgical procedures of the frontal sinus. The associated anatomic variations, proximity of neurovascular structures, angled nature of the dissection, and frequent anatomic distortion from prior procedures support the use of image guidance. The triplanar radiographic display provides critical information throughout the procedure including surgical planning and intraoperative identification of the frontal recess, lamina papyracea, and anterior cranial fossa [2, 14, 23–25, 29]. Multiple angled instruments including suction tips and drills have been adapted for image-guided frontal sinus surgery. Application of image guidance to the EMLP is useful in multiple aspects of the procedure. The sagittal images allow for identification of the area of the frontal recess, frontal beak, and surrounding structures. Image guidance can also be used during open frontal sinus surgery, including the OPF, to delineate the osteotomy sites and identify the surrounding intracranial and orbital compartments [6, 29].

The impact of image guidance on frontal sinus surgery remains incompletely described. Issues in study design such as difficulty obtaining adequate power, ethical issues in randomization, and patient/surgical variability preclude the performance of an appropriate study investigating the impact of image guidance on frontal sinus surgery. However, the existing evidence seems to support its use as an adjunct to the procedure. In a physician survey of 34 physicians, Metson et al. noted increased confidence with the use of image guidance [25]. Our study group noted no major complications in a cohort of 120 patients undergoing image-guided sinus surgery over a 5-year period. The indications in this cohort included revision surgery and frontal sinus surgery [31]. A lower incidence of complications was noted by Sindwani et al. during image-guided versus non-image-guided osteoplastic approaches to the frontal sinus [29]. Finally, Chiu and Vaughan noted a high rate of patency of the frontal recess (86.6%) following revision endoscopic frontal sinus surgery with image guidance [8].

Despite its utility, several issues are associated with the use of image guidance in frontal sinus surgery. The additional information provided by image guidance is used as an adjunct and not a replacement for surgical technique, experience, or intraoperative decision making. Although accuracy rates within 2 mm have been repeatedly described, this may represent a critical distance in surgery of this area. The accuracy may additionally degrade during the course of a case and may therefore provide misleading information. In these situations, surgical judgment is required to interpret the discrepancy between the endoscopic and image guidance information. Finally, data sets based on preoperative imaging alone do not reflect intraoperative changes. Alternative solutions for this issue include intraoperative fluoroscopy and real-time CT scanning [5, 21].

Tips to Avoid Complications

- EMLP is technically complex and requires significant experience in advanced endoscopic sinus procedures.
- A thorough understanding of the patient's disease process and anatomy is required.
- The surrounding anterior ethmoid sinus cells, agger nasi, and uncinate process should be fully dissected prior to the frontal recess portion of the surgery.
- Following identification of the natural recess, the surgical dissection proceeds in a posterior to anterior orientation to avoid entry into the intracranial cavity and the circumferential scarring.
- Long-term patency of the recess requires a large opening at the time of surgery and meticulous postoperative care.

Take-Home Pearls

- Surgery of the frontal recess is challenging and requires a thorough understanding of the patient's anatomy and underlying disease process.
- A stepwise algorithm is useful in frontal sinus surgery.
- The role of the EMLP is evolving and its use may help avoid the issues associated with the OPF procedure.
- Image guidance is a useful adjunct in frontal sinus surgery.

References

1. Anand VK, Kacker A (2000) Value of radiologic imaging and computer-assisted surgery in surgical decisions of the anterior skull base. Rhinology 38:17–22
2. Annon JP, Lipman SP, Oppenheim F, et al.(1994) Computer-assisted endoscopic sinus surgery. Laryngoscope 104:901–905
3. Benoit CM, Duncavage JA (2001) Combined external and endoscopic frontal sinusotomy with stent placement: a retrospective review. Laryngoscope 111:1246–1249
4. Bolger WE, Brown CL, Church CA, et al.(2007) Safety and outcomes of balloon catheter sinusotomy: a multicenter 24-week analysis in 115 patients. Otolaryngol Head Neck Surg 137:10–20
5. Brown SM, Sadoughi B, Cuellar H, et al.(2007) Feasibility of near real-time image-guided sinus surgery using intraoperative fluoroscopic computed axial tomography. Otolaryngol Head Neck Surg 136:268–273
6. Carrau RL, Snyderman CH, Curtin HB, et al.(1994) Computer-assisted frontal sinusotomy. Otolaryngol Head Neck Surg 111:727–732
7. Casiano RR, Livingston JA (1998) Endoscopic Lothrop procedure: the University of Miami experience. Am J Rhinol 12:335–339
8. Chiu AG, Vaughan WC (2004) Revision endoscopic frontal sinus surgery with surgical navigation. Otolaryngol Head Neck Surg 130:312–318
9. Citardi MJ, Javer AR, Kuhn FA (2001) Revision endoscopic frontal sinusotomy with mucoperiosteal flap advancement: the frontal sinus rescue procedure. Otolaryngol Clin North Am 34:123–132
10. Close LG, Lee NK, Leach JL, et al.(1994) Endoscopic resection of the intranasal frontal sinus floor. Ann Otol Rhinol Laryngol 103:952–958
11. Correa AJ, Duncavage JA, Fortune DS, et al.(1999) Osteoplastic flap for obliteration of the frontal sinus: five years' experience. Otolaryngol Head Neck Surg 121:731–735
12. Draf W (1991) Endonasal micro-endoscopic frontal sinus surgery: the Fulda concept. Oper Tech Otolaryngol Head Neck Surg 2:234–240
13. Freeman SB, Blom ED (2000) Frontal sinus stents. Laryngoscope 110:1179–1182
14. Fried MP, Kleefield J Gopal H, et al.(1997) Image-guided endoscopic surgery: results of accuracy and performance in a multicenter clinical study using an electromagnetic tracking system. Laryngoscope 107:594–601
15. Goodale RL, Montgomery WW (1958) Experiences with osteoplastic anterior wall approach to frontal sinus. Arch Otolaryngol 68:185–271
16. Gross WE, Gross CW, Becker D, et al.(1995) Modified transnasal endoscopic Lothrop procedure as an alternative to frontal sinus obliteration. Otolaryngol Head Neck Surg 113:427–434
17. Hardy JM, Montgomery WW (1976) Osteoplastic frontal sinusotomy: an analysis of 250 operations. Arch Otol Rhinol Laryngol 85:523–532
18. Kuhn FA, Bolger WE, Tisdahl RG (1991) The agger nasi cell in frontal recess obstruction: an anatomic, radiologic and clinical correlation. Oper Tech Otolaryngol Head Neck Surg 2:226–231
19. Kuhn FA, Javer AR, Nagpal K, et al.(2000) The frontal sinus rescue procedure: early experience and three-year follow-up. Am J Rhinol 14:211–216
20. Lothrop HA (1914) Frontal sinus suppuration. Ann Surg 59:937–957
21. Manarey CR, Anand VK (2006) Radiation dosimetry of the FluoroCAT scan for real-time endoscopic sinus surgery. Otolaryngol Head Neck Surg 135:409–412
22. McLaughlin RB Jr, Rehl RM, Lanza DC (2001) Clinically relevant frontal sinus anatomy and physiology. Otolaryngol Clin North Am 34:1–22
23. Metson R (2003) Image-guided sinus surgery: lessons learned from the first 1000 cases. Otolaryngol Head Neck Surg 128:8–13
24. Metson R, Gliklich RE, Cosenza M (1998) A comparison of image guidance systems for sinus surgery. Laryngoscope 108:1164–1170
25. Metson RB, Cosenza MJ, Cunningham MJ, et al.(2000) Physician experience with an optical image guidance system for sinus surgery. Laryngoscope 110:972–976
26. Perloff JR, Palmer JN (2004) Evidence of bacterial biofilms on frontal recess stents in patients with chronic rhinosinusitis. Am J Rhinol 18:377–380
27. Samaha M, Cosenza MJ, Metson R (2003) Endoscopic frontal sinus drillout in 100 patients. Arch Otolaryngol Head Neck Surg 129:854–858

27

28. Scott NA, Wormald P, Close D, et al.(2003) Endoscopic modified Lothrop procedure for the treatment of chronic frontal sinusitis: a systematic review. Otolaryngol Head Neck Surg 129:427–438

29. Sindwani R, Metson R (2004) Impact of image guidance on complications during osteoplastic frontal sinus surgery. Otolaryngol Head Neck Surg 131:150–155

30. Stammberger HR, Kennedy DW (1995) Paranasal sinuses: anatomic terminology and nomenclature. The Anatomic Terminology Group. Ann Otol Rhinol Laryngol Suppl 167:7–16

31. Tabaee A, Kacker A, Kassenoff TL, et al.(2003) Outcome of computer-assisted sinus surgery: a 5-year study. Am J Rhinol 17:291–297

32. Ulualp SO, Carlson TK, Toohill RJ (2000) Osteoplastic flap versus modified endoscopic Lothrop procedure in patients with frontal sinus disease. Am J Rhinol 14:21–26

33. Weber R, Draf W, Keerl R, et al.(2000) Osteoplastic frontal sinus surgery with fat obliteration: technique and long-term results using magnetic resonance imaging in 82 operations. Laryngoscope 110:1037–1044

34. Weber R, Mai R, Hosemann W, et al.(2000) The success of 6-month stenting in endonasal frontal sinus surgery. Ear Nose Throat J 79:930–932, 934, 937–938 passim

35. Weber R, Draf W, Kratzsch B, et al.(2001) Modern concepts of frontal sinus surgery. Laryngoscope 111:137–146

36. Wormald PJ (2003) Salvage frontal sinus surgery: the endoscopic modified Lothrop procedure. Laryngoscope 113:276–283

37. Wormald PJ, Ananda A, Nair S (2003) Modified endoscopic lothrop as a salvage for the failed osteoplastic flap with obliteration. Laryngoscope 113:1988–1992

Chapter 28

Granulomatous Diseases of the Sinonasal Tract

28

Glenn B. Williams, Raj Sindwani, and Rakesh K. Chandra

Core Messages

- Granulomatous diseases are rare causes of sinonasal inflammatory disease.
- Patients typically present with non-specific nasal airway obstruction with associated rhinorrhea and epistaxis. Physical examination yields a spectrum of findings ranging from normal appearing mucosa to polypoid nodular changes, adhesion formation, and extensive crusting to marked tissue destruction.
- Histopathology demonstrates the presence of granulomas, which represent foci of chronic inflammation that appear as aggregates of epithelioid macrophages surrounded by a collar of lymphocytes and occasional plasma cells.
- Many of these conditions can be very aggressive and timely diagnosis facilitated by a high index of suspicion, nasal endoscopy with biopsy, and serology where appropriate is critical.
- Advances in endoscopic technology and laboratory evaluation have led to a greater understanding and more appropriate disease-specific care.

Contents

Introduction

Granulomatous diseases are rare causes of sinonasal inflammatory disease. As in many areas of medicine, advances in endoscopic technology and laboratory evaluation have led to a greater understanding and more appropriate disease-specific care. Until the advent of immunohistochemistry, flow cytometry, and advanced molecular techniques, this group of diseases was collectively lumped into a "catch all" category of midline destructive diseases. Typically patients may complain of a non-specific nasal airway obstruction with associated rhinorrhea and epistaxis. Physical examination yields a spectrum of findings ranging from normal-appearing mucosa to polypoid nodular changes, adhesion formation, marked tissue destruction, and excessive crusting. Strictly speaking, histopathologic evaluation of "granulomatous disease" must include the presence of granulomas, which represent foci of chronic inflammation that appear as aggregates of epithelioid macrophages surrounded by a collar of lymphocytes and occasional plasma cells. Giant cells are formed by the fusion of the epithelioid cells in the periphery or sometimes in the center of granulomas and may attain diameters of 40–50 µm. Several disease processes, with and without frank granuloma formation, may exhibit clinical presentation that warrants inclusion in the list of diagnostic possibilities. The goal of this chapter is to describe the salient features of the various disease entities that comprise this differential diagnosis.

Inflammatory

Wegener's Granulomatosis

This rare disease of unknown etiology was first actually described by Klinger in 1931 [44]. A more detailed description by Wegener followed in 1936 and 1939 [98]. The disease is characterized by a necrotizing vasculitis of small and medium-sized vessels, granulomatous lesions of the upper and lower respiratory tracts, and typically there is an associated glomerulonephritis [30, 35]. The male-to-female ratio ranges from 1:1 to 2:1, and the mean age of onset is 45 years, although the disease can present at any age [1].

The disease process initially affects upper respiratory tract organs in 72–99% of individuals diagnosed [36, 59, 72]. Nasal involvement may be present at any stage and gives a good clinical indication of the degree of disease activity [32]. Evidence suggests that Wegener's patients with predominantly otolaryngologic involvement may have a better outcome compared to those with more aggressive systemic vasculitis [53]. The majority of patients will present with nasal crusting (56%), nasal obstruction (54%), serosanguinous discharge (50%), and sinus involvement (33%) [51, 69]. Any structure in the sinonasal cavity, mucosa, septum, turbinates, and sinuses proper, can be involved, although the area of the anterior septum supplied by Kiesselbach's plexus is the most common site of active nasal disease. Vasculitic involvement of these vessels leads to diminished blood flow and subsequent necrosis of all or part of the cartilaginous septum. As the degree of cartilage destruction increases so the nasal suprastructure in the form of a "saddle nose" deformity develops [69].

Diagnosis requires demonstration of granulomatosis in the respiratory tract, where palisading granulomas may be observed as vascular or extravascular lesions [57]. It is also helpful to confirm the diagnosis by demonstration of the cytoplasmic pattern of antineutrophil cytoplasmic antibodies (c-ANCA), which are reactive toward proteinase-3 or myeloperoxidase in plasma [85]. Although both sensitivity and specificity of c-ANCA are high in acute disease (91% and 99%, respectively), sensitivity falls significantly when the disease is quiescent (63%), while the specificity remains high (99.5%) [68]. Imaging findings suggestive of Wegener's disease include bony erosion and destruction of the septum and turbinates, erosion of bone in the ethmoid sinuses, neo-osteogenesis of the maxillary, frontal, and sphenoid sinuses, and complete bony obliteration (Fig. 28.1) of the maxillary, frontal, and sphenoid sinuses [101].

The gold standard for treatment is a combination of corticosteroids and cyclophosphamide, and, since the introduction of immunosuppressive therapy, the 2-year mortality rate has declined dramatically from the previous rate of 93% [53]. Even after the disease is medically controlled and the active inflammatory changes stabilize, permanent damage to the ciliated epithelium may lead to chronic infection and crusting. Septal perforation may result in saddle nose deformity. Additionally, epiphora secondary to lacrimal duct damage can be quite challenging to manage. Nasal hygiene for chronic crusting is best managed with frequent saline irrigation and antibiotic ointments topically to soften crusts with endoscopic debridement as necessary. Chronic nasal carriage of *Staphylococcus aureus* has been associated with higher relapse rates of Wegener's granulomatosis. Therefore superinfections should always include coverage for this organism [88].

Septal perforations are best managed symptomatically for at least 1 year after disease remission. Even thereafter, isolated or mildly symptomatic perforations are best managed conservatively because operative repair is prone to failure secondary to chronic crust formation, chronic nasal carriage of *Staphylococcus aureus*, risk of relapse of active Wegener's disease, and fragile cartilage. Patients in long-term remission who have significant cosmetic sequelae can undergo saddle nose deformity repair with cartilage and bone grafts or facial artery based musculomucosal flaps [18]. Selected patients may also require dacryocystorhinostomy [69].

Sarcoidosis

Sarcoidosis is also a disease of unknown etiology, with a range of incidence of 5–65 cases per 100,000 population. There is a female predominance, and the age at presentation ranges from 20 to 40 years [10, 14, 46]. In North America, sarcoidosis is 10–20 times more common in the black population compared to the white population, with an increased incidence in the southeastern USA [14].

Sarcoidosis affects the respiratory tract in 80–90% of cases, and the most common presentation is as an incidental finding

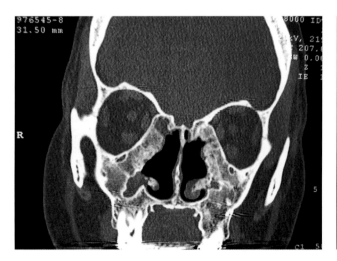

Fig. 28.1 Coronal CT scan revealing marked osteitic changes in a patient with Wegener's granulomatosis who has had multiple endoscopic sinus procedures. Incidentally, she has not undergone Caldwell-Luc, as may be expected from the hypoplastic appearance of her maxillary sinuses

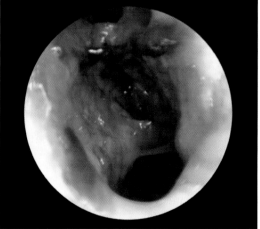

Fig. 28.2 Endoscopic photograph of the left nasal cavity demonstrating edema of the septal and inferior turbinate mucosa with nodular subepithelial deposits characteristic of sarcoidosis. Crusting and adhesions are also present

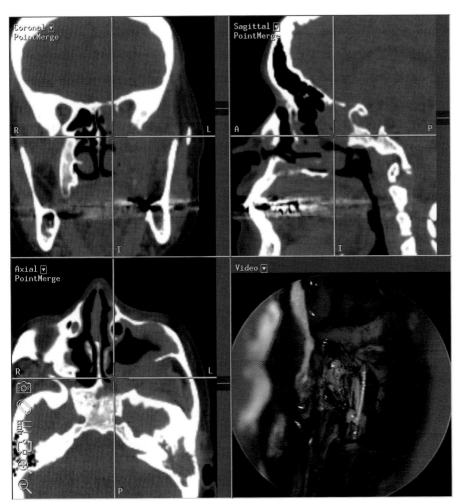

Fig. 28.3 Marked granulomatous inflammation of the skull base in a patient with sarcoidosis. The triplanar CT images reveal erosion of the skull base and orbit, particularly in the coronal plane (*upper left*). The endoscopic image reveals the inflammatory mass. Multiple biopsies revealed non-caseating granulomatous inflammation without evidence of malignancy

of hilar adenopathy on chest x-ray. The reported incidence of head and neck involvement ranges from 3.6% to 9%, with even fewer involving the sinonasal tract [8, 58, 99]. The most common otolaryngologic presentation is posterior triangle cervical adenopathy, but it should be noted that the disease may also involve the larynx (particularly the epiglottis), parotids, eyes (uveitis), and cranial nerves (especially the facial nerve).

Commonly reported signs and symptoms of sinonasal involvement include nasal obstruction, rhinorrhea, nasal crusting, epistaxis, pain, or anosmia [8, 16, 58]. The clinical findings in these patients include erythematous, edematous, friable, hypertrophied mucosa, crusting, studding, plaque-like changes, polyps, or a characteristic submucosal (pale or erythematous) nodularity on the septum or turbinates (Fig. 28.2) [8, 16, 58]. Granulomatous inflammation may also result in sinus obliteration with the inflammatory disease process, and possibly skull base erosion (Fig. 28.3). The perinasal skin may be involved by localized nodular skin lesions or lupus pernio (Fig. 28.4) [8, 37]. This term refers to constellations of red-purplish nodular or plaque-like lesions that occur most often over the nose, cheeks, or ears [37].

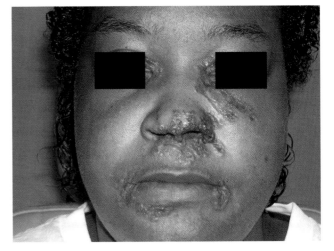

Fig. 28.4 Cutaneous violaceous papules involving the perinasal skin and cheeks (lupus pernio)

The diagnosis of sarcoidosis begins with a thorough history and physical examination. A typical is a history of chronic rhinosinusitis refractory to conventional therapy with radiologic evidence of sinus disease. Additional support for the diagnosis includes discovery of characteristic lesions on sinonasal examination. The diagnosis is strongly suggested by demonstration of non-caseating granuloma (Fig. 28.5) in a biopsy specimen of the nodular deposits. If the diagnosis is suspected, serologic studies should be ordered to measure circulating levels of angiotensin-converting enzyme, which are elevated in 60–80% of patients [8, 46]. Chest radiography should also be done to evaluate hilar adenopathy and pulmonary involvement [8].

The spectrum of treatments described in the literature include watchful waiting of stable or spontaneously regressing lesions, corticosteroids (topical, intralesional, or systemic), surgery, and adjunctive use of medications including hydroxychloroquine, methotrexate, azathioprine, thalidomide, pentoxifylline, or infliximab. The latter medications are often considered to reduce the dose of steroids necessary to control the disease [8].

Krespi et al. developed a staging system and tailored treatment to extent of disease. In this description, stage I patients have limited and reversible disease which manifests as hypertrophic turbinates, mucosal edema, and partial nasal airway obstruction without sinus involvement. These patients are treated with topical nasal saline and topical steroids with good result in 50% of cases. Stage II patients have moderate but reversible disease with findings at presentation that include crusting, epistaxis, limited synechiae, vestibular granulomas, and limited single sinus disease. These patients are treated with a combination of topical saline, topical steroids, and intralesional Kenalog (0.5–1.0 ml), resulting in improvement in 90% of patients. Stage III patients have severe, irreversible disease. At presentation their findings include ulcerations, extensive synechiae, nasal stenosis, cartilage destruction, saddle nose deformity, nasal-cutaneous fistula, and/or extensive sinus involvement. These patients are treated with the above regimen plus 40–60 mg/day of prednisone. Unfortunately, results were poor in this group [46].

The role of endoscopic sinus surgery is limited to diagnosis, lesion biopsy, and relief of nasal obstruction or chronic sinusitis

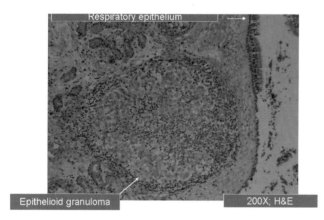

Fig. 28.5 Biopsy specimen demonstrating non-caseating granulomas of sarcoidosis (200×; H&E)

due to anatomic blockage from sarcoid lesions. Surgery does not eradicate disease or prevent recurrence but functions to improve quality of life as an adjunct to medical management [38].

Rheumatoid Arthritis

Rheumatoid arthritis affects all ethnic groups worldwide and can occur at any age. The prevalence increases with age, with peak incidence between decades four and six. Disease prevalence estimates in North America range from 0.3% to 3% with a prevalence 2.5 times greater in women [45].

Necrotizing granulomatous subcutaneous nodules are a common feature in patients with severe, well-established rheumatoid disease and are described in 25% of seropositive patients [103]. They range in size from 0.5 to 3 cm in size and typically are firm and non-tender. Otolaryngologic manifestations of rheumatoid disease include involvement of the larynx, middle ear, nose, cervical spine, and temporomandibular joint. Nasal involvement is typically benign and uncommon. Nasal septal perforation attributed to vasculitic destruction and nasal septal granulomatous nodules have been described in these patients [6, 56].

The American College of Rheumatology revised criteria (1987) are the most widely used scheme for diagnosis, with approximately 90% sensitivity and specificity. Rheumatoid arthritis is defined by the presence of four or more of the following: morning stiffness in and around joints lasting at least 1 h before maximal improvement, soft tissue swelling of three or more joint areas observed by a physician, swelling of the proximal interphalangeal, metacarpophalangeal, or wrist joints, symmetric swelling, rheumatoid nodules, presence of rheumatoid factor, and radiographic erosions and/or periarticular osteopenia in hand and/or wrist joints. The first four must be present for at least 6 weeks to be considered supportive of the diagnosis [2].

Examination of a rheumatoid nodule reveals a smooth, round submucosal nodule. Microscopic examination of biopsy material shows a central area of necrosis containing fibrin and neutrophils, mimicking caseation. Radially oriented histiocytes and fibroblasts surround the central area. Multinucleate giant cells may be present. A marginal zone of vascular connective tissue often infiltrated by lymphocytes surrounds the histiocytic zone [6].

In general the treatment of a rheumatoid nodule is expectant, if asymptomatic. Symptomatic nodules may respond to antirheumatic drugs such as penicillamine, pyridoxine, and hydroxychloroquine, or discontinuing methotrexate therapy [3]. High recurrence rates make excision with primary closure controversial. Local pain, nerve compression, erosion of underlying structures, and infection are indications for surgery [6].

Crohn's Disease

Crohn's disease is a granulomatous inflammatory bowel disease that occurs worldwide. In the USA, the incidence ranges from 3.6 to 8.8/100,000 population. Higher incidence is noted

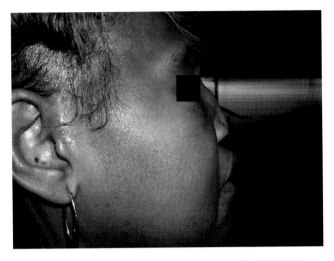

Fig. 28.6 Collapse of the nasal cavity in a patient with Crohn's disease. Other destructive processes such as cocaine abuse, Wegener's granulomatosis, sarcoidosis, or angiocentric T-cell lymphoma may exhibit a similar gross appearance

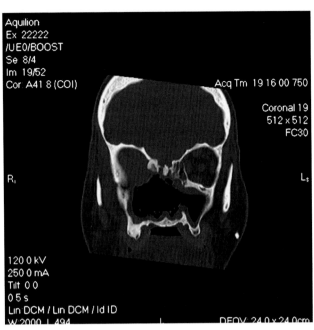

Fig. 28.7 Coronal CT revealing widespread destruction of the midface secondary to cocaine abuse

in the northern latitude [78]. Thirty-six percent of Crohn's patients have extraintestinal involvement [28], and cases of nasal Crohn's disease exist in the literature [19, 43, 65, 93]. Common presenting symptoms include nasal congestion, nasal obstruction, and drainage in patients with a positive history of intestinal Crohn's disease [19, 43, 65, 93]. Physical examination findings can mimic sarcoidosis and may include edematous nasal mucosa with subepithelial deposits, crusting, polypoid pansinusitis, atrophic rhinitis, and areas of granulation [19, 43, 65, 93]. In the long term, saddle nose deformity may be observed as well (Fig. 28.6). The diagnosis is established by performing biopsies of suspicious nasal tissue in a patient with intestinal Crohn's disease with the symptom complex described above. Histopathologic evaluation reveals non-contiguous chronic inflammation and non-caseating granulomas, which may be similar to those observed in sarcoidosis. Reported treatment regimens include topical steroids, systemic steroids, and, for advanced recalcitrant cases, a combination of the above in addition to laser surgery and thiopurine antimetabolite 6-mercaptopurine [93].

Cocaine

Cocaine use is fairly common in the USA. Currently it is estimated that at least 30 million Americans have used cocaine at least once, and 6 million have used it with some regularity (more than once a month) [26]. Chronic intranasal snorting may result in sinonasal destruction secondary to cocaine's intense vasoconstrictive effect and mucosal irritation due to impurities such as talc or powered soap [82, 92].

Early changes include mucosal inflammation followed by ulceration, and septal perforation follows due to ischemic necrosis. Prolonged abuse leads to osteocartilaginous necrosis that can involve any sinonasal structure and may be widespread (Fig. 28.7) [82]. Commonly reported complaints in the history given by the cocaine abuser include nasal airway obstruction, mucopurulent rhinorrhea, epistaxis, crusting, headache, anosmia, nasal regurgitation, dysphonia, and dysphagia [82]. Physical examination may reveal nasal alar collapse, saddle nose deformity, and complete loss of various components of the maxilla including the palatine process and walls of maxillary sinus, with possible oro-nasal fistula. The turbinates, nasal septum, and ethmoid sinus may also exhibit mucosal and bony destruction. Marked crusting is commonly observed [82].

Cocaine abuse must be considered in the differential diagnosis of any destructive sinonasal process. Biopsy specimens are usually non-specific, showing evidence of acute and chronic inflammation, necrosis, and ulceration, and typically no evidence of vasculitis or granuloma [82]. Additionally, macrophages are frequently observed and frank granulomas have been described [27]. For reasons not yet identified, up to 56% of patients have positive immunofluorescence tests for antineutrophilic cytoplasmic antibodies p-ANCA and c-ANCA [82, 92]. Thus the presence of these antibodies does not rule out the diagnosis of cocaine abuse in favor of Wegener's granulomatosis. Arriving at an accurate diagnosis requires a combination of a careful history, serology, biopsy, and drug abuse profile. Treatment is mainly supportive with assistance in cessation of drug use, nasal hygiene, culture-directed antibiotics for any superinfection, and surgical repair after at least 12 months of documented abstinence [82].

Infectious

Tuberculosis

Tuberculosis (TB) is a one of the earliest diseases to affect man and continues to be a significant cause of morbidity and mortality today. The disease is caused by acid- and alcohol-fast bacilli *Mycobacterium tuberculosis* of the family Mycobacteriaceae. According to the CDC, the tuberculosis case rate was 4.8 per 100,000 population during 2005 in the USA. The incidence in foreign-born individuals is eight times that observed in domestic-born patients. From 2001 through 2005, the top five countries of origin of foreign-born persons with tuberculosis were Mexico, the Philippines, Vietnam, India, and China [11].

Tuberculosis involving the head and neck occurs infrequently, and the nasal cavity is an uncommon site of infection. The first report of tuberculosis involving the nose dates back to 1761 when Italian anatomist Giovanni Morgagni first described involvement of the nose, soft palate, and nasopharynx while recording autopsy findings. In 1852, Willigk presented a single case of nasal septal involvement while reviewing 476 tuberculosis cases. In an 1876 address before the Pathological Society of London, Clarke presented the first case of primary tuberculosis of the upper respiratory tract and nose [97]. In a 1997 review, Butt found only 35 cases in the English literature during the preceding 95 years [9]. Cases of nasal tuberculosis are three times more common in women with a median age of 46.5 years [9].

The rarity of nasal involvement is partly explained by the outward-filtering action of the vibrissae and mild bactericidal properties of nasal secretions [9]. There are two forms of tuberculosis classically reported that may involve the nose, lupus vulgaris and granulomatous tuberculosis. Lupus vulgaris describes tuberculous skin infection leading to a destructive lesion that may involve nasal structures. Granulomatous tuberculosis typically involves the anterior nasal septum and produces a range of symptoms [32]. The most common symptom is nasal obstruction followed by discharge. Less commonly reported symptoms are nasal discomfort, mass, epistaxis, crusting, epiphora, postnasal drip, recurrent polyps, ulcerative lesion, or alteration in smell and taste. Atrophic rhinitis is a frequent sequela [9].

Lesions found on nasal examination may be ulcerative, infiltrative, or proliferative. The most common finding is a unilateral bright red exophytic, granular mass or nodular thickening of the mucosa that is soft and bleeds easily when manipulated, and up to one third of cases have bilateral involvement. Nasal polyps and ulcerations are less commonly seen. The cartilaginous septum is the site most commonly involved followed by the inferior turbinate and nasal floor [5].

Definitive diagnosis comes from isolation of *Mycobacterium tuberculosis* from biopsy or surgical specimen. The use of nasal secretions and nasal swabs are low yield. Acid-fast bacilli can be demonstrated on Ziehl-Neelsen staining or auramine-rhodamine staining under fluorescent microscopy of suspicious lesions [63]. Histopathologic demonstration of both caseating and non-caseating granulomas further supports the diagnosis. In any suspected case of nasal tuberculosis, pulmonary tuberculosis should be ruled out. In Butt's review, 59% (17/29) of patients described in the literature had a history of pulmonary

tuberculosis or developed active pulmonary tuberculosis during follow up [9]. Treatment of nasal tuberculosis should follow current guidelines from the American Thoracic Society and Centers for Disease Control and Prevention. These regimens continue to evolve, particularly in the setting of mounting isoniazid resistance [9].

Syphilis

He who knows all of syphilis, knows all of medicine.
(Sir William Osler)

Prior to 1450, syphilis was known as the "great pox", the "Italian Disease", or the "French Disease". Poet-pathologist Fracastorius in 1546 described the symptom complex first recognized in a shepherd by the name of Syphilis [60].

In the USA the rate of both primary and secondary syphilis reached an all time low in 2000 and has since been increasing. The national primary and secondary syphilis rate in 2004 was 2.7 cases per 100,000 population with 7,980 total cases reported. The greatest increase in rates was in men, with the rate of primary and secondary syphilis rising 81% between 2000 and 2004. Congenital syphilis decreased from 10.7 to 8.8/100,000 live births from 2003 to 2004. In 2004, San Francisco had the highest syphilis rate followed by Atlanta, Baltimore, New Orleans, St Louis, Detroit, Washington, Dallas, Jersey City, and Chicago [12].

Syphilis infection falls into two categories acquired and congenital. Acquired syphilis is then further divided into primary, secondary, and tertiary syphilis. Primary syphilis develops after a person has sexual contact with an infected partner. In this scenario there is a one chance in ten of acquiring the disease. Ten to ninety days after inoculation of skin or mucous membrane, a chancre arises at the point of contact at the external genitalia, or the anal or oral mucosa. Chancres are sometimes accompanied by regional lymphadenopathy which is non-tender, non-fluctuant, firm, and may seem disproportionately large in relation to the chancre. Spontaneous resolution of these primary lesions occurs in a few weeks.

The characteristic lesions of secondary syphilis appear asymptomatically, simultaneously with or following the disappearance of the primary lesions. These lesions last 3 weeks to 3 months and include erythematous papulosquamous eruptions, annular lesions or crusted nodules, oral mucous patches, condyloma lata, palmoplantar macules, and moth-eaten alopecia. Twenty-five percent of all untreated patients will undergo relapse of secondary lesions.

Following secondary lesions, the untreated patient will enter a period of latency during which there are no signs or symptoms of disease. One-third of all untreated patients will improve spontaneously, one-third will have latent disease for life, and one-third will develop tertiary syphilis. Of those with tertiary syphilis, one-third will develop cardiovascular syphilis, one-third will develop neurosyphilis, and one-third will have a gummatous form (skin, mucous membrane, bone, or joint).

Untreated or inadequately treated syphilis in pregnant women can profoundly affect fetal outcome. Congenital syphilis occurs due to transplacental infection and may result in perinatal death, prematurity, congenital illness, or illness later in childhood or adulthood. Otolaryngologic manifestations of the infected infant include mucopurulent rhinitis which excoriates the upper lip. Late childhood disease may lead to characteristic stigmata such as rhagades or scars around the mouth or nose, "saddle nose" deformity, a high forehead with frontal bossing secondary to mild hydrocephalus and frontal periostitis, and dental changes consisting of the hutchinsonian incisor (peg-shaped with a central notch) and mulberry molars [21, 22].

Syphilis may have a variety of sinonasal presentations, but primary syphilis within the nasal cavity is rare. The most common presentation includes an erosive, neoplastic-appearing, scabbed, or impetiginous-appearing lesion at the mucocutaneous junction in the nasal vestibule or adjacent septum [60].

Secondary syphilis involving the nose resembles acute rhinitis and often is initially treated as such. Other nasal manifestations which may be noted on examination include scant thick discharge, nasal stenosis, irritation of the anterior nares, mucous patches, or mucosal erythema. The characteristic secondary skin lesions may present as a solitary plaque on the external nose [89] or as a condyloma of the nasolabial fold [23].

In the preantibiotic era, tertiary syphilis of the nose was more common but it is not often seen at the present time. A nasal gumma involving the septum appears as a smooth circumscribed swelling covered by inflamed mucosa. Secondary septal perforation is common with resultant loss of dorsal support leading to a saddle nose deformity. This deformity in syphilis occurs as a result of nasal bone destruction and posterior septal perforation, in contrast to an anterior perforation which is more common in other disease processes [32]. As the disease progresses, ulcerative destruction of the external nose can occur but fortunately is now uncommon.

Definitive diagnostic methods for early syphilis include darkfield examinations and direct fluorescent antibody tests of lesion exudate or tissue. Two types of serologic tests, non-treponemal and treponemal, are available for a presumptive diagnosis. The non-treponemal tests include the Venereal Disease Research Laboratory (VDRL) and rapid plasma reagin (RPR) tests. Treponemal tests include fluorescent treponemal antibody absorbed (FTA-ABS) and *Treponema pallidum* particle agglutination (TP-PA) tests. False-positive non-treponemal test results are sometimes associated with various medical conditions unrelated to syphilis and if positive must be "confirmed" with a treponemal test.

A comprehensive discussion of all syphilis treatment regimens is beyond the scope of this chapter and available elsewhere [100]. Parenterally administered penicillin G is the preferred drug for treatment of all stages of syphilis. Important to note is the Jarisch-Herxheimer reaction that can occur within the first 24 h of treatment, more commonly in patients with early syphilis. It manifests as an acute febrile reaction frequently accompanied by headache, myalgia, and other symptoms. Antipyretics may be used for symptomatic relief. Treatment failure is possible with any regimen so patients must be re-examined clinically and serologically at 6 months and 12 months post-treatment, and more frequently as indicated [100].

Rhinoscleroma

Rhinoscleroma is a chronic granulomatous infectious lesion caused by *Klebsiella rhinoscleromatis*, a gram-negative aerobic coccobacillus, most frequently affecting the respiratory tract mucosa. The disease is endemic to Africa, Central and South America, South Central and Eastern Europe, the Middle East, and China. Sporadic cases have been reported elsewhere, especially in persons who have migrated from the aforementioned areas [42, 81].

The disease was termed "scleroma" or "rhinoscleroma" by Hebra and Kohn in 1870 when the condition was first described and considered a neoplastic growth. The inflammatory nature was later suggested by Gerber and this was followed by Mikulicz's description of foamy cells on biopsy in 1877. Von Frisch isolated the organism, *K. rhinoscleromatis* in 1882. Involvement of both the upper and lower respiratory tracts prompted Belinoff to propose the term scleroma respiratorium in 1932 [81]. Gaafar et al. were able to isolate *K. rhinoscleromatis* from the upper and lower airways after intravenously injecting mice with the organism, demonstrating the affinity for the respiratory tract [25].

The nose is the most commonly affected site of infection [86]. Histologic transition points in the nose serve as sites of predilection for scleroma. The mucocutaneous junction on the floor of the vestibule and points where the epithelium transitions from one type to another are sites commonly affected [81]. Extranasal extension to the hard and soft palate, upper lip, maxillary sinus, pharynx, larynx, trachea, and bronchi can occur [86]. Holinger et al. emphasized the importance of considering lower respiratory tract involvement in patients with chronic destructive granulomatous nasal pathology [31].

Based on clinical and pathologic findings rhinoscleroma can be divided into three stages of disease. The first stage is the catarrhal or atrophic stage in which subepithelial proliferation of the bacilli is followed by the proliferation of capillaries. Neutrophils and histiocytes accumulate in the subepithelium. Biopsy of thickened mucosa, reveals squamous metaplasia and granulation tissue. Clinically in the first stage, the patient has symptoms of a common cold with purulent nasal discharge, headache, variable dyspnea, and fetid odor. Diagnosis is seldom made at this stage, which can last several months. The granulomatous or hypertrophic stage is hallmarked by masses of granulation tissue without ulceration. These masses of tissue are formed by plasma cells, Russell bodies, and Mikulicz cells as demonstrated on histologic examination. Russell bodies are reddish-violet elliptical structures, slightly bigger than plasma cells, and are thought to represent degenerated plasma cells. Mikulicz cells are foamy histiocytes containing *K. rhinoscleromatis*. Clinically, the nasal tip becomes infiltrated, hard, and nodular. As the disease progresses, the nose broadens and becomes firmly fixed to the face. Nasal obstruction progresses during evolution of this stage over months or years. The sclerotic or final stage has the gross and histologic appearance of scar tissue with isolated foci of plasma cells and Mikulicz cells [42, 71].

Biopsy of suspicious lesions is the first step in making the diagnosis after completion of history and physical examination. The maxillary antrum can be involved in up to 60% of cases and is felt to be a possible reservoir for infection [86]. Histopathologic examination reveals a subepithelial dense plasmacytic infiltrate with Russell bodies and Mikulicz histiocytes. These findings are highlighted by Warthin silver, Giemsa, or periodic acid–Schiff (PAS) stains, and these special stains are often required for diagnosis. The phagocytosed bacilli characteristic in Mikulicz histiocytes have an accumulation of antibodies on their surface that are typed based on granular density on electron microscopy. Type A granules are electron-dense granular and fibrillary substances and type B are less electron dense substances, representing bacterial antigen composed of mucopolysaccharides surrounded by antibodies [42, 81].

Treatment includes prompt administration of tetracycline, ciprofloxacin, or rifampin. Surgery and/or laser therapy is reserved for treatment of airway compromise and deformity [42].

Rhinosporidiosis

Rhinosporidiosis (*Rhinosporidium seeberi*) is a chronic granulomatous disease predominately affecting the nose and nasopharynx [40, 75]. In his 1921 doctoral thesis, Argentinean Guillermo Seeber first described the organism isolated from a nasal polyp in an agricultural worker. Ashworth coined the term *Rhinosporidium seeberi* in 1923. The organism was traditionally thought to be fungal but recent molecular studies suggest it to be either a cyanobacterium (bacteria capable of photosynthesis) or a protozoan (parasite that infests fish and amphibians) [40]. On rare occasions it presents as disseminated disease with subcutaneous and pulmonary involvement [66]. Extranasal lesions are believed to be secondary to direct infection or finger-borne autoinoculation [91]. The disease is endemic in India and Sri Lanka where it is commonly found in stagnant waters [66]. Men are more commonly involved in the second to fourth decades of life [70].

Patients commonly present with complaint of nasal obstruction with an associated mass, epistaxis, watery discharge that becomes purulent with secondary infection, or mass projecting from the nose [39, 75]. Nasal examination shows a polypoid, obstructive, fleshy, hemorrhagic (strawberry) mass and hypertrophic mucosa. The characteristic "strawberry" appearance is secondary to increased vascularity punctuated by gray or yellow spots which represent bulging sporangia through the attenuated epithelium [40, 75]. Common points of attachment of the polypoid lesions (in descending order) are the nasal septum, nasal floor, anterior end of the inferior turbinate, middle turbinate, and skin at the junction of the nasal vestibule and upper lip [75].

Diagnosis is confirmed by histopathologic examination of a characteristic polypoid lesion. Microscopic examination shows polypoid structures covered with stratified squamous epithelium and ciliated columnar or transitional epithelium with squamous metaplasia [40, 75]. The stroma contains multiple areas of granulomatous inflammation with numerous large sporangia filled with endospores of *R. seeberi* at different stages of development. Sporangia measure from 120–350 μm and have a cell wall thickness of 5 μm [40, 75]. The organism stains positively for both PAS and Grocotte-Gomori's methenamine silver impregnation technique [39].

Wide local excision of the lesion with electrodessication of the lesion base to reduce recurrence is the optimal form of treatment [40, 66, 75].

Leprosy

Leprosy or Hansen's disease was named after Armauer Hansen of Norway who recognized the bacillus *Mycobacterium leprae* in 1873 [4]. The organism is an acid-fast, obligate intracellular parasite with a generation time of 12.5 days that grows best between 27° to 30°C [33]. The later quality gives it a predilection for the cooler areas of the human body including the nose, ears, upper aerodigestive tract, hands, and feet [33, 50]. It primarily affects the skin, eyes, peripheral nerves, and testes. The most probable route of spread is from nasal secretions of untreated patients as well as from broken skin lesions [49]. The organism is highly infective, but with a low pathogenicity and low virulence [67].

Leprosy is endemic in some developing countries and has recently been reported in the USA, including California, Hawaii, Louisiana, Texas, and New York [55]. Humans are considered the natural reservoir for disease transmission. Leprosy has been found in various animals including wild armadillos in the south-central USA, Texas, and Louisiana. Other animals from which leprosy is naturally acquired include chimpanzees (*Pan troglodytes*), cynomolgus macaque, and sooty mangabey monkey (*Cercocebus torquatus atys*) [94].

Ridley and Jopling described an immunologically based, internationally accepted classification of the spectrum of leprosy [4]. In this scheme, leprosy is classified in a spectrum of five types based on clinical, histopathologic, and immunologic findings. The clinical categories are described as tuberculoid, borderline-tuberculoid, borderline, borderline-lepromatous, and lepromatous. Tuberculoid leprosy represents one end of the spectrum where patients are hyperergic to the organism with nerves primarily affected. Skin lesions and organism presence are less common. Lepromatous leprosy constitutes the other end of the spectrum. In this condition, patients are anergic to the organism and hence organisms are abundant microscopically. The skin is the primarily affected site in the lepromatous state, and nasal mucosa is involved in approximately 95–100% of these patients, typically prior to other manifestations [4, 54].

Nasal symptoms in patients with lepromatous leprosy may include crust formation, nasal obstruction, epistaxis, rhinorrhea, hyposmia, nasal pain, nasal pruritus, headache, sneezing, nasal dryness, cacosmia, and anosmia [4, 54]. Additionally, recent studies using standardized olfactory testing show overall 100% of patients exhibit olfactory dysfunction [62].

The diagnosis of leprosy is made by clinical history and complete physical examination. Suspicious lesions and nasal secretions on nasal examination can be collected for culture and staining. Culture in artificial media is not possible but replication is possible in the armadillo, nude mouse, and to a limited degree in the footpads of mice [54]. Tissue and nasal secretions can be stained with the Ziehl-Neelsen staining procedure and examined for the presence of acid-fast bacilli. There are currently available six effective antileprosy drugs: rifampin, dapsone, clofazimine, minocycline, ofloxacin, and clarithromycin. The first three are most commonly used in a multidrug regimen for 12–24 months [33]. Nasal and systemic symptoms improve rapidly once treatment is initiated, disease progression ceases, and healing begins. Patients typically become non-infectious in 2 weeks, however they should be followed closely until complete resolution occurs [54].

Fungal

Sinonasal fungal infections are divided into two categories, invasive and non-invasive. The two forms of non-invasive are allergic fungal sinusitis and fungal ball. Invasive fungal sinusitis includes the granulomatous "indolent" invasive form, acute fulminant fungal sinusitis, and chronic invasive fungal sinusitis [15]. The present discussion will highlight forms of granulomatous sinonasal fungal disease.

Alternaria is a ubiquitous fungus of the class Deuteromycetes and the family Dematiaceae. It is a common plant pathogen found in the soil and generally regarded as non-pathogenic, however invasion in both immunosuppressed and immunocompetent patients has been reported [84]. Cases described in immunocompetent patients include osteomyelitis involving the premaxilla, hard palate, and anterior nasal septum as well as a sclerosing, destructive, granulomatous process in the ethmoid sinus and nasal cavity with naso-oral fistula formation. Symptoms include intermittent epistaxis, nasal crusting, "moldy" smell, and burning sensation in the palate. Examination of the patient with the sclerosing, destructive granulomatous process may reveal a firm minimally erythematous intranasal mass with deformation of the external nose and naso-oral fistula. Histopathologic examination of involved tissue exhibits non-caseating granuloma with intracellular and extracellular branching filamentous organisms. Treatment includes a combination of surgical debridement and appropriate antifungal therapy [84].

Aspergillus species are associated with two types of granulomatous invasive fungal sinusitis. In both types, the majority of patients are immunocompetent with single sinus involvement and have an overall good prognosis compared to invasive fungal sinusitis in an immunosuppressed host [79]. Nasal examination shows mucosal hypertrophy/hyperplasia and polyposis [79]. Aspergillus flavus is identified in cases of primary paranasal granuloma found in the Sudan [80]. Extensive non-caseating granulomas and fungal tissue invasion are identified on histopathology. Silver staining techniques facilitate recognition of the organism (Fig. 28.8) [80].

The second form is found incidentally on histopathologic examination of surgical specimens in patients with hyperplastic sinus disease, allergic fungal sinusitis, or chronic rhinosinusitis [80]. Fungal hyphae are seen invading superficially through the epithelium into the submucosa where they are well contained by granulomas while bone and vessels are spared [79, 80].

Other fungal organisms that have been associated with granulomatous disease include blastomycosis and histoplasmosis. The former is caused by Blastomyces dermatitidis and is responsible for a spectrum of disease ranging from self-limited primary pulmonary infection, to chronic pulmonary disease, to disseminated infection. Adult males are affected via airborne spread. The disseminated form can involve skin, bones, and the genitourinary tract, and extensive skin lesions can involve the mucous membranes of the nose. Advanced lesion can be mistaken for carcinoma given their proliferative verrucous growth with scarring. Diagnosis is made by identifying single broad-based budding yeast on KOH, PAS, or Gomori methenamine silver staining of specimens. Disseminated histoplasmosis is rare and, when found, it occurs in immunocompromised patients, involving the lung, eye, oral cavity, larynx, nervous system, gastrointestinal tract, and/or sinonasal tract. To date there are four reported cases of sinonasal histoplasmosis in AIDS patients [10, 20, 52]. The disease is caused by inhalation of the dimorphic fungus, Histoplasma capsulatum, found in bat and bird feces worldwide. The sinonasal symptoms described in nasal histoplasmosis are relatively non-specific and histopathologic examination demonstrates macrophages containing endocellular yeast forms.

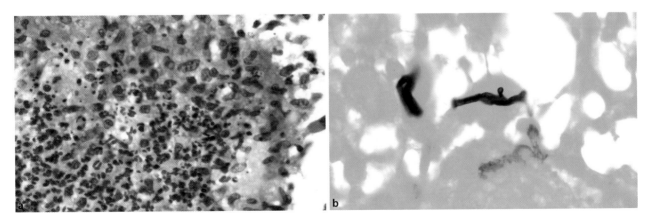

Fig. 28.8 **a** Biopsy specimen revealing non-caseating granulomatous inflammation in a patient with fungal disease (200×; H&E). **b** Gomori's methenamine silver stain demonstrating fungal hyphae in the granuloma (1,000×; oil immersion)

Management of invasive granulomatous fungal disease should include aggressive surgical debridement. Amphotericin B is the drug of choice, and itraconazole or voriconazole can be used in less severe cases. Infectious disease consultation is mandatory.

Nasal-type NK/T-cell Lymphoma

This enigmatic disease has historically been known by many names since the original description by McBride at the 1896 meeting of the Laryngological Society of London. In concert with the evolution of our understanding of the disease process the following terms have been used: malignant granuloma, granuloma gangraenescens, progressive lethal granulomatous ulceration, lethal midline granuloma, Stewart's granuloma, non-healing midline granuloma, midline malignant reticulosis, polymorphic reticulosis, idiopathic midline destructive disease, angiocentric T-cell lymphoma, and now (non-Hodgkin's) nasal-type extranodal NK/T-cell lymphoma. The disease is characterized by a progressive ulceration and destruction of the upper airway with involvement of the nose, the paranasal sinuses, oral cavity, and the soft tissues of the face. In contrast to B-cell lymphoma which predominately involves the sinuses, T-cell and NK/T-cell lymphomas typically originate in the nasal cavity. NK/T-cell lymphomas are known to be highly aggressive with a poorer prognosis than B-cell lymphoma or T-cell lymphoma [41].

Nasal-type NK/T-cell lymphoma, previously angiocentric lymphoma (REAL classification), is one of three major categories of extranodal NK/T-cell tumors recognized in the World Health Organization (WHO) classification [29, 34]. Natural killer (NK)/T-cell lymphoma is characterized by expression of NK cell marker CD56 (poor prognostic significance), absence of surface CD3, presence of cytoplasmic CD3ε and surface CD2 [13]. Other associated characteristics include a T-cell marker germline configuration, presence of azurophilic granules in Giemsa-stained cytologic preparations, and strong association with Epstein-Barr virus (EBV) [13, 34].

The disease is characterized by progressive destruction of midline structures and rapid dissemination occurs if untreated. However, diagnosis is typically made when disease is localized (TNM stage I/II) [13]. Men are predominately affected [13]. Symptoms typically manifest as a non-specific rhinosinusitis with associated nasal obstruction and discharge. Progressive ulceration leading to destruction of sinonasal soft tissue, cartilage, and bone results in a "hollowed out" appearance of the midface. Resultant epistaxis and facial swelling secondary to the disease process serve as signs helpful in diagnosis. Unabated, the destruction continues to surrounding structures; cranial nerves, orbit, and the skull base. Their involvement leads to facial pain and deformity, cranial nerve palsies, diplopia, and proptosis. Extension is not limited to the aforementioned areas and may extend to the oral cavity, the larynx, and the hypopharynx. Cachexia, hemorrhage, meningitis, or secondary infection are typical causes of death [24, 74].

Examination of the nasal cavity may mimic any of the destructive processes mentioned previously in this chapter. The most typical finding on physical examination is a nasal septal perforation (Fig. 28.9). Other possible findings include yellow or gray friable granular lesions on the septum, midline palate, lateral nasal wall, or nasopharynx [74]. Involved structures are marked by extensive necrosis and crusting.

Diagnosis of NK/T-cell lymphomas can be extremely difficult for a variety of reasons. A combination of both clinical and pathologic findings is necessary for diagnosis. Imaging often yields non-specific findings yet gives insight into the extent of destruction (Fig. 28.10) [7, 17, 64, 74, 90]. T-cells and NK cells arise from

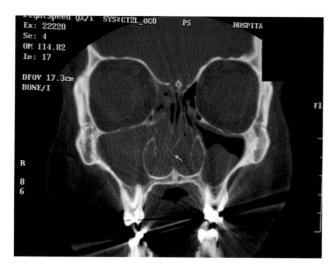

Fig. 28.9 Coronal CT in patient diagnosed with angiocentric T-cell lymphoma may mimic chronic rhinosinusitis. Close inspection reveals discontinuity of the septum (*arrow*) in this patient with no prior history of trauma or surgery

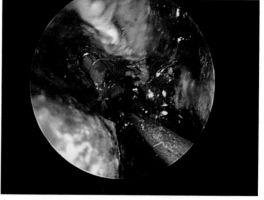

Fig. 28.10 Patient with angiocentric T-cell lymphoma. Note the large septal perforation with ulcerative changes consistent with actively progressive disease. Other destructive conditions such cocaine abuse, sarcoidosis, or Wegener's granulomatosis may take on a similar appearance, but the course is much more fulminant in angiocentric T-cell lymphoma

a common bipotential T/NK precursor; difficulty in separation of the corresponding lineages has led to diagnostic controversy [13, 76, 77]. Extensive necrosis, crusting, and scarcity of malignant cells are further obstacles in obtaining evaluable tissue [29, 83, 96]. The primary role of surgery is de-bridement and obtaining tissue; multiple biopsies are often necessary. Separate tissue samples should be sent in both formalin for light microscopy and immunohistochemistry and fresh for flow cytometry [96]. Ideally the above studies are supplemented by genomic studies seeking the presence of rearrangements of T-cell receptor genes [29]. Histologically, lesions tend to be angiocentric/angiotropic with invasion of blood vessel walls and have a prominent polymorphic inflammatory cell infiltrate (eosinophils, neutrophils, histiocytes, and benign lymphocytes) [34, 48].

Immunohistochemical and flow cytometric diagnosis requires knowledge of tumor biology of these lesions. During T-cell differentiation the T-cell receptor gene undergoes rearrangement such that cytoplasmic CD3ε is lost and surface CD3 emerges. In contrast, during NK cell differentiation neural cell adhesion molecule [N-CAM] CD56 is acquired and cytoplasmic CD3ε is retained [87]. Up to 65% of NK/T-cell lymphomas exhibit an NK cell phenotype including expression of CD2, and cytoplasmic CD3ε and CD56 [13, 47, 74]. These cells also lack T-cell antigens such as CD3, CD4, CD5, and other NK cell markers including CD16 and CD57 [13, 47, 74]. Tissues with high expression of neural cell adhesion molecule (skin, neural tissue, testis, and gastrointestinal tracts) are points of homophilic binding of CD56, giving a possible explanation for the high propensity wide dissemination [13, 47, 74, 83, 95, 96].

Given the rarity of the disease, treatment regimens for nasal NK/T-cell lymphoma are largely derived from retrospective experience. Early stage, localized disease is often treated with single modality radiation therapy. Patients with extensive or disseminated disease warrant more aggressive multimodality therapy, including autologous or allogenic stem cell transplantation [102]. Proposed protocols have included a combination of an anthracycline-based chemotherapy regimen (e. g., CHOP–cyclophosphamide, doxorubicin hydrochloride, vincristine sulfate, and prednisone) with locoregional radiotherapy [61, 74, 96].

The five-year survival for all patients with primary sinonasal lymphoma treated with radiation or combination chemoradiation was 57% in the series published by Kim et al., but, when examined by cell type, T-cell lymphoma was most favorable (80%) followed by B-cell lymphoma (57%). In this series, NK/T-cell lymphoma had the most unfortunate prognosis (37%) [41].

Prognosis is improved in localized disease, with superior results observed in cases treated primarily with radiation versus chemotherapy [73, 102]. These authors hypothesized that NK/T-cell lymphoma may develop resistance to chemotherapy when it is used as a single modality in localized disease.

Conclusion

A multitude of unique biologic processes may present as granulomatous diseases of the sinonasal tract. These disorders must be considered in the context of the full spectrum of inflammatory and destructive lesions that affect the nasal septum, nasal cavity, paranasal sinuses, and midface. Inflammatory, infectious, and neoplastic processes have been implicated in the pathogenesis. Many of these conditions may be rapidly fulminant, particularly if diagnosis is not rendered in a timely fashion, and nasal endoscopy with biopsy is critical in the diagnostic evaluation. It is incumbent upon the otolaryngologist to remain vigilant regarding the head and neck manifestations of systemic disease entities.

References

1. Ahmad I, Lee WC, Nagendran V, et al.(2000) Localised Wegener's granulomatosis in otolaryngology: a review of six cases. ORL J Otorhinolaryngol Relat Spec 62:149–155
2. Arnett FC, Edworthy SM, Bloch DA, et al.(1988) The American Rheumatism Association 1987 revised criteria for the classification of rheumatoid arthritis. Arthritis Rheum 31:315–324
3. Arnold C (1996) The management of rheumatoid nodules. Am J Orthop 25:706–708
4. Barton RP (1976) Clinical manifestation of leprous rhinitis. Ann Otol Rhinol Laryngol 85:74–82
5. Batra K, Chaudhary N, Motwani G, et al.(2002) An unusual case of primary nasal tuberculosis with epistaxis and epilepsy. Ear Nose Throat J 81:842–844
6. Belloso A, Morar P, Estrach C, et al.(2001) Rheumatoid nodule of the nasal septum. J Laryngol Otol 115:853–855
7. Borges A, Fink J, Villablanca P, et al.(2000) Midline destructive lesions of the sinonasal tract: simplified terminology based on histopathologic criteria. AJNR Am J Neuroradiol 21:331–336
8. Braun JJ, Gentine A, Pauli G (2004) Sinonasal sarcoidosis: review and report of fifteen cases. Laryngoscope 114:1960–1963
9. Butt AA (1997) Nasal tuberculosis in the 20th century. Am J Med Sci 313:332–335
10. Butt AA, Carreon J (1997) Histoplasma capsulatum sinusitis. J Clin Microbiol 35:2649–2650
11. CDC (2006) Reported tuberculosis in the United States, 2005. US Department of Health and Human Services, CDC, Atlanta, September 2006
12. CDC (2004) Trends in reportable sexually transmitted diseases in the United States, 2004. National surveillance data for chlamydia, gonorrhea and syphilis. http://www.cdc.gov/std/stats/trends2004 (accessed 12/10/06)
13. Cheung MMC, Chan JKC, Lau WH, et al.(1998) Primary non-Hodgkin's lymphoma of the nose and nasopharynx: clinical features, tumor immunophenotype, and treatment outcome in 113 patients. J Clin Oncol 16:70–77
14. Damrose EJ, Huang RY, Abemayor E (2000) Endoscopic diagnosis of sarcoidosis in a patient presenting with bilateral exophthalmos and pansinusitis. Am J Rhinol 14:241–244
15. deShazo RD, O'Brien M, Chapin K, et al.(1997) A new classification and diagnostic criteria for invasive fungal sinusitis. Arch Otolaryngol Head Neck Surg 123:1181–1188
16. deShazo RD, O'Brien MM, Justice WK, et al.(1999) Diagnostic criteria for sarcoidosis of the sinuses. J Allergy Clin Immunol 103:789–795
17. Drake-Lee AB, Milford CA (1989) A review of the role of radiology in non-healing granulomas of the nose and nasal sinuses. Rhinology 27:231–236

18. Duffy FJ Jr, Rossi RM, Pribaz JJ (1998) Reconstruction of Wegener's nasal deformity using bilateral facial artery musculomucosal flaps. Plast Reconstr Surg 101:1330–1333

19. Ernst A, Preyer S, Plauth M, et al.(1993) Polypoid pansinusitis in an unusual, extra-intestinal manifestation of Crohn's disease. HNO 41:33–36

20. Felix F, Gomes GA, Pinto PC, et al.(2006) Nasal histoplasmosis in the acquired immunodeficiency syndrome. J Laryngol Otol 120:67–69

21. Fiumara NJ (1970) Manifestations of late congenital syphilis. Arch Dermatol 102:78–83

22. Fiumara NJ, Fleming WL, Downing JG, et al.(1952) The incidence of prenatal syphilis at the Boston City Hospital. N Engl J Med 247:48–52

23. Fiumara NJ, Giunta JL, Collins PS (1978) Nasolabial condyloma lata. Report of a case. Sex Transm Dis 5:112–114

24. Friedmann I (1982) McBride and the midfacial granuloma syndrome. J Laryngol Otol 96:1–23

25. Gaafar HA, Bassiouny M, El Mofty M, et al.(2000) Experimental intravenous inoculation of *Klebsiella rhinoscleromatis* bacilli in albino rats: a histopathological and bacteriological study. Acta Otolaryngol 120:279–285

26. Gendeh BS, Ferguson BJ, Johnson JT, et al.(1998) Progressive septal and palatal perforation secondary to intranasal cocaine abuse. Med J Malaysia 53:435–438

27. Gertner E, Hamlar D (2002) Necrotizing granulomatous vasculitis associated with cocaine use. J Rheumatol 29:1795–1797

28. Greenstein AJ, Janowitz HD, Sachar DB (1976) The extra-intestinal complications of Crohn's disease and ulcerative colitis: a study of 700 patients. Medicine (Baltimore) 55:401–412

29. Harris NL, Jaffe ES, Stein H, et al.(1994) A revised European-American classification of lymphoid neoplasms: a proposal from the International Lymphoma Study Group. Blood 84:1361–1392

30. Hoffman GS, Kerr GS, Leavitt RY, et al.(1992) Wegener's granulomatosis: an analysis of 158 patients. Ann Intern Med 116:488–498

31. Holinger PH, Gelman HK, Wolfe CK Jr (1977) Rhinoscleroma of the lower respiratory tract. Laryngoscope 87:1–9

32. Hughes RG, Drake-Lee A (2001) Nasal manifestations of granulomatous disease. Hosp Med 62:417–421

33. Jacobson RR, Krahenbuhl JL (1999) Leprosy. Lancet 353:655–660

34. Jaffe ES, Chan JKC, Su IJ, et al.(1996) Report of the workshop on nasal and related extranodal angiocentric T/natural killer cell lymphomas. Am J Surg Pathol 20:103–111

35. Jennette JC, Falk RJ (1997) Small-vessel vasculitis. N Engl J Med 337:1512–1523

36. Jennings CR, Jones NS, Dugar J, et al.(1998) Wegener's granulomatosis: a review of diagnosis and treatment in 53 subjects. Rhinology 36:188–191

37. Judson MA, Baughman RP, Teirstein AS, et al.(1999) Defining organ involvement in sarcoidosis: the ACCESS proposed instrument. ACCESS Research Group. A Case Control Etiologic Study of Sarcoidosis. Sarcoidosis Vasc Diffuse Lung Dis 16:75–86

38. Kay DJ, Har-El G (2001) The role of endoscopic sinus surgery in chronic sinonasal sarcoidosis. Am J Rhinol 15:249–254

39. Keskin G, Ustundag E, Kacarozkara S, et al.(2004) An erosive mass involving the nasal cavity and maxillary sinus: rhinosporidiosis. Kulak Burun Bogaz Ihtis Derg 13:143–147

40. Khoo JJ, Kumar KS (2003) Rhinosporidiosis presenting as recurrent nasal polyps. Med J Malaysia 58:282–285

41. Kim GE, Koom WS, Yang W-I, et al.(2004) Clinical relevance of the three subtypes of primary sinonasal lymphoma characterized by immunophenotypic analysis. Head Neck 26:584–593

42. Kim NR, Han J, Kwon TY (2003) Nasal rhinoscleroma in a non-endemic area: a case report. J Korean Med Sci 18:455–458

43. Kinnear WJ (1985) Crohn's disease affecting the nasal mucosa. J Otolaryngol 14:399–400

44. Klinger H (1931) Grenzformen der Periarteritis Nodosa. Z Pathol 42:455–480

45. Klippel JH (2001) Rheumatoid Arthritis. In: Primer on the Rheumatic disease, 12th edn. Arthritis Foundation, pp 209–217

46. Krespi YP, Kuriloff DB, Aner M (1995) Sarcoidosis of the sinonasal tract: a new staging system. Otolaryngol Head Neck Surg 112:221–227

47. Kwong YL, Chan ACL, Liang R, et al.(1997) CD56+ NK lymphomas: clinicopathological features and prognosis. Br J Haematol 97:821–829

48. Kwong YL, Chan ACL, Liang RHS (1997) Natural killer cell lymphoma/leukemia: pathology and treatment. Hematol Oncol 15:71–79

49. Lalwani AK, Tami TA, Gelber RH (1992) Lepromatous leprosy: nasal manifestations and treatment with minocycline. Ann Otol Rhinol Laryngol 101:261–264

50. Low WK, Ngo R, Qasim A (2002) Leprosy: otolaryngologist's perspective. Otorhinolaryngology 64:281–283

51. Luqmani RA, Bacon PA, Moots RJ, et al.(1994) Birmingham Vasculitis Activity Score (BVAS) in systemic necrotizing vasculitis. Q J Med 87:671–678

52. Machado AA, Coelho ICB, Roselino AMF, et al.(1991) Histoplasmosis in individuals with acquired immunodeficiency syndrome (AIDS): report of six with cutaneous-mucosal involvement. Mycopathologia 115:13–18

53. Mahr A, Girard, Agher R, Guillevin L (2001) Analysis of factors predictive of survival based on 49 patients with systemic Wegner's granulomatosis and prospective follow-up. Rheumatology 40:492–498

55. Martins ACC, de Carvalho e Castro J, Moreira JS (2005) A ten-year historic study of paranasal cavity endoscopy in patients with leprosy. Rev Bras Otorrinolaringol 71:609–616

55. Mastro TD, Redd SC, Breiman RF (1992) Imported leprosy in the United States, 1978 through 1988: an epidemic without secondary transmission. Am J Public Health 82:1127–1130

56. Mathews JL, Ward JR, Samuelson CO, et al.(1983) Spontaneous nasal septal perforation in patients with rheumatoid arthritis. Clin Rheumatol 2:13–18

57. Matsubara O, Yoshimura N, Doi Y, et al.(1996) Nasal biopsy in the early diagnosis of Wegener's (pathergic) granulomatosis. Significance of palisading granuloma and leukocytoclastic vasculitis. Virchows Arch 428:13–19

58. McCaffrey TV, Mc Donald TJ (1983) Sarcoidosis of the nose and paranasal sinuses. Laryngoscope 19:1281–1284

59. McDonald TJ, DeRemee RA (1993) Head and neck involvement in Wegener's granulomatosis. In: Gross WL (ed) ANCA-associated vasculitides: immunological and clinical aspects. Plenum, New York, pp 309–313

60. McNulty JS, Fassett RL (1981) Syphilis: an otolaryngologic perspective. Laryngoscope 91:899–905

61. Miller TP, Dahlberg S, Cassady JR, et al.(1998) Chemotherapy alone compared with chemotherapy plus radiotherapy for localized intermediate and high-grade non-Hodgkin's lymphoma. New Engl J Med 339:21–26

62. Mishra A, Saito K, Barbash SE, et al.(2006) Olfactory dysfunction in leprosy. Laryngoscope 116:413–416

63. Nayar RC, Kaabi JA, Ghorpade K (2004) Primary nasal tuberculosis: a case report. Ear Nose Throat J 83:188–191

64. Ooi GC, Chim CS, Liang R, et al.(2000) Nasal T-cell/natural killer cell lymphoma: CT and MR imaging features of a new clinicopathologic entity. AJR Am J Roentgenol 174:1141–1145

65. Pochon N, Dulguerov P, Widgren S (1995) Nasal manifestations of Crohn's disease. Otolaryngol Head Neck Surg 113:813–815

66. Rajakannu M, Sri Vengadesh G, Pai D, et al.(2006) Disseminated rhinosporidiosis: an unusual presentation with pulmonary involvement. Int J Dermatol 45:297–298

67. Ramos-e-Silva M, Rebello PF (2001) Leprosy. Recognition and treatment. Am J Clin Dermatol 2:203–211

68. Rao JK, WeinbergerM, Oddone EZ, et al.(1995) The role of anti-neutrophil cytoplasmic antibody (c-ANCA) testing in the diagnosis of Wegener granulomatosis. A literature review and meta-analysis. Ann Int Med 123:925–932

69. Rasmussen N (2001) Management of the ear, nose, and throat manifestations of Wegener granulomatosis: an otorhinolaryngologist's perspective. Curr Opin Rheumatol 13:3–11

70. Ratnakar C, Madhavan M, Sankaran V, et al.(1992) Rhinosporidiosis in Pondicherry. J Trop Med Hyg 95:280–283

71. Razek AA, Elasfour AA (1999) MR appearance of rhinoscleroma. AJNR Am J Neuroradiol 20:575–578

72. Reinhold-Keller E, Beuge N, Latza U, et al.(2000) An interdisciplinary approach to the care of patients with Wegener's granulomatosis: long-term outcome in 155 patients. Arthritis Rheum 43:1021–1032

73. Ribrag V, Ell Hajj M, Janot F, et al.(2001) Early locoregional high-dose radiotherapy is associated with long-term disease control in localized primary angiocentric lymphoma of the nose and nasopharynx. Leukemia 15:1123–1126

74. Rodrigo JP, Suarez C, Rinaldo A, et al.(2006) Idiopathic midline destructive disease: fact or fiction. Oral Oncol 41:340–348

75. Samaddar RR, Sen MK (1990) Rhinosporidiosis in Bankura. Indian J Pathol Microbiol 33:129–136

76. Sanchez MJ, Spits H, Lanier LL, et al.(1993) Human natural killer cell committed thymocytes and their relation to the T cell lineage. J Exp Med 178:1857–1866

77. Sanchez MJ, Muench MO, Roncarolo MG, et al.(1994) Identification of a common T/natural killer cell progenitor in human fetal thymus. J Exp Med 180:569–576

78. Sands BE (2002) Crohn's Disease. In: Feldman M, Friedman LS, Sleisenger MH (eds) Sleisenger & Fordtran's gastrointestinal and liver disease, 7th edn. Saunders, Philadelphia

79. Schubert MS (2001) Fungal rhinosinusitis: diagnosis and therapy. Curr Allergy Asthma Rep 1:268–276

80. Schubert MS (2004) Allergic fungal sinusitis: pathogenesis and management strategies. Drugs 64:363–374

81. Sedano HO, Carlos R, Koutlas IG (1996) Respiratory scleroma: a clinicopathologic and ultrastructural study. Oral Surg Oral Med Oral Pathol Oral Radiol Endod 81:665–671

82. Seyer BA, Grist W, Muller S (2002) Aggressive destructive mid-facial lesion from cocaine abuse. Oral Surg Oral Med Oral Pathol Oral Radiol Endod 94:465–470

83. Sheahan P, Donnelly M, O'Reilly S, et al.(2001) T/NK cell non-Hodgkin's lymphoma of the sinonasal tract. J Laryngol Otol 115:1032–1035

84. Shugar MA, Montgomery WW, Hyslop NE Jr (1981) Alternaria sinusitis. Ann Otol Rhinol Laryngol 90:251–254

85. Slart RH, Jager PL, Poot L, et al.(2003) Clinical value of gallium-67 scintigraphy in assessment of disease activity in Wegener's granulomatosis. Ann Rheum Dis 62:659–662

86. Soni NK (1992) Antroscopy in rhinoscleroma. J Laryngol Otol 106:697–698

87. Spits H, Lanier LL, Phillips JH (1995) Development of human T and natural killer cells. Blood 85:2654–2670

88. Stegeman CA, Tervaert JW, Sluiter WJ, et al.(1994) Association of chronic nasal carriage of Staphylococcus aureus and higher relapse rates in Wegener granulomatosis. Ann Intern Med 120:12–17

89. Sturm HM (1976) Secondary syphilis appearing as a solitary plaque of the nose. Int J Dermatol 15:678–679

90. Teng MMH, Chang CY, Guo WY, et al.(1990) CT evaluation of polymorphic reticulosis. Neuroradiology 31:498–501

91. Thappa DM, Venkatesan S, Sirka CS, et al.(1998) Disseminated cutaneous rhinosporidiosis. J Dermatol 25:527–532

92. Trimarchi M, Nicolai P, Lombardi D, et al.(2003) Sinonasal osteocartilaginous necrosis in cocaine abusers: experience in 25 patients. Am J Rhinol 17:33–43

93. Ulnick KM, Perkins J (2001) Extraintestinal Crohn's disease: case report and review of the literature. Ear Nose Throat J 80:97–100

94. Valverde CR, Canfield D, Tarara R, et al.(1998) Spontaneous leprosy in a wild-caught cynomolgus macaque. Int J Lepr 66:140–148

95. van Gorp J, de Bruin P, Sie-Go D, et al.(1995) Nasal T-cell lymphoma: a clinicopathological and immunophenotypic analysis of 13 cases. Histopathology 27:139–148

96. Vidal RW, Devaney K, Ferlito A, et al.(1999) Sinonasal malignant lymphomas: a distinct clinicopathological category. Ann Otol Rhinol Laryngol 108:411–419

97. Waldman SR, Levine HL, Sebek BA, et al.(1981) Nasal tuberculosis: a forgotten entity. Laryngoscope 91:11–16

98. Wegener F (1939) Über eine eigenartige rhinogene Granulomatose mit besonderer Beteiligung des Arteriensystems und der Nieren. Beitr Pathol Anat 102:36–68

99. Wilson R, Lund V, Sweatman M, et al.(1988) Upper respiratory tract involvement in sarcoidosis and its management. Eur Respir J 1:269–272

100. Workowski KA, Berman SM (2006) Sexually transmitted diseases treatment guidelines 2006. Centers for Disease Control and Prevention. MMWR Morb Mortal Wkly Rep 55(RR-11):1–94

101. Yang C, Talbot JM, Hwang PH (2001) Bony abnormalities of the paranasal sinuses in patients with Wegner's granulomatosis. Am J Rhinol 15:121–125

102. You JY, Chi K-H, Yang M-H, et al.(2004) Radiation therapy versus chemotherapy as initial treatment for localized nasal natural killer (NK)/T-cell lymphoma: a single institute survey in Taiwan. Ann Oncol 15:618–625

103. Ziff M (1990) The rheumatoid nodule. Arthritis Rheum 33:761–767

Chapter 29

Diagnosis, Evaluation and Management of Facial Pain

29

A. Daudia and Nicholas S. Jones

Core Messages

- History taking is the key to accurate diagnosis in patients with facial pain.
- The majority of patients presenting with facial pain as a primary symptom will not have sinusitis, and surgery is very rarely indicated in the treatment of chronic facial pain.
- Sinogenic pain is intermittent and associated with rhinological symptoms.
- Sinus x-rays are not helpful in the diagnosis and management of chronic facial pain and sinusitis. CT scans should not be routinely performed because sinus mucosal thickening is common in asymptomatic patients and management based only on scan findings will result in unnecessary surgery.
- Many patients with chronic facial pain benefit from the appropriate 'neurological' medication.

Contents

Introduction

Patients with facial pain are frequently referred to otorhinolaryngologists. Many have reached the conclusion that the cause of their facial pain lies in their sinuses because most people are aware that their sinuses lie behind the facial bones. The diagnosis has often been reinforced by their primary care physicians or other hospital specialists. However, rhinosinusitis is rarely the cause of facial pain, even in an otorhinolaryngology clinic. An accurate diagnosis, therefore, is essential if inappropriate surgery is to be avoided.

Facial pain has a special emotional significance. This means that symptom interpretation is often influenced by cognitive, affective and motivational factors. For a few patients, facial pain may be the channel by which they express emotional distress, anxiety or the psychological harm associated with disease, trauma or surgery. It may be the means by which they demand attention or obtain secondary gain. The pain, however, is very real to the patient and an empathetic approach is essential. The presence of a marked psychological overlay does not mean that there is no underlying organic problem, but it should make one wary about invasive treatment. If there is a big discrepancy between the patient's affect and the description of the pain, the organic component of the illness may be of relatively minor importance. Pain which remains constant for many months or years, or which extends either across the midline or across defined dermatomes, is less likely to be due to sinusitis. However, pain associated with clear exacerbating or relieving factors, whose onset was clear cut and whose site does not vary between consultations usually has an organic cause.

This chapter aims to assist the reader in the accurate diagnosis of facial pain and the management of this condition.

Taking a History

A careful history is central in establishing a correct diagnosis. It may not be possible to reach a definitive diagnosis at the first visit, and re-taking the history at a subsequent consultation with the patient's diary of their symptoms will often clarify the situation. In making a diagnosis it is helpful to classify facial pain into

29

broad categories, namely rhinological pain, dental pain, vascular pain, neuralgias, pain caused by tumours, midfacial segment pain and atypical facial pain. Although these groups mix both anatomical and pathological criteria, a structured approach to history taking remains a key ingredient to making a diagnosis. Twelve questions form the basis of a mental algorithm that will help draw up a differential diagnosis.

1. *Where is the pain and does it radiate anywhere?*
    Asking the patient to point with one finger to the site of the pain is helpful, not only because it localises the pain, but also because the gesture made often relays information about its nature, and the facial expression indicates its emotional significance to the patient.
2. *Is it deep or superficial?*
    Pain from the skin tends to be sharp and well-defined, while deep pain is dull and poorly localised.
3. *Is the pain continuous or intermittent?*
    The periodicity of symptoms may be a pointer to the diagnosis, e. g. being woken in the early hours by severe facial pain which lasts about 45–120 min suggests cluster headache.
4. *How did the pain begin?*
    An aura preceding unilateral facial pain or headache are typical of classical migraine.
5. *How often does the pain occur?*
    Recurrent bouts of aching of the ear and jaw with sharp twinges is a pattern characteristic of temporomandibular joint dysfunction, whilst monthly premenstrual headaches are typical of migraine.
6. *What is the pattern of the attacks and are they progressing?*
    The relentless progression of a headache, in particular if associated with nausea or effortless vomiting is worrying, and an intracranial lesion should be excluded.
7. *How long is each episode?*
    The stabbing pain of trigeminal neuralgia is short lived with a refractory period.
8. *What precipitates the pain?*
    Trigeminal neuralgia is initiated by a specific trigger point.
9. *What relieves the pain?*
    Tension headaches do not respond to analgesics, whereas patients with migraine often report that lying quietly in a dark room helps.
10. *Are there any associated symptoms?*
    A specific enquiry as to whether nausea accompanies their pain is characteristic, although not diagnostic, of migraine.
11. *What effect does it have on daily life and sleep?*
    Should the patient describe a severe unrelenting pain but have an apparently normal life and pattern of sleep, atypical facial pain should be considered in the differential diagnosis.
12. *What treatment has been tried and with what effect?*
    Tension headache and atypical facial pain fail to respond to analgesics; this in isolation does not clinch the diagnosis but is a useful pointer. Chronic paroxysmal hemicrania specifically responds to indomethacin, and trigeminal neuralgia to carbamazepine.

Rhinological Pain

Sinusitis

The majority of patients who present to an otorhinolaryngology clinic with facial pain and headaches believe they have 'sinus trouble'. However, patients with facial pain secondary to sinusitis, almost invariably have coexisting symptoms of nasal obstruction, hyposmia, and/or a purulent nasal discharge [1] and there are usually endoscopic signs of disease [2].

Acute sinusitis usually follows an acute upper respiratory tract infection and is usually unilateral, severe and associated with pyrexia and unilateral nasal obstruction. In maxillary sinusitis unilateral facial and dental pain are good predictors of true infection confirmed by maxillary sinus aspiration [3]. An increase in the severity of pain on bending forwards has traditionally been thought to be diagnostic of sinusitis but this is non-specific and it can occur in many other types of facial pain. In acute frontal sinusitis the patient is usually pyrexial and has tenderness on the medial side of the orbital floor under the supraorbital ridge where the frontal sinus is thinnest. A normal nasal cavity showing no evidence of middle meatal mucopus or inflammatory changes makes a diagnosis of sinogenic pain most unlikely, particularly if the patient is currently in pain or had pain within the past few days. If the patient is asymptomatic in the clinic it is often useful to review them and repeat the nasendoscopy when they have pain in order to clarify the diagnosis. The key points in the history of sinogenic pain are an exacerbation of pain during an upper respiratory tract infection, an association with rhinological symptoms, worse flying or skiing and a response to medical treatment.

Chronic sinusitis can cause facial pain, particularly during an acute exacerbation, although this diagnosis is often made too readily. Examination of the face is usually normal in patients with chronic sinusitis. Facial swelling is normally due to other pathology such as dental sepsis or more rarely malignancy. Nasendoscopy is mandatory in the diagnosis of sinusitis. A normal nasal cavity showing no evidence of middle meatal mucopus or inflammatory changes makes a diagnosis of sinogenic pain most unlikely, particularly if the patient is currently in pain or had pain within the past few days. Even the presence of inflammatory changes or infection does not indicate with any certainty that the pain is sinogenic and all findings must be considered in conjunction with the history.

Patients who have two or more bacterial sinus infections within 1 year should be investigated for an immune deficiency [4, 5].

The issue of imaging continues to cause controversy. Plain sinus x-rays are used to confirm a diagnosis of acute bacterial sinusitis, however the poor sensitivity and specificity of sinus x-rays make them redundant in the diagnosis of chronic sinusitis [6, 7]. Interpretation of the appearance of the sinuses on computerised tomography (CT) scans must also be treated with caution. Approximately 30% of asymptomatic patients will demonstrate mucosal thickening in one or more sinuses on CT scanning. The presence of this finding is certainly not an indication that pain is sinogenic in origin or that surgery is indicated [8, 9].

Several other clinical observations suggest that a diagnosis of sinusitis causing chronic facial pain should only be made after careful consideration. Chronic rhinosinusitis is common in young children and invariably resolves as the immune system matures. Children very rarely complain of facial pain, even in the presence of florid rhinosinusitis. One must also remember that rhinological symptoms are common, affecting perhaps a fifth of the adult population. These patients suffer from rhinosinusitis due to various conditions including conditions associated with nasal polyps. It is again notable that the vast majority do not complain of significant pain [1]. Headaches are also common in the general population and linking these with unrelated nasal symptoms can lead to an incorrect diagnosis of sinusitis. Vascular pain is frequently associated with autonomic rhinological symptoms such as congestion and rhinorrhoea leading to diagnostic confusion [10].

It is important to stress that surgery should only be considered in the minority of patients where there is good evidence they have sinogenic pain and when medical treatment has failed. It is interesting to note that many patients who undergo inappropriate surgery for non-sinogenic pain experience temporary relief from their symptoms, although the pain normally returns. In some patients surgery does not significantly affect the pain and in a third the pain is made far worse [10, 11]. Patients whose pain is increased by surgery are subsequently particularly difficult to manage with medical treatment.

Pain After Surgery or Trauma

A small minority of patients who have sustained nasal trauma or have undergone surgery continue to experience pain long after the direct effects of the injury or surgery have settled [10, 11]. There is usually little abnormal to find on examination and different theories exist about whether the alteration in the neurological pathway is central or peripheral. These patients often suffer from psychological distress following injury or are dissatisfied with the result of their surgery. This problem seems to be particularly common following cases of assault and on-going litigation may play a part in how quickly the patient's symptoms resolve. Caution is required in the management of such patients, especially if further surgery is being considered.

Dental Pain

Painful Teeth

Usually the diagnosis is clear as the offending tooth is painful to percussion. However, pain originating from the dental pulp may produce poorly localised pain causing misdiagnosis. This pain rarely crosses the midline but can radiate to surrounding structures and in particular the opposite jaw (for example, mandible to maxilla). In contrast, dentinoenamel defects produce a sharp, well-localised pain often caused by decay or a lost or cracked filling. Once the periodontium is involved the pain becomes localised to the area of the affected tooth that throbs and is tender to percussion.

Phantom Tooth Pain

This pain follows a dental extraction although on enquiry there is often a history of some pain that preceded the extraction. A dental extraction has often been performed following pressure from the patient who is convinced they have diseased teeth. Patients may eventually find their way to otorhinolaryngology clinics for the management of 'sinus pain' and unfortunately many subsequently undergo equally inappropriate sinus surgery.

Temporomandibular Joint Dysfunction

The pain of temporomandibular joint (TMJ) dysfunction may be localised to the joint or referred to deep within the ear [12], the periauricular area, the temporoparietal region and along the ramus of the mandible. In the majority of cases the pain is unilateral and whilst chewing often exacerbates the symptoms, clicking is a non-specific sign. Bruxism, poor dental occlusion or poorly fitting dentures may be factors in TMJ dysfunction.

Examination reveals a tender TMJ on direct palpation or lateral jaw movement when the patient is asked to slowly open their jaw from the closed position. Palpation of the lateral pterygoid muscle insertion at the posterior end of the upper buccal sulcus is tender and a sign of TMJ dysfunction. Treatment involves correction of aggravating factors and resting the joint by avoiding yawning and prolonged chewing. Occlusal devices such as bite-raising appliances often help.

Myofascial Pain

This condition is five times more common in postmenopausal women and has a strong association with stress. It has many features in common with TMJ dysfunction. There is a widespread, poorly defined aching in the neck, jaw and ear with tender points in the sternomastoid and trapezoid muscles. The treatment of this condition is controversial but tricyclic antidepressants can play a part in the management.

Vascular Pain

Migraine

Migraine is a common condition affecting approximately 6% of men and 18% of women [13]. It primarily causes severe headache but in a small proportion of patients it can affect the cheek, orbit and forehead. Migraine is a term that is often wrongly used by patients and the diagnosis needs confirmation by precise questioning. The classical variety accounts for 25% of migraine cases and there is often a family history of the condition. In classical migraine an aura precedes the onset of headache and this may include visual disturbances such as fortification, scotomata (blind spots within the field of vision) or visual field defects. The aura may also include unusual tastes and aromas. The headache is usually a throbbing, unilateral pain although it may rarely be

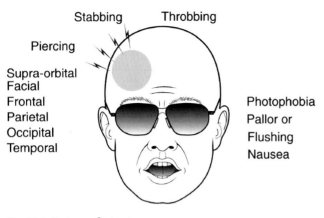

Fig. 29.1 Features of migraine

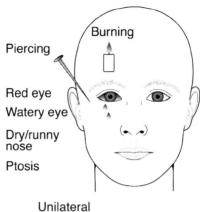

Fig. 29.2 Features of cluster headache

bilateral and constant (Fig. 29.1). Even if the pain is not typically migrainous, patients will normally have nausea, photophobia or phonophobia (sensitivity to sound) [14]. As the name suggests common migraine occurs more frequently than classical migraine accounting for 75% cases. Patients with common migraine have the same throbbing headache and nausea but do not experience the visual aura or other neurological symptoms. Migraine can last up to 72 h [15].

Migraine attacks can be induced by a number of trigger factors including various foods, sleep disturbance and withdrawal of stress ('Saturday morning headaches') and premenstruation. Not infrequently there is an association of migrainous headaches with a woman's menstrual cycle and this finding may point to the aetiology of the pain.

Management of migraine involves avoidance of trigger factors and medical treatment aimed either at the acute episode or prophylactic treatment. Simple treatment in the acute phase includes aspirin and antiemetics. Serotonin agonists such as sumatriptan and rizatriptan are frequently effective in treating acute attacks. Beta-blockers or pizotifen are usually the first-line treatment for prophylaxis provided there are no contraindications to their use. Prophylactic treatment is considered if symptoms occur more than three times a month with a duration of more than 48 h [15, 16]. Referral to a neurologist is recommended for refractory cases. Care must be taken in diagnosing migraine in patients over the age of 50 years as in these patients a central lesion must be excluded.

Cluster Headaches

Cluster headache typically affects men between 20 and 40 years old and typically presents with a very severe unilateral stabbing or burning pain which may be frontal, temporal, ocular, over the cheek or even in the maxillary teeth. Pain is therefore facial and 'headache' is a misnomer. Nausea is absent but frequently there is rhinorrhoea, unilateral nasal obstruction (secondary to vasodilation of the nasal lining), lacrimation and sometimes conjunctival injection, symptoms which can lead to a misdiagnosis of sinusitis (Fig. 29.2). Myosis or facial flushing may be seen. The patient is awakened in the early hours, often walking around the bedroom in distress, with the pain lasting between 30 min and 2 h. Clusters of attacks often continue for several weeks followed by months or years of remission. It may be precipitated by alcohol intake which should be avoided during a cluster period. The treatment is along the same lines as migraine with triptans for acute attacks and pizotifen to prevent recurrent clusters.

Paroxysmal Hemicrania

Paroxysmal hemicrania is an excruciating unilateral pain occurring almost exclusively in women at any time of night or day. It can affect the frontal, ocular, cheek or temporal regions and last 30 min to 3 h. The patient can experience several episodes in 24 h. Nasal congestion, lacrimation and facial flushing can all be a features leading to diagnostic confusion [17, 18]. The first-line treatment is with indomethacin which is usually effective, indeed chronic paroxysmal hemicrania was originally classified on the basis of a response to this drug. More recently the overlap between cluster headaches and chronic paroxysmal hemicrania has been recognised with reports of chronic paroxysmal hemicrania responding to sumatriptan [19, 20].

Temporal Arteritis

Although this condition rarely presents to an otorhinolaryngology clinic, rapid diagnosis is essential to avoid progression of the disease with involvement of the ophthalmic artery and visual loss. It presents with temporal or retro-ocular pain and tenderness of the temporal artery. The majority of patients with temporal arteritis are women aged over 50 years with fever, malaise and severe temporal pain. Examination shows the temporal artery to be thickened and exquisitely tender. Investigation reveals an elevated erythrocyte sedimentation rate (ESR). The diagnosis is confirmed on histological examination of an arterial biopsy that reveals intimal hyperplasia and fragmentation of the internal elastic lamina. Steroids in high doses (60 mg prednisolone daily) should be commenced prior to a diagnostic biopsy if there is a strong clinical suspicion that the condition is present.

Comment on Sluder's Neuralgia and Contact Point Pain

Some workers have hypothesised that rhinological causes other than infection can cause facial pain and these include the presence of contact points and vacuum pain. These theories have been repeatedly quoted in the literature with little critical evaluation.

In 1908 Sluder described 'sphenopalatine neuralgia' as a cause of an ipsilateral, boring, burning facial pain beginning along the lateral side of the nose and in the eye, forehead, orbit, temporal and mastoid regions, constant or paroxysmal, associated with lacrimation, rhinorrhoea, injected conjunctiva and sometimes involving the cheek [21]. Sluder's definition did not describe a single entity but a diverse symptom complex and he never reported a case presenting with a combination of all the features he described. There is no diagnostic test to identify patients with Sluder's description and the criteria used to describe patients in the reported studies often differ from those used by Sluder. Since his description the symptom complex has been categorised as cluster headache [22, 23], hence inclusion in this section, although the name still enters the literature disregarding the efforts of the medical community to rationalise terminology [24]. The term Sluder's syndrome is often used loosely and it is best avoided as his description differs from most clinical entities.

Sluder also described a different type of frontal pain that he attributed to 'vacuum' headaches, which could produce ocular symptoms [25]. These symptoms were not associated with pus or a contact point and the pain was relieved by applying astringents in the area of the middle meatus and in resistant cases he said that removal of the middle turbinate helped, but the pain returned in 2–3 years.

The evidence that a vacuum within a blocked sinus can cause protracted pain is poor. Transient facial pain in patients with other symptoms and signs of rhinosinusitis can occur with pressure changes when flying, diving or skiing but this resolves as the pressure within the sinuses equalises through perfusion with the surrounding vasculature. Silent sinus syndrome that is due to a blocked sinus with resorbtion of its contents to the extent that the orbital floor prolapses into the maxillary sinus causes no pain [26].

Nasal polyposis that is likely to block sinus ostia rarely causes facial pain unless there is coexisting infection with a purulent discharge [1].

The theories that implicate contact points as a cause of facial pain originate from McAuliffe who described stimulating various points within the nasal cavity and paranasal sinuses in five individuals and said that both touch and faradic current caused referred pain to areas of the face [27] that he illustrated in diagrams that have been reproduced in many texts [28]. These findings have been used to support theories which state that mucosal contact points within the nasal cavity can cause facial pain [29] although McAuliffe's studies did not describe contact point induced facial pain. McAuliffe's work has recently been repeated in a controlled study and was found not to produce the referred pain that he described [30]. The prevalence of a contact point has been found to be the same in an asymptomatic population as in a symptomatic population and when they were present in symptomatic patients with unilateral pain, they were present in the contralateral side to the pain in 50% of these patients [31].

Stammberger and Wolf postulated that variations in the anatomy of the nasal cavity result in mucus stasis, infection and ultimately facial pain [32]. They also stated that mucosal contact points might result in the release of the neurotransmitter peptide substance P, a recognised neurotransmitter in nociceptive fibres. Case-controlled studies examining the prevalence of anatomical variations in patients with rhinosinusitis and asymptomatic control groups have shown no significant differences [9, 33]. It seems probable that the majority of the case series in the literature that describe surgery for anatomical variations in patients with facial pain that responded to surgery result from the effect of cognitive dissonance [34] or from surgery altering neuroplasticity within the brainstem sensory nuclear complex [35].

Patients whose primary complaint is headache or facial pain are less likely to have evidence of rhinosinusitis than those who have nasal symptoms [36]. Patients with facial pain or headache without nasal symptoms are very unlikely to be helped by nasal medical or surgical treatment [37].

Neuralgias

Trigeminal Neuralgia

The characteristic presentation of trigeminal neuralgia with paroxysms of severe lancinating pain induced by a specific trigger point is well recognised. In more than one third of sufferers the pain occurs in both the maxillary and mandibular divisions, while in one fifth it is confined to the maxillary division. In a small number of patients (3%) only the ophthalmic division is affected. Typical trigger points are the lips and nasolabial folds, but pain may also be triggered by touching the gingivae. A flush may be seen over the face but there are no sensory disturbances in primary trigeminal neuralgia. Remissions are common but the condition can also increase in severity.

Patients with trigeminal neuralgia, and particularly younger patients should undergo magnetic resonance imaging to exclude other pathology such as disseminating sclerosis. The association of disseminating sclerosis with trigeminal neuralgia is well established. Disseminating sclerosis is identified in 2–4% of patients with trigeminal neuralgia and in a small proportion of these patients trigeminal neuralgia is the first manifestation of the disease. Patients with multiple sclerosis are younger than the general trigeminal neuralgia population and the pain is more frequently bilateral [38]. Tumours such as posterior fossa meningiomas or neuromas are found in 2% of patients presenting with typical trigeminal neuralgia reinforcing the need for imaging to exclude such pathology [39]. Carbamazepine remains the first-line medical treatment, with gabapentin or pregabalin now being employed more frequently. In cases refractory to medical treatment, referral to specialist centres for consideration of other treatment modalities such as microvascular decompression or stereotactic radiotherapy may be appropriate [40].

Glossopharyngeal Neuralgia

This very rare neuralgia is characterised by a severe lancinating pain in the tongue base, tonsillar fossa and posterior pharynx. It may be precipitated by swallowing or yawning and the bouts may last for weeks with a tendency to recur. Treatment is along similar lines to trigeminal neuralgia with imaging to exclude other pathology, including multiple sclerosis. Drug treatment is used initially with surgery reserved for refractory cases [41].

Postherpetic Neuralgia

This is pain following a herpes zoster infection, and is defined as pain recurring or continuing at the site of shingles after the onset of the rash. Up to 50% of elderly patients who have had shingles may develop postherpetic neuralgia. Fortunately most recover during the first year although 8% go on to have protracted severe pain. Antiviral agents may help curtail the pain of acute shingles and the risk of subsequent postherpetic neuralgia [42]. Various medical treatments may be helpful particularly tricyclic antidepressants or carbamazepine or gabapentin.

Pain Caused by Tumours

Although tumours rarely present with facial pain, constant, progressive pain, and if associated with other suspicious symptoms or neurological signs, should alert the clinician. A past history of malignancy may raise the possibility of metastases. A thorough examination and appropriate imaging is mandatory to exclude the possibility of a tumour. One must remember that some lesions such as a neuroma can have a long natural history and that pain may have been present for several years.

Patients with carcinoma of the paranasal sinuses often present with advanced disease. Unilateral blood stained mucus is a common early presentation. Proptosis, epiphora, facial paraesthesia or swelling and a loose tooth or ill-fitting denture may represent more advanced disease. Pain is a usually a late feature.

Tension-type Headache

This is described as a feeling of tightness, pressure or constriction that varies in intensity, frequency and duration. It usually affects the forehead or temple, and often has a suboccipital component (Fig. 29.3). It may be episodic or chronic (>15 days/month, >6 months), and is only occasionally helped by nonsteroidal anti-inflammatory drugs (NSAIDs) but typically pa-

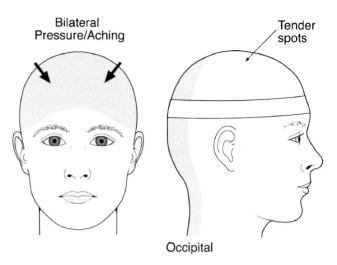

Fig. 29.3 Features of tension-type headache

tients are taking large quantities of analgesics of all kinds but say that they provide little benefit [43]. It is sometimes associated with anxiety, depression or agitated depression. Hyperaesthesia of the skin or muscles of the forehead often occurs, giving the patient the impression they have rhinosinusitis, as they know their sinuses lie under the forehead. It most frequently responds to low-dose amitriptyline, but propranolol, sodium valproate, gabapentin or a change in lifestyle may bring successful relief of symptoms.

Amitriptyline should be given for 6 weeks before judging its effect, and should be continued for 6 months if it has helped [44–46]. The starting dose is 10 mg, and after 6 weeks if pain is not controlled this can be increased to 20 mg (and rarely 75 mg are needed). Patients need to be warned of the sedative effects even at this low dose, but they can be reassured that tolerance usually develops after the first few days. It is our practice to inform patients that amitriptyline is also used in higher doses for other conditions such as depression, but that it is not being given for this reason and its effect is unrelated to its analgesic properties, that would take effect much more quickly and normally require much higher doses. It is often reassuring for patients to know that the dose used for depression is some seven or more times the dose used in tension-type headache and that other antidepressants do not help this condition. Amitriptyline should then be continued for 6 months before stopping it, and in the 20% whose symptoms return when they stop it they need to restart it if the pain returns. In a proportion of patients there are migrainous features, and a triptan may help acute exacerbations as up to 50% of patients have an overlap between tension-type headache and migraine [43].

Midfacial Segment Pain

Midfacial segment pain has all the characteristics of tension-type headache with the exception that it affects the midface. Patients describe a feeling of pressure, heaviness or tightness

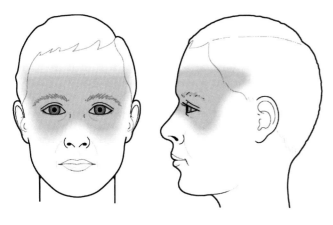

Fig. 29.4 Distribution of the symptoms of pressure in midfacial segment pain

and they may say that their nose feels blocked when they have no airway obstruction. The symptoms are symmetrical and may involve the nasion, the bridge of the nose, either side of the nose, the periorbital region, retro-orbitally or across the cheeks. The forehead and occipital region may also be affected at the same time in about 60% of patients (Fig. 29.4). There are no consistent exacerbating or relieving factors and patients often take a range of analgesics but they have no, or a minimal effect, other than ibuprofen that may help a few to a minor extent. The symptoms are often initially episodic but are often persistent by the time they are seen in secondary care. Patients may be convinced that their symptoms are due to sinusitis as they know that their sinuses lie under this area with the exception of the bridge of the nose. They may have been treated for a long period with antibiotics and topical nasal steroids and a few patients have had some transient response on occasions that may be related to the placebo effect or cognitive dissonance, but these are inconsistent. Patient's symptoms are not worse with routine physical activity, and rarely interfere with the patient getting to sleep.

To make matters more complex, the stimulus of a genuine acute sinus infection may exacerbate the symptoms, with a return to the background faceache on resolution of the infection. It is hardly surprising that patients (and doctors) will interpret all their symptoms as being related to their sinuses. Patients often describe tenderness on touching the areas of the forehead or cheeks leading them to think there is underlying inflammation of the bone. However, on examination there is hyperesthesia of the skin and soft tissues in these areas and gently touching these is enough to cause discomfort and there is no evidence of underlying bony disease. This is similar to the tender areas over the forehead and scalp seen with tension-type headache. It appears that this is an organic disorder as an increase in the pain sensitivity in the central nervous system has been found in tension-type headache [47].

Nasal endoscopy is normal. As approximately 1 in 3 asymptomatic people have incidental changes on their CT this may confuse the picture. A trial of maximal nasal medical treatment

including oral and nasal steroids and a broad-spectrum antibiotic with anaerobic cover fails to help their symptoms. The majority of patients with this condition respond to low-dose amitriptyline as described above. If amitriptyline fails, then relief may be obtained from gabapentin, pregabalin, propranolol, carbamazepine and, occasionally, sodium valproate.

It seems likely that the underlying pathology in midfacial segment pain is similar to tension-type headache. The aetiology of this type of pain is uncertain but Olesen's theory [43, 48] that integrates the effects of myofascial afferents, the activation of peripheral nociceptors and their convergence on the caudal nucleus of trigeminal, along with qualitative changes in the central nervous system, provides one of the best models. There is also a suggestion that there is a downregulation of central inhibition from supraspinal impulses due to psychological stress and emotional disturbances. Other mechanisms have been proposed that include sensitisation of peripheral myofascial receptors, sensitisation of second-order neurons at the spinal or trigeminal level, sensitisation of supraspinal neurons or decreased antinociceptive activity from supraspinal structures [49]. The trigeminal caudal nucleus is the major relay nucleus for head and neck pain, and it appears that supraspinal excitatory input contributes to intense neuronal activation resulting in a generalised increase in sensitivity of the nociceptive pathways, both centrally and peripherally. Midfacial segment pain may be a state of trigeminal neuronal hypersensitivity and pain facilitation. Olesen's model is attractive as it might explain much of the clinical picture of midfacial segment pain [43], for example, the skin and soft tissue hyperaesthesia that accompanies the pain may be due to the above hypersensitivity of the pain pathways. It is of interest that if surgery is mistakenly performed as a treatment for midfacial segment pain, the pain may sometimes abate temporarily, only to return after several weeks to months.

Atypical Facial Pain

This has been a diagnosis of exclusion and care must be taken in reaching this conclusion, even when the patient has received previous opinions and no pathology has been identified. The history is often vague and inconsistent with widespread pain extending from the face onto other areas of the head and neck. The pain may move from one part of the face to another between different consultations and other symptoms such as 'mucus moving' in the sinuses are often described. A number of patients have completely fixed ideas about their condition and they will not be convinced otherwise, whatever the weight of evidence to the contrary. Pain is often described in dramatic terms in conjunction with an excess of other unpleasant life events. Many of these patients have a history of other pain syndromes and their extensive records show minimal progress despite various medications. They may have undergone previous sinus or dental surgery treatment but the onset of their pain usually preceded any intervention and this helps differentiate it from postsurgical neurogenic pain [10]. Many patients with atypical facial pain exhibit significant psychological disturbance or a history of depression and are unable to function normally as a result of their pain. Some project a pessimistic view of treatment, almost

29

giving the impression they do not wish to be rid of the pain that plays such a central role in their lives. A comprehensive examination (including nasendoscopy) is essential to identify significant pathology before the patient is labelled as having atypical pain. The management of such patients is challenging and confrontation is nearly always counterproductive. A good starting point is to reassure the patient that you recognise that they have genuine pain and an empathetic consultation with an explanation should be conducted. Drug treatment revolves around a gradual build-up to the higher analgesic and antidepressant levels of amitriptyline (75–100 mg) at night. Patients should sympathetically be made aware that psychological factors may play a role in their condition and referral to a clinical psychologist may be helpful.

Conclusion

The majority of patients who present to an otorhinolaryngology clinic with facial pain and headaches believe they have 'sinus trouble'. There is an increasing awareness amongst otorhinolaryngologists that neurological causes are responsible for a large proportion of patients with headache or facial pain [50, 51]. We believe that patients with facial pain who have no objective evidence of sinus disease (endoscopy negative, CT negative), and whose pain fails to respond to medical antibiotic/steroid therapy aimed at treating sinonasal disease, are very unlikely to be helped by surgery particularly in the medium and long term. A comprehensive examination (including nasendoscopy) is highly desirable if medical nasal treatment has failed to help in order to identify significant pathology before making or refuting a diagnosis of sinusitis.

Tips to Avoid Complications

- Patients with a normal CT scan are unlikely to have pain due to rhinosinusitis. (NB Approximately a third of asymptomatic patients have incidental mucosal changes on CT so radiographic changes on their own are not indicative of symptomatic rhinosinusitis.)
- Patients with purulent secretions and facial pain are likely to benefit from treatment directed at resolving their rhinosinusitis. Paradoxically only a minority of patients with purulent rhinosinusitis at endoscopy have facial pain.
- If it is not possible to make a diagnosis at the first consultation it is often helpful to ask the patient to keep a diary of their symptoms and have a trial of medical nasal treatment and review the patient.

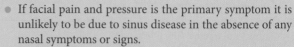

Take-Home Pearls

- If facial pain and pressure is the primary symptom it is unlikely to be due to sinus disease in the absence of any nasal symptoms or signs.
- If a patient has facial pain in addition to nasal obstruction, a loss of sense of smell, and it is associated with the following symptoms: worse with a cold, flying or skiing, their symptoms may be helped by nasal medical or surgical treatment.
- The majority of patients seen in a rhinological clinic with pain are found to have disorders due to causes other than sinusitis [37].
- Patients whose nasal endoscopy is normal are unlikely to have pain due to rhinosinusitis.
- Surgery done for pain in patients with no objective signs of paranasal sinus disease has no effect in one third, makes the pain worse in one third, and whilst it can help reduce the pain of the remaining one third this rarely lasts more than a few months.
- It is important to defer making a diagnosis in studies of facial pain until at least a 12-month period as a response to treatment is often an important aspect of confirming the cause. This is because the effect of cognitive dissonance or surgery altering neuroplasticity within the brainstem sensory nuclear complex may have a temporary effect that can last this long [11].

References

1. Fahy C, Jones NS (2001) Nasal polyposis and facial pain. Clin Otolaryngol 26:510–513
2. Hughes R, Jones NS (1998) The role of endoscopy in outpatient management. Clin Otolaryngol 23:224–226
3. Berg O, Carenfelt C (1988) Analysis of symptoms and clinical signs in the maxillary sinus empyema. Acta Otolaryngol 105:343–349
4. Cooney TR, Huissoon AP, Powell RJ, Jones NS (2001) Investigation for immunodeficiency in patients with recurrent ENT infections. Clin Otolaryngol 26:184–188
5. Chee L, Graham S, Carothers DG, Ballas ZK (2001) Immune dysfunction in refractory sinusitis in a tertiary care setting. Laryngoscope 111:233–235
6. The Royal College of Radiologists Working Party (1993) Making the best use of a Department of Clinical Radiology. Guidelines for Doctors 1993
7. Marshall AH, Jones NS (2003) The utility of radiologic studies in the diagnosis and management of rhinosinusitis. Curr Infect Dis Rep 5:199–204
8. Lloyd GAS (1990) CT of the paranasal sinuses: a study of a control series in relation to endoscopic sinus surgery. J Laryngol Otol 104:447–481

9. Jones NS (2002) A review of the CT staging systems, the prevalence of anatomical variations, incidence of mucosal findings and their correlation with symptoms, surgical and pathological findings. Clin Otolaryngol 27:11–17

10. Khan O, Majumdar S, Jones NS (2002) Facial pain after sinus surgery and trauma. Clin Otolaryngol 27:171–174

11. Jones NS, Cooney TR (2003) Facial pain and sinonasal surgery. Rhinology 41:193–200

12. Booth DF, Hunter MJ (1999) Facial pain and craniomandibular disorders. In: Aranoff GM (ed) Evaluation and treatment of chronic pain. Williams and Wilkins, Baltimore

13. Lipton RB, Stewart WF (1993) Migraine in the United States: a review of epidemiology and health care use. Neurology 43(suppl 3):6–10

14. Goadsby PJ, Oelson J (1996) Diagnosis and management of migraine. BMJ 312:1279–1283

15. Daudia AT, Jones NS (2002) Facial migraine in a rhinological setting. Clinical Otolaryngol 27:251–255

16. Silberstein SD, Goadsby PJ, Lipton RB (2000) Management of migraine: an algorithmic approach. Neurology 55:46–52

17. Fuad F, Jones NS (2002) Paroxysmal hemicrania and cluster headache: two discrete entities or is there an overlap? Clinical Otolaryngol 27:472–479

18. Antonaci F, Sjaastad O (1989) Chronic paroxysmal hemicrania. A review of clinical manifestations. Headache 29:648–656

19. Pascual J (1998) A case of chronic paroxysmal hemicrania responding to subcutaneous sumatriptan. Letters, correspondence, book reviews. J Neurol Neurosurg Psych 65:407

20. Evers S, Husstedt I (1998) Efficacy of sumatriptan in chronic paroxysmal hemicrania. Letter to the editor. Headache 38:630–631

21. Sluder G (1908) The role of the sphenopalatine (or Meckel's) ganglion in nasal headaches. N Y Med J 87:989–990

22. The Headache Classification Committee of the International Headache Society (1988) Classification and diagnostic criteria for headache disorders, cranial neuralgia and facial pain. Cephalalgia 8:1–96

23. Ahmed S, Jones NS (2003) What is Sluder's neuralgia? J Laryngol Otol 117:437–443

24. Puig CM, Driscoll CLW, Kern EB (1998) Sluder's sphenopalatine ganglion neuralgia: treatment with 88% phenol. J Rhinol 12:113–118

25. Sluder G (1919) Headaches and eye disorders of nasal origin. Kimpton, London, pp 57–85

26. Beasley NJP, Jones NS, Downes RN (1995) Enophthalmos secondary to maxillary sinus disease: single-stage operative management. J Laryngol Otol 109:868–870

27. McAuliffe GW, Goodell H, Wolff HG (1943) Experimental studies on headache: pain from the nasal and paranasal structures. Research Publication. New York: Association for Research in Nervous and Mental Disease 23:185–208

28. Wolf HG (1948) Headache and other head pain. Oxford University Press, Oxford

29. Gerbe RW, Fry TL, Fischer ND (1984) Headache of nasal spur origin: an easily diagnosed and surgically correctable cause of facial pain. Headache 24:329–330

30. Abu-Bakra M, Jones NS (2001) Does stimulation of the nasal mucosa cause referred pain to the face? Clin Otolaryngol 26:403–432

31. Abu-Bakra M, Jones NS (2001) The prevalence of nasal contact points in a population with facial pain and a control population. J Laryngol Otol 115:629–632

32. Stammberger H, Wolf G (1988) Headaches and sinus disease: the endoscopic approach. Ann Otol Rhinol Laryngol 143:3–23

33. Jones NS, Strobl A, Holland I (1997) CT findings in 100 patients with rhinosinusitis and 100 controls. Clin Otolaryngol 22:47–51

34. Homer J, Jones NS, Sheard C, Herbert M (2000) Cognitive dissonance, the placebo effect and the evaluation of surgical results. Clin Otolaryngol 25:195–199

35. Sessle BJ (2000) Acute and chronic craniofacial pain: brainstem mechanisms of nociceptive transmission and neuroplasticity, and other clinical correlates. Crit Rev Oral Biol Med 11:57–91

36. Rosbe KW, Jones KR (1998) Usefulness of patient symptoms and nasal endoscopy in the diagnosis of chronic sinusitis. Am J Rhinol 12:167–171

37. West B, Jones NS (2001) Endoscopy-negative, computed tomography-negative facial pain in a nasal clinic. Laryngoscope 111:581–586

38. Hooge CF, Redekop WP (1995) Trigeminal neuralgia in multiple sclerosis. Neurology 45:1294–1296

39. Cheng TMW, Cascino TL, Onofrio BM (1993) Comprehensive study of diagnosis and treatment of trigeminal neuralgia secondary to tumours. Neurology 43:2298–2302

40. Nurmikko TJ, Eldridge PR (2001) Trigeminal neuralgia: pathophysiology, diagnosis and current treatment. Br J Anaesth 87:117–132

41. Patel A, Kassam A, Horowitz M, Chang YF (2002) Microvascular decompression in the management of glossopharyngeal neuralgia: analysis of 217 cases. Neurosurgery 50:705–710

42. Wood MJ, Kay R, Dworkin RH, Soong SJ, Whitely RJ (1996) Oral acyclovir therapy accelerates pain resolution in patients with herpes zoster: a meta-analysis of placebo-controlled trials. Clin Infect Dis 22:341–347

43. Olesen J (1991) Clinical and pathophysiological observations in migraine and tension type headache explained by integration of vascular, supraspinal and myofascial inputs. Pain 46:125–132

44. Schoenen J, Wang W (1997) Tension-type headache. In: Goadsby PJ, Silberstein SD (eds) Headache. Blue books of practical neurology. Butterworth-Heinemann, Boston

45. Bendtsen L, Jensen R, Olesen J (1996) A non-selective (amitriptyline), but not a selective (citalopram), serotonin reuptake inhibitor is effective in the prophylactic treatment of chronic tension-type headache. J Neurol Neurosurg Psych 61:285–290

46. Tomkins GE (2001) Treatment of chronic daily headache with antidepressants: a meta-analysis. Am J Med 111:54–63

47. Ashina A, Bendtsen L, Ashina M, Magrel W, Jensen R (2006) Generalised hyperalgesia in patients with chronic tension-type headache. Cephalgia 26:940–948

48. Jensen R, Olesen J (2000) Tension-type headache: an update on mechanisms and treatment. Curr Opin Neurol 13:285–289

49. Bendtsen L, Jensen R, Olesen J (1996) Quantitatively altered nociception in chronic myofascial pain. Pain 65:259–264

50. Acquadro MA, Salman SD, Joseph MP (1997) Analysis of pain and endoscopic sinus surgery for sinusitis. Ann Otol Rhinol Laryngol 106:305–309

51. Tarabichi M (2000) Characteristics of sinus-related pain. Otolaryngol Head Neck Surg 122:84–87

Chapter 30

Evidence-based Medicine in Rhinosinusitis

30

Seth M. Brown, Abtin Tabaee, and Vijay K. Anand

Core Messages

■ Treatment for rhinosinusitis should be based on the current understanding of the pathology of the disorder, consideration of comorbid conditions, and the various treatment modalities available.

■ There is a scarcity of well-designed studies on the medical management of acute and chronic rhinosinusitis.

Contents

Introduction

In a 2006 study analyzing the medical management, diagnosis, and treatment of rhinosinusitis by United States otolaryngologists, 74% of practitioners reported the basis of their choice for "maximal" medical management was personal clinical experience [32]. Another study in 2007 found the majority of patients receiving medical treatment for chronic rhinosinusitis (CRS) showed only modest improvement in quality of life outcomes [25]. The consensus understanding of the role of various medical treatment modalities for rhinosinusitis remains incomplete. An evidenced-based treatment approach is critical given the incidence, direct and indirect costs, and management challenges associated with rhinosinusitis. The goal of this chapter is to summarize the existing literature on the medical management of acute and chronic rhinosinusitis.

To date, there are no medications that are approved by the United States Food and Drug Administration (FDA) for the indication of CRS and only a few medications, all of them antibiotics, for acute bacterial sinusitis [21]. This is in part due to the lack of an adequate body of well-designed studies investigating the medical treatment of rhinosinusitis. Furthermore, many published studies are inherently biased by financial support of pharmaceutical companies. The paucity of evidence-based data precludes defining a single "best" treatment for rhinosinusitis. Instead, the authors recommend using the existing research as a background to assist in treating patients on an individualized basis. This approach incorporates our current understanding of the pathophysiology of the disorder, consideration of comorbid conditions such as allergy and pulmonary disease, and the role of the various available treatment modalities. An effort is made in this chapter to discuss classes of medications and not individual brands, unless strong support or a specific research study exist supporting one medication over another in the same class.

30

Antibiotics

Oral

Studies have supported the use of oral antibiotics for rhinosinusitis. A meta-analysis of six placebo-controlled studies showed a 30% higher cure rate and a 50% lower rate of treatment failure with the use of antibiotics for acute rhinosinusitis (ARS) [8]. A meta-analysis of pediatric patients also supports higher improvement rates in randomized, controlled studies; 88% cure rate for those patients receiving antibiotics compared to 60% without antibiotics [28]. In comparison, a systemic review by the Cochrane Database on all studies of antibiotic treatment of acute maxillary sinusitis carried out prior to October 1998 showed only mild gains. Looking at all randomized studies of 30 or more adults comparing antibiotics to placebo or comparing different classes of antibiotics, 32 studies met the inclusion criteria. In this review both penicillin and amoxicillin improved cure rates, though were similar to each other. Furthermore, there was no significant difference in cure rates between newer generation non-penicillin antibiotics versus penicillins or between amoxicillin/clavulanate and newer non-penicillin antibiotics [59].

The Cochrane meta-analysis described a relative risk of 1.24, meaning that 7 patients meeting radiographic criteria for acute maxillary sinusitis must be treated with antibiotics to achieve clinical cure in 1 patient [53, 59]. They concluded that this is in large part a function of the high spontaneous rate of cure or improvement in placebo groups (62–69%), as well as the poor specificity of using radiography for identifying bacterial sinusitis [53]. Other studies have found similar results. A meta-analysis in 2005 found a cure rate of approximately two-thirds in patients receiving placebo for ARS [29]. The group did find, however, fewer adverse effects in those patients treated with cephalosporins compared to amoxicillin/clavulanate [59]. They also found relapse rates after successful antibiotic treatment in 7.7% and improvement in radiographic outcomes with the use of antibiotic therapy [59].

One cost analysis of antibiotics in sinusitis looked at simulated data and concluded that newer, expensive antibiotics are of limited value in acute bacterial sinusitis [4]. Another review covering a four-year period (1999–2002), looked at the treatment of ARS and CRS in the USA. The authors concluded that the use of prescription antibiotics far outweighed the predicted incidence of bacterial causes of sinusitis and that the frequency of antibiotic class used was not congruent with reported efficacy of the respective classes [50].

The United States Agency for Healthcare Research and Quality performed a meta-analysis in 2005 investigating antibiotic treatment of acute sinusitis, finding 39 studies meeting the criteria. Looking at the different classes of antibiotics, they concluded that amoxicillin/clavulanate is more effective than cephalosporins for the treatment of ARS with an absolute risk of 1.41 [29]. In this analysis, for every 100 patients treated with a cephalosporin for ARS, 3.5 more would fail as compared to those treated with amoxicillin/clavulanate. Furthermore, the study analysis found no difference between shorter versus longer courses of antibiotics [29].

These findings support the use of culture-directed therapy. However, its use in every patient with ARS may not be cost-effective. It is, therefore, important to understand the usual pathogens in ARS and CRS and use antimicrobials that cover these bacteria (see Chap. 18). Also, it is well known that resistance of bacteria to antibiotics varies not only by country but also by individual regions, communities, and hospitals. An understanding of local resistance patterns provides a key component in the choice of antimicrobials for an individual practitioner. For complicated sinusitis, on the other hand, culture-directed antibiotics are essential. This is particularly true in patients who are immunocompromised. Also, culture-directed therapy should be considered in all hospitalized patients with ARS, as this group carries a much higher rate of resistance. Cultures for sinusitis were traditionally carried out by maxillary sinus taps. Recently, several reports, including a meta-analysis in 2006, have supported the role of endoscopically directed middle meatal cultures based on their high sensitivity and minimally invasive nature [7].

The microbiology patterns differ in patients with a history of previous sinus surgery, affecting the choice of antibiotics. Increased incidences of *Staphylococcus aureus* and *Pseudomonas* species, both with higher frequencies of antibiotic resistance, have been noted in patients with a history of surgery [10]. Furthermore, different pathogens may cause different levels of disease severity. In one study, disease severity was shown to be increased for patients with cultures positive for *Streptococcus pneumoniae* compared to *Haemophilus influenzae* using analysis of symptom severity and radiographic findings [6].

The judicious use of antibiotics is not recommended. In addition to increasing resistance for individual patients and society, one study has shown an increase in fatigue level in patients treated with a higher total number of antibiotic courses and weeks of antibiotic use [9]. Furthermore, the development of resistance in respiratory pathogens is closely related to levels of antibiotic use in the community [39].

Interpretation of studies investigating antibiotics in rhinosinusitis requires an understanding of common limitations. The very definition of "sinusitis" may vary depending on the incorporation of symptom-, imaging-, or culture-based data, each with differing sensitivities and specificities. Additionally, the similarity of clinical and radiographic features between viral upper respiratory infections and acute bacterial sinusitis acts as a confounding variable. Furthermore, most studies have focused on acute maxillary sinusitis and these results may not be applicable to frontal, ethmoid, and sphenoid sinusitis [11]. A common weakness of studies investigating antimicrobial therapy in ARS is the lack of placebo arms, with the majority of reports comparing one antibiotic to another [15].

The funding of antibiotic studies by pharmaceutical companies introduces significant issues including bias. In a 2005 meta-analysis, 34 of the 39 studies determined to be eligible for inclusion were funded by pharmaceutical companies [29]. Additionally, negative studies may not be published secondary to the funding source, raising the issue of publication bias. As a result, although most practitioners would support the use of antibiotics both for acute and chronic rhinosinusitis, significant controversy exists in the protocols that should be fol-

Table 30.1 A sampling of the recent consensus statements on rhinosinusitis

Title	Group	Year	Journal
Update on acute bacterial rhinosinusitis [29]	Agency for Health Care Research and Quality	2005	Online
EAACI position paper on rhinosinusitis and nasal polyps executive summary [18]	Academy of Allergology and Clinical Immunology	2005	Allergy
Antimicrobial treatment guidelines for acute bacterial rhinosinusitis 2004 [2]	Sinus and Allergy Health Partnership	2004	Otolaryngology – Head and Neck Surgery
Acute bacterial rhinosinusitis: patient assessment, risk stratification, referral strategies, and outcome-effective antibiotic selection [11]	Antibiotic therapy for bacterial sinusitis clinical consensus panel	2004	Primary Care Consensus Reports
Clinical practice guidelines: management of sinusitis [56]	Subcommittee on management of sinusitis and committee on quality improvement	2001	Pediatrics
Diagnosis and treatment of uncomplicated acute bacterial rhinosinusitis: summary of the Agency for Health Care Policy and Research evidence-based report [8]	Agency for Health Care Policy and Research	2000	Otolaryngology – Head and Neck Surgery

lowed. Numerous organizations and committees have released consensus statements based on expert opinion and available literature (Table 30.1). Most of these reports conclude that the important first step is to differentiate bacterial sinusitis from viral, and then to treat with high-dose amoxicillin in non-allergic patients, prior to initiating treatment with more expensive and newer alternatives.

Intravenous

Intravenous (IV) antibiotics are used as the mainstay of treatment for acute complicated rhinosinusitis requiring hospitalization. This typically involves initial use of a broad-spectrum agent and subsequent adjustment based on cultures. The indications for IV antibiotics in non-complicated sinusitis are currently evolving and may include CRS refractory to oral therapy, hyperostotic sinusitis and cultures demonstrating resistant organisms, particularly methicillin-resistant *Staphylococcus aureus* (MRSA). In a study of patients with CRS undergoing endoscopically directed cultures in a tertiary referral center, an incidence of 9.22% was found for MRSA. In this study, neither frequency of antibiotic use nor previous endoscopic sinus surgery were found to be contributing factors [38]. Intravenous antibiotics have also been studied in patients with recalcitrant disease either after surgery or after failure of maximal medical therapy with oral antibiotics. In one study of 45 patients, significant improvements in symptoms were seen in patients treated with 6 weeks of culture-directed IV antibiotics after failure of oral antibiotics or surgery [1]. A recent study on safety of ambulatory IV antibiotic therapy with peripherally inserted central

catheters for CRS revealed a 2% incidence of line-related infections and 16% antibiotic-related complications, mostly minor [37]. These studies support further research addressing the role of IV antibiotics in CRS.

Topical

Topical antibiotics delivered as sprays, irrigations, or nebulized treatments are used by many practitioners. However, their efficacy and safety remain controversial. In theory, application of an antibiotic in topical form can work directly on the source of infection with minimal risk of systemic side effects. This is similar to the treatment of otitis externa with ear drops or bacterial conjunctivitis with eye drops. A recent article by Leonard and Bolger support the use of topical ceftazidime (6 g in 60 ml saline then diluted 3 ml into 300 ml of saline). They describe irrigation three times daily in patients with previous sinus surgery and recalcitrant disease. In their experience, the treatment is well tolerated and successful in most patients. They caution the need for patent sinuses for drug delivery, sufficient concentration of the drug, frequent dosing schedule, and the need for adequate antibiotic spectrum of coverage [36]. Despite their success with this treatment, their data are anecdotal and not case controlled. The possibility of a clinical benefit resulting from the mechanical cleansing properties of the carrier medium (saline) and not the dissolved antibiotic exists for these irrigations.

The need for patent postsurgical sinus cavities prior to using topical therapy is supported by a study done by Kobayashi and Baba. The authors examined nebulized fosfomycin and cefmenoxime therapy used three times weekly. In this study they found the medication's main effect to be in the nose and only indirectly working in the maxillary sinus [34]. A randomized, double-blind study in patients with mucopurulent rhinosinusitis was carried out by giving patients nasal sprays of dexamethasone, tramazoline, and neomycin four times daily for 2 weeks. This was compared to controls that used only dexamethasone. The study found no significant differences between the two groups in both symptomatic and objective data [52]. It has been suggested in two reviews that the failure of neomycin to show clinical results in this study was likely a function of the small dose of neomycin, 3,200% less than the standard dose used to treat otitis externa [20, 36].

Another study looked at topical tobramycin solution delivered by a large-particle nebulizer. The study consisted of 20 patients with refractory symptoms after sinus surgery. Patients were randomized into a double-blinded study of tobramycin with saline compared to saline only. The authors found no statistically significant differences in symptoms and objective parameters of rhinosinusitis between the two groups [14]. Furthermore, they found that despite tobramycin giving more rapid resolution of pain for patients, it caused an increase in nasal congestion [14].

Perhaps the most popular topical antibiotic choice for the paranasal sinuses is gentamicin. This is used because of the antibiotic's coverage of many common bacterial causes of sinusitis and its potentially positive effect on cilia function. One recent study has shown that gentamicin can repair gene mutations in cilia of patients with cystic fibrosis [60]. Despite this exciting potential, the literature supporting the use of topical gentamicin remains inadequate. Furthermore, caution should be used when prescribing all topical antibiotics, as serum levels may become detectable, particularly when the medication is used as an irrigation. In one study, a twice daily irrigation of 30 mg gentamicin (80 mg gentamicin mixed in 1 l saline), was found to achieve detectable serum levels in patients, some in the normal range for gentamicin trough [58]. Further studies are warranted in this area before recommendations can be made.

Steroids

Oral

Oral steroids are frequently used to treat CRS. This is particularly true for patients with CRS with nasal polyps and allergic fungal sinusitis (AFS). One recent study looked at systemic corticosteroids for both AFS and CRS with nasal polyps. At a dose of 1 mg/kg prednisone for 10 days prior to surgical intervention, they identified a statistically significant reduction in CT scores on the Lund-MacKay scale, 66% in those patients with AFS and 23% in those patients with CRS and nasal polyps [35].

Another group looked at the treatment of chronic polypoid rhinosinusitis with both systemic and topical steroids. Using nasal budesonide spray twice daily at 0.1 mg/day and either a 12-day oral fluocortolone taper over 12 days for a total steroid dose of 560 mg or over 20 days for a total dose of 715 mg, they found a significant reduction (>30%) in 50% of the patients measured by MRI results. Furthermore, 80% of patients noticed a distinctly diminished decrease in sinus-related symptoms [13]. The durability of this treatment response, however, was not addressed. The use of systemic steroids in patients with CRS must also be weighed against the potential for significant treatment-related complications.

Topical

Over recent years, topical steroids have become a first-line agent for allergic rhinitis and sinusitis. Recent FDA approval in the USA has included both children and pregnant women for certain preparations. A recent study reviewed all randomized, controlled studies on nasal steroids in the English literature. The authors concluded that all four available intranasal steroids were found to be effective and well tolerated in adult patients, with similar efficacy and adverse event profiles [24]. A study looking at increased fatigue in treatments for sinusitis found no increase in fatigue in patients treated with nasal steroids [9].

Although most of the commercial preparations are similar, it is important to note that these agents differ by both the steroid compound and additives. Certain compounds that are present in some formulations, including benzalkonium chloride, may be ciliotoxic in vitro in standard concentrations. The potential for these medications to act as nasal irritants at high doses has been described [47]. Another in vitro study examined the effect of benzalkonium chloride on human neutrophils. The study looked at one sample group treated with nasal saline with the addition of benzalkonium chloride compared to a phosphate-buffered saline. The study found that nasal saline spray with benzalkonium chloride is toxic to human neutrophils even at concentrations far lower than those found in commercially available preparations [12].

One study looked at an alternative application of topical steroids, via nasal drops. In this study, supported by the manufacturer, fluticasone propionate was used in a double-blind, placebo study, in patients meeting criteria for sinus surgery. After treatment for 12 weeks, only 14 of the 27 patients in the study group still met criteria for surgery versus 21 of 27 patients in the control group, making this statistically significant [3].

Another manufacturer-funded study compared nasal steroids (mometasone) versus antibiotics (amoxicillin) and placebo. The authors found a statistically significant improvement in patients treated twice daily with steroids compared to both the antibiotic group and placebo and a statistically superior result in patients treated with steroids once daily compared to placebo when looking at symptom scores [40].

Several studies have looked at topical nasal steroids after endoscopic sinus surgery with conflicting results. One double-blind, placebo-controlled, randomized study looked at the addition of fluticasone propionate aqueous nasal spray after endoscopic sinus surgery for a period of 1 year. Despite twice daily treatment with either 400 or 800 mcg, the study found no difference in recurrent or persistent disease between patients using the nasal steroids or placebo [16]. On the contrary, a different study investigated the efficacy of fluticasone propionate aqueous nasal spray in patients after sinus surgery. In this study, patients were randomized prospectively into a group receiving

200 mcg of medication twice daily 6 weeks after surgery and a group receiving placebo. The study found a decrease in endoscopic polyp score and a higher total nasal volume in the group receiving the medication by a blinded observer at 5 years [49]. Furthermore, they noted that 10 of the 12 patients that required at least one rescue medication course a month for at least 2 consecutive months were in the placebo group [49].

The Cochrane Database was reviewed for success of intranasal corticosteroids for acute sinusitis. After examining the available studies, four double-blinded, placebo-controlled studies were identified. In these studies, 1,943 patients received intranasal corticosteroids for 15 or 21 days. They found that patients treated with the medication were more likely to have resolution or improvement of symptoms than those receiving placebo and that higher doses of steroids had a stronger effect on improvement or complete relief of symptoms [61]. They also found that the median number of days to clinical success in those treated with intranasal corticosteroids was 6 days compared to 9.5 days in those treated with placebo [61].

Saline Rinses/Washes

Nasal saline has been used in the nose and sinuses with several different methods of application including sprays, irrigation, and nebulizer. One study evaluated the distribution of saline by using a contrast material and then evaluating delivery based on imaging. The results demonstrated that irrigation both by positive pressure and negative pressure was far superior to nebulizer for distribution of saline to the ethmoid and maxillary sinuses [42]. Another prospective study using blinded reviewers of endoscopies after using different delivery systems of a dye solution found a bulb syringe to be statistically superior to a nebulizer in all sinonasal sites and superior to an atomizer and spray bottle in the ethmoid sinuses [41].

One study did show promise for a vortex-propelled nebulizer system, showing improved distribution in the sinuses versus a passive nebulizer or a spray bottle. However, this was not tested against a bulb syringe or irrigation [26]. Also of note, although the research was graded by blinded reviewers, the research was funded by the makers of a vortex-propelled nebulizer system.

Another study looked at treatment of various nasal disorders including rhinosinusitis, allergic rhinitis, atrophic rhinitis, and postnasal drip with hypertonic saline administered by a Waterpik device daily for 3–6 weeks. The authors found statistically significant improvements in most nasal symptoms in both patients treated with additional therapies as well as those treated with irrigations alone [54]. Caution must be used when interpreting these results, as this was not a controlled study and many patients may improve simply with time or a placebo effect.

A recent study also found effectiveness of Dead Sea salt nasal irrigation as compared to hypertonic saline. This randomized, prospective, double-blind study found patients treated with the Dead Sea salt solution had significantly better symptom relief and improved scores on the Rhinoconjunctivitis Quality of Life Questionnaire when compared to a group treated with only hypertonic saline [19]. Of note, this study was supported by the makers of a nasal wash and spray.

Decongestants

Randomized, controlled studies on the use of topical decongestants are lacking. One study randomized groups into five different test groups. Patients met criteria for inclusion if they had symptoms of the common cold including runny nose and nasal congestion, but not specifically sinusitis. The groups consisted of two different combinations of ipratropium and xylometazoline, ipratropium alone, xylometazoline alone, and placebo solution. The study found that patients treated with ipratropium, either alone or in combination, had significantly improved scores for rhinorrhea than those patients on other regimens. Conversely, patients treated with xylometazoline had significantly improved scores for congestion than those patients not receiving this medication. Side effects were comparable between groups with the exception of those patients receiving ipratropium alone or in combination, with a higher reporting of blood-tinged mucus, epistaxis, nasal passage irritation, and nasal dryness [17].

Another study examined mucociliary transport times in patients with acute bacterial rhinosinusitis. All study patients received 3 weeks of antibiotics and received one of five additional treatments: fluticasone propionate, oxymetazoline, 3% sodium chloride, 0.9% sodium chloride solution, and no topical treatment. No significant difference in mucociliary transport times was identified among the five groups after 3 weeks of treatment [27]. The authors concluded that the improvement of bacterial rhinosinusitis likely takes longer than 3 weeks [27].

Antifungal Treatment

Topical

The possible role of fungus in CRS has been recently described [23]. Topical antifungal treatment has gained popularity, partially fueled by previous non-randomized studies on topical amphotericin B that showed an excellent safety profile and efficacy [45]. Recent studies on the clinical effects of topical amphotericin B for CRS have been conflicting. In a double-blind, randomized clinical trial using a total daily dose of 4.8 mg of amphotericin B administered as a nasal spray of 3 mg/ml, four times daily in patients with CRS and nasal polyps compared to nasal saline, the study authors found no statistical difference in CT scores between the two groups and a worse symptom score after treatment with amphotericin for 8 weeks [57]. A separate randomized, placebo controlled study of patients with CRS studied the efficacy of 6 months of amphotericin B irrigation of 20 ml per nostril twice daily at a concentration of 250 µg/ml for a total daily dose of 20 mg amphotericin. At this dose, more than 4 times the previous study, the group found an improvement in CT and endoscopic scores, as well as a decrease in intranasal levels of IL-5 and mucus levels of eosinophil-derived neurotoxin [44].

Several explanations exist for the conflicting results. The study by Ponikau et al. used higher dosage of amphotericin B, delivered at larger intervals (twice daily versus four times a day). Other studies have supported higher concentrations of topical amphotericin B. In one in vitro study, nasal fungus continued

30

to grow when exposed to amphotericin B at 100 μg/ml but was arrested in concentrations of 200 and 300 μg/ml [51]. Additionally, the length of treatment was three times as long in the study by Ponikau et al. Finally, the preparations in the two studies were different with the latter using sterile water and the former using sodium deoxycholate and sodium phosphate buffered with 5% glucose.

In addition to these two groups, others have examined antifungal irrigations. Ricchetti et al. investigated the efficacy of amphotericin B lavage on nasal polyposis. Using 20 ml of 1 ml amphotericin B in 1,000 ml distilled water, twice daily for 4 weeks, they found complete resolution of polyps in 39% of patients without a prior history of sinus surgery and 47% of patients with previous surgery [46]. Another non-randomized, non-controlled study showed improvement or stabilization of disease without side effects in patients treated with fluconazole nasal spray in 12 of 16 patients with AFS [30]. Many of these patients were on other medications including steroids and oral itraconazole, but most improved on 100 mg fluconazole in 500 ml normal saline solution administered as five sprays to each nostril twice daily for 3 months [30].

Oral

Oral antifungal treatment is used by some practitioners for the treatment of AFS and CRS. A recent randomized, double-blind, placebo-controlled study investigating the effect of oral terbinafine in patients with CRS failed to show improvement in radiographic scores, investigator therapeutic evaluations, or sinus symptom scores. This study involved 625 mg/day of terbinafine for a period of 6 and 9 weeks of follow up [33].

Intravenous

Although important in the treatment of invasive fungal sinusitis, there is insufficient literature investigating the use of IV antifungal treatment for CRS or AFS.

Complementary Therapy

Herbal Treatments

A recent meta-analysis investigating various herbal remedies used in rhinosinusitis identified ten randomized, controlled studies in the medical literature. The authors concluded that the use of Sinupret and bromelain may improve the symptoms of either chronic or acute sinusitis [22]. They also concluded that four other remedies (Esberitox, Myrtol, Cineole, and Bi Yuan Shu) may have some positive effect [22].

Sinupret, developed in Germany for sinusitis, is an herbal preparation that comes in both tablet and solution form. It consists of five herbal extracts (*Gentiana lutea*, root; *Primula veris*, flower; *Rumex* sp., herb; *Sambucus nigra*, flower; *Verbena officinalis*, herb). Bromelain, on the other hand, is an extract from the stem and fruit of the pineapple (*Ananas comosus*) and contains a concentration of closely related proteinases [22].

Acupuncture

There has been one recently published study comparing Chinese acupuncture with conventional treatment for sinusitis. In this three-armed, single-blinded, randomized controlled study of 65 patients with chronic sinusitis, conventional treatment was compared to Chinese acupuncture and a control group treated with non-acupoints minimal acupuncture. The treatment in the conventional arm consisted of oral antibiotics, corticosteroids, nasal saline, and topical decongestants. The acupuncture groups received ten bilateral acupoints treatments over a 4-week period. Outcome measures included sinus CT scans, evaluation of symptoms, and health-related quality of life. The study found improvement in the soft tissue swelling on the CT in patients treated with conventional therapy. They also found improvement of symptoms in all groups with a non-statistically significant trend toward further improvement in the conventional treatment compared to both the acupuncture group as well as the non-acupoints group at 4 weeks. At 12 weeks and 12 months, no differences were found in the three groups in symptoms. However, a statistically significant improvement in health-related quality of life at 12 weeks was found in the conventional group. There was no improvement in either of the acupuncture groups [48].

Others

Antihistamines

Oral antihistamines are frequently added to the treatment regimens for patients with allergic rhinitis and CRS. Although shown to have positive effects for the treatment of allergies, there is little evidence to support its use in CRS. One study found that using a non-sedating, prescription antihistamine for CRS increased fatigue scores compared to patients on other remedies [9]. An alternative or addition to oral antihistamine treatment is the use of topical antihistamines. Although the supporting studies for oral and nasal antihistamines have investigated their impact on allergic rhinitis and not CRS, these disorders are often coexisting, making the treatment of both conditions important. In patients with mainly allergic nasal symptoms, an advantage would exist for a medication that is applied directly to the source and has little systemic absorption, should treatment response be similar. The analysis of allergic treatment is beyond the scope of this chapter and the reader is referred to Chap. 21.

Leukotriene Inhibitors

Several studies have looked at the effect of leukotriene inhibitors on sinusitis. One study evaluated 40 patients with sinonasal polyposis and sinusitis treated with zileuton or zafirlukast. Patients continued their other medications in the study and in evaluation after at least 1 month of therapy the study found that 72% of patients had subjective improvement in their symptoms, and objective alleviation or stabilization of nasal polyps was found in 50% of patients [43]. Another study looked at antileukotriene therapy in those patients with sinus symptoms and aspirin triad disease. All patients enrolled had previous sinus surgery and did not receive additional medications for sinusitis in the analysis. Retrospectively, the researchers found that after treatment for 1–15 months, there was a statistically significant reduction in both major and minor symptom scores in patients [55]. These studies, although not randomized or controlled, report good results and suggest that further research on antileukotriene medications in sinusitis is warranted.

Immunotherapy

In a study investigating immunotherapy in patients with AFS and a history of sinus surgery, the study authors found that reoperation rates at an average follow up of 4 years were 33% for those not receiving immunotherapy versus 11% for patients receiving immunotherapy [5]. They also found that office visits requiring medical therapy decreased from 4.79 to 3.17 with the addition of immunotherapy [5].

One recent study retrospectively evaluated the addition of exogenous interferon (IFN) gamma in 10 patients with treatment-resistant CRS. These patients all had presumed dysregulated IFN gamma production. They found that sinusitis symptoms improved in all 9 patients that received the treatment for greater than 3 months [31]. However, during the study period 1 patient discontinued the treatment for "presumed" tremor, 1 patient for neutropenia, and 2 patients required hospitalizations for other infections [31]. Although potential benefits of this treatment may exist, readers are cautioned in advising patients this therapy until additional studies are completed evaluating safety.

Vaccines

A meta-analysis on studies examining the effect of the pneumococcal vaccine on acute sinusitis found no relevant studies published prior to September 2004 [29].

Tips to Avoid Complications

- Oral antibiotics play a role in rhinosinusitis and when possible treatment should be culture directed using the narrowest spectrum and most cost-effective antibiotic.
- Resistant organisms are increasing in prevalence and thus need to be considered as pathogens in rhinosinusitis.
- In select situations intravenous and topical antibiotics may be useful.
- Steroids, both oral and topical, likely play a significant role in the treatment of rhinosinusitis and the potential side effects, particularly of oral treatment, need to be weighed against the benefits.
- Antifungal treatments have increased in popularity yet good, controlled studies are still lacking in order to support this treatment in rhinosinusitis.

- Many patients are looking for herbal and alternative therapies and several have shown promising results, thus they should be considered in the treatment algorithm for patients with rhinosinusitis.
- The treatment of allergies both with immunotherapy and medications likely plays a significant role in many patients with rhinosinusitis.

Take-Home Pearls

- Antibiotics are important in the treatment of rhinosinusitis, but are likely overused. Broader spectrum, newer agents should not be used as first-line treatment in routine cases.
- The success rate of antibiotics is high. However, since many patients get better without treatment, this significantly decreases the intention to treat.
- Intravenous antibiotics may play an important role when other medical or surgical options have failed.
- Topical antibiotics, though often used, have little supporting evidence in the literature.
- Steroids, particularly nasal steroids, play an important role in the treatment of CRS.
- There are few data to support the use of nasal saline, washes, or decongestants in sinusitis.
- Fungus has been suggested to be a contributor, if not a cause of CRS, however, initial study results have been conflicting.
- For patients refractory to traditional therapies or reluctant to use prescription medications there may be a role for complementary or alternative remedies, though more research needs to be done to determine the safety and efficacy.
- The treatment of allergy plays an important role in managing patients with CRS.

References

1. Anand V, Levine H, Friedman M, et al.(2003) Intravenous antibiotics for refractory rhinosinusitis in nonsurgical patients: preliminary findings of a prospective study. Am J Rhinol 17:363–358
2. Anon JB, Jacobs MR, Poole MD, Sinus and Allergy Health Partnership (2004) Antimicrobial treatment guidelines for acute bacterial rhinosinusitis. Otolaryngol Head Neck Surg 130:1–45
3. Aukema AAC, Mulder PGH, Fokkens WJ (2005) Treatment of nasal polyposis and chronic rhinosinusitis with fluticasone propionate nasal drops reduces need for sinus surgery. J Allergy Clin Immunol 115:1017–1023

4. Balk EM, Zucker DR, Engels EA (2001) Strategies for diagnosing and treating suspected acute bacterial sinusitis: a cost-effective analysis. J Gen Intern Med 16:701–711

5. Bassichis BA, Marple BF, Mabry RL, et al.(2001) Use of immunotherapy in previously treated patients with allergic fungal sinusitis. Otolaryngol Head Neck Surg 125:487–490

6. Benninger M, Brook I, Farrell DJ (2006) Disease severity in acute bacterial rhinosinusitis is greater in patients infected with *Streptococcus pneumoniae* than in those infected with *Haemophilus influenzae*. Otolaryngol Head Neck Surg 135:523–528

7. Benninger MS, Payne SC, Ferguson BJ, et al.(2006) Endoscopically directed middle meatal cultures versus maxillary sinus taps in acute bacterial maxillary rhinosinusitis: a meta-analysis. Otolaryngol Head Neck Surg 134:3–9

8. Benninger MS, Sedory Holzer SE, Lau J (2000) Diagnosis and treatment of uncomplicated acute bacterial rhinosinusitis: summary of the Agency for Health Care Policy and Research evidence-based report. Otolaryngol Head Neck Surg 122:1–7

9. Bhattacharyya N, Kepnes LJ (2006) Associations between fatigue and medication use in chronic rhinosinusitis. Ear Nose Throat 85:510–515

10. Bhattacharyya N, Kepnes LJ (1999) The microbiology of recurrent rhinosinusitis after endoscopic sinus surgery. Arch Otolaryngol Head Neck Surg 125:1117–1120

11. Bosker G, Armstrong M, Blair E, et al.(2004) Acute bacterial rhinosinusitis: patient assessment, risk stratification, referral strategies, and outcome-effective antibiotic selection. Primary Care Consensus Reports, March 1–20

12. Boston M, Dobratz EJ, Buescher S, et al.(2003) Effects of nasal saline spray on human neutrophils. Arch Otolaryngol Head Neck Surg 129:660–664

13. Damm M, Jungehulsing M, Eckel HE, et al.(1999) Effects of systemic steroid treatment in chronic polypoid rhinosinusitis evaluated with magnetic resonance imaging. Otolaryngol Head Neck Surg 120:517–523

14. Desrosiers MY, Salas-Prato M (2001) Treatment of chronic rhinosinusitis refractory to other treatments with topical antibiotic therapy delivered by means of a large-particle nebulizer: results of a controlled trial. Otolaryngol Head Neck Surg 125:265–269

15. Desrosiers M, Klossek JM, Benninger M (2006) Management of acute bacterial rhinosinusitis: current issues and future perspectives. Int J Clin Pract 60:190–200

16. Dijkstra MD, Ebbens FA, Poublon RM, et al.(2004) Fluticasone propionate aqueous nasal spray does not influence the recurrence rate of chronic rhinosinusitis and nasal polyps 1 year after functional endoscopic sinus surgery. Clin Exp Allergy 34:1395–1400

17. Eccles R, Pedersen A, et al.(2007) Efficacy and safety of topical combinations of ipratropium and xylometazoline for the treatment of symptoms of runny nose and nasal congestion associated with acute upper respiratory tract infection. Am J Rhinol 21:40–45

18. Fokkens W, Lund V, Bachert C, et al.(2005) EAACI position paper on rhinosinusitis and nasal polyps executive summary. Allergy 60:583–601

19. Friedman M, Vidyasagar R, Joseph N (2006) A randomized, prospective, double-blind study on the efficacy of Dead Sea salt nasal irrigations. Laryngoscope 116:878–882

20. Goh YH, Goode RL (2000) Current status of topical nasal antimicrobial agents. Laryngoscope 110:875–880

21. US Food and Drug Administration (2006) Guidance for industry: sinusitis. Designing clinical development programs of nonantimicrobial drugs for treatment. www.fda.gov/Cder/guidance/7316dft.htm

22. Guo R, Canter PH, Ernst E (2006) Herbal medicines for the treatment of rhinosinusitis: a systematic review. Otolaryngol Head Neck Surg 135:496–506

23. Hamilos DL, Lund VJ (2004) Etiology of chronic rhinosinusitis: the role of fungus. Ann Otol Rhinol Laryngol 113:27–30

24. Herman H (2007) Once-daily administration of intranasal corticosteroids for allergic rhinitis: a comparative review of efficacy, safety, patient preference, and cost. Am J Rhinol 21:70–79

25. Hessler JL, Piccirillo JF, Fang D, et al.(2007) Clinical outcomes of chronic rhinosinusitis in response to medical therapy: results of a prospective study. Am J Rhinol 21:10–18

26. Hwang PH, Woo RJ, Fong KJ (2006) Intranasal deposition of nebulized saline: a radionuclide distribution study. Am J Rhinol 20:255–261

27. Inanli S, Ozturk O, Korkmaz M, et al.(2002) The effects of topical agents of fluticasone propionate, oxymetazoline, and 3% and 0.9% sodium chloride solutions on mucociliary clearance in the therapy of acute bacterial rhinosinusitis in vivo. Laryngoscope 112:320–325

28. Ioannidis JPA, Lau J (2001) Technical report. Evidence for the diagnosis and treatment of acute uncomplicated sinusitis in children: a systematic overview. Pediatrics 108:57–65

29. Ip S, Fu L, Balk E, et al.(2005) Update on acute bacterial rhinosinusitis. Evidence report/technology assessment no. 124. Agency for Healthcare Research and Quality 05-E020-2

30. Jen A, Kacker A, Huang C, et al.(2004) Fluconazole nasal spray in the treatment of allergic fungal sinusitis: a pilot study. Ear Nose Throat J 10:692–695

31. Jyonouchi H, Sun S, Kelly A, et al.(2003) Effects of exogenous interferon gamma on patients with treatment-resistant chronic rhinosinusitis and dysregulated interferon gamma production: a pilot study. Arch Otolaryngol Head Neck Surg 129:563–569

32. Kaszuba SM, Stewart MG (2006) Medical management and diagnosis of chronic rhinosinusitis: a survey of treatment patterns by United States otolaryngologists. Am J Rhinol 20:186–190

33. Kennedy DW, Kuhn FA, Hamilos DL, et al.(2005) Treatment of chronic rhinosinusitis with high-dose oral terbinafine: a double blind, placebo-controlled study. Laryngoscope 115:1793–1799

34. Kobayashi T, Baba S (1992) Topical use of antibiotics for paranasal sinusitis. Rhinol Suppl 14:77–81

35. Landsberg R, Segev Y, DeRowe A, et al.(2007) Systemic corticosteroids for allergic fungal rhinosinusitis and chronic rhinosinusitis with nasal polyposis: a comparative study. Otolaryngol Head Neck Surg 136:252–257

36. Leonard DW, Bolger WE (1999) Topical antibiotic therapy for recalcitrant sinusitis. Laryngoscope 109:668–670

37. Lin JW, Kacker A, Anand VK, et al.(2005) Catheter- and antibiotic-related complications of ambulatory intravenous antibiotic therapy for chronic refractory rhinosinusitis. Am J Rhinol 19:365–369

38. Manarey CR, Anand VK, Huang C (2004) Incidence of methicillin-resistant *Staphylococcus aureus* causing chronic rhinosinusitis. Laryngoscope 114:939–941

39. Marple BF, Brunton S, Ferguson BJ (2006) Acute bacterial rhinosinusitis: a review of US treatment guidelines. Otolaryngol Head Neck Surg 135:341–348

40. Meltzer EO, Bachert C, Staudinger H (2006) Treating acute rhinosinusitis: comparing efficacy and safety of mometasone furoate nasal spray, amoxicillin, and placebo. J Allergy Clin Immunol 116:1289–1295

41. Miller TR, Muntz HR, Gilbert E, et al.(2004) Comparison of topical medication delivery systems after sinus surgery. Laryngoscope 114:201–204

42. Olson DE, Rasgon BM, Hilsinger RL (2002) Radiographic comparison of three methods for nasal saline irrigation. Laryngoscope 112:1394–1398

43. Parnes SM, Chuma AV (2000) Acute effects of antileukotrienes on sinonasal polyposis and sinusitis. Ear Nose Throat J 79:18

44. Ponikau JU, Sherris DA, Weaver A, et al.(2005) Treatment of chronic rhinosinusitis with intranasal amphotericin B: a randomized, placebo-controlled, double-blind pilot trial. J Allergy Clin Immunol 115:125–131

45. Ponikau JU, Sherris DA, Kita H, et al.(2002) Intranasal antifungal treatment in 51 patients with chronic rhinosinusitis. J Allergy Clin Immunol 110:862–868

46. Ricchetti A, Landis BN, Maffioli A, et al.(2002) Effect of antifungal nasal lavage with amphotericin B on nasal polyposis. J Laryngol Otol 116:261–263

47. Riechelmann H, Deutschle T, Stuhlmiller A, et al.(2004) Nasal toxicity of benzalkonium chloride. Am J Rhinol 18:291–299

48. Rossberg E, Larsson PG, Birkeflet O, et al.(2005) Comparison of traditional Chinese acupuncture, minimal acupuncture at non-acupoints and conventional treatment for chronic sinusitis. Complement Ther Med 13:4–10

49. Rowe-Jones JM, Medcalf M, Durham SR, et al.(2005) Functional endoscopic sinus surgery: 5 year follow up and results of a prospective, randomized, stratified, double-blind, placebo-controlled study of postoperative fluticasone propionate aqueous nasal spray. Rhinology 43:2–10

50. Sharp HJ, Denman D, Puumala S, et al.(2007) Treatment of acute and chronic rhinosinusitis in the United States, 1999–2002. Arch Otolaryngol Head Neck Surg 133:260–265

51. Shirazi MA, Stankiewica JA, Kammeyer P (2007) Activity of nasal amphotericin B irrigation against fungal organisms in vitro. Am J Rhinol 21:145–148

52. Sykes DA, Wilson R, Chan KI, et al.(1986) Relative importance of antibiotics and improved clearance in topical treatment of chronic mucopurulent rhinosinusitis: a controlled study. Lancet 2(8503):359–360

53. Tang A, Frazee B (2003) Antibiotic treatment for acute maxillary sinusitis. Ann Emerg Med 42:705–708

54. Tomooka LT, Murphy C, Davidson TM (2000) Clinical study and literature review of nasal irrigation. Laryngoscope 110:1189–1193

55. Ulualp SO, Sterman BM, Toohill RJ (1999) Antileukotriene therapy for the relief of sinus symptoms in aspirin triad disease. Ear Nose Throat J 78:604

56. Wald ER, Bordley WC, Darrow DH (2001) Clinical practice guidelines: management of sinusitis. Pediatrics 108:798–808

57. Weschta M, Rimek D, Formanek M, et al.(2004) Topical antifungal treatment of chronic rhinosinusitis with nasal polyps: a randomized, double-blind clinical trial. J Allergy Clin Immunol 113:1122–1128

58. Whatley WS, Chandra RK, MacDonald CB (2006) Systemic absorption of gentamicin nasal irrigations. Am J Rhinol 20:251–254

59. Williams Jr JW, Aguilar C, Cornell J, et al.(2003) Antibiotics for acute maxillary sinusitis. Cochrane Database of Systematic Reviews 2:CD000243

60. Wilschanski M, Yahav Y, Yaacov Y, et al.(2003) Gentamicin-induced correction of CFTR function in patients with cystic fibrosis and CFTR stop mutations. NEJM 349:1433–1441

61. Zalmanovici A, Yaphe J (2007) Steroids for acute sinusitis. Cochrane Database of Systematic Reviews 2:CD005149

Lacrimal Drainage System and Orbit

Chapter 31

Management of Nasolacrimal Duct Obstruction

31

Douglas D. Reh, Ralph B. Metson, and Raj Sindwani

Core Messages

■ Endoscopic surgery for lacrimal outflow obstruction is a safe and effective alternative to traditional external dacryocystorhinostomy (DCR) surgery in most patients, and offers the advantages of excellent visualization, the ability to thoroughly evaluate the location and size of the rhinostomy site, and the avoidance of a facial scar.

■ A variety of endoscopic techniques for DCR have been described, with all focusing on the atraumatic creation of a generous bony rhinostomy on the superolateral nasal wall.

■ Endoscopic DCR offers success rates comparable to those achieved through external approaches.

■ Complications during DCR surgery are best avoided by precisely identifying the location of the lacrimal apparatus intranasally, using key landmarks including the maxillary line and superior middle turbinate attachment.

■ The technical skills and instrumentation required for performing endoscopic DCR are similar to those used for routine endoscopic sinus surgery (ESS).

Contents

Introduction

Intranasal approaches to correct nasolacrimal duct (NLD) obstruction were first described over a century ago [1–3]. These techniques were limited because they provided poor visualization of the lacrimal sac in the superior nasal cavity and lacked effective instrumentation to adequately open the sac. Consequently dacryocystorhinostomy (DCR) was performed predominately with an external approach [4, 5]. With the introduction of endoscopic techniques for surgery of the paranasal sinuses, these limitations have been overcome. Since the early 1990s, there has been renewed interest in performing both primary and revision DCR via an intranasal endoscopic approach [6–8]. In addition to avoiding a skin incision, endoscopic DCR enables the surgeon to identify and correct common intranasal causes of DCR failure, such as adhesions, an obstructing middle turbinate, or an infected ethmoid sinus.

Patient Evaluation

Nasolacrimal duct obstruction can present with a variety of symptoms, including epiphora, dacryocystitis, bloody tears, and medial canthal swelling. Table 31.1 summarizes the causes of NLD obstruction. Primary NLD obstruction was described by Linberg and McCormick in 1986 as a narrowing of the NLD caused by fibrosis or inflammation without any precipitating etiology [9]. Secondary NDL obstruction is caused by a known etiology and can be classified as mechanical, traumatic, inflammatory, infectious, or neoplastic [10]. Not all patients with NLD obstruction have an anatomic obstruction of the NLD. Some patients who present with epiphora will have a patent NLD on irrigation of the duct indicative of a functional obstruction.

Nasal endoscopy is an important part of the preoperative assessment in patients undergoing endoscopic DCR. The inferior meatus is inspected for any masses that could cause obstruction of the NDL orifice. A septal deviation or enlarged middle turbinate which may need to be addressed at the time of endoscopic DCR should also be noted. Computerized tomography (CT) of the paranasal sinuses can be performed prior to endoscopic DCR to delineate sinus anatomy and identify any disease

Table 31.1 Causes of nasolacrimal duct obstruction

Inflammatory	Infectious	Trauma/iatrogenic	Neoplasms
Wegener's granulomatosis	Staphylococcus	Naso-orbito-ethmoid fracture	Eyelid cancer (basal cell carcinoma/squamous cell carcinoma)
Sarcoid	Actinomyces	Functional endoscopic sinus surgery	Benign papillomas
Histiocytosis	Streptococcus	Rhinoplasty	Primary lacrimal sac tumor
Scleroderma	Pseudomonas	Orbital decompression	Transitional cell
Kawasaki disease	Chlamydia	Radiation therapy	Fibrous histiocytoma
	Bacteroides	Chemotherapy (5-fluorouracil)	Lymphoma
	Epstein-Barr virus		
	Human papillomavirus		
	Ascaris		
	Leprosy		
	Tuberculosis		

not recognized on physical examination. Both axial and coronal scans are preferred. Anterior ethmoid air cells which overlie the lacrimal sac and need to be opened at the time of surgery are found in over 90% of patients. Magnetic resonance scans are not generally obtained because they are unable to image the thin bony sinus partitions.

Primary endoscopic DCR may be indicated in the management of either primary or secondary acquired NDL obstruction. Generally, this procedure is indicated when the level of obstruction is determined to be at or distal to the junction of the lacrimal sac and duct. Endoscopic DCR performed on a dilated lacrimal sac yields the best results. Endoscopic DCR is also useful in the management of lacrimal duct injuries associated with sinus surgery or facial trauma as well as in certain patients with atypical forms of congenital dacryostenosis.

Anatomy

Tears pass through the eyelid puncta and enter the superior and inferior canaliculi oriented at right angles to the lid. The vertical portions of the canaliculi course for 2 mm before turning at right angles and moving parallel to the lid for 8 mm. There is some variability in the way that the superior and inferior canaliculi unite. They may join the sac separately or converge into a common canaliculus. At this junction lies the valve of Rosenmüller, a flap of mucosa that prevents reflux of tears back into the canaliculi.

The inferior end of the lacrimal sac tapers to form the lacrimal duct as it enters the nasolacrimal canal formed by the maxillary, lacrimal, and inferior turbinate bones. The NDL runs within this osseous canal for a distance of approximately 12 mm. It continues beneath the inferior turbinate as a membranous duct for an additional 5 mm before opening into the inferior meatus. The duct orifice is found at the junction of the middle and anterior third of the meatus, approximately 8 mm behind the anterior tip of the inferior turbinate and 29 mm from the anterior nasal spine. It is often covered by a flap of mucosa, known as Hasner's valve, which is thought to prevent reflux of nasal secretions. Gentle pressure over the medial canthal region will often produce fluid or bubbles at the duct orifice to confirm its location.

From an endoscopic, intranasal perspective, the lacrimal sac can be found beneath the bone of the lateral nasal wall just anterior to the attachment of the middle turbinate (Fig. 31.1). The long axis of the lacrimal sac is approximately 12 mm in length. The maxillary line is an essential landmark for endoscopic DCR (Fig. 31.2). It is readily identified as a curvilinear eminence along the lateral nasal wall which runs from the anterior attachment of the middle turbinate to the root of the inferior turbinate (Fig. 31.3). Its location corresponds to the suture line between the maxillary and lacrimal bones which runs in a vertical direction through the lacrimal fossa. The maxillary line bisects the lacrimal sac such that the frontal process of the maxilla covers the anterior half of the sac, and the thin lacrimal bone covers the posterior half. The uncinate process lies just medial to the lacrimal sac and must be removed in order to access the thin lacrimal bone covering the posterior portion of the sac. In contrast, exposure of the anterior sac necessitates removal of thicker bone located just anterior to the maxillary line. As the NLD courses inferiorly, it passes an average of 10 mm (range 8–17 mm) anterior to the natural ostium of the maxillary sinus.

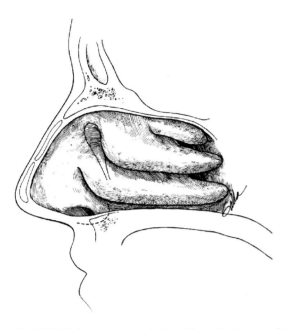

Fig. 31.1 The lacrimal sac can be found beneath the bone of the lateral nasal wall just anterior to the attachment of the middle turbinate

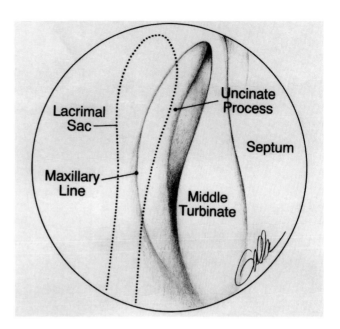

Fig. 31.2 The maxillary line bisects the lacrimal sac such that the frontal process of the maxilla covers the anterior half of the sac, and the thin lacrimal bone beneath the uncinate process covers the posterior half

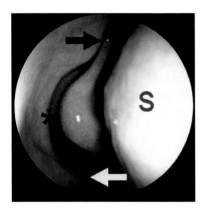

Fig. 31.3 Endoscopic view of right lateral nasal wall showing the maxillary line (*asterisk*), a curvilinear eminence along the lateral nasal wall which runs from the anterior attachment of the middle turbinate (*black arrow*) to the root of the inferior turbinate (*yellow arrow*). S septum

Surgical Technique

Anesthesia and Nasal Preparation

Endoscopic DCR may be performed under either local or general anesthesia, depending on the medical condition of the patient and preference of the surgeon. The authors perform most of their endoscopic DCRs under general anesthesia to ensure patient comfort. A scleral shield is placed over the operative eye at the start of surgery to protect the cornea.

With the patient supine and the head slightly elevated to decrease venous pressure at the operative site, the nose is sprayed with oxymetazoline 0.05% to initiate decongestion of the nasal mucosa. Using a 4-mm-diameter 0-degree endoscope for direct visualization of the lateral nasal wall, endoscopic injection of 1% Xylocaine containing 1:100,000 epinephrine is performed just anterior to the attachment of the middle turbinate. Pledgets soaked in 4% cocaine solution are then placed along the lateral nasal wall and middle meatus to further allow mucosal decongestion.

Mucosal Incision

Surgical dissection is begun with removal of the uncinate process located posterior to the maxillary line (Fig. 31.4). An air space is often entered which corresponds to the infundibulum or an anterior ethmoid air cell overlying the lacrimal sac. Next

31

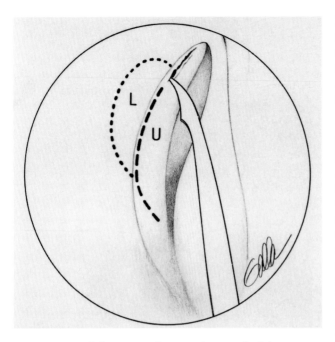

Fig. 31.4 Surgical dissection is begun with removal of the uncinate process (*L*) located posterior to the maxillary line. An incision is next made in the mucosa on the lateral wall along the maxillary line over the lacrimal sac (*L*)

an incision is made in the mucosa on the lateral wall using a sickle knife, blade, or electrocautery and elevated using a Freer elevator. It is helpful to place this incision well anterior to the location of the lacrimal sac to allow for full exposure of the overlying bone. After the mucosa is widely elevated from the underlying bone, Blakesley forceps are used to remove an approximately 1-cm-diameter circle of mucosa along the lateral nasal wall overlying the lacrimal sac.

Bone Removal

To expose the lacrimal sac, the bony lacrimal fossa must be uncovered. Bone removal may be achieved using a variety of instruments and should commence at the maxillary line, proceeding anteriorly. Surgical navigation may be used to identify the location of the lacrimal fossa and sac along the lateral nasal wall, but it is generally not necessary (Fig. 31.5). Although the lacrimal bone, located posterior to the maxillary line, may be taken down with minimal force, the authors recommend the use of a high-speed drill with a cutting burr (supplemented by bone rongeurs) for removal of the dense frontal process of the maxilla which is situated anteriorly (Fig. 31.6). Exposure of the sac is confirmed by movement of a lacrimal probe which has been passed by the assistant through a canaliculus into the sac.

Regardless of the technique selected, a bony rhinostomy of adequate size and location will facilitate a successful outcome.

It is particularly important that the bone overlying the location of the common canaliculus is completely resected. The lacrimal duct probe can be used to palpate the lacrimal sac internally and delineate its boundaries to ensure adequate bone removal. A rhinostomy with a vertical dimension of 8–10 mm is generally achieved in adult patients.

Opening of the Lacrimal Sac

After removal of the overlying bone, the lacrimal sac is incised using a sickle knife (Fig. 31.7). It is often helpful for the assistant to "tent out" the medial wall of the lacrimal sac with the previously inserted lacrimal probe. The medial wall of the lacrimal sac may then be removed with Blakesley forceps and submitted for separate histopathologic examination to rule out neoplasm as an etiology for the NLD obstruction. An adequate rhinostomy should easily permit the passage of lacrimal probes. Removal of the medial wall of the lacrimal sac in the area of the common canaliculus may also be confirmed by direct visualization of the internal common punctum with a 0- or 30-degree endoscope. Exposure and visualization of the common punctum of the lacrimal sac is an essential step for a successful endoscopic DCR.

Lacrimal System Intubation

After the medial sac wall has been resected, a bicanalicular tube is placed by intubating both canaliculi, with subsequent retrieval of the probes from the rhinostomy site endoscopically (Fig. 31.8). The tubing is then tied at the nasal vestibule forming a closed loop and in such a way as to allow the appropriate length and tension of the silicone tubing at the medial canthus. The closed loop acts as a stent for the newly created rhinostomy (Fig. 31.9). The stents are usually removed at 6 weeks postoperatively, but intervals for stent removal ranging from 4 weeks to 6 months have been advocated by others [11–13].

Mitomycin C and Adjunctive Procedures

Some surgeons elect to apply topical mitomycin C to the intranasal rhinostomy site. Mitomycin C is an antimetabolite that inhibits fibroblast function and has been employed to modulate postsurgical fibrosis in a variety of applications. Reports on the utility of mitomycin C in prevention of postoperative mucosal fibrosis and rhinostomy closure have demonstrated mixed results [14–17]. If used, mitomycin C is applied to the rhinostomy site in a concentration of 0.4 mg/ml using a cotton sponge, for a period of 4 min, after which copious saline irrigation is performed.

As noted earlier, concomitant ethmoidectomy may be required to provide adequate access to the anterior lacrimal sac. Other procedures, including uncinectomy, middle turbinectomy, and septoplasty, may also facilitate exposure of the lateral nasal wall. The frequency with which these procedures are performed, as described in several reports, is summarized in Table 31.2.

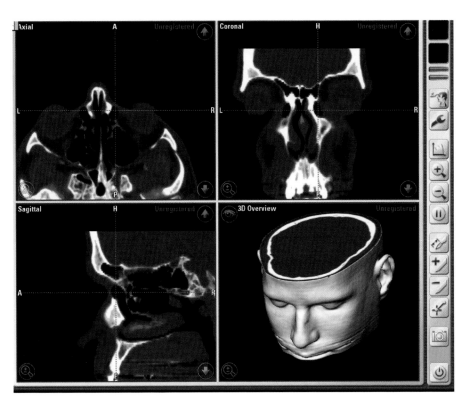

Fig. 31.5 Localization of lacrimal fossa and sac in three dimensions using an image guidance system. (Kolibri system, BrainLAB AG, Munich, Germany)

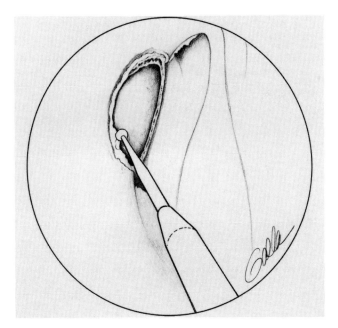

Fig. 31.6 A high-speed drill with a cutting burr is used to remove the dense frontal process of the maxilla which overlies the anterior portion of the lacrimal sac

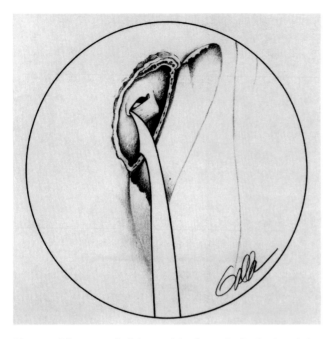

Fig. 31.7 After removal of the overlying bone, the lacrimal sac is incised using a sickle knife

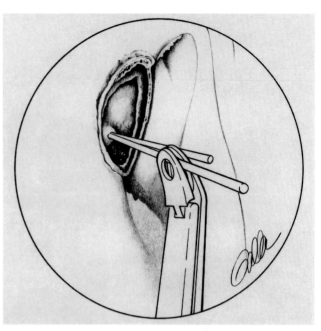

Fig. 31.8 After the medial sac wall has been resected, a bicanalicular tube is placed by intubating both canaliculi, with subsequent retrieval of the probes from the rhinostomy site endoscopically

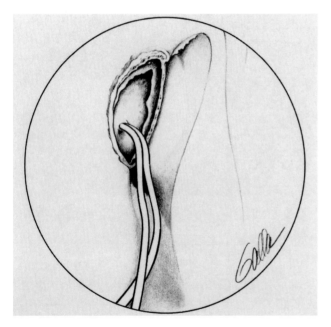

Fig. 31.9 The closed loop acts as stent for the newly created rhinostomy

Table 31.2 Endoscopic DCR adjunctive procedures

Reference	Septoplasty (%)	Ethmoidectomy (%)	Middle turbinectomy (%)
[30]	4	52	24
[27]	NS	NS	24.5
[31]	33	33	58
[13]	5	10	20
[32]	5	78	33

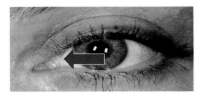

Fig. 31.10 Image of left eye following endoscopic DCR. *Arrow* demonstrates Silastic stent in superior and inferior punctae

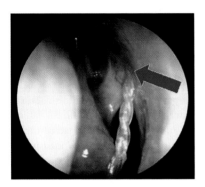

Fig. 31.11 Endoscopic intranasal view 3 weeks postoperatively, showing stent exiting the healed rhinostomy site (*arrow*) along left lateral nasal wall

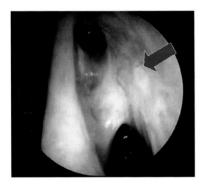

Fig. 31.12 Endoscopic view in same patient after stent removal demonstrating flow of fluorescein through the rhinostomy (*arrow*)

Postoperative Care

If nasal packing is placed for hemostasis at the conclusion of surgery, it is removed the following day. Patients are discharged with instructions to begin twice daily nasal saline irrigations with a bulb syringe. Any remaining intranasal debris is removed from the operative site at the first postoperative visit 1 week following surgery. The Silastic tubing used to stent the surgical ostium is typically removed 6 weeks after surgery by cutting the exposed tubing at the medial canthus and withdrawing it through the nose (Figs. 31.10, 31.11). It may be removed sooner if excessive granulation tissue formation is seen to occur around the tube at the ostium. Patency of the lacrimal drainage system is verified by endoscopic observation of fluorescein dye flowing from the eye through the surgical ostium into the nose (Fig. 31.12).

Surgical Results

The reported outcomes of endoscopic DCR and related procedures are summarized in Table 31.3. The success rates of primary endoscopic DCR in several recent series exceed those obtained in earlier reports, and in some cases match the 85–95% success rates obtained with external DCR [18–20]. The recently reported improvement in surgical outcomes may reflect a collective "learning curve" effect among surgeons performing this procedure. The existence of such a learning curve is supported by a report by Onerci et al., who noted that an endoscopic DCR success rate of 94% in the hands of experienced surgeons drops to only 58% when performed by inexperienced surgeons [21].

Several groups have recently attempted to identify other factors which may influence the success rate of endoscopic DCR in selected patients. A better understanding of the endoscopic anatomy when performing DCR may contribute to improvements in surgical outcomes. Wormald et al. determined that a majority of the lacrimal sac lies above the insertion of the middle turbinate [22]. The authors pointed out that insufficient removal of bone superior to this insertion and a subsequent lack of adequate exposure and opening of the lacrimal sac might represent a primary cause of failure in endoscopic DCR. Exposure of the common canaliculus is an important predictor of success in this surgery.

Wormald and Tsirbas noted a success rate of 97% in patients with anatomic obstruction, but only 84% in patients with functional outflow impairment [23]. Yung and co-workers looked at surgical success as a function of the level of obstruction [24]. They noted success rates of 93% for patients with obstruction at the level of the lacrimal sac or NDL as opposed to 88% and 54% for obstruction at the level of the common canaliculus or canaliculi, respectively.

Surgical Complications

The most common complication of endoscopic DCR is failure of the procedure with persistence of epiphora [25]. This may result from fibrous occlusion of the rhinostomy site or the presence of synechiae between the lateral nasal wall and middle turbinate or nasal septum. In other cases, the ostium may be patent but too small to provide efficient tear drainage. Failure to open the entire portion of the lacrimal sac satisfactorily may result in continued

31

Table 31.3 Results of primary endoscopic DCR

Author(s)	Reference	Year	Number	Success rate (%)
Tripathi et al.	[33]	2002	46	89
Tsirbas and Wormald	[34]	2003	44	89
Massegur et al.	[35]	2004	96	93
Fayet et al.	[25]	2004	300	87
Durvasula and Gatland	[36]	2004	70	92
Wormald and Tsirbas	[23]	2004	70	97
Javate and Pamintuan	[37]	2005	117	98

epiphora due to accumulation of lacrimal debris in the residual sac (lacrimal sump syndrome) [26]. Similarly, an unrecognized lacrimal sac diverticulum that is incompletely drained via the intranasal approach may cause persistent discharge or infection. Other potential complications include orbital injury, postoperative bleeding, and sinusitis.

Revision Endoscopic Dacryocystorhinostomy

Endoscopic revision DCR is indicated in patients in whom primary external or endoscopic DCR has failed. In these patients an endoscopic nasal examination should be performed in order to identify potential causes of failure such as a deviated septum, an obstructing middle turbinate, or adhesions between the middle turbinate and rhinostomy. Patients who have failed DCR should also be evaluated in order to rule out an obstruction proximal to the sac, such as canalicular stenosis. Failure attributable to an obstruction proximal to the lacrimal sac can be corrected by performance of an endoscopic conjunctival DCR in which a Pyrex Jones tube is inserted through an incision in the caruncle at the medial canthus [27].

Endoscopic revision DCR is technically easier to perform than primary DCR because the bone overlying the lacrimal sac has already been removed. For this reason, endoscopic revision DCR is an appropriate initial case for surgeons who wish to become proficient in endoscopic DCR. During revision surgery a fibrous membrane will often be seen occluding the previously created internal DCR ostium. Gentle manipulation of a probe passed through the canaliculus into the sac will usually allow determination of the extent of the previous opening, as well as identification of any residual bone requiring removal. The bony rhinostomy may be further enlarged with rongeurs or a high-speed drill to create a generous bony rhinostomy with adequate exposure of the lacrimal sac. Fibrous tissue occluding the ostium is identified and "tented" into the nasal cavity with probes passed through both canaliculi to provide a broad soft tissue region under tension. This tissue is then incised with a sickle knife and the probes are visualized. The edge of the incised mucosa is grasped with straight or angled Blakesley forceps and removed.

During revision DCR surgery, distinct anatomic structures such as nasal mucosa, the lacrimal sac medial wall, the lateral portion of the lacrimal sac containing the internal common punctum, and orbital soft tissues are often incorporated into a zone of scar tissue occluding the ostium. The surgeon should closely observe the medial commissure while gentle traction is placed on the tissue to be removed at the rhinostomy site. Excessive movement of the medial commissure with this maneuver may signify that deeper tissues than desired are being grasped by the forceps and care must be taken here to avoid injury to the aforementioned structures.

Success rates for endoscopic revision DCR outcomes (75–85%) are lower than those reported for primary endoscopic DCRs (85–95%) and similar to those of external revision DCRs (80–85%) [28, 29].

Conclusions

Endoscopic surgery for lacrimal outflow obstruction is a safe and effective alternative to traditional external DCR surgery in most patients. Endoscopic DCR is particularly advantageous in patients with concomitant sinonasal disease, patients with a previous history of radiation therapy, pediatric patients, and in revision procedures. Advantages include: excellent visualization, the ability to thoroughly evaluate the location and size of the rhinostomy site, and the avoidance of a facial scar. Recent studies suggest that the success rates of endoscopic DCR are comparable to those achieved through external approaches.

Tips to Avoid Complications

- Successful surgery is predicated upon the accurate localization and identification of the lacrimal sac using key landmarks including the maxillary line and superior middle turbinate attachment.

- Tenting the medial wall of the lacrimal sac with intracanalicular probes while the sac is incised avoids damage to the lateral sac wall and deeper elements of the lacrimal apparatus.
- Evaluating the position and integrity of the middle turbinate at the conclusion of the procedure to avoid lateralization of this structure postoperatively is important in avoiding secondary obstruction of the surgical rhinostomy.
- Meticulous surgical technique that minimizes adjacent mucosal trauma which can lead to synechia formation and contribute to poor outcomes. This is especially important during bone removal.

Take-Home Pearls

- Endoscopic surgery for lacrimal outflow obstruction is a safe and effective.
- Advantages of E-DCR include excellent visualization, the ability to thoroughly evaluate the precise location and size of the rhinostomy site, and the avoidance of a facial scar.
- E-DCR offers success rates comparable to those achieved through external approaches.

References

1. Caldwell GW (1893) Two new operations for obstruction of the nasal duct, with preservation of the canaliculi. Am J Ophthalmol 10:189–192
2. West JM (1914) A window resection of the nasal duct in cases of stenosis. Trans Am Ophthalmol Soc 12:654
3. Mosher HP (1921) Re-establishing intranasal drainage of the lacrimal sac. Laryngoscope 31:492–521
4. Toti A (1904) Nuovo metodod conservatore di cura radicale delle suppurazioni croniche del sacco lacrimale (dacriocistorhinostomia). Clin Moderna 10:385–387
5. Dupuy-Dutemps L, Bouquet M (1921) Procede plastique de dacryocystorhinostomie et ses resulats. Ann D'Oculist 158:241–261
6. Metson R (1990) The endoscopic approach for revision dacryocystorhinostomy. Laryngoscope 100:1344–1347
7. Massaro BM, Gonnering RS, Harris GJ (1990) Endonasal laser dacryocystorhinostomy: a new approach to nasolacrimal duct obstruction. Arch Ophthalmol 108:1172–1176
8. McDonogh M (1992) Endoscopic transnasal dacryocystorhinostomy: results in 21 patients. S Afr J Surg 30:107–110
9. Linberg JV, McCormick SA (1986) Primary acquired nasolacrimal duct obstruction. A clinicopathologic report and biopsy technique. Ophthalmology 93:1055–1063
10. Bartley GB (1992) Acquired lacrimal drainage obstruction: an etiologic classification system, case reports, and a review of the literature. Part 1. Ophthal Plast Reconstr Surg 8:237–242
11. Tutton MK, O'Donnell NP (1995) Endonasal laser dacryocystorhinostomy under direct vision. Eye 9:485–487
12. Yung MW, Hardman-Lea S (1998) Endoscopic inferior dacryocystorhinostomy. Clin Otolaryngol Allied Sci 23:152–157
13. Mortimore S, Banhegy GY, Lancaster JL, et al.(1999) Endoscopic dacryocystorhinostomy without silicone stenting. J R Coll Surg Edinb 44:371–373
14. Deka A, Bhattacharjee K, Bhuyan SK, et al.(2006) Effect of mitomycin C on ostium in dacryocystorhinostomy. Clin Exp Ophthalmol 34:557–561
15. Chan KO, Gervais M, Tsaparas Y, et al.(2006) Effectiveness of intraoperative mitomycin C in maintaining the patency of a frontal sinusotomy: a preliminary report of a double-blind randomized placebo-controlled trial. Am J Rhinol 20:295–299
16. Zilelioglu G, Ugurbas SH, Anadolu Y, et al.(1998) Adjunctive use of mitomycin C on endoscopic lacrimal surgery. Br J Ophthalmol 82:63–66
17. Camara JG, Bengzon AU, Henson RD The safety and efficacy of mitomycin C in endonasal endoscopic laser-assisted dacryocystorhinostomy. Ophthal Plast Reconstr Surg 16:114–118
18. Tsirbas A, Davis G, Wormald PJ (2004) Mechanical endonasal dacryocystorhinostomy versus external dacryocystorhinostomy. Ophthal Plast Reconstr Surg 20:50–56
19. Apaydin KC, Fisenk F, Karayalcin B, et al.(2004) Endoscopic transnasal dacryocystorhinostomy and bicanalicular silicone tube intubation. Ophthalmologica 218:306–311
20. Metson R, Woog JJ, Puliafito CA (1994) Endoscopic laser dacryocystorhinostomy. Laryngoscope 104:269–274
21. Onerci M, Orhan M, Ogretmenoglu O, et al.(2000) Long-term results and reasons for failure of intranasal endoscopic dacryocystorhinostomy. Acta Otolaryngol 120:319–322
22. Wormald PJ, Kew J, Van Hasselt A (2000) Intranasal anatomy of the nasolacrimal sac in endoscopic dacryocystorhinostomy. Otolaryngol Head Neck Surg 123:307–310
23. Wormald PJ, Tsirbas A (2004) Investigation of endoscopic treatment for functional and anatomical obstruction of the nasolacrimal duct system. Clin Otolaryngol Allied Sci 29:352–356
24. Yung MW, Hardman-Lea S (2002) Analysis of the results of surgical endoscopic dacryocystorhinostomy: effect of the level of obstruction. Br J Ophthalmol 86:792–794
25. Fayet B, Racy E, Assouline M (2004) Complications of standardized endonasal dacryocystorhinostomy with unciformectomy. Ophthalmology 111:837–845
26. Migliori ME (1997) Endoscopic evaluation and management of the lacrimal sump syndrome. Ophthal Plast Reconstr Surg 13:281–284
27. Metson R (1991) Endoscopic surgery for lacrimal obstruction. Otolaryngol Head Neck Surg 104:473–479
28. Tsirbas A, Davis G, Wormald PJ (2005) Revision dacryocystorhinostomy: a comparison of endoscopic and external techniques. Am J Rhinol 19:322–325
29. El-Guindy A, Dorgham A, Ghoraba M (2000) Endoscopic revision surgery for recurrent epiphora occurring after external dacryocystorhinostomy. Ann Otol Rhinol Laryngol 109:425–430

30. Rice DH (1990) Endoscopic intranasal dacryocystorhinostomy results in four patients. Arch Otolaryngol Head Neck Surg 116:1061

31. Sadiq SA, Hugkulstone CE, Jones NS, et al.(1996) Endoscopic holmium:YAG laser dacryocystorhinostomy. Eye 10:43–46

32. Mortimore S, Banhegy GY, Lancaster JL, et al.(1999) Endoscopic dacryocystorhinostomy without silicone stenting. J R Coll Surg Edinb 44:371–373

33. Tripathi A, Lesser TH, O'Donnell NP, et al.(2002) Local anaesthetic endonasal endoscopic laser dacryocystorhinostomy: analysis of patients' acceptability and various factors affecting the success of this procedure. Eye 16:146–149

34. Tsirbas A, Wormald PJ (2003) Endonasal dacryocystorhinostomy with mucosal flaps. Am J Ophthalmol 135:76–83

35. Massegur H, Trias E, Adema JM (2004) Endoscopic dacryocystorhinostomy: modified technique. Otolaryngol Head Neck Surg 130:39–46

36. Durvasula VS, Gatland DJ (2004) Endoscopic dacryocystorhinostomy: long-term results and evolution of surgical technique. J Laryngol Otol 118:628–632

37. Javate R, Pamintuan F (2005) Endoscopic radiofrequency-assisted dacryocystorhinostomy with double stent: a personal experience. Orbit 24:15–22

31

Chapter 32

Conventional and Endoscopic Approaches to the Orbit and Optic Nerve

32

Kevin Christopher McMains and Stilianos E. Kountakis

Core Messages

- The visual axis can be threatened by several pathologies.
- The options for access to the orbit and optic nerve include intracranial, extracranial open, and extracranial endoscopic approaches.
- Endoscopic approaches may provide access to the orbit and optic nerve with minimal morbidity.

Contents

Introduction

Insults to our visual axis not only threaten that organ system, but also endanger the pathway on which we most rely for contact with the outside world. Threats to this axis can arise from within the globe itself, within the orbit, along the path of the optic nerve, and along the optic tracts to the visual cortex. Possible causes of visual injury include traumatic, infectious, neoplastic, and autoimmune processes. Surgical treatment of several entities has provided opportunity to preserve or improve function of this organ system. This chapter will present several potential surgical approaches to the orbit and optic nerve as well as the significant risks associated with them. It will also review data on traumatic optic neuropathy and discuss the approaches associated with it, as these approaches to the optic nerve can be applied to other clinical entities as well.

Trauma to the Visual Axis

The optic nerve is injured in 0.5–1.5% of cases of closed head injury [1] and between 0.7% and 5% of overall head trauma [2, 3]. Common injuries resulting in traumatic optic neuropathy (TON) include a blow to the ipsilateral brow or forehead, motor vehicle accident (MVA), a bicycle accident, or a fall [4–6]. The incidence of optic canal fracture is reported to be between 6% and 92% of cases of traumatic blindness [5]. Up to one-third of orbital trauma in the USA results from domestic violence or sexual assault [7]. Many authors have suggested theories of the mechanisms and contributing causes, though the precise pathophysiology of and optimal treatment modalities for TON continue to be elusive. Understanding of the regional anatomy, possible mechanisms of injury, imaging and other diagnostic tests, as well as the full range of surgical and non-surgical treatment strategies is essential in forming optimal treatment strategies for specific patient's conditions.

32

Anatomy/Physiology

The optic nerve is a fiber tract of brain white matter, rather than a cranial nerve in the strictest sense. From the retina, afferent fibers course posteriorly into the bony optic canal. This structure begins anteriorly at the posterosuperior bony orbit and courses posteriorly through the lesser wing of the sphenoid. At the anterior entry to the canal, the circumferential fibers of the annulus of Zinn surround the optic nerve. Orbital muscles attach to the annulus of Zinn posteriorly and pass anteriorly through a complicated ligamentous support network within tendinous sheaths to attach to the globe. Contents of the optic canal include the optic nerve, ophthalmic artery, postganglionic sympathetic fibers, and meningeal extensions. Posterior to the bony canal, optic nerves interdigitate at the optic chiasm, then continue posteriorly to the lateral geniculate nuclei and the primary visual cortex. The intraorbital segment of the optic nerve is surrounded by fat and a complex tendinous network allowing some limited motion. However, within the optic canal, the optic nerve dura fuses with the periorbita and fixes the position of the nerve with an intact canal [8]. If shearing forces are applied or swelling occurs, the fixed cross-sectional area of the bony canal places the nerve at risk for secondary ischemic injury [3]. While the ophthalmic artery generally courses laterally to the optic nerve within the optic canal, in 16% of cases it travels medial to the nerve (Fig. 32.1) [9]. Dehiscence of the optic nerve within the sphenoid sinus has been reported in 4% of cases [10], and may be present in up to 25% of cases in which an Onodi cell (posterolateral sphenoid cell) is present [11].

In trauma, injury to the nerve can be either direct or indirect. Direct injuries involve division of the optic nerve by laceration or complete transection. Indirect injury can result from compression, hemorrhage, ischemia, or oxidative damage. Often, direct injury via bony impingement or laceration can be seen in conjunction with indirect mechanisms such as vascular injury. Among patients with fatal traumatic head injuries, 44% suffered shearing of the vascular supply with ischemic necrosis and 36% were found to have interstitial hemorrhage [12]. Among the

subset who suffered interstitial hemorrhage, this injury occurred within the optic canal in approximately two-thirds of cases, suggesting that the tethered position of the nerve within the canal may increase the likelihood of injury via this mechanism.

In recent years, the role of biochemical contributions to traumatic nerve injury has been explored. Excitatory amino acids have a role in free radical production which may potentiate ischemic injury by increasing swelling within areas of tenuous blood supply. The excitatory neurotransmitter glutamate is present in high concentrations within neurons. When these cells sustain damage, glutamate activates N-methyl-d-aspartate (NMDA) receptors, which begin a cascade resulting in the production of free radicals and secondary neuronal damage [13].

Diagnosis

Patient presentations for orbital and optic nerve pathology vary as widely as the etiologies which cause them. Patients may present initially to an ophthalmologist, an endocrinologist, a rheumatologist, a neurosurgeon, or an otolaryngologist. In this era of sophisticated imaging and high-tech laboratory testing, thorough history taking and physical examination remain the mainstay of diagnosis. Elements of the history which are of specific interest include time of disease progression, presence of visual compromise, presence of diplopia, and the mechanism, direction, and relative force of any trauma. Assessment must be made of extraocular muscle action, visual acuity, visual fields, and presence of globe displacement. Specific ophthalmologic examination including funduscopic examination and slit lamp may also be necessary. Often, patients suffering multiple traumatic injuries require intubation and sedation, which limit the depth of clinical examination. The most complete medical history and physical examination that are practical under the circumstances of presentation should be performed. With orbital trauma, the most common abnormality is subconjunctival hemorrhage [14]; however, a significant percentage of patients have no initial physical findings. Despite normal funduscopic

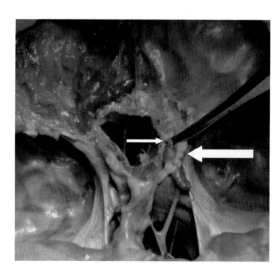

Fig. 32.1 Anatomic dissection demonstrating the relationship of the ophthalmic artery (*small arrow*) medial to the optic nerve (*large arrow*) within the optic canal

examination at presentation, optic atrophy may be noted later in the clinical course [15]. Thus, serial examinations are critical and a high index of suspicion must be maintained.

Similarly, although some degree of visual impairment is present in the majority of cases, patients' visual acuity may range from no light perception to normal vision. Initial visual acuity was correlated with long-term outcomes and, as such, is useful in gauging prognosis [4, 6, 16]. Visual loss can either be global or in specific visual fields. Visual field loss is limited to the lower visual field in 75% of patients which is likely due to greater adherence of the pia and arachnoid in the upper canal wall [4, 6].

Precise imaging can be important in making an accurate diagnosis and can be instrumental in planning the surgical approach. Evaluation of the bony canal is an important component of patient workup since bony impingement on the nerve may require immediate surgical remedy to give the best result. It is important to note that an intact bony canal does not rule out TON [17]. Contrasted computed tomography (CT) is useful in identifying mass lesions within the orbit or impinging on the path of the optic nerves. It is the best initial imaging modality to assess the integrity of the bony canal. Within the bony canal, the most common fracture site in patients with TON is the inferomedial quadrant of the canal within the sphenoid sinus [18]. Some authors recommend cerebral angiography in cases of proven canal fracture in order to rule out cavernous-carotid fistula. In cases in which further detail of the intracanalicular subarachnoid space is required for clinical decision-making, intrathecal contrast study of the region can be useful [19].

For soft tissue lesions within the orbit or optic pathways, magnetic resonance imaging (MRI) may be useful to define tissue characteristics, assess vascularity, and to evaluate tissue planes.

Non-surgical Treatment

Primary therapy for a specific pathology will depend largely on that pathology. In many clinical scenarios involving the visual axis, non-surgical treatment can be effective (e. g., corticosteroid therapy in selected patients with thyroid orbitopathy). Decisions regarding the best therapy for patients suffering TON are clouded by the variance of published clinical outcomes. In patients with TON who receive no therapy directed at this condition, 20–38% can be expected to have spontaneous recovery of vision [4, 20–22]. Because nerve swelling and vasospasm have been implicated in the ischemic component of indirect TON, high-dose corticosteroids (CS) are employed in order to avoid surgical decompression [23]. CS inhibit free radicals, theoretically providing neuroprotection [24].

The multicenter National Acute Spinal Cord Injury Studies (NASCIS I, II, III) demonstrated the benefit to patients with spinal cord injuries of high-dose CS begun within the first 8 h following injury [24–26]. The dosing regimen in the NASCIS was a bolus of 30 mg/kg body weight of methylprednisolone followed by 5.4 mg/kg/h infusion for the subsequent 23 h. Later studies explored increasing doses of methylprednisolone. Surprisingly, an initial loading dose of 60 mg/kg resulted in loss of effect and doses of 90 mg/kg result in increased lipid peroxidation [27].

Another group performed further analysis of the NASCIS data and demonstrated a harmful effect of high-dose CS if begun later than 8 h after the initial injury [28].

Despite the differences in nerve composition between the optic nerve and the spinal cord and the known differences in the response of these tissues to trauma [29], the NASCIS trials gave support for the use of high-dose CS in TON. Because CS carry serious potential risk, including gastrointestinal bleeding, psychomotor agitation, glycemic dysregulation, decreased immune capacity, and cardiac arrhythmia, their use in any clinical situation cannot be undertaken lightly. Risks and benefits must be carefully weighed. Methylprednisolone use carries the additional risk of causing a dose-dependent reduction in optic nerve myelin sheaths following crush injury in a rat model [30]. It is thought that the mechanisms to limit secondary neuronal injury are hindered, allowing increased damage to the nerve.

Clinical efficacy of CS use in TON remains unclear. The variability of treatment initiation clouds any conclusions that could otherwise be drawn from these data. The conclusion drawn by the authors of a recent review of available literature was that the evidence supporting use of CS in TON is "weak at best". They added that withholding CS in these patients is "no longer unethical" [31].

Given the unclear role of CS in TON, researchers have begun to explore other medical therapies. A group of 21-aminosteroids known as the lazaroids possess free-radical scavenging capabilities and may have a superior risk/benefit profile than high-dose CS [26, 32]. MK-801, a non-competitive NMDA receptor antagonist, has been studied in animal models and may prove beneficial to visual performance and ganglion cell survival [33, 34].

Surgical Approaches

Since mass lesions can result in direct pressure on the optic nerve in the orbit or optic canal, a surgical approach to the orbit and optic nerve is often necessary. Several factors must be considered when deciding on a surgical approach: location of lesion, type of lesion, potential morbidity of the approach, training of the surgeon performing the procedure, and any likely adjunctive treatment modalities. Neurosurgical, ophthalmologic, open endonasal, and, more recently, endoscopic endonasal approaches have all been used for pathologies of the orbit and optic canal.

Pringle reported the first optic nerve decompression using an orbital approach [35]. Dandy later described the frontotemporal craniotomy approach to the optic nerve [36]. In the decades which followed, this procedure became the workhorse surgical approach to the optic canal for TON and other pathologies. In 1951, Takahashi described the first endonasal approach to the optic nerve [37]. Niho et al. described transethmoidal approaches to the optic canal in cases of TON [38]. Grade I surgery was performed under local anesthesia and involved complete removal of mucosa from the antrum, ethmoid, sphenoid, and frontal sinus as well as the medial orbital wall. This provided access to the medial canal wall, an area which is difficult to reach via intracranial approaches. If vision did not subjectively improve following grade I surgery, further surgery as undertaken.

32

Grade II surgery consisted of a transfrontal approach to the optic canal roof. This approach provided access to the optic canal with less morbidity than a frontal craniotomy [39]. Recently, Yang et al. described an anterior clinoidectomy approach, demonstrating that interest in improving current practice remains active and that innovation persists [40].

The orbit itself can be approached intracranially via direct frontal craniotomy or frontotemporal craniotomy. This approach allows access to the orbital roof and lesions of the superior orbit.

Understanding the potential for decreased morbidity by avoiding intracranial approaches, several operations have been developed to achieve extracranial access to the orbit and optic nerve.

Several direct approaches to the orbit can be utilized. Selection depends on the specific pathology to be treated. Access to the orbital floor can be achieved via subciliary or transconjunctival approaches. The transconjunctival approach carries less risk of postoperative scarring and ectropion, though the closing stitches have the potential to cause corneal abrasion if not placed carefully. Either approach provides excellent access to the anterior orbital floor and can be extended to address the posterior orbital floor as well. Care must be taken to avoid excessive traction on the globe and to avoid damage to the inferior oblique and lacrimal apparatus. Intranasal endoscopic approaches have been performed to access the orbital floor posterior to the axis of the globe and lateral to the infraorbital canal. Endoscopic removal of the orbital floor avoids threat to the lacrimal apparatus or inferior oblique. This approach requires ethmoidectomy and middle meatal antrotomy as well as the use of angled telescopes.

The medial orbit can be accessed externally via a Lynch incision. Care must be taken to avoid the medial canthus and lacrimal apparatus. Also, anterior and posterior ethmoid arteries must be identified and ligated if dissection continues posteriorly. The medial orbit can be safely approached via an endonasal endoscopic approach involving wide middle meatal antrotomy and ethmoidectomy. The lamina papyracea can be removed from the orbital apex posteriorly to the lacrimal apparatus anteriorly. Care must be taken to avoid direct trauma to the lacrimal system or the ethmoid arteries.

The lateral orbit can be accessed via a lateral canthotomy and cantholysis. Dissection is continued in the subperiorbital plane. Malleable retractors are used to aid visualization, though care must be taken to limit retraction on the globe. High-speed drills can be used in the lateral sphenoid to widen access or expand orbital volume. Due to the proximity of surrounding structures, this presents some risk to the optic nerve as well as the dura overlying the temporal lobe.

The superior orbit can be accessed via a lid-crease incision and a subperiorbital dissection plane. Additional intraconal approaches have been performed externally via one or several approaches. Current work on endoscopic approaches to intraconal lesions is underway. Image guidance systems can be used to good effect for this approach.

For patients with pathology limited to the optic canal, Goldberg and Steinsapir utilized a transethmoid/transorbital approach [41]. Kennerdell's group described a transantral-ethmoidal approach [42]. This technique involved exposure via a Caldwell-Luc with creation of an inferiorly based mucosal flap and ethmoidectomy with mucosa-stripping. Following this, the posterior lamina papyracea and anterior sphenoid are removed under microscopic vision, followed by dissection of the canal.

To improve visibility and increase the angle of incidence with respect to the optic canal, Sofferman introduced the microscopic sublabial sphenoethmoid approach [43]. To achieve this exposure, this technique employs a Caldwell-Luc antrotomy but relies on wider resection of bone than previously described techniques. A posterior septal mucosal flap is preserved and used for reconstruction. This approach allows the optic canal to be dissected inferomedially, preserving a buttress of bone between the optic canal and the internal carotid artery [44].

Call introduced the transorbital-sphenoid decompression. This involved dividing and reflecting the medial canthal tendon and retracting the periorbita laterally. Under microscopic vision, surgery proceeds in a manner similar to Niho's grade I surgery [45]. Lamina defects were reconstructed with silicone to prevent enophthalmos.

Knox's group introduced the lateral facial approach to TON [46]. This procedure addresses patients with multiple facial fractures in whom bony manipulation carries risk of exacerbating optic nerve damage and patients with lateral optic canal fractures. In this approach the temporalis muscle and zygomatic arch are reflected and the greater wing of the sphenoid is removed. The superior orbital fissure is identified and preserved, while the dissection continues via the lesser wing en route to the optic canal.

As fiberoptic technology has improved, completely endoscopic optic nerve decompression has been successfully performed [47]. Ipsilateral total ethmoidectomy and wide sphenoidotomy is performed. Depending on the degree of sphenoid pneumatization, wide sphenoidotomy may be extended far laterally with care to avoid the vidian canal. This exposes the lamina papyracea, orbital apex, and opticocarotid recess. Once fully exposed, a high-speed drill system with diamond burrs can be used to safely thin the bone surrounding the optic nerve. Care must be taken to avoid the carotid inferiorly and the skull base superiorly. The opticocarotid recess is a triangular space in the lateral sphenoid wall separating the carotid imprint from the protruding optic canal, with its base oriented anteriorly (Fig. 32.2). The optic nerve forms the superior side of this triangle, with variable relationship to the skull base, while the carotid artery forms the inferior side. As the dissection is carried posteriorly, the distance between the nerve and the artery narrows considerably. Fully endoscopic techniques hold promise for accomplishing optic nerve decompression with comparatively low morbidity and excellent visualization (Fig. 32.3). Additionally, the ability of angled telescopes to allow off-axis visualization provides a potential benefit over direct, line-of-sight visualization.

Opinions vary as to the utility of incising the optic nerve sheath. The theoretical benefit of nerve sheath incision comes from relieving compression on the swollen nerve. The risk of direct optic nerve damage is supported by the close adherence of the optic nerve to the sheath within the canal. Sofferman states that the benefit of sheath incision is unclear [15]. Some sugges-

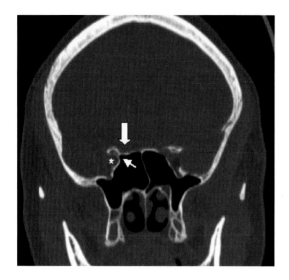

Fig. 32.2 Coronal CT scan demonstrating the anatomy of the optico-carotid recess. The carotid artery (*asterisk*) lies below the optic nerve (*large arrow*), with the intervening opticocarotid recess (*small arrow*)

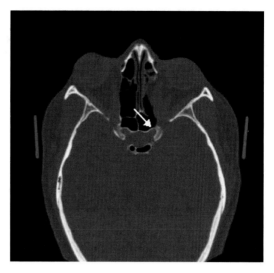

Fig. 32.3 Axial CT scan demonstrating degree of decompression possible via an endoscopic approach. Note proximity to the carotid artery (*arrow*) posteriorly

tion has been made that effective decompression must remove bone from up to 270 degrees around the nerve. The arc of bone that it is necessary to remove in order to sufficiently decrease pressure on the nerve has not been formally studied. In practice, pneumatization patterns of the sphenoethmoid complex dictate the arc of bone that can be safely removed and vary widely among patients.

Surgical Data from Traumatic Optic Neuropathy

Studies that have evaluated the benefits of decompression have produced widely varying results. Reports using surgical decompression by all approaches either as stand-alone therapy or in combination with CS therapy demonstrate benefit in 31–100% of cases [16, 48–56]. Data regarding the time interval before undertaking surgery are, likewise, mixed [14, 57].

Walsh established criteria for surgical decompression of the optic canal via a transcranial approach [3]:
1. In the unconscious patient, surgery is never performed as a selective procedure.
2. In a patient with visual loss, a non-reactive pupil, and immediate visual loss from time of injury, surgery is contraindicated.
3. If visual loss or loss of pupillary response occur after injury, surgery can be considered.
4. If it is unclear whether a lucid interval existed, observation for 4–6 days to allow for recovery can be appropriate.

Lubben and colleagues used a different set of indications for surgery using a frontoethmoidal approach [58] and these are:

1. Post-traumatic visual loss or decrease in acuity (<20/100-20/60)
2. Increasing restriction of visual field
3. Afferent pupillary defect in unconscious patients

Kountakis' group made the additional observation that patients who presented with visual acuity of 20/200 or better improved with CS therapy alone while patients presenting with visual acuity of 20/400 or worse required surgical decompression in addition to CS therapy [16]. Le Fort III fractures, midface fractures, naso-orbital-ethmoid (NOE) fractures, and conchal pneumatization have all been cited as relative contraindications to immediate surgical intervention in cases of TON [16, 51, 59].

With these disparate data from several small studies, the International Optic Nerve Trauma Study (IONTS) was undertaken in order to achieve data of sufficient power that the questions regarding the best pathway for TON management could be answered. Unfortunately, insufficient enrollment resulted in the discontinuation of the IONTS before desired numbers had been achieved. In total, 127 patients were enrolled. No clear benefit was shown from either CS therapy or optic nerve decompression [60].

In an attempt to overcome the power limitations of smaller studies, Cook et al. performed a meta-analysis. They concluded that some intervention, whether CS alone, decompression alone, or a combination of modalities, demonstrated benefit over no intervention at all [49]. In contrast, Steinsapir and Goldberg concluded that the benefit from any type of intervention had not clearly been established [61].

A recent review using the stringent Cochrane Database criteria found no randomized controlled trials that met the threshold

32

for inclusion. Their conclusion was that there was a relatively high rate of spontaneous recovery and there was no evidence that surgical decompression offered benefit in TON [62].

Existing information from patients with variable presentations and time courses and modalities of treatment result in data that are difficult to compare, with conclusions still less clear. CS therapy and optic nerve decompression each carry significant risks. The discouraging natural course of the disease makes expectant management an uncertain choice as well. Considering all these issues, one conclusion is clear: significant questions remain as to the best treatment in cases of TON.

Conclusion

Within the orbit, complex processes and the intricate anatomy allow a patient to interact more fully with his or her surroundings. In this setting, medical and surgical intervention may offer an opportunity to preserve function or remedy a sight-threatening condition. Ultimately, decisions must consider all patient factors and surgeon experience in selecting the best approach for a specific patient's condition.

Tips to Avoid Complications

- Appropriate patient selection.
- Recognize increased risk in patients with facial fractures.
- For intracranial approaches, minimize frontotemporal retraction.
- For external approaches, avoid the lacrimal apparatus and inferior oblique muscle.
- Recognize dehiscent optic nerve in the sphenoid and posterior ethmoid sinuses.
- Use the skull base and opticocarotid recess as landmarks to limit dissection.

Take-Home Pearls

- Carefully weigh risks and benefits of all treatment options.
- In TON, data comparing treatment options are incomplete.
- Endoscopic approaches may provide access to the orbit and optic nerve with minimal morbidity.
- Ultimately, the best approach is the one for which available equipment matches the surgeon's experience and comfort.

References

1. Obenchain TG, Killeffer FA, Stern WE (1973) Indirect injury of the optic nerves and chiasm with closed head injury. Report of three cases. Bull Los Angeles Neurol Soc 38:13–20
2. Kline LB, Morawetz RB, Swaid SN (1984) Indirect injury of the optic nerve. Neurosurgery 14:756–764
3. Walsh FB (1966) Pathological-clinical correlations. I. Indirect trauma to the optic nerves and chiasm. II. Certain cerebral involvements associated with defective blood supply. Invest Ophthalmol 1966:433–449
4. Hughes B (1962) Indirect injury of the optic nerves and chiasma. Bull Johns Hopkins Hosp 3:98–126
5. Noble MJ, McFadzean R (1987) Indirect injury to the optic nerves and optic chiasm. Neuroophthalmology 7:341–348
6. Davidson M (1938) The indirect traumatic optic atrophies. Am J Ophthalmol 21:7–21
7. Hartzell KN, Botek AA, Goldberg SH (1996) Orbital fractures in women due to sexual assault and domestic violence. Ophthalmology 103:953–957
8. Pomeranz HD, Rizzo JF, Lessell S (1999) Treatment of traumatic optic neuropathy. Int Ophthalmol Clin 39:185–194
9. Lang J (1989) Clinical anatomy of the nose, nasal cavity, and paranasal sinuses. Thieme, Stuttgart, pp 85–98, 125–128
10. Fujii K, Chambers SM, Rhoton AL Jr (1979) Neurovascular relationships of the sphenoid sinus. A microsurgical study. J Neurosurg 50:31–39
11. Maniscalco JE, Habal MB (1978) Microanatomy of the optic canal. J Neurosurg 48:402–406
12. Crompton MR (1970) Visual lesions in closed head injury. Brain 93:785–792
13. Farkas RH, Grosskreutz CL (2001) Apoptosis, neuroprotection, and retinal ganglion cell death: an overview. Int Ophthalmol Clin 41:111–130
14. Rajiniganth MG, Gupta AK, Gupta A, Bapuraj JR (2003) Traumatic optic neuropathy: visual outcome following combined therapy protocol. Arch Otolaryngol Head Neck Surg 129:1203–1206
15. Sofferman RA, Harris P (1995) Mosher Award thesis. The recovery potential of the optic nerve. Laryngoscope 105(suppl 72):1–38
16. Kountakis SE, Maillard AA, El-Harazi SM, Longhini L, Urso RG (2000) Endoscopic optic nerve decompression for traumatic blindness. Otolaryngol Head Neck Surg 123:34–37
17. Seiff SR, Berger MS, Guyon J, Pitts LH (1984) Computed tomographic evaluation of the optic canal in sudden traumatic blindness. Am J Ophthalmol 98:751–755
18. Guyon JJ, Brant-Zawadzki M, Seiff SR (1984) CT demonstration of optic canal fractures. AJR Am J Roentgenol 143:1031–1034
19. Jinkins JR (1987) The optic neurogram: evaluation of CSF "block" caused by compressive lesions at the optic canal. AJNR Am J Neuroradiol 8:135–139
20. Lessell S (1989) Indirect optic nerve trauma. Arch Ophthalmol 107:382–386
21. Wolin MJ, Lavin PJ (1990) Spontaneous visual recovery from traumatic optic neuropathy after blunt head injury. Am J Ophthalmol 109:430–435
22. Seiff SR (1990) High dose corticosteroids for treatment of vision loss due to indirect injury to the optic nerve. Ophthalmic Surg 21:389–395

23. Anderson RL, Panje WR, Gross CE (1982) Optic nerve blindness following blunt forehead trauma. Ophthalmology 89:445–455

24. Bracken MB, Collins WF, Freeman DF, Shepard MJ, Wagner FW, Silten RM, Hellenbrand KG, Ransohoff J, Hunt WE, Perot PL Jr, et al (1984) Efficacy of methylprednisolone in acute spinal cord injury. JAMA 251:45–52

25. Bracken MB, Shepard MJ, Collins WF, Holford TR, Young W, Baskin DS, Eisenberg HM, Flamm E, Leo-Summers L, Maroon J, et al (1990) A randomized, controlled trial of methylprednisolone or naloxone in the treatment of acute spinal-cord injury. Results of the second National Acute Spinal Cord Injury Study. N Engl J Med 322:1405–1411

26. Bracken MB, Shepard MJ, Holford TR, Leo-Summers L, Aldrich EF, Fazl M, Fehlings M, Herr DL, Hitchon PW, Marshall LF, Nockels RP, Pascale V, Perot PL Jr, Piepmeier J, Sonntag VK, Wagner F, Wilberger JE, Winn HR, Young W (1997) Administration of methylprednisolone for 24 or 48 hours or tirilazad mesylate for 48 hours in the treatment of acute spinal cord injury. Results of the third National Acute Spinal Cord Injury Randomized Controlled Trial. National Acute Spinal Cord Injury Study. JAMA 277:1597–1604

27. Hall ED (1992) The neuroprotective pharmacology of methylprednisolone. J Neurosurg 76:13–22

28. Bracken MB, Holford TR (1993) Effects of timing of methylprednisolone or naloxone administration on recovery of segmental and long-tract neurological function in NASCIS 2. J Neurosurg 79:500–507

29. Stys PK (1998) Anoxic and ischemic injury of myelinated axons in CNS white matter: from mechanistic concepts to therapeutics. J Cereb Blood Flow Metab 18:2–25

30. Steinsapir KD, Goldberg RA, Sinha S, Hovda DA (2000) Methylprednisolone exacerbates axonal loss following optic nerve trauma in rats. Restor Neurol Neurosci 17:157–163

31. Steinsapir KD, Seiff SR, Goldberg RA (2002) Traumatic optic neuropathy: where do we stand? Ophthal Plast Reconstr Surg 18:232–234

32. Hall ED, Braughler JM, McCall JM (1990) Role of oxygen radicals in stroke: effects of the 21-aminosteroids (lazaroids). A novel class of antioxidants. Prog Clin Biol Res 361:351–362

33. Schmitt U, Sabel BA (1996) MK-801 reduces retinal ganglion cell survival but improves visual performance after controlled optic nerve crush. J Neurotrauma 13:791–800

34. Yoles E, Muller S, Schwartz M (1997) NMDA-receptor antagonist protects neurons from secondary degeneration after partial optic nerve crush. J Neurotrauma 14:665–675

35. Pringle JH (1916–1917) Monocular blindness following diffuse violence to the skull: its causation and treatment. Br J Surg 4:373–385

36. Dandy WE (1922) Prechiasmal intracranial tumors of the optic nerves. Am J Ophthalmol 12:169–188

37. Takahashi R (1951) Exposure of the optic canal. Operation 5:300–302

38. Niho S, Yasuda K, Sato T, et al (1961) Decompression of the optic canal by the transethmoidal route. Am J Ophthalmol 51:659–665

39. Niho S, Niho M, Niho K (1970) Decompression of the optic canal by the transethmoidal route and decompression of the superior orbital fissure. Can J Ophthalmol 5:22–40

40. Yang Y, Wang H, Shao Y, Wei Z, Zhu S, Wang J (2006) Extradural anterior clinoidectomy as an alternative approach for optic nerve decompression: anatomic study and clinical experience. Neurosurgery 59(suppl 2):ONS253–ONS262

41. Goldberg RA, Steinsapir KD (1996) Extracranial optic canal decompression: indications and technique. Ophthal Plast Reconstr Surg 12:163–170

42. Kennerdell JS, Amsbaugh GA, Myers EN (1976) Transantral-ethmoidal decompression of optic canal fracture. Arch Ophthalmol 94:1040–1043

43. Sofferman RA (1979) An extracranial microsurgical approach to the optic nerve. J Microsurg 1:195–202

44. Sofferman RA (1981) Sphenoethmoid approach to the optic nerve. Laryngoscope 91:184–196

45. Call NB (1986) Decompression of the optic nerve in the optic canal. A transorbital approach. Ophthal Plast Reconstr Surg 2:133–137

46. Knox BE, Gates GA, Berry SM (1990) Optic nerve decompression via the lateral facial approach. Laryngoscope 100:458–462

47. Kountakis SE, Maillard AA, Urso R, Stiernberg CM (1997) Endoscopic approach to traumatic visual loss. Otolaryngol Head Neck Surg 116:652–655

48. Fukado Y (1975) Results in 400 cases of surgical decompression of the optic nerve. Mod Probl Ophthalmol 14:474–481

49. Cook MW, Levin LA, Joseph MP, Pinczower EF (1996) Traumatic optic neuropathy. A meta-analysis. Arch Otolaryngol Head Neck Surg 122:389–392

50. Levin LA, Joseph MP, Rizzo JF 3rd, Lessell S (1994) Optic canal decompression in indirect optic nerve trauma. Ophthalmology 101:566–569

51. Li KK, Teknos TN, Lai A, Lauretano A, Terrell J, Joseph MP (1999) Extracranial optic nerve decompression: a 10-year review of 92 patients. J Craniofac Surg 10:454–459

52. Maurer J, Hinni M, Mann W, Pfeiffer N (1999) Optic nerve decompression in trauma and tumor patients. Eur Arch Otorhinolaryngol 256:341–345

53. Luxenberger W, Stammberger H, Jebeles JA, Walch C (1998) Endoscopic optic nerve decompression: the Graz experience. Laryngoscope 108:873–882

54. Schroder M, Kolenda H, Loibnegger E, Muhlendyck H (1989) Optic nerve damage following craniocerebral trauma. A critical analysis of trans-ethmoid decompression of the optic nerve. Laryngorhinootologie 68:534–538

55. Schmidbauer JM, Muller E, Hoh H, Robinson E (1998) [Early trans-sphenoid decompression in indirect traumatic optic neuropathy.] HNO 46:152–156

56. Joseph MP, Lessell S, Rizzo J, Momose KJ (1990) Extracranial optic nerve decompression for traumatic optic neuropathy. Arch Ophthalmol 108:1091–1093

57. Girard BC, Bouzas EA, Lamas G, Soudant J (1992) Visual improvement after transethmoid-sphenoid decompression in optic nerve injuries. J Clin Neuroophthalmol 12:142–148

58. Lubben B, Stoll W, Grenzebach U (2001) Optic nerve decompression in the comatose and conscious patients after trauma. Laryngoscope 111:320–328

59. Weymuller EA Jr (1984) Blindness and Le Fort III fractures. Ann Otol Rhinol Laryngol 93:2–5

32

60. Levin LA, Beck RW, Joseph MP, Seiff S, Kraker R (1999) The treatment of traumatic optic neuropathy: the International Optic Nerve Trauma Study. Ophthalmology 106:1268–1277

61. Steinsapir KD, Goldberg RA (1994) Traumatic optic neuropathy. Surv Ophthalmol 38:487–518

62. Yu Wai Man P, Griffiths PG (2005) Surgery for traumatic optic neuropathy. Cochrane Database Syst Rev. CD005024

Tumors of the Nose, Paranasal Sinuses, Jaws, Skull Base and Related Problems

Chapter 33

Benign Tumors of the Nasal Cavity and Paranasal Sinuses

33

Bernhard Schick and Julia Dlugaiczyk

Core Messages

■ There are two important features of benign tumors of the nose and paranasal sinuses: they are rare and they cover a great variety of different tumor entities.

■ Symptoms of tumors of the nose and paranasal sinuses are unspecific in most cases and mimic the clinical picture of inflammatory disorders. Moreover, many tumors are diagnosed by chance in radiological assessment for other reasons.

■ In case of unilateral symptoms, a tumor of the nose/paranasal sinuses should always be considered in order to make the diagnosis without delay.

■ The endoscopic aspect of unilateral nasal polyposis may be the finding of an inverted papilloma.

■ Magnetic resonance imaging should be added to computed tomography in the radiological assessment of tumors of the nose/paranasal sinuses in order to distinguish between tumor extension and associated inflammatory disorders as well as to determine intracranial/orbital involvement.

Contents

Introduction

The rhinologist is frequently faced with inflammation of the nasal cavity and paranasal sinuses, but only rarely with benign tumors in this location. As a huge number of different entities has to be considered, it is difficult for most rhinologists to gain personal experience in diagnosing and treating many of them. Benign tumors of the nasal cavity and paranasal sinuses may be asymptomatic for a long time. When symptoms arise they often mimic the clinical picture of chronic rhinosinusitis, which is by far more frequent. For these reasons tumor diagnosis is often delayed. Therefore it is of utmost importance to consider a benign tumor especially in case of unilateral symptoms of the nose and paranasal sinuses.

As there is a myriad of different tumor entities, it may be beneficial for the clinician to distinguish between epithelial tumors (e. g., papilloma, pleomorphic adenoma), mesenchymal tumors (e. g., fibromatosis, juvenile angiofibroma, osteoma, ossifying fibroma), neural-related tumors (e. g., schwannoma), and tumor-like lesions (e. g., giant cell granuloma, mucocele). There are certainly further tumor entities not easily fitting into this classification. Among the list of benign lesions of the nasal cavity and paranasal sinuses osteomas, juvenile angiofibromas, and inverted papillomas are highlighted in this chapter (Table 33.1).

Osteoma

Osteomas are regarded as one of the most common benign tumors of the paranasal sinuses. However, the actual incidence of sinus osteoma in the general population is hard to determine, as most of these tumors are asymptomatic. In a series of 3,510 plain sinus radiographs taken for any reason, Childrey (1939) reported an incidence of 0.43% [5]. Mehta and Grewal (1963) found osteomas in 1% of patients who underwent radiographic examination for sinus symptoms [18]. In computed tomography (CT) studies an incidence up to 3% was described [7].

Table 33.1 Characteristics of osteomas, juvenile angiofibromas, and inverted papillomas

	Osteoma	Juvenile angiofibroma	Inverted papilloma
Incidence	0.43% in plain sinus radiographs taken for any reason	< 0,5% of head/neck tumors	0.5–4% of nasal tumors
Typical site of origin	Frontal/ethmoidal sinus	Posterior nasal cavity	Lateral nasal wall/maxillary sinus
Histology	Bone (eburnated vs mature type)	Fibrovascular	Epithelial
Age of presentation	Third to fourth decade	Second decade	Fifth to seventh decade
Male to female ratio	1.5–2:1	Almost exclusively adolescent males	2–3:1
Malignant degeneration	No	No, but often aggressive growth	9.1% (SCC)
Therapy	Observation/operation	Operation first choice (radiation, chemotherapy)	Operation first choice

Clinical Presentation

Sinus osteomas may present at any age, with a peak prevalence in the third and fourth decades of life. Patients from the West Indies and the Middle East tend to present with symptoms at a younger age. Various studies report a male to female ratio of 1.5–2:1 [3]. Ninety-five percent of paranasal sinus osteomas are found in the frontoethmoidal region, with 80% arising from the frontal sinus floor. The ethmoid sinus is involved in 20–30%, whereas the maxillary sinus accounts for less than 5%. Sphenoid sinus osteomas are very rare. Sinus osteomas may be stable in size or grow slowly at different rates. Koivunen et al. (1997) report a growth rate ranging from 0.44 to 6.0 mm/year [12]. A malignant transformation has never been described.

The clinical symptoms of paranasal sinus osteomas depend on location and size of the tumor. Small osteomas are often asymptomatic. The most common symptom is frontal headache or facial pain. In cases where an osteoma blocks the natural drainage of the associated sinus, chronic sinusitis develops. Anterior growth may result in facial deformity. Orbital complications such as proptosis, diplopia, visual disturbance, and epiphora are due to expansion of the tumor into the orbital vault (Fig. 33.1a). Posterior growth of frontal sinus osteomas may lead to intracranial involvement. In case of dura penetration complications such as CSF fistula, meningitis, pneumocephalus, or frontal abscess have to be considered [7, 38].

Osteomas may also be a sign of Gardner's syndrome, an autosomal dominant disorder with multiple osteomas, soft tissue tumors (subcutaneous fibrous tumors, sebaceous cysts), supernumerary teeth, and colorectal polyps that may show malignant transformation [9].

Pathogenesis

The etiology of paranasal sinus osteoma is still a controversial issue. Currently, developmental, traumatic, and infectious theories are discussed. The developmental theory postulates that embryonic stem cells may become trapped at the frontoethmoidal suture during bone maturation and may be the source of uncontrolled bone proliferation later in life. However, this theory does not explain the origin of osteomas in places other than the frontoethmoidal suture [7]. According to Moretti, up to 20% of patients with paranasal sinus osteomas had a positive history of trauma to the skull [23]. The infectious theory sees chronic inflammation as the inciting force for bony tumor formation. A coincidence of chronic rhinosinusitis and osteoma of the paranasal sinuses is often reported. However, it is hard to tell whether the chronic inflammation is the source for osteoma formation or vice versa [7].

Osteomas are benign tumors with a smooth lobulated surface covered by normal sinus mucosa. They are made up of dense lamellar bone with little medullary component. Three histological types can be distinguished. The eburnated osteoma (also known as the ivory or compact type) is very dense, has no haversian canals, and is thought to arise from membranous elements. The mature type (osteoma spongiosum) resembles cancellous bone and is said to originate from cartilaginous elements. The mixed type contains components of eburnated and mature osteomas [3, 7].

Radiology

Osteomas present as well-defined, dense homogenous masses on x-ray and CT. CT is crucial to determine the exact location and size of the tumor as well as its relation to adjacent struc-

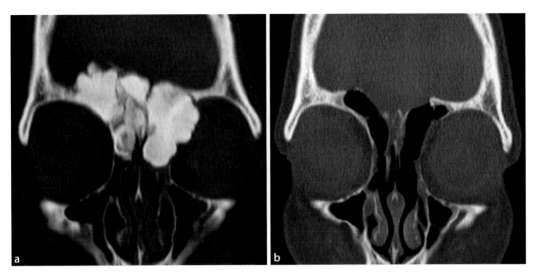

Fig. 33.1a,b Large frontal sinus osteoma with intracranial and orbital tumor extension (**a**) being resected completely (**b**) using an osteoplastic frontal sinus approach

tures. Whenever intracranial involvement is suspected, magnetic resonance imaging (MRI) is recommended [7]. The differential diagnosis has to consider other fibro-osseous lesions such as fibrous dysplasia or ossifying fibroma, which may have a similar radiological appearance to osteomas but with less well-defined borders [40].

Therapy

The first and paramount decision in the management of paranasal sinus osteoma is observation or operation? In case of a newly diagnosed asymptomatic osteoma, CT follow up is suggested to define the osteoma growth pattern. If the tumor stays asymptomatic and no tumor growth is detected, a "wait and scan" policy can be selected. Savic and Djeric (1990) recommend surgical treatment if an osteoma extends beyond the borders of the frontal sinus or if it continues to enlarge [27]. Osteomas of the frontal recess and the ethmoid bone should be resected, as they carry the risk of blocking frontal sinus drainage. Patients with chronic rhinosinusitis or headache should be operated on, after a thorough neurological examination has ruled out other reasons for the headache [27]. According to Smith and Calcaterra (1989), osteomas occupying more than 50% of the frontal sinus should be resected [40]. Orbital and intracranial involvements are indications for surgical intervention. A preoperative endoscopic examination is needed to check for active infection. Any acute infection of the paranasal sinuses should be treated before surgical intervention because of the risk of peri-/postoperative intracranial spread [38].

In general, osteomas of the paranasal sinuses can be addressed by an endonasal, an external, or a combined approach. The choice of technique is determined by the size and location of the tumor. The primary aim of the operation is complete re-

moval of the tumor with minimal trauma to adjacent structures. Large osteomas are debulked with the drill before the remaining tumor parts are removed. The bone at the site of the tumor origin needs to be identified and resected. Applying these principles, nearly all ethmoid and sphenoid osteomas are amendable to endonasal resection. Rare maxillary osteomas mostly require an osteoplastic maxillary sinus operation. In case of frontal sinus osteomas endonasal, external, or combined approaches are chosen. For a complete endonasal removal of frontal sinus osteomas three prerequisites have to be met: (1) the maximum anterior-posterior diameter of the frontal sinus drainage being achievable must ensure adequate access to the tumor; (2) the main part of the tumor must be located medially to a virtual sagittal plane through the lamina papyracea; and (3) the tumor must be attached to the posterior-inferior wall of the frontal sinus [33]. Osteoplastic frontal sinus surgery is an attractive alternative for frontal sinus osteomas that are not suitable for an endonasal approach (Fig. 33.1b). If parts of the anterior frontal sinus wall have to be removed, a coronal incision offers the chance to reconstruct the forehead with split-calvarial bone grafts [31].

Juvenile Angiofibroma

Juvenile angiofibroma is a rare, benign fibrovascular tumor. It accounts for less than 0.5% of all head and neck tumors. Nevertheless juvenile angiofibromas attract much attention due to their typical clinical characteristics. They are believed to arise in the posterior nasal cavity close to the sphenopalatine foramen, and they usually extend into the nasopharynx. Therefore, they have frequently been termed nasopharyngeal angiofibromas. Atypical locations have been described only for a very limited number of juvenile angiofibromas [30].

33

Clinical Presentation

Due to the location of this hypervascular tumor, nasal obstruction and bleeding are the two most frequent clinical symptoms. Typically, this tumor is almost exclusively found in adolescent males. But it may also present within the first decade of life, at an older age, or very rarely in women. Defined blood supply is a characteristic finding in this hypervascular tumor. Juvenile angiofibromas usually derive their blood supply from the spheno-palatine/maxillary artery. The ascending pharyngeal artery and ascending palatine artery are possible further feeders branching off the external carotid artery. Besides both external carotid arteries, the internal carotid arteries (C4 segment of the internal carotid artery, ophthalmic artery, and persistent mandibular artery) have to be considered as an additional source of blood [14, 32]. Tissue architecture is another characteristic tumor feature. Numerous irregularly shaped vessels are embedded in a fibrous stroma. Vessels with an endothelial lining only and vessels with incomplete vascular walls are observed. The inability of these vessels to contract in case of injury explains the risk of profuse tumor bleeding. Furthermore, a significant number of inflammatory cells such as mast cells have been detected within the tumor tissue. Although juvenile angiofibromas are regarded as benign tumors, they often exhibit an aggressive growth pattern with spread through natural fissures and foramens. Even an intracranial tumor extension might be observed [32].

Pathogenesis

Although numerous theories focusing either on the vascular or stromal tumor component have been published, pathogenesis of the tumor is still unknown. A currently attractive assumption based on the irregular vascular architecture is the theory of juvenile angiofibromas as vascular malformations. It considers remnants of the first branchial arch artery to be incorporated into the vascular tumor component [35]. The first branchial arch artery is not only an important connection between the future external and internal carotid arteries in embryological development, but also participates in formation of the spheno-palatine/maxillary artery. Final remnants of the first branchial arch artery are regularly observed close to the sphenopalatine foramen. Thus the assumption of an incomplete regression of the first branchial arch artery would perfectly allow to explain

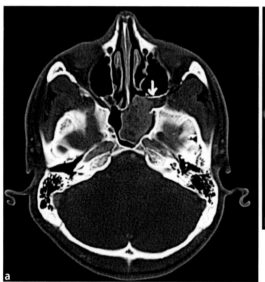

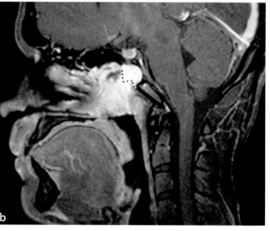

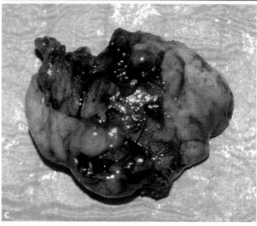

Fig. 33.2a–c Computed tomography (**a**) and sagittal MRI (**b**) indicate a juvenile angiofibroma with widening of the sphenopalatine foramen (*arrow* in **a**) and tumor extension into the sphenoid sinus. Within the sphenoid sinus MRI allows to differentiate between tumor extension and associated inflammatory disorders (*dotted line* in **b**). **c** This tumor could be resected completely using an endonasal approach

Table 33.2 Classification system for juvenile angiofibromas according to Andrews et al. [2]

I	Tumor limited to the nasopharynx and nasal cavity. Bone destruction negligible or limited to the sphenopalatine foramen
II	Tumor invading the pterygomaxillary fossa or the maxillary, ethmoid, or sphenoid sinus with bone destruction
III	a. Tumor invading the infratemporal fossa or orbital region without intracranial involvement
	b. Tumor invading the infratemporal fossa or orbital region with intracranial extradural (parasellar) involvement
IV	a. Intracranial intradural tumor without infiltration of the cavernous sinus, pituitary fossa, or optic chiasm
	b. Intracranial intradural tumor with infiltration of the cavernous sinus, pituitary fossa, or optic chiasm

tumor development close to the sphenopalatine foramen and characteristic tumor blood supply. However, the tumor cell in juvenile angiofibromas has still not been defined.

Genetic and molecular pathological studies have detected numerous chromosomal imbalances so far [37], frequent β-catenin mutations [1], evidence for androgen receptor gene gains [34], c-myc heterogeneity in advanced tumor stages [36], and expression of various growth factors such as TGF-β1 or VEGF [35]. Numerous investigations of hormone receptors in the tumor tissue brought up conflicting results. There is evidence for an increased expression of androgen receptors [11] and estrogen receptor β on the protein level [22]. It might be noteworthy that β-catenin and androgen receptors are translocated into the nucleus together, where they probably stimulate a subset of androgen receptor dependent genes [34]. These are the first findings reflecting the almost exclusive tumor manifestation in adolescent males on a molecular level.

Radiology

Computed tomography, MRI, and angiography are used to define tumor extension and blood supply. Juvenile angiofibromas show specific growth patterns [32]: In early stages, they are usually firmly fixed in the nasopharynx showing bony erosions at the clivus and medial pterygoid plate. In case of tumor growth posterior to the pterygoid base, juvenile angiofibromas may extend to the foramen lacerum. Involvement of the sphenoid sinus is quite common (Fig. 33.2a). Tumor spread into the pterygopalatine fossa is associated with widening of the sphenopalatine foramen (Fig. 33.2b). From the pterygopalatine fossa the tumor may expand into the orbit via the infraorbital fissure or laterally into the infratemporal fossa. Tumor growth through the roof of the infratemporal fossa or the superior orbital fissure may result in intracranial tumor extension. The classification system (Table 33.2) proposed by Andrews et al. [2] is a revision of the system introduced by Fisch [8]. The specific tumor growth pattern and tumor blood supply delineated by CT, MRI, and angiography allow making the diagnosis of a juvenile angiofibroma with high probability. Thus, a biopsy to confirm the diagnosis is not necessary, especially as profuse bleeding has to be considered.

Therapy

The treatment of first choice is tumor resection. With regard to the high tumor vascularity most surgeons propose preoperative tumor embolization to reduce intraoperative blood loss and to improve overall view in the surgical field. Other surgeons recommend avoiding preoperative tumor embolization because of a higher risk of incomplete tumor resection and the risk of severe neurological complications after embolization [24]. The use of cell saver devices and autologous blood donation before surgery are other options to reduce homologous blood transfusion.

Various approaches have been used in angiofibroma surgery (transfacial approaches, midfacial degloving, transnasal approaches). Nowadays, transnasal tumor resection has been established as the mainstay of therapy for most juvenile angiofibromas (Fig. 33.2c). Transnasal surgery provides excellent visualization of the tumor borders. It has been proven to allow tumor resection with at least the same results as obtained by other approaches and low morbidity. Tumor extension into the lateral infratemporal fossa, around the optic nerve, and/or the parasellar region has been reported as limitation for transnasal tumor resection [6]. In case of advanced juvenile angiofibromas, other approaches are selected. If follow up after surgery indicates residual tumor, it remains elusive whether the tumor remnant will show tumor progression, stay stable, or may recede.

If tumor resection is not advisable, radiation or chemotherapy have been recommended. Radiation has been reported to achieve control rates in 85% [16]. However, side effects such as growth retardation, endocrine dysfunction, or malignant transformation have to be considered [16]. There have been individual reports about gamma-knife surgery, but final assessment of this treatment option can not be provided due to limited experience. Chemotherapy has only been used in single advanced tumors so far with promising results [29].

As the tumor is almost exclusively found in adolescent males, hormone treatment in individual patients has been tried. Antiandrogen treatment has been reported to decrease tumor size. A reduction of both tumor size and vascularity has been described after estrogen treatment. These results have been attributed to the antiandrogenic effect of estrogens [15]. However, the application of hormone treatments is limited due to their side effects. Keeping in mind that spontaneous tumor regression has been observed in single juvenile angiofibromas, further development of new therapeutic options such as antihormone treatment with fewer side effects may be highly attractive in the future.

Inverted Papilloma

Sinonasal papillomas are benign epithelial tumors of the sinonasal mucosa (schneiderian mucosa) composed of well-differentiated columnar or ciliated respiratory epithelium with variable squamous differentiation. Columnar, exophytic, and inverted papillomas are distinguished as histological subtypes [39]. Over the years, many different names have been applied for inverted papillomas (schneiderian papilloma, Ewing's papilloma, villiform cancer, papillary sinusitis, transitional cell papilloma), reflecting an initial lack of understanding of the nature and clinical entity of this tumor. Inverted papillomas account for 0.5–4% of primary nasal tumors. The incidence ranges from 0.2 to 0.6/100,000/year. A male to female ratio of 2–3:1 has been reported. The peak prevalence lies between the fifth and seventh decades [19].

Clinical Presentation

The most common site of origin is the lateral nasal wall, followed by the maxillary sinus, ethmoid sinus, the nasal septum, frontal sinus, and sphenoid sinus. Involvement of the sphenoid and frontal sinuses is mostly due to continuous growth of the tumor from the lateral nasal wall. Inverted papillomas usually present with unilateral nasal obstruction and rhinorrhea, as in unilateral chronic rhinosinusitis. Further symptoms include epiphora, epistaxis, facial pain, and headache. A bilateral involvement is seen in 4.9% of cases [13]. The time span between onset of symptoms and diagnosis of the tumor has been reported to range from 27 to 66 months, reflecting the innocuous and unspecific combination of symptoms. The differential diagnosis of an inverted papilloma should therefore be considered in every patient with unilateral symptoms of paranasal sinus disease [19]. The Krouse staging system [13] for inverted papilloma includes tumor location, extent of the disease, and presence of malignancy (Table 33.3).

Grossly, inverted papillomas appear as grey to pink polyps in endoscopic evaluation, albeit with a more fibrovascular structure than inflammatory polyps. Although the surface of these tumors is quite large, they are usually attached to the adjacent mucosa by a small pedicle-like connection (Fig. 33.3). The surface of the tumor bulk rests against adjacent epithelium, which does not show any change or tumor invasion. Inverted papillomas cause clinical problems due to their local invasion, tendency for recurrence, and association with malignancy. Association with squamous cell carcinoma (SCC) has been reported in 9.1% [13]. Inverted papilloma may present with synchronous and less commonly with metachronous malignancy. In case of synchronous malignancy, an inverted papilloma may have foci of SCC within it. Alternatively, a patient may present with two independent nasal tumors—an inverted papilloma and an SCC—at the same time. An SCC developing in an area of prior inverted papilloma resection is termed metachronous malignancy. Due to their possible association with SCC, some authors classify inverted papilloma as a premalignant lesion. However, there are no proven indicators for a malignant degeneration in inverted papilloma today. Also, the number of recurrences is not associated with the malignant potential of an inverted papilloma [19].

Pathogenesis

The term "inverted" papilloma describes the typical growth pattern of this tumor with an invagination of the epithelium into the adjacent stroma [26]. Due to basal cell hyperplasia, the epithelium is thickened compared to normal nasal mucosa. Whereas microcysts containing macrophages and cell debris in the basal cell layers are a characteristic feature, mucus-secreting cells are absent in inverted papillomas. Variable degrees of squamous metaplasia with hyperkeratinization may occur [20].

The etiology of inverted papilloma remains unclear. Allergy as a causative factor has been discounted, and no association with tobacco and alcohol is found [19]. The role of human papillomavirus (HPV) infection in tumor etiology and progression to SCC is still controversial. HPV-DNA subtypes 6, 11, 16, and 18 have been demonstrated in inverted papillomas by in situ hybridization and polymerase chain reaction with a variable prevalence in different studies [4, 10, 17]. However, neither virus particles [20] nor virus proteins [42] have been detected in inverted papillomas.

Table 33.3 Krouse staging system for inverted papilloma [13]

T1	Tumor isolated to one area of the nasal cavity without extension to paranasal sinuses
T2	Tumor involves medial wall of maxillary sinus, ethmoid sinuses, and/or osteomeatal complex
T3	Tumor involves superior, inferior, posterior, anterior, or lateral wall of the maxillary sinus or sphenoid sinus
T4	Tumor with extrasinonasal extent or malignancy

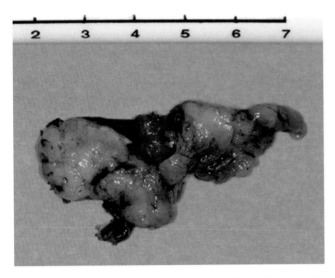

Fig. 33.3 Resection specimen of an inverted papilloma illustrating the different appearance of this tumor compared to inflammatory polyps

Radiology

Although there are classic radiographic findings for inverted papilloma, no unique pathognomonic features can be seen on CT and MRI [28]. Typically, a unilateral soft tissue mass arising from the lateral nasal wall adjacent to the middle turbinate extends into the maxillary sinus. Due to centrifugal tumor growth, the tumor spreads into the paranasal sinuses and the nasopharynx. CT scans delineate the bony changes due to inverted papilloma. As the tumor enlarges, the adjacent bone may be bowed, thinned, eroded, or sclerotic. Bone destruction is seen in up to 30% of cases and is not necessarily a sign of malignancy [41]. Bony changes are most commonly seen along the lateral nasal wall and the lamina papyracea [44]. Furthermore, calcifications of the tumor may be present on CT. This is an unspecific finding, but inverted papilloma and esthesioneuroblastoma are the most common nasal tumors with calcifications [41]. However, CT scans cannot distinguish between inverted papilloma and adjacent inflammatory tissue. Therefore, a preoperative MRI is highly useful to determine the extension of the tumor. Furthermore, MRI is superior to CT in diagnosing intracranial involvement or tumor extension into the orbital vault [45].

Therapy

Surgery is the recommended treatment for inverted papilloma, however the choice of technique is still a controversial issue. Depending on site and extent of the lesion, basically three surgical approaches are possible: (1) complete endonasal resection, (2) an external approach, for example, osteoplastic frontal sinus or osteoplastic maxillary sinus techniques, or (3) a combination of both. The goal of these procedures is an adequate tumor exposure for complete resection. The different surgical

approaches are judged by the freedom of recurrence. Traditionally, lateral rhinotomy or midfacial degloving were described as the gold standard [25]. However, inverted papilloma has been one of the first tumors claimed to be suitable for endonasal resection. Nowadays, many surgeons favor the endonasal approach in the vast majority of cases by pointing out that the recurrence rates are comparable to open procedures, ranging from 0% to 27% [21]. There are two major limitations for an exclusively endonasal approach: (1) involvement of the frontal sinus lateral to a virtual sagittal plane through the lamina papyracea and (2) tumor origin from the lateral or anterior wall of the maxillary sinus. In these cases at least a combined endonasal/osteoplastic approach or a primary osteoplastic approach should be chosen [21]. As the tumor mainly arises from the lateral nasal wall, a medial maxillectomy is performed either by an endonasal or an external approach. Regardless of the selected technique, dissection of the tumor must be carried out in the subperiosteal plane, accomplished by drilling of the underlying bone [43].

Tips to Avoid Complications

- A CT scan cannot distinguish between angiofibromas/inverted papillomas and adjacent inflammatory tissue. MRI is highly useful to determine the extension of the tumor.
- Sinus osteoma is often an "incidentoma". Therefore, the decision for surgery should be made carefully after a thorough ENT/radiological examination and, in case of headache and well-ventilated sinuses, after an additional neurological workup.
- Large osteomas are debulked with the drill before the remaining tumor parts are removed. Pay attention to identify and resect the site of tumor origin.
- Specific growth pattern and tumor blood supply allow diagnosis of a juvenile angiofibroma with high probability. A biopsy to confirm diagnosis is not necessary.
- Preoperative autologous blood donation and the use of a cell-saver device during the operation minimize the need for homologous blood transfusion in juvenile angiofibroma surgery.
- Note that association of inverted papilloma with squamous cell carcinoma has been reported in 9.1% of cases.
- Tumor resection in inverted papillomas should be carried out in the subperiosteal plane, accomplished by drilling of the underlying bone.

References

1.   Abraham SC, Montgomery EA, Giardiello FM, Wu TT (2001) Frequent beta-catenin mutations in juvenile nasopharyngeal angiofibromas. Am J Pathol 158:1073–1078

33

2. Andrews JC, Fisch U, Valavanis A, Aeppli U, Makek MS (1989) The surgical management of extensive nasopharyngeal angiofibromas with the infratemporal fossa approach. Laryngoscope 99:429–437

3. Atallah N, Jay MM (1981) Osteomas of the paranasal sinuses. J Laryngol Otol 95:291–304

4. Buchwald C, Franzmann M-B, Krag Jacobson G, Lindeberg H (1995) Human papillomavirus in sinonasal papilloma: a study of 78 cases using in situ hybridization and polymerase chain reaction. Laryngoscope 105:66–71

5. Childrey JH (1939) Osteomas of the sinuses, the frontal and sphenoid bone. Archives 30:63–72

6. Douglas R, Wormald PJ (2006) Endoscopic surgery for juvenile nasopharyngeal angiofibromas: where are the limits? Curr Opin Otolaryngol Head Neck Surg 14:1–5

7. Eller R, Sillers M (2006) Common fibro-osseous lesions of the paranasal sinuses. Otolaryngol Clin North Am 39:585–600

8. Fisch U (1983) The infratemporal fossa approach for nasopharyngeal tumors. Laryngoscope 93:36–44

9. Gardner EJ, Richards RC (1953) Multiple cutaneous and subcutaneous lesions occurring simultaneously with hereditary polyposis and osteomatosis. Am J Hum Genet 5:139–147

10. Hoffmann M, Klose N, Gottschlich S, et al (2006) Detection of human papillomavirus DNA in benign and malignant sinonasal neoplasms. Cancer Lett 139:64–70

11. Hwang HC, Mills SE, Patterson K, Gown AM (1998) Expression of androgen receptors in nasopharyngeal angiofibromas: an immunohistochemical study of 24 cases. Mod Pathol 11:1122–1126

12. Koivunen P, Löppönen H, Fors AP, Jokinen K (1997) The growth rate of osteomas of the paranasal sinuses. Clin Otolaryngol 22:111–114

13. Krouse JH (2000) Development of a staging system for inverted papilloma. Laryngoscope 110:965–968

14. Lasjaunias P (1980) Angiofibromas: hazards of embolization. Radiology 136:119–123

15. Lee DA, Rao BR, Meyer JS, Prioleau PG, Bauer WC (1980) Hormonal receptor determination in juvenile nasopharyngeal angiofibromas. Cancer 46:547–551

16. Marshall AH, Bradley PJ (2006) Management dilemmas in the treatment and follow-up of advanced juvenile nasopharyngeal angiofibromas. ORL J Otorhinolaryngol Relat Spec 68:273–278

17. McLachlin CM, Kandel RA, Colgan TJ, Swanson DB, Witterick IJ, Ngan BY (1992) Prevalence of human papillomavirus in sinonasal papillomas: a study using polymerase chain reaction and in situ hybridization. Mod Pathol 5:406–409

18. Mehta BS, Grewal GS (1963) Osteoma of the paranasal sinuses along with a case of a fronto-ethmoid osteoma. J Laryngol Otol 77:601–610

19. Melroy CT, Senior BA (2006) Benign sinonasal neoplasms: a focus on inverting papilloma. Otolaryngol Clin North Am 39:601–617

20. Michaels L (1996) Benign tumors of the nose and paranasal sinuses. Semin Diagn Pathol 13:113–117

21. Minovi A, Kollert M, Draf W, Brockmühl U (2006) Inverted papilloma: feasibility of endonasal surgery and long-term results of 87 cases. Rhinology 44:205–210

22. Montag AG, Tretiakova M, Richardson M (2006) Steroid hormone receptor expression in nasopharyngeal angiofibromas. Consistent expression of estrogen receptor beta. Am J Clin Pathol 125:832–837

23. Moretti A, Croce A, Leone O (2004) Osteoma of the maxillary sinus: case report. Acta Otorhinolaryngol Ital 24:219–222

24. Moulin G, Chagnaud C, Gras R, et al (1995) Juvenile nasopharyngeal angiofibromas: comparison of blood loss during removal in embolized group versus nonembolized group. Cardiovasc Intervent Radiol 18:158–161

25. Myers EN, Schramm VL, Barnes EL (1981) Management of inverted papilloma of the nose and paranasal sinuses. Laryngoscope 91:2071–2084

26. Reingertz N (1938) Pathology of malignant tumors arising in nasal and paranasal cavities and maxilla. Acta Otolaryngol Suppl 27:31–42

27. Savic DL, Djeric DR (1990) Indications for the surgical treatment of osteomas of the frontal and ethmoid sinuses. Clin Otolaryngol 15:397–404

28. Savy L, Lloyd G, Lund V, Howard D (2000) Optimum imaging for inverted papilloma. J Laryngol Otol 114:891–893

29. Schick B, Kahle G, Hassler R, Draf W (1996) Chemotherapy of juvenile angiofibromas: an alternative? HNO 44:148–152

30. Schick B, Kind M, Schwarzkopf G, Weber R, Draf W (1997) Angiofibroma with atypical localizations in early childhood. HNO 45:1022–1028

31. Schick B, Hendus J, El Tahan A, Draf W (1998) Reconstruction of the forehead region with tabula externa of the skull. Laryngorhinootologie 77:474–479

32. Schick B, Kahle G (2000) Radiological findings in angiofibromas. Acta Radiol 41:585–593

33. Schick B, Steigerwald C, El Rahman El Tahan A, Draf W (2001) The role of endonasal surgery in the management of frontoethmoidal osteomas. Rhinology 39:66–70

34. Schick B, Rippel C, Brunner C, Jung V, Plinkert PK, Urbschat S (2003) Numerical sex chromosome aberrations in juvenile angiofibromas: genetic evidence for an androgen-dependent tumor? Oncol Rep 10:1251–1255

35. Schick B, Urbschat S (2004) New aspects of pathogenesis of juvenile angiofibroma. Hosp Med 65:269–273

36. Schick B, Wemmert S, Jung V, Steudel W, Montenarh M, Urbschat S (2006) Genetic heterogeneity of the MYC oncogene in advanced juvenile angiofibromas. Cancer Genet Cytogenet 164:25–31

37. Schick B, Wemmert S, Bechtel U, Nicolai P, Hofmann T, Golabek W, Urbschat S (2007) Comprehensive genomic analysis identifies MDM2 and AURKA as novel amplified genes in juvenile angiofibromas. Head Neck 29: 479–487

38. Senior BA, Dubin MG (2005) Benign tumors of the frontal sinuses. In: Kountakis S, Senior B, Draf W (eds) The frontal sinus. Springer, Berlin, pp 153–164

39. Shanmugaratnam K (1991) Histological typing of tumors of the upper respiratory tract and ear. Springer, Berlin, pp 20–21

40. Smith ME, Calcaterra TC (1989) Frontal sinus osteoma. Ann Otol Rhinol Laryngol 98:896–900

41. Som PM, Lawson W, Lidov MW (1991) Simulated aggressive skull base erosion in response to benign sinonasal disease. Radiology 180:755–759

42. Strauss M, Jenson AB (1985) Human papillomavirus in various lesions of the head and neck. Otolaryngol Head Neck Surg 93:342–346

43. Tomenzoli D, Castelnuovo P, Pagella F, Berlucchi M, Pianta L, Delu G, Maroldi R, Nicolai P (2004) Different endoscopic surgical strategies in the management of inverted papilloma of the sinonasal tract: experience with 47 patients. Laryngoscope 114:193–200

44. Woodruff WW, Vrabec DP (1994) Inverted papilloma of the nasal vault and paranasal sinuses: spectrum of CT findings. AJR Am J Roentgenol 162:419–423

45. Yousem DM, Fellows DW, Kennedy DW, Bolger WE, Kashima H, Zinreich SJ (1992) Inverted papilloma: evaluation with MR imaging. Radiology 185:501–505

Chapter 34

Malignant Tumors of the Nose and Paranasal Cavity

34

Gabriel G. Calzada and Randal S. Weber

Core Messages

- Cancers of the nasal cavity and paranasal sinuses are rare, comprising 3% of head and neck malignancies.
- Sinonasal malignancies are seen twice as often in men, are most often diagnosed in the 50s through 70s, and are often associated with occupational exposures.
- Advances in office endoscopy and high-resolution imaging have facilitated more advanced treatment planning.
- Advances in cranial base surgery, microvascular free flaps, delivery of radiotherapy, and new combinations of effective chemotherapy have improved local control rates.

Contents

Introduction

Malignancies of the nasal cavity and paranasal sinuses are rare, accounting for only 3% of head and neck carcinomas and about 0.5% of all malignant disease. The annual incidence rate is 0.5–1.0 per 100,000 population [1, 35].

Treatment of paranasal sinus malignancies remains challenging. The rarity of these tumors, the similarity of their presenting symptoms to common benign nasal conditions, and their propensity for early spread results in most patients presenting with already advanced disease. However, advances in both office endoscopy and high-resolution imaging have allowed earlier detection of disease. In addition, advances in cranial base surgery, microvascular free flaps, delivery of radiotherapy, and new combinations of effective chemotherapy have improved local control rates: survival rates improved from 25% to 40% in the 1960s to 65–75% more recently [10].

Etiology

The cause of sinonasal neoplasms is unknown. Occupational exposure to inhalation of certain metal dusts or aerosols can cause dysplasia of nasal mucosa, and these malignancies are seen more frequently in workers exposed to nickel compounds, alkaline battery manufacture, or to chromium in chromate production [47]. European case-control studies revealed that exposure to leather and wood dust was associated with an excess risk of sinonasal cancer. Wood and leather workers were found to have a higher incidence of sinonasal adenocarcinoma [8, 16, 30]. Both primary and environmental (secondary) tobacco smoke also appear to be related to an increased incidence of sinonasal cancer, particularly squamous cell carcinoma [30].

Patient Evaluation

The goals of patient evaluation for suspected sinonasal cancers include establishing a diagnosis, determining the extent of disease, and developing a treatment plan. The signs and symptoms of early sinonasal tumors can be very subtle and non-specific,

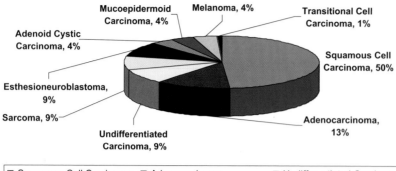

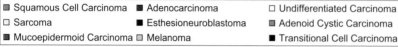

Fig. 34.1 Histology of paranasal sinus malignancies. From: Hanna et al. (1998) Skull Base Surg 8:15

34

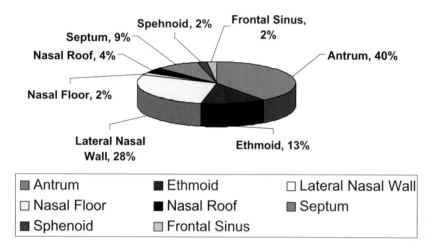

Fig. 34.2 Site of origin of paranasal malignancies. From: Hanna et al. (1998) Skull Base Surg 8:15

and are similar to those of benign conditions, thus requiring a high index of suspicion for proper diagnosis. The failure of common nasal symptoms to respond to medical management and the presence of unilateral signs and symptoms should alert the physician to the possibility of malignancy. A complete history and physical examination is crucial. The physical examination must check for facial asymmetry, limitations of extraocular movements, serous middle ear effusions, hard palate masses, and trismus, all of which can be signs of advanced disease.

Imaging is indicated whenever there is clinical suspicion for a neoplastic process. Both computed tomography (CT) and magnetic resonance imaging (MRI) are complimentary in the pretreatment evaluation of patients with sinonasal tumors. CT is better for evaluating bone destruction, whereas MRI is superior for delineating soft tissue detail [28]. In the future, positron emission tomography (PET) may supplement MRI to distinguish between tumor recurrence and post-treatment fibrosis. Angiography is not indicated in routine assessment of patients with neoplasm of the paranasal sinuses.

Biopsy of suspected malignancies of the paranasal sinuses is important not only to confirm diagnosis, but also to help in the choice of the best treatment options. Biopsies should be performed after high-resolution imaging so that severe bleeding or CSF leak can be avoided. Generously sized biopsies aid the pathologist making an accurate diagnosis. Due to many overlapping cytopathologic features, it is often difficult to distinguish the various tumors with a small sample biopsy (Figs. 34.1, 34.2).

Staging

In 1933, Ohngren proposed a method of classification for cancer of the antrum [39]. He divided the antrum into anterior-inferior and superior-posterior sections by drawing an imaginary line from the angle of the mandible to the medial canthus of the eye. Patients with cancer located above the line had a significantly worse prognosis. Despite this utility, the system was neither reproducible nor precise. Currently, the most widely used system for classifying cancers of the paranasal sinuses is the American Joint Committee on Cancer (AJCC) staging system (see Tables 34.1, 34.2).

Table 34.1 TNM for cancer of the paranasal sinuses. From: AJCC cancer staging manual, 6th edn (2002) published by Springer, New York

Primary tumor (T)	
Tx	Primary tumor cannot be assessed
T0	No evidence of primary tumor
Tis	Carcinoma in situ
Maxillary sinus	
T1	Tumor limited to maxillary sinus mucosa with no erosion or destruction of bone
T2	Tumor causing bone erosion or destruction, including extension into the hard palate and/or the middle nasal meatus, except extension to posterior wall of the maxillary sinus and pterygoid plates
T3	Tumor invades any of the following: bone of the posterior wall of maxillary sinus, subcutaneous tissues, skin of cheek, floor of medial wall of orbit, pterygoid fossa, ethmoid sinuses
T4a	Tumor invades anterior orbital contents, skin of cheek, pterygoid plates, infratemporal fossa, cribriform plate, sphenoid or frontal sinus
T4b	Tumor invades any of the following: orbital apex, dura, brain, middle cranial fossa, cranial nerves other than maxillary division of trigeminal nerve (V2), nasopharynx, or clivus
Nasal cavity and ethmoid sinuses	
T1	Tumor restricted to any one subsite, with or without bony invasion
T2	Tumor invading two subsites in a single region or extending to involve an adjacent region within the nasoethmoid complex, with or without bony invasion
T3	Tumor extends to invade the medial wall or floor of the orbit, maxillary sinus, palate, or cribriform plate
T4a	Tumor invades any of the following: anterior orbital contents, skin of nose or cheek, minimal extension to anterior cranial fossa, pterygoid plates, sphenoid or frontal sinus
T4b	Tumor invades any of the following: orbital apex, dura, brain, middle cranial fossa, cranial nerves other than V2, nasopharynx, or clivus
Regional lymph nodes (N)	
NX	Regional lymph nodes cannot be assessed
N0	No regional lymph node metastasis
N1	Metastasis in a single ipsilateral lymph node, 3 cm or less in greatest dimension
N2	Metastasis in a single ipsilateral lymph node, more than 3 cm but not more than 6 cm in greatest dimension, or in multiple ipsilateral lymph nodes, none more than 6 cm in greatest dimension, or in bilateral or contralateral lymph nodes, none more than 6 cm in greatest dimension
N2a	Metastasis in a single ipsilateral lymph node, more than 3 cm but not more than 6 cm in greatest dimension
N2b	Metastasis in multiple ipsilateral lymph node, none more than 6 cm in greatest dimension
N2c	Metastasis in bilateral or contralateral lymph nodes, none more than 6 cm in greatest dimension
N3	Metastasis in a lymph node, more than 6 cm in greatest dimension
Distant metastasis (M)	
Mx	Distant metastasis cannot be assessed
M0	No distant metastasis
M1	Distant metastasis

Table 34.2 Stage grouping. From: AJCC cancer staging manual, 6th edn (2002) published by Springer, New York

Stage 0	Tis	N0	M0
Stage I	T1	N0	M0
Stage II	T2	N0	M0
Stage III	T3	N0	M0
	T1	N1	M0
	T2	N1	M0
	T3	N1	M0
Stage IVA	T4a	N0	M0
	T4a	N1	M0
	T1	N2	M0
	T2	N2	M0
	T3	N2	M0
	T4a	N2	M0
Stage IVB	T4b	Any N	M0
	Any T	N3	M0
Stage IVC	Any T	Any N	M1

Squamous Cell Carcinoma of the Nasal Cavity and Paranasal Sinuses

Primary squamous cell carcinoma (SCC) of the nasal cavity and paranasal sinuses is a rare condition. It often presents in men between the ages of 60 and 70 years. The majority of SCCs of the paranasal sinuses are keratinizing but tend to be only moderately differentiated. Prognosis is more closely related to size and location than to histologic grade. These tumors often present in the advanced stage and, despite aggressive treatment, the disease remains highly lethal [18, 19, 50]. Cranial base extension can be seen early, most often in superiorly or posteriorly located cancers.

Treatment of SCC of the paranasal sinuses depends on the stage of disease. In general, advanced-stage disease is best treated with multimodal therapy. The most common treatment modality is radical en bloc resection followed by postoperative radiation therapy. The 5-year survival rates associated with this approach range from 55% to 70% [11, 19, 38, 50]. Other treatment options include preoperative radiation and chemotherapy followed by surgical salvage [19]. Optimal treatment strategies for SCC of the paranasal sinuses still need to be defined.

Sinonasal Adenocarcinoma

Adenocarcinoma is the second most common malignant tumor of the sinonasal tract after SCC, accounting for approximately 15% of all sinonasal cancers [18]. The ethmoid sinuses are most frequently involved [45]. Adenocarcinomas exhibit a striking male predominance (75–90%), with a peak age incidence between 55 and 60 years. There is a higher incidence of these tumors in persons involved in wood, leather, textile, and furniture industries [8, 16, 30].

Adenocarcinoma of the sinonasal tract may originate from the surface epithelium, the minor salivary glands, or both. There are three basic growth patterns: papillary, sessile, and alveolar-mucoid, with the papillary type having a better prognosis.

Since most adenocarcinomas present in the ethmoid sinuses, surgical excision frequently involves craniofacial resection. The improvement in the 5-year cancer-specific survival rate, currently between 63% and 73%, when compared to earlier studies, may be associated with increased use of craniofacial resection in the treatment of adenocarcinoma of the sinonasal tract [11, 40]. The use of endoscopic resection for localized low-grade tumors remains controversial, and further study is needed. In Europe, reports of surgical debulking with topical chemotherapy (fluorouracil) in the treatment of adenocarcinoma of the ethmoid sinuses has been reported. The authors concluded that in patients with adenocarcinoma of the ethmoid sinuses, a combination of surgical debulking and repeated topical chemotherapy results in disease control and survival rates that are not different from those obtained by craniofacial resection and postoperative radiotherapy [24]. These contrasting reports in the literature illustrate that optimal treatment for adenocarcinomas of the sinonasal tract remains unclear.

Sinonasal Undifferentiated Carcinoma

In 1986, Frierson and colleagues first described the clinical and pathologic findings of an undifferentiated carcinoma with distinct features arising in the nasal cavity and paranasal sinuses [15]. These tumors were characterized by extensive tissue destruction and frequent involvement of the orbit and anterior cranial fossa [17]. Despite their aggressive behavior, these tumors exhibit a paucity of significant symptoms relative to the extent of disease at the time of diagnosis.

Sinonasal undifferentiated carcinoma (SNUC) is composed of pleomorphic cells with a high nuclear-cytoplasmic ratio, arranged in nests, sheets, and trabeculae [15]. Immunohistochemically, virtually all SNUCs are positive for cytokeratin or epithelial membrane antigen, and many stain for both epithelial markers. Approximately one-half of the tumors are positive for neuron-specific enolase, most lack S-100 immunoreactivity, and all are negative for vimentin [15, 44]. Many SNUCs have shown positive immunostaining for LMP-1, an Epstein-Barr virus (EBV)-related protein, but the role of EBV infection in the pathogenesis of SNUC is still uncertain [6].

There is currently no consensus on the best therapeutic approach to SNUC [13, 34, 36]. In the original case series reported by Levine et al., the overall cause-specific survival for this series was 9% [26]. In 2002, Musy et al. published a follow-up study in which 10 patients were treated with curative intent with neo-adjuvant chemoradiotherapy followed by craniofacial resection. Their recommendation for patients with good performance status and limited intracranial or intraorbital disease was initial treatment with chemoradiotherapy followed by craniofacial resection. Patients whose disease is deemed inoperable as a result of advanced disease should be treated with palliative chemoradiotherapy only [36].

Olfactory Neuroblastoma (Esthesioneuroblastoma)

Olfactory neuroblastoma (ONB) is a rare tumor of the nasal cavity, with approximately 945 cases having been described in the world literature [4]. Its incidence is 3% of all intranasal tumors [31]. The sex distribution is roughly equal [4] and it is predominantly a disease of white individuals [43]. No etiologic basis has been determined. Several authors have demonstrated a bimodal distribution in age of diagnosis, showing peaks in age groups 11–20 years and 51–60 years [12, 46]. Other authors noted unimodal distribution mainly in the fifth decade of life [43].

Diagnosis tends to be late, because early lesions are largely asymptomatic. The most common presenting symptoms are unilateral nasal obstruction and epistaxis. Esthesioneuroblastoma is a tumor of neuroectodermal origin, arising from olfactory epithelium. It is usually a polypoid mass high in the nasal cavity with paranasal sinus extension, in close proximity to the cribriform plate. ONB is a locally aggressive malignancy that frequently invades the skull base and orbit. The incidence of metastasis is reportedly 10–33% at the time of diagnosis, with the most common metastatic site being the cervical lymph nodes. Distant metastasis occurs in 12–25% of patients, with lung, brain, and bone being the most common sites [12, 22, 43, 46].

Several staging systems have been proposed for ONB. The Kadish system [22] is most commonly used; however, Biller et al. presented an alternate system based on the more standard TNM system [3]. A third classification system proposed by Dulguerov and Calcaterra is based on the TNM system and incorporates high-resolution imaging before therapy [10].

The most significant advance in the treatment of ONB occurred in the 1970s. In 1976, at the University of Virginia, Drs. Jane and Fitz-Hugh introduced craniofacial resection for the treatment of ONB. Their 5-year survival improved from 37.5% to 82% when extracranial surgical excision and craniofacial resection were compared [25]. However, no consensus exists regarding the treatment of ONB: it is agreed that ONB is a surgical disease, but the role of adjuvant therapies remains uncertain, although the advent of craniofacial resection has clearly improved disease-free survival. Radiotherapy alone has been proposed as primary treatment in ONB, since it is believed that ONB is a radiosensitive tumor. However, recurrence rates of up to 67% have been cited when radiation alone was used [10, 12].

Numerous authors have commented on the effectiveness of chemotherapy in the treatment of ONB. Most authors report partial responses with preoperative or salvage chemotherapy [7, 43]. McElroy et al. reviewed a 20-year experience of chemotherapy for ONB at the Mayo Clinic, and found that only two of eight patients responded, both of whom had high-grade tumors. They recommend chemotherapy in patients with advanced, high-grade lesions, but cautioned that it is not curative. Even though these high-grade tumors were sensitive to chemotherapy, overall survival of those patients was still shorter [32].

A recent review of the MD Anderson Cancer Center experience highlighted the fact that surgery with postoperative radiation therapy is still the standard of care for all these lesions. Using this approach, the overall 5-year and 10-year survival was 89% and 81%, respectively. All incidences of recurrence were found in patients whose disease was initially stage C. Patients with stage C disease tend to have both local and regional recurrences developing during long-term follow-up, thus warranting long-term follow-up with routine imaging [9].

Sinonasal Adenoid Cystic Carcinoma

Adenoid cystic carcinoma (ACC) is a rare tumor in the sinonasal tract. Sinonasal ACC accounts for 10–25% of all head and neck ACC [21]. It is slightly more common among women, and approximately 90% of patients are between 30 and 70 years of age, with a peak incidence in the fifth and sixth decades of life.

Adenoid cystic carcinoma exhibits three histologic subtypes based on tumor architecture: cribriform, tubular, and solid. The most common subtype is the cribriform, but the solid subtype is known to have the worst prognosis among the three subtypes [48]. Pathologic subtype has not been shown to serve as an independent prognosis-determining factor in sinonasal ACC.

Among the various malignancies of salivary gland origin originating in the sinonasal tract, ACC shows a peculiar biologic characteristic. It exhibits a slow-growing, locally aggressive, relentless progression of disease. It tends to recur locally long after remission by initial treatment. Recurrence can occur 10–20 years after the initial treatment, and, thus, 5-year survival rates may give an erroneous indication of absolute survival [23]. Sinonasal ACC most often arises from the maxillary sinus, and frequently has delayed distant metastasis. Perineural spread, the hallmark of adenoid cystic carcinoma, is usually evident and provides avenues of spread to the cranial base and the central nervous system. Perineural invasion in ACC has been considered as one of the determining factors for locoregional recurrence or distant metastasis [49]. Lymphatic spread of ACC is uncommon. The incidence of lymph node metastasis from ACC detected at presentation or developing later in the course of the disease ranges from 10% to 30% [21]. Distant hematogenous dissemination is considerably more frequent than lymphatic metastasis, with an average incidence of 40%. The lungs and bones are the sites most frequently involved in systemic metastasis.

The treatment for ACC of the sinonasal tract has traditionally been surgical resection with postoperative adjuvant radiation therapy. Due to perineural spread, achievement of negative surgical margins in cases of ACC of the sinonasal tract can be difficult, which provides an explanation as to why ACC of the si-

34

nonasal tract has the worst prognosis of all sites in the head and neck [23]. In a recent report from the University of Pittsburgh of 35 patients with ACC of the sinonasal tract treated with craniofacial resection and postoperative radiation, the local control rate was 64%. This high rate of local disease control, however, did not translate to an improvement in disease-free survival, probably because of the high incidence of distant metastasis [41]. In the University of Michigan experience with patients with ACC of the sinonasal tract, the 6-year survival for patients treated with surgery and radiation was 73% compared with 50% for those treated with radiation alone [37]. Currently, the use of chemotherapy in the treatment of ACC is investigational. Over the past decade, there has been growing evidence that fast-neutron radiation therapy provides higher rates of locoregional control of unresectable or recurrent ACC compared with photon or electron radiation therapy, and perhaps should be considered the initial treatment of choice in some cases [20].

Sinonasal Melanoma

Mucosal melanoma of the head and neck is an uncommon condition. Sinonasal tract mucosal melanomas account for approximately 3% of sinonasal cancers [18]. Mucosal melanoma occurs most frequently in the nasal cavity. The anterior portion of the nasal septum (33%) and the lateral nasal wall (28%) are the most common sites of development of the tumors, followed by the middle and inferior turbinates (15%), and nasal vestibule (10%). In the paranasal sinuses, the most common site of origin is the maxillary sinus, followed by the ethmoid (6%), frontal, and sphenoid sinuses (1%) [14]. The peak age of incidence is between the fifth and eighth decades. Patients with sinonasal melanoma commonly present with epistaxis and nasal obstruction as well as unilateral polyposis with or without pigmentation. Concurrent nasal and paranasal lesions are infrequent.

Histologic appearance of sinonasal melanoma is varied. High mitotic rate and vascular invasion, absence of tumor-infiltrating lymphocytes, and regression are features shared by all sinonasal melanomas. Special stains and electron microscopy are used to establish the diagnosis. Cytokeratin differentiates melanoma from undifferentiated carcinoma. S-100 protein is usually expressed, but with variable staining intensity. HMB45 is strongly and uniformly expressed in over 80% of all undifferentiated small blue cell sinonasal melanomas. In poorly differentiated amelanotic malignant melanomas, antibody to HMB45 has proved to be a superb diagnostic marker [42].

Mucosal melanomas of the paranasal sinuses are rapidly lethal neoplasms [33]. Long-term survival is unusual to rare; 5-year survival is poor, and the 10-year survival is dismal [2].

In 1999 Lund and associates published their experience with sinonasal mucosal melanoma. In 72 patients with sinonasal mucosal melanoma treated with radical surgery with and without adjuvant radiation therapy, overall 5-year actuarial survival was 28%, and overall 10-year survival was 20%, with a median survival of 21 months. There was no statistical difference in local control or survival between patients receiving surgery alone and those receiving surgery and radiotherapy. The addition of chemotherapy had no impact on survival, nor did the site of the tumor, the surgical procedure, the presence of lymph node metastases, or the age of the patient [29]. Future work on mucosal melanomas will focus on biologic and immunomodulatory treatments.

Sinonasal Sarcomas, Lymphomas, and Metastasis to the Sinonasal Tract

The most common head and neck sarcoma is rhabdomyosarcoma. Rhabdomyosarcoma involving the sinonasal tract accounts for approximately 10% of head and neck rhabdomyosarcomas. Sinonasal rhabdomyosarcomas involving the non-orbital parameningeal sites demonstrate a more aggressive behavior than do those arising in other sites. A study for MD Anderson Cancer Center reported the outcome of 37 pediatric and adult patients with sinonasal rhabdomyosarcomas. Overall 5-year survival was 44%. For patients treated with a combination of chemotherapy and radiotherapy with or without surgery, 5-year survival was 60%, compared with 19% for patients treated with other forms of therapy. Factors associated with poorer survival were adult onset of disease, alveolar histology, and treatment with systemic chemotherapy for less than 1 year [5]. Other forms of sarcoma in the sinonasal tract include: chondrosarcomas, chordomas, angiosarcomas, and osteogenic sarcomas.

Extranodal non-Hodgkin's lymphoma (NHL) of the head and neck is relatively uncommon. Various staging systems, different modality of therapy, and small cohorts of populations make comparisons between different studies difficult. Most treatment plans include various combinations of radiation therapy and chemotherapy.

Sinonasal T-cell lymphoma is a distinct clinicopathologic entity and has a strong association with EBV infection. This disorder is rare in Western populations and occurs more commonly among Asians, Mexicans, and South Americans, accounting for 2.6–8.0% of all NHLs [51]. Sinonasal T-cell lymphomas are characterized clinically by progressive destruction of nasal or midline facial structures, and patients are prone to massive nasal bleeding. These lymphomas have a relative higher resistance to combination treatment modalities, and currently more aggressive systemic therapy is under investigation [27].

Renal cell carcinoma is the most common source of distant metastasis to the sinonasal tract. Other metastatic lesions include lung, breast, and ovarian malignancies. Treatment is usually palliative and often radiation therapy.

Take-Home Pearls

- Sinonasal tumors comprise a variety of neoplasms with diverse biologic behavior, ranging from slow-growing and indolent to highly aggressive and lethal.
- Understanding the biologic behavior of these tumors is paramount to selecting the optimal treatment strategy.

- The signs and symptoms of early-stage sinonasal malignancy are similar to those of benign conditions and require a high index of suspicion for their proper diagnosis.
- Both CT and MRI are complimentary in the pretreatment evaluation of patients with sinonasal tumors.
- Treatment of sinonasal tumors is frequently multimodal, and requires close ongoing multidisciplinary cooperation.
- Major prognostic factors include stage of the disease, surgical margins, and mode of therapy.
- Future research should focus on quality of life and biologic markers of aggressive behavior.

References

1. Ayiomamitis A, Parker L, Havas T (1988) The epidemiology of malignant neoplasms of the nasal cavities, the paranasal sinuses and the middle ear in Canada. Arch Otorhinolaryngol 244:367–371
2. Batsakis JG, Suarez P, El-Naggar AK (1998) Mucosal melanoma of the head and neck. Ann Otol Rhinol Laryngol 107:626–630
3. Biller HF, Lawson W, Sachdev VP, et al.(1990) Esthesioneuroblastoma: surgical treatment without radiation. Laryngoscope 100:1199–1201
4. Broich G, Pagliaria A, Ottaviani F (1997) Esthesioneuroblastoma: a general review of the cases published since the discovery of the tumor in 1924. Anticancer Res 17:2683–2706
5. Callender TA, Weber RS, Janjan N, et al.(1995) Rhabdomyosarcoma of the nose and paranasal sinuses in adults and children. Otolaryngol Head Neck Surg 112:252–257
6. Cerilli LA, Holst VA, Brandwein MS, et al.(2001) Sinonasal undifferentiated carcinoma. Am J Surg Pathol 25:156–163
7. Chao KSC, Kaplan C, Simpson JR, et al.(2001) Esthesioneuroblastoma: the impact of treatment modality. Head Neck 23:749–757
8. Demers PA, Kogevinas M, Boffetta P, et al.(1995) Wood dust and sinonasal cancer: pooled reanalysis of twelve case-control studies. Am J Ind Med 28:151–166
9. Diaz EM, Johnigan RH, Pero C, et al.(2005) Olfactory neuroblastoma: the 22-year experience at one comprehensive cancer center. Head Neck 27:138–149
10. Dulguerov P, Calcaterra T (1992) Esthesioneuroblastoma: the UCLA experience 1970–1990. Laryngoscope 102:843–849
11. Dulguerov P, Jacobsen MS, Allal AS, et al.(2001) Nasal and paranasal sinus carcinoma: are we making progress? Cancer 92:3012–3029
12. Elkon D, Hightower SI, Linn ML, et al.(1979) Esthesioneuroblastoma. Cancer 44:1087–1094
13. Enepekides DJ (2005) Sinonasal undifferentiated carcinoma: an update. Curr Opin Otolaryngol Head Neck Surg 13:222–225
14. Freedman HM, DeSanto LW, Devine KD, et al.(1973) Malignant melanoma of the nasal cavity and paranasal sinuses. Arch Otolaryngol 97:322–325
15. Frierson HF Jr, Mills SE, Fechner RE, et al.(1986) Sinonasal undifferentiated carcinoma: an aggressive neoplasm derived from schneiderian epithelium and distinct from olfactory neuroblastoma. Am J Surg Pathol 13:947–954
16. Gordon I, Boffetta P, Demers PA (1998) A case study comparing a meta-analysis and a pooled analysis of studies of sinonasal cancer among wood workers. Epidemiology 9:518–524
17. Gorelick J, Ross D, Marentette L, et al.(2000) Sinonasal undifferentiated carcinoma: case series and review of the literature. Neurosurgery 47:750–755
18. Hanna E, Vural E, Teo C, et al.(1998) Sinonasal tumors: the Arkansas experience. Skull Base Surg 8:15
19. Hayashi T, Nonaka S, Bandoh N, et al.(2001) Treatment outcome of maxillary sinus squamous cell carcinoma. Cancer 92:1495–1503
20. Huber PE, Debus J, Latz D, et al.(2001) Radiotherapy for advanced adenoid cystic carcinoma: neutrons, photons or mixed beam? Radiother Oncol 59:161–167
21. Jones AS, Hamilton JW, Rowley H, et al.(1997) Adenoid cystic carcinoma of the head and neck. Clin Otolaryngol 22:434–443
22. Kadish S, Goodman M, Wang CC (1976) Olfactory neuroblastoma. A clinical analysis of 17 cases. Cancer 37:1571–1576
23. Kim GE, Park HC, Keum KC, et al.(1999) Adenoid cystic carcinoma of the maxillary antrum. Am J Otolaryngol 20:77–84
24. Knegt PP, Ah-See KW, vd Velden LA, et al.(2001) Adenocarcinoma of the ethmoidal sinus complex: surgical debulking and topical fluorouracil may be the optimal treatment. Arch Otolaryngol Head Neck Surg 127:141–146
25. Levine PA, McLean WC, Canrell RW (1986) Esthesioneuroblastoma: the University of Virginia experience 1960–1985. Laryngoscope 96:742–746
26. Levine PA, Frierson HF, Stewart FM, et al.(1987) Sinonasal undifferentiated carcinoma: a distinctive and highly aggressive neoplasm. Laryngoscope 97:905–908
27. Li CC, Tien HF, Tang JL, et al.(2004) Treatment outcome and pattern of failure in 77 patients with sinonasal natural killer/T-cell or T-cell lymphoma. Cancer 100:366–375
28. Loevner LA, Sonners AI (2002) Imaging of neoplasms of the paranasal sinuses. Magn Reson Imaging Clin N Am 10:467–493
29. Lund VJ, Howard D, Harding L, et al.(1999) Management options and survival in malignant melanoma of the sinonasal mucosa. Laryngoscope 109:208–211
30. Mannetje A, Kogevinas M, Luce D, et al.(1999) Sinonasal cancer, occupation, and tobacco smoking in European men and women. Am J Ind Med 36:101–107
31. McCormack LJ, Harris HE (1955) Neurogenic tumors of the nasal fossa. JAMA 157:318–321
32. McElroy EA, Buckener JC, Lewis JE (1998) Chemotherapy for advanced esthesioneuroblastoma: the Mayo Clinic experience. Neurosurgery 42:1023–1028
33. Medina JE, Ferlito A, Pellitteri PK, et al.(2003) Current management of mucosal melanoma of the head and neck. J Surg Oncol 83:116–122

34

34. Mendenhall WM, Mendenhall CM, Riggs CE, et al.(2006) Sinonasal undifferentiated carcinoma. Am J Clin Oncol 29:27–31

35. Muir CS, Nectoux J (1980) Descriptive epidemiology of malignant neoplasms of nose, nasal cavities, middle ear and accessory sinuses. Clin Otolaryngol 5:195–211

36. Musy PY, Reidel JF, Levine PA (2002) Sinonasal undifferentiated carcinoma: the search for a better outcome. Laryngoscope 112:1450–1455

37. Naficy S, Disher MJ, Esclamado RM (1999) Adenoid cystic carcinoma of the paranasal sinuses. Am J Rhinol 13:311–314

38. Ogawa K, Toita T, Kakinohana Y, et al.(2001) Postoperative radiotherapy for squamous cell carcinoma of the maxillary sinus: analysis of local control and late complications. Oncol Rep 8:315–319

39. Ohngren LG (1933) Malignant tumors of the maxillo-ethmoidal region. Acta Otolaryngol 19:476

40. Orvidas LJ, Lewis JE, Weaver AL, et al.(2005) Adenocarcinoma of the nose and paranasal sinuses: a retrospective study of diagnosis, histologic characteristics, and outcomes in 24 patients. Head Neck 27:370–375

41. Pitman KT, Prokopakis EP, Aydogan B, et al.(1999) The role of skull base surgery for the treatment of adenoid cystic carcinoma of the sinonasal tract. Head Neck 21:402–407

42. Regauer S, Anderhuber W, Richtig E, et al.(1998) Primary mucosal melanoma of the nasal cavity and paranasal sinuses. A clinicopathological analysis of 14 cases. APMIS 106:403–410

43. Resto VA, Eisele DW, Forastiere A, et al.(2000) Esthesioneuroblastoma: the Johns Hopkins experience. Head Neck 22:550–558

44. Righi PD, Francis F, Aron BS, et al.(1996) Sinonasal undifferentiated carcinoma: a 10-year experience. Am J Otolaryngol 17:167–171

45. Roush GC (1979) Epidemiology of cancer of the nose and paranasal sinuses: current concepts. Head Neck Surg 2:3–11

46. Spaulding CA, Kranyak MS, Constable WC, et al.(1988) Esthesioneuroblastoma: a comparison of two treatment eras. Int J Radiat Oncol Biol Phys 15:581–590

47. Sunderman FW (2001) Nasal toxicity, carcinogenicity, and olfactory uptake of metals. Ann Clin Lab Sci 31:3–24

48. Szanto PA, Luna MA, Tortoledo ME (1984) Histologic grading of adenoid cystic carcinoma of the salivary glands. Cancer 54:1062–1069

49. Teymoortash A, Pientka A, Schrader C, et al.(2005) Expression of galectin-3 in adenoid cystic carcinoma of the head and neck and its relationship with distant metastasis. J Cancer Res Clin Oncol 24:1–6

50. Tiwari R, Hardillo JA, Mehta D, et al.(2000) Squamous cell carcinoma of maxillary sinus. Head Neck 22:164–169

51. Van GJ, Liu WP, Jacobse K, et al.(1994) Epstein-Barr virus in nasal T-cell lymphomas in Western China. J Pathol 173:81–87

Chapter 35

Benign Cysts and Tumors of the Jaw Bones

Pushkar Mehra

35

Core Messages

- Contemporary surgical treatment of benign pathology of the jaws must be based on evidence-based concepts related to the principles of specific cyst and tumor biology.
- Most benign lesions of the jaws are odontogenic in origin and, thus, it is imperative to have a sound understanding of surgery as well as dentistry for appropriate treatment of these lesions.
- Unlike their malignant counterparts, most benign pathologic lesions of the jaws do not require extensive resection-type surgical procedures. Although many lesions appear large on clinical and radiographic presentations, most can adequately be treated with enucleation and/or curettage.

Contents

Introduction

The diagnosis and management of benign lesions of the jaws is one of the most exciting and challenging areas in head and neck pathology. The intricate and detailed anatomy of this region make diagnosis and treatment of jaw bone diseases an extremely complex science. The maxilla and mandible are associated with bone, odontogenic epithelium, developmental remnants, salivary and seromucous glands, sinonasal and dermal epithelia, and nerve tissue elements besides other structures; thus, one can only imagine that a very diverse array of pathologic lesions can arise within the upper and lower jaws.

Definitive diagnosis of jaw lesions requires close interaction between the surgeon, radiologist, and pathologist because clinical presentations, radiographic interpretations, and microscopic features of many jaw lesions have striking similarities. This chapter is a concise description of common jaw diseases. It has been divided into two broad sections: cysts of the jaws and tumors of the jaws. The aim is to familiarize the reader with a combination of basic and advanced principles required to optimally treat benign jaw pathology.

Cysts of the Jaws

Cystic lesions are pathologic cavities remarkable for the presence of an epithelial lining. Cysts are commonly encountered in the jaws and oral cavity, and the epithelial lining of oral cystic lesions may be derived from a variety of sources including residua of epithelium persisting following odontogenesis, from glandular tissue such as salivary and seromucous glands, from the sinonasal tract, and from dermal epithelial tissue. Although the pathogenesis of cysts of the oral cavity is incompletely understood, appropriate clinicopathologic correlation typically makes it possible to diagnose and treat the lesions.

The classification of maxillofacial cystic lesions is somewhat controversial. In the text that follows, the classification of cysts will be divided into cysts of either odontogenic or non-odontogenic origin. Additionally, lesions of a "pseudocystic" nature are described, and these are remarkable for the absence of a true epithelial lining. The following discussion is written with an aim to delineate the characteristic clinical and histologic features of some common cysts of the oral cavity, and to provide pertinent information for the clinician to render an appropriate diagnosis and provide optimal treatment for these cystic lesions.

Odontogenic Cysts

An odontogenic cyst develops from remnants of odontogenic epithelium that may persist in the oral cavity following tooth development. Although the pathogenesis of odontogenic cysts is incompletely understood, stimulation and proliferation of these odontogenic epithelial residua are thought to result in cyst development [1, 2]. Bone resorption is frequently associated with expansion of a cystic lesion; this expansion gives rise to a radiolucent bony defect. Often, a thin radiopaque border is appreciated at the periphery of a cystic radiolucency on plain films; this sclerotic border is the result of reparative bone developing at a faster rate at the periphery as compared to the rate of bone resorption occurring centrally due to cystic growth.

Developmental Odontogenic Cysts

Dentigerous Cyst

In the final stages of tooth development, the outer and inner enamel epithelial tissues merge to form the reduced enamel epithelium. Proliferation of this epithelial lining and subsequent expansion of the subjacent follicular space leads to cyst formation. Although the exact pathogenesis is uncertain, differing theories suggest methods whereby accumulation of luminal fluid leads to cyst formation and expansion [3, 4]. Although these cysts are considered to be developmental in nature, some appear to arise secondary to an inflammatory stimulus.

By definition, a dentigerous cyst is associated with the crown of an unerupted tooth and is adherent to the cementoenamel junction. Dentigerous cysts comprise approximately 20% of all cystic lesions of the jaws [5, 6], and are found in highest frequency associated with impacted third molar and canine teeth. Most dentigerous cysts are asymptomatic and discovered on routine radiographic examination presenting as a well-circumscribed unilocular to multilocular radiolucency around the crown of an unerupted tooth (Fig. 35.1a). Large lesions may compromise the integrity of the mandible (Fig. 35.1b). Since many other odontogenic cysts and tumors can present in a dentigerous configuration, histologic evaluation is required in order to make a definitive diagnosis.

Histologic examination shows stratified squamous epithelium and fibromyxomatous connective tissue in cystic configuration. The cystic epithelial lining is thin and may occasionally contain "Rushton" bodies. Foci of lining cells exhibiting mucous differentiation or a ciliated luminal surface can be observed. When inflammation is present, the epithelial lining is typically hyperplastic with a complicated, anastomosing rete ridge ar-

chitecture. Occasional discrete odontogenic epithelial rests and dystrophic calcifications may be found in the cyst wall. Rare cases of mucoepidermoid carcinoma and clonal transformation of the cystic epithelial lining to squamous cell carcinoma have been reported [7].

Diagnostic Workup and Treatment

Dentigerous cysts can vary in size; if allowed to enlarge, they may, over time, cause significant bony expansion and destruction of large portions of the jaws (Fig. 35.1b). A panoramic radiograph is usually sufficient for treatment planning of most cases, but computed tomography (CT) scans can be valuable, especially when treatment planning large cysts.

For large lesions, especially those with an aggressive behavior, an incisional biopsy may be indicated to rule out other cysts and tumors. Aspiration of all lesions is recommended to rule out vascular lesions. This can easily be accomplished with a 14- or 16-gauge needle under local anesthesia. If the aspirate contains straw-colored fluid, a diagnosis of a cystic lesion is more likely, versus a situation with a lack of aspirate, which may lead the practitioner to think in terms of solid lesions such as ameloblastomas, which can have very similar radiographic and clinical appearances (Fig. 35.1c).

The preferred treatment for dentigerous cysts is complete removal of the lesion via enucleation. Surgery is usually performed through an intraoral approach. A full thickness mucoperiosteal flap is raised and, if required, bone is removed to access the cyst. The round back edge of a surgical curette is then used to lift the thick-walled cyst from its bony cavity. Even if the cyst is in close proximity to the inferior alveolar neurovascular bundle, it can generally be separated from the bundle with careful dissection. The associated tooth is extracted concurrently. Adjacent teeth do not need to be extracted unless a specific indication for tooth sacrifice exists (example: inability to remove the complete cyst because of lack of surgical access, severe external root resorption, etc.) (Fig. 35.1d–f).

Marsupalization of large dentigerous cysts can also be performed, and may be indicated in certain cases depending on patient preference or surgeon experience. It does not decrease the chance of pathologic fracture or infection. The clinician must understand that although it involves prolonged treatment time and carries the theoretical risk of neoplastic transformation, it has the advantage of naturally shrinking the lesion over time, thereby making the definitive surgery less invasive and less complicated.

In certain selected cases of large cysts, additional treatment including intermaxillary fixation and bone grafting may be indicated. Recurrence is extremely rare unless incomplete removal of the cyst was performed during initial surgery.

Eruption Cyst

Representing a soft tissue counterpart to the dentigerous cyst, an eruption cyst occurs within the alveolar mucosa and arises

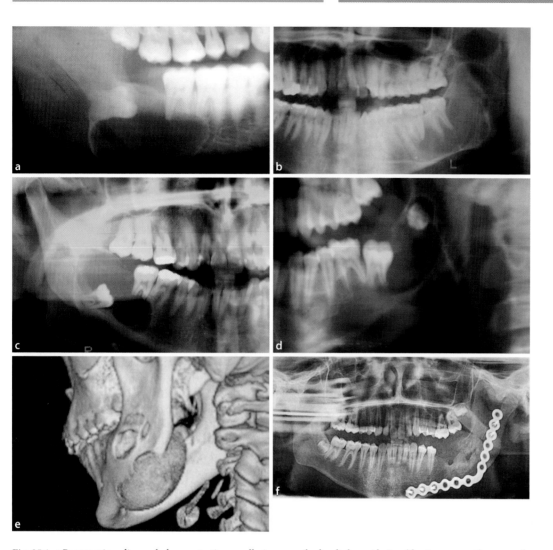

Fig. 35.1 **a** Panoramic radiograph demonstrating a well-circumscribed radiolucent lesion (dentigerous cyst) surrounding the crown of an impacted third molar. Note that the lesion has caused resorption of adjacent teeth roots. **b** A large dentigerous cyst involving the left mandible body, angle, and ascending ramus areas. **c** Unilocular cystic lesion similar to a dentigerous cyst, which was found to be an ameloblastoma. **d** Preoperative panoramic radiograph showing a large dentigerous cyst in a 18-year-old man. The lesion caused significant facial expansion and destruction of the left mandible. **e** Preoperative CT scan showing dentigerous cyst and associated mandibular expansion. **f** Postoperative panoramic radiograph after mandibular resection with nerve preservation, and jaw reconstruction with cancellous marrow bone grafts. Note the large amount of bone volume that has successfully been built following resection

following formation of a cleft between the crown of an erupting tooth and its associated dental follicle. This cystic lesion presents clinically as a translucent swelling of the alveolar mucosa superficial to an erupting tooth. Frequently, hemorrhage into the cystic cavity may impart a bluish color to the lesion.

Eruption cysts are typically seen in young children, generally between the ages of five and nine, and are commonly found in the permanent dentition with the first molars and maxillary anterior teeth most frequently affected [8]. Occasionally patients with multiple eruption cysts are encountered, and some cases have been linked to use of medications such as cyclosporin A and diphenylhydantoin. Histologically, the eruption cyst is located within the connective tissue in close approximation to the surface mucosa and is lined by unremarkable stratified squamous epithelium.

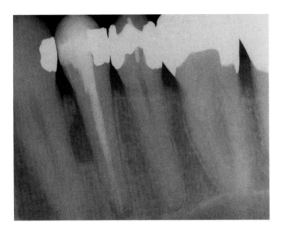

Fig. 35.2 Radiolucent lesion in between the canine and premolar teeth which was diagnosed to be a lateral periodontal cyst. It is not uncommon for odontogenic keratocysts to have a similar presentation

35

Treatment

Most eruption cysts do not require surgery, and resolve without intervention. Occasionally, an eruption cyst may prevent eruption of the underlying tooth and, in these cases, "de-roofing" of the cyst may be indicated to allow for eruption. Localized incision and drainage with antibiotic treatment may be required in infected cysts. Care should be taken during any surgery as overzealous instrumentation may cause damage to the underlying erupting tooth.

Lateral Periodontal Cyst

The lateral periodontal cyst is presumed to originate from residual remnants of dental lamina retained within the alveolar bone following tooth development [9]. It presents clinically as a well-circumscribed solitary "teardrop-shaped" radiolucency in between the roots of vital teeth (Fig. 35.2). These lesions have a predilection for occurring in the mandible, and are most frequently encountered in the premolar region [9, 10]. A variant of the lateral periodontal cyst called the botryoid (resembling a cluster of grapes) odontogenic cyst typically presents in a multilocular configuration. A higher recurrence rate has been reported for the botryoid variant, which may be related to difficulties encountered in completely removing the multilocular lesion in its entirety.

Histologic examination of the lateral periodontal cyst reveals a stratified squamous epithelial lined cavity remarkable for focal areas of nodular intraluminal proliferation. Glycogenated clear cells are commonly dispersed throughout the lining epithelium and may comprise a significant component of the nodular epithelial foci. In contrast to the conventional lateral periodontal cyst, the botryoid variant typically shows multiple independent epithelial-lined cavities, which are histologically identical to the conventional counterpart. Both the solitary and multilocular lesion lack remarkable significant inflammation, unless secondarily infected. One rare case of squamous cell carcinoma arising from the lining of a lateral periodontal cyst has been documented in the literature [11].

Treatment

Enucleation of the lesion is the treatment of choice for a true lateral periodontal cyst. Bone regeneration within the surgical defect occurs spontaneously. A broad-based full-thickness mucoperiosteal flap is recommended as it allows for adequate coverage of the bony defect and minimizes the chances of postoperative periodontal disease. Most lesions are accessed via a labial or buccal approach. Recurrence is not expected, and most recurrences often related to incomplete removal of the original cyst. Multilocular lesions should also be treated with enucleation, but, as the epithelial lining is thin, the potential for incomplete removal and thus recurrence is greater. Follow up for approximately 10 years is recommended for multilocular "botryoid" lesions because of the limited number of reported cases and lack of complete understanding of its behavior.

Odontogenic Keratocyst

The odontogenic keratocyst is believed to arise from remnants of the dental lamina retained within the alveolar bone following tooth development. It is remarkable for an aggressive infiltrative growth pattern and a high rate of recurrence similar to a benign cystic neoplasm [12]. Odontogenic keratocysts occur both in a sporadic fashion and as a component of the nevoid basal cell carcinoma syndrome, in which patients may develop multiple lesions. Recently, the gene for nevoid basal cell carcinoma syndrome was mapped to chromosome 9q22.3 and shown to be the human homologue to the *Drosophila* segment polarity gene ptc patched (PTCH) [13, 14]. This tumor suppressor gene functions as a component of the Hedgehog signaling pathway and has

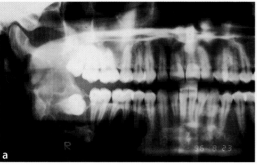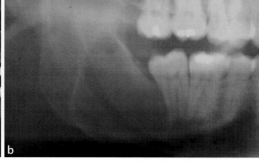

Fig. 35.3a,b Odontogenic keratocysts can present with a multilocular (**a**) or unilocular appearance (**b**)

been isolated in both sporadic and syndrome-associated odontogenic keratocysts [15].

The odontogenic keratocyst can present over a wide age range with the most common age range being patients around 30 years of age [16]. Most often, these lesions occur in the posterior mandible in a dentigerous configuration associated with the crown of an unerupted tooth. Our experience has shown a significant number of odontogenic keratocysts may also present in the mandibular canine and first premolar regions and mimic a lateral periodontal cyst. Maxillary lesions are less frequently seen. Odontogenic keratocysts may reach a large size prior to detection, and may show either a unilocular or multilocular radiographic appearance (Fig. 35.3a, b). Patients usually become symptomatic only when the lesions are large enough to cause pain and expansion [16, 17]. A review of the literature reports a wide recurrence rate, ranging from 1% to 56% [18].

Histologically, the odontogenic keratocyst characteristically has a uniformly thin stratified squamous cystic epithelial lining, approximately six to eight cell layers in thickness. The luminal surface exhibits parakeratosis with focal surface corrugations akin to corrugated cardboard when viewed on-end. Parakeratotic debris may be appreciated within the cystic lumen. The basal epithelial layer of the cystic lining exhibits nuclear palisading and hyperchromaticity. In the presence of inflammation, the cystic epithelial lining often loses these characteristic features and demonstrates a more hyperplastic appearance with transformation to a non-keratinizing stratified squamous morphology. Cell proliferation markers and cytokeratin expression patterns are altered in odontogenic keratocysts in the context of inflammation [19, 20]. This alteration has been demonstrated in cysts undergoing marsupalization (decompression and irrigation) prior to surgical removal. This alteration in composition suggests that marsupalization techniques have the potential to transform aggressive lesions into less proliferative cysts with reduced recurrence [20].

Treatment

Although gains in knowledge in recent years have improved the understanding of these lesions, the odontogenic keratocyst remains an enigma for clinicians and researchers. The aims of treatment include the lowest rate of recurrence with the least degree of morbidity to the patient, and ruling out the presence of nevoid basal cell carcinoma syndrome. Enucleation of the lesion, by itself, is not an acceptable form of treatment. The cystic lining of these lesions is very friable and will tend to fragment during enucleation, thereby leading to an increased incidence of incomplete removal of lesions. Root canal therapy is not required for teeth that test negative to electric and thermal vitality testing, but these teeth should be monitored closely. If the lesion invaginates around teeth roots, it should be curetted out completely. The teeth that are instrumented in their radicular portions may become denervated but are not devitalized, and most regain responsiveness to pulp testing within 1–2 years.

The general approach for treating these lesions is enucleation and curettage. The most commonly employed method of curettage after enucleation is "mechanical curettage" in the form of a "peripheral ostectomy" using hand or rotary instruments. Some authors recommend use of additional "chemical curettage" using Carnoy's solution. This is a chemical fixative that is applied to the bony cavity following enucleation and curettage, and it has been demonstrated that after a 5-min application the chemical penetrates bone up to a depth of 1.54 mm [21, 22]. Thermal curettage with cryotherapy has also been shown to be effective [23], but is not very popular as cryotherapy equipment is not universally available. Alternative therapies for treatment include marsupalization and resection. Marsupalization of large lesions has been shown to be effective, and is gaining in popularity. Proponents of marsupalization claim that the cystic lining becomes thicker and easier to remove after prolonged irrigations, and a significant reduction in the size of the lesion (including complete elimination of cysts) can be attained. It has also been shown that irrigation and decompression techniques can trans-

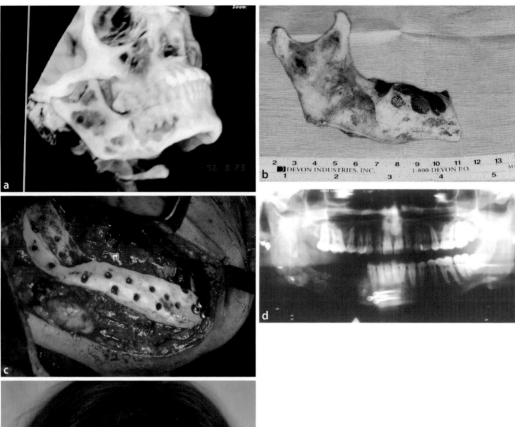

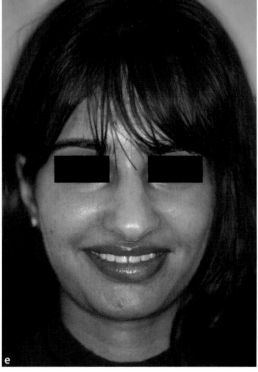

Fig. 35.4 **a** Three-dimensional CT scan showing a large odontogenic keratocyst of the right mandible. **b** The mandible including the condylar and coronoid processes has been resected. This is termed a disarticulation resection as part of the temporomandibular joint is included in the resection specimen. **c** Concomitant reconstruction of the resected area with a cadaveric rib and iliac crest bone grafts. Cancellous bone grafts have many advantages as they are easy to harvest with minimal morbidity, can be conformed to facial contours and are ideal for reconstruction following ablative surgery for benign lesions. **d** Postoperative panoramic radiograph showing reconstructed right mandible. Note how bone grafting has successfully been used to completely re-form the condyle and coronoid processes with adequate bone height in the alveolar bone area. **e** Postoperative photograph showing the effectiveness of modern reconstruction procedures in obtaining extremely esthetic results

form an aggressive cyst to a histologically more benign cyst. In contrast, opponents of this technique contend that it may lead to a higher rate of recurrence, especially in multilocular cases, and that the treatment has the disadvantages of a protracted course which does not decrease the incidence of pathologic fracture or infection.

Resection is indicated in two instances: (1) multiple recurrences after enucleation and curettage procedures, and/or (2) large multilocular keratocysts in which an enucleation and curettage procedure would result in near continuity loss by itself. Initial resection margins should be approximately 0.5–1.0 cm based on panoramic radiographs. Intraoperative radiographs of a resected specimen can be invaluable tools as they can help the clinician with intraoperative clinical decision making for deciding final surgical margins. Figure 35.4a–e shows treatment of an odontogenic keratocyst of the mandible treated by one-stage mandibular resection and reconstruction. Traditionally, resection has often been performed in en bloc fashion, with sacrifice of the inferior alveolar neurovascular bundle. However, newer modifications to this surgery are being used whereby the inferior alveolar nerve can be preserved despite resection procedures.

Location of an odontogenic keratocyst also influences treatment philosophies. Some surgeons recommend more aggressive treatment for maxillary odontogenic keratocysts as compared to mandibular lesions. This philosophy is based on the fact that there is a lack of thick cortical boundaries in the maxilla, and large lesions can rapidly extend into soft tissues and "dangerous" areas like the orbit and infratemporal fossa. However, for small lesions, enucleation and curettage is very effective. In this area, a sinus communication will often result, but this will readily heal with good primary closure. The presence of the maxillary sinus should not intimidate the clinician into being less thorough in this location and thereby invite recurrence.

The author of this chapter has used all the above treatment modalities. Each case must be individually assessed, and treatment rendered with the aims of performing the least morbid surgery with the lowest rate of recurrence. In addition to the primary mode of treatment, we also advocate the practice of removal of a rim of keratinized gingival tissue (especially on the lingual aspect) as it is believed that recurrences may arise from the residual odontogenic tissue (epithelial rests) that is found in this area.

Prognosis

A wide variance in recurrence rates has been reported in the literature [18]. However, a critical analysis of the recurrence literature reveals a wide array of treatment methods with limited scientific stratification of data regarding size, location, origin, and recurrence. Many reasons for recurrence have been proposed including [24, 25]: (a) collagenase production, (b) daughter or satellite cysts, (c) budding, (d) incomplete removal, and (e) increased mitotic activity.

Nevoid Basal Cell Carcinoma Syndrome

Nevoid basal cell carcinoma syndrome represents a condition of autosomal dominant inheritance remarkable for marked variability in expressivity. The gene for this syndrome has been mapped to chromosome 9q22.3, the human homologue to the *Drosophila* segment polarity gene ptc patched (PTCH) [13, 14]. Patients with this syndrome have widespread involvement affecting the jaws, skin, axial skeleton, and central nervous system. Although a diverse array of clinical features may be seen in association with the syndrome including enlarged occipitofrontal circumference, calcification of the falx cerebri, rib anomalies, spina bifida, epidermal cysts and palmar/plantar pits of the skin, and mild ocular hypertelorism, the most serious manifestation of the syndrome is the proclivity to develop multiple basal cell carcinomas. With regard to the jaws and oral cavity, patients with nevoid basal cell carcinoma syndrome often develop multiple odontogenic keratocysts. In contrast to the sporadic cases of odontogenic keratocysts, syndrome-associated odontogenic keratocysts typically present in a younger patient population.

Diagnostic Workup

Plain radiographs should include: (a) skull films including A-P and panoramic radiographs to visualize intracerebral calcifications and keratocysts, respectively, (b) chest radiographs to assess rib abnormalities, and (c) lumbosacral views to evaluate for spina bifida. Skin examination with biopsy of suspicious lesions should be performed. Palmar and plantar pits can be easily seen if they are coated with an iodine solution. Measurements of the occipitofrontal circumference and intercanthal distance are also important. Figure 35.5a–e shows a patient with nevoid basal cell carcinoma syndrome. The maxillary odontogenic keratocysts were treated with enucleation and curettage, and the large mandibular keratocysts necessitated mandibular resection. Simultaneous mandibular reconstruction was performed with iliac crest bone grafts and platelet-rich plasma.

Treatment

Genetic counseling is recommended for all patients since the inheritance pattern is autosomal dominant. However, approximately 40% of cases are new mutations. Treatment should follow the same general principles that are used for treating isolated odontogenic keratocysts. Although multiple cysts are the characteristic finding, some patients may only have solitary lesions. Most patients are young in age and most odontogenic follicles may have functionally usable teeth; thus, marsupialization and orthodontics to guide eruption may be options for treatment. Skin lesions are usually basal cell carcinomas, but the type of lesions seen in these patients is usually not as aggressive as the ones seen from actinic damage. It has been suggested that only those lesions with ulceration, rapid growth, bleeding, or encrustment be removed, and all others be observed, but this is controversial. Long-term follow up of syndromic patients is recommended.

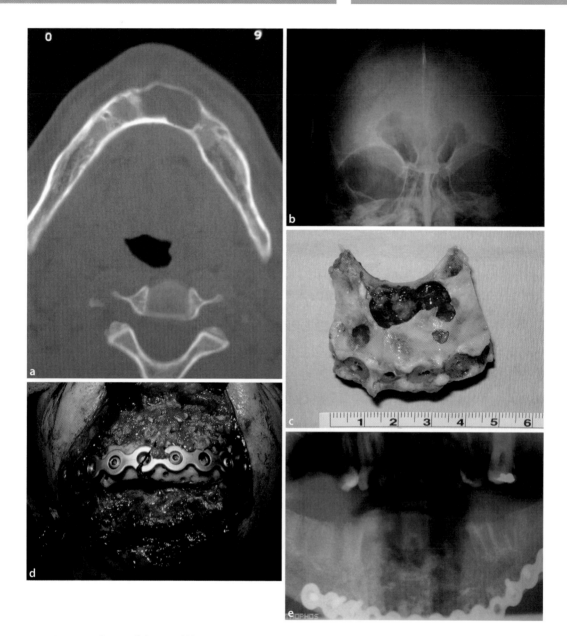

Fig. 35.5 **a** Axial view of the mandible in a patient with Gorlin's syndrome showing radiolucent lesions in the anterior mandible (odontogenic keratocysts). **b** Plain film of the skull showing a calcified falx cerebri, which is one of the characteristic features of this syndrome. **c** The anterior mandible including the multiple keratocysts has been resected. **d** Intraoperative view showing stabilization of resected mandible with a reconstruction plate and placement of iliac crest cancellous bone grafts. Platelet-rich plasma has been mixed with the grafts and this adds bone growth factors and also makes intraoperative handling of the cancellous graft easier. **e** Postoperative panoramic radiograph showing reconstructed anterior mandible. Use of cancellous bone grafts harvested from the iliac crest has many advantages including the ability to obtain excellent height and width of bone, and perform the surgery with minimal morbidity. Most patients ambulate the same day and leave the hospital within 1–2 days after surgery

Orthokeratinizing Odontogenic Cyst

Historically, the orthokeratinizing odontogenic cyst was thought to represent a variant of the odontogenic keratocyst, but it is now understood to simply represent an odontogenic cyst that exhibits orthokeratosis. Typically discovered on routine radiographic examination, orthokeratinizing odontogenic cysts present as solitary well-circumscribed radiolucencies. Most frequently presenting in the posterior mandible and often found in a dentigerous configuration around the crown of an unerupted tooth, orthokeratinizing odontogenic cysts have a predilection for occurring in men and present over a wide age range [26]. Unlike the parakeratinized odontogenic keratocyst, orthokeratotic odontogenic cysts do not exhibit an aggressive character and seldom recur. Differences in expression patterns of cytokeratins and extracellular matrix proteins between orthokeratinizing odontogenic cysts and the odontogenic keratocyst further support the distinction between the two entities and the differences in biologic behavior [27].

Histologic examination of an orthokeratinizing odontogenic cyst shows a cystic cavity lined by orthokeratinized stratified squamous epithelium. Orthokeratotic debris may be appreciated within the cystic lumen. A prominent keratohyaline granular cell layer is present just below the orthokeratotic surface. The epithelium is uniformly thin; approximately six to eight cell layers in total thickness. The basal epithelial cell layer is typically flattened cuboidal, and lacks the characteristic nuclear palisading observed in parakeratinized odontogenic keratocysts.

Treatment

Simple enucleation is recommended and recurrence is not expected following complete removal of the lesion.

Glandular Odontogenic Cyst

The term glandular odontogenic cyst is a recently described developmental odontogenic cyst remarkable for an often-aggressive biologic behavior [28]. Most lesions present in the anterior mandible. The cysts occur over a wide age range, but are typically encountered in adults over the age of 20 years. Pain and expansion are common presenting symptoms [29]. This lesion classically presents as radiolucency apical to vital teeth but, rarely, it may assume a dentigerous configuration, and unilocular, multilocular, and even multicentric lesions unassociated with tooth structure have been reported [29]. The recurrence rate is reported to be greater than 21% [29, 30].

Histologically, the glandular odontogenic cyst is lined by stratified squamous epithelium. The luminal aspect of the epithelial lining is remarkable for the presence of eosinophilic cuboidal to columnar cells that may assume an irregular subtle papillary configuration. Surface cilia, scattered mucous cells, and cells with clear cytoplasm are often noted. Foci of epithelial proliferation are frequently encountered and pools of mucicarmine-positive material surrounded by cuboidal eosinophilic

cells are seen yielding a duct-like appearance. The basal epithelial cell layer is often hyperchromatic, and the epithelial–connective tissue interface is flat without demonstrable rete ridge architecture.

Treatment

Controversy continues to surround this lesion, and until more clear-cut data from longer follow up studies is available, in the author's opinion, enucleation and curettage is the recommended treatment. Recurrence has been reported if enucleation alone is performed. It may be prudent to obtain a second opinion from an experienced oral pathologist, who could study serial sections of the specimen. There have been some reports of low-grade mucoepidermoid carcinomas arising in patients approximately 3–5 years after the lesions were originally diagnosed as glandular odontogenic cysts. Controversy exists as to the validity of these reports since they may have represented initially underdiagnosed mucoepidermoid carcinomas. Theoretically, since the potential for such malignant transformation exists, all patients with this diagnosis should be closely monitored.

Calcifying Odontogenic Cyst

The calcifying odontogenic cyst represents an uncommonly encountered developmental odontogenic cyst occurring with equal frequency in the maxilla and mandible. It is very common to see this lesion together with an odontogenic tumor such as an odontoma, ameloblastic fibroma, adenomatoid odontogenic tumor, or ameloblastoma.

The calcifying odontogenic cyst may present exclusively within bone or peripherally as a soft tissue mass within the alveolar mucosa. A more aggressive, solid variant (dentinogenic ghost cell tumor) is also known. The varied presentation of the calcifying odontogenic cyst has historically made the classification scheme for this entity cumbersome. While some support the idea that the calcifying odontogenic cyst exists in two clinical-pathologic forms – one as a cystic lesion and the other as a neoplastic lesion [31, 32] – others suggest the lesion simply represents a neoplasm with the potential for cyst formation.

The intraosseous calcifying odontogenic cyst typically presents in the second decade of life, while the peripheral and neoplastic solid variants have a later onset. The intraosseous lesions have a predilection for occurring anterior to the first molar and are well circumscribed with either a unilocular or multilocular configuration on radiographic examination. Occasionally, the lesions contain radiodensities consistent with foci of calcification (Fig. 35.6). Peripheral lesions present on the alveolar mucosa and show a nodular proliferation clinically indistinguishable from other common benign gingival nodules, and may have erosion of the subjacent alveolar bone. If the lesion is located proximal to the apices of teeth, divergence of roots and marked root resorption are not uncommon.

The calcifying odontogenic cyst shares histologic resemblance to the craniopharyngioma and the pilomatrixoma of

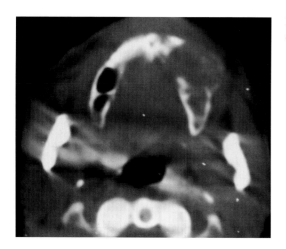

Fig. 35.6 CT scan of the mandible showing a large calcifying odontogenic cyst containing foci of calcification

the skin. Interestingly, each of these lesions has been shown to harbor a somatic β-catenin mutation. Histologically, the cystic lesions consist of a cavity lined by epithelial cells showing a columnar basal epithelial cell layer exhibiting reversed nuclear polarity with overlying stellate reticulum-like epithelium yielding a distinct resemblance to the ameloblastoma. So-called ghost cells characteristic of the lesion are present in variable amounts and consist of polygonal eosinophilic cells with central pale-staining regions representing absence of nuclei. Dysplastic dentin if seen, is thought to result from induction by proximal odontogenic epithelium. The neoplastic solid form of the calcifying odontogenic cyst shows a mature fibrous stroma with islands of odontogenic epithelium exhibiting columnar peripheral cells with reversed nuclear polarity surrounding a stellate reticulum-like core. The epithelial islands contain sheets of ghost cells, variable foci of calcification, and dentinoid formation. An invasive growth pattern, atypical mitoses, and cellular pleomorphism may suggest an aggressive or malignant variant [33].

Treatment

There is no consensus regarding the biologic behavior of these lesions. While most researchers believe that these lesions have limited biologic behavior, some feel that many variants of these lesions exist, and that some of these variants have neoplastic potential [33]. When one reads contemporary surgical literature, recommendations for treatment of calcifying odontogenic cysts are generally confined to either enucleation or enucleation with curettage for central cystic lesions, and simple excision for peripheral variants [33, 34].

Inflammatory Odontogenic Cysts

Buccal Bifurcation Cyst

It is hypothesized that at the time of initial eruption of the first molars, a focus of inflammation just apical to the epithelial attachment stimulates epithelial proliferation [35], leading to development of the buccal bifurcation cyst. Although an inflammatory etiology is most likely, genetic predisposition may also play a role as the lesion has also been reported in identical twins [36]. The buccal bifurcation cyst is an uncommon lesion presenting in children typically preceding eruption of the mandibular first molar. Clinically, the following are characteristic of the lesion [35]: (a) cystic lesion that is associated with vital teeth having a radiographically normal periodontal ligament and lamina dura, and (b) expansion of the cystic lesion on the buccal surface of the tooth causing tipping of the root apices toward the lingual cortical plate making the apices visible lingual to the crown when viewed on an occlusal radiograph.

Histologically, the buccal bifurcation cyst is characterized by a cystic cavity lined by hyperplastic, stratified squamous epithelium. A prominent chronic inflammatory cell infiltrate is found within the cyst wall and marked exocytosis of inflammatory cells can be appreciated within the epithelial lining. Treatment usually involves simple enucleation similar to dentigerous cysts. It is recommended that teeth in association with these lesions be preserved.

Periapical Cyst

The periapical cyst typically develops secondary to sustained antigenic stimulation from the pulp canal of a non-vital tooth. Keratinocyte growth factor produced by connective tissue fibroblasts is thought to stimulate transformation of odontogenic epithelial rests of Malassez within the alveolar bone from a quiescent epithelial rest into a cystic epithelial lining [37]. Unless secondarily infected, periapical cysts present clinically as asymptomatic lesions that are discovered on routine radiographic examination. Associated with the apex of a tooth containing necrotic pulpal tissue, the periapical cyst presents as a well-circumscribed radiolucency indistinguishable from a periapical granuloma (Fig. 35.7a). Elimination of the inciting inflammatory stimulus by treatment of the infected tooth with either a root canal procedure or extraction typically leads to resolution. If lesional tissue persists within the alveolar bone following extraction of the affected tooth, a residual cyst may result. Over

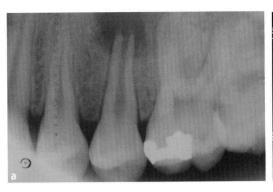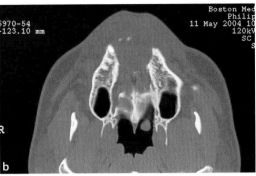

Fig. 35.7 **a** Periapical cysts present well-circumscribed radiolucencies at the apex of teeth. The offending teeth test negative to pulp testing (non-vital teeth). **b** If allowed to enlarge, periapical cysts can increase in size to large dimensions and compromise jaw integrity due to extensive bone destruction

time, these residual lesions often regress secondary to lack of an inflammatory stimulus.

Histologically, the periapical cyst consists of a cystic cavity lined by hyperplastic, stratified squamous epithelium. A mixed inflammatory infiltrate is noted within the cyst wall with inflammatory cell exocytosis appreciated throughout the epithelium. Calcified "Rushton" bodies may often be seen. Cholesterol cleft formation and dystrophic calcification may be observed within the cyst wall. Additionally, the cyst wall may also contain amorphous eosinophilic hyaline rings that represent fibrosed inflammatory exudates in association with multinucleated giant cells.

Treatment

Treatment of most periapical (radicular) cysts involves removal of the offending cause, i.e., tooth pulp infection. In general, every effort should be made to preserve the tooth. If the tooth can be salvaged, endodontic therapy (root canal therapy) is indicated; conversely, if the tooth is non-salvageable, then extraction of the tooth is recommended. If the endodontic treatment is not adequately performed or if the root canals are not optimally sealed, the inflammatory process perpetuates, and the cyst may continue to enlarge. Surgical curettage with apicoectomy and retrofill may be indicated in these cases. In cases where extraction of the tooth is performed, but the cyst is not removed, one should expect cyst involution with time. If spontaneous involution does not occur within a reasonable period of time, further treatment may be indicated. Occasionally, untreated periapical cysts can increase significantly in size and cause extensive bone destruction (Fig. 35.7b).

Selected Cysts of the Jaws of Non-odontogenic Origin

Nasopalatine Duct Cyst

The nasopalatine duct cyst is believed to be derived from residua of embryonic ductal structures that persist within the incisive

canal, and is the most common jaw cyst of non-odontogenic origin. Although the exact etiology is unknown, local trauma, focal inflammatory events such as infection, and spontaneous proliferation have been hypothesized to initiate the process of cyst development [38].

Nasopalatine duct cysts typically present in patients in the fifth to seventh decades of life. Common presenting symptoms include pain and swelling in the anterior palate posterior to the maxillary central incisors (Fig. 35.8a, b). Secondary infection may yield intermittent drainage of purulent exudate with associated waxing and waning of symptoms. Radiographic examination reveals a well-circumscribed radiolucency between the apices of the maxillary central incisors. Occasionally the radiolucency is remarkable for a heart shape, which may result from superimposition of the nasal spine on radiographic imaging or a true invagination of the cystic lesion by the nasal septum. Pure soft tissue lesions that do not involve the underlying bone occasionally occur and are referred to as cysts of the incisive papilla.

Histologic examination of the lesion reveals an epithelial-lined cystic cavity. The composition of the epithelial lining is variable, most typically showing pseudostratified ciliated columnar and/or stratified squamous differentiation. Mucous cells are frequently noted within the cystic epithelial lining. The cyst wall generally contains contents of the incisive canal including numerous neurovascular bundles, mature hyaline cartilage, and minor salivary gland lobules. The cyst wall may contain variable numbers of inflammatory cells.

Treatment

Simple enucleation is the recommended treatment for these cysts. The maxillary anterior teeth must be pulp tested to rule out the possibility of odontogenic origin, but clinicians must be aware that there may be false-negative results. If bone erosion is seen labially on CT scanning, access via a labial approach is recommended. However, many lesions requires a palatal approach. A posteriorly based full-thickness flap is raised, and the lesion enucleated. Care should be taken while performing surgery on

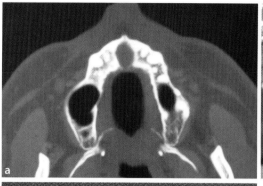
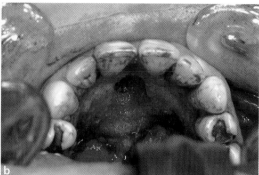
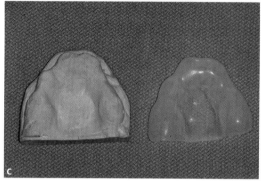

Fig. 35.8 **a** Nasopalatine cysts frequently appear as a "heart-shaped" radiolucency at the anterior palate in the midline region. **b** Intraoperative view of the palate. A full-thickness flap has been reflected, and the cyst with bone destruction is seen in the nasopalatine canal area. c A dental impression of the maxilla and teeth is taken and a model made (*left*); a customized soft-thermoplastic splint (*right*) can be fabricated to act as a full-coverage palatal splint

large lesions, as the cyst is frequently found to be adherent to the palatal mucoperiosteum. These areas may require careful, and often sharp dissection to avoid palatal tissue tears during surgery.

The author recommends the use a soft thermoplastic splint (Fig. 35.8c) if a palatal surgical approach is utilized. The splint can be secured with screws, wires, or sutures, and has the following advantages: (a) increased patient comfort, (b) provides protection to those areas with iatrogenic tears that have been repaired, and (c) provides support to palatal soft tissue which can otherwise dehisce from hematoma formation in the bony cavity. In the author's experience, bone grafting is not needed as the bony cavity will spontaneously generate bone. Recurrence is not expected after complete removal.

Nasolabial Cyst

The nasolabial cyst is a developmental cyst thought to either be derived from rests of epithelium persisting after incomplete degeneration of the embryonic nasolacrimal duct or from epithelium entrapped during fusion of the medial and lateral nasal processes. The lesion presents as a swelling of the upper lip lateral to the ala of the nose with intraoral obliteration of the maxillary labial vestibule. Occasionally, a bony defect secondary to pressure erosion of the subjacent bone may be seen.

Histologic examination of the nasolabial cyst shows a cystic cavity typically lined by pseudostratified ciliated columnar epithelium containing scattered mucous cells, but squamous, cuboidal, and columnar differentiation can be seen.

Treatment

Classically, a nasolabial cyst does not have bony involvement and is non-odontogenic in origin. However, large cysts can result in secondary bone erosion due to pressure (nasoalveolar cysts). Pulp testing of the maxillary anterior teeth should be performed to rule out an odontogenic source of the swelling. Treatment involves simple excision, and recurrence is not expected. Perforation into the nasal cavity can be expected during surgery.

Gingival Cysts of the Adult

The gingival cyst of the adult is thought to be derived from residua of dental lamina persisting within the alveolar mucosa following tooth development. Typically presenting on the buccal surface of the alveolar mucosa in the mandibular premolar and canine region, the gingival cyst of the adult commonly occurs in patients from 40 to 60 years of age. The lesion represents a swelling that may exhibit a slight blue to gray coloration. A resorptive defect of the alveolar bone may be appreciated subjacent to the soft tissue lesion. Treatment involves simple excision and primary closure. Recurrence is not seen.

Palatal Cysts of the Newborn

Palatal cysts of the newborn are thought to be derived from either entrapment of epithelium along embryonic lines of fusion or from embryonic epithelial residua of developing minor salivary gland lobules. Common lesions discovered in neonates, palatal cysts present as small yellow-white single or clustered nodules on the palate often in the midline at or near the junction of the hard and soft palate.

Histologic examination of a palatal cyst of the newborn shows an epithelial-lined cavity, which often contains keratin. The cystic epithelial lining shows a stratified squamous differentiation and may communicate with the surface mucosa.

No treatment except parental reassurance is needed. Typically, palatal cysts spontaneously involute or rupture into the oral cavity by 3–4 months of age.

Dermoid Cyst

The dermoid cyst represents a developmental non-odontogenic cystic lesion thought to derive from pluripotential cells entrapped within tissues. These cells possess the capacity to develop into tissues from each representative germ layer. The term "dermoid" cyst is an inclusive term with further subclassification of cystic variants into three categories defined by the constituent germ layers represented within the cystic lesion:

1. Epidermoid cyst: Cystic lesions comprised of an epithelial lining and surrounded by an unremarkable fibrous connective tissue wall without dermal adnexa.
2. Dermoid cyst: When the cystic lesion consists of both an epithelial lining and contains dermal adnexa in the cyst wall such as sebaceous glands and hair appendages.
3. Teratoid cyst: Reserved for complex lesions comprised of an epithelial-lined cavity with both epithelial and non-epithelial elements within the cyst wall such as bone, muscle, and gastrointestinal tissue.

Clinically, the dermoid cyst typically presents as a fluctuant midline swelling of the floor of the mouth (Fig. 35.9a), but its location may be paramidline and it may also occur in the tongue and mandible. If the lesion develops above the geniohyoid muscle, dyspnea and dysphagia may develop. Lesions occurring below the geniohyoid muscle yield a characteristic "double chin" appearance. Although these lesions typically present in patients in the second and third decades of life, occasional congenital lesions have been reported.

Histologic examination of a dermoid cyst shows a cystic epithelial lining that may show pseudostratified ciliated columnar or orthokeratinized stratified squamous epithelial differentiation. The contents of the cystic cavity often contain abundant keratinous debris. Variable apocrine and eccrine dermal appendages and pilosebaceous structures may be found within the cyst wall. In addition to dermal adnexal structures, complex teratoid cystic lesions may contain variable amounts of mesenchymal tissue including muscle, gastrointestinal, respiratory, and bone within the cyst wall.

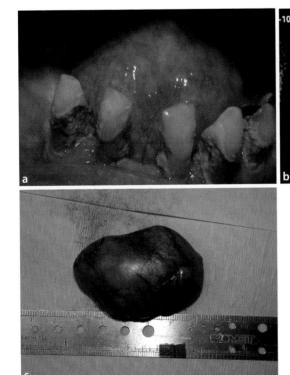

Fig. 35.9 **a** Intraoral view showing dome-shaped raised lesion in the floor of the mouth. **b** MRI scan showing a large well-defined fluid filled mass in the floor of the mouth region. **c** The mass has been resected via an intraoral approach. This lesion was diagnosed to be a dermoid cyst due to the presence of dermal adnexal structures within the cyst wall

Treatment

These lesions can vary tremendously in size and location. Aspiration will usually show return of straw-colored fluid with keratin-like material. Small lesions in easily accessible surgical sites may be excised in an office setting under local anesthesia or intravenous sedation. However, larger and deeper lesions and those in surgically "difficult" areas will require wider access, possible transcutaneous incisions, and general anesthesia in a hospital setting. CT scan or MRI examination is very useful (Fig. 35.9b).

Care should be taken to preserve the salivary gland ducts and lingual nerves during surgery. Treatment usually involves excision of the lesion from surrounding tissue via a transoral and/or transcutaneous approach. If adherent to adjacent tissues, it is often necessary to use blunt and sharp dissection for optimal removal. If the cyst is large (Fig. 35.9c), removal will often leave a significant defect with large dead space and, thus, layered closure of the wound with drain placement is recommended. Even if the surgery was performed transorally, it may be prudent to place a drain through a transcutaneous stab incision in the submental crease to allow for dependent drainage.

Pseudocysts of the Jaws

Simple Bone Cyst

The simple bone cyst represents a non-neoplastic intraosseous cavity devoid of an epithelial lining. Although the etiology may likely be different for each lesion, the simple bone cyst is currently thought to represent a focal vasodynamic abnormality. This vascular irregularity may result from increased regional blood flow at the site of bone remodeling giving rise to a hydrodynamic anomaly with secondary venous obstruction and bone cyst formation [39, 40]. The simple bone cyst most frequently presents in the mandible in patients under the age of 20 years. Radiographically, the simple bone cyst traditionally presents as a unilocular radiolucent lesion with possible interdental "scalloping" between the roots of vital teeth without cortical expansion. Multilocular lesions, lesions presenting in a dentigerous configuration, and multiple lesions have been reported.

Histologically, a simple bone cyst cavity consists of fragments of fibrous connective tissue and extravasated erythrocytes, granulation tissue, and spicules of vital bone from the cavity wall. Since this lesion does not represent a true cyst, no epithelial lining is appreciated.

Treatment

Most lesions are diagnosed only during surgical exploration. Aspiration reveals some initial air bubbles, followed by some straw-colored fluid, and then by blood. The continued negative pressure of aspiration disturbs the medullary capillaries, and initiates bleeding from them. It is important to rule out vascular lesions, and a thorough examination should be performed for any cystic lining. On surgical exploration, an empty bony cavity with scant fibrinous material is expected. The bony walls should be curetted, and usually this exploration surgery stimulates bony fill and remodeling within the lesion in most cases.

Aneurysmal Bone Cyst

The aneurysmal bone cyst typically presents as a central osteolytic lesion in patients younger than 20 years, has a predilection for occurring in the posterior mandible, and a propensity for recurrence [41–43]. The etiology of this lesion is incompletely understood, but recent genetic evidence leans toward a true neoplastic process. "Secondary" aneurysmal bone cyst-like areas have been described in association with other benign and malignant neoplasms.

The clinical presentation often consists of pain and swelling. Radiographic findings include a unilocular to multilocular, soap-bubble or honeycomb radiolucency with bony expansion and occasional cortical perforation. Histologic examination reveals multiple sinusoidal spaces filled with erythrocytes and surrounded by a cellular fibrous connective tissue stroma. Multinucleated osteoclast-type giant cells, osteoid, woven bone, and fine, reticular calcifications are often found at the periphery of the blood-filled spaces.

Treatment

Curettage of the cyst and its bony cavity is recommended. Many surgeons also recommend cryotherapy or cauterization of the bony cavity following curettage as adjunctive measures as, historically, there has been a high recurrence rate in the literature for aneurysmal bone cysts in the general skeleton. Recurrent or large lesions that risk pathologic fracture may require en bloc resection with 0.5- to 1.0-cm margins, followed by jaw reconstruction. The surgeon can expect significant hemorrhage until the pathologic tissue is entirely removed, especially in large lesions. Although recurrence has been reported, it is rare if treatment has been performed during initial surgery. Solid lesions are virtually indistinguishable from central giant cell "lesions."

As non-surgical treatment is gaining in popularity for the treatment of many giant cell lesions of the jaws, it is possible that one or more of these medical treatments may play some role in treatment of such giant cell lesions. Examples of such treatments include corticosteroids, calcitonin hormone, and, more recently, antiangiogenic pharmaceutical therapy [44–46].

Benign Jaw Tumors

Odontogenic Tumors

Most tumors of the jaws are benign tumors of odontogenic origin, and this chapter will mainly focus on diagnosis and management of these lesions. Although non-odontogenic tumors (example: maxillary sinus tumors) and malignant tumors (rarely odontogenic and more commonly non-odontogenic in origin) can affect the maxilla and mandible, these are rare and are discussed elsewhere in the textbook.

Traditionally, odontogenic tumors are divided into three categories based on the neoplastic component:
1. Epithelial tumors: the neoplastic component is comprised of odontogenic epithelium without ectomesenchymal proliferation.
2. Ectomesenchymal tumors: derived from ectomesenchymal elements and although odontogenic epithelium may be seen, it does not participate in the neoplastic process.
3. Mixed tumors: both odontogenic epithelial and ectomesenchymal elements contribute to neoplastic proliferation.

Due to the known complexity of odontogenic tumors, their specific biologic behavior and proliferative capacity interact to determine clinical outcome and prognosis. Treatment guidelines are aimed to eradicate lesional tissue with the principles of least morbidity and maximum preservation with restoration of function.

Epithelial Odontogenic Tumors

Adenomatoid Odontogenic Tumor

This tumor is believed to originate from neoplastic transformation of dental lamina residua that persist within the alveolar bone following tooth development [47]. Incompletely understood events stimulate these odontogenic epithelial rests to proliferate with subsequent tumor formation. The adenomatoid odontogenic tumor most commonly presents in the anterior maxilla in female patients under the age of 20 years, most often in association with the crown of an impacted canine. Alternatively, lesions can sometimes present in an extrafollicular location, independent of an unerupted tooth, and peripheral lesions,

clinically indistinguishable from other benign gingival nodules, have also been reported.

Patients present with a chief complaint of delayed eruption of teeth and lesions are discovered on diagnostic radiographs. The adenomatoid odontogenic tumor most commonly presents as a radiolucent lesion with a distinct radiopaque border surrounding the crown of an unerupted tooth and extending beyond the cementoenamel junction (Fig. 35.10). Small radiopaque foci, so-called snowflake calcifications, are frequently present within the lesion.

Histologic examination of the adenomatoid odontogenic tumor shows an encapsulated proliferation of spindled epithelial cells oriented in sheets and whorls. Although, primary glandular tissue is present within the lesion, the adenomatoid odontogenic tumor is remarkable for variable numbers of duct-like structures. Columnar odontogenic epithelial cells exhibiting nuclear polarization away from the pseudolumina line the duct-like structures. Rosette-like structures containing amyloid-positive material may also be appreciated. Abortive enamel and dentin formation within the tumor generates small foci of calcification that may be apparent on radiographic examination.

Treatment

Differential diagnosis includes lesions such as dentigerous cyst, calcifying odontogenic cyst, calcifying epithelial odontogenic tumor, and desmoplastic ameloblastoma. Aspiration will usually draw out straw-colored fluid. Surgical enucleation is the recommended treatment. A full-thickness mucoperiosteal flap is raised, and a bony window is made through the thinned out cortex to access the lesion. The thick-walled nature of the tumor lends itself to easy removal from its bony crypt. Recurrence is very rare. The impacted tooth is generally present within the cyst lumen, and is removed with the specimen.

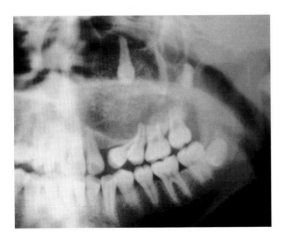

Fig. 35.10 Radiographic presentation of a calcifying epithelial odontogenic tumor usually shows a radiolucent lesion in association with an impacted tooth. Variable amounts of radiopacities are present within the lesion

Squamous Odontogenic Tumor

The squamous odontogenic tumor is an uncommon benign odontogenic neoplasm remarkable for its locally infiltrative behavior. Central and peripheral variants are recognized: Central lesions most likely arise from neoplastic transformation of odontogenic epithelial rests of Malassez retained within the periodontal ligament space following tooth root development, and peripheral lesions are thought to originate from rests of dental lamina that persist within the gingival tissues.

The squamous odontogenic tumor is most commonly encountered in the third decade of life, and can present anywhere in the jaws [48]. Typically, it presents as a wedge-shaped radiolucency within the inter-radicular alveolar bone. It is a slow-growing neoplasm, which often develops asymptomatically and is discovered only during routine radiographic examination. Patients with lesions that are large in size and of long duration may present with swelling, periodontal defects, tooth mobility, and pain [48]. Peripheral lesions confined exclusively to the soft tissue are impossible to distinguish clinically from other benign gingival nodules. Pressure resorption of the underlying alveolar bone may create a saucer-shaped radiolucent defect subjacent to the soft tissue neoplasm. Rare examples of the squamous odontogenic tumor involving multiple quadrants and multifocal lesions occurring within individuals of the same family have also been described.

Histologic examination of the squamous odontogenic tumor shows squamous epithelial islands of irregular size and shape within a mature fibrous connective tissue stroma. The epithelial islands are characterized by smooth, rounded borders with fluid lines, the peripheral cells of which are generally cuboidal or markedly flattened. Within the epithelial islands single cell dyskeratosis and central cystic degeneration are often noted. Additionally, foci of dystrophic calcific material and laminated calcifications are frequently appreciated.

Treatment

The squamous odontogenic tumor is a rare tumor. Because most tumors present as well-circumscribed, unilocular radiolu-

cencies, serious consideration must be given to the thought that the lesion may represent a more common cyst or tumor such as an odontogenic keratocyst, lateral periodontal cyst, ameloblastoma, or odontogenic myxoma. An incisional biopsy is indicated to confirm the diagnosis. It is important that the specimen be submitted for histologic diagnosis to an experienced oral pathologist, since the histologic presentation can resemble an ameloblastoma or squamous cell carcinoma to an individual unfamiliar with the lesion.

Recommended surgical treatment usually involves enucleation and curettage. Peripheral ostectomy is recommended by some practitioners. Because the lesion is benign but infiltrative, the surgical treatment approach must be based on individual case consideration. If the presence of tooth roots interferes with a thorough curettage, tooth removal may be required. Occasionally, resection of the alveolus without creating a continuity defect may be needed to permit complete removal of the tumor. If the lesion perforates bony cortices, removal of the overlying soft tissue should be considered. Recurrence is rare after complete removal.

Calcifying Epithelial Odontogenic Tumor

The calcifying epithelial odontogenic tumor is a rare odontogenic neoplasm of controversial origin. Historically, the neoplasm is considered to be derived from reduced enamel epithelium [49], but recent investigation leans toward origins from neoplastic transformation of dental lamina residua persisting within the alveolar bone following tooth formation [50]. The calcifying epithelial odontogenic tumor most commonly presents in the posterior mandible of patients in their third to fifth decades of life but can also involve other sites throughout the maxilla and mandible. Typically, the tumor presents centrally within bone as a slow-growing, expansile, painless mass surrounding the crown of an unerupted tooth. A peripheral variant of the calcifying epithelial odontogenic tumor confined exclusively to the soft tissue has been reported. This variant is clinically indistinguishable from other benign gingival nodules.

Radiographically, the central calcifying epithelial odontogenic tumor presents as a unilocular or multilocular radiolucent

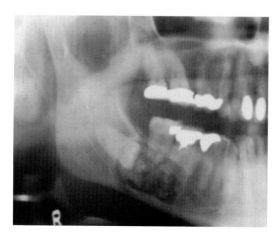

Fig. 35.11 Radiographic presentation of a calcifying epithelial odontogenic tumor usually shows a radiolucent lesion in association with an impacted tooth. Variable amounts of radiopacities are present within the lesion

lesion with scalloped margins and variable foci of radiopacity (Fig. 35.11). Lesions often show foci of calcification in close proximity to the crown of the involved tooth. Peripheral lesions may occasionally produce pressure resorptive defects on adjacent alveolar bone.

Histologic examination of the calcifying epithelial odontogenic tumor reveals sheets of polyhedral epithelial cells remarkable for deeply eosinophilic cytoplasm and conspicuous intercellular bridges in a mature fibrous connective tissue stroma. Nuclear pleomorphism is often seen within the epithelial component of the lesion; however, this variability in nuclear morphology does not suggest malignant biologic behavior. Foci of amorphous extracellular eosinophilic product exhibiting the tinctorial and ultrastructural features of amyloid may be seen in the lesion. Calcific foci are appreciated in varying abundance throughout the lesion. The small, droplet-like calcific foci frequently unite to form large syncytial conglomerations.

Treatment

These tumors may present as radiolucent or more commonly, as mixed radiolucent-radiopaque lesions. With the radiolucent presentation, differential diagnosis must include common odontogenic lesions such as a dentigerous cyst, odontogenic keratocyst, ameloblastoma, or an odontogenic myxoma. For mixed-density lesions, the differential diagnosis should include such entities as the calcifying odontogenic cyst, ameloblastic fibro-odontoma, desmoplastic ameloblastoma, and fibro-osseous lesions.

Surgical treatment should be addressed in a case-specific fashion. Although the 1992 World Health Organization (WHO) conference describes the calcifying epithelial odontogenic tumor as a benign, locally invasive neoplasm without a recurrence pattern, there are reports of up to 30% recurrence within 2–3 years. A review of the recurrent cases shows that most were originally treated by enucleation and curettage. Based on the paucity of reported cases and the high rate of recurrence with conservative management, it is recommended that resection with 1.0- to 1.5-cm margins should be performed for this tumor. Immediate or delayed bone reconstruction can be performed.

Ameloblastoma

The ameloblastoma is one of the most "well-known" jaw tumors. It is a benign odontogenic tumor with a locally aggressive behavior and high recurrence rate. Both these characteristics are attributed to its tendency to extend into surrounding tissues. Although the exact pathogenesis remains uncertain, it is likely that the ameloblastoma arises from neoplastic transformation of dental lamina residua persisting within the alveolar bone following tooth development. Three variants of ameloblastoma are recognized and are notable for differing clinical characteristics and biologic behavior:
1. Conventional "solid" variant
2. Unicystic variant
3. Peripheral variant

The conventional ameloblastoma usually presents in patients over the age of 20 years and has a predilection for occurring in the posterior mandible. Typically, it presents as a slow-growing, painless, expansile mass. Radiographically, it classically appears as a multilocular radiolucency with a "soap bubble" or "honeycomb" appearance (Fig. 35.12a), however unilocular lesions are also encountered (Fig. 35.12b). A specific variant of this tumor is termed a desmoplastic ameloblastoma. This variant is remarkable for a mixed radiolucent-radiopaque appearance and has a predilection for occurring in the anterior maxilla. Histologically, the conventional follicular ameloblastoma shows infiltrative islands of odontogenic epithelium on a mature fibrous connective tissue stroma. The epithelial islands consist of a central stellate reticulum-like core rimmed by columnar epithelial cells exhibiting palisading and reversed nuclear polarity with cytoplasmic vacuolization proximal to the basement membrane.

Histologic variants in which the stellate reticulum-like area is composed of either squamous epithelium or granular cells are seen. Other histologic variants include the plexiform pattern in which the proliferating odontogenic epithelium forms anastomosing cords rimmed by peripheral cuboidal to columnar ameloblast-like cells. The desmoplastic ameloblastoma shows a densely collagenized fibrous connective tissue stroma with condensed islands and cords of odontogenic epithelium. Peripheral

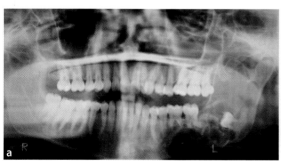
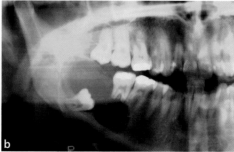

Fig. 35.12a,b Classically, ameloblastomas present as soap-bubble, multilocular radiolucencies (**a**), but it is not uncommon for these tumors to present as unilocular lesions (**b**) that can radiographically resemble dentigerous cysts

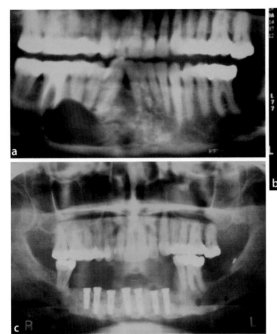

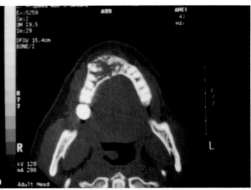

Fig. 35.13 **a** Panoramic radiograph showing a large radiolucent lesion in the anterior mandible causing tooth migration and bone expansion. The lesion was biopsied and found to be an ameloblastoma. **b** Axial CT scan of the mandible showing the bone expansion and destruction associated with the lesion. **c** The tumor has been removed, and the mandible reconstructed with cancellous marrow grafts and dental implants. Picture courtesy of Dr. David Cottrell, Boston, Mass

columnar cells with characteristic palisading and reversed nuclear polarity are not easily seen. A rarely encountered basal cell pattern has also been described.

The unicystic ameloblastoma also most commonly develops in the posterior mandible during the second and third decades of life. The unicystic ameloblastoma most frequently presents as a unilocular radiolucency surrounding the crown of an unerupted tooth. Based on this tendency to occur in a pericoronal configuration, the unicystic ameloblastoma is often diagnosed clinically as a dentigerous cyst with the definitive diagnosis made only after submission of lesional tissue for histologic examination. Rare extrafollicular lesions are occasionally encountered. Occasionally, mural extension of the process into the cyst wall is appreciated. Here, isolated islands of odontogenic epithelium with the histologic features of the conventional follicular ameloblastoma are seen infiltrating the surrounding fibrous connective tissue stroma. The biologic behavior of a unicystic ameloblastoma with mural involvement is similar to that of the conventional ameloblastoma. Thus, it is imperative that the clinician clearly distinguishes whether a unicystic ameloblastoma is with or without mural involvement. Specimens with histologic features suspicious for unicystic ameloblastoma should be thoroughly evaluated for mural involvement by an experienced oral pathologist.

The peripheral variant of ameloblastoma is confined exclusively to the alveolar mucosa and is clinically indistinguishable from other benign gingival nodules. Like the conventional variant, the peripheral ameloblastoma is thought to arise from rests of dental lamina; however, it is possible that some lesions may arise from oral mucosal epithelium. Large lesions may cause some pressure-related resorption of adjacent bone. Histologic examination of the peripheral ameloblastoma shows unremarkable oral mucosa overlying a mature fibrous connective tissue stroma. Within the fibrous connective tissue, infiltrative islands

of odontogenic epithelium are seen remarkable for a central stellate reticulum-like core surrounded by columnar epithelial cells exhibiting hyperchromaticity, reversed nuclear polarity, and cytoplasmic vacuolization. Occasionally, the stellate reticulum-like areas are replaced by stratified squamous epithelium. A plexiform pattern showing anastomosing cords of odontogenic epithelium rimmed by peripheral cuboidal to columnar epithelial am[e]loblast-like cells is also seen. A rare basal cell pattern has been reported, however no significant difference in biologic behavior is appreciated amongst the histologic variants.

Ameloblastic Carcinoma and Malignant Ameloblastoma

Ameloblastic carcinoma is a rare malignancy characterized by overt cytologic atypia within a lesion that is otherwise histologically indistinguishable from ameloblastoma. Although occasional mitotic activity is noted in benign lesions, abundant atypical mitotic figures in conjunction with nuclear pleomorphism, calcific foci, necrosis, and robust cellularity are features of malignant transformation. The so-called malignant ameloblastoma represents an unusual situation in which a cytologically benign ameloblastoma metastasizes to a distant locale. The incidence of malignant ameloblastoma is rare and the pathogenesis is poorly understood.

Treatment

a. Conventional ameloblastoma: Resection using 1.0- to 1.5-cm margins and removal of one uninvolved anatomic barrier is indicated. If enucleation and curettage is employed as the treatment modality, one can expect a recurrence in 70–85%

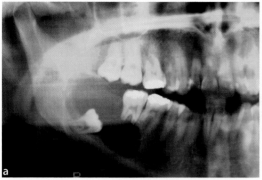
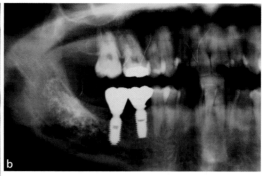
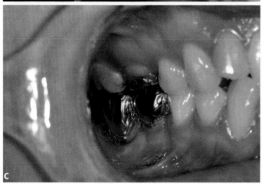

Fig. 35.14 **a** Radiographic appearance of a unicystic ameloblastoma without mural involvement of the right posterior mandible. Note that this radiographic appearance is virtually indistinguishable from many other common odontogenic cysts and tumors. **b** The lesion has been removed via an intraoral approach with enucleation and curettage with peripheral ostectomy, and the bone defect reconstructed with particulate bone. Delayed placement of implants is performed approximately 5 months after bony reconstruction of the jaw. **c** Intraoral photograph demonstrating result of functional dental rehabilitation with fixed, implant-supported restorations

of cases, but it may take approximately 5 years for the recurrences to become apparent. Ameloblastomas treated by adequate resection do not usually recur. Figure 35.13a–c shows a 51-year-old female patient with an ameloblastoma of the left mandible. The tumor was resected and the mandible was reconstructed simultaneously with iliac crest bone grafts. Functional rehabilitation was achieved with implant supported dental restorations.

b. Unicystic ameloblastoma (without mural extension): These tumors should be treated more conservatively with enucleation and thorough curettage. Fig. 35.14a–c shows a patient with unicystic ameloblastoma who was treated with enucleation and curettage of the lesion, simultaneous bone grafting of the defect, and delayed placement of dental implants.

c. Unicystic ameloblastoma (with mural extension): These tumors should be treated in a manner similar to conventional ameloblastomas.

d. Peripheral ameloblastoma: These tumors lack the aggressiveness and biologic behavior of a central conventional ameloblastoma. They can usually be treated by excision of the soft tissue lesion with a rim of soft tissue tumor-free margins. The exact margin of soft tissue to be excised beyond the tumor is controversial, but generally, 1.0- to 1.5-cm margins are considered adequate. Recurrence after adequate treatment is rare.

e. Recurrent ameloblastoma: A review of the literature supports the fact that most recurrent tumors arise as a result of inadequate treatment during initial surgery. Recurrences are seen approximately 5–10 years after initial treatment, and are best managed by resection with 1.5-cm margins. The author recommends that, for predictable results, the resection should

be based on initial radiographs and not on those which demonstrate the recurrence; this philosophy is based on experience and the hypothesis that if one determines the resection margin on the "new" recurrent tumor radiograph, it would treat only the isolated recurrent lesion, and this approach risks further recurrences in the other areas of the original tumor which have been under-treated initially.

Ectomesenchymal Odontogenic Tumors

Odontogenic Fibroma

The central odontogenic fibroma is a benign odontogenic neoplasm that presents clinically as a painless, expansile, slow-growing mass. The occurrence has a slight female predilection, and the tumor presents with equal frequency in the maxilla and mandible, with the anterior maxilla and posterior mandible being the most commonly involved sites. Radiographically, either a unilocular or multilocular radiolucency can be seen, but most often the lesion is present around the crown of an unerupted tooth. Peripheral lesions confined exclusively to the soft tissue are occasionally encountered and are clinically indistinguishable from other benign gingival nodules. Some cases where the tumor contains calcific foci that are evident on radiographic imaging have been encountered.

Histologic examination of the odontogenic fibroma shows a proliferation of mature fibrous connective tissue of variable cellularity. Additionally, foci of inactive odontogenic epithelium may be appreciated in variable amounts throughout the lesion. A classification based on two distinct histologic variants exists:

the simple type and the WHO type. The simple type shows a delicate collagenous stroma with scattered stellate-shaped fibroblasts, nests of odontogenic epithelium in variable amounts, and foci of dystrophic calcification. The WHO pattern consists of a densely cellular fibrous connective tissue stroma with abundant foci of odontogenic epithelium oriented in nests or cords. Dysplastic dentin or cementum-like calcification may be appreciated. Although the existence of the distinct histologic variants is debated extensively in the literature, the discussion is essentially academic as the biologic behavior between the histologic variants is indistinguishable.

Treatment

Recurrences or re-growth of residual lesions has been reported; this is perhaps a result of inadequate initial treatment. There are also some very rare reports of a highly aggressive and infiltrative behavior similar to a fibrosarcoma.

Generally speaking, it is agreed that most of these lesions should be treated with enucleation and curettage. The lesions readily separate from their bony cavity, and should not show any evidence of bony infiltration. The inferior alveolar nerve bundle should be preserved, whenever possible. Teeth in the lesion should be removed. Peripheral soft tissue lesions should be excised down to bone with a 3- to 5-mm rim of soft tissue margin. Recurrence is rare and should warrant a review of the histopathologic examination of the original specimen.

Cementoblastoma

The cementoblastoma is a benign ectomesenchymal odontogenic tumor derived from neoplastic cementoblasts. This slow-growing lesion originates from and insinuates itself within the tooth root apparatus. Clinically, the cementoblastoma demonstrates dramatic growth potential and has the capacity to overrun the root structure of adjacent teeth as the lesion expands. Although rare cases involving the deciduous dentition have been reported, the cementoblastoma typically involves the erupted mandibular permanent molar or bicuspid teeth of patients in their second and third decades of life. Frequently pain, expansion of the cortical plates, and displacement of teeth are described. Radiographically, the cementoblastoma typically presents as a well-circumscribed radiopacity intimately fused to

and obscuring tooth root structure (Fig. 35.15). A radiolucent rim frequently surrounds the radiopaque lesion, but completely radiolucent lesions are known to occur.

Histologic examination of the cementoblastoma shows a proliferation of plump cementoblasts embedded in a stroma of haphazardly arranged calcified matrix exhibiting prominent basophilic reversal lines and disorderly lacunae. A fibrovascular connective tissue stroma and variable numbers of multinucleated osteoclast-type giant cells are also appreciated. Poorly mineralized trabeculae of eosinophilic matrix arranged in radiating cords are often noted at the periphery of the lesion.

Treatment

The cementoblastoma is a localized benign lesion and, thus, the primary recommended treatment is enucleation with curettage. The lesion has a distinct fibrous connective tissue wall, and is usually easy to separate from bone. The offending tooth is generally extracted with the lesion attached.

Odontogenic Myxoma

The odontogenic myxoma is a benign ectomesenchymal odontogenic tumor characterized by the replacement of bone with a grossly gelatinous tissue composed of delicate collagen fibers and abundant glycosaminoglycans. Typically presenting in the posterior mandible of patients in the second to fourth decades of life, the odontogenic myxoma is a slow-growing neoplasm remarkable for tooth displacement, pain, expansion, perforation of the bony cortex, and the capacity to extend itself into the surrounding soft tissues. This aggressive behavior may be attributed to the dysregulation of antiapoptotic proteins and the secretion of matrix metalloproteinases within the tumor. The lesion presents as either a unilocular (Fig. 35.16) or more commonly, a multilocular radiolucency similar to a "soap bubble" or "honeycomb" appearance. Residual bony trabeculae persisting within the lesion are oriented at right angles to each other and may yield an appearance akin to the strings of a tennis racket.

Histologic examination shows a background of myxomatous connective tissue and finely dispersed stellate and spindle-shaped cells. The myxomatous stroma is predominantly composed of glycosaminoglycans. Occasional foci of odontogenic epithelium may be appreciated within the lesion, however the

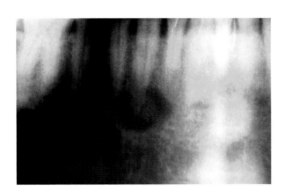

Fig. 35.15 Radiographic view of a cementoblastoma showing a radiopaque mass attached to the root of a tooth. Many lesions have a radiolucent rim around the main lesion as is seen in this radiograph

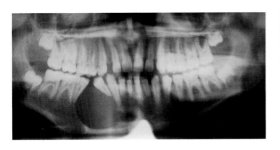

Fig. 35.16 Although odontogenic myxomas frequently have a multilocular, honey-combed appearance, it is not unusual to find that many lesions present as unilocular radiolucencies on plain films

epithelium is not always encountered and is uninvolved with the neoplastic process. Immunohistochemical stains are positive for vimentin and focally positive for muscle-specific actin within the tumor cell population.

Treatment

Definitive treatment involves resection with 1.0- to 1.5-cm tumor-free bony margins, and one uninvolved anatomic barrier. Primary or secondary jaw reconstruction can be performed as per surgeon preference. Some surgeons advocate enucleation with curettage for small (1- to 2-cm-sized), unilocular lesions; however, a review of most recurrent cases shows that they were initially treated by this modality. The author of this chapter does not recommend enucleation and curettage as a form of treatment for odontogenic myxomas. This "conservative" treatment should be reserved for those individuals who specifically prefer or request palliative correction over curative resection, or for those individuals whose general anesthetic risk is too great to undergo curative surgery.

Mixed Odontogenic Tumors

Odontoma

This is the most commonly encountered odontogenic tumor. Many believe it to be a developmental hamartoma rather than

a true neoplastic process. The odontoma represents a so-called mixed lesion exhibiting a proliferation of both odontogenic epithelium and mesenchymal tissue. Odontomas can be classified into two distinct types: the compound variant and the complex variant. Both types basically consist of a proliferation of odontogenic tissues in variable amounts and arrangements.

The compound odontoma most commonly presents in the first or second decades of life and has a site predilection for occurring in the anterior maxilla (Fig. 35.17a, b) [51, 52]. These lesions demonstrate proliferation of odontogenic tissues in appropriate odontogenic configuration. There are multiple small crudely formed tooth-like structures circumscribed by a radiolucent rim usually in association with an impacted regular tooth or supernumerary tooth. The lesions frequently remain asymptomatic and are only discovered on routine radiographic examination or when investigating the chief complaint of delayed eruption. Histologically, the compound odontoma consists of multiple small crudely-formed single-rooted "toothlets" comprised of overlying enamel matrix with underlying dentin and a central pulp chamber.

The complex odontoma typically also presents in the first or second decades of life. In contrast to the compound type, here the proliferation of odontogenic tissues is in a haphazard arrangement. Bony expansion is more common and it most commonly occurs in the posterior mandible. Radiographically, the complex odontoma presents as a well-demarcated focus of radiopacity surrounded by a peripheral radiolucent rim. The radiodensity of the radiopaque mass is consistent with that of tooth structure. Histologic examination of a complex odon-

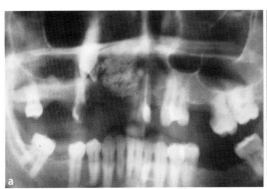
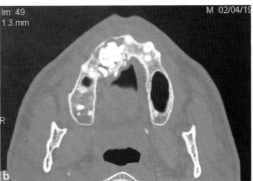

Fig. 35.17 **a** Panoramic radiograph showing a large, radiopaque mass in the anterior right maxilla, lateral to the nasal region. Compound odontomas have a predilection for occurring in the anterior maxillary region. **b** CT scan of the same lesion as in **a**, showing multiple small radiopaque masses within the lesion. Clinically, odontomas consist of multiple tooth-like structures

35

toma shows a proliferation of odontogenic tissues oriented in a haphazard configuration. Typically, variable amounts of dentin, enamel matrix, pulpal tissues, and cementum are seen juxtaposed with each other in an indiscriminate fashion. Primitive lesions may show multiple foci of early odontogenesis.

Treatment

Excision of the lesion with enucleation and curettage is curative. These lesions are usually removed via an intraoral approach. A full-thickness flap is made, and bone is removed to expose the lesion. The calcified masses are generally not adherent to bone, and are often easily removed with usual exodontia instruments or hand curettes. If the lesions are extremely large, they may be need to be cut into smaller sections to permit adequate removal without jaw fracture. Spontaneous bone formation is generally sufficient to avoid bone grafting in most cases, but is dependent on the extent of surgery, age, and systemic health of the patient. Corticocancellous marrow grafts may be needed if dental implants are planned in the area of surgery, or if the mandible is atrophic and requires bone augmentation for strengthening. Significantly large lesions may also benefit from intermaxillary fixation or, rarely, placement of a bone plate to prevent jaw fracture.

Ameloblastic Fibroma

The ameloblastic fibroma represents a rarely encountered benign odontogenic tumor that arises as a result of neoplastic proliferation of both odontogenic epithelial and mesenchymal tissues. Although documented to occur over a wide age range, the ameloblastic fibroma typically presents in the posterior mandible of patients in the first or second decades of life. It is known to occur with slightly greater frequency in male patients and is typically associated with the crown of an unerupted permanent toot. Lesions of long-standing duration may present as painless expansile masses; but asymptomatic lesions are also common. Radiographically, the ameloblastic fibroma presents as either a unilocular or multilocular radiolucency with well-defined margins.

Histologic examination of the ameloblastic fibroma shows a proliferation of primitive cell-rich mesenchymal tissue with interspersed islands and anastomosing cords of odontogenic epithelium lined by columnar cells exhibiting reversed nuclear polarity and cytoplasmic vacuolization. Frequently, a rim of hyalinization cuffs the epithelial islands. The primitive cell-rich stroma shares a resemblance to the dental papilla, and its presence aids to distinguish the lesion from the ameloblastoma in which a mature fibrous connective tissue stroma is noted.

Occasionally, there are some lesions that are clinically indistinguishable from ameloblastic fibroma except for a mixed radiolucent-radiopaque appearance; the radiopaque component possessing the radiodensity of tooth structure. Histologic examination reveals features of an ameloblastic fibroma with variable amounts of calcified tissue comprised of dentin and enamel matrix. Occasionally, crudely formed tooth structures are appreciated. These lesions are referred to as the ameloblastic fibro-odontoma, and are considered to be a variant of the ameloblastic fibroma by some and a variant of odontoma by others.

Malignant transformation of an ameloblastic fibroma or de novo malignant lesions sharing features of the ameloblastic fibroma are referred to as ameloblastic fibrosarcoma. Often encountered as a recurrent lesion at the site of a pre-existing benign ameloblastic fibroma, the ameloblastic fibrosarcoma presents as a destructive expansile mass with ill-defined radiographic boundaries. Histologically, these lesions are characterized by atypia within the mesenchymal component of the lesion remarkable for dense cellularity, nuclear pleomorphism, hyperchromaticity, and abundant atypical mitotic figures. Interestingly, only the mesenchymal component of the lesion shows features of malignancy with the associated epithelial component demonstrating nondescript cytomorphology.

Treatment

Enucleation and curettage is the first treatment of choice for ameloblastic fibromas. Most lesions tend to be encapsulated. The tumor does not invade the inferior alveolar canal or the neurovascular bundle, so nerve preservation is readily achieved. Most recurrences perhaps result from incomplete removal. Extensive lesions may require mandibular resection with or without continuity defects. Mandibular defects can usually be reconstructed with bone grafts, and maxillary defects are usually covered by custom-made obturators if radical surgery is performed. Since most patients are very young, bone grafting may not be required, especially for non-continuity defects, as some spontaneous bone regeneration is expected.

Some studies have shown that approximately 45% of fibrosarcomas evolve from previously diagnosed ameloblastic fibromas, and hence, long-term clinical and radiographic follow up is recommended for all lesions. All recurrent lesions must be closely examined.

Benign Non-odontogenic Lesions of the Jaws

Benign Fibro-osseous Lesions

Benign fibro-osseous lesions represent those lesions characterized by the replacement of normal bone by fibrovascular connective tissue and woven bone or cementum-like calcification. Three major categories of benign fibro-osseous lesions involve the maxillofacial bones: fibrous dysplasia, cemento-ossifying fibroma, and cemento-osseous dysplasia. Histologic examination of benign fibro-osseous lesions shows replacement of normal bone with fibrovascular connective tissue and variable amounts of woven bone or cementum-like calcification. As there are histologic similarities amongst all fibro-osseous lesions, clinical, radiographic, and histologic features must be correlated to arrive at a definitive diagnosis.

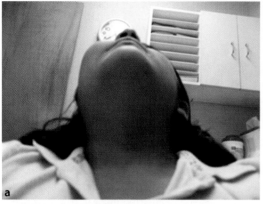

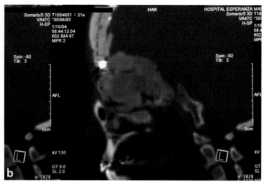

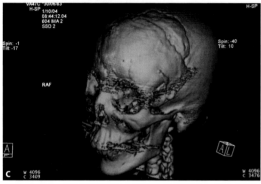

Fig. 35.18 **a** Caudal view of a 12-year-old female patient with fibrous dysplasia of the maxilla. Note severe facial deformity and bone expansion. **b, c** Axial (**b**) and 3-D (**c**) CT scans of the skull of a patient affected with craniofacial fibrous dysplasia; note diffuse involvement of the frontal, nasal, and ethmoid bones

Fibrous Dysplasia

Fibrous dysplasia is considered to be a benign, hamartomatous growth of unknown etiology. It is characterized by a mutation in the guanine nucleotide-binding protein, α-stimulating activity polypeptide 1 (GNAS 1) gene. Four types of disease are known:
1. Monostotic: only a single bone is involved.
2. Polyostotic: multiple bone involvement throughout the body.
3. McCune-Albright syndrome: multiple bone involvement with hyperpigmentation and endocrinal abnormalities such as precocious puberty and hyperthyroidism.
4. Craniofacial fibrous dysplasia: multiple bones of the craniofacial complex are affected (Fig. 35.18a–c).

Fibrous dysplasia usually presents in the first and second decades of life and is more common in the maxilla and in female patients. It is a slow-growing process that often causes painless expansion and deformity. The gradual expansion and bone deposition can cause impingement on vital anatomic structures such as the optic canal. Radiographically, fibrous dysplasia is remarkable for a so-called ground glass mixed radiolucent-radiopaque appearance. The process possesses the tendency to blend itself into adjacent normal bone and, thus, the radiographic margins of the lesion can be poorly defined. One distinctive feature of fibrous dysplasia involving the mandible is a tendency for superior displacement of the inferior alveolar canal.

Treatment

The best treatment is periodic observation. Surgical treatment is usually limited to osteoplasty for bone recontouring in symptomatic cases. If elective, this should be performed only during quiescent phases of the disease and not during phases of active growth. Medications including intravenous bisphosphonate therapy have been effectively used for control of extensive and generalized disease.

Ossifying Fibroma

Ossifying fibroma, also known as cemento-ossifying fibroma, is also a neoplasm whose exact origins are unclear. It occurs over a wide age range, and usually occurs as a solitary lesion in the form of a painless expansile mass in the posterior mandible with a predilection for occurring in female patients. Radiographically, the cemento-ossifying fibroma is a well-demarcated mixed radiolucent-radiopaque lesion that frequently has well-defined sclerotic borders (Fig. 35.19a). Sometimes, a bowing defect of the mandibular inferior cortical bone and marked tooth displacement are seen. An aggressive variant of the cemento-ossifying fibroma is occasionally seen and is termed the juvenile aggressive ossifying fibroma (Fig. 35.19b). Remarkable for an aggressive biologic behavior including a tendency to invade local structures, the lesion typically presents at a younger age,

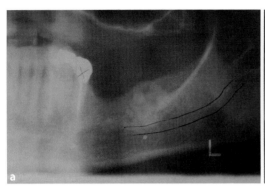
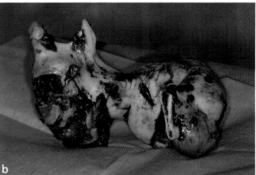

Fig. 35.19 **a** The ossifying fibroma usually presents as a mixed, radiolucent-radiopaque lesion with well-defined borders. **b** The juvenile ossifying fibroma is a rare, but very aggressive variant of an ossifying fibroma which can have relatively rapid growth. This tumor involved almost the entire mandible and was causing significant functional and respiratory problems due to its extensive size

during the first to second decades of life, with a predilection for maxillary involvement. Clinical presentations can include symptoms such as significant facial asymmetry, proptosis, visual disturbances, and nasal obstruction.

Treatment

Complete surgical excision is advised. Enucleation with curettage/peripheral ostectomy is recommended for smaller lesions and this can be accomplished via an intraoral approach. Extensive tumors require a more invasive approach and resection-type procedures. High recurrence rates approaching 50% have been reported.

Cemento-osseous Dysplasia

Cemento-osseous dysplasias are the commonest types of fibro-osseous disease seen in the alveolar part of the jaws. As a group, they generally are asymptomatic, are of diagnostic significance only, and occur due to a mismatched and disordered production of bone and cementum. There are three distinct clinical subtypes: periapical, focal, and florid cemento-osseous dysplasia.

Periapical cemento-osseous dysplasia presents clinically as an asymptomatic lesion typically discovered on routine radiographic examination (Fig. 35.20). It has a propensity to occur in middle-aged black women, and commonly presents as a multifocal process involving the apices of vital mandibular anterior teeth. As the lesion matures, a spectrum of radiographic

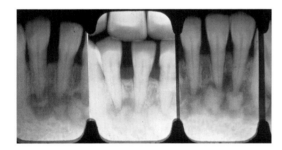

Fig. 35.20 Periapical cemento-osseous dysplasia presents as multiple radiolucencies around the apices of the mandibular anterior teeth. With time, lesions become more radiopaque as is seen on the radiographs. Bone expansion is absent and the teeth are vital on pulp testing

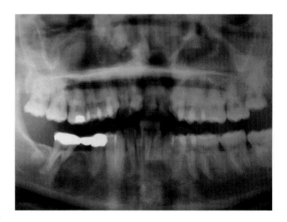

Fig. 35.21 Focal cemento-osseous dysplasia generally occurs in the posterior mandible as a solitary lesion. It usually presents as a radiopaque mass surrounded by a radiolucent rim

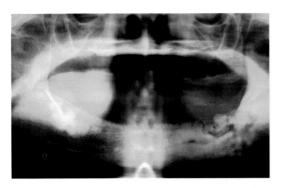

Fig. 35.22 Florid osseous dysplasia must be differentiated from chronic diffuse sclerosing osteomyelitis. Multiple mixed lesions with varying degrees of radiopacities are common and present bilaterally in the mandible

changes can be appreciated ranging from early lesions that are entirely radiolucent to lesions of long standing that are purely radiopaque. In the absence of expansion or other changes in the character of the process, periapical cemento-osseous dysplasia only requires periodic clinical and radiographic observation.

Focal cemento-osseous dysplasia presents clinically as an asymptomatic lesion typically discovered on routine radiographic examination (Fig. 35.21). It is more common in Caucasian women, and presents as a solitary lesion at the apex of a vital tooth most commonly located in the posterior mandible. Occasionally, lesions are encountered in edentulous regions of the alveolar bone. As the focal process undergoes maturation, a spectrum of radiographic changes ranging from early lesions that are entirely radiolucent to lesions of long standing that are purely radiopaque may be appreciated. A peripheral rim of radiolucency is typically noted to circumscribe the lesion. In the absence of clinical expansion or a change in character of the lesion, periodic clinical and radiographic observation is all that is required.

Florid cemento-osseous dysplasia presents as a multifocal process involving more than one quadrant of the maxilla and/or mandible. More common in middle-aged black women, the process is typically asymptomatic. Radiographic examination reveals multiple foci of mixed radiolucencies that are often bilateral and symmetric (Fig. 35.22). Florid cemento-osseous lesions exhibit a spectrum of radiographic changes ranging from early lesions that are entirely radiolucent to lesions of long standing that are purely radiopaque, and must be clinically differentiated from chronic diffuse sclerosing osteomyelitis as treatment is different. In the absence of clinical expansion, or change in character, only periodic clinical and radiographic observation is required.

Osteoblastoma and Osteoid Osteoma

Both these tumors seem to be essentially the same neoplastic process, with the osteoblastoma representing the larger variant (greater than 2 cm in size). There have been some reports of regression after biopsy, which has led some to believe that these may represent a reactive process. The hallmark of these tumors is pain and they occur much more commonly in long bones than in the jaws. Osteoid osteoma is known for nocturnal pain, which is relieved with anti-inflammatory medications while osteoblastoma has more severe pain, often not relieved with medications. Radiographically, both present as well-defined radiolucent-radiopaque lesions. A "sun-ray" pattern of new bone formation similar to malignant tumors has been described. Treatment is complete surgical removal with curettage or local excision, which is generally performed with an intraoral approach.

Synovial Chondromatosis and Osteochondroma

Synovial chondromatosis is a very rare condition that can affect temporomandibular joints (TMJ). The exact etiology is unknown, but trauma has been proposed as a contributing factor. Histologically, it consists of small particulate tissue that resembles individual chondromas. Treatment involves simple excision of the lesion and synovial tissues via standard TMJ surgical approaches.

Osteochondroma is a rare tumor of the TMJs. It presents as an exophytic growth on the mandibular condyle (Fig. 35.23a). The lesions can be broad-based or pedunculated and are histologically similar to osteochondromas of the long bones. Clinically, the tumor can cause growth in a vertical, horizontal, or combination vectors. Patients often present with facial asymmetry, changes in occlusion, chin deviation to contralateral side (horizontal growth vector), and bowing of the ramus (vertical vector growth) (Fig. 35.23b, c). Histologically, the lesional tissue

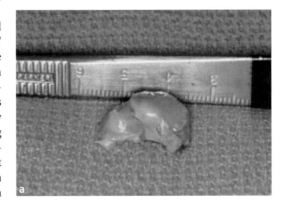

Fig. 35.23 **a** Resected specimen showing an osteochondroma of the mandibular condyle. Note the exophytic growth on the condylar cartilage cap **b,c** *see next page*

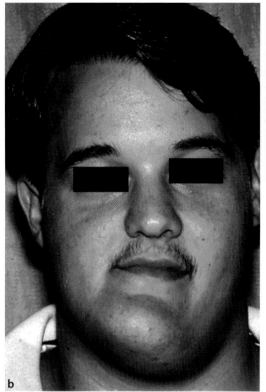

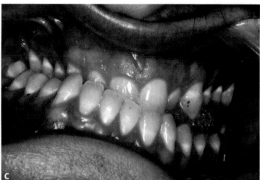

Fig. 35.23 (*continued*) **b** Facial view of a patient with osteochondroma of the left mandibular condyle. The tumor has caused significant facial asymmetry including deviation of the chin to the contralateral side. **c** Intraoral view showing significant malocclusion and open bite due to the growth of the tumor in the TMJ/condylar region which has displaced the mandible inferiorly and laterally. Picture courtesy of Dr. Douglas Dingewerth, Dallas, Texas

reveals a cellular, hyaline cartilaginous cap covered by perichondrium. Deeper layers of the cartilage have endochondral ossification with bone or cartilage deposition. The recommended treatment is conservative excision using a high- to medium-level condylectomy [53]. For large tumors, a low-level condylectomy can be performed with concomitant TMJ reconstruction using costochondral or sternoclavicular bone grafts [53]. Recurrence after adequate removal is rare.

Osteoma

Osteomas are benign tumors of compact and cancellous bone. The etiology is unknown, but a history of prior trauma accompanies some lesions. Two distinct types are recognized, periosteal (present on the bone surface) and endosteal (central within bone) osteomas. Clinically, most patients are asymptomatic, and the lesions are discovered on routine radiographic examination. Endosteal lesions can remain quiescent while periosteal osteomas grow on the bony surface and maybe more evident as bone masses. Patients with osteomas must be screened for Gardner's syndrome. This syndrome consists of multiple osteomas of the jaws, intestinal polyps, skin lesions, and multiple impacted teeth. Diagnosing this syndrome is significant as the intestinal polyps are premalignant.

Radiographic examination generally reveals well-defined, dense, sclerotic radiopaque masses. Histologically, some lesions are composed of dense, compact, mature lamellar bone and relatively sparse marrow spaces. Other lesions contain lamellar trabeculae of cancellous bone with interspersed fibrofatty tissue. Osteoblastic activity is prominent. Once a diagnosis has been established, asymptomatic lesions can be observed with periodic radiographic examination if one desires. Surgical treatment involves excision, which is accomplished with intraoral approaches. Recurrence is not expected.

Neurofibroma and Neurilemmoma

These two tumors are of nerve tissue origin and will be considered together as they are extremely rare in the jaws. Both tumors are more common in soft tissues but can occur in bone when they arise from the nerve sheath tissue of the inferior alveolar nerve. The neurofibroma can present as solitary lesion or as part of generalized neurofibromatosis (Von Recklinghausen's disease of skin), an autosomally dominant condition. Radiographically, they present as well-defined radiolucent lesions. Clinically, paresthesia, dysesthesia, or pain in distribution of the affected nerve can result. Histologically, neurilemmoma (schwannoma) consists of spindle cells in either Antoni A (palisaded arrangement) or Antoni B (haphazard arrangement) pattern. Treatment involves localized surgical excision. Malignant transformation of neurofibromas has been reported.

Giant Cell Lesions

Giant Cell Granuloma

The giant cell granuloma represents a proliferative vascular lesion characterized by the replacement of normal bone with cellular fibrous connective tissue containing numerous multinucleated giant cells, extravasated erythrocytes, hemosiderin-laden macrophages, and trabeculae of reactive bone. The exact pathogenesis is incompletely understood, but genetic abnormalities may have a role in some lesions. The giant cell granuloma presents centrally within bone, however histologically identical lesions are frequently seen that arise peripherally in the alveolar mucosa confined exclusively to the soft tissue. The central giant cell granuloma occurs over a wide age range typically presenting in the first three decades of life. Current literature supports the division of central giant cell granulomas into either non-aggressive, intermediate, or aggressive categories based on biologic behavior using features such as: a size greater than 5 cm, cortical perforation or thinning, root resorption, pain, marked growth rate, and recurrence after conservative treatment to indicate aggressive tendencies [54]. The central giant cell granuloma has a predilection for occurring in the mandible, frequently presenting in the anterior region, and often crossing the midline. Peripheral lesions are clinically indistinguishable from other benign gingival nodules and are not known for aggressive behavior (Fig. 35.24a). Although recurrence is occasionally reported in peripheral giant cell granulomas, the lesion may represent a focal reactive process and recurrence is most likely related to persistence of local inciting factors and/

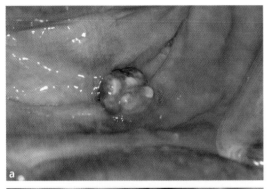

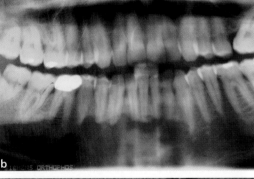

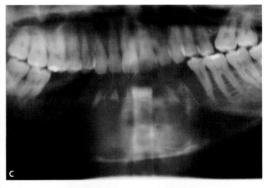

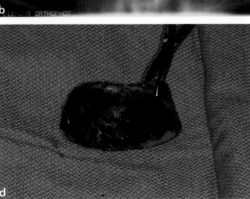

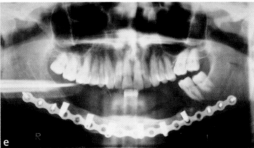

Fig. 35.24 **a** Peripheral giant cell granulomas are confined to the gingiva and present as variable colored gingival nodules or masses. An incisional or excisional biopsy is required for an accurate diagnosis. Recurrence potential is high and curettage of bone must be performed after removal of lesions to decrease chances of recurrence. **b** The central giant cell granuloma usually presents as a well-defined radiolucency of the jaw. **c** Large lesions can cause extensive bone destruction and pathological fractures of the mandible. **d** Intraoperative photograph showing resected central giant cell granuloma of the anterior mandible. The large size of the lesion necessitated resection. **e** Postoperative panoramic radiograph of same patient shown in **c**. Endosseous dental implants have been placed in the reconstructed mandible

or incomplete removal. Radiographically, the central giant cell granuloma presents as a well-delineated unilocular to multilocular radiolucency (Fig. 35.24b). Peripheral lesions often show a saucer-shaped resorptive defect in the alveolar bone subjacent to the soft tissue neoplasm.

Histologically, the giant cell granuloma consists of multinucleated giant cells on a cellular fibrovascular stroma of ovoid mesenchymal cells. Extravasated erythrocytes, hemosiderin-laden macrophages, and trabeculae of reactive bone are appreciated in varying amounts. Although a point of some controversy, the multinucleated giant cells within the giant cell granuloma are most likely osteoclastic in nature and derived from cells of the monocyte/macrophage lineage. The mesenchymal cellular component of the lesion represents the proliferative constituent of the process serving to recruit monocytes and subsequently encourage their differentiation into osteoclast-type giant cells. A correlation between the presence of large multinucleated giant cells and marked stromal cellularity with the tendency for aggressive biologic behavior has been suggested. It is important to note that the histological features of the giant cell granuloma and the so-called brown tumors of hyperparathyroidism are indistinguishable, and that this condition should be considered in the differential diagnosis of all giant cell lesions.

Treatment

Given that the histologic features of this lesion are indistinguishable from the so-called brown tumor of hyperparathyroidism, evaluation of serum calcium, phosphate, and parathyroid hormone levels is essential prior to treatment. The most commonly used treatment modality is aggressive curettage. Large lesions that risk pathologic fracture may require resection (Fig. 35.24c). If surgery is contemplated, the surgeon must be prepared to encounter significant intraoperative hemorrhage until the entire lesion has been curetted. Although surgery has historically been the mainstay of treatment (Fig. 35.24d, e), intralesional corticosteroid therapy, calcitonin therapy, and more recently antiangiogenic therapy have also been shown to be effective in treating these lesions [44–46].

Cherubism

Cherubism is a rare genetic condition where the bone is replaced by fibrous and vascular elements containing multinucleated giant cells. The clinical presentation is variable and can range from asymptomatic lesions to large and symptomatic lesions. The term "cherubism" was coined from the word "cherubs," which was used to describe young holy angels who were historically pictured in the Renaissance period with their eyes turned up toward heaven; in cherubism, gradual replacement of bone with fibrovascular tissue results in a filled-up, rounded facial appearance with scleral show, which gives the appearance as if the eyes are turned up! The disease manifests itself during childhood, but may not be discovered until later, depending on the degree and rate of bone involvement. A classification has been proposed depending on the areas of involvement, but is

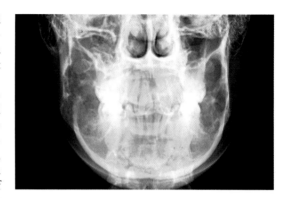

Fig. 35.25 Plain skull film of a 16-year-old boy with cherubism. Note bilateral mandibular soap-bubble radiolucencies in the mandibular posterior body and ascending ramus areas

does not have much clinical significance in reference to treatment and prognosis. The mandible is more commonly affected than the maxilla. Common clinical features of extensive disease include premature exfoliation of deciduous teeth, displacement of permanent teeth, alteration in tooth eruption patterns, and bone expansion. Figure 35.25 shows a radiograph of a 16-year-old boy with cherubism.

Histologically, the lesions are very similar to a central giant cell granuloma. Perivascular cuffing may be prominent. Treatment is reserved for large and rapidly growing lesions. Small and/or asymptomatic lesions should be observed as the disease is usually self-limiting. Some authorities believe that no surgery should be performed during active phases of the disease as it may cause an increased rebound growth postsurgically, but this is controversial. Calcitonin, which is quite effective for treatment of central giant cell granulomas, is not very effective in treating cherubism. Children with large lesions causing psychological and functional problems may occasionally require early procedures like debulking and/or recontouring in an attempt to direct teeth eruption and improve facial esthetics.

Aneurysmal Bone Cyst

This entity has been discussed earlier in the chapter.

Hyperparathyroidism

This systemic medical disorder causes calcium mobilization from the bones in an attempt to maintain a balance in the blood calcium levels with the increased renal excretion of calcium. Three distinct types of hyperparathyroidism are recognized:

1. Primary hyperthyroidism: There is increased activity of parathyroid glands (increased parathormone secretion) resulting in hypercalcemia.
2. Secondary hyperparathyroidism: Renal failure results in excessive loss of calcium and thus, hypocalcemia, which in turn

signals the normal parathyroid glands to release parathormone.

3. Tertiary hyperparathyroidism.

Calcium is mobilized from the jaws from localized areas and produces multiple radiolucent lesions. Histologically, hyperparathyroidism lesions are very similar to a central giant cell granuloma. Thus, diagnosis is based on laboratory investigations and treatment is aimed at medically correcting the hyperparathyroidism, which results in resolution of the associated jaw disease.

Miscellaneous Bony Lesions of the Jaws

Tori

These are well-rounded bony projections than can occur in the maxilla (torus palatinus) and the mandible (torus mandibularis). The incidence is quite common. A maxillary torus is located in the midline of the palate and depending on the size, may have lobulations and variable extension into adjacent paramidline regions (Fig. 35.26a). In contrast, mandibular tori are usually bilateral and occur on the lingual aspect of the premolar and molar teeth. They are generally small in size but at times, smaller tori may coalesce to form larger nodules (Fig. 35.26b). Radiographic examination is limited due to overlap of dental structures. Diagnosis is made by clinical examination, and no treatment is required unless the lesions increase in size or interfere with function or prosthetic dental rehabilitation. Caution must be exercised during surgical removal/reduction of these lesions to prevent damage to important anatomic structures such as the nasal cavity and sinus (maxilla) and lingual nerve (mandible). A suck-down thermoplastic splint is very useful in the immediate postoperative phase after maxillary torus surgery (Fig. 35.8c).

Langerhans Cell Disease

Langerhans cell disease (LCD) is a rare disease. It mainly occurs in children and the pathogenesis includes proliferation of monoclonal CD1a-positive cells of unknown origin. Although the exact etiology is unknown, a theory labeling viral etiology as the cause is most common. Historically, the disease was known as histiocytosis X and three distinct variants were described [55]:

1. Hand-Schüller-Christian disease: The chronic disseminated form of the disease involves skin, multiple organs, and bone. A typical triad of bone lesions, exophthalmos, and diabetes insipidus is pathognomonic.
2. Letterer-Siwe syndrome: Acute disseminated form of the disease which occurs in infants and is usually fatal due to widespread visceral involvement.
3. Eosinophilic granuloma: Chronic focal disease limited to bone involvement.

Relative to bony involvement, the skull, mandible, vertebrae, ribs, and long bones are the most commonly involved sites. Clinical signs and symptoms include pain and swelling, loose teeth, and inflamed periodontal tissues. Pathologic mandibular fractures can result. Radiographic examination reveals single or multiple radiolucent lesions resulting in extensive bone loss giving the appearance of "floating teeth" (Fig. 35.27a). Diagnosis should be made only after histologic examination of the biopsy specimen, and additional techniques such as electron microscopy and immunochemical staining can further aid in confirming the diagnosis. Treatment is dependent on extent of disease and options include surgery (curettage), intralesional medications (corticosteroids), systemic chemotherapy (reserved for extensive multisystem disease), and low-dose radiation treatment (Fig. 35.27b, c).

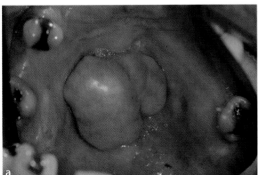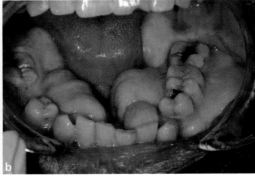

Fig. 35.26 **a** Intraoral photograph showing a large palatal torus that interfered with function including mastication and speech. **b** Intraoral photograph showing extremely large bilateral mandibular tori. Care must be taken during removal or reduction of such large tori as there is risk of jaw fracture and possible damage to the lingual nerve which runs in the lingual soft tissues adjacent to the mandible

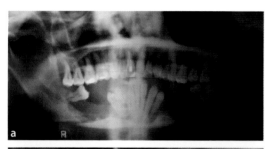

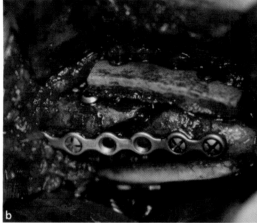

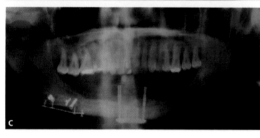

Fig. 35.27 **a** Panoramic radiograph of a 29-year-old man with bilateral mandibular fractures. The dentulous portion of the mandible shows "floating teeth." **b** The patient was initially treated for his mandibular fractures with cranial bone grafts and rigid fixation. Bone biopsies were taken to confirm the presence of Langerhan's cell disease. **c** Complete regeneration of the mandible is seen after low-dose radiation therapy. A transosteal bone plate (transmandibular implant) has been placed in preparation for dental prosthetic rehabilitation

Paget's Disease

Also known as osteitis deformans, Paget's disease is a benign, slow-growing disease of bone. It usually presents after 50 years of age and there is a male preponderance. Although the exact etiology is unknown, the most common theory revolves around a viral infection. Clinical symptoms occur due to varied bone deposition the results of which give rise to patient complaints such as caps, hats, gloves, and dentures no longer fitting them. Headaches, vascular compression, pain, and bone deformities can also occur, and the maxilla is more often involved than

the mandible. The disease course includes alternating phases of bone resorption and deposition, and changes in vascularity. Radiographically, a "cotton-wool" appearance of the skull and maxilla is classically described. Dental radiographs reveal loss of lamina dura and hypercementosis, which complicates exodontic procedures. Histologic examination reveals reversal lines due to alternate bone deposition and resorption. Definitive diagnosis is based on clinical, radiographic, and histologic examination and elevated alkaline phosphatase levels. Paget's disease is considered to be a premalignant condition with up to a 15% incidence of sarcoma development [56]. Treatment includes use of medications such as calcitonin and bisphosphonates. Surgical recontouring for functional or cosmetic purposes can be undertaken if required, but the surgeon should expect significant bleeding in view of the vascular nature of the disease process. Prognosis is poor and patients die due to osteosarcoma development or due to vascularity-related hemodynamic complications.

Surgical Management of Benign Jaw Pathology

General Considerations

Jaw tumors vary greatly in their biologic behavior. Clinical signs and symptoms can be variable. While some lesions are extremely slow growing, others can be extremely destructive; some lesions have defined boundaries and others are locally aggressive. Thus, correlation of clinical, radiographic, and histologic analysis is essential to prevent over- or under-treatment.

The panoramic radiograph is a useful initial film and helps in development of an initial working differential diagnosis. It gives an overall view of the jaws and its structures. For larger lesions requiring complex treatment planning, a CT scan is recommended. MRI is indicated in specific instances, especially for soft tissue imaging.

An incisional biopsy is usually performed for most lesions. However, excisional biopsies may be indicated in some circumstances, for instance small radiopaque lesions or for other lesions less than 1.0–1.5 cm in size. Multiple biopsy specimens may be needed in some cases to make a definitive diagnosis, particularly if the lesion shows unusual characteristics (e.g., slow-growing cystic lesion with root resorption). The specimens should be appropriately labeled, oriented, and sent to a pathologist experienced in odontogenic pathology. It is well established that odontogenic tumors can be very complex; most head and neck tumor surgeons agree that if there is any question, it may be prudent to consult with an oral pathologist before embarking on definitive surgical treatment.

It is the responsibility of the surgeon to diagnose the specific lesion and provide appropriate treatment. Unfortunately, even today, when our understanding of most tumors has significantly increased, many surgeons continue to perform inappropriate surgical procedures. This is perhaps due to lack of a rationalized tumor-biology-based approach. It should be noted that almost no benign odontogenic neoplasm requires surgery as extensive as microvascular reconstruction. These patients are not cancer patients, and the rule of cure with least morbid surgery must be followed.

Based on the known biology of benign odontogenic tumors, it seems as if, out of all primary odontogenic benign cysts and tumors, only the following neoplasms have continued growth potential and invasive properties and require resection: ameloblastoma, odontogenic myxoma, and calcifying epithelial odontogenic tumor. Although controversial, all other benign lesions can usually be treated with enucleation and curettage. The reader should note that, at present, there are no absolute guidelines for management of many odontogenic tumors, and treatment of some lesions continues to be controversial.

Resection Procedures for Surgical Treatment of Benign Mandibular Neoplasms

In general, resection with 1.0- to 1.5-cm margins, removal of one uninvolved anatomic barrier, and frozen sections demonstrating tumor-free margins are standard principles.

Intermaxillary fixation must be applied to maintain the relationship of the jaws to each other. The mandible can be approached via a transoral or transcutaneous approach depending on surgical access and surgeon experience. As these are benign lesions and no neck dissections are needed, the usual dissection plane is deep to the superficial layer of deep cervical fascia, deep to the common facial vein, and deep to the marginal mandibular nerve. It is superficial to the submandibular gland, digastric muscles, and the sternocleidomastoid. If the CT scan shows no cortical perforation, then the periosteum is lifted off the bone in subperiosteal fashion; if cortical perforation is noted on the CT scan, then supraperiosteal dissection is performed as the periosteum becomes the uninvolved anatomic barrier that is removed with the tumor specimen.

The tumor is identified and a mandibular reconstruction plate (locking or non-locking rigid plate) should be adapted to mimic the normal mandibular contour. If possible, it is recommended that the plate extend three holes beyond the anticipated tumor margins on either side of the resected specimen. The plate is temporarily fixed to the mandible prior to resection in order to maintain control of the proximal and distal segments. If the mandibular condyle is to be resected with the specimen, a condyle replacement must be used. Common options include TMJ reconstruction with autogenous tissues such as costochondral grafts, sternoclavicular grafts, or condylar prostheses. The TMJ disc is usually left in place as the autogenous TMJ reconstruction grafts articulate quite well with it.

Mandibular resection can either be complete (continuity defect results) or marginal/peripheral (inferior border is left so that there is no continuity defect). The resection margins should be planned so that adequate bone (3–5 mm) remains in between the mandibular margins and the adjacent tooth. This will prevent bone resorption, periodontal disease, and infection.

Peripheral/marginal resection procedures also require some additional caveats. It is recommended that at least 1 cm of native inferior border of the mandible be left as if it is less than 1 cm it could pose a higher risk for postsurgical fracture. Additionally,

instead of the routine 90-degree angles, a gentle rounded curve shape should be employed as this will distribute biting forces more evenly.

Resection Procedures for Surgical Treatment of Benign Maxillary Neoplasms

Indications for resection of the maxilla remain the same as for the mandible. The surgery usually involves a subtotal or partial maxillectomy depending on the tumor extent. Generally, 1.0- to 1.5-cm margins are used for most tumors as in mandibular tumors. Most tumors are approached transorally, but certain large tumors may require transcutaneous access via a Weber-Ferguson or other approaches.

Unlike cancer surgery, mucosa is only removed if it is infiltrated by the tumor. Thus, dissection is usually performed in a subperiosteal plane and the infraorbital nerve can usually be preserved for most tumors. In the author's experience, extensive bone grafting is not needed routinely as most maxillary defects are easily closed by custom-made obturators.

Jaw Bone Reconstruction

There has been significant advancement in mandibular reconstruction techniques over the last few years. While microvascular reconstructive surgery is the most common procedure performed for reconstruction of cancer patients, cancellous bone graft reconstruction remains the workhorse and procedure of choice for reconstruction following resection of benign neoplasms.

The surgical wound consists of a bone clot, which is hypoxic, and creates a steep oxygen gradient from the wound center to the periphery of the tissue bed. When cancellous bone grafts harvested from the iliac crest are placed into this surgical site, there is transfer of viable osteogenic cells into the wound. The bone graft is initially dependent on this tissue gradient for diffusion of nutrients and survival. Platelets aggregated in the blood clot secrete bone growth factors that additionally attract other cells into the site. Continued hypoxia and lactic acidosis within the surgical wound are potent physiochemotactic agents that recruit macrophages into the area, and these macrophages secrete angiogenic factors. This results in revascularization of the bone graft which, although initiated immediately within hours of bone grafting, takes approximately 14 days to be complete. Once revascularization is complete, the bone graft is ready for independent survival.

The surviving endosteal cells of the cancellous bone graft initially form woven bone on each trabecula. This initial woven bone is laid down randomly and is referred to as phase 1 bone. The woven bone bridges the continuity defect and is gradually replaced by more mineralized, mature, lamellar, phase 2 bone, with the replacement process starting at about 4 weeks postoperatively. The amount of phase 1 bone formed is directly dependent on the number of osteoprogenitor cells transplanted. Thus, it is advisable to compact bone as much as possible as a denser graft would most likely have more osteoprogenitor cells transferred. Syringes are often used intraoperatively to compact bone grafts. Ultimately, all phase 1 bone is completely resorbed by osteoclasts. The osteoclasts release bone morphogenic protein (BMP) during the resorption process, and this BMP release induces stem cells within the graft (transplanted osteogenesis) and in the surrounding tissues (periosteum, muscles, etc.) to form phase 2 bone (osteoinduction) across the biologic or alloplastic framework (osteoconduction).

Cancellous bone grafts for maxillofacial reconstruction are usually harvested from the iliac crest via an anterior or posterior approach as the iliac crest yields the maximum volume of osteoprogenitor cells in an adult human patient. Approximately 10 cc of non-compacted bone is required for reconstruction of each 1 cm of continuity defect of the mandible. While the anterior iliac crest yields approximately 50 cc of bone, a posterior approach may yield two to three times that amount.

As our understanding of bone physiology and regeneration improves, many recent advances are taking place in the area of

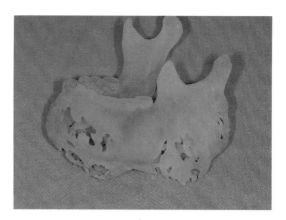

Fig. 35.29 Three-dimensional stereolithographic models can be obtained prior to surgery. They are very accurate and help in treatment planning. Preparatory surgery can be performed on the model itself, and many models can also be sterilized for intraoperative use. They clearly define the relationship of the pathology to adjacent structures, and allow for pre-bending of reconstruction plates thereby reducing operating time

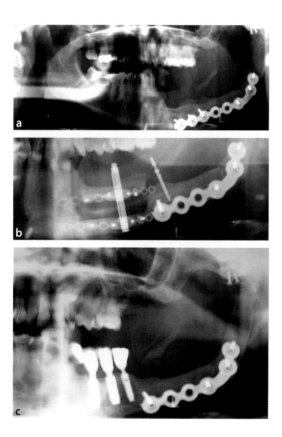

Fig. 35.28 a Panoramic radiograph showing reconstructed atrophic mandible. Due to the significant soft and hard tissue defect, dental rehabilitation is not possible. b Alveolar distraction osteogenesis has been used to augment the atrophic jaw. Note height of osteotomized mandibular alveolus and distraction using a plate-type distraction device. c Postoperative panoramic radiograph showing placement of three dental implants and implant-supported fixed restorations in the distracted segment

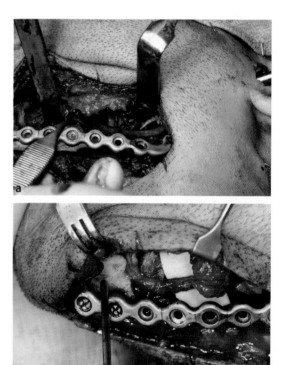

Fig. 35.30a,b The mandible is laterally decorticated posterior to the posterior resection margin to identify the nerve. Anteriorly, the nerve is transected at the mental foramen. a The resection is performed, and the nerve is freed out by pulling it out of the specimen posteriorly. b Once the nerve is pulled out of the specimen, it can be anastomosed in standard fashion using epineural sutures. Approximately 85–90% of return of sensation is expected, which is better than alternative nerve graft procedures

bone reconstruction. Examples of such concepts include distraction osteogenesis (Fig. 35.28a–c), use of three-dimensional stereolithographic models fabricated with computer-aided design–computer-aided manufacture (CAD-CAM) technology for treatment of complex cases (Fig. 35.29), and preservation and/or reconstruction of vital soft tissue structures, for example the inferior alveolar nerve, which need not be sacrificed in surgery for benign pathology (Figs. 35.30a, b, 35.31c). Knowledge, development, and clinical use of bone growth factors (BMPs, platelet-rich plasma, etc.) are adding a new dimension to the science and art of jaw reconstruction. Restoration of form and function with implant-supported dental prostheses (Fig. 35.31a–e) should be considered the benchmark and standard of care after jaw-bone reconstruction.

In the twenty-first century, removal of a jaw cyst or tumor should only be considered a starting point; likewise, stabilizing continuity defects and jaw segments with rigid plates and adding bone to deficient areas should not be considered as the ending point; instead, the journey must only be considered complete once we have achieved "comprehensive esthetic and functional jaw reconstruction" (Fig. 35.31e).

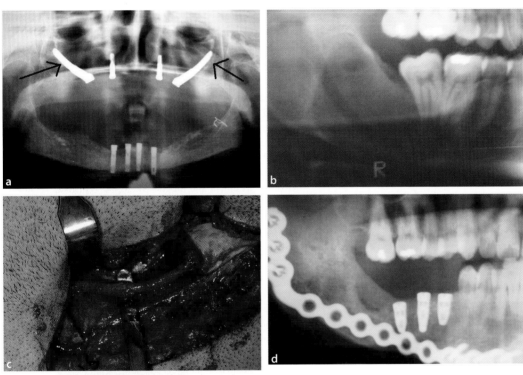

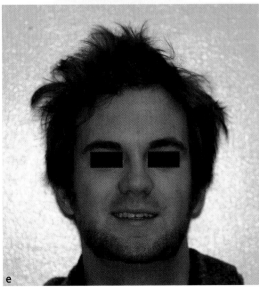

Fig. 35.31 **a** Dental restorations supported by zygomatic implants are now being used; these allow for implant-supported restorations in the maxilla without the need for bone grafting of the posterior resected areas. **b** Recurrent odontogenic keratocyst of the right posterior mandible in a 19-year-old man. **c** Mandibular resection with inferior alveolar nerve preservation. The cyst was removed and bone resected without transection of the nerve, thereby maintaining normal lip and chin sensation. **d** Panoramic radiograph showing results of jaw reconstruction with cancellous marrow grafts harvested from the iliac crest. Normal height of bone can be achieved using this technique. **e** Postoperative photograph 2 years after fixed dental restorations with dental implants placed in grafted bone showing results of functional and esthetic jaw reconstruction. Dental restorations supported by implants placed in grafted bone are extremely esthetic, maintain alveolar height and width, and give patients long-term predictable service

Tips to Avoid Complications

- It is recommended surgeons involve a pathologist experienced in oral pathology to review histopathologic slides prior to surgery. The area of oral and maxillofacial pathology is extremely complex and many clinical and/or histopathologic presentations are similar in appearance but warrant differing treatment(s).
- The rule of "least morbid surgery for cure" must be followed. It is generally agreed that most odontogenic lesions, irrespective of their size and location, can often be managed conservatively with intraoral approaches.

35

Acknowledgements

In the writing of this chapter the following textbooks were referred to for concepts and general guidelines:

a. Marx RE, Stern D (2003) In: Oral and maxillofacial pathology: a rationale for diagnosis and treatment. Quintessence, Illinois
b. Williams TP, Stewart JCB (2000) In: Fonseca R (ed) Oral and maxillofacial surgery: surgical pathology. Saunders, Philadelphia
c. Neville BW, Damm DD, Allen CM, Bouquot JE (2002) Oral and maxillofacial pathology. Saunders, Philadelphia
d. Barnes L (2001) Surgical pathology of the head and neck. Dekker, New York

References

1. Toller PA (1972) Newer concepts of odontogenic cysts. Int J Oral Surg 1:3–16
2. Ten Cate AR (1972) The epithelial rests of Malassez and the genesis of the dental cyst. J Oral Surg 34:956–964
3. Main DMG (1970) The enlargement of epithelial jaw cysts. Odontol Rev 21:29–49
4. Browne RM (1975) The pathogenesis of odontogenic cysts: a review. J Oral Pathol 4:31–46
5. Mourshed F (1964) A roentgenographic study of dentigerous cysts. I. Incidence in a population sample. Oral Surg Oral Med Oral Pathol 18:47–53
6. Dreidler JF, Raubenheimer EJ, van Heerden WF (1993) A retrospective analysis of 367 cystic lesions of the jaw: the Ulm experience. J Craniomaxillofac Surg 21:339–341
7. Yasuoka T, Yonemoto K, Kato Y, Tatematsu N (2000) Squamous cell carcinoma arising in a dentigerous cyst. J Oral Maxillofac Surg 58:900–905
8. Aguilo L, Cibrian R, Bagan JV, Gandia JL (1998) Eruption cysts: retrospective clinical study of 36 cases. ASDC J Dent Child 65:102–106
9. Wysocki G, Brannon R, Gardner D, Sapp P (1980) Histogenesis of the lateral periodontal cyst and the gingival cyst of the adult. Oral Surg Oral Med Oral Pathol 50:327–334
10. Cohen D, Neville B, Damm D, White D (1984) The lateral periodontal cyst: a report of 37 cases. J Periodontol 55:230–234
11. Baker RD, D'Onofrio ED, Corio RL (1979) Squamous cell carcinoma arising in a lateral periodontal cyst. Oral Surg Oral Med Oral Pathol 47:495–499
12. Ahlfors E, Larsson A, Sjogren S (1991) The odontogenic keratocyst: a benign cystic tumor? J Oral Maxillofac Surg 20:362–365
13. Wicking C, Bale AE (1997) Molecular basis of the nevoid basal cell carcinoma syndrome. Curr Opin Pediatr 9:630–635
14. Cohen MM Jr (1999) Nevoid basal cell carcinoma syndrome: molecular biology and new hypotheses. Int J Oral Maxillofac Surg 28:216–223
15. Barreto DC, Gomez RS, Bale AE, Boson WL, De Marco L (2000) PTCH gene mutations in odontogenic keratocysts. J Dent Res 79:1418–1422
16. Myoung H, Hong SP, Hong SD, Lee JI, Lim CY, Choung PH, Lee JH, et al (2001) Okct: review of 256 cases for recurrence and clinicopathologic parameters. Oral Surg Oral Med Oral Pathol Oral Radiol Endod 91:328–333
17. Brannon RB (1976) The odontogenic keratocyst: a clinicopathologic study of 312 cases. I. Clinical features. Oral Surg Oral Med Oral Pathol 42:54–72
18. Blanas N, Freund B, Schwartz M, Furst I (2000) Systematic review of the treatment and prognosis of the odontogenic keratocyst. Oral Surg Oral Med Oral Pathol Oral Radiol Endod 90:553–558
19. de Paula AMB, Carvalhais JN, Domingues MG, Barreto DC, Mesquita RA (2000) Cell proliferation markers in the odontogenic keratocyst: effect of inflammation. J Oral Pathol Med 29:477–482
20. August M, Faquin WC, Troulis MJ, Kaban LB (2003) Dedifferentiation of odontogenic keratocyst epithelium after cyst decompression. J Oral Maxillofac Surg 61:678–683
21. Voorsmit RACA (1984) The incredible keratocyst. Thesis, University of Nijmegan, The Netherlands
22. Voorsmit RACA, Stoelinga PJ, Van Haelst UJGM (1981) The management of keratocysts. J Maxillofac Surg 9:228–235
23. Schmidt BL, Pogrel MA (2001) The use of enucleation and liquid nitrogen cryotherapy in the management of odontogenic keratocysts. J Oral Maxillofac Surg 59:720–725
24. Browne RM (1971) The odontogenic keratocyst: histological features and their correlation with clinical behavior. Br Dent J 131:249–259
25. Rud J, Pindborg JJ (1961) Odontogenic keratocysts: a follow-up study of 21 cases. J Oral Surg 27:323–330
26. Wright JM (1981) The odontogenic keratocyst: orthokeratinized variant. Oral Surg Oral Med Oral Pathol 51:609–618
27. da Silva MJA, de Sousa SO, Correa L, Carvalhosa AA, de Araujo VC (2002) Immunohistochemical study of the orthokeratinized odontogenic cyst: a comparison with the odontogenic keratocyst. Oral Surg Oral Med Oral Pathol Oral Radiol Endod 94:732–737
28. Gardner DG, Kessler HP, Morency R, Schaffner DL (1988) The glandular odontogenic cyst: an apparent entity. J Oral Pathol 17:359–366

29. Koppang HS, Johannessen S, Haugen LK, Haanaes HR, Solheim T, Donath K(1988) Glandular odontogenic cyst (sialo-odontogenic cyst): report of two cases and review of 45 previously reported cases. J Oral Pathol Med 27:455–462

30. Ramer M, Montazem A, Lane SL, Lumerman H (1997) Glandular odontogenic cyst: report of a case and review of the literature. Oral Surg Oral Med Oral Pathol Oral Radiol Endod 84:54–57

31. Toida M (1998) So-called calcifying odontogenic cyst: review and discussion on the terminology and classification. J Oral Pathol Med 27:49–52

32. Praetorius F, Hjorting-Hansen E, Gorlin RJ, Vickers RA (1981) Calcifying odontogenic cyst. Range, variations and neoplastic potential. Acta Odontol Scand 39:227–240

33. Lu Y, Mock D, Takata T, Jordan RC (1999) Odontogenic ghost cell carcinoma: report of four new cases and review of the literature. J Oral Pathol Med 28:323–329

34. Buchner A, Merrel PW, Hansen LS, Leider AS (1991) Peripheral (extraosseous) calcifying odontogenic cyst: a review of forty-five cases. Oral Surg Oral Med Oral Pathol 72:65–70

35. Stoneman DW, Worth HM (1983) The mandibular infected buccal cyst: molar area. Dent Radiogr Photogr 56:1–14

36. Shohat I, Buchner A, Taicher S (2003) Mandibular buccal bifurcation cyst: enucleation without extraction. J Oral Maxillorfac Surg 32:610–613

37. Gao Z, Flaitz CM, Mackenzie IC (1996) Expression of keratinocyte growth factor in periapical lesions. J Dent Res 75:1658–1663

38. Abrams AM, Howell FU, Bullock WK (1963) Nasopalatine cyst. Oral Surg Oral Med Oral Pathol 16:306–332

39. Watanabe H, Arita S, Chigira M (1994) Aetiology of a simple bone cyst. A case report. Int Orthop 18:16–19

40. Abdel-Wanis ME, Tsuchiya H (2002) Simple bone cyst is not a single entity: point of view based on a literature review. Med Hypotheses 58:87–91

41. Vergel De Dios AM, Bond JR, Shives TC, McLeod RA, Unni KK (1992) Aneurysmal bone cyst: a clinicopathologic study of 238 cases. Cancer 69:2921–2931

42. Rapidis AD, Vallianatou D, Apostolidis C, Lagogiannis G (2004) Large lytic lesion of the ascending ramus, the condyle, and the infratemporal region. J Oral Maxillofac Surg 62:996–1001

43. De Silva MVC, Raby N, Reid R (2003) Fibromyxoid areas and immature osteoid are associated with recurrence of primary aneurysmal bone cysts. Histopathology 43:180–88

44. Tajima Y, Yokose S, Sakamoto E, Yamamoto Y, Utsumi N (1992) Ameloblastoma arising in calcifying odontogenic cyst. Oral Surg Oral Med Oral Pathol 74:776–779

45. Zeitoun IM, Dhanrajani PJ, Mosadomi HA (1996) Adenomatoid odontogenic tumor arising in a calcifying odontogenic cyst. J Oral Maxillofac Surg 54:634–637

46. Yoon JH, Kim HJ, Yook JI, Cha IH, Ellis GL, Kim J (2004) Hybrid odontogenic tumor of calcifying odontogenic cyst and ameloblastic fibroma. Oral Surg Oral Med Oral Pathol Oral Radiol Endod 98:80–84

47. Philipsen HP, Samman N, Ormiston IW, Reichart PA (1992) Variants of the adenomatoid odontogenic tumor with a note on tumor origin. J Oral Pathol Med 21:348–352

48. Philipsen HP, Reichart PA (1996) Squamous odontogenic tumor (SOT): a benign neoplasm of the periodontium: a review of 36 reported cases. J Clin Periodontol 23:922–926

49. Pindborg JJ (1958) A calcifying epithelial odontogenic tumor. Cancer 11:838–843

50. Philipsen HP, Reichart PA (2000) Calcifying epithelial odontogenic tumor: biological profile based on 181 cases from the literature. Oral Oncol 36:17–26

51. Hisatomi M, Asaumi J-I, Konouchi H, Honda Y, Wakasa T, Kishi K (2002) A case of complex odontoma associated with an impacted lower deciduous second molar and analysis of the 107 odontomas. Oral Dis 8:100–105

52. Philipsen HP, Reichart PA, Praetorius F (1997) Mixed odontogenic tumors and odontomas. Considerations on interrelationship. Review of the literature and presentation of 134 new cases of odontomas. Oral Oncol 33:86–99

53. Wolford LM, Mehra P, Franco P (2002) Use of conservative condylectomy for treatment of osteochondroma of the mandibular condyle. J Oral Maxillofac Surg 60:262–268

54. Chuong R, Kaban LB, Kozakewich H (1986) Central giant cell lesions of the jaws: a clinicopathologic study. J Oral Maxillofac Surg 44:708–712

55. Lichenstein L (1953) Histiocytosis X: integration of eosinophilic granuloma of bone, "Letterer-Siwe disease" and "Schuller-Christian disease" as related manifestations of a nosologic entity. AMA Arch Pathol 56:84–102

56. Whyte MP (2006) Clinical practice. Paget's disease of bone. N Engl J Med 355:593–600

Chapter 36

Midfacial Degloving Approach to the Nose, Sinuses, and Skull Base

36

Daniel M. Zeitler and Gady Har-El

Core Messages

■ The midfacial degloving approach provides wide and comfortable exposure to the midfacial skeleton, all paranasal sinuses, and the anterior skull base.

■ The midfacial degloving approach can be employed for a variety of procedures including but not limited to benign tumor resection, malignant neoplasm en bloc resection, reconstructive procedures, and repair of cerebrospinal fluid leaks.

■ Midfacial degloving can be combined with endoscopic or neurosurgical techniques in order to perform anterior craniofacial resection.

■ While the technique of midfacial degloving was originated decades ago, new modifications exist which reduce postoperative complications as well as improve cosmetic results.

Contents

Introduction

The concept of the midfacial degloving (MFD) procedure was first introduced in the French literature in 1927 by Portmann and Retrouvey when they described a transoral sublabial incision approach for a maxillectomy [32]. This technique was modified by Converse in 1950 when he described unilateral exposure of the midfacial skeleton via a sublabial incision with subperiosteal elevation [8]. Casson et al. were the first to use the MFD procedure as it is known and applied today when they extended their dissection to combine a sublabial incision with an intercartilaginous and full transfixion incisions of the nose allowing for bilateral soft tissue elevation of the middle one-third of the face [6]. Since the 1970s, MFD has been popularized by Conley [7], Price [33–35], and Maniglia [28] among others [4, 15–18, 20].

Until the popularization of MFD in the USA and Europe, the gold standard exposure for en bloc excision of paranasal sinus and nasal cavity tumors has been through an external approach such as a lateral rhinotomy or a Weber-Fergusson incision. Despite the ease with which these approaches are performed, they invariably result in facial scars and can lead to disfiguring complications such as alar retraction, asymmetry of the upper lip and nasolabial groove, and medial canthal deformity [41]. MFD combines the surgical principles of sublabial sinus surgery with the cosmetic principles of rhinoplasty to provide wide exposure of the external and internal nose, all paranasal sinuses, orbits, and nasopharynx while sparing external facial incisions [1, 7, 10, 15–18, 28, 33–35].

In the majority of the literature on MFD, inverted papilloma has proven to be the most common indication for the procedure [4, 12, 24, 31]. However, this technique is also particularly advantageous in the management of locally aggressive, but histologically benign lesions such as juvenile angiofibroma [15, 16, 20, 37]. A wide variety of other nasal cavity or paranasal sinus conditions have been treated via MFD including ameloblastoma, odontogenic keratocysts, vascular lesions, benign fibro-osseous conditions, as well as for exposure prior to performing reconstructive surgery and bone grafting [19, 20, 28, 29]. Additionally, as many gain experience with MFD, its uses have expanded into the treatment of midface and naso-orbito-ethmoid (NOE) fractures as well as orbital floor resection and reconstruction [2, 3, 9]. Recently, authors have shown MFD to be useful in the removal of congenital lesions of the midface in infants and children with no subsequent disturbance in the growth centers of the midface or facial skeleton development despite previous concerns over the possibility of such outcomes [14, 27, 38, 40].

One area of debate concerning MFD is its feasibility in the resection of malignant sinonasal neoplasms. Given the prognostic importance of complete oncologic clearance and en bloc resection of malignant tumors, many surgeons do not feel adequate exposure is possible via MFD. Howard and Lund state that while MFD can be used in cases of sinonasal malignancy, the technique should only be attempted in select cases in which the tumor can be successfully encompassed by the exposure [19, 20]. Others contend that MFD is indicated for small or slow-growing malignancies (i. e., low-grade salivary gland neoplasms) as long as clean margins can be obtained [19, 21]. We believe that the MFD approach can provide the surgeon with an exposure equal to that obtained with lateral rhinotomy in most cases, and wider than endoscopic approaches for malignancies.

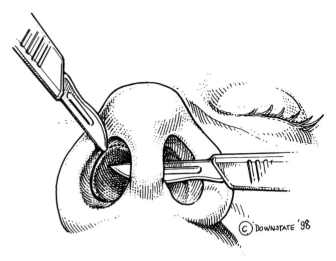

Fig. 36.1 Bilateral complete circumvestibular incisions are created by combining a standard complete transfixion incision with bilateral intercartilaginous and nasal floor incisions. Reprinted with permission from: Har-El G, The midfacial degloving approach. In: De Souza C (ed) Head and neck surgery. Longman Orient, Hyderabad

Technique

Although the technique we use for MFD is described elsewhere in the literature, we have included a few modifications. After general orotracheal intubation is accomplished, eye ointment is placed on the cornea and 6-0 nylon sutures are used to perform temporary tarsorrhaphies bilaterally through the conjunctival aspect of the eyelids. One must take care not to place the stitch through the skin side of the eyelid as this can cause inversion of the lashes and potential corneal abrasion.

We begin the procedure with injection of a vasoconstrictive solution through the intercartilaginous space bilaterally. Infiltration is achieved in the area of the nasal bones, the midline, the glabella, the nasomaxillary grooves, and both medial canthal regions through this single portal. Transcutaneous infiltration of the frontal bone as well as both medial orbital walls is performed in addition to transoral injection of the greater palatine foramen. Finally, the planned incision line in the sublabial region is infiltrated.

A standard complete transfixion incision is made and connected, at the dome of the nose, with intercartilaginous incisions allowing separation of the septum and upper lateral cartilages (ULC) from the lower lateral cartilages (LLC) and columella (Fig. 36.1). Extensive undermining of the nasal dorsum to the level of the medial canthus on each side is performed. The dissection is carried laterally in a subperiosteal plane to include the anterior wall of the maxillary sinus on the ipsilateral and contralateral side as well as medially to include the frontal bone. Once all adhesions between the nasal skeleton and soft tissue envelope are released, the intercartilaginous incision is extended laterally and caudally as a full-thickness incision through the periosteum of the nasal floor and pyriform margin and connected to the transfixion incision. This completes the bilateral circumvestibular 360-degree incision.

Attention is then directed toward the sublabial incision, which is usually made between the first molars, about 4 mm above the teeth leaving a generous cuff of gingiva to facilitate closure. However, the incision may be extended on the ipsilateral side to the third molar in anticipation of requiring lateral exposure or if ligation of the internal maxillary artery is anticipated or planned. Periosteal elevators are used to elevate the soft tissues off the anterior maxillary wall and connect this with the previous intranasal incisions. Care must be taken to identify and protect both infraorbital nerves while elevation is continued superiorly to the level of the orbital rim. Once complete, the midfacial skin is now separated from the maxilla and nasal pyramid. A Penrose rubber drain is placed through each nostril and around the upper lip in order to retract the midfacial flap superiorly. Our habit is to release one of these drains every 20–30 min allowing reperfusion of the central lip area, or sooner should the vermillion mucosa become dusky.

The "degloving" portion of the procedure is now complete (Fig. 36.2). At this point, one has gained adequate exposure of many of the bones of the midface should repair of midfacial and/or periorbital traumatic injuries be necessary. For example, in the case of Le Fort fractures, open reduction and rigid fixation may be achieved with excellent exposure of the alveolar ridge, maxillary bones, and the inferior, lateral, and medial orbital rims. Additionally, the nasal and frontal bones may also be easily accessed. One may also gain access to the medial aspect of the superior orbital rim through this exposure.

One of the most common procedures we performed via the MFD approach is a medial maxillectomy. Medial maxillectomy is the gold standard for surgical resection of inverted papillomas, but its other indications include wide exposure and en bloc excision of sinonasal malignancies, benign tumors of the nasal cavity or paranasal sinuses, tumors of the oral cavity that extend into the hard palate, or as the first step in the wide exposure of deeper spaces and structures such as the pterygopalatine fossa,

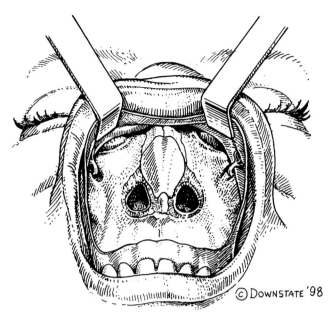

Fig. 36.2 The "degloving" portion of the procedure is complete. The bony midface is exposed including the nasal pyramid, pyriform apertures, infraorbital rims, orbits, and the glabella. It is important that each infraorbital nerve be identified early in the procedure and protected throughout. Reprinted with permission from: Har-El G, The midfacial degloving approach. In: De Souza C (ed) Head and neck surgery. Longman Orient, Hyderabad

sphenoid sinus, nasopharynx, and anterior and middle skull base.

To begin the medial maxillectomy, the anterior wall of the maxillary sinus should be removed. Anterior wall removal is performed while taking care to preserve and protect the infraorbital neurovascular bundle. This part of the procedure is best done with a set of Kerrison rongeurs of different sizes and angulations. Bone removal continues superomedially toward the ethmoid complex and superolaterally toward the zygomatic buttress. Once anterior maxillary bone removal is complete, but before starting the resection itself, the nasolacrimal sac/duct (NLSD) must be addressed. A variety of management techniques for the NLSD have been described elsewhere in the literature ranging from simple transection of the sac at the level of the periorbita with or without stenting to a complete drill-out of the nasolacrimal canal with preservation of the entire NLSD along its length. The time-saving technique we have found most efficient is to perform a transection of the NLSD with subsequent marsupialization. Using a mastoid drill, approximately 10–15 mm of the anterior wall of the bony nasolacrimal canal is removed starting from the orbital rim (Fig. 36.3a). Once the NLSD has been mobilized, distal transection is performed and the NLSD is removed from the canal. In the distal portion of the duct, two short opposing cuts are made creating two semicircular flaps (Fig. 36.3b). The flaps are everted and sutured to the proximal duct or periorbita with absorbable sutures thereby preventing stenosis and post-surgical epiphora.

Osteotomies for medial maxillectomy are performed at this point in a fashion similar to that performed via lateral rhinotomy (Fig. 36.4). To begin, a cut is made along the nasal bone from the pyriform aperture toward the glabella several millimeters anterior to the nasomaxillary groove and another cut in a horizontal orientation just below the glabella directed toward the frontoethmoid suture line. Following these cuts, an osteotomy running below and parallel to the frontoethmoid suture line is made in an anterior-posterior direction. This cut can be tailored to the specific lesion being removed or the desired exposure as the posterior limit can extend as far as the optic canal. The next cut begins at the orbital rim anteriorly (medial to the infraorbital foramen) in an oblique direction to join with the posterior limit of the frontoethmoid cut in the posterior ethmoid area. Finally, an inferior cut starting at the pyriform aperture anteriorly and extending posteriorly to the posterior wall of the maxillary sinus is made which separates the maxillary sinus from its floor. Upon the completion of the bony osteotomies, soft tissue cuts are made in an identical fashion to begin to free the specimen. The final maneuver involves freeing the posterior aspect of the specimen along the posterolateral nasal wall and ascending palatine bone with osteotomes and/or scissors. Specimen removal will expose a bleeding sphenopalatine artery either within its foramen or as it exits the foramen. While the artery can be clamped and ligated, improved access for proximal control of the internal maxillary artery in the pterygopalatine fossa can be gained by removing the ascending process of the palatine bone.

Sessions and Larson first described the "classic" medial maxillectomy in 1977 [39]. Since then, many authors have proposed modifications in an effort to improve postoperative cosmesis. While the classic operation includes the removal of the bone along the lateral nasal wall, superolateral pyriform aperture, and 25–35% of the orbital floor and rim, Anand describes a technique in which the inferior and medial orbital rim, including a rim of bone around the pyriform aperture, is preserved [1]. Another modification described uses miniplates to reattach the bony framework of the maxillary sinus and pyriform aperture to the alveolar ridge, orbital rim, and glabella [10]. Despite these and other modifications on the classic maxillectomy technique, our opinion is that by maintaining the nasomaxillary angle by preserving the nasal bone, alveolar bone, and up to three-quarters of the orbital rim, satisfactory cosmetic results can be achieved while saving time and avoiding complicated procedures.

One modification on the original procedure which we invariably perform is to develop an 8- to 12-mm-wide bipedicled flap of inner nasal vestibular skin before the removal of the anterior face of the maxillary sinus and lateral nasal wall. This flap, just caudal to the bony pyriform aperture, is created by extending an incision from the edge of the pyriform aperture at the junction of the ULC to the nasal floor (Fig. 36.5a, b). At the completion of the MFD, this bipedicled flap is sutured to the free edge of the circumvestibular incision. In our experience, we have found this to be an excellent maneuver to prevent postoperative nasal valve stenosis.

Following the completion of the medial maxillectomy, one may gain access to other compartments of the facial skeleton

36

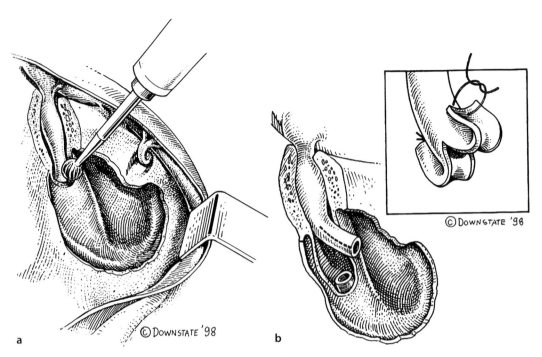

a   © Downstate '98   b   © Downstate '98

Fig. 36.3 a Using a mastoid drill, the anterior wall of the nasolacrimal bony canal is removed exposing the NLSD. Reprinted with permission from: Har-El G, The midfacial degloving approach. In: De Souza C (ed) Head and neck surgery. Longman Orient, Hyderabad. **b** The NLSD is transected distally using a #11 blade and elevated off its bony canal. *Inset* The two distal semicircular flaps are everted, folded, and sutured to the proximal sac (or periorbita) using absorbable sutures. Reprinted with permission from: Har-El G, The midfacial degloving approach. In: De Souza C (ed) Head and neck surgery. Longman Orient, Hyderabad

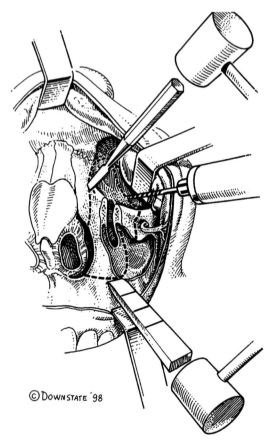

© Downstate '98

Fig. 36.4 Bone cuts for medial maxillectomy (see text for details). Reprinted with permission from: Har-El G, The midfacial degloving approach. In: De Souza C (ed) Head and neck surgery. Longman Orient, Hyderabad

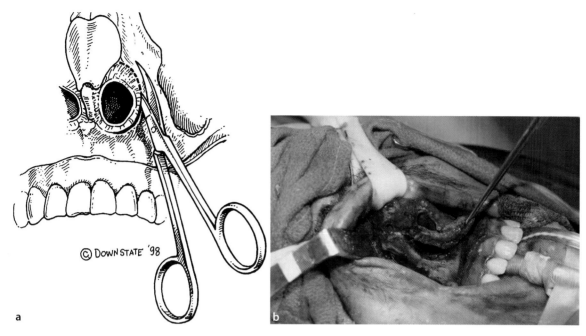

a

b

Fig. 36.5 **a** An 8- to 12-mm-wide bipedicled flap of inner nasal vestibular skin is created just caudal to the bony pyriform aperture by extending an incision from the edge of the pyriform aperture at the junction of the ULC to the nasal floor. Reprinted with permission from: Har-El G, The midfacial degloving approach. In: De Souza C (ed) Head and neck surgery. Longman Orient, Hyderabad. **b** Bipedicled vestibular skin flap. Reprinted with permission from the American Journal of Rhinology [18]

and skull base. The orbital contents are widely exposed and the optic nerve may be drilled out of its bony canal and followed throughout its length. Portions of the posterior and lateral maxilla can be resected allowing access to the pterygopalatine and infratemporal fossae including the foramen ovale as well as the central aspect of the middle cranial fossa (foramen lacerum). An anterior sphenoidotomy can give access to the cavernous carotid artery and the sella. Finally, the fovea ethmoidalis is well exposed, and with middle turbinectomy, the cribriform plate and anterior cranial fossa are easily visualized.

On completion of the procedure, the surgical cavity is packed with antibiotic-soaked gauze that is passed superiorly to the bipedicled flap and brought out via the nostril. The soft tissues are allowed to return to their anatomic position. Meticulous care is taken to close all intranasal incisions with 4-0 absorbable sutures while preserving and restoring preoperative projection and rotation of the nose. The sublabial incision is closed with 3-0 absorbable sutures. A dorsal nasal splint may be applied to reduce edema. The packing is removed in 1–3 days and aggressive nasal irrigation is initiated.

Technical Considerations

Anterior Craniofacial Resection with Midfacial Degloving

Prior to any MFD procedure, CT scanning is paramount to assess the bony integrity of the anterior skull base. If the bony in-terface is intact and en bloc resection would not mandate bony resection, or if partial tumor removal is an acceptable surgical option (i. e., benign lesions), an MFD procedure alone may be sufficient [3]. However, many lesions in the nasal cavity and paranasal sinuses are destructive lesions involving the skull base and/or dura and demand greater exposure than MFD alone can offer. In such cases, MFD can be combined with a conventional frontal craniotomy or with the subcranial approach through the posterior wall of the frontal sinus and anterior ethmoid complex [13, 17]. Additionally, MFD can be combined with the subcranial preauricular infratemporal fossa (SPIF) for tumors extending into the infratemporal fossa or those tumors with involvement of the middle cranial fossa or lateral portion of the cavernous sinus [30]. These adjunctive approaches not only aid in providing excellent exposure of the anterior skull base and middle cranial fossa, but also avoid external facial incisions.

Endoscopic-assisted Procedures

With the recent technical advances in endoscopic sinus surgery (ESS), surgeons can now perform endonasal surgery with visual quality rivaling the exposure of an open procedure. This had led many to combine ESS with MFD for tumors extending onto the anterior skull base within the posterosuperior nasal cavity. El-Banhawy et al. have described the successful use of endoscopic-assisted MFD (EAMFD) for juvenile angiofibroma located at the skull base, base of the pterygoid process, the vaginal process of the sphenoid bone, and in the medial and inferior aspect of the orbit and olfactory fossa [11]. Other uses for EAMFD include the removal of midface congenital lesions in infants and young children with underdeveloped or maldeveloped bony architecture [40], addressing processes involving the lamina papyracea or orbital contents [21], and dissection in narrow fields adjacent to vital neurovascular structures [3]. EAMFD also offers a particular advantage with iatrogenic cerebrospinal fluid (CSF) leaks. Using rigid endoscopes allows easy identification of the site of the CSF leak.

Frontal Sinus Involvement

Some authors believe MFD does not provide adequate exposure to the frontal sinus for tumors and lesions involving this area [25, 34–36]. However, our experience is different [15, 16, 18]. Through the classic medial maxillectomy and ethmoidectomy via MFD as described, the frontal sinus outflow tract is easily identified in the surgical field anterior to the anterior ethmoid air cells and anterior ethmoid artery. Additionally, if more exposure of the frontal sinus is desired, the medial canthal tendon (MCT) can be transected and separated from the medial orbital wall to allow for superior retraction of the midfacial flap. Care must be taken on completion of the operation to meticulously reattach the MCT to its bony insertion as failure to do so can result in telecanthus, disruption of the normal angular contour of the eye, ectropion, and/or epiphora. Krause described a modification of MFD in which bilateral nasal osteotomies and septal transection are performed, thereby enabling the ULC and nasal bones to be retracted superiorly [23]. This technique allows improved visualization of the frontal sinus outflow tract. However, with gross tumor involvement of the frontal sinus many authors would recommend MFD in combination with an osteoplastic flap with or without an extended subcranial approach, further obviating the need for external facial incisions [13].

Complications

Following MFD, many patients have crusting present within the surgical cavity. While this is an inevitable and expected operative sequela, patients often complain of nasal congestion or difficulty with breathing. Lindemann et al. showed that aggressive removal of the turbinates and lateral nasal wall via MFD, as is often performed for aggressive inverted papilloma, disturbed humidification and heating of respiratory air in the nasal cavity thereby contributing to nasal crusting and dryness [26]. Once the nasal packing has been removed, meticulous attention to nasal debridement in the office setting and continuous nasal saline irrigation can be started, with resolution of crusting occurring with mucosal regeneration.

The most common complication of the MFD technique, affecting 60–80% of patients, is temporary facial hypesthesia or anesthesia in the region supplied by the infraorbital nerve [3, 5, 9, 21, 29, 31, 33, 36, 41]. While retraction of the infraorbital nerve is unavoidable in order to achieve adequate exposure of the surgical field, direct trauma to the nerve and prolonged com-

pression of the nerve must be avoided. While almost all patients have complete recovery of midfacial sensation in 1–4 months, they should be made aware of this complication preoperatively. In our experience, the rate of prolonged infraorbital anesthesia is less than 1%.

Other less common complications include oroantral fistula, aesthetic changes in the nasal structure, epiphora, and vestibular stenosis (VS). While VS is a rare complication, its occurrence has prompted many surgeons to modify the MFD technique. Jeon et al. describe a hemifacial degloving approach for unilateral medial maxillectomy [22]. This unilateral approach avoids the circumvestibular incision thought to contribute to VS while providing adequate exposure for the ipsilateral medial maxillectomy. Krause also describes a technique whereby the intercartilaginous incision is not performed to avoid the circumvestibular incision. Instead, a lateral osteotomy is performed to mobilize the entire nasal pyramid [23]. Finally, by using a bipedicled nasal vestibular skin flap as described above, our rate of symptomatic nasal valve stenosis is 0.5%. When MFD is combined with adjunctive neurosurgical procedures, more serious complications such as cranial nerve injuries, dural disruption, and CSF leak can occur; however, these are beyond the scope of this chapter.

Tips to Avoid Complications

- Development and preservation of the bipedicled vestibular skin flap during the procedure will prevent postoperative nasal vestibular stenosis.
- Meticulous marsupialization of the nasolacrimal sac/duct system will prevent duct stenosis and epiphora.
- Careful attention to the closure of the bilateral circumvestibular nasal incisions will preserve cosmesis and symmetry of the face.
- If detachment of the medial canthal tendon is necessary for increased exposure during the procedure, careful reattachment should be performed to prevent subsequent telecanthus.

Take-Home Pearls

- Careful attention to wide infiltration with the vasoconstricting solution will result in a relatively bloodless procedure.
- Aggressive undermining toward both zygomatic buttresses and high on the frontal bone will allow wide exposure of the midfacial skeleton.
- Medial maxillectomy can serve as the approach to deeper structures such as the pterygopalatine fossa, nasopharynx, clivus, and both the anterior and middle skull base.

References

1. Anand VK, Conley JJ (1983) Sublabial surgical approach to the nasal cavity and paranasal sinuses. Laryngoscope 93:1483–1484

2. Baumann A, Ewers R (2001) Midfacial degloving: an alternative approach for traumatic corrections in the midface. Int J Oral Maxillofac Surg 30:272–279

3. Browne JD (2001) Skull base tumor surgery: the midfacial degloving procedure for nasal, sinus, and nasopharyngeal tumors. Otolaryngol Clin North Am 34:1095–1201

4. Buchwald C, Franzmann MB, Tos B (1995) Sinonasal papillomas: a report of 82 cases in Copenhagen County, including a longitudinal epidemiological and clinical study. Laryngoscope 105:72–79

5. Cansiz H, Güvenç MG, Şekercioğlu N (2006) Surgical approaches to juvenile nasopharyngeal angiofibroma. J Craniomaxillofac Surg 34:3–8

6. Casson PR, Bonnano PC, Converse JM (1974) The midfacial degloving procedure. Plast Reconstr Surg 53:102–103

7. Conley JJ, Price JC (1979) Sublabial approach to the nasal and nasopharyngeal cavities. Am J Surg 138:615–618

8. Converse JM (1950) Restoration of facial contour by bone grafts introduced through oral cavity. Plast Reconstr Surg 6:295–300

9. Cultrara A, Turk JB, Har-El G (2004) Midfacial degloving approach for repair of naso-orbito-ethmoid and midfacial fractures. Arch Facial Plast Surg 6:133–135

10. Draf W (1993) Juvenile angiofibroma. In: Sekhar LN, Janecka IP (eds) Surgery of cranial base tumors. Raven, New York

11. El-Banhawy OA, El-Dien AEHS, Amer T (2004) Endoscopic-assisted midfacial degloving approach for type III juvenile angiofibroma. Int J Pediatr Otorhinolaryngol 68:21–28

12. Esteban F, Jurado A, Cantillo E, et al (1997) Facial degloving as a versatile approach to paranasal sinus tumors. Acta Otorrhinolaringol Esp 48:457–460

13. Fliss DM, Zucker G, Amir A, et al (2000) The combined subcranial and midfacial degloving technique for tumor resection: report of three cases. J Oral Maxillofac Surg 58:106–110

14. Handley GH, Reilly JS (1989) Nasal obstruction in children. Otolaryngol Clin North Am 22:383–396

15. Har-El G (1999) Medial maxillectomy via midfacial degloving approach. Op Tech Otolaryngol Head Neck Surg 10:82–86

16. Har-El G (1999) Management of juvenile angiofibroma via midfacial degloving with medial maxillectomy. Op Tech Otolaryngol Head Neck Surg 10:107–108

17. Har-El G (2004) Anterior craniofacial resection without facial skin incisions: a review. Otolaryngol Head Neck Surg 130:780–787

18. Har-El G, Lucente PE (1996) Midfacial degloving approach to the nose, sinuses, and skull base. Am J Rhinol 10:17–22

19. Howard DJ, Lund VJ (1992) The midfacial degloving approach to sinonasal disease. J Laryngol Otol 106:1059–1064

20. Howard DJ, Lund VJ (1999) The role of midfacial degloving in modern rhinological practice. J Laryngol Otol 113:885–887

21. Ikeda K, Suzuki H, Oshima T, et al (1998) Midfacial degloving approach facilitated by endoscope to the sinonasal malignancy. Auris Nasus Larynx 25:289–293

22. Jeon SY, Jeong JH, Kim HS, et al (2003) Hemifacial degloving approach for medial maxillectomy: a modification of midfacial degloving approach. Laryngoscope 113:754–756

23. Krause GE, Jafek BW (1999) A modification of the midface degloving technique. Laryngoscope 109:1781–1784

24. Lawson W, Kaufman MR, Biller HF (2003) Treatment outcomes in the management of inverted papilloma: an analysis of 160 cases. Laryngoscope 113:1548–1556

25. Lenarz T, Keiner S (1992) Midfacial degloving: an alternative approach to the frontobasal area, nasal cavity, and paranasal sinuses. Laryngorhinootologie 71:381–387

26. Lindemann J, Leiacker R, Sikora T, et al (2002) Impact of unilateral sinus surgery with resection of the turbinates by means of midfacial degloving on nasal air conditioning. Laryngoscope 112:2062–2066

27. Lund VJ, Neijens H, Clement P, et al (1995) The treatment of chronic sinusitis: a controversial issue. Int J Pediatr Otorhinolaryngol 32(suppl):S21–S35

28. Maniglia AJ (1986) Indications and techniques of midfacial degloving: a 15-year experience. Arch Otolaryngol Head Neck Surg 112:750–752

29. Maniglia AJ, Phillips DA (1995) Midfacial degloving for the management of nasal, sinus, and skull-base neoplasms. Otolaryngol Clin North Am 28:1127–1143

30. Paris J, Guelfucci B, Moulin G, et al (2001) Diagnosis and treatment of juvenile nasopharyngeal angiofibroma. Eur Arch Otorhinolaryngol 258:120–124

31. Peng P, Har-El G (2006) Management of inverted papillomas of the nose and paranasal sinuses. Am J Otolaryngol Head Neck Med Surg 27:233–237

32. Portmann G, Retrouvey H (1927) Le cancer du nez. Doin, Paris

33. Price JC (1986) The midfacial degloving approach to the central skull base. Ear Nose Throat J 65:46–53

34. Price JC (1987) The midfacial degloving approach. In: Goldman JL (ed) The principles and practice of rhinology. Churchill Livingstone, New York

35. Price JC, Koch WM (1991) The midfacial degloving approach to the paranasal sinuses and skull base. In: Blitzer A, Lawson W, Friedman WH (eds) Surgery of the paranasal sinuses, 2nd edn. Saunders, Philadelphia

36. Price JC, Holliday MJ, Johns ME, et al (1988) The versatile midfacial degloving approach. Laryngoscope 98:291–295

37. Radkowski D, McGill T, Healy GB, et al (1996) Angiofibroma: changes in staging and treatment options (see comments). Arch Otolaryngol Head Neck Surg 122:122–129

38. Reilly JR, Koopman CF, Cotton R (1992) Nasal mass in a pediatric patient. Head Neck 14:415–418

39. Sessions RB, Larson DL (1977) En bloc ethmoidectomy and medial maxillectomy. Arch Otolaryngol 103:195–202

40. Uretzsky ID, Mair EA, Schoem SR (1998) Endoscopically guided midfacial degloving in infants for removal of congenital and acquired midfacial masses. Int J Pediatr Otorhinolaryngol 46:145–158

41. Zaghloul AS, Nouh MA, El Fatah HA (2004) Midfacial degloving approach for malignant maxillary tumors. J Egypt Nat Cancer Inst 16:69–75

Chapter 37

Craniofacial Approaches to the Anterior Skull Base

37

Jannis Constantinidis

Core Messages

- The proper selection of the surgical approach to the anterior skull base will allow adequate exposure of the pathology, safe resection, and reconstruction of the resulting defect including the dura mater.
- Preoperative imaging (high-resolution CT scan, MRI, angiography) provides information about the location and the extent of the disease which is necessary for the selection of the surgical approach.
- The placement of the incision should incur the least possible functional and cosmetic deficits.
- A high degree of versatility in selecting and modifying the proper surgical approach will accommodate individual variations of anatomy and pathology.
- Craniofacial approaches are favorable in that they allow spatial isolation, interruption of vascular supply, and complete resection of the tumor while identifying and preserving neighboring structures.
- Cooperation within an interdisciplinary team (neurosurgery, neuroradiology, ophthalmology, head and neck surgery, maxillofacial and facial plastic surgery) is a fundamental prerequisite to manage these complex cases.

Contents

Introduction

The anterior skull base is in close topographic vicinity to the nose, the paranasal sinuses, the nasopharynx, the orbita, and the intracranial contents. The diagnosis and treatment of various neoplastic diseases of the skull base is complex and requires an interdisciplinary team approach. Thorough knowledge of the complex three-dimensional anatomy of the anterior skull base will allow the experienced surgical team to obtain functionally and aesthetically pleasing surgical results. Prior to the development of the combined craniofacial approaches to the skull base, the anterior skull base, and, in particular, the area of the cribriform plate, fovea ethmoidalis, and the planum sphenoidale were relatively difficult to access. Smith et al. [44], Ketcham et al. [20], Shah and Galicich [42], and Schramm [40] have contributed substantially to the early development of craniofacial approaches to the anterior skull base, followed by others who further modified and enhanced these approaches [2, 18, 24, 37]. Today the anterior craniofacial approaches are the treatment of choice for the resection of tumors of the anterior skull base. These approaches can be classified into extracranial, intracranial, and combined extra- and intracranial approaches (Table 37.1). The placement of the incision line should induce minimal functional and cosmetic deficits particularly in pediatric patients. It is of major importance to consider the possible growth abnormalities in pediatric patients; trauma to growth zones should be avoided if possible. It has been observed that osteoplastic procedures with meticulous reconstruction of the bony flaps interfere less with growth than less extensive approaches which involve resection of bone without reconstruction.

Anterior Skull Base Approaches

Extracranial Approaches

The access for extracranial approaches is through the facial skeleton. Infiltrated bone of the skull base can be removed through these approaches, if necessary. Indications for the extracranial approaches include tumors where their exposure and resection with safe margins is impossible through less extensive ap-

Table 37.1 Craniofacial approaches to the anterior skull base

Extracranial	Intracranial	Combined
Midfacial degloving	Transfrontal	Transfacial-transcranial
Transfacial	Frontotemporal	
With preservation of the orbit		
With orbital exenteration		
Le Fort I osteotomy		
Bilateral		
Unilateral		
Midfacial split		
Facial translocation		
Lateral (infratemporal fossa approach)		

proaches. Limitations of extracranial approaches are extensive infiltration of the dura and intracranial extension of the tumor. In such cases the extracranial approaches are combined with intracranial ones.

Midfacial Degloving

Midfacial degloving represents an extended sublabial rhinotomy. This allows good exposure of the deep midface, and in particular the nasal cavity, paranasal sinuses, and anterior skull base posterior to the cribriform plate. This approach is applicable to a variety of tumors in this region as long as these have no intracranial extension or anterior extension past the foramen cecum toward the glabella [10]. Limitations of this technique include tumor invasion into the orbit and the infratemporal fossa. The midfacial degloving approach can easily be combined with other intracranial or lateral approaches. The surgical technique is discussed in detail in Chap. 36.

Transfacial Approaches

Important principles of facial plastic surgery should be respected when transfacial approaches are utilized. Incisions should be well hidden parallel to the relaxed skin tension lines, with respect to the aesthetic units or subunits or the midline (Fig. 37.1). Dissection should be performed in a subperiosteal plane or subfascially in order to preserve the neurovascular supply of the dissected area [25].

External Frontoethmoidectomy

The external frontoethmoidectomy approach allows access to the frontal sinus, the ethmoid sinuses, the anterior skull base, and the medial orbit. An infrabrow incision exposes the anterior wall and floor of the frontal sinus as well as the frontal process of the maxilla and the nasal bones. These structures are then resected, giving the surgeon excellent exposure of the cribriform plate and the fovea ethmoidalis. Moreover this approach offers better exposure of the dura mater of the anterior skull base making possible its resection and reconstruction. It is important to preserve the supraorbital rim in order to avoid contour deformities [19].

Lateral Rhinotomy

The incision starts inferior to the medial aspect of the eyebrow and incorporates a broken line or w-plasty. It follows the junction between the nasal side wall and the aesthetic unit of the cheek and may be continued around the vertical alar crease to the philtrum (Fig. 37.2a–c). Subciliary incisions have been combined with this approach in order to gain access for a simultaneous maxillectomy. The periosteum is then exposed and the skin soft tissue envelope is carefully dissected off the periosteum for about one centimeter in each direction. The periosteum is sharply transected and elevated. This preserves a separate periosteal flap that allows reconstitution of the previous bony contour after resection of the underlying bones. The skin soft tissue envelope is elevated in a subperiosteal plane over the cheek, elevating the lacrimal sac if required. The lateral nasal wall and cribriform plate as well as the inferior aspect of the interior wall of the frontal sinus and its floor are removed. This approach offers exposure and resection of tumors that may extend into the sphenoid sinus [39, 40]. The anterior wall of the maxillary sinus may be included in the resection allowing excellent exposure of the maxillary sinus, the orbital floor, and the pterygopalatine fossa [1, 9]. In most cases a part of the tumor needs to be resected under microscopic control in order to visualize the aspects of the tumor which are in close contact or have invaded

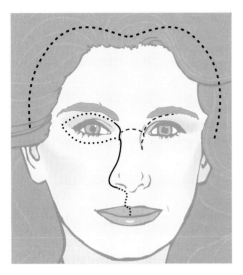

Fig. 37.1 Craniofacial incisions for accessing anterior skull base. Note the lateral rhinotomy incision (*solid line*) and the options of extensions (*dotted lines*) of a lateral rhinotomy incision which can include a lip split for cheek rotation (Weber-Ferguson incision) and orbital exenteration access. Also note an external frontoethmoidectomy incision (*interrupted line*) and a coronal incision (*squared line*)

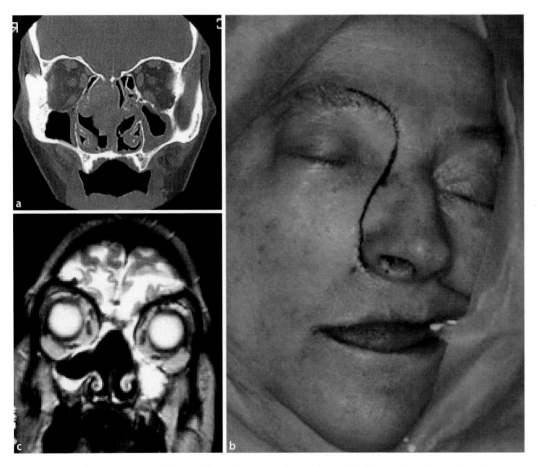

Fig. 37.2a–c Adenocarcinoma of the middle turbinate involving ethmoidal cells, nasal cavity, and nasal septum. **a** Preoperative coronal computed tomography scan. **b** Lateral rhinotomy incision. **c** Postoperative coronal magnetic resonance image showing complete tumor removal

the skull base. A cutting burr may be used to resect the bony skull base around the tumor which is then carefully dissected off the dura mater. If the dura is invaded, it is resected in adequate margins.

The lateral rhinotomy approach provides a safe access to the nasal cavity, the lateral nasal wall, the ethmoid sinuses, the maxilla, the medial orbital wall, the floor of the frontal sinus, and the anterior skull base including the sella turcica and the pterygopalatine fossa. The advantage of this technique is that dissection proceeds in a plane parallel to the skull base and the medial orbital wall, a fact which optimizes visualization. The incision may be extended across the nasion to the contralateral side. Through a contralateral deep lateral osteotomy the entire nose can be rotated out of the field offering maximal exposure [30].

Intraoperatively, one must determine whether the tumor has infiltrated the orbit and whether an orbital exenteration is required. In such cases, the orbital wall and periorbita are dissected free in with a wide margin around the infiltrated area. Biopsies of the orbital wall and periorbita are obtained and sent for frozen section histologic examination. Infiltration and penetration of the periorbita by high-grade malignancies may be an indication to exenterate the orbita [27]. The extent of the tumor toward the medial canthus and the medial orbit determines whether the upper and lower lids need to be resected. Skin from the upper and lower lids may also be harvested as a thin full-thickness skin graft to line the remaining orbital cavity. The periorbita is completely dissected off the orbital walls, and thus the tumor is entirely enclosed within the orbital contents. The optic nerve is ligated and transected with appropriate instrumentation. Exenteration of the orbit, removal of the lateral nasal wall, and complete ethmoidectomy provide a broad access to the anterior skull base from below [10]. If the tumor originates primarily from the maxillary sinus or has infiltrated the maxillary sinus, a partial or complete maxillectomy is also necessary. This requires an extension of the incision as described by Weber-Ferguson. This incision has been modified by Janecka and incorporates a modification of the incision along the nasal vestibule and upper lip resulting in improved aesthetic appearance [18].

Le Fort Osteotomy

Bilateral maxillary osteotomy was first described by Langenbeck in 1859 [23] and by Cheever in 1867 [3]. More recently bilateral as well as modified unilateral horizontal maxillary osteotomies have been described [5, 14, 38]. These approaches can be performed through a mid-facial degloving approach. The horizontal osteotomy is performed slightly above the level of the nasal floor for preservation of the tooth roots. The nasal septum is sharply divided off the nasal floor and the perpendicular plate of the pterygoid is divided off the maxilla with a curved chisel. Subsequently the maxilla may be fractured down and freed up from the remaining soft tissue attachments. This provides a broad access and visualization from the posterior ethmoid to the atlas. After removal of the tumor the previously mobilized maxilla is repositioned and fixated with plates. The mucosal incisions are carefully reapproximated with absorbing sutures.

An endonasal pack is placed. A soft diet is initiated in the early postoperative period and additional moisturizing treatment to the nasal mucosa is begun. This approach is used for access to tumors located along the posterior frontal skull base, in particular tumors of the posterior ethmoid sinus, the sphenoid sinus, and the clivus. The dura can be resected in a controlled fashion and reconstructed using autologous fascia, a mucoperiosteal nasal septal flap, or a temporalis muscle flap [5]. Limitations of this approach include reduced visualization of the anterior skull base and nasal cavity.

Midfacial Split

The midfacial split approach allows access to the central skull base and anterior cranial fossa including the sphenoid sinus, nasopharynx, and clivus up to the craniocervical transition [17]. The cutaneous incisions include a median rhinotomy which is extended cranially into an infrabrow incision bilaterally and inferiorly into a paramedian lip split. Nasal and maxillary osteotomies allow temporary removal of the bony structures of the midface. The cartilage of the nasal septum is lateralized. A particularly wide access to the anterior skull base is provided with this approach. Substantial cosmetic deformities can occur with this approach, thus the midfacial split is reserved for very extensive cases where other approaches do not allow adequate exposure.

Facial Translocation

The facial translocation approach allows temporary translocation of the facial skin soft tissue envelope. Wide craniofacial osteotomies allow broad exposure of anterior and lateral skull base including the nasopharynx, clivus, and intratemporal fossa [15, 16]. The incision begins at the vermillion and is extended along the nasal ala into a lateral rhinotomy incision. At the level of the medial canthus a transconjunctival incision is performed and extended laterally into the preauricular sulcus. The frontal branch of the facial nerve is transected and will be repaired at the end of the procedure. The soft tissues of the cheek are elevated and orbita-maxillary osteotomies are performed which allow temporary removal of the anterior wall of the maxillary sinus, the inferior and lateral orbital rim, and the orbital floor together with the zygoma. The temporalis muscle is transposed after the coronoid process is transected. This approach may be combined with a frontotemporal craniotomy and allows additional extra- and intradural dissection along the anterior and middle cranial fossae [15, 16].

Lateral Approach (Infratemporal Fossa Approach)

If the pathology extends from the paranasal sinuses and the anterior skull base into the nasopharynx, intratemporal fossa, apex of the orbit, and middle cranial fossa, the infratemporal fossa approach may be required [12, 29, 41]. In cases requiring visualization and dissection of the internal carotid artery, a transfacial access should be combined with lateral approaches. The line of incision starts with a coronal incision which is extended past the midline. Laterally this is extended toward the root of the zygoma and the preauricular sulcus which is followed similar to a facelift incision around the ear lobe. The incision is then extended inferiorly behind the mandible similar to a parotidectomy incision. The scalp is dissected in a supraperiosteal plane and joined with the plane of loose areola tissue between the temporoparietal fascia and the deep temporal fascia in the temporal fossa. This allows elevation and preservation of the frontal branch of the facial nerve. Over the zygoma the dissection plane is transitioned into the subdermal plane which is carried all the way down to the inferior part of the dissection over the platysma. The insertion of the masseter muscle is dissected off the zygomatic arch and the zygomatic arch is removed. The ascending ramus of the mandible is dissected and an osteotomy behind the coronoid process is performed. A temporary transection of the ascending ramus of the mandible may be helpful. In some cases the ascending ramus of the mandible is completely removed. The main trunk of the facial nerve is identified and the facial nerve is dissected free which results in a superficial parotidectomy. The facial nerve branches are mobilized. The skull base can then be approached through the infratemporal fossa and the pterygopalatine fossa, also providing access to the nasopharynx. A middle fossa craniotomy may be combined with the infratemporal fossa approach, a fact which allows simultaneous intra- and extracranial dissection.

Intracranial Approaches

Intracranial approaches allow extradural dissection of the cranial contents from above the skull base. This allows removal of the pathology of the anterior skull base while the brain is protected, minimizing the risk of neurologic complications. Multiple variations of frontal and frontotemporal craniotomies are used to approach pathologic processes of the paranasal sinuses [4, 28, 45]. The skin soft tissue envelope over the frontal bones is reflected anteriorly from one lateral canthus to the other by means of a coronal incision. The galea is dissected carefully and the supraorbital and supratrochlear neurovascular bundles are preserved, offering a vascularized pericranial flap for later reconstruction. An adequate length of the pericranial flap can be secured when the coronal incision is placed further posteriorly [29]. Most frequently a bifrontal craniotomy is performed. This craniotomy is performed slightly above the superior orbital rims [7, 11]. Some authors describe a subcranial extended anterior approach with inclusion of the supraorbital rims and the nasion into a temporarily dissected block [33, 34]. This allows a broad access to the entire anterior skull base, sphenoclival region, nose, and paranasal sinuses.

In addition this approach combines the craniotomy with the surrounding paranasal sinuses and the nasal cavity in such a way that no additional transfacial approach is needed [32, 35]. The subcranial extended anterior approach is used for traumatic injuries of the anterior skull base as well as for the treatment of congenital malformations and tumors [13, 33, 35]. In frontal sinus fracture repair of the anterior and posterior wall, surgeons must determine whether the frontal recess will allow adequate drainage of the frontal sinus after the frontal osteoplastic flap reinsertion. If larger parts of the anterior and posterior wall are resected or absent, the complete removal of all frontal sinus mucosa and obliteration of the frontal sinus with free abdominal fat transplants may be indicated. Alternatively the frontal sinus may be cranialized after removal of the entire posterior wall [6, 8]. The frontotemporal craniotomy provides a lateral access to the anterior and middle cranial fossae after careful retraction of the frontal and temporal lobes. In addition the optic canal and lateral orbit can be approached through this access from laterally. The resulting dural defect is closed with temporalis fascia, fascia lata, or a pericranial flap. The pericranial flap is preferred since it provides well-vascularized tissue for repair especially in previously irradiated patients or patients who require postoperative radiation treatment. The bony skull base may also be reinforced with cartilage of the cavum conchae or calvarial bone grafts, if required.

Combined Approaches

Multiple combined approaches are reported in the literature. These may be categorized as combined extradural approaches and combined extra- and intradural approaches. For extradural approaches a transfacial and transcranial procedure may be combined. The term craniofacial surgery has been coined for the combination of a lateral rhinotomy and a bifrontal craniotomy approach [37, 43]. Other combinations include transfacial approaches with any craniotomy [21, 31]. A mini-craniotomy carries less risk of delayed wound healing after radiation therapy when compared to larger osteoplastic flaps. In addition retraction of the frontal lobe is minimized with this technique.

Postoperative Care and Complications

Wound Healing

Procedures of the skull base are associated with a risk of delayed wound healing as well as infection and loss of skin grafts or other flaps. Application of broad-spectrum antibiotics and careful debridement of the intranasal wounds may reduce the risk of infection. Vital structures such as the internal carotid artery and the brain should be covered with well-vascularized flaps. After orbital exenteration, the walls of the orbit should be lined with epithelium. Hemorrhage from the internal maxillary artery or the anterior and posterior ethmoid arteries may require ligation of these vessels. In particular when well-vascularized tumors are present, preoperative angiography with embolization may substantially reduce intraoperative bleeding as well as the risk of postoperative hemorrhage [10].

Skull Base

A CSF leak is a quite frequent complication after craniofacial approaches to the anterior skull base, and are reported to occur in 2–14% of cases [22]. Associated meningitis has been observed in 1–5% of the cases [22, 26, 36]. Rarely an intracranial abscess, tension pneumocephalus, or osteomyelitis may occur. To minimize the risk of these complications a meticulous reconstruction of the various layers of the skull base (dura, bone, soft tissue) is crucial. Autologous materials should be preferred when available. Especially with previously irradiated patients, osteonecrosis of a temporarily removed osteoplastic flap is possible. Well-vascularized flaps may contribute to reduce this risk. Hyperbaric oxygen therapy has been used in the treatment of osteoradionecrosis. Injury or resection of the upper cranial nerves may entail a number of functional problems (visual changes, diplopia, anosmia, facial paresthesias). Injuries of the cerebral parenchyma from resection, retraction, or reduced hemoperfusion may result in stroke or seizures.

Orbita

During transfacial approaches the nasolacrimal duct may be injured with resulting epiphora. Intraoperative dacryocystorhinostomy with stenting of the lacrimal system for 3 months is recommended if the lacrimal sac and the entire lateral nasal wall have been resected. When transfacial osteotomies are performed, extraocular muscles may be injured with resulting diplopia. If this complication occurs, an ophthalmologic consultation should be obtained. The optic nerve may also be injured by bony fragments or be compressed by a hematoma. This may require intravenous administration of high-dose corticosteroids and decompression of the optic nerve. Hypoglobus and enophthalmus may result from deficits of the medial and inferior orbital wall or a resection of orbital fat. This can be repaired with the standard surgical techniques for these complications.

Tips to Avoid Complications

- When dissecting the pericranial flap, the supraorbital nerve should be preserved in order to preserve sensation of the forehead skin.
- The dissection plane of the scalp flap within the temporal fossa should be below the temporoparietal fascia and on top of the deep temporal fascia for the protection of the frontal branch of the facial nerve.
- For reconstruction of the bony skull base autologous grafts should be used. In cases of previously irradiated patients, free microvascular or other vascularized flaps should be utilized.
- Careful postoperative debridement of the nasal cavity may reduce the risk of infections.

Take-Home Pearls

- Tumors of the nasal cavity and the paranasal sinuses can be effectively treated through craniofacial approaches. These approaches allowed more radical removal of paranasal sinus malignancies and may increased survival of these patients.
- Opening of the dura increases the complication rate. The limit margins of resection are dictated by vital structures such as the internal carotid artery, cavernous sinus, optic nerve, and frontal lobe.
- The optimal visualization and exposure of the pathology should be obtained through the simplest possible approach with the least associated morbidity.
- Detailed frozen section pathology assessment is mandatory since tumor margins cannot be easily estimated intraoperatively.

Acknowledgement

The author would like to thank Prof. of Art Anatomy Sourvalis Dimitrios for the medical illustrations.

References

1. Bagatella F, Mazzoni A (1995) Microsurgery in juvenile nasopharyngeal angiofibroma: a lateronasal approach with nasomaxillary pedicle flap. Skull Base Surg 5:219–226
2. Cheesman AD, Lund VJ, Howard DJ (1986) Craniofacial resection for tumors of the nasal cavity and paranasal sinuses. Head Neck Surg 8:429–435
3. Cheever DW (1867) Nasopharyngeal polypus attached to the basilar process of occipital and body of the sphenoid bone successfully removed by a section, displacement, and subsequent replacement and reunion of the superior maxillary bone. Boston Medical and Surgical Journal 8:162
4. Close LG, Mickey B (1992) Transcranial resection of ethmoid sinus cancer involving the anterior skull base. Skull Base Surg 2:213–218
5. Cocke EW, Robertson JH Jr (1998) Extended unilateral maxillotomy approach. In: Donald PJ (ed) Surgery of the skull base. Lippincott-Raven, Philadelphia
6. Constantinidis J, Steinhart H, Schwerdfeger K, Zenk J, Iro H (2001) Therapy of invasive frontal sinus mucoceles. Rhinology 39:33–38
7. Constantinidis J, Steinhart H, Koch M, Buchfelder M, Schänzer A, Weidenbecher M, Iro H (2004) Olfactory neuroblastoma: the University of Erlangen-Nuremberg experience 1975–2000. Otolaryngol Head Neck Surg 130:567–574
8. Donald PJ, Bernstein L (1978) Compound frontal sinus injuries with intracranial penetration. Laryngoscope 88:225–232
9. Donald PJ (1998) Anterior fossa approaches: transfacial approach. In: Donald PJ (ed) Surgery of the skull base. Lippincott-Raven, Philadelphia

37

10. Draf W, Berghaus A (1993) Tumoren und Pseudotumoren der frontalen Schädelbasis – Rhinochirurgisches Referat. Eur Arch Otolaryngol (Suppl) 1:105–186

11. Fahlbusch R, Neubauer U, Wigand M, Weidenbecher M, Rockelein G, Thierauf P, Sauer R (1989) Neuro-rhinosurgical treatment of aesthesioneuroblastoma. Acta Neurochir 100:93–100

12. Fisch U, Mattox DE (1988) Microsurgery of the skull base. Thieme, Stuttgart

13. Fliss DM, Zucker G, Cohen A, Amir A, Sagi A, Rosenberg L, Leiberman A, Gatot A, Reichenthal E (1999) Early outcome and complications of the extended subcranial approach to anterior skull base. Laryngoscope 109:153–160

14. James D, Crockard HA (1991) Surgical access to the base of the skull and upper cervical spine by extended maxillotomy. Neurosurgery 29:411–416

15. Janecka IP, Sen CN, Sekhar LN, Arriaga M (1990) Facial translocation: a new approach to the cranial base. Otolaryngol Head Neck Surg 103:413–419

16. Janecka IP, Sen CN, Sekhar LN, Nuss DW (1991) Facial translocation for cranial base surgery. Keio J Med 40:215–220

17. Janecka IP, Ness DW, Sen CN (1991) Midfacial split for access to the central base. Acta Neurochir Suppl 53:199–203

18. Janecka IP, Sen CN, Sekhar LN, Ramasastry S, Curtin HD, Burnes EL, DAmico F (1994) Cranial base surgery: results in 183 patients. Otolaryngol Head Neck Surg 110:539–546

19. Kaplan MJ, Jane JA, Park TS, Cantrell RW (1984) Supraorbital rim approach to the anterior skull base. Laryngoscope 94:1137–1139

20. Ketcham AS, Wilkins RH, Vanburen JM, Smith RR (1963) A combined intracranial approach to the paranasal sinuses. Am J Surg 106:699–703

21. Ketcham AS, Chretien PB, van Buren JM (1973) The ethmoid sinuses: a re-evaluation of surgical resection. Am J Surg 126:469–476

22. Kraus DH, Shah JP, Arbit E, Calicich JH, Strong EW (1994) Complications of craniofacial resection for tumors involving the anterior skull base. Head Neck 16:307–312

23. Langenbeck v B (1859) Beiträge zur Osteoplastik: die osteoplastische Resektion des Oberkiefers. In: Goschen A (ed) Deutsche Klinik. Reimer, Berlin

24. Lund VJ, Howard DJ, Wei WI, Cheesman AD (1998) Craniofacial resection for tumors of the nasal cavity and paranasal sinuses: a 17-year experience. Head Neck 20:97–105

25. Lydiatt DD, Hollins RR (1993) Vascular considerations in approaches to the deep midface. Head Neck 15:164–168

26. McCaffrey TV, Olsen KD, Yohanan JM, Lewis JM, Ebersold MJ, Piepgras DG (1994) Factors affecting survival of patients with tumors of the anterior skull base. Laryngoscope 104:940–945

27. McCary W, Levine P, Cantrell R (1996) Preservation of the eye in the treatment of sinonasal malignant neoplasms with orbital involvement. Arch Otolaryngol Head Neck Surg 122:657–659

28. Nuss DW, Janecka IP, Sekhar LN, Sen CN (1991) Craniofacial disassembly in the management of skull-base tumors. Otolaryngol Clin North Am 24:1465–1497

29. Osguthorpe JD, Patel S (1995) Craniofacial approaches to skull base malignancies. Otolaryngol Clin North Am 28:1239–1257

30. Osguthorpe JD, Patel S (2001) Craniofacial approaches to tumors of the anterior skull base. Otolaryngol Clin North Am 34:1123–1142

31. Panje WR, Dohrmann WJ, Pitcock JK, Scher N, Weichselbaum RR, Sutton HG, Vokes E, Moss J (1989) The transfacial approach for combined anterior craniofacial tumor ablation. Arch Otolaryngol Head Neck Surg 115:301–307

32. Pinsolle J, San-Galli F, Siberchicot F, Caix P, Emparanza A, Michelet FX (1991) Modified approach for ethmoid and anterior skull base surgery. Arch Otolaryngol Head Neck Surg 117:779–782

33. Raveh J, Vuillemin T (1988) The surgical one-stage management of combined cranio-maxillo-facial and frontobasal fractures: advantages of the subcranial approach in 374 cases. J Craniomaxillofac Surg 16:160–172

34. Raveh J, Laedrach K, Speiser M, Chen J, Vuillemin T, Seiler R, Ebeling U, Leibinger K (1993) The subcranial approach for fronto-orbital and anteroposterior skull base tumors. Arch Otolaryngol Head Neck Surg 119:385–393

35. Raveh J, Laedrach K, Lizuka T, Leibinger F (1998) Subcranial extended anterior approach for skull base tumors: surgical procedure and reconstruction. In: Donald PJ (ed) Surgery of the skull base. Lippincott-Raven, Philadelphia

36. Richtsmeier WJ, Briggs RJS, Koch WM, Eisele DW, Loury MC, Price JG, Mattox DE, Carson BS (1992) Complications and early outcome of anterior craniofacial resection. Arch Otolaryngol Head Neck Surg 118:913–917

37. Samii M, Draf W (1989) Surgery of the skull base. Springer, Berlin

38. Sasaki CT, Lowlitcht RA, Astrachan DI (1990) LeFort I osteotomy approach to the skull base. Laryngoscope 100:1073–1076

39. Schramm VL, Myers EN, Maroon JC (1979) Anterior skull base surgery for benign and malignant disease. Laryngoscope 89:1077–1091

40. Schramm VL Jr (1987) Anterior craniofacial resection. In: Sekhar LN, Schramm VL Jr (eds) Tumors of the cranial base: diagnosis and treatment. Futura, New York

41. Sekhar LN, Schramm VL, Jones NF, Yonas H, Horton J, Latchaw RE, Curtin H (1986) Operative exposure and management of the petrous and upper cervical internal carotid artery. Neurosurgery 19:967–982

42. Shah JP, Galicich JH (1977) Craniofacial resection for malignant tumors of ethmoid and anterior skull base. Arch Otolaryngol Head Neck Surg 103:514–517

43. Shah JP, Kraus DH, Arbit E, Galicich JH, Strong EW (1992) Craniofacial resection for tumors involving the anterior skull base. Otolaryngol Head Neck Surg 106:387–393

44. Smith RR, Klopp CT, Williams JM (1954) Surgical treatment of cancer of the frontal sinus and adjacent areas. Cancer 7:991–994

45. Zappia JJ, Garroll WR, Wolf GT, Thornton AF, Ho L, Krause CJ (1993) Olfactory neuroblastoma: the results of modern treatment approaches at the University of Michigan. Head Neck 15:190–196

Chapter 38

Surgical Procedures for the Treatment of Malignant Neoplasms of the Nose and Paranasal Sinuses

38

Christopher N. Prichard, Gabriel G. Calzada, and Randal S. Weber

Core Messages

- The anatomic relationship of the sinuses to the orbit, anterior cranial fossa, and face makes complete tumor removal with preservation of form and function challenging.
- Goals of resection include oncologically sound tumor removal with minimal compromise of critical function.
- Endoscopic approaches facilitate diagnosis and may complement traditional open resection.

Contents

Introduction

Malignancies of the nose and paranasal sinuses represent a challenging dilemma to the head and neck surgeon. Several clinical features contribute to the overall difficulty in successful management of sinonasal cancers. Most commonly, these tumors present with symptoms which are synonymous with benign inflammatory sinus disease. Patients frequently present with persistent nasal congestion, sinusitis, and recurrent epistaxis. Subsequently, there is frequently a delay from 6 to 8 months from the onset of symptoms which results in a relatively advanced stage of disease at the time of diagnosis. This contributes to an overall poor prognosis of sinonasal malignancy, with 5-year survival rates traditionally ranging from 30% to 40% [1–4]. In addition, sinonasal tumors are relatively rare, accounting for approximately only 3% of upper aerodigestive tract malignancies [5]. As a result, most research is retrospective and compiling sufficient numbers of cases to compare between treatment modalities is not practically possible. Also, the sum total of sinonasal malignancy is actually comprised of several different pathologic types of tumors, which further compounds the difficulty in generalizing the results of clinical studies to a given patient. Hence, an evidence-based approach to optimal treatment is impractical in treating these cancers. Finally, the close relationship of critical structures to the nose and paranasal sinuses, including the orbit and anterior and middle cranial fossae, makes wide oncologic resection challenging without compromising function such as smell, vision, speech, and swallowing. The fragility of the ethmoid labyrinth also makes en bloc resection of tumor difficult, if not impossible. Ultimately, all of these dilemmas make the successful surgical management of sinonasal malignancy challenging.

Surgical procedures for the management of malignant tumors of the nose and paranasal sinuses include traditional open surgery, endoscopically assisted open surgery, and endoscopic resection alone. Adequacy of exposure for complete and safe tumor resection should never be compromised for the sake of avoiding a facial incision. Each procedure entails both an approach (incision) for visualization and extent of resection. The lateral rhinotomy may be used for a variety of tumor types and locations; however, both the approach and extent of resection should be tailored to each patient's tumor to maximize cosmesis, function, and, most importantly, oncologically sound resection. For the purposes of this chapter, we will combine a description of commonly used approaches with, when possible, the ablative procedure most commonly used through that approach.

Caldwell-Luc Approach (Anterior Antrostomy)

The anterior antrostomy approach was described separately, yet independently, by the American George Caldwell (1893) and the Frenchman Henri Luc (1895) [6]. This approach has traditionally been applied to inflammatory sinus disease but may be a useful adjunct for tumors of the maxillary sinus, inferior orbit, or medial maxilla. The approach may assist in the complete resection of benign tumors. The Caldwell-Luc approach should be avoided for diagnostic biopsies if access can be achieved transnasally.

Lateral Rhinotomy Approach/Medial Maxillectomy

The lateral rhinotomy was first described by Michaux in 1848, though formally presented by Moure of Bourdeaux in 1902 [7, 8]. The approach consists of an incision halfway between the medial canthus and nasal dorsum along the lateral nasal sidewall to the alar crease. The lateral rhinotomy approach has the benefit of a typically excellent, almost unnoticeable, cosmetic result as well as visualization of the lateral nasal wall (medial maxillary wall), ethmoids, nasal septum, and skull base.

The medial maxillectomy is the ablative procedure most commonly performed through the lateral rhinotomy approach [9–11]. The medial maxillectomy was initially described by Sessions and Larson in 1977 as a method of en bloc resection of tumors of the nasoethmoid region [9]. The resection is performed through a lateral rhinotomy combined with a generous Caldwell-Luc. To expose the lamina papyracea, the medial canthal tendon is elevated off the anterior lacrimal crest along with the bony periosteum followed by transection of the lacrimal duct. The orbital contents are reflected laterally and the anterior and posterior ethmoidal arteries are controlled with bipolar cautery. The procedure consists of a series of osteotomies: anterior to posterior to divide the lateral wall of the nose from the palate, anterior to superior from the floor of the maxillary sinus to the superior aspect of the lacrimal fossa, from the posterior medial floor of the maxillary sinus superiorly to the frontal ethmoidal suture line, and from the medial orbit through the orbital floor medial to the infraorbital canal. Ultimately the soft tissue attachments of the middle and inferior turbinates are transected [10–12]. The procedure results in en bloc resection of the medial maxillary wall.

Care must be taken to stay inferior to the frontoethmoid suture line to avoid CSF leak. Osteotomies should not be carried too far posteriorly in order to avoid optic nerve injury. Dacryocystorhinostomy needs to be performed to avoid epiphora or dacryocystitis after transection of the lacrimal duct. Precise reapproximation of the medial canthal tendon to the anterior lacrimal crest prevents telecanthus or diplopia secondary to medial canthal tendon release.

Midfacial Degloving Approach

Another versatile open surgical approach for the resection of sinonasal malignancy is the midfacial degloving approach [13, 14]. The approach technique was first reported by Casson and Converse in 1974 [15], and in 1979 Conley and Price reported their 10-year experience with midfacial degloving [16]. This approach offers excellent exposure to tumors of the lower nasal cavity, maxillary sinus, and nasopharynx. When combined with a Lynch incision exposure of the orbit, ethmoid and sphenoid sinuses, superior septum, and anterior skull base is possible. Midfacial degloving offers the advantage of a bilateral approach for sinonasal malignancies crossing the midline. It avoids palatal dysfunction or risk of oroantral fistula. Because no external incisions are necessary an excellent cosmetic result is achievable. The midfacial degloving approach has traditionally been used for a wide spectrum of benign masses of the nose and paranasal sinuses. Its application for sinonasal malignancy is more limited, but in selected cancers that can be completely encompassed by this approach it adds a valuable tool to the surgeon's armamentarium. The midfacial degloving approach would be contraindicated in any tumor which extends to the facial soft tissues and skin, requiring their resection en bloc with the tumor.

The midfacial degloving approach consists of the bilateral combination of a number of incisions. Bilateral gingivobuccal sulcus incisions, bilateral gingivolabial sulcus incisions, and bilateral intercartilaginous incisions are performed. A single septocolumellar transfixion incision connects the two sides, and the periosteum is elevated off the anterior maxilla bilaterally. Subsequently, the facial soft tissues are elevated from the bony framework of the midface and suspended superiorly.

Despite its advantages, the midfacial degloving procedure also possesses several potential pitfalls which need to be considered. Of paramount importance in tumor surgery is adequate exposure for safe and complete resection. The midfacial degloving may not provide optimal exposure in some circumstances. Most commonly, transient or rarely permanent infraorbital nerve anesthesia can occur from traction injury to the infraorbital nerves bilaterally. Frequently patients experience transient nasal crusting, which usually responds to aggressive local hygiene and diminishes over time. Injury to the tooth roots and denervation can occur. Finally, patients may experience nasal vestibular stenosis due to the intercartilaginous incisions. This is of particular concern in patients who undergo postoperative radiotherapy after midfacial degloving procedures. Meticulous closure of intercartilaginous incisions must be carried out to avoid stenosis, and nasal packing for 3–4 days postoperatively may help maintain vestibular patency as incisions heal. Postoperative taping and Aquaplast splint immobilization help minimize tip edema.

Transoral Approach/Infrastructure Maxillectomy

Certain tumors are amenable to a transoral approach, which obviously possesses the cosmetic benefit of avoiding external incisions. Specifically, tumors that are limited to the hard palate or the floor of the maxillary antrum are amenable to this procedure. Tumors that extend posterior to the maxillary tuberosity should not be resected transorally due to the potential for extension into the masticator space. Whereas there is significant cosmetic benefit, there is also significant functional challenge to speech and swallowing due to resection of the palate. Close collaboration is required with the prosthodontist or oncologic dentist for construction with an obturator to avoid significant functional sequelae; this collaboration cannot be overemphasized. Preoperative dental impressions are mandatory and a temporary surgical obturator is prepared for immediate insertion in the operating room.

The infrastructure maxillectomy can be performed unilaterally or bilaterally, depending on the extent of tumor involvement. For tumors isolated to the maxillary antrum, the soft palate is preserved and facilitates prosthetic rehabilitation.

The infrastructure maxillectomy is carried out through a gingivobuccal incision. A Caldwell-Luc is performed if necessary to assess tumor extent and the appropriateness of the infrastructure maxillectomy. Bony cuts can be made using the oscillating saw across the anterior lateral face of the maxilla to include the pyriform aperture if necessary. The posterior wall of the sinus is transected with an osteotome either through the Caldwell-Luc or by continuing the lateral osteotomy posteriorly and medially. The final bony cut to release the maxilla is division of the pterygoid plate. This may be performed with the osteotome placed perpendicular to the attachment of the plates or vertically just behind the posterior wall of the maxillary sinus depending on the location of the tumor. The integrity of the lacrimal system must be maintained to avoid epiphora. The medial maxillary wall is included en bloc with the specimen, as resection of the inferior turbinate facilitates seating the prosthetic obturator [17]. For unilateral hard palate or maxillary lesions, a shelf of bone can be preserved adjacent to the nasal septum on the resected side which functions as a shelf on which a obturator may be seated.

The residual maxillary sinus mucosa is removed and the sinus and exposed pterygoid muscles are resurfaced with a split-thickness skin graft. The cavity is packed with Xeroform gauze that is secured by the placement of a temporary surgical obturator. The packing is removed on postoperative day 5 and an interim obturator is placed. Once final complete healing and epithelialization has occurred a definitive obturator is placed with dentition.

Weber-Ferguson Approach/ Total and Radical Maxillectomy

Lazars offered the first description of a procedure to resect the maxilla and sinuses in 1826, but his initial attempt at performing the procedure in 1827 was halted because of blood loss [18]. Joseph Gonsol of Lyon successfully performed the operation in 1827, but offered credit to Lazars for his initial description [19]. In 1828, Syme reported a successful total maxillectomy with orbital exenteration [18]. Larger tumors of the maxillary sinus with or without orbital involvement may be resected via a Weber-Ferguson incision. This incision is contraindicated with tumor invasion of the overlying skin, which requires more advanced free-flap reconstruction. The extent of resection is dic-

tated by the extent of tumor extirpation necessary. For tumors which spare the orbit but involve the entire maxillary antrum, total maxillectomy is performed. For more extensive tumors which invade the orbital floor or periorbita, this operation is extended to a radical maxillectomy, which includes orbital exenteration with preservation of the superior and superolateral orbital rims. If the periorbita is free of tumor, the orbital contents may be spared with resection of the floor of the orbit, followed by reconstruction to support the orbital contents. This will minimizes enophthalmos or diplopia. In situations in which the floor of the maxillary sinus is spared but orbital contents are involved, a suprastructure maxillectomy is possible.

The Weber-Ferguson approach consists of an extended lateral rhinotomy incision which splits the ipsilateral upper lip along the philtrum and may be extended with the addition of a subciliary incision. This begins at the level of the medial canthus in the naso-orbital groove, and is extended inferiorly just medial to the nasofacial groove. It is carried around the nasoalar groove and down through the ipsilateral philtrum. A gingivobuccal sulcus incision is fashioned and the flap reflected laterally in the subperiosteal plane, avoiding injury to the infraorbital nerve if possible.

If the orbital contents are spared, dissection is carried out reflecting the periorbita and exposing the anterior and posterior ethmoid arteries. The anterior ethmoid artery is frequently coagulated with bipolar electrocautery; however, the posterior ethmoid artery should be ligated or coagulated with caution due to its proximity to the optic nerve. Osteotomies are carried out through the zygoma and along the medial maxilla. An anterior-posterior osteotomy is performed just inferior to the frontoethmoid suture line on the medial orbital wall and connected with a lateral orbital osteotomy across the inferior orbital fissure. The hard palate is divided near the midline. The maxillectomy specimen is freed from the pterygomaxillary fissure using an osteotome to divide the pterygoid plates and delivered en bloc [18–20].

As in infrastructure maxillectomy, preoperative consultation with a prosthodontist is crucial as the defect will require obturator reconstruction. The cheek flap is lined with a split-thickness skin graft, as is the periorbita and pterygoid musculature. A rim of medial hard palate bone facilitates a secure prosthesis. The procedure is routinely carried out under relative hypotension to minimize blood loss [19, 20]. Dacryocystorhinostomy can avoid postoperative epiphora.

Transcranial/Craniofacial Resection

Tumors extending superiorly to the roof of the ethmoids and cribiform plate usually require a combined craniofacial resection [21–31]. While skull base resection may at times be performed through a transfacial approach, in most instances a separate craniotomy incision is necessary. The craniofacial approach provides excellent and safe exposure to the subfrontal area, dura, and medial orbital regions. Smith et al. first described the transcranial approach to sinus tumors in 1954 [30]. Ketcham et al. introduced the concept of combined craniofacial resection in 1963 [31]. The University of Texas MD Anderson Cancer Center has reported its experience of 76 patients with malignant tumors of the paranasal sinuses requiring some form of transcranial approach for resection. In this series, patients with involvement of the floor of the maxillary sinus, invasion of the base of the nasal septum, involvement of the soft tissues of the face, or orbital involvement requiring exenteration necessitated a transfacial approach in addition to bifrontal craniotomy—hence, a craniofacial approach. Of the 76 patients, 47 required a craniofacial approach. However, 29 patients were amenable to resection via a solely transcranial approach. Interestingly, the complication rate was higher in the patients undergoing craniotomy alone (13/29 patients) when compared with craniofacial resection (15/47 patients). Hemostasis seems a particular challenge to the craniotomy alone group compared with the craniofacial resections, evidenced by rates of hematoma requiring evacuation of 14% versus 4%, respectively. The improved access by the combined craniofacial approach may reduce hematoma. In addition, the 2 patients experiencing bifrontal cerebral injury underwent craniotomy alone. Limiting retraction on the frontal lobes can help prevent cerebral injury. Four out of 5 patients with symptomatic pneumocephalus underwent craniofacial resection [27].

Early experience with the craniofacial approach was plagued by major infectious complications, with a 42% infection rate in the first 31 patients reported by Ketcham et al. [31]. This intuitively results from communication between the nose and sinuses and the CSF space. Subsequently, CSF leak posed an early challenge in the development of the craniofacial technique. However, the advent of more advanced broad-spectrum antibiotics in the 1980s as well as the introduction of anterior skull base reconstruction with a pericranial flap [24] have greatly reduced the incidence of postoperative infections and CSF leak. In the MD Anderson series, only 1 significant infectious complication and 3 CSF leaks were reported [27].

Endoscopic Approach

Technological advances over the past decade in powered instrumentation as well as angled endoscopes have resulted in increased sophistication in the surgical management of inflammatory sinus disease as well as benign sinonasal tumors [32, 33]. As a natural extension, there has been increasing experience in the application of endoscopic techniques to malignant sinonasal tumors. Endoscopic approaches are applicable toward sinonasal malignancy for: (1) endoscopic biopsy for tumor diagnosis, (2) endoscopically assisted resection in combination with conventional approaches, and (3) total endoscopic resection [34–37].

Complete resection of malignancy by endoscopic techniques alone has been a controversial issue. Advocates of endoscopic approaches cite the advantages of improved cosmesis, better postoperative surveillance, diminished bleeding, less pain, and better ability to preserve uninvolved structures in support of endoscopic resection. Critics of the endoscopic approach note that it involves piecemeal resection of tumor as well as a questionable ability to resect the tumor with an obvious clear margin. Moreover, it marks a clear shift in paradigm, as the surgeons

who develop the advanced endoscopic skills ideal for endoscopic resection (rhinologists) differ from those who classically manage head and neck malignancy (head and neck surgical oncologists).

Given the relatively new application of endoscopic techniques to sinonasal malignancy, the data in support of its use are relatively sparse. The majority of the experience with endoscopic techniques has been in the application to benign neoplasms. In a meta-analysis reviewing the rates of recurrence of traditional versus endoscopic techniques for resection of inverting papilloma, Busquets and Hwang noted an improved recurrence rate for tumors resected endoscopically compared with traditional techniques (12% versus 20%, respectively, $p = 0.001$) [32].

The largest reported experience with the endoscopic management of sinonasal malignancy reported on 19 patients, 15 patients treated with curative intent, and 6 of these were a combined endoscopic approach with bifrontal craniotomy. All patients were presented at a multidisciplinary tumor board and given informed consent regarding endoscopic approaches.

They reported overall and disease-free survival rates of 78.9% and 68.4%, respectively, with over 32 months of follow-up. There were two major complications, pneumocephalus in a patient undergoing craniotomy and one major intraoperative hemorrhage [35]. These early data lend support that, in certain selected cases, endoscopic resection offers a viable treatment modality for sinonasal tumors. However, the oncologic principles of complete tumor resection should be followed. Image guidance may help prevent complications due to anatomic distortion secondary to tumor.

Conclusions

Sinonasal malignancy represents a difficult clinical entity. Surgical resection remains critical to the multimodality management of these tumors. The anatomic relationship of the nose and paranasal sinuses to the orbit, brain, and face makes adequate tumor resection with minimal morbidity extremely challenging. Knowledge of the various surgical approaches for the management of sinonasal malignancies is an important skill for the head and neck surgical oncologist to acquire.

Take-Home Pearls

- Sinonasal malignancies are best managed with multimodality care. Advancements in cranial base surgery, microvascular free flaps, delivery of radiotherapy, and new combinations of effective chemotherapy have improved outcomes.
- Endoscopic approaches facilitate diagnosis and may complement traditional open resection.
- Goals of resection include oncologically sound tumor removal with minimal compromise of critical function.

References

1. Waldron J, Witterick I (2003) Paranasal sinus cancer: caveats and controversies. World J Surg 27:849–855
2. Kondo M, Ogawa K, Inuyama Y, et al.(1985) Prognostic factors influencing relapse of squamous cell carcinoma of the maxillary sinus. Cancer 55:190–196
3. Giri SP, Reddy EK, Gemer LS, et al.(1992) Management of advanced squamous cell carcinomas of the maxillary sinus. Cancer 69:657–661
4. Alvarez I, Suarez C, Rodrigo JP, et al.(1995) Prognostic factors in paranasal sinus cancer. Am J Otolaryngol 16:109–114
5. Osguthorpe JD, Richardson M (2001) Frontal sinus malignancies. Otolaryngol Clin North Am 34:269–281
6. Macbeth R (1971) Caldwell, Luc and their operation. Laryngoscope 81:1652–1657
7. Mertz JS, Pearson BW, Kern EB (1983) Lateral rhinotomy: indications, technique, and review of 226 patients. Arch Otolaryngol 109:235–239
8. Weisman R (1995) Lateral rhinotomy and medial maxillectomy. Otolaryngol Clin North Am 28:1145–1156. PMID: 8927390
9. Sessions RB, Larson DL (1977) En bloc ethmoidectomy and medial maxillectomy. Arch Otolaryngol 103:195–202
10. Sessions RB, Humphreys DH (1983) Technical modifications of the medial maxillectomy. Arch Otolaryngol 109:575–577
11. Osguthorpe JD, Weisman RA (1991) "Medial maxillectomy" for lateral nasal wall neoplasms. Arch Otolaryngol 117:751–756
12. Myers EN (1997) Medial maxillectomy. In: Myers EN (ed) Operative otolaryngology: head and neck surgery, vol I. Saunders, Philadelphia
13. Maniglia AJ, Phillips DA (1995) Midfacial degloving for the management of nasal, sinus, and skull-base neoplasms. Otolaryngol Clin North Am 28:1127–1143
14. Ikeda K, Suzuki H, Oshima T, Nakatsuka S, Takasaka T (1998) Midfacial degloving approach facilitated by endoscope to the sinonasal malignancy. Auris Nasus Larynx 25:289–293
15. Casson PR, Bonnano PC, Converse JM (1974) The midface degloving procedure. Plast Reconstr Surg 53:102–103
16. Conley JJ, Price JC (1979) Sublabial approach to the nasal and nasopharyngeal cavities. Am J Surg 138:615–618
17. Johnson JT (1997) Inferior maxillectomy. In: Myers EN (ed) Operative otolaryngology: head and neck surgery, vol I. Saunders, Philadelphia
18. Rice DH Stanley RB (1999) Surgical therapy of tumors of the nasal cavity, ethmoid sinus, and maxillary sinus. In: Thawley SE, Panje WR, Batsakis JG, Lindberg RD (eds) Comprehensive management of head and neck tumors, vol I. Saunders, Philadelphia
19. Harrison DFN (1971) The management of malignant tumors of the nasal sinuses. Otolaryngol Clin North Am 4:159–177
20. Close LG (1996) Weber-Ferguson approach with subtotal maxillectomy and total maxillectomy with orbital preservation. In: Bailey BJ, Calhoun KH, Coffey AR, Neely JG (eds) Atlas of head and neck surgery: otolaryngology. Lippincott-Raven, Philadelphia
21. Catalano PJ, Hecht CS, Biller HF, Lawson W, Post KD, Sachdev V, Sen C, Urken ML (1994) Cranial facial resection. Arch Otolaryngol Head Neck Surg 120:1203
22. Chapman P, Carter RL, Clefford P (1981) The diagnosis and surgical management of olfactory neuroblastoma: the role of craniofacial resection. J Laryngol Otol 95:795
23. Conley J, Baker DL (1979) Management of the eye socket in cancer of the paranasal sinuses. Arch Otolaryngol 105:702
24. Johns ME, Winn HR, McLean WC, Cantrell RW (1981) Pericranial flap for the closure of defects of craniofacial resection. Laryngoscope 91:952
25. Sisson GA, Bytell DE, Becker SP, et al.(1976) Carcinoma of the paranasal sinuses and craniofacial resection. J Laryngol Otol 90:59
26. Terz JJ, Young HF, Lawrence W (1980) Combined craniofacial resection for locally advanced carcinoma of the head and neck. II. Carcinoma of the paranasal sinuses. Am J Surg 140:618
27. McCutcheon IE, Blacklock JB, Weber RS, DeMonte F, Moser RP, Byers M, Goepfert H (1996) Anterior transcranial (craniofacial) resection of tumors of the paranasal sinuses: surgical technique and results. Neurosurgery 38:471–479
28. Blacklock JB, Weber RS, Lee YY, Goepfert H (1989) Transcranial resection of tumors of the paranasal sinuses and nasal cavity. J Neurosurg 71:10–15
29. Ketcham AS, Chreien PB, Van Buren JM, Hoye RC, Beazley RM, Herdt JR (1973) The ethmoid sinuses: a re-evaluation of surgical resection. Am J Surg 126:469–476
30. Smith RR, Klopp CT, Williams JM (1954) Surgical treatment of cancer of the frontal sinus and adjacent areas. Cancer 7:991–994
31. Ketcham AS, Wilkins RH, Van Buren JM, Smith RR (1963) A combined intracranial facial approach to the paranasal sinus. Am J Surg 106:698
32. Busquets JM, Hwang PH (2006) Endoscopic resection of sinonasal inverted papilloma: a meta-analysis. Otolaryngol Head Neck Surg 134:476–482
33. London SD, Schlosser RJ, Gross CW (2002) Endoscopic management of benign sinonasal tumors: a decade of experience. Am J Rhinol 16:221–227
34. Poetker DM, Toohill RJ, Loehrl TA, Smith TL (2005) Endoscopic management of sinonasal tumors: a preliminary report. Am J Rhinol 19:307–315
35. Roh HJ, Batra PS, Citardi MJ, Lee J, Bolger WE, Lanza DC (2004) Endoscopic resection of sinonasal malignancies: a preliminary report. Am J Rhinol 18:239–246
36. Banhiran W, Casiano RR (2005) Endoscopic sinus surgery for benign and malignant nasal and sinus neoplasm. Curr Opin Otolaryngol Head Neck Surg 13:50–54
37. Batra PS, Citardi MJ (2006) Endoscopic management of sinonasal malignancy. Otolaryngol Clin North Am 39:619–637

Chapter 39

Combined Approaches for Excision of Complex Anterior Skull-Base Tumors

39

Ziv Gil and Dan M. Fliss

Core Messages

- A comprehensive algorithm for resection of complex skull-base tumors is presented.
- Anterior skull-base tumor: the craniofacial of subcranial approaches.
- Benign tumors extending to the maxillary sinus compartment: the subcranial-midfacial degloving approach or endoscopic approach.
- Malignant tumors extending to the maxilla: the craniofacial approach or the subcranial approach.
- Extension to the lateral skull base: the subcranial-orbitozygomatic approach.
- Tumors extending to the lower clival region: the subcranial-LeFort I approach.
- Tumors with orbital apex or intraorbital extension: The subcranial-transorbital approach.

Contents

Introduction

The subcranial or craniofacial approaches are single-stage procedures used in those with tumors involving the anterior skull base. Craniofacial resection (CFR) is a well-established technique for the removal of tumors involving the anterior skull base and paranasal sinuses [1–3]. This technique requires a frontal craniotomy along with a transfacial approach to allow broad exposure of the anterior cranial fossa and subcranial compartment. Another access to the anterior skull-base is via the subcranial approach [4–7]. The extent of exposure in the subcranial approach includes the frontal sinus anteriorly, the clivus posteriorly, the frontal lobe superiorly, and the paranasal sinuses inferiorly. Laterally, the boundaries of this approach are both superior orbital walls. The subcranial approach has several major advantages over the traditional CFR: (1) it affords a broad exposure of the anterior skull base from below rather than through the transfrontal route; (2) it provides an excellent access to the medial orbital walls and to the sphenoethmoidal, nasal and paranasal cavities; (3) it allows simultaneous intradural and extradural tumor removal and safe reconstruction of dural defects; (4) it does not require facial incisions; and (5) It is performed with minimal frontal lobe manipulation.

Although the subcranial approach allows complete tumor resection in the majority of cases, there are still situations in which the inferior, lateral or posterior aspects of the tumor are not adequately exposed. These include neoplasms with extension to the maxillary antrum and palate caudally, to the cavernous sinus posteriorly and to the orbital apex, pterygopalatine fossa (PPF) or infratemporal fossa (ITF) laterally, and involvement of the nasopharynx and inferior aspect of the clivus inferoposteriorly. Such cases require a combination of other approaches in addition to the classical subcranial approach as a one-stage procedure.

In this chapter we describe combinations of the subcranial approach which are used for extirpation of complex tumors extending out from the anterior fossa compartment to involve adjacent compartments. The surgical, oncological and quality-of-life (QOL) characteristics of the patients were evaluated and compared to those treated using classical subcranial approach.

Surgical Approaches

The route of spread of tumors originating in the anterior skull base and paranasal sinuses is determined by the complex anatomy of the craniofacial compartments. These tumors may invade laterally to the orbit and middle fossa, inferiorly to the maxillary antrum and palate, posteriorly to the nasopharynx and PPF, and superiorly to the cavernous sinus and intracranial space [2]. Recent improvements in endoscopic technology now allow the resection of mostly benign neoplasms or early malignant tumors with minor dural involvement. For larger tumors, the classical subcranial approach has emerged as an excellent surgical technique, allowing extirpation of tumors involving the anterior skull-base and midfacial region. In cases of tumor extension caudal or lateral to these areas, however, the subcranial approach alone cannot provide adequate exposure of the tumor, and other supplementary techniques are needed to provide vascular control and preserve vital structures, thereby allowing safe resection of the tumor.

In this chapter we propose a comprehensive algorithm for excision of multicompartment tumors, based on the exact anatomical localization of the lesion (Table 39.1). All cases presented in this series involved tumors originating in the anterior skull-base area and all the tumors extended to an adjacent anatomical compartment laterally, inferiorly or posteriorly.

The Classical Subcranial Approach

The conventional exposure of the infra- or suprastructure of the maxilla involves lateral rhinotomy or Weber-Fergusson incisions along with bifrontal craniotomy (the craniofacial approach). This technique carries several limitations: lateral rhinotomy with or without Dieffenbach or Lynch incisions may be associated with contractures of the lateral margins of the nostrils and ectropion. A Weber Ferguson incision also may lead to upper lip retraction and asymmetry. To avoid facial incisions in order to improve cosmesis, the authors suggest two modification of the subcranial approach. A unilateral or bilateral medial

maxillectomy may be performed from above via the subcranial approach in order to allow direct visualization of the maxillary antrum, the maxillary floor and the lateral maxillary walls. By means of this approach, it is possible to safely and reliably access benign tumors involving the medial or superior walls of the maxilla and even resect selected malignant lesions that were not invading the hard palate. Complete resection of tumors which extend to the middle maxillary wall, such as hemangiopericytoma, squamous cell carcinoma (SCC) and esthesioneuroblastoma, can be achieved using this approach.

The surgical technique of the classical subcranial approach has been described in detail elsewhere [5–7]. Briefly, following anesthesia, the skin is incised above the hairline and a bicoronal flap is created in a supraperiosteal plane. A flap is elevated anteriorly beyond the supraorbital ridges and laterally superficial to the temporalis fascia. The pericranial flap is elevated up to the periorbits, and the supraorbital nerves and vessels are carefully separated from the supraorbital notch. The lateral and medial walls of the orbits are then exposed, and the anterior ethmoidal arteries are clipped or ligated. The pericranium is elevated above the nasal bones, and the flap is rotated forward and held over the face throughout the rest of the procedure. Titanium miniplates are applied to the frontal bones and removed before the osteotomies to ensure the exact repositioning of the bony segments at the end of the operation. An osteotomy of the anterior or the anterior and posterior frontal sinus walls, together with the nasal bony frame, part of the medial wall of the orbit, and a segment of the superoposterior nasal septum, is then performed. For a *type A* osteotomy, the anterior frontal sinus wall as well as the nasal frame are osteotomized and removed in one block. If a *type B* osteotomy is planned, burr holes are made and the posterior frontal sinus wall is resected after the dura has been detached from the frontal, orbital and ethmoidal roofs. A part of the distal nasal bone is preserved in order to support the nasal valve. In cases of lateral invasion of a tumor, the osteotomy lines can be extended to include segments of the orbital roofs. After the nasofrontoorbital (NFO) bone segment is osteotomized, it is stored in saline until the reconstructive procedure. A bilateral ethmoidectomy and a sphenoidotomy are then performed: this

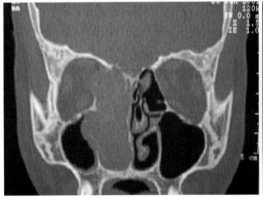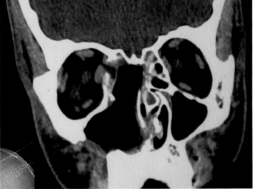

Fig. 39.1 CT images of a 20-year-old patient with juvenile nasopharyngeal angiofibroma (*left* preoperative, *right* postoperative)

approach enables the exposure and assessment of the tumor in its entire circumference. The tumor is extirpated at this stage and the dura or brain parenchymas are also resected when involved by tumor. Frozen sections are taken during surgery in order to ensure tumor-free margins. One or both sides of the cribriform plate and olfactory filaments are preserved whenever possible.

Medial Maxillectomy via the Extended Subcranial Approach

A unilateral or bilateral maxillectomy is performed via the subcranial approach for tumors infiltrating the medial or superior walls of the maxilla. A radical ethmoidectomy and sphenoidectomy are performed following removal of the NFO segment and cribriform plate. Removal of the ethmoidal cells opens an entrance to the nasal cavity and medial maxillary wall from above, allowing exposure of the caudal aspect of the tumor. A medial maxillectomy is than performed, exposing the maxillary antrum. This approach is also recommended for benign tumors extending to the maxillary antrum as well as for selected malignant lesions without palatal infiltration.

The Subcranial-Transfacial Approach

Malignant tumors infiltrating the lower, lateral, anterior or posterior maxillary walls cannot be fully exposed via a combination of the subcranial and midfacial degloving approach, and therefore should be resected via the subcranial-transfacial approach or with the conventional CFR. These approaches offer wide exposure of the tumor and its circumference, allowing *en bloc* resection of the intracranial and inframaxillary extensions of the tumors with free margins. For tumors involving the intraorbital content, the resection is performed via a subcranial-transfacial-transorbital approach in a similar manner. These approaches also allow proper reconstruction of the palate and skull base after tumor resection, with the use of composite free flaps.

The Subcranial Midfacial-Degloving Approach

In order to expose larger tumors which impinge upon the infrastructure (i.e. the maxillary compartment and orbital floor), a combined midfacial degloving is combined with the subcranial approach [8]. This permits the surgeon to expose the entire circumference of the tumor from below and from above in a single operation, without the need for facial incisions. This combined approach is used mainly for benign vascular tumors such as juvenile nasopharyngeal angiofibromas (Figs. 39.1 and 39.2).

Following resection of the tumor from above, a bilateral gingivolabial incision is made, extending to the maxillary tuberosity on each side. The soft tissue of the cheek is raised from the anterior surface of the maxilla, taking care to preserve the infraorbital nerves and vessels. Intracartilaginous incisions are made, similar to the classical closed rhinoplasty, and continued into a full transfixion incision around the limen vestibulae cir-

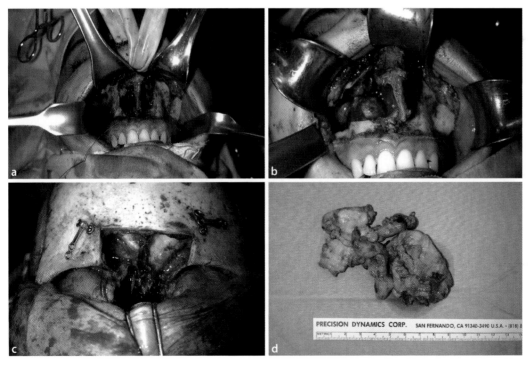

Fig. 39.2a–d Intraoperative photographs of the same patient as in Fig. 39.1. The tumor was extirpated via the combined subcranial-midfacial degloving approach. **a, b** Exposure of the tumor from below using the midfacial degloving approach. **c** Exposure from above via the subcranial approach. **d** The surgical specimen

cumferentially. The nasal skeleton is then undermined, allowing degloving of the soft tissue of the lower face and exposure of the anterior maxillary walls bilaterally. It is then possible to perform partial maxillectomy (i.e. medial and/or anterior maxillary walls), gaining access to the inferior aspect of the tumor both in the lower nasal cavity and in the maxillary sinus. This approach is used for highly vascular tumors infiltrating into the maxillary sinus.

Similarly, the orbitozygomatic-midfacial degloving approach is used for tumors involving the paranasal sinuses superolaterally towards the cavernous sinus.

The Subcranial-Orbitozygomatic Approach

The subcranial approach offers limited access for tumors infiltrating lateral to the orbital roofs, as well as for tumors involving the cavernous sinus, greater sphenoid wing, PPF and ITF. For such cases, retraction of the frontal lobes is necessary when utilizing the classical subcranial approach, which may cause postoperative encephalomalacia and brain edema. Combining the orbitozygomatic approach with the subcranial approach, however, extends visibility to the operative field, gaining access to areas that were not accessible via the subcranial approach alone, eliminating the need of frontal lobe retraction.

This approach is a combination of the subcranial approach and the orbitozygomatic approach [9]. A coronal incision is performed and the skin flap elevation continues down to the level of the fat pad overlying the zygoma, above the temporalis fascia. On the ipsilateral side, the remainder of the dissection dips below the level of the temporalis fascia from the horizontal line above the arch and continues as a fasciocutaneous flap, as described by Yasargil et al. [10]. The muscle is detached anteriorly and superiorly, exposing the temporal fossa. The next stage includes osteotomies in both the frontal and pterional regions. The osteotomy line includes the anterior and the posterior table of the frontal sinus, part of the medial orbital walls, and the superior aspect of the nasal septum. The osteotomy can be extended laterally as required to include a portion of the orbital roof. The bone segment is then removed in one or two pieces, exposing the orbital, ethmoid and sphenoid roofs, the cribriform plate, the temporal fossa and the parasellar area. The osteotomized segment may be removed as one large frontolateral bone flap or as two separate bone flaps.

In this way, a unilateral pterional approach is added to the subcranial approach to expose the more lateral aspect of the orbit, the retroorbital region, the cavernous sinus, the PPF, the chiasmatic region or the ITF [11]. Large central nervous system tumors with extracranial extent, such as meningiomas involving the orbit or upper nasal and sinus cavities, can also be resected via this combined approach.

The Subcranial-Transorbital Approach

For tumors infiltrating the periorbit, the subcranial approach alone offers an excellent exposure from above and below the or-

bit, allowing thorough resection of the tumor from the underlying orbital fat and muscles. Massive orbital involvement, with or without orbital apex infiltration, however, mandates orbital exenteration. In this case, a combined subcranial-transorbital approach allows safe exposure of tumor margins from both sides of the bicoronal flap, and permits reconstruction with a temporalis muscle rotational flap within the same surgical field.

A combined subcranial-transorbital approach is used for tumors that extend to the anterior orbital content (T4a) or orbital apex (T4b). The subcranial approach is performed as described earlier, and the orbit is exenterated using a meticulous dissection from both sides of the bicoronal-facial flap. The upper and lower lids may be spared if they are not involved by tumor, allowing an improved cosmetic result and future insertion of an orbital implant. A combined *subcranial-transorbital-transfacial approach* is performed with a total maxillectomy, allowing *en bloc* resection when the tumor extends from the orbit to the maxilla.

The Subcranial-LeFort I Approach

Tumors involving both the anterior skull base and the clivus are resected using the classical subcranial approach which allows simultaneous exposure of both compartments from above, avoiding the need of facial incisions. For tumors which extend to the lower margin of the clivus, however, the subcranial approach alone is not sufficient. For such cases a LeForte I down-fracture is added to the subcranial approach. One patient with a dedifferentiated chordoma involving the clivus and cavernous sinus was operated upon using the combined subcranial-LeFort I approach.

Following the subcranial approach, an osteotomy and downfracture of the upper alveolus is performed via a gingivobuccal incision. In the combined approach, it is also possible to perform a partial maxillectomy (i.e. medial and/or anterior maxillary walls) in order to gain access to the inferior aspect of the tumor and its extension to the lower nasal cavity and clival region. This is the approach we use to extirpate large chordomas/chondrosarcomas originating in the clivus, with intracranial extension. Specifically, the subcranial approach offers excellent exposure of anterior skull-base tumors which involve the sphenoid clivus. A combination of the subcranial approach with a LeFort I down-fracture osteotomy is used when the tumor extends from the anterior skull base inferoposteriorly to involve the lower part of the clivus.

Combinations of the craniofacial approach with the transfacial approach (i.e. Weber-Ferguson, lateral rhinotomy, Lynch, subciliary or transconjunctival incisions), facial degloving, transorbital and middle fossa approaches have been described in detail by Shah for large malignant tumors of the anterior skull base and paranasal sinuses [2]. A combined facial translocation approach has also been described and safely used by Hao et al. for both malignant and benign tumors [12]. Our algorithm is the first to include the use of the classical subcranial approach in combination with other conventional surgical techniques in such settings.

Reconstruction

Dural and anterior skull-base reconstructions are performed with the double-layer fascia lata technique or with a pericranial flap. Fibrin glue is used to provide additional protection against CSF leakage. Reconstruction of the medial orbital walls is performed only in cases in which the total removal of this segment is necessary or if the periorbit has been resected. In such cases, a split calvarial bone graft, a fascia lata sling or three-dimensional titanium mesh covered by pericranium may be used. Septal cartilage can be used for reconstruction of a limited defect of the inferior orbital wall.

A temporalis muscle flap and a split-thickness skin graft to cover the orbital socket are used in cases of orbital exenteration. In cases of radical maxillectomy with or without orbital exenteration, a lateral thigh free flap or a rectus abdominus musculocutaneous free flap may be utilized to obliterate this large defect and to support the obturator.

After surgery, the patient is immediately transferred to the critical care unit for 24 hours. The lumbar drain is removed 3–5 days after the operation and the nasal packing is removed on the 8th postoperative day.

Surgical Results and Survival

Surgical Results

The surgical outcomes in 120 patients who had undergone skull-base tumor resections via the subcranial approach, alone or in combination with other approaches, were analyzed by Gil and colleagues. In 34% of the patients a second approach or a modification of the classical subcranial approach was used for tumor resection. A combined approach was used for tumors involving more than one compartment apart from the anterior skull base (i.e. lateral skull base, clivus and maxillary sinuses). Most patients (66%) had malignant tumors. The most common tumor was SCC (in 20% of patients). Most patients had stage III/IV disease. Most patients (58%) underwent perioperative radiation therapy and one-third of them had undergone at least one previous operation. The subcranial approach was combined with a midfacial degloving procedure in 14 patients, a medial maxillectomy in 13, an orbitozygomatic approach in 6, a transorbital approach in 5, a transfacial approach in 2, and a LeForte I downfracture in 1. The specific approaches used for each neoplasm are shown in Table 39.1.

Complete tumor resection was achieved in 92% of the patients. The tumor extended to the dura mater in 20 of these patients. If the tumor involved the cavernous sinus, orbital nerve or trigeminal ganglion with intracranial extension partial resection was achieved.

The principal skull-base reconstruction procedure was performed by means of a double-layer fascia lata. A temporalis muscle flap was used for cases in which orbital exenteration was performed and used the same method of double-layer fascial flap for anterior skull-base reconstruction in these patients. A bony reconstruction was required if tumor resection produced a significant bony defect of the orbital walls, nasal bone or anterior frontal sinus wall. This was achieved by applying a split calvarial bone graft or posterior sinus wall. A titanium mesh covered with a pericranial flap was utilized for reconstruction of the medial orbital walls and to cover extensive calvarial defects. In patients with significant defects in the maxilla and anterior skull-base reconstruction was performed with a rectus abdominis muscle as a free graft.

Complications

Postoperative complications occurred in one-third of the patients and included intracranial related complications, bone necrosis and orbital complications. For comparison, postoperative

Table 39.1 Surgical approaches used for excision of multicompartment anterior skull-base tumors

Tumor extension	Surgical approach
Anterior skull base, frontal/ethmoidal/sphenoidal sinuses, sphenoid clivus, planum sphenoidale	Classical subcranial
Medial or superior maxillary walls and periorbit	Subcranial with ipsilateral/bilateral partial maxillectomy
Benign tumors extending to the maxillary sinus compartment ± pterygopalatine fossa or nasopharynx	Subcranial-midfacial degloving
Malignant tumors extending to the inferior/anterior/lateral maxillary walls	Subcranial-transfacial
Lateral skull base, cavernous sinus, middle fossa or infratemporal fossa	Subcranial-orbitozygomatic
Lower clival region	Subcranial-LeFort I
Orbital apex or intraorbital extension	Subcranial-transorbital
Malignant tumors extending to the maxillary sinus with intraorbital extension	Subcranial-transfacial-transorbital

complications occurred in 35% of patients operated upon via the classical subcranial approach alone. There was no statistically significant difference between the two groups. The complication rate encountered in patients operated upon via the combined approaches was similar to that following the subcranial approach alone, despite the extensive resections required in cases of multicompartment tumor involvement. An international study group recently published three papers on different characteristics of patients after craniofacial surgery [3, 13, 14]. Their 36% rate of postoperative complications (433/1,100 patients) is similar to the complication rate found in our study. Nevertheless, Ganly et al. reported 4.7% mortality rate [13], compared to 0% in our series.

Survival

Gil and Fliss analyzed the overall and disease-free survival of all patients with malignant tumors operated upon by combinations of the subcranial approach. The mean follow-up time was 33±4 months. The 2-year overall and disease-free survival was 66% and 60%, respectively. The disease-free and overall survival rates of patients operated upon via the combinations of the subcranial approaches did not differ from the survival of patients operated upon by the subcranial approach alone (as reported by the same group [15]), and they were also similar to the results of other studies of patients with malignant tumors [13, 14].

Quality of Life

In order to gain an insight into the QOL of patients operated upon via the combined subcranial approach Gil et al. analyzed their QOL using a disease-specific questionnaire. The QOL of these patients may be lower than that of patients operated upon via the classical subcranial approach alone, due to a larger extirpation and increased morbidity. Therefore the authors compared the QOL scores of the two groups. The QOL of 13 patients operated upon via combinations of the subcranial approach and that of 23 patients operated by the classical subcranial approach alone was assessed retrospectively using the ASBS QOL ques-

tionnaire [16–18]. The results are summarized in Table 39.2. The overall QOL of the two groups was similar (p=0.40). The scores for the role of performance, physical function, vitality, pain and impact upon emotions domains were very similar for the two groups. There was, however, a significant difference in the disease-specific domain between the two groups (p<0.0004). Similar results were found in a prospective analysis of 17 patients operated upon via the classical approach and 12 patients operated upon via a combined approach, before and 6 months after the operation.

Most of our patients reported that the surgical procedure improved or did not affect their overall QOL. The only domain that showed a significantly lower QOL score was the specific symptoms domain which includes questions on the function of taste and smell, mastication, appearance, nasal secretions and visual function, which would be expected to be affected by wide resections involving the hard palate (subcranial with radical or partial maxillectomy), the orbit (subcranial-transorbital approach) or both.

Conclusions

The techniques presented in this chapter are innovative combinations of various commonly used procedures. This chapter proposes a comprehensive approach for the resection of complex anterior skull-base tumors with multicompartment invasion. Figures 39.3 and 39.4 summarize our algorithm for extirpation of large tumors with multicompartment involvement in the skull base. Using these combined approaches, tumors that previously might have been resected in multiple stages can be approached in a single-stage *en bloc* fashion, with reliable reconstruction and excellent cosmetic and functional results. The incidence and severity of perioperative complications, QOL and survival associated with these techniques are similar to those encountered following the classical subcranial approach alone.

Continuing improvement of the proposed approaches along with adjuvant therapy and improved imaging methods will better surgical and functional results for patients with anterior skull-base tumors.

Table 39.2 QOL domain score for the classical and combined subcranial approaches

Approach	No. of patients	QOL domain						
		Role of performance	Physical function	Vitality	Pain	Specific symptoms	Impact on emotions	Overall
Combined approaches	13	2.4±0.6	2.5±0.3	2.4±0.7	2.83±0.3	2.2±0.7	2.7±0.8	2.55±0.4
Classical subcranial	23	2.7±0.67	2.7±0.4	2.8±0.6	2.81±0.3	2.8±0.4	2.6±0.7	2.88±0.6
P value	NS	NS	NS	NS	NS	0.004	NS	NS

NS not statistically significant.

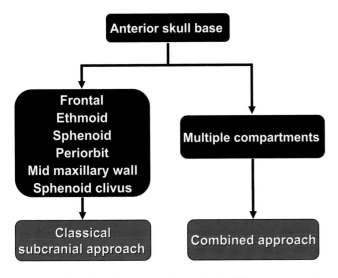

Fig. 39.3 Algorithm for excision of anterior skull-base tumors using open approaches. The classical subcranial approach is used for tumors originating in the central compartment. The combined approaches are used for tumors involving multiple compartments. *Mid* Middle.

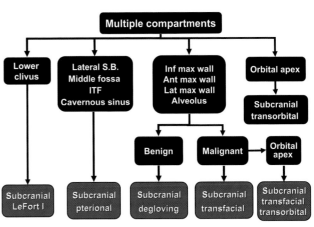

Fig. 39.4 Algorithm for excision of tumors involving multiple compartments. *S.B.* skull base, *ITF* infra temporal fossa, *Inf* inferior, *Ant* anterior, *Lat* lateral.

Tips to Avoid Complications

- Perform detailed preoperative physical and radiological evaluation.
- Use a multidisciplinary team approach.
- Tight dural seal using fascia lata or vascular flaps is crucial to prevent CSF leakage and meningitis.
- Postoperative monitoring in the intensive care unit.
- Avoid excessive CSF drainage (should not exceed approximately 10 cc per hour).
- Treat infection promptly and thoroughly using broad-spectrum antibiotics.

Take-Home Pearls

- Using combined approaches; tumors that previously might have been resected in multiple stages can be approached in a single-stage *en bloc* fashion.
- The surgical results of the combined approaches are good, with good quality of life and survival.

References

1. Ketcham AS, Wilkins RH, Vanburen JM, Smith RR (1963) A combined intracranial facial approach to the paranasal sinuses. Am J Surg 106:698–703
2. Shah JP (2003) Head and neck surgery and oncology. Mosby, New York, pp 57–93
3. Patel SG, Singh B, Polluri A et al (2003) Craniofacial surgery for malignant skull base tumors: report of an international collaborative study. Cancer 98:1179–1187
4. Raveh J (1979) Gesichtsschadelverletzungen: Eigene Erfahrungen und modificationen. Aktuel Probl ORL 3:145–154
5. Fliss DM, Zucker G, Cohen A et al (1999) Early outcome and complications of the extended subcranial approach to the anterior skull base. Laryngoscope 109:153–160
6. Raveh J, Laedrach K, Speiser M et al (1993) The subcranial approach for fronto-orbital and anteroposterior skull-base tumors. Arch Otolaryngol Head Neck Surg 119:385–393
7. Raveh J, Turk JB, Ladrach K et al (1995) Extended anterior subcranial approach for skull base tumors: long-term results. J Neurosurg 82:1002–1010
8. Casson PR, Bonanno PC, Converse JM (1974) The midface degloving procedure. Plast Reconstr Surg 53:102–103
9. Al Mefty O (1987) Supraorbital-pterional approach to skull base lesions. Neurosurgery 21:474–477
10. Yasargil MG, Reichman MV, Kubik S (1987) Preservation of the frontotemporal branch of the facial nerve using the interfascial temporalis flap for pterional craniotomy. Technical article. J Neurosurg 67:463–466

11. Fliss DM, Zucker G, Amir A et al (2001) The subcranial approach for anterior skull base tumors. Oper Techn Otolaryngol Head Neck Surg 11:238–253

12. Hao SP, Pan WL, Chang CN, Hsu YS (2003) The use of the facial translocation technique in the management of tumors of the paranasal sinuses and skull base. Otolaryngol Head Neck Surg 128:571–575

13. Ganly I, Patel SG, Singh B et al (2005) Complications of craniofacial resection for malignant tumors of the skull base: report of an International Collaborative Study. Head Neck 27:445–451

14. Ganly I, Patel SG, Singh B et al (2005) Craniofacial resection for malignant paranasal sinus tumors: report of an International Collaborative Study. Head Neck 27:575–584

15. Fliss DM, Gil Z, Spektor S et al (2002) Skull base reconstruction after anterior subcranial tumor resection. Neurosurg Focus 12:1–7

16. Gil Z, Abergel A, Spektor S et al (2004) Patient, caregiver, and surgeon perceptions of quality of life following anterior skull base surgery. Arch Otolaryngol Head Neck Surg 130:1276–1281

17. Gil Z, Abergel A, Spektor S et al (2004) Development of a cancer-specific anterior skull base quality-of-life questionnaire. J Neurosurg 100:813–819

18. Abergel A, Gil Z, Spektor S et al (2004) Quality-of-life following anterior skull base surgery. Harefuah 143:489–493

Chapter 40

Skull-Base Reconstruction Following Oncological Procedures

Ziv Gil and Dan M. Fliss

Core Messages

■ Tumor resection may create extensive skull-base defects requiring meticulous reconstruction.

■ There is no single "gold standard" technique for anterior cranial base reconstruction.

■ The fascia lata offers a versatile and reliable method of dural reconstruction.

■ Neovascularization of the fascia lata graft provides long-term viability without an overlying vascularized flap.

■ Reconstruction of the medial orbital wall is performed only after extensive resections.

■ For extensive orbital resections and exenterations use a temporalis muscle rotational flap.

■ For a radical maxillectomy use a musculocutaneous free flap supported by an obturator.

■ Use pericranial wrapping if adjuvant radiation therapy is planned in order to prevent osteoradionecrosis.

Contents

Introduction

Considerable progress has been made during the last decade in our understanding of the complex anatomy of the anterior skull base. Anatomical and clinical studies have contributed extensively to the development of new surgical approaches, while new imaging tools have significantly increased the accuracy of preoperative evaluation and postoperative follow-up of patients. Finally, the concept of cooperation between multidisciplinary teams has been adopted for the treatment of these tumors allowing complete eradication of large tumors involving the skull base and craniofacial regions.

When tumors arising in the anterior skull base invade both soft and hard tissues of the skull base, tumor resection may create extensive skull-base defects and produce a free conduit between the paranasal sinuses and the intracranial space. Following tumor extirpation, skull-base defects require precise and durable reconstruction in order to (1) form a fluid-tight dural seal, (2) provide a barrier between the contaminated sinonasal space and the sterile subdural compartment, (3) prevent air flow into the intracranial space, (4) maintain a functional sinonasal system, and (5) provide a good cosmetic outcome.

A variety of approaches have been developed to accomplish these goals. A split calvarial bone graft, hydroxyapatite paste or titanium mesh may be utilized for bony reconstruction. Autologous flaps (pericranial or galeal flaps) and artificial substitutions are often used for reconstruction of the skull base. Unfortunately, these methods bear significant disadvantages. Local flaps are often insufficient in size for reliable restoration of extensive anterior skull-base defects [1]. Synthetic substitutions of dura and bone can induce chronic inflammation, carry a high risk of infection and are inferior to biological sources in terms of strength and sealing quality [2].

Recent progress in microvascular and surgical techniques has enabled the development and implementation of free tissue transfer. Following skull-base resection, free flaps may be used for massive defects, with excellent surgical results and low complication rates [1, 3, 4]. Free tissue transfer is, however, a relatively complex surgical procedure that requires high technical qualifications. Another drawback of this method is the bulk of the muscular free flap, which may mask local recurrence and make radiological follow-up more difficult [5].

Autografts, such as fascia lata and temporalis fascia, have been used in the past for skull-base reconstruction, but they are usually covered with a vascularized flap (i.e. free muscular flaps, pericranial or galeal flaps), assuming that an overlying vascular tissue is essential in order to preserve long-term viability of the fascial graft [6].

In any situation, failure to create adequate reconstruction harbors significant complications, among them cerebrospinal fluid (CSF) leakage, meningitis, brain herniation, and tension pneumocephalus [7]. Although the subcranial or craniofacial approaches have become an established procedures for management of anterior skull base tumors [8], surgeons commonly use combinations of methods in order to accomplish satisfactory anterior skull-base reconstruction. Thus, there is no single "gold standard" technique that is both simple and reliable for reducing the morbidity and mortality associated with anterior cranial base operations.

This chapter describes a reliable and reproducible algorithm for cranial base reconstruction, with low rates of intra- and extracranial complications. The healing process of the reconstructed base of skull is described and evidence is provided to show that long-term viability of the graft is achievable without an overlying vascularized flap.

Types of Reconstruction

Regional Flaps

This reconstruction modality has been shown to be a reasonable option for dural reconstruction [1]. This technique is often sufficient to form a barrier separating the dura from the nasopharynx, and the pericranial and galeal flaps are the most common regional flaps chosen for this purpose [9]. They are readily available, easily harvested, and can be used to repair various dural defects. Galeal flaps may, however, not always be fit for use, particularly after radiation therapy or previous operations. They can also cause functional and cosmetic complications, including sensorimotor loss and regional alopecia [10]. Furthermore, galeal or pericranial flaps may be too small to cover defects of the frontal bone (e.g., burr holes and craniotomy bone cuts). Loss of galea and frontalis muscle from the undersurface of the frontal scalp means that there will be a very thin and poorly vascularized flap of skin for covering the bone flap, and therefore its use after radiation therapy could be problematic.

Free Avascular Flaps

The double layer fascia lata is often used as the standard material for anterior skull-base reconstruction. We have previously described a simple technique for harvesting large fascia lata sheaths which affords a low complication rate and low donor limb morbidity [11]. The thin and low mass properties of the fascia lata enable the surgeon to cover large dural defects with a single fascial sheath. Furthermore, the flexibility of the fascia lata enables coating of extensive cranial defects, including parts

of the orbit and paranasal sinuses. Large cranial base defects and prior surgery and radiotherapy (previously considered indications for free flap reconstruction [12]) can be managed by fascia alone, and free flaps, autologous fat, or skin grafts are not necessary in our opinion for achieving a reliable anterior skull-base reconstruction.

Several authors believe that bony reconstruction of the skull base is necessary to support the newly reconstructed skull base and to prevent herniation of the cranial contents [13]. However, recent reports indicate that reconstruction with a double-layer fascia does not require a rigid support of bone or synthetic materials. In the authors' hands not one brain herniation occurred in a series of 120 procedures. Furthermore, this procedure does not require the high technical qualifications which are essential for free muscle transfer. Finally, the overall duration of the reconstructive procedure described here is not longer than that for a pericranial flap [14], and takes considerably less time than free tissue transfer procedures [15].

Routine postoperative radiological follow-up of patients after extirpation of malignant anterior skull base tumors is required in all cases. The relatively low bulk of the fascia lata facilitates radiological follow-up in patients with an increased risk of local recurrence. The use of fascial flaps does not require the utilization of skin grafts or muscle flaps for covering the nasopharyngeal space. Transnasal endoscopic examination several weeks postoperatively reveals that the exposed nasal surface of the fascial flap has been completely covered by the neighboring sinonasal mucosa.

Free Flaps

Free flaps are usually used for reconstruction in cases which require anterior skull-base tumor resection and radical maxillectomy with or without orbital exenteration. The rectus abdominis is the most commonly used free flap in this anatomical area, followed by the lateral thigh, radial forearm and latissimus dorsi flaps. Free tissue transfer promises flexibility in flap content and design, and provides the opportunity to introduce a large quantity of well-vascularized tissue to the reconstructed area in a single-stage operation. In our study, the rectus abdominis or lateral thigh free flaps also allowed adequate support to the obturator, with good cosmesis and functional outcome.

Bony Reconstructions

Bony reconstruction is used for orbital, nasal and anterior frontal sinus wall reconstruction. This can be achieved with the use of biological tissue, such as a split calvarial bone graft or the posterior wall of the frontal sinus, or with artificial materials, such as 3D titanium mesh or BoneSource. These materials are wrapped with a pericranial flap if postoperative radiation is planned. Obliteration of the frontal sinus is indicated following extirpation of small benign tumors confined to the frontal sinus (Fig. 40.1a), and can be easily achieved with free abdominal fatty tissue. On the other hand, resection of the posterior frontal sinus and frontal sinus cranialization is mandatory if the tumor invades the intracranial space (Fig. 40.1b). In this

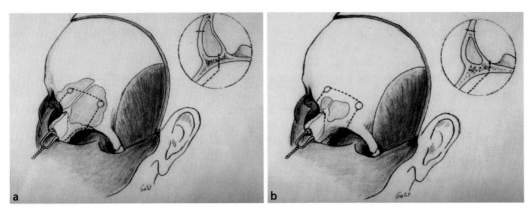

Fig. 40.1a,b Surgical approach to the anterior skull base. **a** Following extirpation of small benign tumors confined to the frontal sinus the anterior base of skull is preserved. In this case obliteration of the frontal sinus is required. **b** Following resection of the anterior and posterior frontal sinus, frontal sinus cranialization is performed requiring reconstruction of the anterior base of the skull

Table 40.1 Reconstruction modalities following anterior skull-base tumor resection

Type of defect	Reconstructive modality
Minimal dural tear	Primary closure
Small dural defect	Temporalis fascia
Moderate-to-large dural defect	Fascia lata
Bony defect: orbital wall, nasal and frontal bones	Posterior frontal sinus wall graft
	Split calvarial bone graft
	Titanium mesh
Posterior sinus wall intact	Frontal sinus obliteration with abdominal fat, if needed
Posterior sinus wall involved	Frontal sinus cranialization
Orbital exenteration	Temporalis muscle flap and split thickness skin graft
Orbitomaxillary resection	Rectus abdominus free flap and obturator
Orbital wall resection	Titanium mesh
	Fascia lata sling
	Septal cartilage
Orbital wall resection or medial maxillectomy	Dacryorhinocystostomy
Perioperative radiotherapy	Pericranial wrapping of all osteotomized bony segments or titanium mesh

case, the outer layer of the fascia lata serves as the roof of the paranasal cavity.

gorithm for skull-base reconstruction according to the type of craniobasal defect is shown in Table 40.1.

A Comprehensive Algorithm for Skull-Base Reconstruction

The surgical technique of the anterior skull base resection is described in chapter 39 of this book [16–19]. The reconstruction technique is tailored to the type and size of the cranial defect, based on radiological and intraoperative calculations. Our al-

Dural Reconstruction

Primary closure of the dura is performed whenever possible. A graft of temporalis fascia is used if the defect is small. If tumor resection results in an extensive skull-base defect, a second surgical team simultaneously harvests a large fascia lata sheath. The size of the fascia used for reconstruction is tailored according to the dimension of the dural and skull base defects. The fascia is tacked under the edges of the dura and carefully sutured in place. The dural repair is then covered with a second layer of fascia that is applied against the entire undersurface of the ethmoidal roof, the sella and the sphenoidal area. Fibrin glue is used to provide additional protection against CSF leakage. Following dural repair, Vaseline gauze is applied below the dura and into the paranasal cavity in order to provide additional support against pulsation.

Frontal Sinus Reconstruction

A *type A* osteotomy is performed for a limited, benign frontal sinus lesion. We suggest performing obliteration of the frontal sinus with abdominal fat in such cases or to leave the sinus intact (Fig. 40.1a). Alternatively, for malignant tumors, posterior sinus wall violations or major dural tears, we routinely perform a *type B* osteotomy, with frontal sinus cranialization ex vivo (Fig. 40.1b). After removing all the mucosa from the sinus, the earlier osteotomized segment is repositioned in its original anatomical place and fixed with prebent titanium plates.

Bony Reconstruction

Hydroxyapatite paste (BoneSource) or 3D titanium mesh can be used for small defects of the calvarium following removal of the frontal sinus outer table. Alternatively, biological materials, such as a split calvarial bone graft or a posterior frontal sinus wall graft, are used for the same purpose. A split calvarial bone graft or posterior frontal sinus wall can be used for reconstruction when the tumor involves the nasal bone or an adjacent frontoorbital segment. A bone graft can be also used for dorsal nasal support if the nasal septum has been violated. Medpor biometrical implant (Porex Corporation, Fairburn, GA) is used in cases of a large frontal or temporal bone defect and only when postoperative radiotherapy is not planned. The same material is

used for cosmetic reconstruction of large temporal defects following rotation of a temporalis muscle flap.

Orbital Reconstruction

Reconstruction of the medial orbital wall is performed only in cases in which a total removal of this segment is necessary or if the periorbit is excised. In these situations, a split calvarial bone graft, fascia lata sling or 3D titanium mesh covered with pericranium can be utilized (Fig. 40.2). Septal cartilage can be used for reconstruction of a limited defect of the inferior orbital wall. For extensive orbital wall resections and if eye globe exenteration is performed, a temporalis muscle flap and a split-thickness skin graft can be used. For a radical maxillectomy with or without orbital exenteration, we use a lateral thigh free flap or a rectus abdominis musculocutaneous free flap to obliterate this large defect and to support the obturator from above (Fig. 40.3). A dacryorhinocystostomy (DCR) is performed on all patients undergoing orbital wall resection or medial maxillectomy.

Following tumor resection and reconstruction, a centripetal compression of both globes is performed to reduce telecanthus. This method involves guiding two threads through the medial canthal ligament and driving them underneath the nasofrontoorbital (NFO) segment. The threads are tightened and fixed to the contralateral frontal plates in order to enable medial compression and alignment, thereby avoiding telecanthus altogether.

Pericranial Wrapping

For patients undergoing extirpation of malignant tumors and for whom adjuvant radiation therapy is planned, Gil and Fliss suggest wrapping the NFO segment with a pericranial flap in order to prevent osteoradionecrosis [20]. A pericranial flap is also used in cases of orbital wall reconstruction in order to cover the bone-graft segments or the titanium mesh, and we wrap the

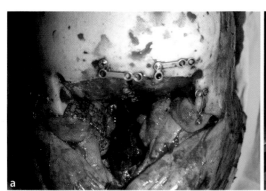
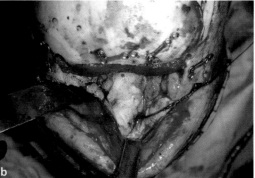

Fig. 40.2a,b Orbital reconstruction following subcranial resection in a patient with squamous cell carcinoma. **a** The periorbit was reconstructed with titanium mesh. **b** Wrapping of the frontonasoorbital segment and mesh was accomplished with a pericranial flap

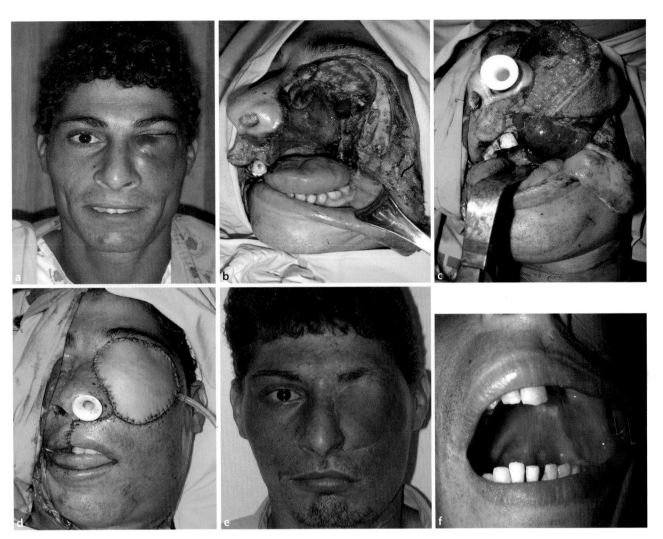

Fig. 40.3a–f Reconstruction following resection of an anterior skull-base malignant peripheral nerve sheath tumor, including orbital exenteration and radical maxillectomy. **a** Preoperative picture of the patient showing left orbital involvement. **b** The surgical defect following resection of the tumor. **c** Reconstruction of the orbita and maxilla is achieved using a rectus abdominus free flap. **d** Postoperative result. A nasal airway is placed for preservation of nasal breathing. **e** 6 months after surgery. **f** Epithelialization of the hard palate

NFO segment with a rotational temporoparietal fascia bilaterally (Fig. 40.3). This procedure begins with the removal of all the mucosa from the under surface of the earlier osteotomized bone segment. The frontal sinus bone is cranialized and the NFO segment is repositioned in its original anatomical position. Wrapping is accomplished by a double-sided covering of the bone segment with the pericranial flap. This vascularized tissue is guided underneath the bony segment to cover the intranasal surface and then it is externalized over the entire frontal area. The NFO segment and its overlying pericranial flap are fixed with prebent titanium plates.

Surgical Results and Complications

Reconstruction of the anterior skull base is technically challenging and may be further complicated by several factors. First, there is a paucity of local tissue that is available for transfer into the defect. Second, previous radiation treatment significantly reduces tissue perfusion and so delays normal wound healing. Finally, many of these patients have undergone earlier surgical interventions prior to the index operation, thus increasing its complexity and decreasing tissue perfusion, secondary to scar tissue formation.

In a recent study, Gil et al. evaluated the results of their reconstruction algorithm performed on 109 patients who had undergone 120 procedures for anterior skull-base tumor resections. Of their patients, 50% had undergone at least one previous operation and one-third had undergone perioperative radiation therapy. The principle skull-base reconstruction method performed was by means of the double layer fascia lata. The tumor extended to the dura mater in most of these patients. They used the temporalis muscle flap in the six procedures involving orbital exenteration and employed the same method of double layer fascial flap for anterior skull-base reconstruction. A craniofacial reconstruction was required if tumor resection produced a significant bony defect of the orbital walls, nasal bone or anterior frontal sinus wall. This was achieved by applying a split calvarial bone graft or posterior sinus wall. A titanium mesh covered with a pericranial flap was utilized for reconstruction of the medial orbital walls and to cover extensive calvarial defects. A hydroxyapatite paste was seldom used to fill defects in the calvarium after harvesting the outer table for reconstruction. A rectus abdominis free flap was utilized for reconstruction of large defects following subcranial resection and radical maxillectomy.

The overall complication rate in their series was 38%, but the incidence of CSF leakage, intracranial infection and tension pneumocephalus was less than 5%. One patient who was operated upon for a pituitary adenoma and who suffered from meningitis died 42 days after surgery. The overall postoperative complications associated with skull-base and cranial reconstructions are listed in Table 40.2. Seven of the eight patients who had osteoradionecrosis with fistula had undergone perioperative radiotherapy. Because of the risk of osteoradionecrosis of the NFO segment in patients who undergo perioperative radiation therapy, Gil and Fliss utilized a new method for wrapping the frontal bone segment with pericranial flap [20]. Bone flap necrosis did not occur in any of the 26 patients who underwent this procedure. Wound dehiscence in two patients associated with temporalis muscle transfer following orbital exenteration was successfully treated with local flaps several days after surgery. The complication rates in the patients with benign and malignant tumors were similar.

Table 40.2 Complications of skull-base reconstruction procedures

Complication	n	%
Telecanthus	9	7.5
Osteoradionecrosis and fistula	8	6.6
Epiphora	7	5.8
Wound infection	6	5
Deep vein thrombosis	6	5
Meningitis	4	3.3
Tension pneumocephalus	1	0.8
Mucocele	2	1.6
Intracranial hematoma	2	1.6
Pneumonia	2	1.6
CSF leakage	1	0.8
Total	45	

Healing Processes in Avascular Flap Reconstruction

The healing process in fascia lata grafts was investigated in seven patients. Fragments of the fascia lata that had previously been used for skull-base reconstruction and were not involved with the index tumor were excised and submitted for histopathological evaluation (H&E). Microscopic examination revealed that the entire graft was composed of viable dense fibrocollagenous tissue (Fig. 40.4). The bipolar, wavy-shaped nuclei of the fibroblasts were embedded in a collagenous stroma in large areas. Immunohistochemical staining for endothelial cells with CD31 and factor VIII showed proliferation of neovascular channels lined by plumped endothelial cells in the specimens of four patients. The histological findings demonstrated an almost complete fibrous replacement of the fascia lata allograft.

We also studied the histopathology of the reconstructed fascia lata in order to investigate the healing process of the reconstructed area in patients who had undergone a second operation. Our histological analysis of previously harvested human fascial flaps showed evidence of integration of a vascularized fibrous tissue into the fascial graft. The fascial flap was uniformly coated by fibrous tissue, and invasion of blood vessels had occurred without the presence of an overlying vascularized flap in all fascial flaps that were examined. Using an animal model, Tachibana et al. [2] demonstrated a tight connection between the fascial graft and the dura within 1 week of surgery, in agreement with our findings. They reported that the fascial graft had been completely replaced by durable fibrous tissue 2 weeks following the surgical repair, and speculated that fibroblast growth factor b plays a significant role in the healing process of free fascial grafts [21].

Thus, our current work and this animal model confirm that excellent skull-base reconstruction can be achieved without the need for blood supply from an overlying regional flap or free muscular flap. Moreover, the rapid healing process of the fascial reconstruction provides a robust physiological barrier between the nasopharynx and the intracranial space within days following surgery, no small advantage in its use.

New Frontiers in Skull-Base Reconstruction

During the last decade laser tissue welding systems have moved from the laboratory to accepted clinical practice. The efficacy of a temperature-controlled CO_2 laser soldering technique for skull-base reconstruction has recently been described in reports from the Tel Aviv University Skull Base Surgery and Applied Physics Groups. In a recent work, Gil et al. developed an animal model for dura–fascia repair using a novel laser apparatus that enables the control of surface temperature, thereby affording protection to the brain parenchyma during dural soldering [22]. The authors investigated this tissue-closure technique for immediate sealing of the dura mater. Dura–fascia laser soldering should provide five primary physiological and technical benefits: (1) a high-quality seal to provide a fluid-tight and air-tight barrier; (2) the ability to withstand considerable shearing forces and the ability to support a CSF pressure greater than 20 mmHg

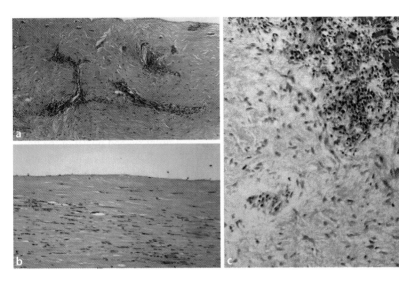

Fig. 40.4a–c Neovascularization of the fascia lata graft 12 months after surgery in a case with recurrent tumor (H&E staining). **a** Low magnification of the fascia lata shows that the graft has been replaced with a viable dense fibrocollagenous tissue. **b** High magnification shows fibroblasts embedded in a dense collagenous stroma. **c** High magnification shows the presence of neovascularized channels lined by endothelial cells

during the postoperative period; (3) a biophysical strength and elastic properties of the soldered tissue that is close to those of intact tissue within seconds of fusion; (4) the avoidance of artificial material, which should reduce the incidence of dehiscence and infection; and (5) simplicity in application and a reduction in the time required for the procedure. It should also make dural closure possible in situations in which space constraints make traditional suture closure difficult, as in anterior skull-base procedures. Gil et al. used a welding system for heating spots on tissues to approximately 70°C with an accuracy of several degrees. The laser beam is moved along the reconstructed dura during welding. The CO_2 laser was chosen because its radiation is highly absorbed by water, soft tissues, and albumin. The laser energy heats only the top (roughly 20 mm) of the albumin layer, and the underlying dura–fascia layers are heated by conduction. Heat, therefore, does not penetrate deep into the tissue. This procedure greatly reduces the risk of thermal damage to underlying tissues. In vivo results from our laboratory performed on live pigs showed no neurological or surgical complications (e.g., CSF leakage) after dura soldering [23, 24]. Histological examination of the surgical specimen showed a fluid-tight seal with no evidence of brain tissue damage. Furthermore, bonding of the fascia and dura was complete, without necrosis or excessive inflammation. This laser system has the potential to be used in endoscopic surgery. Laser soldering therefore offers an alternative to

for endoscopic dural reconstruction. Moreover, soldering can be done in deep and narrow areas of the skull base (e.g., the sphenoid and sellar region) where suture placement is difficult, providing the surgeon with another tissue bonding technique for dural reconstruction in those areas.

Conclusions

We have reviewed our experience of skull-base reconstruction after extirpation of tumors and propose a comprehensive ap-

proach to complex defects in the anterior craniobasal compartment. Our "dray horse" for dural reconstruction is the double layer fascia lata, which provides a simple and versatile means of skull-base reconstruction after resection of advanced tumors. The other reconstruction methods we use according to need are bone grafts, titanium mesh, temporalis muscle flap, free flaps and pericranial wrapping. The incidence and severity of perioperative complications associated with our double layer fascia lata technique are comparable to other reconstructive methods. Histological findings indicate that free fascial grafts survive via local proliferation of a newly formed vascular layer embedded within the fascial sheath. Future developments of biomedical materials will probably bring with them continuing improvement in current techniques for skull-base reconstruction with fewer complications and the promise of a better quality of life for the patients.

Tips to Avoid Complications

- Perform detailed preoperative physical and radiological evaluation.
- Note that previous surgery or radiotherapy significantly delays normal wound healing.
- Because of the risk of osteoradionecrosis in patients undergoing perioperative radiotherapy, wrap the frontal bone segment with a pericranial flap.
- Postoperative monitoring in the intensive care unit.
- Treat infection promptly and thoroughly using broad-spectrum antibiotics.
- Use combinations of methods in order to accomplish satisfactory anterior skull-base reconstruction.

Take-Home Pearls

- The "dray horse" for dural reconstruction is the double layer fascia lata.
- Other reconstruction methods are used according to surgical need; they include bone grafts, titanium mesh, temporalis muscle flap, free flaps and pericranial wrapping.
- The incidence and severity of perioperative complications associated with our double layer fascia lata technique are low compared to other reconstructive methods.
- Histological findings indicate that free fascial grafts survive via local proliferation of a newly formed vascular layer embedded within the fascial sheath.

References

1. Neligan PC, Mulholland S, Irish J et al (1996) Flap selection in cranial base reconstruction. Plast Reconstr Surg 98:1159–1166
2. Tachibana E, Saito K, Fukuta K, Yoshida J (2002) Evaluation of the healing process after dural reconstruction achieved using a free fascial graft. J Neurosurg 96:280–286
3. Clayman GL, DeMonte F, Jaffe DM et al (1995) Outcome and complications of extended cranial-base resection requiring microvascular free-tissue transfer. Arch Otolaryngol Head Neck Surg 121:1253–1257
4. Califano J, Cordeiro PG, Disa JJ et al (2003) Anterior cranial base reconstruction using free tissue transfer: changing trends. Head Neck 25:89–96
5. Kiyokawa K, Tai Y, Inoue Y et al (2000) Efficacy of temporal musculopericranial flap for reconstruction of the anterior base of the skull. Scand J Plast Reconstr Surg Hand Surg 34:43–53
6. Hasegawa M, Torii S, Fukuta K, Saito K (1995) Reconstruction of the anterior cranial base with the galeal frontalis myofascial flap and the vascularized outer table calvarial bone graft. Neurosurgery 36:725–731
7. Boyle JO, Shah KC, Shah JP (1998) Craniofacial resection for malignant neoplasms of the skull base: an overview. J Surg Oncol 69:275–284
8. Fliss DM, Zucker G, Amir A et al (2001) The subcranial approach for anterior skull base tumors. Oper Techn Otolaryngol Head Neck Surg 11:238–253
9. Fukuta K, Potparic Z, Sugihara T et al (1994) A cadaver investigation of the blood supply of the galeal frontalis flap. Plast Reconstr Surg 94:794–800
10. Snyderman CH, Janecka IP, Sekhar LN et al (1990) Anterior cranial base reconstruction: role of galeal and pericranial flaps. Laryngoscope 100:607–614
11. Amir A, Gatot A, Zucker G et al (2000) Harvesting of fascia lata sheaths: a rational approach. Skull Base Surg 10:29–34
12. McCutcheon IE, Blacklock JB, Weber RS et al (1996) Anterior transcranial (craniofacial) resection of tumors of the paranasal sinuses: surgical technique and results. Neurosurgery 38:471–479
13. Derome P (1988) The transbasal approach to tumors invading the base of the skull. In: Schmidek H, Sweet W (eds) Current techniques in operative neurosurgery. Grune and Stratton, New York, p 629
14. Sundaresan N, Shah JP (1988) Craniofacial resection for anterior skull base tumors. Head Neck Surg 10:219–224
15. Nibu K, Sasaki T, Kawahara N et al (1998) Complications of craniofacial surgery for tumors involving the anterior cranial base. Neurosurgery 42:455–461
16. Raveh J (1979) Gesichtsschädelverletzungen: Eigene Erfahrungen und Modifikationen. Aktuel Probl ORL 3:145–154
17. Raveh J, Laedrach K, Iizuka T et al (1998) Subcranial extended anterior approach for skull base tumors: surgical procedure and reconstruction. In: Donald PJ (ed) Surgery of the skull base. Lippincott-Raven, New York, pp 239–261
18. Raveh J, Laedrach K, Speiser M et al (1993) The subcranial approach for fronto-orbital and anteroposterior skull-base tumors. Arch Otolaryngol Head Neck Surg 119:385–393
19. Raveh J, Turk JB, Ladrach K et al (1995) Extended anterior subcranial approach for skull base tumors: long-term results. J Neurosurg 82:1002–1010
20. Gil Z, Fliss DM (2005) Pericranial wrapping of the frontal bone after anterior skull base tumor resection. Plast Reconstr Surg 116:395–398
21. Folkman J, Klagsbrun M (1987) Angiogenic factors. Science 235:442–447
22. Gil Z, Shaham A, Vasilyev T et al (2005) Novel laser tissue-soldering technique for dural reconstruction. J Neurosurg 103:87–91
23. Forer B, Vasilyev T, Brosh T et al (2006) Dural defect repair with fascia by a CO2 laser system in a porcine model. Laryngoscope 116:1002–1006
24. Forer B, Vasilyev T, Brosh T et al (2005) Repair of pig dura in vivo using temperature controlled CO(2) laser soldering. Lasers Surg Med 37:286–292

40

Chapter 41

Skull-Base Surgery in Children and Adolescents

41

Ziv Gil and Dan M. Fliss

■ There are several differences between adults and children with regard to skull-base anatomy.

■ In the pediatric population, benign tumors are threefold more common than malignant tumors.

■ Most common skull-base approaches can be used for children and adolescents.

■ In general, sarcomas occurring in children and young adults tend to be chemotherapy-sensitive.

■ Skull-base procedures produce a negligible net effect on the cosmetic and functional outcomes in children.

Contents

Introduction

Technical developments in the fields of head and neck surgery and neurosurgery have had a major impact on the long-term survival and quality of life of patients with lesions involving the skull base [1–6]. The variety of approaches that have been developed have been applied mainly to adult patients, and little is known about their feasibility in children.

There are several differences between cranial base tumors in adults and children. First, skull-base tumors are relatively uncommon in children. Second, the types of tumors as well as the oncological management and prognosis of patients vary between adults and children. Third, anatomical differences, such as the size of the cranial fossa and paranasal sinuses or stage of tooth eruption, may also influence the choice of surgical approach [7]. A major concern in skull-base procedures in children is the potential impact of osteotomies on the subsequent development of the face and paranasal sinuses. The feasibility of standard skull-base procedures in the pediatric population and their potential effect on the long-term esthetic results in these patients have not been established.

This chapter presents the recent developments in the surgical approach to pediatric skull-base tumors. We describe a variety of approaches and their postoperative results, and discuss the feasibility and versatility of these procedures.

Anatomy

There are several differences in skull-base anatomy between adults and children. The most significant anatomical difference between children and adults is the size of the cranial base and maxillofacial complex. Another difference is the inconsistency of specific anatomical landmarks in children in comparison with the fully developed cranium of adults. The mastoid air cells are also not fully pneumatized in very young children since the mastoid and middle fossa reach adult size only after the age of 10 years [8]. The superior orbital fissure, which serves as a landmark for orbital and orbitozygomatic approaches, may also be absent in children younger than 8 years [7]. Another important anatomical discrepancy is the developmental stage of the paranasal sinuses: the frontal sinus starts to develop from the age of 6 years and reaches its full size at the end of puberty [8]. The surgeon must cautiously consider the variability in size of the frontal sinus if a frontal craniotomy is required. For example, osteotomy of the anterior frontal sinus wall should be tailored according to the size and degree of development of the sinus. In such a case, an intraoperative transnasal illumination of the frontal sinus is used, in order to outline its borders before the osteotomies are carried out.

Pathology

In the pediatric population, benign tumors are three times more common than malignant tumors [9]. This is most probably the reason for the prognosis being more favorable in children (80% 2-year survival) than in adults (45–80%) [10, 11]. Gil et al. recently presented the surgical outcomes in 67 children who had undergone skull-base tumor resection [12]. Benign tumors were twice as common as malignant tumors (Fig. 41.1). The most common tumor was craniopharyngioma (15%). The most common malignant tumor was sarcoma (13.4%). Table 41.1 summarizes the underlying pathologies in the children in this study.

Two of the most characterized benign tumors that originate in the skull base are schwannomas and neurofibromas. Neurofibroma type 2 (NF2) is an autosomal dominant disorder that is frequently associated with bilateral vestibular schwannomas along with other tumors in the central nervous system. These tumors are more common in adults and adolescents. After vestibular schwannomas, the second most common disease associated with mutation of the *NF2* gene is meningioma. In the pediatric population, approximately 40% of the meningiomas are associated with *NF2*, which must be ruled out in any child with meningioma, especially if it is multifocal. Other less common genetic syndromes associated with meningioma are non-*NF2*-associated meningiomas, Cowden's syndrome, Gorlin's nevoid basal cell syndrome, Li-Fraumeni syndrome, Turcot's/ Gardener's syndrome and von Hippel-Lindau disease. Juvenile

nasopharyngeal angiofibroma (JNA) is a benign tumor that occurs exclusively in adolescent and young adult males. This is a locally invasive fibrovascular tumor that originates in the sphenopalatine foramen area. A gain of chromosome X leads to androgen receptor gene gain and may suggest that JNA is an androgen-dependent tumor [13]. This is supported by the finding that beta-catenin, known to be over expressed in JNAs, acts as a coactivator of the androgen receptor. Its most common presenting symptom is epistaxis. Biopsy should be avoided in patients with suspected JNA and diagnosis should be performed using imaging modalities including magnetic resonance imaging, and angiography.

Table 41.1 Histopathology of skull-base tumors

Pathology	*n*	%
Craniopharyngioma	10	15
Sarcoma	9	13.4
Juvenile nasopharyngeal angiofibroma	8	12
Chiasmatic glioma	8	12
Encephalocele	4	6
Epidermoid	4	6
Esthesioneuroblastoma	3	4.5
Germinoma	2	3
Juvenile pilocytic astrocytoma	2	3
Acoustic schwannoma	2	3
Neurofibroma	2	3
Eosinophilic granuloma	1	1.5
Aneurysmal bone cyst	1	1.5
Schwannoma	1	1.5
Fibrous dysplasia	1	1.5
Mucocele	1	1.5
Meningioma	1	1.5
Chondroma	1	1.5
Ependymoma	1	1.5
Squamous cell carcinoma	1	1.5
Hypothalamic hematoma	1	1.5
Gangliocytoma	1	1.5
Chordoma	1	1.5
Total	67	100

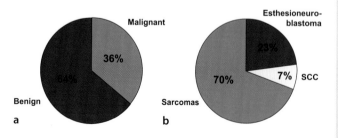

Fig. 41.1a,b Pathological features of pediatric skull base tumors. **a** Benign tumors are twice as common as malignant tumors. **b** Among malignant tumors, sarcomas are the most common (*SCC* squamous cell carcinoma). Sarcomas included: rhabdomyosarcoma, Ewing's sarcoma and osteogenic sarcoma

Soft-tissue sarcomas are infrequently found in the head and neck region in the mature population. These tumors are more common in childhood where up to 40% of them occur in the head and neck. Histologically, it is difficult to distinguish between skull-base soft-tissue tumors based on conventional pathological and cytological measures. For example, distinguishing between Ewing's sarcoma, embryonal rhabdomyosarcoma (RMS), small-cell osteogenic sarcoma and lymphoma may be challenging. RMS is the most common soft-tissue sarcoma of childhood, and also the most common skull-base malignant tumor in the pediatric population. RMS is divided into two major histologic subtypes: embryonal RMS and alveolar RMS. Embryonal RMS typically occurs in children <10 years of age and most frequently in the head and neck or skull-base regions. In contrast, alveolar RMS most commonly occurs in adolescents and young adults and typically in the trunk and extremities. The prognosis of embryonal RMS is generally favorable compared to alveolar RMS, which portends a poor prognosis.

Osteosarcoma is an uncommon tumor of skeletal origin that may involve the skull base and craniofacial area. In children, this is the most common nonhematological malignant tumor of bone, comprising more than half of the cases of bone malignancy among the pediatric population. Most osteosarcomas are high-grade tumors with a propensity to metastasize, resulting in a less than 10% long-term disease-free survival. Osteosarcoma is more common in children previously treated with radiotherapy for retinoblastoma. Retinoblastoma by itself is the most common malignant tumor of the orbit. Nevertheless, if treated early, this tumor rarely infiltrates the orbital roof and therefore is not considered a skull-base tumor by many. Among the common malignant skull-base tumors of neuroectodermal origin are esthesioneuroblastomas, Ewing's sarcoma, Askin's tumor, and malignant peripheral nerve sheath tumor (MPNST). Conventional histopathological classification of these tumors may be complicated since these neoplasms have similar morphological and cytological features. Esthesioneuroblastoma is a relatively uncommon tumor that arises from the olfactory epithelium in the upper nasal cavity and often shows an intracranial extension. It is rare in young children and is more frequent in adolescents. Esthesioneuroblastomas closely resemble Ewing's sarcoma and other peripheral primitive neuroectodermal tumors and therefore present a diagnostic challenge to the pathologist. Malignant peripheral nerve sheath tumor, also known as neurofibrosarcoma, malignant schwannoma or neurogenic sarcoma, is a rare neoplasm of Schwann cell origin. It is a rare tumor in both adults and the young.

Surgical Techniques

Various surgical techniques for extirpation of skull-base tumors have been established during the past 30 years [12, 14–16]. Most of the publications on base-of-skull surgery pertain to its applicability to adult patients since tumors located in this anatomical area are infrequent in the pediatric population. In contrast, very few reviews have been published in the English language literature on skull-base procedures in children [17, 18]. The first

advance in the techniques of transfacial approaches in children emerged from the work of Tessier et al. [19] on reconstruction of facial birth defects. This was later adopted and modified by Bruce et al. [20] for midline lesions. Teo et al. [9] reported the first retrospective analysis of skull-base operations in 26 patients younger than 21 years, and Brockmeyer et al. [7] and Hanbali et al. [21] recently reported their experience in 55 and 24 skull-base operations in children, respectively. Most of the children described in these reports had anterolateral, medial or posterior skull-base tumors, and the main approach to the anterior skull base and paranasal sinuses was the craniofacial/transfacial approach.

Approaches to the Anterior Skull Base

A bifrontal or unilateral subfrontal approach is used for tumors originating in the anterior skull base with intracranial involvement [22–24]. A subcranial approach is used for tumors involving the cribriform plate, the frontal sinus and for lesions extending far into the paranasal sinus, nasal cavity or orbits (Fig. 41.2 and 41.3a). This approach has been described in detail [25]. Following anesthesia, the skin is incised above the hairline and a bicoronal flap is created in a supraperiosteal plane. A flap is elevated anteriorly beyond the supraorbital ridges and laterally superficial to the temporalis fascia. The pericranial flap is elevated up to the periorbits, and the supraorbital nerves and vessels are carefully separated from the supraorbital notch. The lateral and medial walls of the orbits are then exposed, and the anterior ethmoidal arteries are clipped or ligated. The pericranium is elevated above the nasal bones, and the flap is rotated forward and held over the face throughout the rest of the procedure. Titanium micro- or miniplates are applied to the frontal bones and removed before the osteotomies to ensure the exact repositioning of the bony segments at the end of the operation. An osteotomy of the anterior frontal sinus wall alone or the anterior and posterior frontal sinus walls, together with the nasal bony frame, part of the medial wall of the orbit, and a segment of the superoposterior nasal septum is then performed. This approach provides an immediate and direct route to the cribriform plate and olfactory grooves, ethmoid sinuses, sphenoid sinuses, nasal cavities and both orbits. The optic canals may be exposed entirely if necessary, revealing the optic nerves.

Medial maxillectomy may also be performed from above through the subcranial approach if indicated. In cases of massive involvement of the lower segments of the maxilla or the pterygomaxillary fossa, a maxillectomy is performed using the transfacial approach (via a Weber Fergusson incision), the facial translocation technique or the midfacial degloving approach [26]. Large tumors which involve the maxilla and anterior cranial fossa require a combined approach (subcranial-transfacial, subcranial-transorbital, subcranial-degloving or pterional-degloving). Figures 41.2 and 41.3 show a combined transfacial transcranial approach and radical maxillectomy of a child with Ewing's sarcoma.

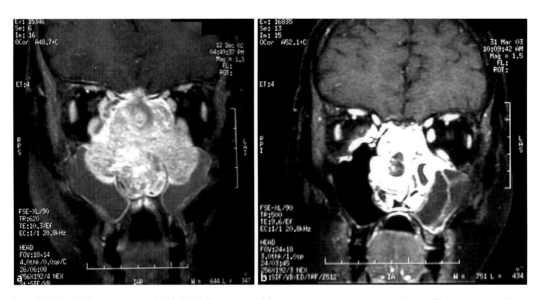

Fig. 41.2a,b A 14-year-old child with Ewing's sarcoma of the paranasal sinuses and anterior skull base. **a** Coronal MR image with gadolinium enhancement prior to treatment. **b** MR image after four courses of neoadjuvant chemotherapy with etoposide, ifosfamide, vincristine, Adriamycin and cyclophosphamide.

41

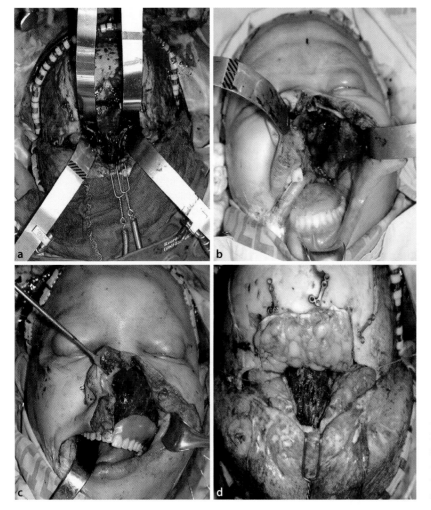

Fig. 41.3a–d Surgical resection of the tumor in the same patient as in Fig. 41.2. **a,b** Surgical approach which included a combined transfacial, subcranial approach. **c,d** Reconstruction of the defect with a double layer fascia lata, rectus abdominus free flap and obturator

Approaches to the Lateral and Posterior Skull Base

The authors utilize the pterional or orbitozygomatic approaches if the tumor extends to the middle cranial fossa or for lesions involving the cavernous sinus. A question mark skin incision is performed and a thick pericranial flap is dissected as a separate layer. The zygomatic process along with the lateral orbital wall is osteotomized and removed and the temporalis muscle is displaced inferiorly. Care is than taken not to injure the frontal branch of the facial nerve. This allows exposure of the pterional and infratemporal area. A single bone flap craniotomy is then performed which allows access to the middle cranial fossa [27]. A two-piece craniotomy (i.e. a low frontal craniotomy followed by an osteotomy of the roof of the orbit, the zygomatic process of the frontal bone and part of the glabella across the midline) may also used for patients with a large craniopharyngioma.

A retrosigmoid approach is used for tumors involving the cerebellopontine angle. In this approach, a craniotomy is performed behind the sigmoid sinus, near the angle of the sigmoid and lateral sinuses. The petrous bone is removed, allowing exposure and visualization of the internal auditory meatus. This approach may be combined with a radical mastoidectomy with or without a labyrinthectomy (i.e. retrosigmoid and translabyrinthine approach, respectively). Parietooccipital, transsphenoidal, posterolateral and temporal approaches are used for tumors involving the middle and posterior cranial fossa.

Reconstruction

The technique for reconstruction of the anterior skull base is designed according to the size of the cranial defect, based on radiological and intraoperative calculations and is not different from that in adult patients. Primary closure of the dura is performed whenever possible. A graft of temporalis fascia is used if the defect is limited. A double layer of fascia lata is used in cases with extensive skull-base defects. A split calvarial bone graft or posterior frontal sinus wall is used when the tumor involves the nasal bone or other frontoorbital segments. A bone graft can also be used for dorsal nasal support if the nasal septum has been resected. Reconstruction of the medial orbital walls is performed with a split calvarial bone graft or by a three-dimensional titanium mesh covered by pericranium. Hydroxyapatite paste (BoneSource) is used for small or medium defects of the calvarium following removal of the outer table (performed for grafting purposes).

A composite rectus abdominous free flap can be utilized to cover the orbital socket in cases of eye globe exenteration with radical maxillectomy, as well as in cases of a large anterior skull-base tumor resection which also requires radical maxillectomy. In patients undergoing extirpation of malignant tumors and for whom adjuvant radiation therapy is planned, we wrap the frontonasoorbital segment with a pericranial flap in order to prevent osteoradionecrosis [28, 29]. A pericranial flap is also used in cases of medial orbital wall reconstruction to cover the bone-graft segments or the titanium mesh.

After surgery, patients are immediately transferred to the pediatric critical care unit for 48–72 hours. All the patients in the current study were followed on a regular basis for a period of 3–60 months following discharge (average follow-up period of 2.5 years).

Surgical Results

Gil and Fliss recently reported total removal of tumors (>99%) in 49 of 67 children (73%), near-total removal (95–99%) in 6, and partial removal in 12. Following a mean follow-up of 3 years, 8% of the children had died of their disease, and 12.5% were alive with disease. The overall long-term complication rate was 32%, and included: panhypopituitarism, obesity, hemiparesis, osteoradionecrosis of the maxillary complex, ascites, learning disabilities, wound infection, visual-field defects, intraoperative carotid injury, syndrome of inappropriate ADH secretion, and air embolism due to atrioventricular shunt (one patient each). There were no cases of cerebrospinal fluid (CSF) leakage, intracranial infection or tension pneumocephalus. The complication rate in our pediatric series is also significantly lower than in the adult population following similar procedures. We recently published our experience with skull-base operations performed by the same surgeons [26, 28–30]. We found a 43% complication rate, including two patients with meningitis, one with CSF leakage and one with tension pneumocephalus. In our pediatric series, we encountered no such complications. It is possible that comorbidity, multiple surgical procedures and preoperative radiation increased the complication rate in the adults.

One of our key observations during pediatric skull-base procedures is that a child's brain is somewhat tighter than an adult's [12]. For example, in a few patients neither ventriculostomy nor opening the basal cisterns was effective in reducing brain tightness during surgery. In contrast, similar measures carried out in an adult patient would have provided a marked improvement in brain relaxation. We could not find any data relating to the differences in brain elasticity in various age groups. We hypothesize, however, that the pediatric brain may be tighter because the sulci, fissures, and cisterns that comprise the subarachnoid space are generally smaller, leaving a relatively larger portion of the intracranial volume for the parenchyma. In addition, neurovascular elements in children are thinner and more fragile than in adults. Therefore, CSF drainage results in less brain relaxation than in adults. We suggest that utilizing the subcranial or orbitozygomatic approaches can reduce brain retraction in the pediatric population, which might be even more significant than in adult neurosurgery.

Adjuvant Treatment

In general, sarcomas occurring in children and young adults tend to be chemotherapy-sensitive, particularly osteogenic sarcoma, rhabdomyosarcoma and Ewing's sarcoma [31]. On the other hand, in the more common situation of adult sarcomas, tumor resistance to chemotherapy occurs because of a high incidence of multidrug resistance [32, 33]. Except for the tumors mentioned above, the use of chemotherapy as a postoperative adjuvant or in a preoperative setting in an effort to decrease the extent of locoregional treatment is not yet completely established as standard management [34, 35].

Postoperative radiotherapy has been shown to improve local control of malignant skull-base tumors of various origins, but the benefit of radiation therapy for treatment of pediatric skull-base malignancies has not yet been evaluated. Regardless of the lack of prospective studies regarding the benefit of radiotherapy for head and neck or skull-base tumors, there has been a significant increase in the use of adjuvant radiation therapy for the treatment of this disease, especially high-grade tumors [36]. At our institutions, we generally recommend adjuvant radiotherapy for patients who have undergone a marginal surgical resection or for patients with a high-grade tumor.

Effect of Skull-Base Surgery on Facial Growth in Children

A major issue in pediatric craniofacial surgery is the need to avoid disruption of the permanent dentition within the maxillary complex during maxillotomy, since permanent tooth eruption does not take place before the age of 10 years [37]. Therefore we suggest that the use of the LeFort I down-fracture approach be avoided for this reason. In order to prevent injury to the tooth buds, a dental panoramic radiograph or coronal CT scan is required for presurgical planning of the osteotomies. The

midfacial degloving and transmaxillary approaches are suitable for wide exposure and extirpation of tumors originating in the paranasal sinuses and nasal cavity with preservation of normal tooth eruption.

Little is known on the effect of skull-base and craniofacial surgery on facial growth and development in the pediatric age group. Because the frontonasal suture is an active growth center of the anterior skull base up to the age of 16 years, one can speculate that osteotomies performed in that region might have an undesirable effect on midface development, and possibly affect both vertical and horizontal maxillary growth. Lowlicht et al. found the effect of LeFort I maxillary osteotomy on maxillary growth in a group of pediatric patients to be negligible [38].

In a recent study we evaluated the maxillary and midfacial development in a group of growing patients who had undergone excision of anterior skull-base tumors via the subcranial approach [12]. Cephalometric parameters were used for estimating facial growth in this population (Fig. 41.4). All subjects had superiorly positioned maxilla. The upper incisor teeth were proclined relative to the cranial base reference planes. Nevertheless, all cephalometric changes were within 10% of normal values. This study also compared two age groups: those with a growing facial skeleton (6–16 years old) and those no longer growing (17–18 years old). The cranial base relationship, the mandible-cranial relationship, the mandibular length and dental development (maxilla and mandible) were similar in these

41

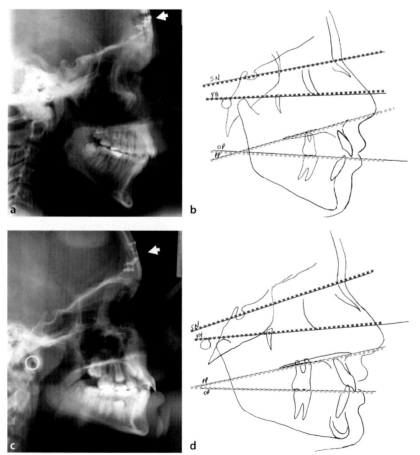

Fig. 41.4a–d Cephalometric analysis of two patients who underwent subcranial resection of a skull-base tumor: **a,b** a 6-year-old child; **c,d** an 18-year-old boy. The pictures show postoperative cephalograms (**a,c**) and an analysis of the radiographic images (**b,d**). *Red lines* cranial base relationship (angle between the anterior cranial base and Frankfurt horizontal). *Green lines* mandibula to maxilla angle. *White arrows* (**a,c**) miniplates of the reconstruction area

groups. However, small differences were recorded in the maxillary-cranium relationship and the maxillary length. Although not significantly different, our analysis suggested a counterclockwise rotation of the palatal plane that, in turn, resulted in a more superiorly situated anterior nasal spine. Also, there was a delay in the sagittal maxillary growth in the younger age group. Overall, the vertical cephalometric changes were within 10% of normal values. Such minor changes produce a negligible net effect on the cosmetic and functional outcomes, which are also clinically acceptable. These are critically important elements in the quality of life of the patients in the younger age group [39, 40].

Conclusions

We have reviewed our experience of skull-base surgery for extirpation of tumors in children. The surgical techniques we describe are suitable for skull-base resections of both malignant and benign tumors. Collaboration of a multidisciplinary team, including head and neck surgeons, neurosurgeons, plastic surgeons, intensive care pediatricians and pediatric anesthesiologists is essential to the safety and success of these complex procedures. The long-term cosmetic effect of the subcranial approach is negligible.

Tips to Avoid Complications

- Perform detailed preoperative physical and radiological evaluation.
- Use a multidisciplinary team approach.
- Avoid extensive frontal lobe retraction.
- Use frozen sections to evaluate surgical margins intraoperatively.
- Postoperative monitoring in the pediatric intensive care unit.
- Treat infection promptly and thoroughly using broad-spectrum antibiotics.
- Use pain control medication without restriction.

Take-Home Pearls

- The surgical techniques described here are suitable for skull-base resections in children and adolescents.
- Collaboration of a multidisciplinary team, including head and neck surgeons, neurosurgeons, plastic surgeons, intensive care pediatricians and pediatric anesthesiologists is essential to the safety and success of complex skull-base procedures.
- The long-term cosmetic effect of the subcranial approach is negligible.

References

1. Cheesman AD, Lund VJ, Howard DJ (1986) Craniofacial resection for tumors of the nasal cavity and paranasal sinuses. Head Neck Surg 8(6):429–435
2. Donald PJ (1992) Skull base surgery. Otolaryngol Head Neck Surg 106(1):10–11
3. Irish JC, Gullane PJ, Gentili F et al (1994) Tumors of the skull base: outcome and survival analysis of 77 cases. Head Neck 16(1):3–10
4. McCutcheon IE, Blacklock JB, Weber RS et al (1996) Anterior transcranial (craniofacial) resection of tumors of the paranasal sinuses: surgical technique and results. Neurosurgery 38(3):471–479
5. Sekhar LN, Nanda A, Sen CN et al (1992) The extended frontal approach to tumors of the anterior, middle, and posterior skull base. J Neurosurg 76(2):198–206
6. Sundaresan N, Shah JP (1988) Craniofacial resection for anterior skull base tumors. Head Neck Surg 10(4):219–224
7. Brockmeyer D, Gruber DP, Haller J et al (2003) Pediatric skull base surgery. 2. Experience and outcomes in 55 patients. Pediatr Neurosurg 38(1):9–15
8. Gruber DP, Brockmeyer D (2003) Pediatric skull base surgery. 1. Embryology and developmental anatomy. Pediatr Neurosurg 38(1):2–8
9. Teo C, Dornhoffer J, Hanna E, Bower C (1999) Application of skull base techniques to pediatric neurosurgery. Childs Nerv Syst 15(2-3):103–109
10. Porceddu S, Martin J, Shanker G et al (2004) Paranasal sinus tumors: Peter MacCallum Cancer Institute experience. Head Neck 26(4):322–330
11. Suarez C, Llorente JL, Fernandez De Leon R et al (2004) Prognostic factors in sinonasal tumors involving the anterior skull base. Head Neck 26(2):136–144
12. Gil Z, Constantini S, Spektor S et al (2005) Skull base approaches in the pediatric population. Head Neck 27(8):682–689
13. Schick B, Rippel C, Brunner C et al (2003) Numerical sex chromosome aberrations in juvenile angiofibromas: genetic evidence for an androgen-dependent tumor? Oncol Rep 10(5):1251–1255
14. Donald PJ (1999) Complications in skull base surgery for malignancy. Laryngoscope 109(12):1959–1966
15. Kellman RM, Marentette L (2001) The transglabellar/subcranial approach to the anterior skull base: a review of 72 cases. Arch Otolaryngol Head Neck Surg 127(6):687–690
16. Roux FX, Moussa R, Devaux B et al (1999) Subcranial fronto-orbito-nasal approach for ethmoidal cancers surgical techniques and results. Surg Neurol 52(5):501–508
17. Kennedy JD, Haines SJ (1994) Review of skull base surgery approaches: with special reference to pediatric patients. J Neurooncol 20(3):291–312
18. Shah MV, Haines SJ (1992) Pediatric skull, skull base, and meningeal tumors. Neurosurg Clin N Am 3(4):893–924
19. Tessier P, Guiot G, Rougerie J et al (1969) Hypertelorism: cranio-naso-orbito-facial and subethmoid osteotomy. Panminerva Med 11(3):102–116
20. Bruce D, Munro I, Shapiro K (1994) Techniques of skull base surgery. In: Cheek WR (ed) Pediatric neurosurgery: surgery of developing nervous system. Saunders, Philadelphia, pp 598–613

21. Hanbali F, Tabrizi P, Lang FF, DeMonte F (2004) Tumors of the skull base in children and adolescents. J Neurosurg 100 [2 Suppl Pediatrics]:169–178

22. Hassler W, Zentner J (1989) Pterional approach for surgical treatment of olfactory groove meningiomas. Neurosurgery 25(6):942–945

23. Ojemann GA (1991) Cortical organization of language. J Neurosci 11(8):2281–2287

24. Turazzi S, Cristofori L, Gambin R, Bricolo A (1999) The pterional approach for the microsurgical removal of olfactory groove meningiomas. Neurosurgery 45(4):821–825

25. Raveh J, Turk JB, Ladrach K et al (1995) Extended anterior subcranial approach for skull base tumors: long-term results. J Neurosurg 82(6):1002–1010

26. Fliss DM, Zucker G, Amir A et al (2001) The combined subcranial-midfacial degloving approach. Oper Techn Otolaryngol Head Neck Surg 11:279–285

27. Siomin V, Spektor S, Beni-Adani L, Constantini S (2001) Application of the orbito-cranial approach in pediatric neurosurgery. Childs Nerv Syst 17(10):612–617

28. Gil Z, Fliss DM (2005) Pericranial wrapping of the frontal bone after anterior skull base tumor resection. Plast Reconstr Surg 116(2):395–398

29. Fliss DM, Gil Z, Spektor S et al (2002) Skull base reconstruction after anterior subcranial tumor resection. Neurosurg Focus 12(5):e10

30. Gil Z, Cohen JT, Spektor S et al (2003) Anterior skull base surgery without prophylactic airway diversion procedures. Otolaryngol Head Neck Surg 128(5):681–685

31. Adelstein DJ (2000) The role of chemotherapy for skull base carcinomas and sarcomas. Neurosurg Clin N Am 11(4):681–691

32. Keohan ML, Taub RN (1997) Chemotherapy for advanced sarcoma: therapeutic decisions and modalities. Semin Oncol 24(5):572–579

33. Steward WP (1997) Chemotherapy for metastatic soft tissue sarcomas. Cancer Treat Res 91:157–172

34. Antman KH (1997) Adjuvant therapy of sarcomas of soft tissue. Semin Oncol 24(5):556–560

35. Lewis JJ, Benedetti F (1997) Adjuvant therapy for soft tissue sarcomas. Surg Oncol Clin N Am 6(4):847–862

36. Wanebo HJ, Koness RJ, MacFarlane JK et al (1992) Head and neck sarcoma: report of the Head and Neck Sarcoma Registry. Society of Head and Neck Surgeons Committee on Research. Head Neck 14(1):1–7

37. Bell W (1980) Timing of treatment in growing patients. In: Bell W (ed) Surgical correction of dental facial deformities. Saunders, Philadelphia

38. Lowlicht RA, Jassin B, Kim M, Sasaki CT (2002) Long-term effects of Le Fort I osteotomy for resection of juvenile nasopharyngeal angiofibroma on maxillary growth and dental sensation. Arch Otolaryngol Head Neck Surg 128(8):923–927

39. Gil Z, Abergel A, Spektor S et al (2003) Quality of life following surgery for anterior skull base tumors. Arch Otolaryngol Head Neck Surg 129(12):1303–1309

40. Gil Z, Abergel A, Spektor S et al (2004) Development of a cancer-specific anterior skull base quality-of-life questionnaire. J Neurosurg 100(5):813–819

41

Chapter 42

Diagnosis, Evaluation and Management of CSF Rhinorrhea

42

Jeffrey B. LaCour and Brent A. Senior

Core Messages

- The etiologies of CSF fistulae include accidental trauma, iatrogenic causes, tumors, encephaloceles, and spontaneous leaks.
- A thorough head and neck evaluation including nasal endoscopy must be performed if suspicious for a CSF leak. If able to collect rhinorrhea, the fluid should be sent for a beta-2-transferrin assay.
- Select the appropriate imaging modality when working-up a leak. High-resolution CT demonstrates the bony skull base and its defects. If suspicious for encephalocele, MRI (magnetic resonance imaging) should be performed.
- Consider the etiology of the leak when deciding the treatment. Conservative measures such as bed rest, stool softeners, and head of bed elevation may resolve a traumatic leak. Acetazolamide (Diamox) and lumbar drain placement are other alternatives which may negate the need for surgical repair.
- Endoscopic repair of CSF fistulae has become the method of choice in most clinical scenarios.

Contents

Introduction

Misunderstanding of the physiology of cerebrospinal fluid (CSF) and the anatomy of the CSF-containing spaces characterized medical history for nearly 2,000 years. In the 4th century BC, CSF was thought by Hippocrates to be a pathological condition known as "fluid on the brain." Until the 17th century, it was believed that CSF communicated freely with the nose via the pituitary and ethmoid sinuses [1]. Understanding began to improve, however, when Versalius helped depict the ventricular system through his careful dissections in the 1500s, and subsequently in the 1700s when Cotugno accurately described the relationships of CSF and its flow throughout the brain.

Willis was the first to describe anterior skull-base CSF fistulae into the nasal/sinus cavity in 1862, while Dandy described the first surgical repair via frontal craniotomy in 1926. This was then followed by Dohlman's first report of an extracranial approach to repair CSF fistulae (via nasoorbital incision) in 1948. Vrabec and Hallberg then described an intranasal approach to repair cribriform plate CSF fistulae. Finally, Wigand in 1981 in describing his approach to endoscopic surgery of the sinuses, noted the successful endoscopic repair of iatrogenic CSF fistulae occurring in this setting. Since then, numerous reports have confirmed a low complication rate combined with a high success rate with endoscopic repair, so that most CSF fistulae of the anterior skull base are now being managed via transnasal endoscopic techniques.

Normal CSF Physiology

Most of the CSF (80–90%) is produced in the choroid plexuses of the ventricular system with the lateral ventricles being the bulk producers. CSF flows from the lateral ventricles medially to the third ventricle via the foramina of Munro. From there it passes in the midline through the narrow aqueduct of the midbrain (Sylvian or cerebral aqueduct) into the fourth ventricle. CSF leaves the fourth ventricle medially from the foramen of Magendie and laterally from the two foramina of Luschka just above the foramen magnum into the subarachnoid space under the cerebellum: the cisterna magna [2].

Through an active process requiring adenosine triphosphate, the ependymal cells of the choroid plexuses secrete CSF at a rate of 0.3–0.4 ml per minute. The active transport system causes a divergence in the concentrations of various solutes in CSF compared with plasma. The amount and types of protein differ in the CSF and plasma, a fact that aids identification of a CSF leak. The total CSF volume is 140 ml with 22 ml residing in the ventricular system and 118 ml in the subarachnoid space. Absorption of CSF occurs at the arachnoid villi where a pressure gradient of 2–3 cm H_2O drives CSF into the sagittal sinus.

Normal intracranial pressure (ICP) in an adult is in the range 5–15 cm H_2O and varies with respiratory phase, body positioning, activity level and multiple other factors. Homeostatic mechanisms regulate ICP with transient elevations being associated with coughing, sneezing, or Valsalva maneuvers. Increased ICP is considered a sustained pressure between 20–30 cm H_2O and can occur from a mass lesion obstructing the CSF pathway, over-production of CSF, or decreased absorption of CSF such as in the setting of venous sinus thrombosis and increased venous pressure. Global symptoms of elevated ICP include headache, depressed consciousness, balance problems, vomiting, papilledema, cranial nerve VI palsies, and Cushing's triad of bradycardia, respiratory depression and hypertension. Continuous progression of ICP could eventually lead to herniation of the brainstem with compression of the respiratory centers in the medulla oblongata and death. Intraventricular, intraparenchymal, subarachnoid, and epidural monitors are available for monitoring ICP with intraventricular monitors being the gold standard. In patients with elevated ICP CSF fistulae are more likely to develop and successful fistula repair is more likely to fail [3].

Pathophysiology

Hydrocephalus is defined as a disturbance of formation, flow, or absorption of CSF resulting in an increased volume in the central nervous system. Hydrocephalus associated with increased ICP can be classified as either noncommunicating or communicating. Noncommunicating hydrocephalus occurs when CSF flow within the ventricular system or the outlet foramina is obstructed by a pathological process. In communicating hydrocephalus, there is an overproduction of CSF or, more commonly, defective absorption at the arachnoid villi. Normal pressure hydrocephalus refers to pathologically enlarged ventricles with normal opening pressures on lumbar puncture. These patients present with Hakim's triad of gait apraxia, incontinence, and dementia. ICP may also be elevated in the absence of ventricular enlargement in a condition known as benign intracranial hypertension which we discuss later in the chapter. Elevated ICP or hydrocephalus appreciated on preoperative imaging may influence the surgeon's decision to use CSF diversion at the time of fistula repair.

The two main concerns associated with CSF fistulae are the development of life–threatening meningitis and pneumocephalus. The risks of developing meningitis with an untreated CSF fistula is unknown, but has been cited as 10% annually and 40% long-term [4]. Because of this risk, we recommend pneumococ-

cal vaccination for patients suspected of having a fistula as well as for those who have undergone repair. Pneumocephalus is another serious concern with an untreated fistula, having been first described by Dandy. It is a particular risk in patients with obstructive sleep apnea who require a continuous positive airway pressure machine at night.

The etiologies CSF fistula can be divided into accidental trauma, surgical trauma, tumors causing direct erosion of the skull base with or without noncommunicating hydrocephalus, congenital encephaloceles, or spontaneous with or without an associated increased in ICP.

In most case series, accidental trauma associated with a closed head injury accounts for 60–70% of CSF leaks with 1–3% of all closed head injuries being associated with a leak. Approximately 66% of leaks will be evident within 48 hours of injury with 95% apparent within 3 months [5]. Common locations of injury include the ethmoid roof and cribriform plate where olfactory neurons, surrounded by dura and arachnoid, penetrate into the nasal cavity. Conservative treatments for these injuries include bed rest, laxatives, head of bed elevation, and, in some situations, placement of a lumbar drain. While 70% of these leaks will close spontaneously with conservative measures, the incidence of ascending meningitis has been reported as high as 40% in long-term follow-up for this nonsurgical treatment group. This high incidence combined with the evidence that antibiotic prophylaxis has not been effective in preventing meningitis in these patients may prompt the surgeon to perform early endoscopic exploration and repair [6, 7].

Iatrogenic causes of CSF leaks comprise the second most common etiology and account for 20–30% of leaks. Surgical procedures associated with this risk include endoscopic or open sinus surgery, transsphenoidal pituitary surgery, endoscopic or open resection of skull-base tumors, and transcranial approaches to cavernous carotid or optic chiasm. The two most common sites injured during endoscopic sinus surgery are the lateral lamella of the cribriform plate and the posterior ethmoid roof near the face of the sphenoid. The lateral lamella of the cribriform plate may be injured during dissection of the anterior ethmoid or frontal recess or when resecting the middle turbinate close to the skull base. Posterior ethmoid injuries typically occur when the maxillary sinus is highly pneumatized and expands superomedially resulting in a relatively decreased superior to inferior dimension of the posterior ethmoid [8]. CSF leaks in the cribriform region have been reported to be more common on the right side due to the tendency of right hand surgeons to drift medially towards the thin and often low-lying lateral lamella. Overall, the risk of a CSF leak has been reported to be <1% during endoscopic sinus surgery [9]. The neurological surgery associated with the highest risk of a CSF leak is pituitary surgery when the sellar diaphragm is disrupted.

Tumors may cause CSF leaks via direct erosion of the skull base. These lesions may arise intranasally, intracranially, or may be a metastatic lesion from another primary. Treatments for these tumors, such as surgery, radiation or chemotherapy, may create a bony dehiscence and devascularized wound bed resulting in a CSF leak. Tumors may also obstruct normal CSF flow and cause noncommunicating hydrocephalus with a constant elevated ICP leading to an eventual bony dehiscence with a CSF leak. In these patients, it is imperative to identify and treat the underlying lesion before correcting the CSF leak as the leak acts as a safety valve for the elevated ICP and intracranial hypertension. These patients may ultimately require CSF diversion if the lesion does not respond to treatment.

Congenital encephaloceles may also result in CSF fistulae. Although the occipital type account for 75% of encephaloceles, the sincipital and basal types account for most anterior skull-base fistulae. The nasofrontal and nasoethmoidal subtypes of sincipital encephaloceles arise from a patent fonticulus nasofrontalis and foramen cecum, respectively, and present externally along the glabella or dorsum of the nose. The transethmoidal, sphenoethmoidal, and transsphenoidal subtypes of basal encephaloceles present intranasally and result from a defect along the cribriform plate, ethmoid roof or sphenoid [10]. It is imperative that these lesions not be biopsied in the office. Appropriate diagnosis begins with imaging including a CT scan which may demonstrate bifidity of the crista galli or a patent foramen cecum, and an MRI scan to evaluate intracranial extension of the lesion [11]. In addition to an encephalocele, the differential diagnosis for a midline nasal mass includes a dermoid, glioma, hemangioma, or teratoma. An encephalocele may also be acquired particularly in the setting of a spontaneous leak due to chronic hydrostatic forces from the elevated ICP. The presence of an encephalocele may influence the surgeon's technique of repair and decision to use CSF diversion postoperatively. It is also associated with an increased risk of postoperative complications, which should be discussed with the patient [12].

Spontaneous CSF fistulae have recently been suggested to be a likely variant of benign intracranial hypertension (BIH). Schlosser et al. found that over 70% of their patients with spontaneous leaks or encephaloceles met the modified Dandy criteria for BIH used by neuroophthalmologists. BIH, also known as idiopathic intracranial hypertension or pseudotumor cerebri, typically occurs in obese middle-aged women (BMI >30 kg/m²) with signs and symptoms suggestive of increased ICP: pressure headaches, pulsatile tinnitus, balance abnormalities, visual disturbances, papilledema and a high incidence of empty sella syndrome. The suspected etiology of the increased ICP is impaired absorption of CSF at the arachnoid villi which leads to the exertion of hydrostatic forces along the skull base. Inherently weak structures such as the natural perforations along the cribriform, the sellar diaphragm, and other areas with significant paranasal sinus pneumatization are prone to bony thinning from these forces leading to CSF leaks and acquired encephaloceles. This increased ICP may explain why spontaneous leaks have the highest incidence (50–100%) of meningoencephalocele formation compared to other fistula etiologies. The increased ICP may also explain why spontaneous leaks have the highest rate of surgical failure with 25–87% failure reported after successful initial repair compared to 10% for most other causes [8].

Diagnosis of CSF Fistula

Patients with a CSF leak will usually present with unilateral watery rhinorrhea. The drainage may be continuous or intermittent with a possible increase in flow elicited with straining or the head in a downward position. A low-pressure headache may be associated with an acute or chronic leak. A halo sign on linen or tissue may also be present. Good history taking will help steer the physician towards potential etiologies. Over 50% of traumatic leaks will present as rhinorrhea within 48 hours. These patients may also have hyposmia or anosmia. Iatrogenic injury should be suspected in patients who have undergone endoscopic sinus surgery or excision of skull-base lesions. Recurrent bacterial meningitis in immunologically competent individuals should raise suspicion for a CSF leak. Middle-aged obese females presenting with pressure headaches, pulsatile tinnitus, balance abnormalities, or visual disturbances may have a spontaneous leak associated with benign intracranial hypertension. An intranasal mass that enlarges with straining may indicate the presence of an encephalocele.

All patients should have a thorough head and neck examination, and the rhinorrhea should be provoked by having the patient lean forward. Nasal endoscopy is then performed paying special attention to the sphenoethmoidal recess, middle meatus, cribriform plate, and eustachian tube. A Valsalva maneuver may increase the flow of CSF and help with leak detection. If a patient is able to produce the rhinorrhea, a sample should be taken to test for the presence of the protein, beta-2-transferrin (β-2-trf). Transferrin is an iron-binding glycoprotein found in several polymorphic forms in the serum and other body fluids. Beta-2-trf, also known as the "tau" isoform, is a neuraminidase-induced desialated isoform highly specific to CSF, perilymph, and aqueous humor. This helps differentiate CSF from serum where the fully sialated beta-1 transferrin is found [13]. Requiring only 0.17 ml of nasal fluid for diagnosis, this test can be performed and completed in less than 3 hours by immunofixation electrophoresis. The test is highly sensitive and specific although false-positive results may occur in patients with chronic liver disease such as from alcoholism or in patients with genetic variants of transferrin [14]. Some authors feel that detection of β-2-trf should be mandatory before surgery considering the number of unnecessary surgical procedures for presumed CSF rhinorrhea when the β-2-trf was negative [15].

Beta trace protein analysis has been offered as an alternative to β-2-trf testing. Beta trace protein is prostaglandin-D synthase, the second most abundant protein in the CSF after albumin. Produced primarily in the meninges and choroid plexus, it may also be detected in urine, amniotic fluid, seminal plasma, breast cyst fluid, milk of lactating women, breast tumor extracts, placental extracts, fetal brain, and fetal heart tissues, perilymph, and serum [16]. Although beta trace protein testing has been reported to take less time and be less expensive, it is currently not widely available, and most authors utilize the β-2-trf test to diagnose CSF fistulae.

High-resolution computed tomography (CT) scanning is extremely useful as a screening tool when evaluating for a CSF leak. This test delineates the skull-base bony anatomy and may demonstrate a dehiscence of bone or fracture. Stone et al. noted a bony defect on CT scans in 71% of patients with a CSF leak [17]. Shetty et al. found extensive pneumatization of the sphenoid sinus lateral recess to be associated with a sphenoid CSF leak. In their series, 91% of patients with sphenoid CSF leaks had extensive lateral pneumatization compared to 23% in the control group [18].

Identifying the location of the leak can be enhanced using CT cisternography. Prior to CT scan, a water-soluble, nonionic contrast agent such as metrizamide or iohexol is injected into the intrathecal space via lumbar puncture. The patient is then placed in a prone kneeling or prone Trendelenburg position for several minutes before being scanned. Although the precise location of the leak may be identified, an active leak is required for a positive test leading to a high false-negative rate. Further disadvantages to this test include the need for an invasive procedure and poor soft-tissue definition when evaluating for a concomitant encephalocele.

Magnetic resonance imaging (MRI) is the modality of choice to detect the presence of an encephalocele. Although a poor imaging modality for bony anatomy, an MRI scan is best for soft-tissue anatomy and best identifies empty sella syndrome (ESS). ESS is associated with spontaneous CSF leaks where the increased ICP causes a weakness of the sellar diaphragm and an eventual herniation of dura through the diaphragm into the sella turcica. The CSF compresses the pituitary gland and gives the appearance of an empty sella on MR images [19].

MRI cisternography is an alternative study for detecting CSF fistulae which avoids the need for lumbar puncture. This is important for individuals with a high ICP in whom lumbar puncture would be contraindicated. This test relies on heavy T2-weighting and high spatial resolution, the suppression of all flow phenomena, and a short examination time in the prone or head-down position to demonstrate a CSF fistula. This test has been shown to be better than CT cisternography at detecting dural lesions less than 2 mm in size [20]. Detractors of MRI cisternography point to the lack of fine bony detail which limits the accuracy for localizing the leak.

Radionuclide cisternography is another method for detecting a CSF leak. Radioactive isotopes are injected into the CSF via a lumbar puncture. Multiple agents have been used and include: iodine-131, radioactive serum albumin (RISA), ytterbium (Yb) diethylene triamine pentaacetic acid (DTPA), indium-111 (^{111}In) DTPA, technetium (Tc-99m) serum albumin, and TC-99m pertechnetate. After injecting the isotope, cottonoid pledgets are placed in the nasal cavity in the middle meatus, sphenoethmoidal recess, and at the eustachian tube. After several hours, the pledgets are removed and counts are taken from each of them to determine if a leak is present. This method of detection may be beneficial in a slow or intermittent leak. Disadvantages of this test include an invasive lumbar puncture, exposure of the patient to radioactive material, absorption of the isotope into the circulatory system with contamination of extracranial tissue, and the inability to identify the exact location of the leak.

Sodium fluorescein has been used to help identify the exact location of a leak either preoperatively or intraoperatively. A mixture of 0.1 ml 10% fluorescein and 9.9 ml sterile saline is injected into the intrathecal space during lumbar puncture. Its distinguishing yellow–green color is helpful in detecting CSF drainage, and the use of a blue light filter further enhances detection. Although tinnitus, nausea, headache, seizures, and death have been reported with the use of intrathecal sodium fluorescein, several large studies involving hundreds of intrathecal injections of sodium fluorescein have shown only minimal complications [21]. Complications appear to be dose-dependent with few side effects experienced with less than 25 mg administered. It is extremely important to have a detailed discussion with the patient regarding the potential side effects as the product is not FDA-approved for use in this manner. Recently, Saafan et al. have advocated the topical intranasal application of 5% fluorescein for the preoperative and intraoperative localization of the leak site. A change in the color of the fluorescein from yellow to green denotes the presence of CSF [22].

Treatment Modalities

It is necessary to consider the etiology of the CSF leak when determining appropriate treatment modalities. Patients with more severe injuries with large skull-base defects may go directly for surgical repair. Conservative measures such as bed rest, stool softeners, and avoidance of straining or nose-blowing may lead to closure in most patients with a small bony defect following accidental trauma. A lumbar drain may be utilized should a leak persist after 2–3 days of conservative observation. A rough guideline is the removal of 150–250 ml of CSF per day. Lumbar puncture should not be performed in patients with increased ICP or cerebral edema, so brain imaging by either CT or MRI scan is mandatory prior to tapping. Acetazolamide (Diamox) has been shown to decrease CSF production by as much as 48% and may play an adjunctive role when increased ICP contributes to an ongoing leak. Increased ICP may also respond to steroids and mannitol. Surgical intervention should be considered if there is still a leak after 3–4 days of CSF diversion via lumbar drainage or after failed medical management, though each case needs to be considered separately before deciding on a surgical plan. An understanding of the etiology and pathophysiology of the fistula is necessary for successful surgery. Factors such as presence of increased ICP, location and extent of the bony defect, previous repair attempts, and coexisting medical conditions should all be taken into account.

Four techniques have been described for the endoscopic repair of CSF fistulae:

1. The *overlay* technique involves denuding the mucosa from around the leak site and placing a graft, usually free, over the dural lesion and the exposed bony margins. The graft is then supported in place with layers of absorbable and nonabsorbable packing. In a meta-analysis, Hegazy et al. found that the overlay technique was used in 79% of patients compared to the underlay technique in 12% [23].

2. The *underlay* technique is often used for large skull-base defects. It involves elevating the dura intracranially around the skull-base defect. A harvested piece of bone, cartilage, or other graft material is then placed intracranially with its edges overlapping the bony defect. An overlay graft is then placed followed by intranasal packing for extra support.

3. The *bath plug* technique utilizes abdominal or ear-lobe fat to occlude the fistula. After the defect is identified, a Vicryl suture is placed through the harvested fat and the fat is placed intracranially. Traction on the suture then seals the fat into

the bony defect. An overlay mucosal free graft can then be placed on the suture to support the fat graft. Intranasal packing is then placed for support.

4. The *sinus obliteration* technique is most commonly utilized for fistulae of the frontal sinus and sphenoid sinus lateral recess. After the mucoperiosteum is stripped from the sinus in the region of the defect, the sinus is partially or completely obliterated with either muscle or fat. With sphenoid leaks, the face of the sphenoid can then be reconstructed with bone, cartilage, or an absorbable plate.

Graft materials can be classified as free or pedicled and self or nonself. Free grafts include, but are not limited to, local mucoperichondrium or mucoperiosteum from the adjacent septum or turbinates, abdominal fat, temporoparietal fascia, and temporalis muscle. Pedicled grafts are usually from the adjacent turbinate or septum and may include cartilage or bone. A number of nonself graft materials have been used and include: acellular dermal matrix (AlloDerm; LifeCell, Branchburg, NJ), absorbable gelatin (Gelfoam; Pharmacia and Upjohn, Kalamazoo, MI), and hemostatic matrix (FloSeal; Baxter, Deerfield, IL).

Although most authors use prophylactic antibiotics perioperatively, there is no evidence that antibiotics reduce the risk of meningitis in the setting of a CSF leak. Indeed, some neurosurgeons feel that the risk of meningitis with a resistant bacteria is sufficiently elevated that they should not be used. However, antibiotics should be used while intranasal packing is in place in order to reduce the risk of toxic shock syndrome.

The use of lumbar drainage for CSF diversion is controversial. In the meta-analysis of Hegazy et al., 48% of 204 leak repairs utilized a lumbar drain [23]. In a survey of the American Rhinologic Society, 67% of the members reported the use of lumbar drains for an average of 4 days after the repair of CSF fistulae or encephaloceles [12]. Lumbar drains would appear to be most beneficial for those patients in whom initial leak repair has failed and for those middle-aged obese females with spontaneous leaks who likely have a variant of benign intracranial hypertension. Clearly, lumbar drainage should only be performed in skilled hands with skilled nurses adroit at handling lumbar drains postoperatively. Indeed, the risks of lumbar drainage are not insignificant and include headache, meningitis, radicular pain, and vocal fold dysfunction. Other reported risks include posterior lateral infarction of the left occipital lobe secondary to kinking of the posterior cerebral artery across the tentorium cerebelli and L5 inflammation, both attributed to lumbar drainage of CSF [24]. Particularly concerning is the risk of "air-siphoning" with lumbar drainage in the presence of large skull-base defects. As noted previously, in all patients in whom lumbar drainage is considered, brain imaging should be performed beforehand in order to assess for significantly increased ICP, mass effect, or cerebral edema.

Schlosser et al. have documented the benefit of postoperative ICP monitoring via lumbar drain to guide the future management of those with increased ICP. All eight patients in their series were obese females with a mean age of 49.9 years and spontaneous CSF leak. Knowledge of ICP after repair may direct the initiation of diuretic therapy or the consideration of a shunt placement for those with benign intracranial hyperten-

sion [25]. Intraoperative measurement of ICP may be falsely low and should be repeated postoperatively for a truer indication of elevated pressures.

Frontal Sinus Leaks For leaks involving the frontal sinus, the surgical approach usually involves the use of an osteoplastic flap with or without complete or partial sinus obliteration (Fig. 42.1). Incision options include coronal, pretrichial, brow, or midbrow depending on the patient's hairline and the location of the leak. Access may also be obtained going through preexisting frontal

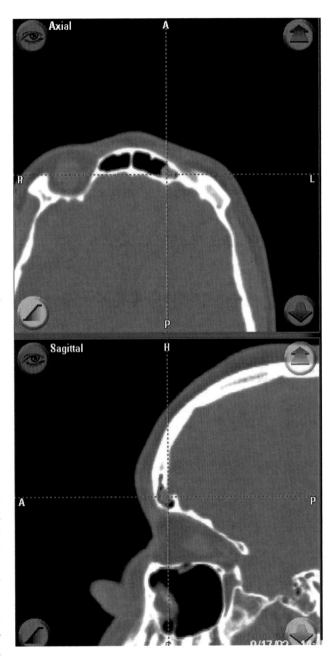

Fig. 42.1 Frontal sinus encephalocele which was treated with an open osteoplastic flap with obliteration of the lateral component of the sinus only

lacerations sustained in an accident. Bony cuts are made with an osteotome or drill with the use of frontal sinus transillumination, six-foot Caldwell films, or CT image guidance with great care not to cut outside the sinus limits with resultant possible dural injury. CT image guidance has been shown to be more accurate than the other two methods and least likely to overestimate the size of the sinus [26].

Fistulae may be repaired using the techniques outlined above. After repairing a fistula, particularly in the setting of trauma, the status of the frontal sinus outflow tracts is determined. This combined with the condition of the frontal sinus mucosa and the reliability of the patient help steer our decision to obliterate the sinus. Preservation or restoration of the normal sinus anatomy and function is ideal and in some cases will be augmented with an endoscopic frontal sinusotomy to reestablish outflow. Life-long follow-up with CT and endoscopic examinations are necessary because of concern for late mucocele formation in this setting.

Ethmoid Roof and Cribriform Leaks For leaks involving the ethmoid roof and cribriform, surgical approaches include transnasal endoscopic, external ethmoidectomy, or frontal craniotomy. The most common sites of ethmoid leaks include the posterior ethmoid roof, where injury occurs when the surgeon fails to recognize the downward sloping of the skull base posteriorly, and even more commonly, the lateral lamella of the cribriform plate, where the dura is tightly adherent and the anterior ethmoid artery perforates causing a natural weakening of the bony wall. In endoscopic sinus surgery, this risk appears to be heightened in the presence of a deep olfactory fossa as defined by Keros. Additionally, there is a trend toward right-handed surgeons causing a right-sided ethmoid leak by drifting medially towards the thin and potentially low-lying lateral lamella during surgery.

External ethmoidectomy approaches can also be performed to expose the skull base and defect. In this approach, the frontoethmoid suture line is used as a landmark for the cribriform, and the anterior ethmoid artery is ligated. Once the leak is identified, a pedicled turbinate or septal mucosal flap can be used for closure.

Less commonly performed today, frontal craniotomy approaches were well outlined by Ray and Bergland in 1969. Utilizing a coronal incision with removal of a frontal bony plate, the frontal lobe is retracted with the olfactory tract divided behind the bulb. The anterior portion of the falx cerebri may be divided for exposure. The leak may be sealed by reflecting dura from the roof of the orbit or by mobilizing a portion of the falx [27].

Currently, the preferred method of treatment of ethmoid roof and cribriform leaks is endoscopic. A total sphenoethmoidectomy is performed to expose the entire anterior skull base. After identifying the leak with the assistance of intrathecal fluorescein (if necessary), edges of the defect are freshened and an overlay, underlay, or bath plug graft is placed. Intranasal absorbable packing is placed followed by nonabsorbable packing to bolster the repair site. Special efforts should be made to preserve the middle turbinate as a landmark for revision surgery and to prevent lateralization of the turbinate remnant which could cause frontal recess outflow obstruction.

Sphenoid Sinus Leaks Sphenoid sinus leaks can be approached with craniotomy, endoscopically, or via a transseptal approach (Fig. 42.2). The craniotomy approach is similar to that discussed by Ray and Bergland for ethmoid leaks. After exposing the anterior skull base, the dura over the tuberculum sellae is removed and some of the bone is removed to identify the mucosa of the sphenoid sinus roof. Rather than removing the sinus mucosa, they described pushing the mucosa away and packing the sinus with muscle. A flap of dura is then cut and turned back over the tuberculum defect [27].

A transseptal approach to the sphenoid utilizes a sublabial or transnasal incision followed by a transfixion incision to rotate the septum rostrally. A Hardy speculum is then inserted and the rostrum and intersinus septum are removed. The sinus mucosa is removed and the leak repaired. The rostrum is then reconstructed with either bony or septal cartilage.

The endoscopic technique has become a popular technique and is a safe alternative for leaks of the sphenoid sinus and is analogous to that used for ethmoid leak repair. For leaks involving the lateral recess of the sphenoid, 70° endoscopes are utilized to help visualize the area. Extreme care is needed as the carotid artery and the optic nerve are running along this lateral wall inferiorly and superiorly, respectively, and often have a dehiscent bony covering. Once the leak is identified, it can be repaired using a technique similar to that used for an ethmoid leak. In some cases, partial or complete sphenoid obliteration may be performed using abdominal fat. After removing the mucoperiosteum from the sinus, the fat is placed to fill the sinus, and the face of the sphenoid is then repaired using cartilage, bone, or a bioabsorbable plate.

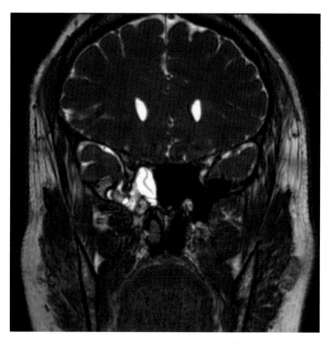

Fig. 42.2 Patient with a right lateral sphenoid sinus CSF leak and associated encephalocele which was repaired endoscopically with the use of the 45° and 70° endoscopes

An alternative approach to access the lateral recess of the sphenoid sinus has been described by Bolger and Osenbach, and is termed the "transpterygoid" approach. Following a large maxillary antrostomy, the posterior wall of the maxillary sinus is exposed and the mucosa stripped. A wide sphenoidotomy is then performed in routine fashion. Proceeding through the maxillary sinus, the bone of the posterior wall is removed and a hemaclip is used to ligate the sphenopalatine artery. The vidian nerve, infraorbital nerve, and pterygopalatine ganglion are preserved. The lateral recess of the sphenoid sinus is then accessed by removing the bone of the pterygoid process [28].

- Consider the etiology of the leak and choose conservative management initially if there is a small traumatic defect.
- Each patient should be managed individually when deciding the method of repair or the use of a lumbar drain.
- Endoscopic repair of CSF leaks should only be performed in the hands of skilled surgeons who have appropriate training to handle this entity.

Conclusions

Endoscopic repair of CSF fistulae has become the method of choice in most clinical scenarios. Success rates are approximately 90% on first attempt with 96% for a second attempt. Patients with increased ICP or leaks of the lateral recess with a well pneumatized sphenoid sinus have an greater failure rate. This is compared to craniotomy approaches with success rates of approximately 60–80% and extracranial open procedures with reported success rates of 86–100% on first attempt [27, 29]. Besides sparing the patient an open procedure, complication rates of endoscopic repair are low with an overall incidence of 2.5%. The most common complication is meningitis (1.1%) with all other complications being less than 1%. Endoscopic encephalocele repair carries a higher complication rate of 8.6% with seizures being the highest at 3.1% followed by meningitis 2.3%.

Tips to Avoid Complications

- CT image guidance is least likely to overestimate the size of the frontal sinus compared to transillumination or a six-foot Caldwell film when making bony cuts.
- A total sphenoethmoidectomy should be performed to expose the entire skull base when repairing ethmoid and sphenoid leaks.
- When repairing a leak of the sphenoid sinus lateral recess, the surgeon must be cognizant of a potential bony dehiscence over the carotid artery or optic nerve.
- If lumbar drainage is considered, brain imaging should be performed beforehand to rule out significantly increased ICP, mass effect, or cerebral edema.

Take-Home Pearls ⬇

- A high suspicion of CSF leak is necessary to make the diagnosis. Confirming the presence of a leak with an imaging study and a beta-2-transferrin assay will help avoid unnecessary surgery.

References

1. Calcaterra TC (1980) Extracranial repair of cerebrospinal rhinorrhea. Ann Otol Rhinol Laryngol 89:108–116
2. Hendleman W (2005) Atlas of functional neuroanatomy, 2nd edn. CRC Press, Boca Raton, pp 64–65
3. Tindall GT, Cooper PR, Barrow DL (eds) (1995) The practice of neurosurgery. Williams & Wilkins, Baltimore, pp 35–69
4. McMains KC, Gross CW, Kountakis SE (2004) Endoscopic management of cerebrospinal fluid rhinorrhea. Laryngoscope 114:1833–1837
5. Zlab MK, Moore GF, Daly DT et al (1992) Cerebrospinal fluid rhinorrhea: a review of the literature. Ear Nose Throat J 72:314–317
6. Klastersky J, Sadeghi M, Brihaye J (1976) Antimicrobial prophylaxis in patients with rhinorrhea or otorrhea: a double blind study. Surg Neurol 6:111–114
7. MacGee EE, Cauthen JC, Brackett CE (1970) Meningitis following acute traumatic cerebrospinal fluid fistula. J Neurosurg 33:312–316
8. Schlosser RJ, Woodworth BA, Wilensky EM et al (2006) Spontaneous cerebrospinal fluid leaks: a variant of benign intracranial hypertension. Ann Otol Rhinol Laryngol 115:495–500
9. Stankiewicz JA (1991) Cerebrospinal fluid fistula and endoscopic sinus surgery. Laryngoscope 101:250–256
10. Suwanwela C, Suwanwela N (1972) A morphological classification of sincipital encephalomeningoceles. J Neurosurg 36:201–211
11. Denoyelle F, Ducroz V, Roger G, Garabedian EN (1997) Nasal dermoid sinus cysts in children. Laryngoscope 107:795–800
12. Senior BA, Jafri K, Benninger M (2001) Safety and efficacy of endoscopic repair of CSF leaks and encephaloceles: a survey of the members of the American Rhinologic Society. Am J Rhinol 15:21–25
13. Normansell D, Stacy E, Booker C et al (1994) Detection of beta-2 transferrin in otorrhea and rhinorrhea in a routine clinical laboratory setting. Clin Diagn Lab Immunol 1:68–70
14. Papadea C, Schlosser RJ (2005) Sensitive detection of beta-2 transferrin in cerebrospinal fluid leakage using an automated immunofixation electrophoresis method, Clin Chem 51:464–470
15. Bateman N, Jones NS (2000) Rhinorrhoea feigning cerebrospinal fluid leak; nine illustrative cases, J Laryngol Otol 114:462–464

16. Meco C, Oberascher G, Arrer E et al (2003) Beta-trace protein test: new guidelines for the reliable diagnosis of cerebrospinal fluid fistula. Otolaryngol Head Neck Surg 129:508–517

17. Stone J, Castillo M, Neelon B et al (1999) Evaluation of CSF Leaks: high-resolution CT compared with contrast-enhanced CT and radionuclide cisternography. Am J Neuroradiol 20:706–712

18. Shetty PG, Shroff MM, Fatterpekar GM et al (2000) A retrospective analysis of spontaneous sphenoid sinus fistula: MR and CT findings. Am J Neuroradiol 21:337–342

19. Schlosser RJ, Bolger WE (2003) Significance of empty sella in cerebrospinal fluid leaks. Otolaryngol Head Neck Surg 128(1):32–38

20. Eberhardt KE, Hollenbach HP, Deimling M et al (1997) MR cisternography: a new method for the diagnosis of CSF fistulae. Eur Radiol 7:1485–1491

21. Keerl R, Weber RK, Draf W et al (2004) Use of sodium fluorescein solution for detection of cerebrospinal fluid fistulas: an analysis of 420 administrations and reported complications in Europe and the United States. Laryngoscope 114:266–272

22. Saafan ME, Ragab SM, Albirmawy OA (2006) Topical intranasal fluorescein: the missing partner in algorithms of cerebrospinal fluid fistula detection. Laryngoscope 116:1158–1161

23. Hegazy HM, Carrau RL, Snyderman CH et al (2000) Transnasal endoscopic repair of cerebrospinal fluid rhinorrhea: a meta-analysis. Laryngoscope 110:1166–1172

24. Roland PS, Marple BF, Meyerhoff WL et al (1992) Complications of lumbar spinal fluid drainage. Otolaryngol Head Neck Surg 107:565–569

25. Schlosser RJ, Wilensky EM, Grady S et al (2003) Cerebrospinal fluid pressure monitoring after repair of cerebrospinal fluid leaks. Presented at the Annual Meeting of the American Academy of Otolaryngology – Head and Neck Surgery. 21–24 September

26. Melroy CT, Dubin MG, Hardy SM, Senior BS (2006) Analysis of methods to assess frontal sinus extent in osteoplastic flap surgery: transillumination vs. six foot Caldwell vs. image guidance. Am J Rhinol 20:77–83

27. Ray BS, Bergland RM (1969) Cerebrospinal fluid fistula: clinical aspects, techniques of localization, and methods of closure. J Neurosurg 30:399–405

28. Bolger WE, Osenbach R (1999) Endoscopic transpterygoid approach to the lateral sphenoid recess. Ear Nose Throat J 78:36–46

29. Aarabi B, Leibrock LG (1992) Neurosurgical approaches to cerebrospinal fluid rhinorrhea. Ear Nose Throat J 71:300–305

Chapter 43

Conventional and Endoscopic Approaches to the Pituitary

43

Karen A. Kölln and Brent A. Senior

Core Messages

- Conventional and endoscopic approaches to the pituitary both lead to satisfactory treatment of pituitary disease, with endoscopic approaches resulting in fewer endonasal complications.
- A multidisciplinary approach should be utilized when treating individuals with pituitary lesions secondary to the vast array of endocrine, neurosurgical, ophthalmological and otolaryngological sequelae that arise.
- Patients with Cushing's disease and acromegaly require special consideration due to increased perioperative morbidity.

Contents

Introduction

Over the past 100 years pituitary surgery has evolved greatly, with otolaryngologists contributing significantly as the approaches have become progressively less invasive in nature. Pituitary lesions were initially treated with a traditional craniotomy but there was great interest in accessing the sella via the sphenoid due to the high morbidity of the subfrontal or middle fossa approaches. As techniques were first explored, extensive facial incisions were used with wide resection of intranasal structures, including a transglabellar-nasal approach [1]. Schloffer introduced the transsphenoidal approach in 1907 and in 1914 Cushing described a sublabial approach obviating the need for facial incisions. Cushing later largely abandoned this strategy as the visualization and illumination were poor, and he was concerned about increased mortality and incomplete tumor resection. Approximately 40 years later Guiot introduced radiofluoroscopy to assist with gauging the depth of instrumentation during the procedure and subsequently, in 1969, Hardy first utilized the operating microscope which greatly enhanced visualization and lighting. The sublabial transseptal approach first described by Cushing with the modification of Hardy is still utilized and is considered the "traditional" approach to the sella [2]. The next major advance in pituitary surgery came in 1992 when Jankowski et al. first reported the successful use of 0° and 30° endoscopes in the resection of pituitary adenomas in three patients, paving the way for the endoscopic endonasal transsphenoidal hypophysectomy [3]. The aim of this chapter is to describe pituitary anatomy, traditional and endoscopic approaches, and compare complications and outcomes associated with these procedures.

Pituitary Anatomy

The pituitary gland (hypophysis cerebri) is the central regulatory endocrine gland and comprises the anterior lobe (adenohypophysis) and posterior lobe (neurohypophysis or pars nervosa). The anterior lobe is formed from an evagination of oropharynx known as Rathke's pouch, whereas the posterior gland is formed from an evagination of neural crest cells from the third ventricle.

Rathke's pouch is reduced to a cleft-like remnant and delineates the separation between the anterior and posterior lobes.

The pituitary fossa at the base of the skull holds the gland, and is limited anteriorly, posteriorly and inferiorly by the sella turcica, a depression in the sphenoid bone. The sphenoid sinus lies inferiorly, and as pneumatization of the sinus increases, the amount of the floor it comprises increases as well. The pituitary gland is an extradural structure and a fold in the dura, the diaphragma sella, forms an incomplete roof over the gland and allows the transmission of the pituitary stalk and blood supply, and also separates the pituitary from the optic chiasm which lies superiorly. Cerebrospinal fluid (CSF) may leak around the diaphragma causing the pituitary gland to become compressed, known as an "empty sella." Lateral to the pituitary fossa lie the cavernous sinuses which comprise venous channels, the internal carotid artery, as well as numerous cranial nerves (oculomotor, trochlear, first and second divisions of the trigeminal, and abducens). Key landmarks within the sphenoid sinus include the internal carotid artery lying posterolaterally and the optic chiasm which courses anterosuperiorly, which can be dehiscent in 10% and 4% of individuals, respectively. A firm understanding of this anatomy is vital in the surgical management of pituitary pathology.

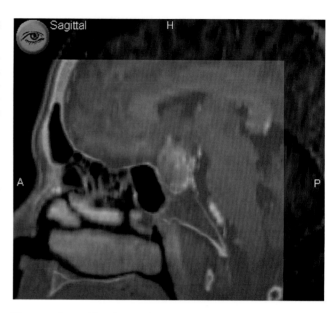

Fig. 43.1 Sagittal fused CT and MRI image. This technique maximizes the benefits of both imaging modalities: the bony definition seen in the CT image and the soft-tissue detail in the MR image. Also note the sellar mass

Surgical Indications

Surgical intervention is generally recommended for pituitary adenomas which cannot be controlled by medical management, pituitary masses that are causing visual impairment and lesions that are shown to be increasing in size on serial imaging. Pituitary apoplexy is considered a surgical emergency; this is when necrosis or hemorrhage into a pituitary lesion causes abrupt vision loss, headache, cranial neuropathies and sometimes acute adrenal insufficiency.

Preoperative Evaluation

It is recommended that all patients be evaluated in a multidisciplinary fashion, with complete evaluation by an endocrinologist, neuroophthalmologist, neurosurgeon and otolaryngologist. Preoperative anesthesia consultation should also be considered, especially in patients with Cushing's disease and acromegaly. Patients with Cushing's disease have numerous comorbidities including obesity, obstructive sleep apnea (OSA), hypertension and diabetes, leading to increased intraoperative anesthetic risk. Excessive growth hormone in acromegaly affects the heart leading to cardiac myopathy and pharyngeal tissue leading to hypertrophy of the base of the tongue and redundant mucosa creating a potentially difficult intubation. Perioperative stress dose steroids are routinely given in our institution because of concern for disruption in endogenous steroid production.

OSA is very common in these patients, particularly in those with acromegaly, and great care with perioperative management of the airway is needed. Consideration should be given to temporary tracheotomy in patients with severe OSA, as the use of continuous positive airway pressure in the postoperative period is not possible.

History regarding sinonasal complaints including facial pressure and pain, nasal congestion or obstruction, hyposmia/anosmia, rhinorrhea, postnasal drip, past nasal trauma, and headache should be elicited, as well as any other medical illnesses. A thorough physical examination should be performed specifically to evaluate for visual field loss, decreased visual acuity, stigmata of endocrine dysfunction, and cranial nerve palsies. Sinonasal endoscopy should be performed to evaluate for septal deviation, nasal polyposis and sinusitis. Imaging is utilized during preoperative evaluation for surgical planning as well as intraoperatively for stereotactic guidance. Imaging should include a noncontrast computed tomography (CT) scan of the paranasal sinuses (to better define bony anatomy, pneumatization of the sphenoid, location of the intersinus septum, position and possible dehiscence of the internal carotid artery, and presence of Onodi cells) and magnetic resonance imaging (MRI) of the brain with special focus on the pituitary gland (to define the extent and location of the tumor, any vascular abnormalities, involvement of the cavernous sinus or impingement on the optic nerve/chiasm). We routinely fuse these images for intraoperative stereotactic guidance, which is especially helpful in revision procedures which can be complicated by scar and altered anatomy (Fig. 43.1). Laboratory data including complete blood count, comprehensive metabolic panel and a thorough endocrine evaluation should be obtained. Coagulation studies including partial thromboplastin time (PTT), prothrombin time (PT) and international normalized ratio (INR) should be performed if there is a family history of bleeding disorders [4].

Tips to Avoid Complications

- Obtain preoperative anesthesia evaluation in patients with Cushing's disease and acromegaly due to increased anesthetic risk.
- Patients with acromegaly can have a difficult airway because of hypertrophy of the base of the tongue and redundancy of the pharyngeal mucosa.
- Consider tracheostomy in patients with severe OSA, since CPAP cannot be utilized in the postoperative period.
- Perioperative steroids are critical given the patient's disruption in endogenous steroid production.

Conventional Approaches to the Pituitary

Conventional approaches to the pituitary that are still used today include the sublabial transseptal and endonasal transseptal approaches. The sublabial transseptal approach utilized today has not been altered much since Cushing's description in 1912. The patient is positioned with the head elevated and the nose is decongested with pledgets soaked in oxymetazoline. A hemitransfixion incision is made in the caudal edge of the septum using a scalpel, the dissection is carried down to the cartilage and around the caudal end and a complete mucoperichondrial and mucoperiosteal flap is elevated. The cartilaginous septum is displaced off its bony junction and inferior tunnels are elevated bilaterally. A sublabial incision is then made and connected to the intraseptal space. A Hardy speculum is placed through the sublabial incision and the posterior septum is removed exposing the sphenoid rostrum. In some cases, the patient is then placed in the Trendelenburg position, the patient's neck is extended and the surgeon operates from the head of the table utilizing the operating microscope. At this time the sphenoid rostrum is removed, along with the intersinus septae and the mucosal lining of the sphenoid sinus. The sella anterior wall is taken down and the tumor is removed with neurosurgical curettes. Traditionally the sella has then been packed with fat, the septum reconstructed and the nose packed after the incisions have been closed with 5.0 chromic cat gut (hemitransfixion incision) and 3.0 Vicryl (sublabial incision) [5].

In the endonasal transseptal approach pledgets soaked in oxymetazoline are used for decongestion and 1% lidocaine with 1:100,000 epinephrine is injected into the nasal septum. A Killian incision is made in the right nasal septal mucosa, approximately 2–3 mm posterior to the mucocutaneous junction, and a mucoperichondrial flap is raised on the right. In order to raise a similar flap on the opposite side an incision is made in the quadrangular cartilage 1–2 cm posterior to the rostral margin. Utilizing ethmoid forceps and cutting Jansen-Middleton forceps the posterior portion of the quadrangular cartilage and the perpendicular plate of the ethmoid are removed. The mucosa on the rostrum of the sphenoid is elevated bilaterally until the sphenoid ostia are identified. A Hardy speculum is then placed

and the operating microscope is appropriately positioned. A Kerrison punch is then used to open the sphenoid ostium and to remove the intersinus septum. Care must be taken when removing the septum as it can insert on the carotid canal or optic nerve. The face of the sella is then taken down and tumor removal is performed with neurosurgical curettes. At the conclusion of the procedure the speculum is removed and the mucosal flaps are reapproximated. The incision is closed with 5.0 chromic gut sutures and the flaps are sutured together with a whip stitch, easily performed with a 4.0 chromic on a Keith needle. Nasal packing and/or nasal splints may or may not be used depending on the surgeon's preference [1].

Endoscopic Approach to the Pituitary: Minimally Invasive Pituitary Surgery

After Jankowski first introduced endoscopes into the surgical treatment of pituitary disease, numerous authors have reported on the operative technique [3, 6–8]. We report here our technique of minimally invasive pituitary surgery (MIPS). Standard length 0° 4-mm endoscopes fitted with scope irrigation provide the best visualization and illumination while approaching the sella; however, longer scopes and angle (45° and occasionally 70°) scopes can aid in tumor resection and exploration of the sella. In contrast to the technique described above, the sella is approached off the midline. The side of the approach is primarily determined by nasal factors: the presence of septal deviation, the degree of nasal congestion and location of the sphenoid intersinus septum. If all other nasal factors are equal, the contralateral side usually confers the better angle of approach in lesions that are off the midline or extend into the cavernous sinus. Frequently both nasal cavities are utilized with one side for the endoscopes and the other for instrumentation. This is necessary in patients with unusually thin nasal cavities or if more than one instrument is necessary during tumor removal.

The patient is positioned in the "beach-chair" position with the torso elevated and the knees slightly bent. The patient's head rests in a foam or gel donut and the head is rotated fifteen degrees toward the surgeon. We routinely use stereotactic computer guidance to aid in identification of landmarks and safe tumor removal, and at this point the patient is registered with the computer software. The abdomen is sterilely prepped and draped so that a fat graft can be harvested if required, whereas the face is not, as the instruments are passed through a contaminated nasal cavity. Greater palatine blocks are routinely performed to aid in hemostasis by transorally injecting 1.5 ml 1% lidocaine with 1:100,000 epinephrine into each greater palatine canal. Under endoscopic guidance pledgets soaked in a solution of 0.05% oxymetazoline hydrochloride are placed for decongestion and then additional anesthetic is injected in the region of the sphenopalatine foramen, at the junction of the horizontal portion of the basal lamella and lateral nasal wall, to obtain a sphenopalatine artery block.

The sphenoid ostium is identified in the sphenoethmoid recess, which is bound by the skull base, superior turbinate and septum. To gain access to the recess the middle turbinate may need to be gently lateralized and rarely a concha bullosa

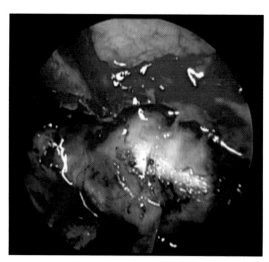

Fig. 43.2 Endoscopic view of the sella after cauterization at the point of incision into the dura with a sickle knife

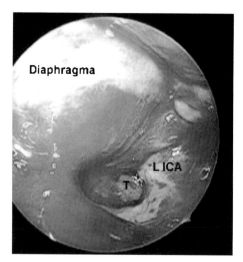

Fig. 43.3 Endoscopic view within the sella utilizing the 45° telescope. Residual tumor (*T*) is seen next to the left internal carotid artery (*L ICA*). This image demonstrates the high optical quality of the endoscopes and the ability to ensure complete tumor removal laterally within the sella

resected. However, the advantage of this approach lies in the fact that the sinuses lateral to the middle turbinate are largely untouched, maintaining the functionality of these sinuses. The posterior-inferior third of the superior turbinate is then conservatively resected and the ostium is identified medial to the turbinate, just posterior to its inferior edge. After the ostium is identified, it is enlarged with a mushroom punch or Kerrison punch in an inferior and medial direction until the nasal septum is encountered. The posterior part of the nasal septum is then resected using back-biting forceps until the contralateral sphenoid is widely exposed. The intersinus septum is then resected with great care as it can attach over the carotid canal in 10% and over the optic nerve in 4% of individuals.

Once adequate sellar exposure is obtained the endoscope is attached to a fixed pneumatic holder or an assistant can hold the scope for the surgeon, allowing the operating surgeon both hands for instrumentation. The mucosa on the posterior wall of the sphenoid sinus is coagulated with a bipolar cautery. The sella is then usually entered by creating a window with a 4-mm chisel. Alternatively, in the case of a thickened sellar face, a high-speed drill can be used to enter the sella. Once an opening is created it is enlarged with a Kerrison punch. The dura is then cauterized with bipolar cautery and a sickle knife is used to make a cruciate incision as widely as possible (Fig. 43.2). The tumor generally bulges through the opening and samples are taken and sent for frozen sectioning. The remaining tumor is then removed using suction and neurosurgical ring curettes and is usually easily differentiated from normal pituitary by its orange/yellow color and firmer texture.

In order to ensure complete tumor removal the endoscope can be inserted inside the sella and angled telescopes can be used to examine the lateral crevices of the sella, one of the advantages of the endoscopic technique (Fig. 43.3). However, this may be difficult if the normal pituitary tissue descends down

into the newly created space. The technique of "hydroscopy" can therefore be essential in obtaining complete tumor removal. A system of normal saline irrigation under pressure is attached to the endoscope which floods the sella and improves visualization by pushing the diaphragma up and washing away debris and clot.

After complete tumor removal hemostasis is obtained by placing a hemostatic substance, such as microfibrillar collagen in thrombin, over the operative field. This is then washed away and no additional packing is placed. If no CSF leak is encountered at the end of the procedure we have found that reconstruction of the sella is not necessary. In our first 28 procedures no reconstruction of the sella was performed, and postoperatively there was no increase in the rate of leak (0.4% compared to reported rates of 0.8 to 6.4%) and there were no cases of meningitis or empty sella syndrome [9]. If CSF leak is encountered at the completion of the procedure we typically reconstruct the sella using microfibrillar collagen, and a fat graft bolstered by an absorbable miniplate cut to fit under the edges of the sella.

Tips to Avoid Complications

- Always remove the intersinus septum with care as this can insert on the carotid canal or optic nerve.
- Utilize intraoperative stereotactic guidance to help in the identification of anatomical landmarks.
- Care must be taken when opening the Hardy speculum during the conventional approach to the pituitary to avoid fracture of the optic foramen or orbit.

Outcomes

The major aims of pituitary surgery are to obtain endocrinological remission and gross tumor removal. The rate of surgical removal and the ability to achieve an endocrinological cure are similar in patients undergoing MIPS and in those undergoing a transseptal procedure. There is no measured or perceived disadvantage to performing an endoscopic procedure in terms of the treatment of pituitary disease [10]

Complications

There are numerous complications that are common to pituitary surgery independent of the approach. The reported mortality rate of pituitary surgery is less than 1%, with the most common causes of death being medical complications such as deep vein thrombosis or myocardial infarction [11].

Serious complications include meningitis, carotid injury, intracranial hemorrhage and ophthalmoplegia. Meningitis occurs with an incidence of 0.15–1.2% and is associated with preoperative sinusitis and postoperative CSF leak. Acute sinusitis preoperatively should be treated aggressively and if the procedure is elective in nature, should be postponed until the infection has resolved [12]. Chronic sinusitis without acute purulence probably does not increase the risk of meningitis, but cultures of any suspicious mucus in the nasal cavity in this situation should be obtained.

The carotid artery is at risk during pituitary surgery due to its tortuous and variable course along the skull base and within the cavernous sinus. and it is dehiscent in 10% of individuals [13]. Intraoperative damage to the carotid artery occurs with an incidence of 0.78–1.16% [14], and if it occurs the area should be packed and angiography should be performed emergently. If the initial angiogram is normal, angiography should be repeated on postoperative day 6 to 10. The same holds true if a patient presents with delayed massive epistaxis to ensure there is no false aneurysm or carotid–cavernous fistula [15, 16]. Intracranial hemorrhage occurs with an incidence of 0.4–3% and most often occurs in the setting of incomplete removal of a macroadenoma, underscoring the need for meticulous and complete tumor removal [17].

Ophthalmoplegia and loss of vision occur rarely with an incidence of 0.3–1.4%. This can be caused by damage to the nerves coursing through the cavernous sinus, as a result of compression from hematoma, herniation into an empty sella or direct injury to the optic nerve. Unique to the transseptal approach, when the Hardy speculum is used, the force created when the speculum is opened can dissipate through the orbit causing a fracture of the optic foramen or orbit [18].

The most common major complication following transsphenoidal pituitary surgery is CSF leak. This can occur intraoperatively or postoperatively and most commonly occurs when there are large suprasellar tumors where extensive dissection is required, and where the diaphragma becomes thin and incompetent, or in revision surgery. If noted intraoperatively the leak should be repaired immediately to decrease the risk of postoperative meningitis. When the CSF leak occurs postoperatively it can be treated conservatively with bed-rest and head elevation,

lumbar puncture and/or surgical re-exploration. Some authors advocate early surgical intervention, citing the benefits of decreased risk of developing meningitis for those in whom conservative management fails, avoiding the risk associated with a lumbar drain, and potentially a decreased hospital stay [19].

Endocrine complications are also common in the postoperative period, with diabetes insipidus occurring with the most frequency. Most commonly diabetes insipidus is transient in nature, occurring in the first 24 to 72 hours postoperatively but complicates up to 31% of pituitary surgery. Most individuals are able to sustain enough oral intake to not require medical management; however, if it becomes permanent or symptomatic desmopressin is used. Factors associated with developing transient diabetes insipidus include macroadenoma, Rathke's cleft cyst, craniopharyngioma, and occurrence of intraoperative CSF leak [20].

Endonasal complications vary greatly between conventional and minimally invasive techniques. We compared the first 50 MIPS procedures with the last 50 transseptal procedures at our institution and found that postoperative epistaxis and upper lip anesthesia were significantly more common in the transseptal group, whereas there was no difference in the number of CSF leaks. Septal perforation can occur as a result of both techniques; however, the perforations in the endoscopic technique occur at the face of the sphenoid and will not result in symptoms for the patient, as opposed to those that occur in the transseptal group. The patient's quality of life is also significantly better following an endonasal procedure. The patients' mean stay in the hospital was decreased from 5.4 days to 3.7 days in the endoscopic group in our study [21]. Patients who had a revision endoscopic hypophysectomy after having a prior sublabial approach stated that the endonasal procedure overall had an easier recovery, less pain with better nasal airflow. Also patients who had nasal packing placed postoperatively had a significantly worse postoperative experience than those who did not ($p = 0.001$) [22].

Conclusions

Pituitary surgery has come full-circle over the past century. Transsphenoidal surgery was initially abandoned, but as technology has caught up with this less invasive procedure it has become the favored approach to the sella. Transseptal procedures have been performed for years with good outcomes, but with the advent of endoscopic surgery, the complications have become even fewer. The advantage to performing an endoscopic procedure is the decrease in endonasal complications, shorter hospital stay and increased patient satisfaction. Further advances in technology, including intraoperative CT or MRI may further aid in safe and effective tumor removal.

Take-Home Pearls

- Pituitary apoplexy is a surgical emergency.
- Repair of the sella is only indicated if CSF leak is visualized at the completion of the procedure.

▼

- Endoscopic endonasal transsphenoidal pituitary surgery is associated with a lower risk of intranasal complications.
- Intracranial hemorrhage most often occurs in the setting of incomplete resection of a macroadenoma.
- Airway management in the patient with acromegaly or Cushing's disease is paramount.

References

1. Couldwell WT (2004) Transsphenoidal and transcranial surgery for pituitary adenomas 69:237–256

2. Carrau RL, Kassam AB, Snyderman CH (2001) Pituitary surgery. Otolarygol Clin North Am 34:1143–1155

3. Jankowski R, Auque J, Simon C et al (1992) Endoscopic pituitary surgery. Laryngoscope 102:198–202

4. Nemergut EC, Dumont AS, Barry UT et al (2005) Perioperative management of patients undergoing trasspehnoidal pituitary surgery. Anesth Analg 101:1170–1181

5. Kennedy DW, Cohn ES, Papel ID et al (1984) Transsphenoidal approach to the sella: the Johns Hopkins experience. Laryngoscope 94:1066–1074

6. Cappabianca P, Cavallo LM, de Divitiis E (2004) Endoscopic endonasal transsphenoidal surgery. Neurosurgery 55:933–941

7. Jho HD, Carrau RL, Ko Y et al (1997) Endoscopic pituitary surgery: an early experience. Surg Neurol 47:213–223

8. Rosen MR, Saigal K, Evans J et al (2006) A review of the endoscopic approach to the pituitary through the sphenoid sinus. Curr Opin Otolaryngol Head Neck Surg 14:6–13

9. Sonnenburg RE, White D, Ewend MG et al (2003) Sellar reconstruction: is it necessary? Am J Rhinol 17:343–346

10. Zada G, Kelly DF, Cohan P et al (2003) Endonasal transsphenoidal approach for pituitary adenomas and other sellar lesions: an assessment of efficacy, safety and patient impressions. J Neurosurg 98:350–358

11. Ciric I, Ragin A, Baumgartner C et al (1997) Complications of transsphenoidal surgery: results of a national survey, review of the literature and personal experience. Neurosurgery 40:225–237

12. van Aken MO, Feelders RA, de Marie S et al (2004) Cerebrospinal fluid leakage during transsphenoidal surgery: postoperative external lumbar drainage reduces the risk for meningitis. Pituitary 7:89–93

13. Renn WH, Rhoton AL Jr (1975) Microsurgical anatomy of sellar region. J Neurosurg 43:288–298

14. Laws ER (1999) Vascular complications of transsphenoidal surgery. Pituitary 2:163–170

15. Ahuja A, Guterman L, Hopkins LN (1992) Carotid cavernous fistula and false aneurysm of the cavernous carotid artery: complications of transsphenoidal surgery. Neurosurgery 31:774–779

16. Raymond J, Hardy J, Czepko R et al (1997) Arterial injuries in transsphenoidal surgery for pituitary adenoma: the role of angiography and endovascular treatment. AJNR Am J Neuroradiol 18:655–665

17. Woollons AC, Balakrishnan V, Hunn MK et al (2000) Complications of transsphenoidal surgery: the Wellington experience. Aust N Z J Surg 70:405–408

18. Barrow DL, Tindall GT (1990) Loss of vision after transsphenoidal surgery. Neurosurgery 27:60–68

19. Shiley SG, Lionadi F, Delashaw JB et al (2003) Incidence, etiology and management of cerebrospinal fluid leaks following trans-sphenoidal surgery. Laryngoscope 113:1283–1288

20. Nemergut EC, Zuo Z, Jane JA et al (2005) Predictors of diabetes insipidus after transsphenoidal surgery: a review of 881 patients. J Neurosurg 103:448–454

21. White DR, Sonnenburg RE, Ewend MG et al (2004) Safety of minimally invasive pituitary surgery (MIPS) compared with a traditional approach. Laryngoscope 114:1945–1948

22. Dusick JR, Esposito F, Mattozo CA et al (2006) Endonasal trasspehnoidal surgery: the patient's perspective – survey results from 259 patients. Surg Neurol 65:332–342

43

Section II

Endonasal Endoscopic Surgery

Bernhard Schick (Editor) and
Wolfgang Draf (Senior Editor)

Anatomy and Imaging

Chapter 44

Nasal and Paranasal Sinus Anatomy for the Endoscopic Sinus Surgeon

44

Andreas Prescher

Core Messages

- The nomenclature of the anatomy of the nasal cavity and of the paranasal sinuses is often used arbitrarily. Therefore only terms that have been precisely defined should be used in order to avoid further confusion.
- Endonasal sinus surgery requires exact and detailed anatomical knowledge, including that of the numerous morphological variations. This knowledge must be acquired by thorough cadaver dissections.
- The ethmoidal complex can be divided into the anterior and the posterior ethmoid. The separation line is the basal lamella of the middle turbinate. Cells located anterior to this lamella belong to the anterior ethmoid, while those located posterior to this lamella belong to the posterior ethmoid.
- The middle turbinate on the lateral nasal wall is a physiologically essential structure as well as an important landmark for orientation. Laterally beneath this structure, both the uncinate process and the ethmoidal bulla must be identified with precision. It is important that the dangerous ethmoidal formations classified as Keros types II and III be kept in mind to avoid perforation of the lateral wall of the olfactory groove.
- Accessory ethmoidal pneumatizations may occur: Onodi-Grünwald cells are crucial due to their physically close relationship with the optic canal and optic nerve. Frontal bullae are important for the morphology of the frontal infundibulum; the infraorbital cells (Haller cells) may include the infraorbital nerve.

Contents

Introduction

The first endonasal surgery of the maxillary sinus is regularly attributed to von Mikulicz-Radecki in 1886 [32, 56]. Von Mikulicz-Radecki [33] published his method for draining an empyema of Highmore's cave in 1887 in the famous "Archiv für Klinische Chirurgie", but it must be said that he developed this technique using the ideas and cadaver experiments of Hunter, Jourdain (a dentist in Paris) and the anatomist Emil Zuckerkandl. After these early beginnings, endoscopic sinus surgery was essentially developed and publicized by Draf [6–9], Messerklinger [27, 28, 30, 31], and Wigand [50–55, 57, 58]. Nowadays endoscopic paranasal sinus surgery has become an established method for the surgical therapy of most pathologies of the paranasal sinus system [39].

Whereas the nasal cavity presents a relatively clear anatomical situation, the paranasal sinuses are problematic structures. In humans the paranasal sinuses include the ethmoidal cells, the frontal sinus, the maxillary sinus and the sphenoidal sinus. The latter is not a paranasal sinus in narrow sense, because it develops by narrowing and separating from the main nasal cavity and not by an active process of resorption by the mucosal lining. The functional aspects of the paranasal sinuses have only been incompletely elucidated. At first Hippocrates of Kos assumed that a mucous secretion produced by the brain is drained by the paranasal sinuses into the nose. In contrast to this ancient view, modern physiology provides several hypotheses for the function of the paranasal sinuses, as summarized in Table 44.1.

Due to their complicated three-dimensional structure with many morphological variations, the paranasal sinuses are very important structures for the rhinologist. For sinus surgery, and endoscopic sinus surgery in particular, therefore, a very detailed anatomical and topographical knowledge is necessary. This precise knowledge is not only necessary for the normal-appearing structures, but also for the many anatomical variations that can be observed during endoscopy, and which must be classified and differentiated from pathological entities [9, 29]. It must be stated at this point that detailed anatomical and topographical knowledge of the paranasal sinus system can only be achieved by doing numerous anatomical preparations. Draf [9] in this sense recommends performing numerous endoscopic cadaver operations.

Table 44.1 Hypothetical functions of the paranasal sinuses

Structural functions	Weight reduction Harmonization of skull architecture Skull surface enlargement for muscle origin Stability enhancement Substitution of function-free bone material
Physiological functions	Warming and humidification of the inhaled air Reservoir for olfactory molecules Resonance Thermal isolation of the cranial cavity Production of nitric oxide
Without function	Relic of former osteoclast activity within the skull Relic of an archaic swimming ability of primates ("aquatic ape theory")

The description of the paranasal sinuses is essentially complicated by an inconsistent terminology that is rich in synonyms and different definitions and views [42]. The aim of this chapter is to provide a short anatomical overview with a consistent, clearly defined terminology, enabling the surgeon to recognize and describe the characteristic landmarks for his orientation, especially in the endoscopic keyhole-like view.

Nasal Cavity

The nasal cavity is divided by the septum nasi into a right and a left half. Each half must be further divided into a small anterior part, called the nasal vestibule, and a larger dorsal part, the nasal cavity in its narrowest sense.

Vestibulum Nasi

The vestibulum nasi is distinguished from the nasal cavity by a small curved elevation, the limen nasi. This elevation is produced by the upper margin of the lateral crus of the major alar cartilage. The vestibule is lined with stratified squamous epithelium. Furthermore, thick, coarse hairs, the vibrissae, can be found in this region. The base of these hairs lacks the smooth muscles called arrectores pilorum muscles, which can be found in other skin hairs. The skin of the vestibulum contains typical sebaceous and sudiferous glands.

Cavum Nasi

The nasal cavity is bordered by a floor, a roof, and a lateral and medial wall. The floor is formed by the hard palate. Merkel termed the roof the carina nasi [26]. This part can be divided into an anterior section (pars nasalis), a middle section (pars

ethmoidalis), and a dorsal section (pars sphenoidalis). The medial wall is established by the nasal septum. The morphology of the lateral wall is very important for endoscopic sinus surgery. The relief of the lateral wall is structured by three nasal conchae or turbinates. The superior and the middle turbinate belong to the ethmoidal bone, whereas the inferior turbinate has lost its connection to the ethmoidal complex and forms a separate bone, which is therefore often called the maxilloturbinate bone. In some cases the small supreme concha of Santorini, positioned above the superior turbinate, may occur. The supreme concha, which can be seen more frequently in foetal and newborn specimens, belongs to the second ethmoturbinal [37]. This supreme concha was observed by Lang [19] in 17% of his cases, whereas other authors present a remarkably much higher incidence (e.g. van Alyea: 67%) [46]. These differences may be explained by the different definitions of the supreme concha used by different authors, or by misinterpretation of the folded or crenated middle turbinates.

The middle turbinate is the crucial structure for the endoscopic surgeon because it can be considered a signpost to the ethmoidal complex. After careful medial mobilization of the middle turbinate the other typical landmarks, the uncinate process, the ethmoidal bulla, and the hiatus semilunaris between these structures can be easily identified. It is also possible to first identify and then remove the uncinate process, laterally, so as to avoid harming the structures of the middle turbinate. This also allows enough space for further orientation. The morphological details of the uncinate process, the ethmoidal bulla, and the hiatus semilunaris are discussed later (see ethmoidal sinus). The nasal cavity is separated dorsally from the epipharynx by an artificial line, which runs perpendicular through the dorsal ends of the nasal conchae.

Septum Nasi

The medial limitation of the nasal cavity is formed by the septum nasi, which is a complicated structure consisting of three parts: the osseous septum, the cartilaginous septum and the mobile septum. The osseous septum is composed by the perpendicular lamina of the ethmoidal bone, the vomer, and the nasal cristae of the maxillary and the palatine bone. This osseous septum is completed by the septal cartilage, which presents a posterior process, which is intercalated between the perpendicular lamina and the vomer. In the anterior region the cartilaginous septum is fixed to the anterior nasal spine only by connective tissue. This small part is termed as the mobile part of the septum. The whole septum is lined by mucosa, which covers nerves (especially the nasopalatine nerve of Scarpa), arteries and veins. Two additional structures must be mentioned at the septum nasi: the vomeronasal torus, which represents a developmental relict, and Kiesselbachs' locus, where bleeding often occurs from the small, thin veins that lie within the papillae of the corium directly beneath the epithelium. Both structures are positioned in the inferior region of the nasal septum and are not very important for endoscopic surgery.

44

Nerves and Vessels of the Nasal Cavity and the Paranasal Sinuses

Principally, the septum nasi and the lateral wall present a superior part and an inferior part with respect to the vessel and nerve supply. The arterial supply was exhaustively described by Zuckerkandl [60]. The arteries of the superior part arise from the ophthalmic artery and therefore from the internal carotid artery, whereas the inferior part is supplied by the maxillary artery and therefore by the external carotid artery. There are four essential arteries: the anterior ethmoidal artery, the posterior ethmoidal artery, the sphenopalatine artery, and the descending palatine artery, which together continue as the greater palatine artery. With lateral rami, the anterior ethmoidal artery supplies the lateral wall of the nasal cavity, parts of the ethmoidal labyrinth, and the frontal sinus [22]. Medial rami supply the anterior superior part of the septum nasi. The posterior ethmoidal artery supplies the posterior ethmoidal sinus and the posterior superior part of the lateral wall. The sphenopalatine artery is a great vessel, which reaches the nasal cavity through the sphenopalatine foramen.

The topography of the sphenopalatine foramen is important for the surgeon, and the ethmoidal crest of the palatine bone is the principle landmark for identifying the foramen [41]. The ethmoidal crest is a rough, horizontally orientated osseous line to which the posterior end of the middle turbinate is fixed. For practice, this crest can be identified as the horizontal elongation of the posterior end of the middle turbinate. This crest belongs to the palatine bone and points to the posteriorly located sphenopalatine foramen. According to Wareing and Padgham [48], three different situations must be considered:

1. Type I (35%): the sphenopalatine opening lies within the ethmoidal crest and opens purely into the superior meatus (Fig. 44.1a).
2. Type II (56%): the foramen spans the ethmoidal crest and opens into both the superior and middle meatus (Fig. 44.1b).
3. Type III (9%): this is characterized by two separate openings positioned in the superior and the middle meatus (Fig. 44.1c). This type is of great importance because the inferior foramen contains vessels that supply the inferior turbinate. If the surgeon is not aware of this situation, in cases of severe epistaxis it may result in failure of the endonasal ligation of all important vessels (see Chap. 59). Therefore, both the superior and the medial meatus should be investigated in order to identify all relevant vessels of the sphenopalatine foramen.

The sphenopalatine artery divides into the posterior nasal lateral branches and the septal branches. According to Lang [19] and Simmen and Jones [41], this ramification can take place before or within the sphenopalatine foramen. The surgeon must

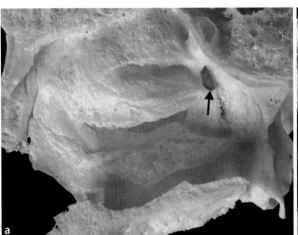
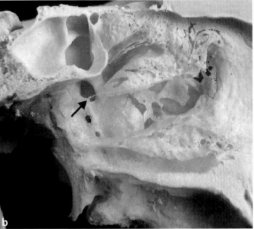
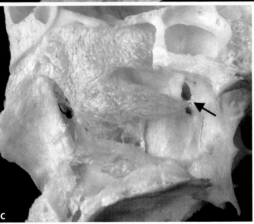

Fig. 44.1a–c The location of the sphenopalatine foramen can be classified into three types (shown in a–c, respectively) according to Wareing and Padgham [48]. **a** The foramen opens completely in the superior meatus and lies above the ethmoidal crest, which is marked by an *arrow*. **b** The foramen opens partly into the superior and partly into the middle nasal meatus. The *arrow* points towards the ethmoidal crest. Some dehiscences in the medial wall of the greater palatine canal, seen beneath the *arrow*, are also frequently observed anatomical peculiarities, especially in the older patient. **c** The third type is characterized by two completely separated openings into the middle as well as the superior nasal meatus. The *arrow* marks the osseous bridge representing the ethmoidal crest, which divides the foramen

therefore be prepared to find more than one vessel in the plane of the sphenopalatine foramen. The anterior branch of the sphenopalatine artery can be identified above the posterior nasal fontanella. The septal branches, also termed the nasopalatine artery, run over the sphenoid body towards the septum. The rami of the major palatine artery run through the foramen incisivum and then communicate with the arterial net of the septum nasi. All of these arteries are accompanied by veins [49]; the drained venous areas are thus concordant with the arterial areas.

The olfactory, anterior ethmoidal, posterior ethmoidal and maxillary nerves are particularly important. The olfactory nerves supply a small area, about 1 cm², in the cranial part of the septum nasi and on the opposite superior turbinate. It must be noted, however, that the precise distribution of the human olfactory neuroepithelium is not yet clearly understood. According to the investigations of Leopold et al. [25], the olfactory epithelium can also be found in the region of the fixation of the anterior middle turbinate. The sensory innervation comes from the anterior ethmoidal nerve, which divides into the lateral nasal rami, medial nasal rami and an external nasal branch on the posterior side of the nasal bone. The posterior ethmoidal nerve supplies the posterior ethmoidal cells and posterior parts of the lateral wall. Furthermore, different groups of nerves arise from the maxillary nerve: the posterior superior lateral nasal nerves for the lateral wall of the nasal cavity, and posterior superior medial nasal nerves for the septum. One of these medial nerves on the septum is longer and runs towards the foramen incisivum. This nerve is termed the nasopalatine nerve (of Scarpa). The inferior turbinate is supplied by posterior inferior nasal branches splitting from the major palatine nerve. These nerves often spread out with the vessels.

Somewhat more complicated and not entirely established are the lymphatics of the nasal cavity and of the paranasal sinuses, although overviews have been published by different authors [1, 36, 49]. In the olfactory region two important special lymphatic systems exist beside the normal one: the lymphatic sheaths surrounding the olfactory nerves, which present a communication between the nose and the endocranium, and another web [5, 35, 36], which also communicates with the meningeal lymphatics and the endocranial spaces. This specialized web must be seen, for example, as an analogue of the perioptic lymphatics [36]. In the nasal mucosa there are two different webs, a superficial web and a profound web, and these communicate with each other [49]. Furthermore, the density of lymphatic vessels is high at the inferior turbinate and diminishes in the cranial direction [35]. Similarly, the lymphatic vessels are more concentrated in the posterior parts of the turbinates and diminish towards the anterior parts [49]. In general it can be said that the concentration of lymphatic vessels is dependent upon the tension and thickness of the mucous layer; a thick and loosely arranged mucous layer contains more vessels than a thin and tightly arranged one [43]. The localization of lymphatic collectors is also important for the surgeon, because their destruction may cause disturbances of the lymphatic drainage system. For the nasal cavity these collectors are localized mainly in the mucous layer of the floor, the basal septum, and on the inferior and middle turbinates [49]. The most anterior parts of the nasal cavity drain to the lymphatics of the outer nose, which then run with the facial vein to the

submandibular nodes. The lymphatics of the dorsal parts of the nasal cavity run through the choanae and form a large stem in the region of the pharyngeal tubal ostium. More detailed topography is not important for the topic of this chapter.

The lymphatics of the paranasal sinuses run in an osteumorientated direction and drain into the lymphatics of the nasal cavity [49]; thus they also run to the lateral retropharyngeal nodes and to the deep cervical nodes. It must be noted, especially for the maxillary sinus, that many lymphatic vessels perforate the osseous walls and drain into the lymphatics of the face, and therefore into those of the submandibular nodes [1].

Paranasal Sinuses

Maxillary Sinus

The maxillary sinus, also termed Highmore's cave (according to the classical description of the English practitioner Nathanael Highmore in 1651) [14], represents the largest pneumatic cave of the skull. Furthermore, its morphology is quite constant, exhibiting only few anatomical variations. The first, but unpublished description was done by Leonardo da Vinci. The maxillary sinus lies within the body of the maxillary bone beneath the orbita. According to this typical topography the floor of the orbita is simultaneously the roof of the maxillary sinus. For traumatology it is very important to know that the orbital floor has no support or strengthening. These anatomical facts explain a typical injury, which was first described in 1889 by Lang [24] in the Transactions of the Ophthalmologic Society of the United Kingdom as a "blowout fracture". This injury is characterized by a bursting out of the orbital floor into the maxillary sinus, and this bursting out is often accompanied by a herniation of adipose tissue as well as the inferior rectus muscle, which explains the subsequent diplopia (see Chap. 60).

Two hypotheses have been developed to explain the development of a blowout fracture. The first is called the hydraulic pressure hypothesis, according to which the force is transmitted to the orbital content, which is more or less incompressible, and thus the force is transmitted to the osseous boundaries of the orbit. The weakest point will break out, which is the orbital floor. The second hypothesis is known as buckling force hypothesis. According to this explanation, the force is transmitted to the osseous orbital frame, which is elastically deformed. Due to the suddenly increased pressure within the orbital compartment, the orbital floor is wrinkled and breaks out into the maxillary sinus.

The dorsal wall of the maxillary sinus is bordered by the infratemporal fossa on the lateral side and the pterygopalatine fossa on the medial side (see Chap. 64). This typical topographical relationship is important for the transmaxillary approach to the sphenopalatine artery and to the pterygopalatine ganglion. The recesses of the maxillary sinus can be described according to the grade of pneumatization (Table 44.2). The alveolar recess is particularly important because in cases of excessive pneumatization the apices of the roots of the teeth can project into the maxillary sinus and cause a maxilloantral fistula during extraction. Furthermore, the plexuses of dental nerves and ves-

Table 44.2 Recessus of the maxillary sinus

Recessus infraorbitalis
Recessus palatinus
Recessus zygomaticus (Reschreiter)
Recessus praelacrimalis
Recessus ossis palatini
Recessus alveolaris

Table 44.3 The ground lamella of the middle turbinate

Part	Orientation	Attachment
Anterior	Vertical	Lamina cribrosa
Middle	Frontal	Lamina papyracea
Posterior	Horizontal	Lamina papyracea and dorsal medial wall of the maxillary sinus

sels supplying the dental root structure lie directly beneath the mucosal lining of the maxillary sinus, so that these structures can be easily damaged [40]. Septations are also not rare events. Irregular septa can often be observed in the region of the alveolar recess that separates the molar region from the premolar region. These septa are called Underwood's septa [45]. Rarely, horizontally or sagittally extending septa are observed as well as complete vertical septa, separating an anterior from a posterior maxillary sinus. The infraorbital nerve and the infraorbital artery are located within the roof of the maxillary sinus. These structures often are included in the infraorbital recess, so that they run in an osseous trabecular structure.

Ethmoid Sinus

The ethmoid sinus represents the most complicated part of the paranasal sinus system, so that it is also called the ethmoidal labyrinth (see Chap. 51). It comprises several minor pneumatic cells located bilaterally beside the upper part of the nasal cavity. These ethmoidal cells are separated from the orbita by the very thin lamina orbitalis ossis ethmoidalis, which is also termed the lamina papyracea. This very thin structure is stabilized by the walls of the ethmoidal cells. Cranially, the ethmoid labyrinth reaches the anterior cranial fossa beside the olfactory groove and forms a part of the so called rhinobasis. The ethmoid complex is bordered dorsally by the sphenoid sinus, and caudally it

reaches the maxillary sinus and the nasal cavity. It is bordered anteriorly by the frontal and nasal bones.

The line of fixation of the middle turbinate, called the basal lamella of the middle turbinate, is highly essential (Fig. 44.2). This basal lamella can be divided into three parts (Table 44.3): the first part is orientated vertically, the medial part frontally, and the posterior part horizontally. These three parts present a constant attachment at the osseous structures of the lateral wall of the nasal cavity. The vertical part is fixed at the lateral edge of the lamina cribrosa; it is often termed the lamina conchalis [19]. The medial part is fixed at the lamina orbitalis and the posterior part also at the lamina orbitalis and additionally at the medial wall of the maxillary sinus. This complicated fixing line provides a three-dimensional stabilization and therefore contributes essentially to the stability of the middle turbinate. Furthermore, this constant osseous attachment of the middle turbinate is used to subdivide the ethmoidal complex (Fig. 44.2). The anterior ethmoidal cells are located in front of the line, whereas the posterior ethmoidal cells are found behind it. The openings of the anterior cells are located before and beneath the basal lamella, whereas the posterior ethmoidal cells open behind and above the basal lamella. The middle ethmoidal cells should not be classified any further, because there are neither topographical nor developmental arguments for doing so [42]. Furthermore, the middle turbinate can be pneumatized, and thus contains a large cavity. This condition is termed "concha bullosa", appears in about 8% of us [12], and may cause symptoms (Fig. 44.3).

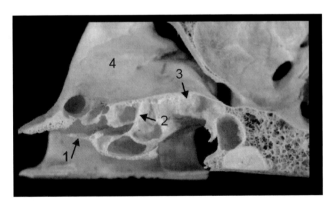

Fig. 44.2 Horizontal section through the middle turbinate, presenting the three different parts of the ground lamella (view from above). *1* Anterior, vertical part; *2* frontal, middle part; *3* sagittal, posterior part; *4* orbital floor

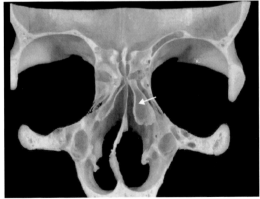

Fig. 44.3 Frontal section of the viscerocranium. The *arrow* points to a large concha bullosa. The opposite middle turbinate is also pneumatized

Two osseous structures of the ethmoidal complex are very important for the endoscopic orientation at the lateral wall of the nasal cavity: the uncinate process (Fig. 44.4) and the prominent ethmoidal bulla. The sickle-shaped uncinate process was first described by Johann Friedrich Blumenbach in 1790 [2]. This structure represents a thin, brittle, osseous lamella, which is sagittally oriented and has quite a dorsal concave margin and an anterior convex one. The uncinate process is attached to the perpendicular lamina of the palatine bone and at the ethmoidal process of the inferior turbinate. The uncinate process may be fixed cranially at different structures so that three systematically different topographical situations can be classified:

1. Type A: the uncinate process inserts at the lamina papyracea.
2. Type B1: the uncinate process inserts at the skull base.
3. Type B2: the insertion takes place at the middle turbinate.

It is important to mention that osseous dehiscences, termed anterior nasal fontanelles (Zuckerkandl's fontanelles), may occur at the anterior margin (Fig. 44.4). Posterior nasal fontanelles are located above the dorsal end of the uncinate process where it is fixed at the perpendicular lamina of the palatine bone. The nasal fontanelles are often closed by the mucous membrane, but in about 10% of these positions [18] accessory openings of the maxillary sinus may occur, which lead directly to the lumen of the maxillary sinus (see Chap. 50). In some cases the uncinate process is bent into the nasal cavity and often reaches the lateral surface of the medial turbinate. This anatomical variation can be seen as an atavism and was called "doubled medial turbinate" by Kaufmann in 1890 [15]. In rare cases the uncinate process can be pneumatized.

The term "ethmoidal bulla" was introduced by Zuckerkandl in 1893 [59], although this structure was well-known before. Samuel Thomas Sömmering described it as "pars turgida ossis ethmoidalis", and in 1870, Zoja called it "eminentia fossae nasalis". The ethmoid bulla is the largest and most constant anterior

ethmoidal cell, and is positioned with a broad base on the lamina papyracea. Lang [19] noted that about 30% of the ethmoidal bullae lack pneumatization, so an osseous torus is formed. This variation should be termed "torus ethmoidalis". The topographical relationship to its neighbouring structures is important. If the ethmoidal bulla reaches the skull base, the bulla forms the posterior border of the frontal recess (Fig. 44.4). If it does not reach the skull base, an accessory recess is formed above the ethmoidal bulla, which is termed the suprabullar recess. If the dorsal border of the ethmoidal bulla does not reach the middle turbinate a retrobullar recess will be established (Chap. 51). Grünwald [12] termed the irregular spaces of the suprabullar and the infrabullar recesses together as the "lateral sinus".

The semilunar hiatus is located between the uncinate process and ethmoidal bulla (Fig. 44.4). This structure exhibits a sagittally oriented cleft, which represents the entrance into the ethmoidal infundibulum. The ethmoidal infundibulum – a term introduced by Boyer in 1805 – forms an atrium in the maxillary sinus. The frontal sinus can discharge into the ethmoidal infundibulum, usually in the region between the medial and posterior thirds.

If an exhaustive pneumatization takes place, some accessory cells or cell groups may be formed within the ethmoidal labyrinth. The following accessory cells may develop from the anterior ethmoidal complex: lacrimal cells, agger cells and frontal cells or bullae frontales. The lacrimal cells are located within the lacrimal bone (see Chap. 58). If pneumatizations occur in the region of the agger nasi, agger cells are formed. According to van Alyea [46] these cells are present in about 89% of cases and are therefore considered to be part of a normal anatomical condition. These cells are in direct contact with the laterally positioned nasolacrimal duct. This topography should be borne in mind during operations. On the other hand, a dacryocystorhinostomia can be easily performed at this location. The frontal cells or bullae frontales occur in about 20% of cases (Fig. 44.5). These cells are typical anterior ethmoidal cells that bulge into the floor of the frontal sinus and distort the frontal infundibu-

44

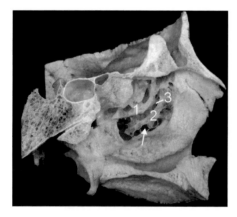

Fig. 44.4 Lateral wall structure. The *arrow* marks the anterior nasal fontanelles (Zuckerkandl's fontanelles). *1* Bulla ethmoidalis, *2* uncinate process, *3* hiatus semilunaris

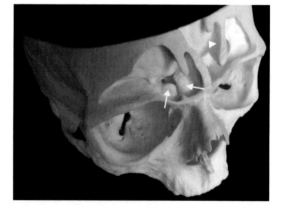

Fig. 44.5 Frontal sinus. The *arrows* point to two frontal bullae, which are narrowing the frontal infundibulum of Killian. The *arrowhead* marks a typical incomplete septulum

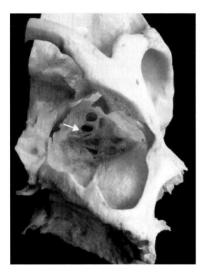

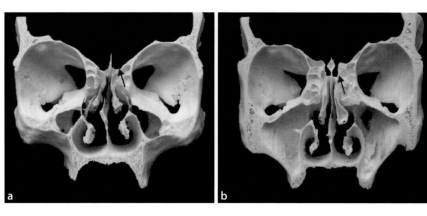

Fig. 44.7 Keros-type 1 (**a**) and Keros-type 2 (**b**). **a** The *arrow* points towards the short lateral wall of the olfactory groove. **b** The *arrow* marks the high lateral wall of the olfactory groove

Fig. 44.6 Maxillary sinus. The *arrow* points towards the infraorbital cells (Haller cells)

lum of Killian, so that a considerable narrowing of the outlet structure of the frontal sinus takes place (see Chap. 52).

Accessory pneumatizations may also occur in the medial infraorbital region (Fig. 44.6). These cells are called "infraorbital ethmoidal cells (Haller cells)". Albrecht von Haller first described these cells in 1743. The infraorbital ethmoidal cells may originate from either the anterior or posterior ethmoid and are therefore transitional structures between the anterior and the posterior ethmoid. The infraorbital cells are important for the orientation during operation. If they are not established, a false route can be taken and the orbita can be damaged (see Chap. 54). In some cases the infraorbital cells involve the infraorbital nerve, which can also be a dangerous topographical situation. Largely developed infraorbital cells narrow the ethmoidal infundibulum and can therefore be responsible for pathologies of the maxillary sinus. The sphenoethmoidal cells of Onodi-Grünwald are derived from the posterior ethmoid, and these are in close connection to the optic canal; in rare cases the whole optic canal can be surrounded by pneumatic cells. If a close relationship between the optic nerve and a sphenoethmoidal cell is present, the optic nerve can bulge into the posterior ethmoidal pneumatic space. This bulging structure is termed the optic nerve tubercle (see Chap. 61). According to Lang [20], Onodi-Grünwald cells occur in about 11.4% of cases. These cells are very important because of the very close topographical relationship between them and the content of the optic canal, which means that the optic nerve is at risk of damage during surgical procedures in the posterior ethmoidal labyrinth. In addition, inflammations of the cells can spread readily into the optic canal, especially if there are dehiscences in the osseous wall of the optic canal.

The ethmoidal labyrinth is crossed by two important arteries, the anterior ethmoidal artery and the posterior ethmoidal artery, which are accompanied by small veins and nerves. Both

arteries arise from the ophthalmic artery and therefore belong to the area supplied by the internal carotid artery. Two foramina can be found at the medial border of the orbita and the superior margin of the lamina papyracea: the anterior ethmoidal foramen and the posterior ethmoidal foramen. Both foramina can be doubled and exhibit a high degree of anatomical variability [23]. The anterior foramen leads into the orbitocranial canal and the posterior one into the orbitoethmoidal canal. The orbitocranial canal normally lies in the gusset between the first orbital ethmoidal cell and the frontal sinus [34]. This canal is often not a complete osseous canal, but shows dehiscences in its walls, so that the periosteal tube may be located directly under the mucous lining of the ethmoidal cells. Its internal opening into the endocranium is located just above the lamina cribrosa of the olfactory groove. In this region, often still in the orbitoethmoidal canal, the anterior ethmoidal artery splits off the anterior meningeal artery, which fans out anteriorly, becoming embedded in slight osseous sulci. The posterior ethmoidal artery supplies the posterior ethmoidal labyrinth, some posterior parts of the nasal cavity, and the posterior septum. The ethmoidal arteries are of great surgical importance because they run transversely through the ethmoidal labyrinth, where they can easily be damaged. If a laceration occurs, the artery will retract into the orbit, and a retrobulbar haematoma occurs, which threatens the optic nerve as a result of stretching (see Chap. 54).

Three general ethmoidal types of ethmoidal labyrinth were defined by Keros in 1965 [16] according to the phenotype of the olfactory groove (types I–III; Fig. 44.7a, b). Type I is defined by a lateral wall height of 1–3 mm, type II by a lateral wall height of between 4 and 7 mm and type III by a lateral wall height of 8–16 mm. The risk of an incidental perforation of the lateral wall from the ethmoidal side is severely increased with increasing depth of the olfactory groove (see Chap. 62).

Frontal Sinus

The frontal sinus is a bilaterally expressed cavitation within the frontal bone that presents many anatomical variations. Hypoplasias and aplasias can be observed, with racial differences; for example, 52% of Eskimos do not present with a frontal sinus [19]. If the frontal sinus is largely pneumatized, it will extend into the orbital roof, resulting in a double-layered structure (Fig. 44.8). Only in rare cases does the septum of the frontal sinus lie in the median–sagittal plane; it is often asymmetric, bent to one side. According to Boege [3] small, incomplete accessory septal ridges called "septula" can frequently be seen (Fig. 44.8). Gerber states that the left sinus is usually larger than the right [11]. If the frontal sinus extends largely to the dorsal region, it will reach the olfactory groove, the anterior borders of which will then form a prominent ridge, projecting into the frontal sinus. These ridges consist of a fragile, thin, osseous substance and are termed "crista olfactoria". This typical situation, which results from excessive pneumatization, was termed "dangerous frontal bone" by Boenninghaus [4]. The crista olfactoria can easily be damaged during surgical procedures, resulting in opening of the endocranium. In cases of a dangerous frontal bone, the crista galli is often also pneumatized and contains a pneumatic cell, termed "recessus cristae galli" or "recessus of Palfyn". In these cases the pneumatization originates from the frontal sinus. It must also be mentioned that the pneumatization of the crista galli can also be established from the bullae ethmoidales. It is important that cases of a pneumatized crista galli must not be combined with an asymmetrically expressed interfrontal septum, as shown clearly by Tonndorf [44].

An important structure of the frontal sinus is the funnel-shaped outlet structure, called the frontal sinus infundibulum [17], which opens into the frontal recess (see Chap. 52). According to the developmental history of this region the frontal recess must be considered an anterior ethmoidal cell. This cell was responsible for the pneumatization of the frontal bone and therefore for the development of the frontal sinus [17, 37]. The frontal recess can be seen as the cranially directed continuation of the ethmoidal infundibulum and presents typical anatomical boundaries: it lies dorsal to the agger nasi and ventral to the ethmoidal bulla. The lateral border is the lamina papyracea and the medial border is formed by the lateral lamella of the middle turbinate. Lang [19] differentiates two main conditions: if the outlet duct is longer than 3 mm he describes it as a nasofrontal duct (77.3%); if the duct is shorter he prefers the term "frontal ostium" (22.7%). Various surgeons stressed, however, that the term "nasofrontal duct" does not adequately describe the funnel-shaped structure of the frontal recess and should therefore no longer be used. Unfortunately there are many different definitions in this region that cannot be discussed in detail in this overview. It should be borne in mind that the term "nasofrontal duct" is not a synonym for the frontal recess, a point that was also stressed by Stammberger et al. [42]. According to Vogt and Schrade [47], a simple connection between the frontal sinus and the nose can only be found in one-third of cases. In the other two-thirds the drainage route is divided between the passages of the ethmoidal cell system and therefore complicated topographical situations occur. Also, aberrant olfactory fibres may occur in the region of the frontal recess anterior and lateral to the middle turbinate [44]. This is a dangerous variation because damage to these fibres opens the lymphatic sheaths and produces a continuation with the subarachnoid space, so that meningitis may develop.

Sphenoid Sinus

The sphenoid sinus is a structure that presents a large number of anatomical variations as a result of different grades of pneumatization. According to Hardy [13], three types of sphenoid sinus can be differentiated: the conchal type, the presellar type and the sellar type. In rare cases, according to Grünwald in about 1.5% of cases, a complete aplasia of the sphenoid sinus can be observed. The bilaterally expressed sphenoid sinuses are separated from each other by the septum sinuum sphenoidalium. This septum is rarely a symmetrical structure, in most cases being asymmetrically bent to the right or the left side. If a horizontal septum seems to be present, this must be explained with a

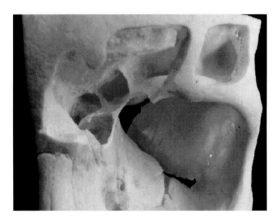

Fig. 44.8 Frontal sinus, largely pneumatized and extending into the orbital roof, so that a double-layered structure results

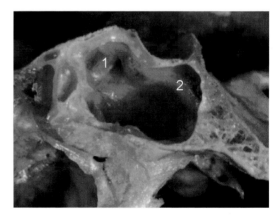

Fig. 44.9 Median-sagittally sectioned sphenoid sinus. *1* Prominentia nervi optici, *2* Prominentia arteriae carotidis

Table 44.4 Recessus of the sphenoid sinus

Recessus septalis
Recessus ethmoidalis
Recessus lateralis superior/inferior
Recessus palatinus
Recessus pterygoideus
Recessus posterior
Recessus posterior superior

posterior ethmoidal cell lying above the sphenoid sinus. Incomplete additional septa can often occur in addition to the main septum, which may complicate the architecture of the sphenoid sinus remarkably. The asymmetrically expressed septum may be a dangerous structure because it can be connected to the carotid prominence. In such cases, fracture of the septum can cause damage to the osseous carotid prominence and therefore to the carotid artery itself, resulting in severe bleeding (see Chap. 54). If a large pneumatization has taken place, several additional recesses may occur (Table 44.4); in such cases it is important to note that essential neighbouring structures can bulge into the sphenoid sinus. The internal carotid artery forms the prominentia arteriae carotidis, and the optic nerve forms the prominentia nervi optici, both on the lateral side (Fig. 44.9). The maxillary nerve can also produce a slight prominence just above the floor. In older patients with rarefying osseous processes, dehiscences may occur in the region of these prominences, so that these important structures are not covered by bone, but are lying directly beneath the mucosa. It is therefore essential to open the sphenoid sinus in the middle part of its anterior wall so as to avoid the dangerous lateral structures (see Chap. 53). The posterior end of the middle turbinate marks the level of the perforation, to avoid laceration of the posterior septal branches (nasopalatine ramus) of the sphenopalatine artery. It should be further noted that in rare cases an aneurysm of the internal carotid artery may bulge into the sphenoid sinus [9]. In yet other rare cases the so-called "kissing carotids" may protrude into the sella turcica and therefore reach the midline [38]. In these pathological cases osseous dehiscences are often present, so that the arterial structures lie directly under the mucosal lining of the sphenoid sinus. The nerve of the pterygoid canal (Vidian's nerve) is often observed heading towards the pterygoid fossa in the floor of the sphenoid sinus. If there is a large pneumatization of the sphenoid sinus the superior osseous wall of the pterygoid canal can be resorbed, so that the nerve is in direct contact with the mucosal membrane of the sphenoid sinus.

The sphenoid sinus opens with a round or elliptic aperture into the sphenoethmoidal recess behind the superior turbinate. The relationship between the sphenoidal aperture and the floor of the sphenoid sinus is quite variable. In most cases the aperture lies within the upper half of the anterior wall of the sphenoid sinus only a few millimetres under the nasal roof. Since the sphenoethmoidal recess is inclined against the sagittal plane (the superior part lies more laterally than the inferior one) and the sphenoid sinus aperture is positioned in the superior, more lateral part, the aperture is often hidden behind the superior

turbinate in the anterior view. The sphenoethmoidal recess does not appear to have a typical appearance, and Lang and Sakals [21] found an obvious recess in about only 48.3% of cases. This recess can be important for bleeding, because a small arterial ramus can be present in this region. According to Forschner [10], this artery arises consistently from the nasopalatine ramus (posterior septal branches) of the sphenopalatine artery, runs upwards towards the sphenoethmoidal recess and lies in the lateral part of this location.

Take-Home Pearls

- The sphenopalatine foramen is located at the posterior end of the middle turbinate. The ethmoidal crest of the palatine bone can be used as a landmark.
- The sphenopalatine artery is often already divided in the plane of the sphenopalatine foramen, so the surgeon must be aware that he or she may find several vessels belonging to this artery.
- It should be kept in mind that the nerves and vessels supplying the superior teeth lie directly under the mucosal sheet of the maxillary sinus, so that these structures can easily be damaged.
- The ethmoidal complex is penetrated by the anterior and posterior ethmoidal vessels. Laceration should be carefully avoided, because a retrobulbar haematoma may occur, which may cause stretching of, and ultimately damage to the optic nerve.
- The morphological situation of the "dangerous frontal bone" should be borne in mind to avoid an unexpected opening of the cranial cavity.
- The anterior wall of the sphenoid sinus should be opened near the midline and at the level of the middle turbinate, because surgically threatened structures are located at the lateral wall of the sphenoid sinus. An opening inferior to the middle turbinate may cause bleeding from the nasopalatine branches of the sphenopalatine artery.

References

1. Bartels P (1909) Das Lymphgefäßsystem. In: von Bardeleben K (ed) Handbuch der Anatomie des Menschen, vol 3, 4. Fischer, Jena
2. Blumenbach JF (1790) Decas collectionis suae craniorum diversarium gentium illustrata. Göttingen
3. Boege K (1902) Zur Anatomie der Stirnhöhle: Sinus frontales. Diss. Königsberg
4. Boenninghaus G (1923) Die Operationen an den Nebenhöhlen der Nase. In: Katz L, Preysing H, Blumenfeld F (eds) Handbuch der speziellen Chirurgie des Ohres und der oberen Luftwege. vol 3, 3. edn. Kabitzsch, Würzburg; Leipzig
5. Cuneo B, André M (1905) Relations des espaces périmenigés avec des lymphatiques des fosses nasales. Bull Soc Anat Paris 80:58

6. Draf W (1975) Die Endoskopie der Nasennebenhöhlen. Diagnostische und therapeutische Möglichkeiten. Laryngol Rhinol Otol 54:209–215

7. Draf W (1978) Therapeutic endoscopy of paranasal sinuses. Endoscopy 10:247–254

8. Draf W (1978) Endoskopie der Nasennebenhöhlen. Technik – Typische Befunde – Therapeutische Möglichkeiten. Springer, Berlin

9. Draf W (1982) Die chirurgische Behandlung entzündlicher Erkrankungen der Nasennebenhöhlen. Indikation, Operationsverfahren, Gefahren, Fehler und Komplikationen, Revisionschirurgie. Arch Otorhinolaryngol 235:133–305

10. Forschner L (1950) Über die Gefahr von Blutungen bei Eingriffen am Keilbein. Arch Ohren Nasen Kehlkopfheilk 158:270–275

11. Gerber PH (1909) Die Komplikationen der Stirnhöhlenentzündungen. Karger, Berlin

12. Grünwald L (1925) Deskriptive und topographische Anatomie der Nase und ihrer Nebenhöhlen. In: Denker A, Kahler O (eds) Handbuch der Hals-Nasen-Ohrenheilkunde, vol. 1,1. Springer, Berlin, pp 1–95

13. Hardy J (1967) La chirurgie de l'hypophyse par voie trans- sphenoidale – étude comparative de deux modalités techniques. Union Med Can 96:702–712

14. Highmore N (1651) Corporis Humani disquisitio anatomica. Haga comitibus

15. Kaufmann E (1890) Über eine typische Form von Schleimhautgeschwulst (laterale Schleimhautgeschwulst) an der äußeren Nasenwand. Monatsschr Ohrenheilk 24:13, 35, 75, 106, 143, 171, 208, 238

16. Keros P (1962) Über die praktische Bedeutung der Niveauunterschiede der Lamina cribrosa des Ethmoids. Z Laryngol Rhinol Otol Grenzgeb 41:808–838

17. Killian G (1895) Zur Anatomie der Nase menschlicher Embryonen. II. Arch Otorhinolaryngol 3:17–25

18. Krmpotic-Nemancic J, Draf W, Helms J (1985) Chirurgische Anatomie des Kopf-Hals-Bereiches. Springer, Berlin, Heidelberg, New York, Tokyo

19. Lang J (1988) Klinische Anatomie der Nase, Nasenhöhle und Nebenhöhlen. Thieme, Stuttgart, New York

20. Lang J (1988) Über die Cellulae ethmoidales posteriores und ihre Beziehungen zum Canalis opticus. HNO 36:49–53

21. Lang J, Sakals E (1982) Über den Recessus spheno-ethmoidalis, die Apertura nasalis des Ductus nasolacrimalis und den Hiatus semilunaris. Anat Anz 152:393–412

22. Lang J, Schäfer K (1979) Arteriae ethmoidales: Ursprung, Verlauf, Versorgungsgebiete und Anastomosen. Acta Anat (Basel) 104:183–197

23. Lang J, Schlehahn F (1978) Foramina ethmoidalia und Canales ethmoidales. Verh Anat Ges 72:433–435

24. Lang W (1889) Injuries and diseases of the orbit 1. Traumatic enophthalmos with retention of perfect acuity of vision. Transact Ophthalmol Soc U K 9:41–45

25. Leopold DA, Hummel T, Schwob JE, Hong SC, Knecht M, Kobal G (2000) Anterior distribution of human olfactory epithelium. Laryngoscope 110:417–421

26. Merkel F (1885–90) Handbuch der topographischen Anatomie zum Gebrauch für Ärzte, vol 1. Vieweg, Braunschweig, pp 333–339

27. Messerklinger W (1970) Die Endoskopie der Nase. Monatsschr Ohrenheilk 102:451–456

28. Messerklinger W (1972) Nasenendoskopie: Der mittlere Nasengang und seine unspezifischen Entzündungen. HNO 20:212–215

29. Messerklinger W (1973) Zur endoskopischen Anatomie der menschlichen Siebbeinmuscheln. Acta Otolaryngol 75:243–248

30. Messerklinger W (1978) Endoscopy of the nose. Urban Schwarzenberg, München

31. Messerklinger W (1979) Das Infundibulum ethmoidale und seine entzündlichen Erkrankungen. Arch Otorhinolaryngol 222:11–22

32. Mikulicz J (1886) Zur operativen Behandlung des Empyems der Highmorshöhle. Prager Z Heilk 7:257–259

33. Mikulicz J (1887) Zur operativen Behandlung des Empyems der Highmorshöhle. Arch Klin Chir 34:626–634

34. Minnigerode B (1966) Zur Anatomie und klinischen Bedeutung des Canalis ethmoidalis. Z Laryngol Rhinol Otol 45:554–559

35. Most A (1901) Ueber den Lymphapparat von Nase und Rachen. Arch Anat Physiol Anat Abt pp 75–94

36. Most A (1917) Chirurgie der Lymphgefäße und der Lymphdrüsen. Enke, Stuttgart

37. Peter K (1913) Atlas der Entwicklung der Nase und des Gaumens beim Menschen mit Einschluß der Entwicklungsstörungen. Fischer, Jena

38. Prescher A, Brors D (1994) A rare variety of the course of the internal carotid artery and rarefying hyperostosis of the cranial vault. Surg Radiol Anat 16:93–96

39. Rauchfuss A (1990) Komplikationen der endonasalen Chirurgie der Nasennebenhöhlen. Spezielle Anatomie, Pathomechanismen, operative Versorgung. HNO 38:309–316

40. Schicketanz H-W, Schicketanz W (1961) Mittelbare und unmittelbare Zahnschädigungen nach Kieferhöhleneingriffen. HNO 9:169–175

41. Simmen D, Jones N (2005) Chirurgie der Nasennebenhöhlen und der vorderen Schädelbasis. Thieme, Stuttgart

42. Stammberger H, Hosemann W, Draf W (1997) Anatomische Terminologie und Nomenklatur für die Nasennebenhöhlenchirurgie. Laryngorhinootologie 76:435–449

43. Teichmann L (1861) Das Saugadersystem. Engelmann, Leipzig

44. Tonndorf W (1926) Zur Anatomie der Lamina cribrosa und der Crista olfactoria. Beitr Anat Physiol Ohr Nase 23:654–667

45. Underwood AS (1910) An inquiry into the anatomy and pathology of the maxillary sinus. J Anat Physiol 44:354–369

46. Van Alyea OE (1939) Ethmoid labyrinth; anatomical study, with consideration of the clinical significance of its structural characteristics. Arch Otolaryngol 29:881–902

47. Vogt K, Schrade F (1979) Anatomische Varianten des Ausführungsgangsystems der Stirnhöhle. Laryngol Rhinol Otol (Stuttg) 58:783–794

48. Wareing MJ, Padgham ND (1998) Osteologic classification of the sphenopalatine foramen. Laryngoscope 108:125–127

49. Werner JA (1995) Untersuchungen zum Lymphgefäßsystem der oberen Luft- und Speisewege. Shaker, Aachen

50. Wigand ME (1981) Transnasale, endoskopische Chirurgie der Nasennebenhöhlen bei chronischer Sinusitis. I. Ein biomechanisches Konzept der Schleimhautchirurgie. HNO 29:215–221

44

51. Wigand ME (1981) Transnasale, endoskopische Chirurgie der Nasennebenhöhlen bei chronischer Sinusitis. II. Die endonasale Kieferhöhlen-Operation. HNO 29:263–269

52. Wigand ME (1981) Transnasale, endoskopische Chirurgie der Nasennebenhöhlen bei chronischer Sinusitis. III. Die endonasale Siebbeinausräumung. HNO 29:287–293

53. Wigand ME (1981) Transnasal endoscopical surgery of the anterior skull base. Proceedings of the XIIth ORL World Congress, Budapest Hung. Acad Sci, pp 137–140

54. Wigand ME (1981) Transnasal ethmoidectomy under endoscopic control. Rhinology 19:7–15

55. Wigand ME (1981) Ein Saug-Spül-Endoskop für die transnasale Chirurgie der Nasennebenhöhlen und der Schädelbasis. HNO 29:102–103

56. Wigand MW (1989) Endoskopische Chirurgie der Nasennebenhöhlen und der vorderen Schädelbasis. Thieme, Stuttgart, New York

57. Wigand ME, Steiner W (1977) Endonasale Kieferhöhlenoperation mit endoskopischer Kontrolle. Laryngol Rhinol Otol 56:421–425

58. Wigand ME, Steiner W, Jaumann MP (1978) Endonasal sinus surgery with endoscopical control: from radical operation to rehabilitation of the mucosa. Endoscopy 10:255–260

59. Zuckerkandl E (1893/1892) Normale und pathologische Anatomie der Nasenhöhle und ihrer pneumatischen Anhänge, vol 1, 2. Braumüller, Wien Leipzig

60. Zuckerkandl E (1885) Ueber den Circulationsapparat in der Nasenschleimhaut. Denkschrift Akad Wiss Wien 49:121–151

Chapter 45

Radiology of the Nose and Paranasal Sinuses for the Endoscopic Sinus Surgeon

45

Erich Hofmann

Core Messages

- Plain films are almost obsolete in the diagnostic workup of paranasal sinus disease. Acute sinusitis is a clinical, not a radiologic diagnosis. Chronic recurrent sinusitis, trauma, neoplastic disease, and malformations require more sophisticated (i.e., specific and sensitive) imaging techniques.

- Computed tomography (CT) is the workhorse in paranasal sinus imaging. CT depicts not only the complex three-dimensional anatomy, but also the extent of disease and the wide range of anatomic normal variations that are of great importance to the endoscopic surgeon.

- Magnetic resonance imaging (MRI) is needed in selected cases. Its superb soft-tissue contrast makes it an ideal tool for searching for mucoceles, the delineation of tumors, and the degree of involvement of neural structures in malformations. In addition, plain MRI is able to show injury to the brain and dura mater in trauma patients.

- Intrathecal administration of contrast medium (CT-cisternography, magnetic resonance cisternography) may be necessary to pinpoint the location of dural leaks, especially in complex cases of cerebrospinal fluid rhinorrhea.

- Digital subtraction angiography is rarely needed for diagnostic purposes, but is employed for the preoperative devascularization of tumors that are prone to bleed at surgery, and for embolization of intractable epistaxis.

Contents

Introduction

In comparison to conventional open surgical access, the endoscopic surgeon has a rather limited and specific view of the operating field. He is therefore dependent upon precise preoperative information regarding the anatomy and pathology that awaits him at surgery. Endoscopic surgery has been made possible by, among others, the dramatic progress of modern imaging techniques, especially computed tomography (CT) and magnetic resonance (MR) imaging (MRI), which have become important complementary procedures to sinus endoscopy [2]. This chapter gives a brief introduction to these individual imaging modalities, their respective advantages, and their drawbacks, and may serve as a guideline for their rational application.

Plain Films

These are cheap, fast, and give a good survey of the region under consideration. Plain films were once the mainstay of diagnosis of sinus disease. However, manifold superpositions of the complex facial structures significantly limit their diagnostic value. For example, the ethmoid labyrinth and the sphenoid bone are impossible to assess adequately and much pathology is prone to be overlooked on conventional films (Fig. 45.1). Plain films do not provide critical information necessary to guide endoscopic surgery [6]. Polytomography can, to some degree, cope with the superpositions of plain film; however, it is time consuming, indistinct, and associated with a comparatively high radiation exposure. It is no longer in use in most radiologic institutions.

Conventional X-ray films may play some role in therapy planning (e.g., in the creation of templates in osteoplastic fontal sinus surgery).

Computed Tomography

Imaging of the nose and paranasal sinuses has benefited from recent advancements in CT technology. Modern CT scanners employ helical technology, enabling them to scan large volume ranges by constantly moving the patient past a rotating tube/

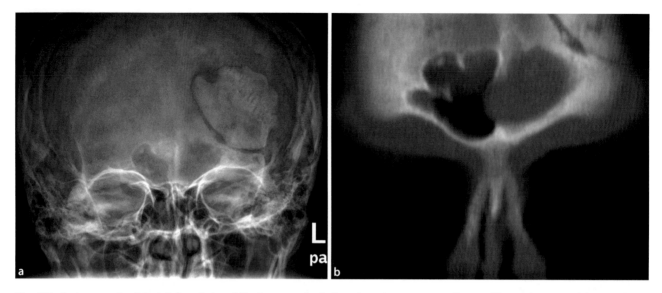

Fig. 45.1a,b A mucocele of the left frontal sinus following osteoplastic frontal craniotomy is virtually invisible on plain X-ray (**a**) but is clearly depicted on computed tomography (CT; **b**) The examinations were performed one day apart

45

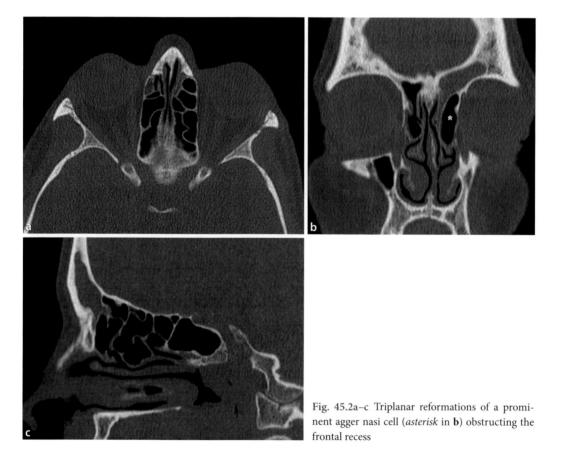

Fig. 45.2a–c Triplanar reformations of a prominent agger nasi cell (*asterisk* in **b**) obstructing the frontal recess

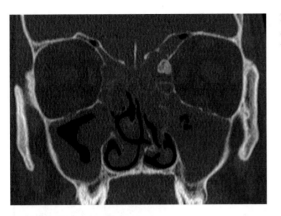

Fig. 45.3 Specific diagnosis using CT: spongiform osteoma of the left ethmoid in addition to a severe bilateral polyposis

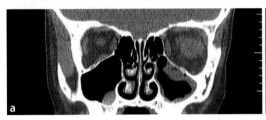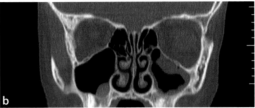

Fig. 45.4a,b Reduced blowout fracture of the left orbital floor ("trapdoor" fracture) with herniation and incarceration of the inferior rectus muscle

detector array. Speed of examination and/or spatial resolution is further increased by multislice detectors, which generate data sets with a high resolution in all three dimensions of space. From such nearly isotropic high-resolution data sets, high-quality multiplanar reformations can be obtained at the user's discretion, either automatically or interactively. Secondary (coronal/sagittal) reformation of data sets obtained with axial scanning geometry are not degraded by dental filling artifacts, which is usually the case in primary coronal scans [5]. Crossregistration, available at workstations, contributes significantly to the understanding of complex anatomy (Fig. 45.2).

CT should be employed routinely prior to endoscopic surgery. Chronic sinusitis is confirmed and staged with CT. Beyond the extent of disease and the definition of bony landmarks (frontal recess, ethmoid infundibulum and ostiomeatal unit, sphenoethmoidal recess) in chronic inflammation, the images are checked for important anatomic variations (concha bullosa, Haller and Onodi cells, deviation and spurs of the bony septum) [1, 5]. Preoperative workup of the following checklist is a must before every endoscopic paranasal surgery in order to avoid complications (see Chap. 44):
1. High or low position of the olfactory groove.
2. Symmetry or asymmetry and thickness or dehiscence of the foveae ethmoidales.
3. Thickness and dehiscence of the lamina papyracea.
4. Protrusion of the carotid sulcus into the sphenoid sinus.
5. Bony covering of the carotid artery sulcus and the optic nerve canal.

The CT scan should always include the alveolar ridge so as not to overlook disease of the dental apparatus and the dental origin of any maxillary sinus inflammation. Hyperintense contents of an opacified sinus and calcifications that are hyperdense, like metallic foreign bodies, point to a mycotic etiology of inflammation.

In tumors of the paranasal sinuses the CT images are scrutinized for osteolytic destructions. Occasionally, calcifications or bone sclerosis can give diagnostic hints for a specific diagnosis of some neoplasms and tumor-like lesions (ossifying fibroma, fibrous dysplasia, meningioma, osteoplastic metastasis, compact and spongiform osteoma; Fig. 45.3).

CT is indispensable in trauma of the midface and the paranasal sinuses. Description and classification of fractures is based on CT, which shows not only the extent of osseous trauma, but also involvement of soft-tissue structures (e.g., in the anterior/middle cranial fossa or in the orbit and optic canal; Fig. 45.4).

Laceration of the dura and traumatic leakage of cerebrospinal fluid (CSF) are difficult to assess on plain CT alone. Intradural air bubbles can only give vague locational hints. Unless a patient with traumatic CSF rhinorrhea is revised surgically, the search for a dural leak may necessitate a CT-cisternography following intrathecal administration of water-soluble iodinized contrast medium.

Malformations of the paranasal sinuses need a very subtle diagnostic workup by CT. Minute bony dehiscences leading to arachnoid herniations as well as rudimentary bony channels and cele formations are easily depicted by CT (Fig. 45.5).

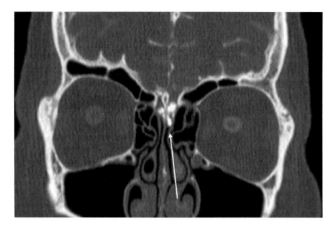

Fig. 45.5 CT cisternography of a female with idiopathic intracranial hypertension and proven cerebrospinal fluid rhinorrhea. Arachnoid herniation can be seen along the sheath of an olfactory filum (*arrow*)

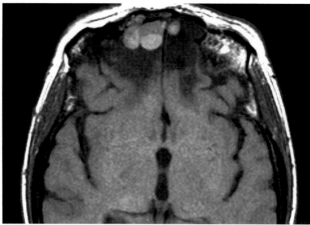

Fig. 45.6 Mucocele of the right frontal sinus following oteoplastic surgery. The high signal on T1-weighted magnetic resonance imaging (MRI) indicates desiccated retained mucus secretion

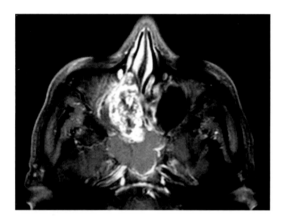

Fig. 45.7 Adenocarcinoma of the right ethmoid in a carpenter. On this contrast-enhanced, T1-weighted MRI scan, the strongly and irregularly enhancing tumor can be outlined against secondary mucus retention in the sphenoid sinus

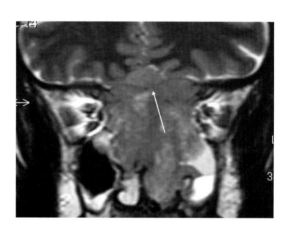

Fig. 45.8 Esthesioneuroblastoma with transdural extension (*arrow*) into the anterior cranial fossa

45

Magnetic Resonance Imaging

MRI is not routinely employed in paranasal sinus disease despite its superb soft-tissue contrast. Another advantage of MRI over CT is the absence of ionizing radiation. Shortcomings of MRI over CT are the inability to depict delicate bony septa, the comparatively long examination time, and the hazards caused by metallic foreign bodies, implants, and pacemakers. A routine MRI protocol of the nose and paranasal sinuses should include multiplanar T2-weighted scans (fluid-sensitive) and T1-weighted scans before and after contrast medium (good anatomical depiction). Additional "short tau inversion recovery" (STIR) sequences are used in search of lymphadenopathy. In inflammatory disease, however, CT is the method of choice as it demonstrates the relevant osseous details better than MRI.

However, the search for T1-hyperintense desiccated secretions in a mucocele warrants the employment of MRI as a primary screening method (Fig. 45.6).

Neoplastic disease is less reliably assessed by CT (see Chap. 63). When there is a suspicion of tumor, MRI can distinguish between retained mucus secretion and a solid tumor, the latter usually exhibiting enhancement following application of contrast medium (Fig. 45.7). Tumor tissue specificity is rarely possible on MR criteria alone: in malignant melanoma, T1-hyperintense paramagnetic melanin in melanotic melanoma gives important clues. Inverted papilloma can exhibit a typical puff-paste structure due to the tubular growth of the tumor undermining the mucosal surface [4].

In tumors adjacent to the skull base, involvement of the dura mater is an important issue. High-resolution T2-weighted im-

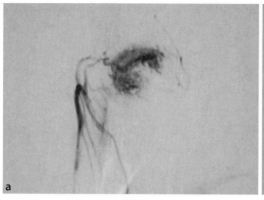 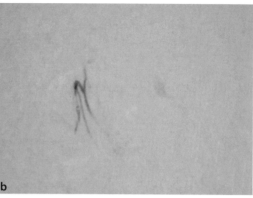

Fig. 45.9a,b Juvenile angiofibroma. Digital subtraction angiography with injection into a branch of the ascending pharyngeal artery before (**a**) and after (**b**) embolization using gelatin-coated trisacryl particles

ages created perpendicular to the skull base can depict the dura as a delicate, linear, hypointense structure that is interrupted as the tumor breaches past this layer (Fig. 45.8). MRI is better than CT for establishing perineural spread of a tumor as well as extension beyond the outlines of the paranasal sinuses into the orbit and the intracranial compartment. However, CT and MRI play complementary roles in the assessment of sinus neoplasms [3].

In selected patients with CSF rhinorrhea due to malformations or following trauma (see Chap. 62), intrathecal injection of paramagnetic contrast medium for MRI (MR-cisternography), similar to CT-cisternography, may be necessary to analyze very complex situations that cannot be solved otherwise, especially when leaking opacified CSF cannot be distinguished from bone on CT-cisternography. It should be borne in mind that intrathecal injection of paramagnetic contrast medium is an off-label procedure that should be carried out only by radiologists who have experience in this field. The indication for MR-cisternography has to be established using very strict criteria.

Patients should not be exposed to the unnecessary risk of nephrogenic systemic sclerosis, a potentially lethal disease, which may occur in patients with renal failure and appears to be associated with the prolonged dwelling time of gadolinium in the organism.

Digital Subtraction Angiography

Diagnostic angiography is an invasive procedure and plays only a minor role in the diagnostics of sinus disease. Rarely, however, the evaluation of vascular pathology or anatomy warrants DSA. In patients with highly vascular tumors (e.g., angiofibroma), DSA aids in the differentiation between postoperative scar tissue and residual tumor.

Interventional endovascular techniques, however, are routinely employed in the preoperative embolization of highly vascularized neoplasms of the nose and sinuses. A typical example is juvenile angiofibromas (see Chap. 63). Subtle and thorough devascularization, even in more than one session, can help to reduce the perioperative blood loss and can even turn inoperable tumors into operable ones [5]. It is essential to bear in mind that the goal of embolization is the devascularization of the tumor parenchyma, not occlusion of the feeding arteries. This goal can best be achieved using particles that are injected through microcatheters, superselectively into the tumor vessels (Fig. 45.9). Any attempts to proximally occlude the feeding arteries, although in some cases very tempting, can create an even worse situation than before and should be regarded as malpractice. Furthermore, DSA may be used for embolization of intractable epistaxis (see Chap. 59).

Take-Home Pearls

- Plain radiography and polytomography are obsolete in most situations.
- CT with multiplanar reformations is the method of choice for inflammatory disease.
- In neoplastic disease, CT and MRI play a complementary diagnostic role. Preoperative embolization of highly vascularized tumors reduces intraoperative blood loss.
- Trauma requires high-resolution multiplanar CT. MR- and CT-cisternography help to assess dural leaks.
- In malformations, high-quality CT and MRI are necessary for a subtle analysis. CT-and MR-cisternography may become necessary in complex malformations with involvement of the skull base and dura mater.

References

1. Earwaker J (1993) Anatomic variants in sinonasal CT. Radiographics 13:381–415
2. Laine FJ, Smoker RK (1992) The ostiomeatal unit and endoscopic surgery; anatomy, variations, and imaging findings in inflammatory disease. Am J Roentgenol 159:849–857

3. Loevner LA, Sonners AI (2002) Imaging of neoplasms of the paranasal sinuses. Mag Reson Imaging Clin N Am 10:467–493

4. Rao VM, el-Noueam KI (1998) Sinonasal imaging. Radiol Clin N Am 36:921–939

5. Schuknecht B, Simmen D (2002) Stellenwert radiologischer Bildgebung der Nasennebenhöhlen. Laryngorhinootologie 81:126–146

6. Zinreich SJ (2006) Progress in sinonasal imaging. Ann Otol Rhinol Laryngol Suppl 196:51–6

45

Instrumentation

Chapter 46

Instrumentation for Endonasal Sinus Surgery. From Basic to Advanced

46

Amir Minovi and Dominik Brors

Core Messages

- Most sinus surgeries can be carried out with the 0° endoscope, which has the advantage of excellent orientation, especially for beginners.
- For any work "around the corner", such as middle-meatus antrostomy, 30° or 45° telescopes are very useful.
- Frontal-sinus surgery should be performed with the help of 45° and/or 70° endoscopes.
- The 70° curved drills are beneficial for median drainage (frontal sinus Draf type III drainage according).
- In experienced hands, the soft-tissue shaver is a very helpful instrument, especially for removal of polyps with minimal trauma to the mucosa.

Contents

Introduction

A new era in sinus surgery began in the early 1970s with the development of different-angled endoscopes based on the new Hopkins rod lens technology and its use in the evaluation of the paranasal sinuses [2, 13]. Messerklinger investigated the anatomy and pathophysiology of the nose and its relationship to chronic sinusitis, and Draf examined the different sinuses systematically and directly; he was the first person to perform endoscopy of the frontal and the sphenoid sinus. His primary goal was to establish more solid indications for sinus surgery, thereby avoiding unnecessary radical surgeries, especially because at that time imaging techniques were still poor, offering only plain x-ray and sometimes conventional tomography. Soon after, he started like Messerklinger to perform endoscopic treatment of inflammatory diseases. Nasal endoscopy with rigid instruments and computed tomography (CT) of the paranasal sinuses enabled the surgeon to approach the ostiomeatal complex (OMC) more precisely. Concomitantly, the use of the binocular operating microscope was introduced in sinus surgery as an additional instrument [3, 4, 9, 18]. In this chapter we would like to present the most commonly used instruments in endonasal sinus surgery, from basic to advanced.

Basic Instrumentation

Endoscopes and Microscopes

Endonasal sinus surgery is performed mostly with the help of different-angled endoscopes (see Chap. 47) or with the operation microscope, or a combination of both, named micro-endoscopic surgery. Most surgeons prefer to perform the entire surgery endoscopically. The rigid fibre-optic nasal telescope provides superb visualisation of the operative field [10–12, 17]. The 0°, 4-mm rigid telescope is used for the major part of the surgery. In children one can use the 2.7-mm rigid endoscope. Most of the paranasal sinuses can be visualised with the 0° scope. Beginning endoscopic sinus surgeons in particular should perform almost the whole surgery with the 0° scope. As the angle of the telescope rises, so does the risk of disorientation. Therefore

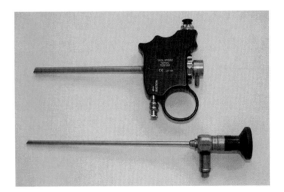

Fig. 46.1 Combined irrigation/suction handle with a 45° rigid endoscope

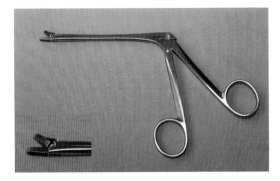

Fig. 46.3 Straight through-cutting forceps, which allow tearless removal of tissue

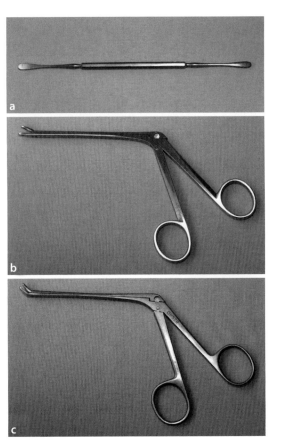

Fig. 46.2 **a** Freer elevator for gentle medialisation of the middle turbinate or incision of the uncinate process. **b** Straight Blakesley forceps for removal of polyps. **c** The 45° upturned Blakesley forceps for working around the frontal recess

46

the 30°, 45° and 70° telescopes are only used for work in areas "around the corner" like the frontal recess and the maxillary sinus. With the 30° endoscope one is able to achieve an orientation over the middle-meatal antrostomy, whereas the 45° is a very helpful instrument judging the frontal recess. A camera is usually attached to the eyepiece of the endoscope and the endoscopic view is transmitted to a monitor. The surgeon may thus perform the surgery while looking through the endoscope or at the monitor, or a combination of both. Most surgeons nowadays look at the monitor. Combined endonasal micro-endoscopic surgery is performed mainly by using an operating microscope with a 250- or 275-mm objective lens and a 45 rigid telescope with a suction/irrigation handle (Fig. 46.1).

Freer Elevator and Sickle Knife

It is most commonly the Freer elevator (Fig. 46.2a) that is used to medialise the middle turbinate and gain a better view of the uncinate process and bulla ethmoidalis. One can also use it for incision and removal of the uncinate process. Most surgeons use the sickle knife for this part of procedure. This manoeuvre

should be done in a sagittal way because of the risk of perforating the lamina papyracea.

Blakesley Forceps

Blakesley forceps are most commonly used to remove mobilized polyps or tissue. The straight forceps (Fig. 46.2b) are particularly appropriate for removing loose pieces of bone from the surgical area. They are also helpful for opening the ethmoidal bulla. One should gently push the forceps into the bulla and carefully open it within the bulla. With this manoeuvre the bulla is prepared with minimal trauma to the mucosa. This forceps cannot cut tissue; hence, one should not remove attached tissue and polyps with this instrument, particularly around the middle turbinate. Careless handling can easily lead to perforation of the lamina papyracea or skull base, with possible damage to the dura. The 45° upturned Blakesley forceps (Fig. 46.2c) are very useful instruments for work around the frontal recess. With its help one can remove polyps in the frontal sinus. One try to work strongly lateral of the middle turbinate. Special delicate forceps like the ethmoid forceps (after Draf) were developed for surgery around the skull base; these are available in several sizes and allow precise work in the skull-base area.

Through-Cutting Instruments

Nowadays, through-cutting instruments belong to the basic equipment of the rhinosurgeon, since these instruments allow the controlled removal of tissue without tearing the mucosa. The straight, through-cutting forceps (Fig. 46.3) can be used in several steps of sinus surgery, whereas the 45° upturned forceps are used around the frontal recess. The through-cutting forceps after Moriyama, which are delivered as straight, up-cutting and up-curved forms in different sizes, allow a particularly exact manipulation at anatomically critical places. These instruments allow for atraumatic dissection, resulting in less bleeding and less postoperative scar tissue formation.

Suckers

Most of the surgery is performed with straight-ended suckers. For identification of the sphenoid sinus entrance one can use the 1-mm sucker. A 2-mm sucker is selected if there is more bleeding in the surgical field. Different types of curved suckers are taken for work performed mainly in the maxillary sinus. They are also used to access the frontal sinus.

Back Biters

Back biters (Rhinoforce Stammberger Antrum Punch) are best used for removal of the uncinate process. There are left, right and intermediate back biters. A big advantage is that one can take about three bites with these instruments before they need to be cleaned. They can also be used to widen the middle antrostomy in an anterior direction.

Soft-Tissue Shavers

Before their introduction for endonasal sinus surgery, soft-tissue shavers were used for many years by orthopaedic surgeons for knee arthroscopy. The original instrument was called a "vacuum rotatory dissector" and the patent was held by Dr. J.C. Urban. Setliff and Parsons were the first, in 1994, to introduce the use of soft-tissue shavers in endonasal sinus surgery

[16]. Since that time, soft-tissue shavers (Fig. 46.4) have become one of the most commonly used power instruments in endonasal surgery, especially in the treatment of nasal polyposis. Soft-tissue shavers consist mainly of three parts: a small light and ergonomic hand piece, an outer blunt cannula with a lateral opening at the end and an oscillating or rotating cutting inner blade. Oscillation of the blade is realised by continuous suction, which removes permanently soft tissue, blood and debris from the operative area. The soft-tissue shavers are available in various sizes and shapes and can oscillate at at least 1000 rpm [7]. They are most commonly used for the removal of nasal polyps. The soft-tissue shavers can also be used in narrowed areas. Most surgeons generally prefer a diameter of between 3.5 mm and 5.5 mm. The length of the blades varies between 8 cm to 13.3 cm (see Chap. 47).

The major advantage of shavers is that polyps can be removed without pulling at their attachment (and thereby sometimes causing a cerebrospinal fluid fistula). Another advantage is their continuous suction and ability to maintain a bloodless surgical field. They are also used for outpatient removal of nasal polyps without any need of nasal packing [8]. Nevertheless, this instrument requires careful handling and experienced surgeons. One disadvantage of shavers is that the surgeon looses to some degree the ability to palpate, which may lead to a greater chance of perforation into the periorbital area and suction of the periorbital fat. Knowledge of anatomy (see Chap. 44) and detailed preoperative study of the CT scans (see Chap. 54) are mandatory, as these instruments can be aggressive. One should also keep in mind that for histological examination, some pathological tissue should be removed with conventional instruments.

Bone-Cutting Drills

The bone-cutting drills used in endonasal sinus surgery were also adapted from arthroscopy as performed by orthopaedic surgeons. They usually consist of an oval-shaped or spherical burr that is affixed to a shaft. The backside of the burr may be protected by a shaft shield. These drills allow for the precise removal of bone. Rotation speed lies around 10,000 rpm and also allows the removal of thicker bony areas. Suction is permanently applied through the sheath so that burred bone can be quickly removed from the surgical area. Drills without protecting shields, and thus with a wider action radius, are also available (see Chap. 47).

Bone-cutting burrs are most commonly used in endonasal frontal sinus surgery when extended frontal sinus drainage is

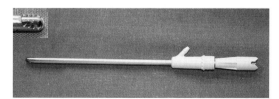

Fig. 46.4 In experienced hands, power instruments like the soft-tissue shaver allow fast and satisfactory removal of polyps

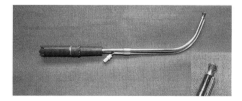

Fig. 46.5 A 70° angled diamond bur for performing resection work on the floor and septum of the frontal sinuses

required. For performing frontal sinus type-IIb or frontal sinus type-III drainage according to Draf [4], the surgeon needs to remove the frontal sinus floor and the septum sinuum frontalium with the burr (see Chap. 26). As in ear surgery, two different kinds of burr can be distinguished: sharp-cutting burrs are used when removal of a thick bone, like osteoma, is needed; they should be used only by experienced surgeons. Most parts of the sinus surgery can be performed with diamond burrs, which are safer. Of great help for drilling in the frontal sinus are the new straight and differently curved drills used with the shaver, providing simultaneous suction and irrigation and thus reducing fogging of the telescopes. A 70 -angled diamond burr is very useful for resection at the floor and septum/septa of the frontal sinuses (Fig. 46.5) [5, 6]. Furthermore, the cutting burrs are used in endonasal surgery for different kinds of tumour, especially for endonasal removal of osteomas, inverted papillomas and malignant tumours [1]. The surgical strategy in the management of inverted papilloma in particular is to identify and widely remove the tumour origin along the subperiosteal plane and drill the underlying bone [14, 15]. With the help of these instruments one can safely remove these tumours completely.

Conclusion

A new era in sinus surgery started almost 30 years ago with the development of different-angled endoscopes, sometimes used in combination with the operating microscope. The surgeon today gains access to almost any part of the sinuses. Powered instruments have gained widespread use in endonasal sinus surgery. These instruments allow a precise and less traumatic removal of pathology with maximum preservation of healthy mucosa. Nevertheless, they should be handled with care, since if incorrectly used they could be dangerous. Curved drills and bony shavers are useful instruments in the expanded application of sinus surgery as, for example, in the treatment of benign and malignant tumours.

Tips to Avoid Complications with Microdebriders and IGS

- For avoiding a laceration of the periorbit, incision of the uncinate process with the sickle knife should be used in a sagittal direction.
- Do not, or only very carefully, pull on attached tissue or polyps with the Blakesley forceps.
- Soft-tissue shavers should only be used by experienced surgeons.
- Frontal recess work demands a 45° or 70° endoscope.
- For endonasal removal of tumours, the combination of endoscope and microscope is helpful, particularly in cases of more severe bleeding.
- Curved drills are almost indispensable for removing the septum/septa sinuum frontalium.

References

1. Bockmuhl U, Minovi A, Kratzsch B, et al (2005) Endonasal micro-endoscopic tumor surgery: state of the art. Laryngorhinootologie 84:884–891
2. Draf W (1983) Endoscopy of the paranasal sinuses. Springer, Berlin Heidelberg New York (German edition 1978: Die Endoskopie der Nasennebenhöhlen)
3. Draf W (1990) Operating microscope for endonasal sinus surgery. First International Symposium: Contemporary Sinus Surgery, November 1990, Pittsburgh, Pennsylvania
4. Draf W (1991) Endonasal micro-endoscopic frontal sinus surgery: the Fulda concept. Oper Tech Otolaryngol Head Neck Surg 2:234–240
5. Draf W (2005) Endonasal frontal sinus drainage Type I–III according to Draf. In: Kountakis S, Senior B, Draf W (eds) The Frontal Sinus. Springer Berlin Heidelberg New York, pp219–232
6. Draf W, Minovi A (2006) The frontal T in the refinement of endonasal frontal sinus type III drainage. Oper Tech Otolaryngol Head Neck Surg 17:121–125
7. Gross CW, Becker DG (1996) Power instrumentation in endoscopic sinus surgery. Oper Tech Otolaryngol Head Neck Surg 7:236–241
8. Hawke WM, McCombe AW (1995) How I do it: nasal polypectomy with an arthroscopic bone shaver: the Stryker "Hummer". J Otolaryngol 24:57–59
9. Heermann H (1958) Ueber endonasale Chirurgie unter Verwendung des binocularen Mikroskopes. Arch Ohren-Nasen-Kehlkopfheilkd 171:295–297
10. Howard DJ, Lund VJ (1986) Endoscopic surgery in otolaryngology. Br Med Bull 42:234–239
11. Kennedy DW (1985) Functional endoscopic sinus surgery: technique. Arch Otolaryngol 111:643–649
12. Kennedy DW, Zinreich SJ, Shaalan H, et al (1987) Endoscopic middle meatal antrostomy: theory, technique, and patency. Laryngoscope 97:1–9
13. Messerklinger W (1978) Endoscopy of the Nose. Urban und Schwarzenberg, Baltimore
14. Minovi A, Kollert M, Draf W, et al (2006) Endonasal micro-endoscopic resection of sinonasal inverted papilloma. Laryngorhinootologie 85:421–425
15. Minovi A, Kollert M, Draf W, et al (2006) Inverted papilloma: feasibility of endonasal surgery and long-term results of 87 cases. Rhinology 44:205–210
16. Setliff RC, Parsons DS (1994) The "Hummer": new instrumentation for functional endoscopic sinus surgery. Am J Rhinol 8:275–278
17. Stammberger H (1986) Endoscopic endonasal surgery – new concepts and treatment of recurring rhinosinusitis. I. Anatomic and pathophysiologic considerations. II. Surgical technique. Otolaryngol Head Neck Surg 94:143–156
18. Weber R, Draf W, Keerl R, et al (1997) Micro-endoscopic endonasal pansinus operation in chronic sinusitis. Results and complications. Am J Otolaryngol 18:247–253

46

Chapter 47

Powered Instrumentation and Image Guidance Technology: State of the Art

47

Joshua C. Demke, Farhad Ardeshirpour, and Brent A. Senior

Core Messages

- The introduction of endoscopes, computed tomography, and powered instrumentation has revolutionized modern-day sinus surgery, and remarkable technological innovations continue to advance the field of rhinology.
- Endoscopes are important diagnostic and therapeutic tools that provide entry to otherwise difficult-to-reach areas and make minimally invasive surgery feasible.
- Microdebriders combine cutting and suction in a single tool, enabling accurate and precise tissue removal without damaging the surrounding mucosa. There is the potential for rapid and drastic complications when used along the orbits and skull base.
- Drill burrs come in various angles and sizes, which prove useful not only in inflammatory disease, but also in the resection of osteitic bone and soft-tissue tumors.
- Image-guided surgery has the potential to improve efficiency and safety, especially in complicated or revision cases; however, it is important to be familiar with general sinus anatomy and individual anatomic landmarks to avoid complications.

Contents

Introduction

In the latter part of the 20th century, the introduction of endoscopes and high-resolution computed tomography (CT), and subsequently powered instrumentation and CT image guidance revolutionized modern-day sinus surgery [24]. Surgical management for sinus disease has evolved from scarring external procedures and relatively blind intranasal procedures into minimally invasive endoscopic procedures [9, 24, 33]. With these changes came a fundamental shift in the goals of sinus surgery. Sinus surgery has transformed from aggressive removal of all mucosa and bone to a more "functional" approach, involving mucosal preservation and restoration of sinus function [33]. Powered instrumentation, which was developed after endoscopic instruments, has drastically improved the visualization and efficiency of the surgery, while CT image guidance has provided the potential for increased surgical safety and surgeon confidence.

In the 1970s, Messerklinger pioneered techniques utilizing endoscopes in the sinuses, and these techniques were later refined by Draf and Stammberger [15, 17, 43, 55]. In 1985, Kennedy's work on functional endoscopic sinus surgery (FESS) became instrumental to the understanding and evolution of endoscopic sinus surgery in the USA [31, 34, 43].

Today, endoscopic sinus surgery is performed routinely for chronic rhinosinusitis. Rapidly occurring advances in powered instrumentation and computer-aided technology now allow otolaryngologists to endoscopically manage mucoceles, frontal sinus fractures, cerebrospinal fluid (CSF) leaks, aspects of septorhinoplasty, encephaloceles, orbital decompression, choanal atresia, anterior skull-base lesions, and extirpation of neoplasms, to name just a few [14, 43].

Powered instrumentation began with the invention of the vacuum dissector for otologic surgery in 1968 [43]. By the 1980s, orthopedic surgeons were using microdebriders for joint dissections. In 1995, the use of powered instrumentation in endoscopic sinus surgery gained recognition when Setliff and Parsons highlighted the benefits of continuous suctioning, precision, and the ability to preserve surrounding mucosa [53]. In 1996, Christmas and Krouse described further applications and techniques of powered instrumentation in FESS [12] along with

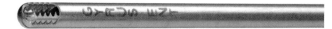

Fig. 47.1 Close-up straight microdebrider tip (courtesy of Gyrus)

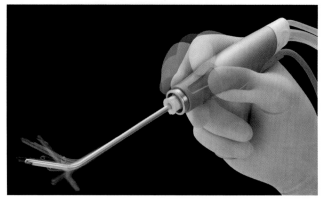

Fig. 47.2 Rotating angled microdebrider tip (courtesy of Gyrus)

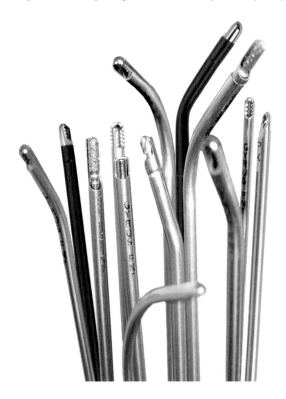

Fig. 47.3 Various straight and angled drills and microdebrider tips (courtesy of Gyrus)

an outcomes study concluding that the use of microdebriders in FESS provides excellent outcomes with fewer complications and faster healing than with use of conventional tools [36, 43].

Over the past two decades, image-guided surgery (IGS) systems have evolved from cumbersome, challenging systems requiring an intraoperative technologist to run them, to systems that are small and portable, and rapidly and easily applied to a wide variety of endoscopic sinus procedures. Otolaryngologists are hopeful that IGS will help reduce complication rates and improve outcomes related to endoscopic skull-base and sinonasal procedures.

The objectives of this chapter are to outline the basics of powered instrumentation and computer image guidance as well as current and future technical innovations that seek to improve efficacy and outcomes while minimizing morbidity. Surgical pearls and pitfalls will be discussed. When used correctly and judiciously, these tools can improve efficiency and efficacy and are a valuable complement to endoscopic surgery of the sinuses and skull base.

Endoscopes

Some of the pioneers in nasal endoscopy include the likes of Hirschmann and Reichart in the early 20th century. The improvements in optics in the 1960s came in large part from contributions by Harold Hopkins, the inventor of the telephoto lens

for cameras as well as the rigid rod endoscope. These inventions subsequently enabled Messerklinger to use these superior optics and enhanced light rod endoscopes to study mucociliary function and anatomic variation. His work resulted in the seminal text on endoscopy of the nose in the late 1970s. Early pioneers in the field, such as Messerklinger, Draf, and Wigand, then began using endoscopes in the surgical management of disease. Later, with the advent of angled scopes such as 30, 45, and 70 telescopes, a wider angle of view and improved lighting became available. Recently, multifunctional endoscopes, including a 90 angled scope, have been described that incorporate separate channels for viewing, suction, and irrigation, and an additional operating port through which specially fitted drills or forceps can be channeled. While this may free up the contralateral hand to maneuver a separate instrument, this comes at the expense of generally decreased optics and, at times, impaired visibility [6].

One of the disadvantages of the endoscope has been monocular vision. Efforts to develop three-dimensional endoscopes have been in large part imperfect, although dual-channel endoscopes may provide an improved view. Alternatively, oblique-viewing scopes allow for the viewing direction to change by rotating the scope cylinder, although these scopes present challenges for camera calibration [59]. In addition, multidirectional endoscopes have been described in the neurosurgery literature, enabling a 360 view via an integrated joystick [3]. The future will surely bring further advances such as rigid endoscopes with flexible tips.

47

Microdebriders

The concept of mucosal sparing, as advocated by Hilding [25] and others, was later confirmed through the work of early surgeons who noted that mucosal loss led to increased postoperative scarring, neo-osteogenesis, and persistent pain [32,44,45]. This led to the development of mucosal-preserving instrumentation such as through-cutting instruments. The original rotary dissector developed by Jack Urban for acoustic neuroma surgery was modified and applied to orthopedic surgery, and subsequently modified again in the mid 1990s, and popularized by Setliff, for intranasal use [52].

Newer microdebriders (or soft-tissue shavers as they are often termed) use disposable blades and concurrent suction, thereby optimizing visualization in the face of persistent bleeding. The design, a suction-based, powered instrument with a blunt end and guarded inner oscillating or rotating blade, affords excellent control and precision for resection of soft tissue, cutting and removing only tissue suctioned into the rotating blades of the guarded opening, while preserving the surrounding tissue (Fig. 47.1) [52]. Single-use disposable blades remain sharp, thus minimizing unwanted mucosal injury. Newer-generation debriders are available in a variety of angles and have the capability of 360 degrees of rotation relative to the handpiece (Fig. 47.2). These devices support variable speeds ranging generally from 6,000 to 12,000 rpm. Lower speeds often prove more effective in resecting larger amounts of tissue in a time-efficient manner, and thus should be employed with bulky diseased tissues, while higher speeds reduce the suction time in which tissue is pulled into the port, thereby reducing the size of the fragment removed.

Microdebriders are particularly useful in resecting polyps, polypoid mucosa, and bulky soft-tissue tumors. In addition, the wide variety of blades and drill burrs (Fig. 47.3) available make powered instrumentation useful in many situations including ethmoidectomy, frontal sinusotomy, antrostomy, antralchoanal polypectomy, inferior-turbinate reduction, choanal atresia repair, nasal hump reduction, debulking of recurrent respiratory papillomatosis, benign and malignant sinonasal or skull-base tumors, complicated adenoidectomies, septal spurs, and dacryocystorhinostomies [46].

Special mention should be made with regard to dissection of the frontal recess in FESS with soft-tissue shaver tips available in 40, 60, 65, 90, and 120 angles. Surgeons have achieved unrivaled potential to preserve mucosa and resect polypoid mucosa in this often otherwise difficult-to-reach area. Similar advantage has been seen with these tips in the deep recesses of the maxillary sinus.

Several authors have concluded that FESS with the microdebrider results in decreased scarring, decreased blood loss, and a faster healing time [5, 36]. However, in a recent prospective randomized study comparing FESS with the microdebrider versus conventional instruments, in which patients served as their own controls, there was no difference noted at 13 months between either method with regard to polyp recurrence, access to the ethmoid complex, patency of the middle meatal antrostomy, synechiae, or symptoms [51]. A recent prospective audit of over 3,128 patients in England and Wales in which the microdebrider was used for nasal polyposis and chronic rhinosinusitis in 16.5%, concluded that the rate of complications increased with severity of disease as determined by symptom severity, extent of polyposis, and opacification of the CT scan, regardless of the use of conventional techniques or powered instrumentation. Interestingly, 31% of these procedures were performed without endoscopes, and over 33% of these were performed without a preoperative CT scan [26].

One additional potential advantage of powered instrumentation is that it theoretically reduces operative time because of the high efficiency of dissection and ability to accurately spare unintended structures, although the question of efficiency has not been studied thoroughly. Conversely, it has been suggested that tactile feedback, sometimes referred to as "haptic feedback", is lost with microdebriders because of their weight, vibration, and flexibility [24].

Microdebriders are of particular benefit in soft-tissue tumor resection, such as inverted papillomas. The constant suction helps clear blood and tumor cells, theoretically decreasing the risk of tumor seeding, while the use of multiple traps may help to compartmentalize and thereby map the tumor [4]. Tumors may be quickly and efficiently debulked back to their area of origin. While such resections are not performed "en bloc," most endoscopists argue that the superior visualization gained and the resection provided with the aid of powered instruments more than compensate for the lack of an "en bloc" resection.

Differences between microdebriders exist with regard to suction orientation through the device (straight or angled) and the orientation of the motor to the blade (straight or angled). These distinctions, combined with shaft stiffness, vibration, and blade design lead to variability in the effectiveness of different devices. Surprisingly, little research has been done comparing microdebriders. In one early study, Ferguson et al. made comparisons using an oyster model, suggesting that the XPS Straight Shot (Xomed, Jacksonville, FL, USA) was the most efficient aspirator [18]. Dave et al. later expanded on this work comparing the Diego Powered Dissector (Gyrus, Bartlett, TN, USA) and the XPS 3000 (Medtronic Xomed), by comparing not only rate of aspiration, but also clog frequency and clearance. The conclusion was that with straight blades the two were statistically equivalent, but the XPS 3000 aspirated more tissue when using angled blades. The investigators in this study found the revolving nose cone, which facilitates blade manipulation, and the ergonomically shaped handle to be advantages of the Gyrus Diego [16].

The literature is somewhat limited regarding the complications of powered instrumentation and specifically whether the rate of complications is any different compared to standard instruments. Some have argued that the ability to maintain a clean field and cut precisely with such instruments reduces complications. However, there have been case reports of orbital injury and skull-base injury, suggesting the potential for increased complication severity, greater difficulty of repair, and rapid, sudden injury occurrence; complications occurring in large part because of the ability of the powered suction to draw material, when misdirected, into the rotating blades with great speed and efficiency where it is quickly severed and aspirated. This thereby compounds injury by aspirating the dura and periorbita, as well as potentially the underlying brain, muscle, or fat [23,24]. As an example, with conventional instrumentation, exposure of

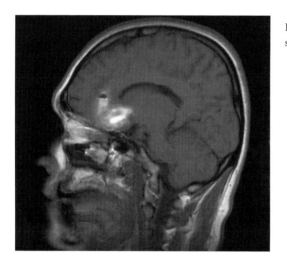

Fig. 47.4 Sagittal T1-weighted magnetic resonance imaging (MRI) scan demonstrating intracranial injury as a result of microdebrider use

periorbital fat is uncommon and is generally without sequelae if appreciated and avoided during the remainder of the procedure. With a microdebrider, however, the threat of serious injury in this setting is greater, with rapid suctioning and cutting of the fat and adjacent orbital structures, resulting in greater risk of injury to the medial rectus, inferior rectus muscle, or even the optic nerve.

Intracranial injury (Fig. 47.4) is also potentially more dramatic with resultant rapid and extensive injuries to the skull base and brain parenchyma. Whereas such injuries to the skull base certainly can and do happen with conventional instruments, the scale of injury is often more severe and extensive with microdebriders [23]. Surprisingly, a recent survey found that one-third of participants were unaware that powered instruments could be involved in orbital injury and 50% were unaware that cranial injuries could occur as a result of powered instrumentation [57].

Drills

The introduction of microdebriders has led to the development of simultaneous powered drills designed specifically for intranasal use. Most microdebrider systems allow for the removal of the blade, which may be replaced with a variety of drill burrs. Simultaneous suction and irrigation, combined with a wide variety of burr designs, make these devices particularly valuable in the narrow confines of the nasal cavity. Initially drills were used only in cases of inflammatory disease, but they have also proven useful in the resection of benign intranasal tumors, such as osseous and fibro-osseous neoplasms, and inverting papillomas.

Powered drills allow the removal of thickened osteitic bone more easily than conventional instruments. Curettes are frequently unsuccessful in removing thickened bone in a controlled manner, whereas forceps can be imprecise, thus making powered drills useful adjuncts. Some have reported the use of drilling to thin osteitic bone, while a hand punch may complete the removal in an atraumatic and mucosally sparing approach [8].

Newer powered instrumentation supports drill rotation speeds of 12,000 rpm or greater. Such speeds are critical for the rapid but controlled removal of bone [4]. The coupling of such drills with improved endoscopic visualization has aided in significantly reducing the need for an osteoplastic flap with frontal sinus obliteration in the setting of chronic frontal sinusitis. Angled drills have been developed to improve visualization and technical capabilities when extensive drilling of the frontal recess is required, such as in Draf types IIb and III (modified Lothrop) sinusotomies (see Chap. 52).

Chandra et al. [8] observed that the 4-mm burr size at a 70 angle allows for bone removal yet permits visualization with 45 or 70 angled scopes. They found that fine diamond burrs may resist skipping at relatively low speeds of 6,000 rpm, thereby decreasing mucosal trauma. The trajectory of the 70 drill allows good access, control, and efficacy, with significantly reduced collateral trauma compared with the straight drill in the frontal recess. However, we have found that coarser cutting or diamond burrs, in addition to weaker drill shafts, result in greater skipping and mucosal trauma.

In 2004, Hosemann et al. [27] compared the advantages and shortcomings of different types of burrs in performing Draf type IIb frontal sinusotomies in cadavers. Complementary use of the right-angled burr with the straight burr allowed easier bone removal, particularly in spacious anatomic specimens. Solo use of the straight drills revealed significant collateral damage, while use of the curved frontal sinus burr was stopped prematurely because of difficulties with the flexible axle.

Image-Guided Surgery

Sterotactic IGS, also called computer-assisted surgery, allows preoperative CT or magnetic resonance imaging (MRI) data to be correlated or "registered" with fixed anatomic points. This allows the surgeon to accurately determine an instrument's position within the sinonasal cavity relative to corresponding triplanar reconstructed images, thereby aiding intraoperative localization and allowing, in theory, a more complete and

47

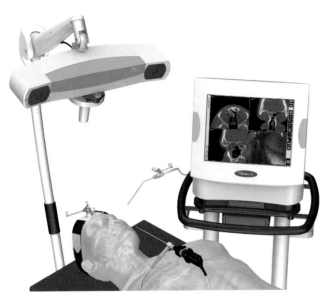

Fig. 47.5 BrainLAB optical-tracking image-guidance system (courtesy of BrainLAB)

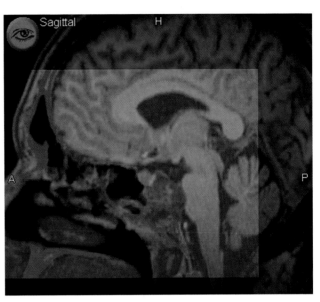

Fig. 47.6 MRI/computed tomography fusion demonstrating clival chordoma

safe dissection [4]. IGS has been shown to assist the surgeon in formulating a more effective surgical plan and in performing the procedure with greater comfort, confidence, and safety [1, 4, 39, 48].

While the concepts of IGS go back to the 1950s, clinically useful image-guided systems have only been available since the late 1980s. Initially, devices by the Aachen group and ISG Technologies used electromagnetic (EM) technology, which was easily distorted by the minimal magnetic fields and metallic instruments that are common in operating rooms [33]. In addition, they were unwieldy, difficult to set up, required head fixation, and were often inaccurate. Today's IGS systems are based on either optical or EM technology [13] and are much more reliable and user-friendly. However, they still involve a learning curve by otolaryngologists and operating-room staff [33].

All clinically available systems for sinus surgery feature relatively simple registration and compensation for any head movement during surgery without the need for head fixation [58]. EM systems have the disadvantage of signal distortion of the EM field by large metal objects, and the necessity for the patient to wear a specialized headset during image acquisition [39,42]. Optical tracking systems utilize infrared light to track optical markers on a head piece worn by the patient during surgery. These optical markers are also placed on probes and suctions, and with current adapter technology, virtually any surgical instrument can be tracked (Fig. 47.5) [41]. Surface and landmark registration techniques eliminate the need for a headset to be worn during preoperative imaging, as required in EM. However, these units have line-of-sight issues whereby if objects block the view of the overhanging infrared camera, image guidance is temporarily disabled [39,42].

IGS is most useful in cases with distorted anatomy or loss of anatomic landmarks, such as in revision cases, cases of extensive nasal polyposis, or when bony landmarks are lost or altered. IGS is certainly not needed for all endoscopic surgical procedures [13]. Currently, guidelines from the American Academy of Otolaryngology/Head and Neck Surgery [14] support IGS for:

1. Revision sinus surgery.
2. Distorted sinus anatomy of development, postoperative, or traumatic origin.
3. Extensive sinonasal polyposis.
4. Pathology involving the frontal, posterior ethmoid, and sphenoid sinuses.
5. Disease abutting the skull base, orbit, optic nerve, or carotid artery.
6. CSF rhinorrhea or conditions where there is a skull-base defect.
7. Benign and malignant sinonasal neoplasms.

Retrospective reviews by Loehrl et al. [40], Gibbons et al. [21], and Fried et al. [19], while not significantly powered, have all reported decreased complications with image-guided sinus surgery, although rates of revision are not different. Chiu and Vaughan [10] and Kacker et al. [30] have reported that IGS is of great benefit in revision of frontal sinus surgery, with a lower rate of complications compared to non-IGS revision [29]. There are currently no randomized, prospective studies with adequate follow up that investigate the comparative efficacy and safety of IGS in various clinical situations [30].

Adding recently to the functionality of IGS is fusion technology, which allows the combination of preoperative CT and MRI images for use during navigation. This is particularly advantageous in skull-base procedures in close proximity to neurovascular structures such as the carotid arteries, enabling the surgeon to see both bony anatomy and soft-tissue structures, and to better delineate the extent of the tumors (Fig. 47.6) [11,37–39].

As imaging technology continues to evolve, additional capabilities may develop such as three-dimensional fly-through imaging, which mimics the point of view of the endoscopist [7].

The accuracy of most of these systems with both CT or MRI is limited by the slice thickness of the preoperative scan, usually 1–2 mm, which may mean the difference between an intranasal versus an intracranial location if reliance is solely on such systems and not clinical judgment and a sound understanding of skull-base and sinus anatomy [1,2,14,19,41,49,50,54]. The technology is susceptible to displacement of the headpieces and instrument adapters, or even computer malfunction. Registration inaccuracies may occur if the patient's facial anatomy has changed since obtaining the preoperative imaging, as evident in cases of facial edema as a result of steroid use. Similarly, progression of pathology may occur, invalidating the accuracy of the preoperative images. We recommend that in the setting of inflammatory disease, images for navigation be no older than 6 months to avoid these problems. In addition, as the surgery progresses, changes to the anatomy occur that may also invalidate the preoperative images utilized in navigation. This is particularly significant when objects surrounded by soft tissue are removed, resulting in shifting of those soft-tissue margins, such as in pituitary adenoma surgery or orbital surgery. In all cases, repeated visual confirmation of anatomic accuracy should be performed during the surgery to reduce the likelihood of error and complications [35].

Despite the new technology and the computer-based navigation systems, there is certainly no substitute for thorough knowledge of surgical anatomy [13], and it is imperative that surgeons be cognizant of the limitations of IGS. Indeed, the greatest danger of image-guided systems, as in any new technology, is over reliance.

Intraoperative imaging technology has recently been introduced that can dynamically demonstrate surgical progression through an operative case [14,39]. MRI is the predominant intraoperative imaging modality used and has proven itself valuable in neurosurgery and skull-base surgery. However, implementing intraoperative MRI is very expensive, and using nonferromagnetic instrumentation for this technology is both expensive and surgically limiting [33]. An alternative is intraoperative CT scanning or fluoroscopically updated images. While much less expensive than MRI, radiation exposure is a concern. In addition, attempting to update the images during the procedure often results in poorer-quality images, a problem also seen with lower-magnetic-strength, intraoperative MRI [20,28,33].

An alternative to intraoperative imaging is digital subtraction software, such as "Eraser" (BrainLAB, Heinstetten, Germany), technology that attempts to digitally modify the preoperative images during surgery, creating a digital "real-time" image. The concept is analogous to the digital eraser technology used in photo manipulation. Rather than tracking the instrument in the field, the instrument becomes an eraser on the images, removing structures from the pictures. While this is particularly beneficial in sinus surgery, where the margins of dissection remain static, the problem of soft-tissue shift in pituitary surgery remains.

Until recently, the disadvantages of intraoperative imaging, such as higher costs, repeated exposure to radiation, and

prolonged anesthesia, have outweighed the potential benefits. While using this technology for standard sinus and skull-base surgery is not currently recommended, this will likely change with the introduction of smaller scanners with lower radiation exposure and improved images. Such technology has recently come online, including xCAT (Xoran, Ann Arbor, MI, USA), and Tomoscan M (Philips, Amsterdam, The Netherlands), and CereTom (Neurologica, Danvers, MA, USA) [56]. However, problems with these units still exist that need to be overcome, including blood artifact, the distinction between scar and polyp, increased time required for patient positioning and data acquisition, increased space requirement, higher costs, repeated exposure to radiation, and prolonged anesthesia [39].

Still in the preclinical phase, the Mobile C-arm (Siemens Medical Systems, Erlangen, Germany) is an intraoperative imaging system that combines low-dose fluoroscopy and fully three-dimensional CT. It has been used to assist the surgical approach to the frontal recess in six cadavers [47]. This portable system provides near-real-time CT guidance, generating intraoperative, volumetric CT changes with acceptably low radiation exposure.

Tips to Avoid Complications with Microdebriders and IGS

- Exercise heightened vigilance when using in areas of potential injury such as along the skull base or the lamina. Angle the rotating blade 90 away from areas of potential injury such as the lamina, and dissect superior to inferior along the lamina.
- Overzealous use of powered instrumentation will lead to denuded surfaces and excessive bleeding, thereby obscuring visualization. Use in short, discrete bursts to minimize mucosal injury and bleeding [22].
- Suction traps should always be used for collection of pathologic specimens and should be changed with each side or subsite to aid in the localization and lateralization of trap contents should an unexplained lesion be identified pathologically [22].
- The use of microdebriders in the sphenoid sinus or in a sphenoethmoidal cell has the potential to result in direct trauma to the optic nerve and/or the internal carotid artery. Careful handling is therefore indicated in these locations.
- Low threshold for use of stereotactic image guidance when difficult anatomy, revision cases, and sinonasal tumors are encountered. If there is confusion regarding structures, reassess and reorient based on known landmarks and compare known structures with their stereo-tactic localization. Confirm registration often, and reregister the IGS if concerned about changes in localization.
- Have a thorough understanding of general sinonasal anatomy, as well as individual case-by-case anatomy, taking advantage of triplanar imaging for preoperative planning and intraoperative guidance.

- Leave the eyes exposed to allow for intraoperative examination for subconjunctiva edema or hemorrhage and pupil activity in suspected orbit injury. Gentle ballottement to help with visualization of the lamina and potential periorbital fat exposure may also be performed.

Take-Home Pearls

- A thorough understanding of general sinus anatomy as well as individual anatomic landmarks, as well as judicial use of stereotactic CT guidance is essential in preoperative planning and intraoperative execution.
- Special care needs to be employed in revision surgery in which natural landmarks or bony landmarks may be altered or destroyed. The narrow frontal recess also requires particular attention if powered instrumentation is to be used, as does the sphenoid sinus.
- Powered instrumentation has the potential to improve efficiency, but the potential for dramatic and quick complications is great if caution is not exercised.

References

1. Anderson TD, Kennedy DW (2001) Surgical intervention for sinusitis in adults. Curr Allergy Asthma Rep 1:282–288
2. Anon JB (1998) Computer-aided endoscopic sinus surgery. Laryngoscope 108:949–961
3. Aryan HE, Hoeg HD, Marshall LF, Levy ML (2005) Multidirectional projectional rigid neuro-endoscopy: prototype and initial experience. Minim Invasive Neurosurg 48:293–296
4. Batra PS, Citardi MJ (2006) Endoscopic management of sinonasal malignancy. Otolaryngol Clin North Am 39:619–637, x–xi
5. Bernstein JM, Lebowitz RA, Jacobs JB (1998) Initial report on postoperative healing after endoscopic sinus surgery with the microdebrider. Otolaryngol Head Neck Surg 118:800–803
6. Bumm K, Wurm J, Bohr C, Zenk J, Iro H (2005) New endoscopic instruments for paranasal sinus surgery. Otolaryngol Head Neck Surg 133:444–449
7. Cartellieri M, Vorbeck F (2000) Endoscopic sinus surgery using intraoperative computed tomography imaging for updating a three-dimensional navigation system. Laryngoscope 110:292–296
8. Chandra RK, Schlosser R, Kennedy DW (2004) Use of the 70-degree diamond burr in the management of complicated frontal sinus disease. Laryngoscope 114:188–192
9. Chiu AG (2006) Frontal sinus surgery: its evolution, present standard of care, and recommendations for current use. Ann Otol Rhinol Laryngol Suppl 196:13–19
10. Chiu AG, Vaughan WC (2004) Revision endoscopic frontal sinus surgery with surgical navigation. Otolaryngol Head Neck Surg 130:312–318
11. Chiu AG, Palmer JN, Cohen N (2005) Use of image-guided computed tomography-magnetic resonance fusion for complex endoscopic sinus and skull base surgery. Laryngoscope 115:753–755
12. Christmas DA Jr, Krouse JH (1996) Powered instrumentation in functional endoscopic sinus surgery. I: Surgical technique. Ear Nose Throat J 75:33–36, 39–40
13. Citardi MJ, Batra PS (2005) Image-guided sinus surgery: current concepts and technology. Otolaryngol Clin North Am 38:439–452, vi
14. Cohen NA, Kennedy DW (2005) Endoscopic sinus surgery: where we are – and where we're going. Curr Opin Otolaryngol Head Neck Surg 13:32–38
15. Danielsen A, Olofsson J (2006) Endoscopic endonasal sinus surgery: a review of 18 years of practice and long-term follow-up. Eur Arch Otorhinolaryngol 263:1087–1098
16. Dave SP, Polak M, Casiano RR (2005) Microdebriders used in functional endoscopic sinus surgery: secondary analysis and validation of a new tissue model. Laryngoscope 115:1641–1645
17. Draf W, Weber R (1993) Endonasal micro-endoscopic pansinusoperation in chronic sinusitis. I. Indications and operation technique. Am J Otolaryngol 14:394–398
18. Ferguson BJ, DiBiase PA, D'Amico F (1999) Quantitative analysis of microdebriders used in endoscopic sinus surgery. Am J Otolaryngol 20:294–297
19. Fried MP, Moharir VM, Shin J, Taylor-Becker M, Morrison P (2002) Comparison of endoscopic sinus surgery with and without image guidance. Am J Rhinol 16:193–197
20. Fried MP, Topulos G, Hsu L, Jalahej H, Gopal H, Lauretano A, Morrison PR, Jolesz FA (1998) Endoscopic sinus surgery with magnetic resonance imaging guidance: initial patient experience. Otolaryngol Head Neck Surg 119:374–380
21. Gibbons MD, Gunn CG, Niwas S, Sillers MJ (2001) Cost analysis of computer-aided endoscopic sinus surgery. Am J Rhinol 15:71–75
22. Graham SM (2006) Complications of sinus surgery using powered instrumentation. Oper Tech Otolaryngol Head Neck Surg 17:73–77
23. Graham SM, Nerad JA (2003) Orbital complications in endoscopic sinus surgery using powered instrumentation. Laryngoscope 113:874–878
24. Hackman TG, Ferguson BJ (2005) Powered instrumentation and tissue effects in the nose and paranasal sinuses. Curr Opin Otolaryngol Head Neck Surg 13:22–26
25. Hilding A (1932) The physiology of drainage of nasal mucus. Arch Otolaryngol 17:760–8
26. Hopkins C, Browne JP, Slack R, Lund VJ, Topham J, Reeves BC, Copley LP, Brown P, van der Meulen JH (2006) Complications of surgery for nasal polyposis and chronic rhinosinusitis: the results of a national audit in England and Wales. Laryngoscope 116:1494–1499
27. Hosemann W, Herzog D, Beule AG, Kaftan H (2004) Experimental evaluation of drills for extended frontal sinusotomy. Otolaryngol Head Neck Surg 131:187–191
28. Hsu L, Fried MP, Jolesz FA (1998) MR-guided endoscopic sinus surgery. AJNR Am J Neuroradiol 19:1235–1240
29. Jiang RS, Hsu CY (2002) Revision functional endoscopic sinus surgery. Ann Otol Rhinol Laryngol 111:155–159

30. Kacker A, Tabaee A, Anand V (2005) Computer-assisted surgical navigation in revision endoscopic sinus surgery. Otolaryngol Clin North Am 38:473–482

31. Kennedy DW (1985) Functional endoscopic sinus surgery. Technique. Arch Otolaryngol 111:643–649

32. Kennedy DW (2001) Functional endoscopic sinus surgery: concepts, surgical indications, and instrumentation. In: Kennedy DW, Bolger WE, Zinreich SJ (eds) Diseases of the Sinuses: Diagnosis and Management. BC Decker, Ontario, pp 197–210

33. Kennedy DW (2006) Technical innovations and the evolution of endoscopic sinus surgery. Ann Otol Rhinol Laryngol Suppl 196:3–12

34. Kennedy DW, Zinreich SJ, Rosenbaum AE, Johns ME (1985) Functional endoscopic sinus surgery. Theory and diagnostic evaluation. Arch Otolaryngol 111:576–582

35. Koele W, Stammberger H, Lackner A, Reittner P (2002) Image guided surgery of paranasal sinuses and anterior skull base – five years experience with the InstaTrak-System. Rhinology 40:1–9

36. Krouse JH, Christmas DA Jr (1996) Powered instrumentation in functional endoscopic sinus surgery. II: A comparative study. Ear Nose Throat J 75:42–44

37. Leong JL, Batra PS, Citardi MJ (2005) Three-dimensional computed tomography angiography of the internal carotid artery for preoperative evaluation of sinonasal lesions and intraoperative surgical navigation. Laryngoscope 115:1618–1623

38. Leong JL, Batra PS, Citardi MJ (2006) CT-MR image fusion for the management of skull base lesions. Otolaryngol Head Neck Surg 134:868–876

39. Ling FT, Kountakis SE (2006) Advances in imaging of the paranasal sinuses. Curr Allergy Asthma Rep 6:502–507

40. Loehrl TA, Toohill RJ, Smith TL (2000) Use of computer-aided surgery for frontal sinus ventilation. Laryngoscope 110:1962–1967

41. Metson R, Gliklich RE, Cosenza M (1998) A comparison of image guidance systems for sinus surgery. Laryngoscope 108:1164–1170

42. Metson R, Cosenza M, Gliklich RE, Montgomery WW (1999) The role of image-guidance systems for head and neck surgery. Arch Otolaryngol Head Neck Surg 125:1100–1104

43. Mirante JP, Christmas DA Jr, Yanagisawa E (2001) History and development of powered instrumentation in otolaryngology – head and neck surgery. In: Yanagisawa E, Christmas DA, Jr, Mirante JP (eds) Powered Instrumentation in Otolaryngology – Head and Neck Surgery. Singular Thomson Learning, San Diego, pp 1–3

44. Moriyama H, Ozawa M, Honda Y (1991) Endoscopic endonasal sinus surgery. Approaches and post-operative evaluation. Rhinology 29:93–98

45. Moriyama H YK, Ohtori N, Asai K, Fukami M (1996) Healing process of sinus mucosa after endoscopic sinus surgery. Am J Rhinol 10:61–66

46. Parsons DS (1996) Rhinologic uses of powered instrumentation in children beyond sinus surgery. Otolaryngol Clin North Am 29:105–114

47. Rafferty MA, Siewerdsen JH, Chan Y, Moseley DJ, Daly MJ, Jaffray DA, Irish JC (2005) Investigation of C-arm cone-beam CT-guided surgery of the frontal recess. Laryngoscope 115:2138–2143

48. Reardon EJ (2005) The impact of image-guidance systems on sinus surgery. Otolaryngol Clin North Am 38:515–525

49. Reittner P, Tillich M, Luxenberger W, Weinke R, Preidler K, Köle W, Stammberger H, Szolar D (2002) Multislice CT-image-guided endoscopic sinus surgery using an electromagnetic tracking system. Eur Radiol 12:592–596

50. Roth M, Lanza DC, Zinreich J, Yousem D, Scanlan KA, Kennedy DW (1995) Advantages and disadvantages of three-dimensional computed tomography intraoperative localization for functional endoscopic sinus surgery. Laryngoscope 105:1279–1286

51. Selivanova O, Kuehnemund M, Mann WJ, Amedee RG (2003) Comparison of conventional instruments and mechanical debriders for surgery of patients with chronic sinusitis. Am J Rhinol 17:197–202

52. Setliff R (1995) New concepts and the use of powered instrumentation (the "Hummer") for functional endoscopic sinus surgery. In: Stankiewicz JA (ed) Advanced Endoscopic Sinus Surgery, 1st edn. Mosby, St. Louis, p 176

53. Setliff R, Parsons D (1994) The Hummer – new instrumentation for functional endoscopic sinus surgery. Am J Rhinol 8:275–278

54. Snyderman C, Zimmer LA, Kassam A (2004) Sources of registration error with image guidance systems during endoscopic anterior cranial base surgery. Otolaryngol Head Neck Surg 131:145–149

55. Stammberger H, Posawetz W (1990) Functional endoscopic sinus surgery. Concept, indications and results of the Messerklinger technique. Eur Arch Otorhinolaryngol 247:63–76

56. Stieve M, Schwab B, Haupt C, Bisdas S, Heermann R, Lenarz T (2006) Intraoperative computed tomography in otorhinolaryngology. Acta Otolaryngol 126:82–87

57. Surgery, American Academy of Otolaryngology, Head and Neck (2004) Committee on Devices: miniseminar on powered instrumentation and ESS. Annual Meeting of the American Academy of Otolaryngology. New York, NY,

58. Wise SK, DelGaudio JM (2005) Computer-aided surgery of the paranasal sinuses and skull base. Expert Rev Med Devices 2:395–408

59. Yamaguchi T, Nakamoto M, Sato Y, Konishi K, Hashizume M, Sugano N, Yoshikawa H, Tamura S (2004) Development of a camera model and calibration procedure for oblique-viewing endoscopes. Comput Aided Surg 9:203–214

47

Chapter 48

Image-Guided Surgery of the Paranasal Sinuses

48

Dary Costa, Thomas Sanford, and Raj Sindwani

Core Messages

- The application of image-guidance technology to endoscopic sinus surgery improves surgeon confidence, but is associated with increased costs and operation room time.
- In addition to providing real-time localization in all three orthogonal planes during surgery using the preoperative imaging, these systems are very useful in preoperative planning.
- There are two commercially available platforms for navigation: (1) optical-based systems, which use infrared technology for tracking, and (2) electromagnetic systems, which use radiofrequency. The accuracy (within 2 mm) and general functioning of the systems are considered to be materially equivalent.
- Navigation systems continue to evolve. There is a noted trend toward cheaper, smaller, more powerful machines that are easier to use.
- This technology has established itself as a valuable adjunctive tool for the endoscopic surgeon and its continued proliferation seems certain, although the proper role and indications for its application remain incompletely defined.
- Image-guided surgery is not currently standard of care.

Contents

Introduction

Functional endoscopic sinus surgery (FESS) using rigid endoscopes was first described in the mid 1980s and quickly became the standard of care for opening obstructed outflow tracts of the paranasal sinuses. Well over 200,000 cases of endoscopic sinus surgery (ESS) are estimated to be performed annually in the United States [1]. Rigid endoscopes permit visualization of surface anatomy and provide a means to safely operate within the confines of the nasal cavity without the use of a headlight. Unfortunately, the rigid-lens system provides only a two-dimensional view, requiring surgeons to localize instruments based in part on their depth of penetration and tactile sensation. Orientation and localization within the sinonasal tract can be problematic, especially in the setting of extensive disease, revision surgery, or bleeding. Due to the close proximity of intracranial structures and the orbit, complications from sinus surgery, although rare, can be devastating.

Image-guidance systems were developed to provide assistance with real-time intraoperative localization of surgical anatomy. These systems function to identify surgical instruments, calculate the location of the instrument tip in relation to the patient, and project the instrument location onto a previously obtained imaging study (usually a computed tomography, CT, scan). The operator can use this information for intraoperative surgical navigation or preoperative planning using the computer workstation, which displays the patient's images simultaneously in all three anatomic planes (coronal, axial, and sagittal). Navigation technology can determine, with great accuracy, the precise location of key landmarks and critical structures during the course of an operation. The use of surgical navigation in paranasal sinus surgery has become pervasive since the introduction of this technology in the 1990s. In a remarkably short time, navigation systems have gone from being a curious novelty to a near-necessity in some complex skull-base procedures. Early studies investigated the technology, demonstrated its accuracy, and confirmed its utility for ESS [1, 2]. Commercially available navigations systems have improved considerably over the past several years, as is evidenced by their current widespread use in otolaryngology. A recent survey demonstrated that 73% of otolaryngologists use image guidance, with over 80% of respondents agreeing that it provides safer surgery [3].

This technology has established itself as a valuable tool for the endoscopic surgeon and its continued growth seems certain, although the proper role and indications for its application remain undefined. Obtaining maximal benefit from these systems requires a general understanding of how they work, and an appreciation of their limitations. Image-guidance technology is an adjunct in the operating room and does not substitute for basic anatomic knowledge and surgical skill. Image-guided surgery (IGS) has also been called computer-assisted surgery, computer-guided surgery, and surgical navigation; in this chapter we will use the term IGS.

History of Image Guidance

Image guidance was first developed for neurosurgical applications to assist with the intraoperative localization of intracranial lesions and nearby structures. Initial efforts were described by Horsley and Clark in the early 1900s using skull landmarks to identify specific targets within a monkey brain. In 1947, Spiegel and Wycis published data on a system of operative framed stereotaxy [2]. A metal frame was placed on the patient's head and the instrument distance and trajectory from specific points on the frame were measured. Instrument location within the cranial cavity could then be calculated using known anatomic relationships from a surgical atlas and plain-film x-rays. The frames provided a stable reference that had limited use, such as draining abscesses and creating small lesions in the brain parenchyma. Progress with this technique was stifled by the need for accurate surgical atlases, undistorted anatomy, and complicated calculations of angles and distances from the frame reference points.

Stereotactic surgery with CT scanning was described in 1976 by Bergstrom and Greitz [4]. A rigid headset was fixed to the patient's head and a CT scan was performed, followed by surgery with the headset still in place. The stereotactic surgical frames, however, obstructed surgical access and operator range of motion and there was no real-time imaging. In addition, the measurements proved too inaccurate to provide useful information, and widespread use was not practical [2].

Advances in CT imaging and registration techniques progressed such that instruments could be localized without a rigid frame, but tracking technology using early electromagnetic systems was too inaccurate to be useful. Thus, early systems required instruments to be attached to a computer with articulated arms; the computer recognized joint angles to calculate instrument location in space. Early systems from ISG (ISG Technologies, Mississauga, Ontario, Canada) and the Aachen Group (University of Technology and University Hospital, Aachen, Germany) were successful in neurosurgical applications, but these devices still used mechanical arms and required head fixation (using cranial pins) [2].

Although IGS was developed for neurosurgical usage, navigating through the soft tissue structures of the cranial cavity has significant limitations. Limited bony landmarks and invariable intraoperative soft-tissue shift reduce the sustained accuracy of intracranial applications of image guidance. Roberts et al. [5] compared points on the cerebral cortex both preoperatively and intraoperatively and reported a 10-mm average change (or drift) in point location. In stark contrast, the sinonasal cavities are an ideal environment for the application of image-guidance technology. First, the bony borders of the sinonasal tract provide a constant framework that prevents extensive shift of tissues and loss of accuracy. Furthermore, several of these borders are "fixed" landmarks that are not to be violated or altered during the course of surgery, such as the lamina papyracea, skull base, and sphenoid face. Thus, even though portions of the surgical field may change due to surgical manipulation (and therefore no longer be represented accurately by a static preoperative CT scan), the outer bony boundaries of the sinonasal tract that are conserved during routine surgery should still localize well throughout the procedure.

The use of IGS in ESS was delayed by prohibitive cost and reliability. Anon et al. [6] first described computer-assisted ESS in 1994 using a frameless stereotaxy system with articulated arms of the ISG Viewing Wand (ISG Technologies). The Viewing Wand was found to be accurate to within 2 mm and assisted in the localization of instruments in frontal sinus surgery, revision surgery, sphenoid disease, sinonasal carcinoma, and skull-base procedures [7]. As in neurosurgical applications, the wand system required rigid head fixation using cranial pins, and the articulated arms were found cumbersome by some surgeons [8], prompting developments in alternative tracking devices. One of the first basic advances that made application of this to technology to ESS practical was to remedy the need for rigid head fixation. Head fixation using cranial pins was not tolerated by patients undergoing more routine "quality of life" surgery for chronic sinus disease. Improvements in accuracy were next to be addressed. Early attempts at electromagnetic calibration and tracking in the 1980s were too inaccurate to be useful. The technology improved sufficiently such that in the late 1990s, accurate and easy-to-use electromagnetic and optical-based tracking systems became available. Studies at that time demonstrated the feasibility and utility of image-guidance systems in the identification of sinonasal landmarks and adjacent structures [9].

The innovations in registration that have followed have eliminated the need for patients to wear fiducial markers between the time when the CT scan is obtained and surgery. Registration techniques have been simplified for ease of application, the surgeon–machine interface has become more user-friendly,

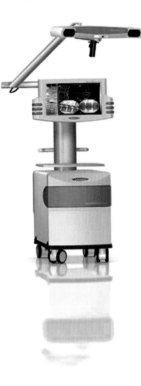

Fig. 48.1 Example of an optical-based image-guidance system (VectorVision by BrainLAB, Munich, Germany) showing a computer workstation, video display, and infrared source and camera

and systems have become much more powerful, affordable, and compact (Fig. 48.1). Recent studies have demonstrated that image-guidance systems are highly accurate and improve surgeon confidence [10]. As computer power, image quality, and tracking technology improves, IGS will become more accurate and the applications will continue to expand.

Imaging of the Paranasal Sinuses

Advances in imaging of the paranasal sinuses have been critical to the development of IGS. In many ways, the evolution of IGS has mirrored advances in imaging techniques. Prior to the advent of ESS, plain films were used to identify disease in the frontal and maxillary sinuses, but were inaccurate in demonstrating the extent of disease within the sinuses and had limited anatomic detail necessary for preoperative planning [11]. As the understanding of sinus physiology progressed and therapy was directed toward widening of the natural sinus ostia and resection of ethmoid cells, the limited detail provided by plain films rendered this imaging modality obsolete [12]. The evolving concepts of sinus function were supported by advances in rigid nasal endoscopy and CT imaging. For the first time, key functional areas such as the ethmoid labyrinth could actually be identified on CT cuts, and mucociliary clearance and sinus obstruction could be visualized through rigid telescopes, further consolidating modern-day concepts.

CT scans are still the imaging modality of choice when evaluating the paranasal sinuses, and are therefore used routinely for IGS. The early CT scanners were single-channel machines that required 2 s to generate one image with one rotation of the

detector. The development of multislice spiral scanners allowed for multiple images to be captured in one rotation with less artifact. Currently, 64-channel scanners are commonly available and can obtain images of the entire body with 0.2 mm section thickness in 60 s [13]. A slice thickness of 3 mm or less provides optimal data for evaluation of the paranasal sinuses. The unit of data (voxel) in CT scans is cuboidal and this allows for reconstruction of images in any plane. The coronal plane is the view of choice because the patency of the osteomeatal complex, frontal recess, and sphenoethmoid recess can be evaluated. The coronal view also corresponds with the endoscopic view experienced during surgery. CT images are routinely reformatted to provide all anatomic planes (axial, coronal, and sagittal), allowing for localization in all three planes when using image guidance.

The radiation exposure from CT scanning is variable and increases with increasing tube current milliamp-seconds (mAs). Lower mAs may decrease image detail and increase noise. Using 50–80 mAs at 120 kV peak provides reasonable radiation exposure without compromising image quality [13]. The current recommendations are to limit a patient to a maximum of two CT scans per year to minimize radiation exposure, and special precautions should be used in children and in women of child-bearing age [13]. The speed of contemporary multislice CT scanners and the reduced radiation and cost associated with them have rendered the once popular "limited sinus CT" (providing fewer, thicker CT cuts) unnecessary.

Magnetic resonance (MR) imaging (MRI) provides excellent soft-tissue resolution and can be used as an adjunct for imaging the paranasal sinuses. The extent of soft-tissue and inflammatory processes can be delineated without the radiation exposure from a CT scan. Fungal sinusitis has a characteristic low signal intensity on T2-weighted MRI images (causing a "dropped signal" on T2 when compared to T1). MRI is also extremely useful in the evaluation of possible neoplasia; precisely detailing the site and extension of benign and malignant sinonasal tumors. This modality can also be useful in evaluating cerebrospinal fluid (CSF) leaks, as the high intensity signal of CSF in the sinuses on T2-weighted imaging can suggest the presence of a leak. Subtle findings of an encephalocele would also be illustrated.

The main issue limiting use of MRI in IGS of the sinuses is that MRI does not provide adequate detail of bony anatomy, particularly the thin bones of the anterior skull base and ethmoid labyrinth. In addition, inflammatory tissue may be difficult to distinguish from the nasal cycle. Moreover, MRI is associated with higher costs and longer acquisition times than conventional CT imaging. For complex lesions involving the sinonasal tract and anterior cranial fossa, however, it may be useful to navigate with MRI and CT, to further characterize anatomy for the surgical approach.

IGS Components

The IGS system is composed of a computer workstation with registration/tracking software, imaging data, video display, tracking system and surgical instrumentation (Fig. 48.2). The imaging data can come in many forms, with CT data being the most common. The image data set is transferred to the IGS

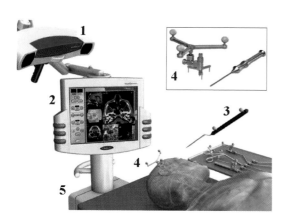

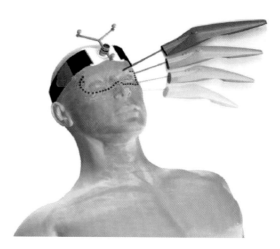

Fig. 48.2 Optical-based image-guidance system (VectorVision by BrainLAB) demonstrating the application of a skull fixation reference array that permits external approaches. Components: *1* boom with infrared source and camera, *2* video display, *3* standard navigation probe, *4* percutaneous skull fixation array, *5* computer workstation

Fig. 48.3 Illustration showing contour-based registration, identifying multiple surface points using the Z-Touch laser and headset (Brain-LAB). Points are identified over bony structures such as orbital rims and nasal dorsum to reduce error

computer through digital storage media, or more recently, it can be directly downloaded via high-speed Internet or wireless Ethernet connections. The IGS system will only work as well as the quality of imaging study applied to the system. The optimal CT scan is an axial 1-mm CT with a 512×512-pixel matrix. Because the registration process involves the surface of the patient's face it is important to have the entire head and skin surface captured within the study. The slice thickness sets the lower limit for accuracy. A CT scan with 3-mm slices will only have an accuracy of 3 mm at best, even when registration is 100% accurate.

The operating system on the computer workstation is dependent on the manufacturer. Windows 2000, Windows XP, and Linux platforms are available. The software has become easier to use and a variety of configurations to view the data set are used including three-dimensional model reconstruction and cut-out view reconstruction. The display is a high-resolution flat-panel monitor and several systems have touch-screen capability, although the standard computer mouse and keyboard may be used for data entry.

Registration Paradigms

Accuracy during surgical navigation hinges upon the registration process. Registration is the establishment of a rigid relationship between two coordinate systems: that by which the images were obtained and an arbitrary system employed to describe every point within the surgical field. After registration has been performed, a navigation system is capable of translating from any point either in the images or the patient, to the same point on the other entity using a transformation matrix created by the registration process. Registration allows translation freely between the three-dimensional space of the images

(a virtual space) and the anatomical structure of the patient (a real space).

All image-guidance systems require some form of registration in order to employ preoperatively obtained images of the patient's anatomy for use by the surgeon within the operating room. If the registration tightly maps the imaging data set to the operative field, the fidelity of the navigational system will be optimal. In reality, all registration methods are less than ideal. Bone-anchored fiducial markers provide the best results with regard to accuracy and the lowest rate of systematic errors; however, this invasive strategy is impractical in most rhinology patients. All other registration paradigms sacrifice varying amounts of accuracy for improvements in the user-friendliness of the technology.

There are currently three types of registration available depending on the manufacturer of the IGS system used for sinus surgery. They are paired-point registration, automatic registration, and contour-based registration [14]. Multiple clinical trails have shown these three systems to be reliable with accuracies of 1–2 mm [15,16]. The paired-point method requires the surgeon to designate fiducial points on both the patient and imaging data. These points can be markers placed prior to imaging or anatomic landmarks such as the tragus and lateral canthus. Accuracy can be improved by increasing the number of points and using a distribution of fiducial points to encompass the three-dimensional area of surgical interest. Therefore, a greater number of paired points is desirable; however, a greater number of points increases the time for registration and does not significantly improve accuracy. Most surgeons recommend 6–10 paired points in a nonlinear distribution around the surgical area [14]. Automatic registration employs a headset that is placed on the patient at the time of CT or MRI. The headset is designed to fit the patient in a reproducible fashion and it must be reapplied and worn dur-

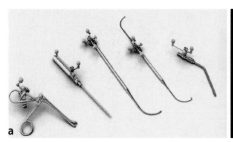 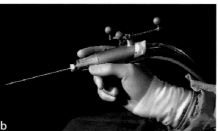

Fig. 48.4a, b Using current image-guided surgery (IGS) technology, almost any rigid surgical instrument can be tracked. As shown in **a**, examples include: Blakesley forceps, pointer, curettes, and different types of suction cannulae. The position of the reflective spheres is adaptable to allow for more ergonomic handling. **b** A microdebrider (Gyrus Diego, Memphis, TN, USA) being tracked with removable reflective spheres

ing surgery. The IGS system recognizes points within the headset and uses these as fiducial points for registration. The accuracy of this "automatic" method is dependent on consistent placement of the headset, which is not guaranteed. Contour-based registration requires the IGS system to build a three-dimensional model of surface contours of the patient's face using the imaging data. A standard probe or reflected laser light can then be used to define the surface contour of the patient at the time of surgery (Fig. 48.3). This technique defines a large number of registration points (40–500) in a short period of time. The contour method loses accuracy if the patient's surface contour changes from the time of image collection to the time of surgery due to edema, weight gain, and stretching from surgical drapes. While early registration paradigms were difficult to follow [17], recent features such as touch screens, autoregistration, and surface registration have simplified the process significantly. It is important to remember that the navigation process is dynamic and a small change in the initial registration may cause a significant change in the projected location of the instrument on the IGS display.

Tracking Technology

The technology for tracking and calibration of the IGS instruments has been refined in two forms using either optical- or electromagnetic-based systems. Both systems are highly accurate to within 2 mm and both systems account for intraoperative head movement by fastening a headset to the patient. Electromagnetic systems track by utilizing a radiofrequency transmitter within the headset and a receiver positioned within the instrument. The headset and instrument are attached via wires to the system hardware. The same headset must be worn during the preoperative CT scan, and again intraoperatively. Electromagnetic tracking may be susceptible to interference from metal instruments within the field or the metal operating-room table. Thus, metal devices and anesthesia equipment must be placed an appropriate distance away from the operating field (the patient's head), and some authors recommend placing extra padding between the patient and the table [18].

Optical systems use infrared light and a camera tracking system positioned 6 feet (approximately 1.8 m) above the patient's head to track instruments affixed with reflective spheres. This provides a wireless mechanism for instrument localization, but requires a clear pathway between the tracking device and the instruments. Equipment must be placed carefully and draping performed to avoid line-of-site obstruction. When optical and electromagnetic systems were compared by Metson et al. [18], no significant difference was found in blood loss or complications. The accuracy and general functioning of the systems are considered to be materially equivalent.

Some specialized equipment and instruments are needed for both types of systems. Optical tracking systems require light-reflecting spheres (also referred to as "stars" or "glions") attached to the proximal end of surgical instruments. Electromagnetic platforms require the attachment of a wired probe to the instruments. Both systems allow for a wide variety of instruments to be tracked including probes, a variety of straight and angled suctions and curettes, drills, and microdebriders (Fig. 48.4). The computer workstation integrates the data set with information from the tracking system and projects the location of the instrument tip simultaneously on all three CT views [19].

During the course of surgery it is important that the surgeon corroborates the accuracy of the IGS frequently using obvious surface and intranasal landmarks such as the tip of the nose or the posterior wall of the maxillary sinus. Shifting of the registration platform is a risk, especially during a long procedure or a challenging case where movement of the head or neck may be required. The calibration of the instruments can also change, particularly if unusual positions of the instruments are required to reach a surgical site. A change in the angle of the instrument facing an optical tracking device can change the projected location [15].

Today, several systems are available for IGS of the paranasal sinuses. Major vendors in the surgical navigation market include BrainLAB (Munich, Germany), General Electric (Waukesha, WI, USA), Medtronic Xomed (Jacksonville, FL, USA), and Stryker (Kalamazoo, MI, USA). The General Electric system is the only commercially available system that is based on electromagnetic

Table 48.1 Image-guided surgery (IGS) manufacturers and products

Manufacturer	Platform	Instrument tracking	Registration
BrainLAB	VectorVision	Infrared	Contour-based
	Kolibri ENT	Infrared	Contour-based
General Electric	InstaTrak 3500	Electromagnetic	Automatic
	ENTrak	Electromagnetic	Automatic
Medtronic Xomed	LandmarX Element	Infrared	Contour or paired-point
	LandmarX Evolution	Infrared	Contour or paired-point
Stryker	Stryker Navigation System	Infrared	Contour or paired-point

technology, while the others employ optical-based platforms. Table. 48.1 compares several features of current IGS systems. Each system has its own advantages and disadvantages and it is beyond the scope of this chapter to contrast such details. All four systems have a record of excellent reliability and accuracy.

Multimodal Navigation and Fusion Technology

For the vast majority of sinus procedures, the preoperative CT scan is downloaded into the IGS computer and used effectively for intraoperative navigation. Recent advances in IGS technology, however, permit the surgeon to navigate using CT images, MR images (common for intracranial approaches), or a combination of these two data sets fused together or superimposed [20]. The technique of relating one type of imaging modality to another is simply a manifestation of the overall concept of registration. Instead of relating images to the anatomy of the patient, two image data sets, taken with respect to two different coordinate systems, are related to each other such that any point in one image data set can be depicted in the other data set [21]. One common way to display two image datasets coregistered to each other is to overlay them on top of one another, frequently with one image data set in color, and the other in grey scale (Fig. 48.5). The act of relating two image datasets to each other, and then to the patient's anatomy, to arrive at a composite image that has more information than either of the combined images, is called image fusion.

A common procedure that is ideally suited for navigation employing CT and MR image fusion is transsphenoidal pituitary surgery. Otolaryngologists providing access to the sphenoid sinus during these procedures are interested in the bony anatomic details of the sinuses, which are provided optimally by CT images. In contradistinction, our neurosurgical colleagues are more concerned with the soft-tissue extension of the tumors arising out of the sella turcica, and hence prefer the use of MR images (Fig. 48.6). Navigation can proceed with a single-modality view or a unique hybrid CT-MR fusion view can also be employed. Leong et al. [20] studied CT-MR fusion and demon-

strated accuracy within 2 mm as well as facilitation of preoperative planning by better defining anatomic relationships.

Other imaging modalities may also be incorporated to provide even more information to further enhance localization. Fusion technology need not refer only to the fusion of CT and MRI images, as other data sets can also be combined; including digital angiography or ultrasound. Although infrequently encountered, there are situations where navigation using several of these modalities may prove advantageous, such as utilizing CT-angiography or MR-angiography during extended intracranial/skull-base procedures for lesions in close proximity to the internal carotid or basilar arteries. Accurate localization of vasculature with fusion of angiographic datasets could also be potentially helpful in endoscopic sphenopalatine artery ligation, pituitary surgery, and endoscopic tumor resections (e.g., juvenile nasopharyngeal an-

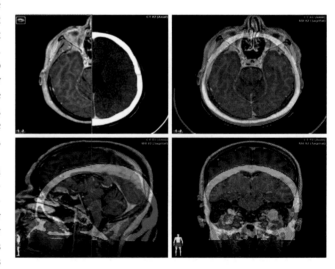

Fig. 48.5 Navigation using computed tomography (CT) and magnetic resonance imaging (MRI) fusion to simultaneously display soft tissue and bony anatomic detail. The CT data is colored *blue* to accentuate the two imaging modalities

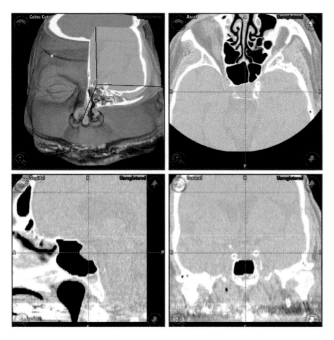

Fig. 48.6 Standard IGS video display (Kolibri by BrainLAB) showing localization of a pituitary tumor on orthogonal views and three-dimensional computer reconstruction with advanced cut-out mode (top left panel)

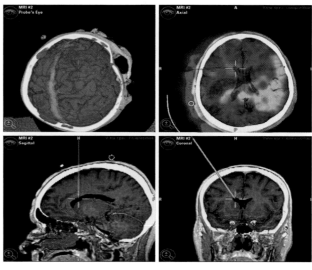

Fig. 48.7 Display of multiple fused datasets from a patient with a left parietal lesion. The *upper left* image demonstrates cortex segmentation viewed in advanced three dimensions with bone-volume rendering. The *upper right* image shows positron emission tomography, MRI, and CT fusion. The *bottom two* panels show CT (*yellow color*), MRI, and digital angiography datasets superimposed (VectorVision by BrainLAB)

giofibroma). As more challenging and invasive intracranial and lateral skull-base procedures are performed endoscopically, the demand for better and more thorough localization modalities such as fusion techniques will become evident.

Newer imaging techniques, such as positron emission tomography (PET) scanning, studying functional changes rather than structural abnormalities, are emerging that may become useful to endoscopic surgeons. This modality detects metabolic activation of specific areas of the body while the patient being imaged performs a specific task. In this regard, IGS is evolving into "*information* guided surgery," as we incorporate multimodal datasets, some of which are based on functional information. This type of functional data is already employed during intracranial surgery (Fig. 48.7), and may eventually find a role in advanced endoscopic surgery of the lateral skull-base temporal bone, intracranial lesions, or surgery in the region of the olfactory cleft or orbital apex.

IGS Indications and Applications

The role of image guidance has not been completely defined, but most surgeons feel that it is best applied when additional information beyond the endoscopic or surgical view is beneficial to the surgical procedure. Some authors have suggested that the utility of IGS can be determined by categorizing patients into three groups [22]: (1) IGS not needed, (2) IGS maybe useful but not necessary, and (3) IGS is preferred or needed.

Group 1: IGS not Needed

This group includes patients with minimal disease or disease localized to the maxillary and ethmoid sinuses. Image guidance is not necessary if these patients have well-defined anatomic landmarks and endoscopic procedures can be performed safely with standard equipment. In fact, the use of IGS in these patients may be considered an unnecessary effort and expense.

Group 2: IGS may be Useful but not Necessary

These are patients with intermediate disease and include patients with disease of the frontal or sphenoid sinuses. The complex anatomy of the frontal recess can be difficult to appreciate endoscopically and identification and enlargement of the frontal ostium may be greatly enhanced with image guidance. The proximity of the sphenoid sinus to the carotid artery, optic nerve, and skull base requires a high degree of precision when operating in this area. IGS can assist with identification of the sphenoid face and ostium as well as avoidance of adjacent critical structures (Fig. 48.8). Diffuse polyposis may obscure surgical landmarks that could be better appreciated with IGS. Similarly, patients with previous sinus surgery may have absent or obscure anatomic landmarks and may benefit from the use of navigation.

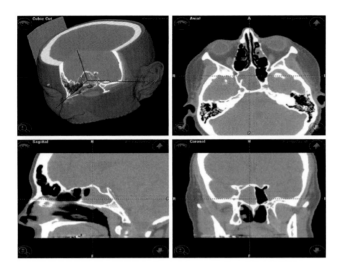

Fig. 48.8 IGS video display showing isolated sphenoid disease

Group 3: IGS is Preferred or Needed

Patients with advanced disease or unusual pathology are included in this group. These patients often have unusual pathology or disease in unusual locations, often resulting in significantly altered anatomy (Fig. 48.9). Patients with lesions requiring extended endoscopic approaches to the skull base or parasinus regions fall into this category. IGS can be very useful to avoid critical structures and determine the extent of resection. Examples include sinonasal neoplasia, petrous apex lesions, and pathology involving the skull base, orbit, or sella. In addition to the navigational advantage with IGS, the display of the imaging data in three simultaneous planes can be a very powerful tool for preoperative planning in these cases.

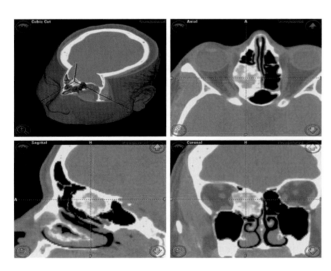

Fig. 48.9 Display of a complex fibro-osseous lesion attached to the skull base and lamina papyracea that was removed endoscopically with the aid of IGS

Revision ESS may be complicated by loss of anatomic landmarks and the presence of synechiae. IGS may help the surgeon identify structures such as the orbit and skull base in the absence of anatomic landmarks. Thus, the risk of complications is theoretically lowered and the number of diseased sinus cells that are entered may be increased [23]. Tabaee et al. [24] studied 85 patients who underwent revision surgery with IGS and they reported no serious complication within this group. These results stand in contrast to data published by Jiang and Hsu [25], who reported a 9.9% complication rate in cases of revision ESS without IGS. However, this study was retrospective from 1988 to 1998 and there are likely to have been other improvements in ESS since that review.

Frontal sinus surgery, with close proximity to the orbit and skull base, may also be simplified by IGS, particularly in revision procedures when scar tissue obstructs key areas of the frontal outflow tract. IGS imaging data greatly facilitates the preoperative evaluation and planning of approaches to the complex anatomy of the frontal recess. The ability to rapidly and simultaneously scroll through all three planes promotes a better sense of the three-dimensional relationships of the frontal sinus outflow tract (Fig. 48.10). The sagittal cuts are extremely

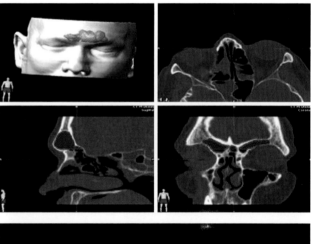

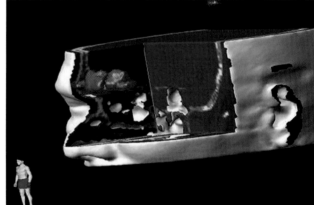

Fig. 48.10 Complex three-dimensional frontal sinus reconstructions for enhanced preoperative planning and localization

Table 48.2 Indications for IGS

Revision sinus surgery
Distorted sinus anatomy of development, postoperative or traumatic origin
Extensive sinonasal polyposis
Pathology involving the frontal, posterior ethmoid, and sphenoid sinuses
Disease abutting the skull base, orbit, optic nerve, or carotid artery
Cerebrospinal fluid rhinorrhea or conditions where there is a skull-base defect
Benign and malignant sinonasal neoplasms

valuable in evaluating the anatomy of the frontal recess region. During frontal sinusotomy, an IGS instrument such as a curved frontal sinus probe can be passed through the dissected recess and directly into the ostium, while its correct location can be confirmed on the IGS display. This can be useful in differentiating the frontal sinus ostium from an adjacent supraorbital ethmoid cell, which can be challenging. In a review of 800 sinus procedures done at a community hospital, Reardon noted a significant increase in the number of frontal sinuses entered after the introduction of an IGS system [26]. When an IGS system is used for drillout surgery of the frontal sinus, the calibrated curved probe can be used to assist in the identification of the frontal ostium and to ensure that drilling is preformed in a safe direction. Without an IGS system, initial drilling is often blind until the frontal sinus can be visualized. Success rates for complex procedures such as frontal drillout surgery with and without IGS are statistically comparable, although there appears to be a trend toward higher surgical success rates when the IGS system is employed [26].

The indications for the use of image guidance endorsed by the American Academy of Otolaryngology – Head and Neck Surgery [27] are listed in Table 48.2. These are settings in which the Academy suggests that the application of IGS could be considered. Although not specified as an indication by the American Academy of Otolaryngology – Head and Neck Surgery, image guidance also assists in teaching cases by improving the ability of the surgeon to teach anatomical relationships and monitor the progress of residents. It should also be noted that when first becoming familiar with this technology, surgeons are advised to use IGS on cases where they do not actually think it will be "needed," so that they may gain confidence and understanding of its uses and limitations in a safe environment. It should be emphasized that at the present time, the use of image-guidance technology for ESS is *not* considered standard of care [28].

Expanded Applications

Recently, external approaches to the sinuses have also been augmented through the use of IGS technology. Frontal sinus obliteration via the osteoplastic flap technique is a prime example. Obliteration of the frontal sinus is considered when endoscopic attempts to establish frontal sinus ventilation and drainage fail. Traditionally, a radiographic template has been used to guide osteotomies through the frontal bone around the perimeter of the frontal sinus to expose the sinus interior. A high rate of complications has been encountered historically, including inadvertent orbital or intracranial penetration as a result of misdirected osteotomies [29]. A major obstacle to the application of IGS to external frontal sinus surgery was the standard headset. The headsets of all commercially available navigations systems sit on and obstruct access to the forehead area. Through the use of a skull fixation array positioned in an unobtrusive location away from the forehead, the need for a standard headset is obviated, and IGS can be used to accurately demarcate the perimeter of the frontal sinus once the frontal bone is exposed. This information can then be used to direct cuts through the anterior table in a very precise manner. The use of IGS for frontal sinus localization during the obliteration procedure has been demonstrated to be safer than traditional non-IGS methods [30, 31]. More recently, a less invasive endoscopic method for obliteration of the frontal sinus using IGS has also been described [32]. In this very novel approach, an incision is made over the inferomedial eyebrow, IGS is used to verify the location of the frontal sinus, and it is entered at the lateral aspect of the sinus floor. The mucosa is then elevated under endoscopic guidance through a generous trephine, the sinus walls are drilled to remove any mucosal remnants, and the frontal ostium and sinus are carefully obliterated.

Previous maxillofacial trauma or congenital anomalies may also distort sinonasal anatomy. Image guidance provides additional data about the borders of the operative field and may assist in defining altered structures. With the refinement of the endoscopes and surgical equipment, otolaryngologists have been applying endoscopic transnasal techniques to skull-base and even intracranial surgery. IGS can assist in the localization of tumors and determine the extent of inflammatory diseases involving the skull base. Challenging skull-base tumors are now being biopsied or removed entirely using endoscopic approaches. The IGS systems are more ideally suited to bony tumors, but also aid in the endoscopic resection of soft-tissue tumors [33]. Endoscopic management of encephaloceles and/or CSF rhinorrhea is a well-appreciated indication for IGS. As shown in Fig. 48.11, IGS can help define the extent of the skull-base defect and help avoid adjacent vital intracranial structures. Tabaee et al. [34] concluded that IGS is a valuable adjunct in the endoscopic management of CSF rhinorrhea, but did not statistically improve rates of successful closure.

Endoscopic orbital procedures such as dacryocystorhinostomy, orbital decompression, and optic nerve decompression may also be enhanced with image guidance. During orbital and optic nerve decompression, key landmarks in the area of the orbital apex, including the lateral sphenoid face, sphenoethmoid angle, and opticocarotid recess can be identified with near certainty to avoid injury [35]. In addition, the preoperative IGS evaluation will help identify the association between the sphenoid architecture, optic canal, and the proximity of the carotid artery. Variants such as sphenoethmoid cells (or Onodi cells) with possible dehiscence of either the carotid artery or optic nerve are better characterized by the three-plane images of IGS.

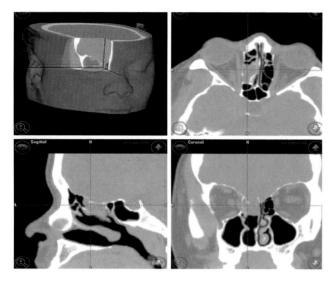

Fig. 48.11 Localization of a right ethmoid encephalocele that was repaired using IGS

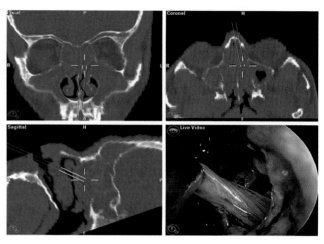

Fig. 48.12 Intraoperative view of the display during image-guided ESS for allergic fungal sinusitis. Note classic allergic mucin being suctioned from left maxillary sinus on endoscopic view in the *right lower panel*

48

Removal of optic canal bone can be done with greater confidence with simultaneous visualization of the carotid path and intracranial border [35].

IGS has also positively influenced pediatric sinonasal surgery. The definition of pediatric sinusitis and the surgical approaches utilized have been evolving over the last decade. Certain sinus conditions found in the pediatric population are especially amenable to the use of IGS. Examples include the extensive polyposis of cystic fibrosis, allergic fungal sinusitis (Fig. 48.12), and endoscopic choanal atresia repair (Fig. 48.13).

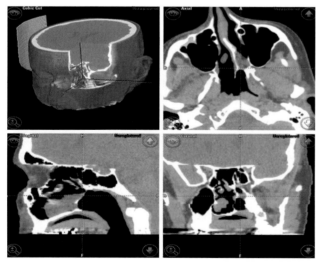

Fig. 48.13 Left choanal atresia repaired endoscopically with image-guidance to identify the bony obstructive component

IGS and Preoperative Surgical Planning

Detailed preoperative evaluation of the patient's imaging for surgical planning provides a significant advantage to the surgeon, and offers a tremendous benefit to resident education and surgical training. Powerful and easy-to-use software programs allow interactive preoperative evaluation and surgical planning through the simultaneous view of coordinated axial, coronal, and sagittal projections of the patient's anatomy. Computerized image reconstruction, three-dimensional model simulation, three-dimensional cut-view reconstruction, as well as distance and volume measurement capabilities are other system features. These software tools allow review of preoperative images in a manner that facilitates understanding of complex anatomic relationships, enabling the surgeon to formulate a detailed surgical plan. Advances in the display of this information and in the detailed computer reconstructions will continue to corroborate the important role of the navigation system in preoperative evaluation and planning.

Surgical planning is especially critical in complex skull-base and intracranial procedures, especially when performed endoscopically. In conjunction with conventional image-guidance systems, devices such as the Dextroscope (Volumetric Interactions, Princeton, NJ, USA) may be used to further enhance the surgeon's appreciation of the targeted anatomy. This sophisticated virtual reality system uses computer software to integrate tomographic images from CT, MRI, and nuclear medicine into true three-dimensional volumetric objects that can be viewed stereoscopically. It allows surgeons to take patient-specific images reconstructed three-dimensionally, and virtually hold them, turn them, and even operate on them using virtual drills to evaluate different surgical approaches. As demonstrated in Fig. 48.14, the system utilizes two, six-degrees-of-freedom po-

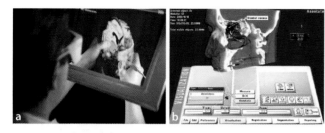

Fig. 48.14 **a** Surgeon using Dextroscope (Volumetric Interactions, Princeton, NJ, USA) for image manipulation and preoperative planning of the surgical approach for a complex skull-base lesion. **b** Three-dimension cut-away view demonstrating the anatomic detail of the frontal recess

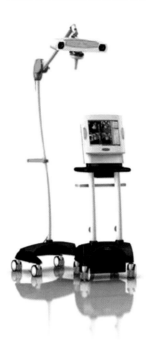

Fig. 48.15 Example of a compact optical-based image-guidance system that can be useful in ambulatory surgery centers. This device offers the advantages of a smaller size and lower cost. (Kolibri System, BrainLAB)

sitional controllers, one in each hand, that work as extensions of the surgeon's hands, providing the ability to interact with the patient's virtual anatomy.

Cost of Image Guidance

In making the decision to use image guidance for each procedure and for each surgeon, there is a dynamic balance between the demands for accurate localization and tolerance for the costs and time required to utilize this technology [10]. This benefit versus cost estimation is a difficult problem for almost all new medical technologies, and is decided without input from prospective randomized clinical studies designed to achieve a true measure of the benefit of a proposed technology. Generally speaking, the "costs" of using IGS are: increased time expenditure, a disruption in the "flow" of the operation, and financial. The increased monetary costs associated with using IGS are difficult to measure precisely as they come from many different sources; for example capital expenses, upkeeping expenses and repair of hardware, disposables (reflective spheres), longer operating room times (impacts personnel, surgeon, and anesthesia-related costs), and radiology-related expenditure. Metson et al. [36] demonstrated an average increase in operative time of 17.4 min/case, commenting that this will likely improve as the learning curve associated with this new technology plateaus over time. Based on operating room and anesthesia, charges, this increase in time resulted in an additional charge of approximately US$500/case. However, selection bias may account for some of these findings as operations involving image guidance are usually more complex and therefore possibly of longer duration. It is also possible, however, that as a result of the application of IGS, the surgeon could improve his efficiency, which may actually decrease the operative length,

not to mention possibly avoiding complications. Another consideration is that as software and computing power have evolved, image-guidance systems have become much more user-friendly, resulting in shorter set-up times and minimizing lengthy trouble-shooting episodes.

Separate from the operative costs of IGS is the initial capital expenditure for an IGS system. Most typical IGS systems can be purchased for around US$200,000, depending on the level of sophistication and upgrades selected. Compact "basic units" promoted for the ambulatory surgery center (ASC) market are offered by several companies for about half of this amount (Fig. 48.15). Through the development of these smaller and less expensive models, image-guidance technology is no longer limited to large academic centers. Many ASCs, a major trend in surgical care in the USA, also offer IGS technology to their sinus patients. Professional reimbursement for the use of IGS is possible using the 61795 CPT code for surgeons, and there is a facility fee allotted to the institution. As the technology improves and image-guidance systems become more widely used, the cost will continue to decrease.

Limitations of IGS

IGS has several important limitations that must be recognized. First, the introduction of any new technology is and will continue to be problematic at times. There is a significant learning curve associated with the use of IGS, and the surgeon–machine interface presented must be respected and reconciled. A certain amount of technology *savvy* is beneficial, although software advances are making these devices much more user-friendly and simpler to use. Patient headsets worn intraoperatively allow for real-time tracking but are prone to movement while the patient is manipulated, thus decreasing accuracy and introducing drift. Frequent corroboration with the clinical landmarks and evaluation of the headset for possible movement during a case will allow this to be identified and addressed early (e.g., through re-registration). As discussed, the design of current headsets also restricts external access to the frontal sinus.

For the optical-based systems, maintaining a clear line of sight from the camera to the instruments can be challenging, especially during complex procedures where the endoscope may block the reflective spheres on the instruments or if the instruments are being used at unconventional angles/positions, making the spheres difficult to see. Although unbound from issues related to line of sight, electromagnetic systems have their own limitations including problems with too many cords looping over the surgical field and encountering interference from nearby metal objects.

Patients with complex pathology often have studies obtained prior to recognition of the need for image guidance. Until very recently, most available IGS systems required a special CT protocol for the dataset to be incorporated into the software, and CT scans performed elsewhere (so-called "foreign data sets") were not usable for navigation. This of course mandated repeat imaging, exposing the patient to further radiation and increasing cost, solely for the purpose of employing navigation. This issue has recently been significantly improved by the manufacturers of most systems, such that the majority (but not all) of foreign data sets are now accepted provided they are available in electronic format (on a CD or flash drive). Finally, it should be stressed that although highly accurate, navigation systems are fallible and not perfect. These systems are simply an adjunct to clinical expertise and experience.

The Future of IGS

The future of image guidance holds great potential, and the application of this technology to endoscopic sinus and skull-base surgery will continue to expand. Although not presently the case, IGS will one day become the standard of care for complicated ESS cases. There is no perfect navigation system on the market. Considering the current role of image-guidance technology in rhinology, Table 48.3 highlights some of the characteristics that an ideal navigation system might possess [21]. Automatic reregistration during a procedure could minimize drift and ensure that the surgical accuracy of systems is maintained. One limitation of current devices is the relatively large size of the physical system. Many systems are limited by bulky equipment with a relatively large footprint in the operating room. A new market has developed for stations that are more compact and portable, potentially even allowing for transport between ASCs or servicing more remote rural communities. As ASCs increase in popularity, they will provide significant market pressure for smaller and cheaper systems. In the foreseeable future, all of the hardware components of IGS will become integrated into the endoscopic operating room suite, and will become invisible to the surgeon. Incorporation of robotic technology and voice-activated controls for IGS also seems likely.

Table 48.3 Characteristics of the ideal navigation system

- Highly accurate, maintenance of accuracy throughout the procedure
- Physically unobtrusive, easily integrated into the procedure
- Affordable and user-friendly
- Not restricted by line-of-sight issues
- Permits preoperative evaluation and detailed surgical planning
- Allows seamless intranasal and external navigation with a variety of equipment
- Incorporates any existing image datasets for navigation
- Allows intraoperative updates of preoperative image data set(s)
- Permits multimodal navigation
- Permits extended applications and robotic integration

Rapid development in other hardware components has already permitted the integration of display systems into the operating room and wireless data transfer. Universal instrument registration, at least for optical-based systems, has expanded the range of instruments that can be used for navigation, such that almost any rigid instrument can be tracked. The electromagnetic system, due to its platform, is not currently as amenable to such variations. A significant advance in navigation will be the ability to track nonrigid, flexible instruments such as catheter tips placed deep within body cavities or structures. This will invariably utilize electromagnetic technology. Software advances will also allow for more complex three-dimensional modeling of patient anatomy for preoperative surgical planning. Options and indications for multimodal navigation will undoubtedly grow.

A major limitation of IGS today is that navigation occurs based upon static preoperative images that do not reflect intraoperative changes. Effective real-time intraoperative imaging and dataset update likely represents the next major step in the evolution of IGS technology. One way that this caveat could be overcome is by using software to identify operative changes and to display a revised preoperative data set. However, high computer processing power as well as continuous intraoperative calibration would be required for real-time updates to the data set to occur in any useful fashion [21]. Furthermore, the surgeon would still be navigating using old (albeit modified) preoperative data. It would be advantageous in some complex cases (tumor removal, for example) to gage the extent and success of surgery by reimaging a patient intraoperatively to evaluate whether the goals of the operation (complete tumor removal, for example) have been accomplished. This aim would be most effectively and directly served through repeat imaging in the operating room during surgery. Recent attempts to do this using fluoroscopy (as a more practical proxy for CT image data) and MRI have had considerable drawbacks. The use of intraoperative MRI is currently being used in selected neurosurgical procedures in some centers and has been described for ESS [37]. Unfortunately, intraoperative imaging complicates the operation by adding significant time and increasing cost. In addition, the quality of intraoperative imaging is almost invariably inferior to images obtained with scanners designed purely for diagnosis [38]. As imaging systems become smaller, faster, and less expensive, repeat intraoperative imaging is sure to find its way into the operating theater.

Conclusion

IGS is safe, accurate, and holds considerable promise for improving patient care. The application of image guidance can be viewed as one way to improve overall visualization during the course of a procedure, but is no substitute for surgical expertise. Commercially available navigation systems have improved considerably over the past several years, as is evidenced by their current widespread use in endoscopic sinonasal surgery. Indeed, this technology has established itself as a valuable adjunctive tool for the endoscopic surgeon and its continued proliferation seems certain, although the proper role and indications for its application remain incompletely defined. IGS is not currently standard of care.

Tips to Avoid Complications

- The best way to avoid complications is to understand the workings, benefits and limitations of navigation systems and use them as they are meant to be used. Fortunately, ESS is associated with a low complication rate. May et al. [39] reported that major complications of FESS occur in 0.85% of cases. The most common major complication is CSF leak and the sequelae of this condition can be devastating. Other major complications include injury to the orbit, major hemorrhage or death. Minor complications are identified in 6.9% of FESS cases and include middle turbinate adhesions, epistaxis, anosmia, and periorbital emphysema. A study by Metson [36] reviewed 121 cases and found no significant difference in complication rate between operations performed with and without image guidance. Although it would take a very large-scale effort to demonstrate that navigation systems reduce complications in routine ESS, reports have shown that the complication rate of some sinus procedures may be significantly reduced by employing this technology [31,40].
- Another study reviewed 1,000 cases performed using image guidance and described several tips to avoid complications [41]. Surgeons should start with relatively easy cases when learning to use an image-guidance system. There is of course a learning curve when using new technology. Initially using IGS for routine procedures establishes familiarity with the equipment so that the surgeon will feel comfortable using the system on more challenging cases. Initial assistance from the vendor representative may also help instruct the surgeon on the proper setup, registration, and calibration techniques.

- The accuracy of image guidance has been well documented, but the image-guidance system should not be used to make millimeter decisions about how to proceed during surgery. IGS is best used when evaluating large spaces. For example, IGS can be used to identify the sphenoid face and ensure complete removal of posterior ethmoid cells. IGS can also help delineate the course of the optic nerve and carotid artery when performing endoscopic orbital surgery [42]. The surgeon should frequently reevaluate the instrument location and determine if the projected instrument location is consistent with the appearance and palpation of structures based on clinical judgment.
- When information from the image-guidance system conflicts with clinical judgment, trust your judgment. Loss of accuracy due to anatomic drift or intraoperative changes may be easy to identify if the instrument location is clearly in a different location from that shown on the monitor. Reregistration can mitigate these errors; however, if the location in question is flush with a critical structure or the discrepancy is unclear, the surgeon may be better off leaving that area undisturbed.
- It should be underscored that technology is not a substitute for technique. The increased level of confidence gained from using image-guidance should not serve as justification for performing procedures the surgeon would not otherwise perform, or is not sufficiently trained to perform. IGS does not change the nature of the procedure and will not substitute for lack of training or experience. Despite the benefits of image guidance and increasing availability of this technology, the standard of care does not yet include the use of image guidance for ESS [28].

Take-Home Pearls

• Image-guidance systems are relatively accurate and reliable. Accuracy within 2 mm is currently achievable with all contemporary methods of instrument tracking and registration. Loss of accuracy is usually due to headset movement intraoperatively and instrument location should be frequently verified by clinical correlation. Repeat registration is necessary if the fidelity of the system appears suspect. The use of an image-guidance system is associated with increased operative time and expense. Image-guidance systems enhance surgeon confidence. A survey of otolaryngologists demonstrated that 85% of surgeons reported increased confidence when using image-guidance [24]. Using IGS, surgeons can definitively identify key anatomic landmarks during surgery, and by identifying disease that has not yet been addressed may possibly perform a more thorough operation [43]. Despite increased levels of confidence among surgeons using IGS, these systems are not meant for every surgeon. Most surgeons are comfortable performing certain procedures and the addition of image guidance may serve as a distraction from the case. In addition, occasional equipment failure should be expected and the surgeon should be willing to accept such difficulties with minimal frustration.

• Image-guidance systems are also not meant for every patient or procedure. The cost and increased operative time of IGS for patients with conserved landmarks and limited disease may not be justified. Image guidance may not enhance the procedure if the surgeon is comfortable performing difficult cases based on his expertise and experience using traditional instruments. Interestingly, the impact of image guidance on clinical outcomes from routine sinus surgery is unknown. One study examined quality of life after ESS and found no significant difference in patients who underwent image-guided or non-image-guided ESS [44]. Some studies have suggested a statistical trend in reducing navigation errors [26], but the low complication rate associated with sinus surgery would require very large studies to demonstrate a statistically significant reduction in complications with navigation.

References

1. Anon JB, Rontal M, Zinreich SJ (1995) Computer-assisted endoscopic sinus surgery – current experience and future developments. Oper Tech Otolaryngol Head Neck Surg 6:163–170
2. Palmer JN, Kennedy DW (2005) Historical perspective on image-guided sinus surgery. Otolaryngol Clin North Am38:419–428
3. Hepworth EJ, Bucknor M, Patel A, Vaughan WC (2006) Nationwide survey on the use of image-guided functional endoscopic sinus surgery. Otolaryngol Head Neck Surg 135:73–75
4. Bergstrom M, Greitz T (1976) Stereotaxic computed tomography. AJR Am J Roentgenol 127:167–170
5. Roberts DW, Hartov A, Kenned FE, Miga MI, Paulsen KD (1998) Intraoperative brain shift and deformation: a quantitative analysis of cortical displacement in 28 cases. Neurosurgery 43:749–758
6. Anon JB, Lipman SP, Oppenheim D, Halt RA (1994) Computer-assisted endoscopic sinus surgery. Laryngoscope 104:901–905
7. Carrau RL, Snyderman CH, Curtin HD, Janecka IP, Stechison M, Weissman JL (1996) Computer-assisted intraoperative navigation during skull base surgery. Am J Otolaryngol 17:95–101
8. Freysinger W, Gunkel AR, Martin A, Bale RJ, Vogele M, Thumfart WF (1997) Advancing ear, nose, and throat computer-assisted surgery with the arm-based ISG viewing wand: the stereotactic suction tube. Laryngoscope 107:690–693
9. Fried MP, Kleefield J, Gopal H, Reardon E, Ho BT, Kuhn FA (1997) Image-guided endoscopic surgery: results of accuracy and performance in a multicenter clinical study using an electromagnetic tracking system. Laryngoscope 107:594–601
10. Hemmerdinger SA, Jacobs JB, Lebowitz RA (2005) Accuracy and cost analysis of image-guided sinus surgery. Otolaryngol Clin North Am 38:453–460
11. Aygun N, Uzuner O, Zinreich SJ (2005) Advances in imaging of the paranasal sinuses. Otolaryngol Clin North Am 38:429–437
12. Zinreich JS (2006) Progress in sinonasal imaging. Ann Otol Rhinol Laryngol Suppl 196:61–65
13. Aygun N, Zinreich SJ (2006) Imaging for functional endoscopic sinus surgery. Otolaryngol Clin North Am 39:403–416
14. Citardi M, Batra P (2005) Image-guided sinus surgery: current concepts and technology. Otolaryngol Clin North Am 38:439–452
15. Fried MP, Kleefield J, Gopal H, Reardon E, Ho BT, Kuhn FA (1997) Image-guided endoscopic surgery: results of accuracy and performance in a multicenter clinical study using a electromagnetic tracking system. Laryngoscope 107:594–601
16. Anon JB (1998) Computer-aided endoscopic sinus surgery. Laryngoscope 108:949–961
17. Metson R, Cosenza MJ, Cunningham MJ, Randolph GW (2000) Physician experience with an optical image-guidance system for sinus surgery. Laryngoscope 110:972–976
18. Metson R, Gliklich RE, Cosenza M (1998) A comparison of image-guidance systems for sinus surgery. Laryngoscope 108:1164–1170
19. Reardon EJ (2005) The impact of image-guidance systems on sinus surgery. Otolaryngol Clin North Am 38:515–525
20. Leong JL, Batra PS, Citardi MJ (2006) CT-MR image fusion for the management of skull base lesions. Otolaryngol Head Neck Surg 134:868–876
21. Sindwani R, Bucholz RD (2005) The next generation of navigational technology. Otolaryngol Clin North Am 38:551–562
22. Metson R, Gray S (2005) Image-guided sinus surgery: practical considerations. Otolaryngol Clin North Am 38:527–534

48

23. Kacker A, Tabaee A, Anand V (2005) Computer-assisted surgical navigation in revision endoscopic sinus surgery. Otolaryngol Clin North Am 38:473–482

24. Tabaee A, Kacker A, Kassenoff TL, Anand V (2003) Outcome of computer assisted sinus surgery; a 5-year study. Am J Rhinol 17:291–297

25. Jiang RS, Hsu CY (2002) Revision functional endoscopic sinus surgery. Ann Otol Rhinol Laryngol 111:155–159

26. Reardon EJ (2002) Navigational risks associated with sinus surgery and the clinical effects of implementing a navigational system for sinus surgery. Laryngoscope 112:1–19

27. American Academy of Otolaryngology – Head and Neck Surgery (AAO–HNS) (2004) AAO–HNS policy on intra-operative use of computer-aided surgery. Approved 2004 Sep 12. Accessed Nov 2, 2006. Available at URL address: http://www.entlink.net/practice/rules/image–guiding.cfm

28. Dubin MG, Kuhn FA (2005) Stereotactic computer assisted navigation: state of the art for sinus surgery, not standard of care. Otolaryngol Clin North Am 38:535–549

29. Weber R, Draf W, Keerl R, Kahle G, Schinzel S, Thomann S, Lawson W (2000) Osteoplastic frontal sinus surgery with fat obliteration: technique and long-term results using magnetic resonance imaging in 82 operations. Laryngoscope 110:1037–1044

30. Carrau RL, Snyderman CH, Curtin HB, Weissman JL (1994) Computer-assisted frontal sinusotomy. Otolaryngol Head Neck Surg 111:727–732

31. Sindwani R, Metson R (2004) Impact of image-guidance on complications during osteoplastic frontal sinus surgery. Otolaryngol Head Neck Surg131:150–155

32. Ung F, Sindwani R, Metson R (2005) Endoscopic frontal sinus obliteration: a new technique for the treatment of chronic frontal sinusitis. Otolaryngol Head Neck Surg 133:551–555

33. Schlosser R, Bolger W (2005) Image-guided procedures of the skull base. Otolaryngol Clin North Am 38:483–490

34. Tabaee A, Kassenoff TL, Kacker A, Anand VK (2005) The efficacy of computer assisted surgery in the endoscopic management of cerebrospinal fluid rhinorrhea. Otolaryngol Head Neck Surg 133:936–943

35. Pletcher S, Sindwani R, Metson R (2006) Endoscopic orbital and optic nerve decompression. Otolaryngol Clin North Am 39:943–958

36. Metson R, Cosenza M, Gliklich RE, Montgomery WW (1999) The role of image-guidance systems for head and neck surgery. Arch Otolaryngol Head Neck Surg 125:1100–1104

37. Fried MP, Hsu L, Topulos GP, Jolesz FA (1996) Image-guided surgery in a new magnetic resonance suite: preclinical considerations. Laryngoscope 106:411–417

38. Cartellieri M, Vorbeck F (2000) Endoscopic sinus surgery using intraoperative computed tomography imaging for updating a three-dimensional navigation system. Laryngoscope 110:292–296

39. May M, Levine HL, Mester SJ, Schaitkin B (1994) Complications of endoscopic sinus surgery: analysis of 2108 patients – incidence and prevention. Laryngoscope 104:1080–1083

40. Sindwani R, Metson R (2005) Image-guided frontal sinus surgery. Otolaryngol Clin North Am 38:461–471

41. Metson R (2003) Image-guided sinus surgery; lessons learned from the first 1000 cases. Otolaryngol Head Neck Surg 128:8–13

42. Chow JM, Stankiewicz JA (2005) Application of image-guidance to surgery of the orbit. Otolaryngol Clin North Am 38:491–503

43. Fried MP, Moharir VM, Shin J, Taylor-Becker M, Morrison P (2002) Comparison of endoscopic sinus surgery with and without image guidance. Am J Rhinol 16:193–197

44. Tabaee A, Hsu AK, Shrime MG, Rickert S, Close LG (2006) Quality of life and complications following image-guided endoscopic sinus surgery. Otolaryngol Head Neck Surg 135:76–80

Endoscopic Surgery of the Nose, Paranasal Sinuses, and Orbit

Chapter 49

Endoscopic Management of Inferior Turbinate Hypertrophy

49

Iordanis Konstantinidis and Jannis Constantinidis

- The main cause of turbinate dysfunction is allergic rhinitis. Other causes include vasomotor rhinitis, drug-induced rhinitis, and acute and chronic rhinosinusitis.
- Dynamic assessment of the nose (before and after decongestion) should always be part of the preoperative evaluation, as the results of the examination can change the treatment strategy (e.g., bony part hypertrophy). Computed tomography scan is not recommended for the assessment of turbinate disease alone.
- The ideal turbinate reduction procedure would be one that effectively reduces the turbinate volume, preserves physiologic function, and avoids complications.
- The philosophy of inferior turbinate surgery is that a submucous resection is preferable, resecting bone and/or turbinate submucosal tissue in the process.
- Our knowledge regarding the role of the turbinates in nasal physiology and the long-term effects of turbinate surgery/interventions in patients is limited. This should lead surgeons toward less aggressive interventions, preventing long-standing problems.
- No single technique has established itself as the gold standard for inferior turbinate reduction. Several methods continue to be practiced and each patient should be assessed individually in order to determine which method might provide the best result.

Contents

Introduction

Turbinate surgery is commonly practiced; however, there is disagreement over its clinical effectiveness and long-term benefit as there is a lack of randomized control trials [5]. Actual research in this field is strongly influenced by the development of new technologies. The current literature mainly analyzes submucosal conventional methods, laser techniques, radiofrequency reduction, and powered instrumentation.

The inferior turbinate is a predominant structure in the anterior part of the nose that contributes to nasal valve formation [27]. As the internal nasal valve accounts for 50% of total airways resistance [27], the inferior turbinate has a significant contribution in nasal airways resistance. Turbinate reduction surgery is based on the idea that an increase in nasal airway volume leads to better functional nasal airflow, and this fact will be translated as an improvement in patients' subjective symptoms. Furthermore, it has been shown that inferior turbinate hypertrophy can significantly influence the distribution of topical steroids and antihistamines to the superior nasal cavity, having a negative impact on the medical management [18]. Thus, surgical reduction of the inferior turbinate can indirectly improve the symptoms of rhinitis, helping the proper application of nasal sprays into the nasal cavities.

The philosophy underlying inferior turbinate surgery is that a submucous resection is preferable, resecting bone and/or turbinate submucosal tissue in the process. A main question, thus, is to what extent inferior turbinate surgery affects one of the turbinate functions. The ideal turbinate-reduction procedure would be one that effectively reduces turbinate volume, preserves physiologic function (conduction, filtration, heating, humidification, and chemosensation), and avoids complications [2]. The main idea of less invasive surgery is that it helps to avoid nonreversible, long-standing pathologic conditions of the nose (e.g., atrophic rhinitis, empty nose syndrome).

Causes of Turbinate Disease

The most common cause of inferior turbinate hypertrophy is allergic rhinitis [5, 14] (Table 49.1). Allergic rhinitis is characterized by nasal obstruction with itchy nose, sneezing, and rhinorrhea. Nasal assessment demonstrates pale, edematous mucosa, and nasal smear demonstrates eosinophilia. The histopathology of hypertrophied turbinates is characterized by mast-cell abundance in the lamina propria [14]. In patients with a long history of allergic rhinitis, there is seromucous gland proliferation, and fibrosis. Vasomotor rhinitis is another cause, which is characterized by congestion and rhinorrhea without sneezing, and eosinophilia on nasal smear. Drug-induced rhinitis is characterized by a history of topical use of decongestants (e.g., oxymetazoline), which presents with edematous and often erythematous, fragile mucosa. Acute rhinosinusitis, usually caused by viral infection, is characterized by clear rhinorrhea, fever, sneezing, and nasal obstruction with or without pain. Nasal exam is similar to that in allergic rhinitis, but nasal smear findings may demonstrate lymphocytes and neutrophils. Chronic rhinosinusitis presents the same symptoms with a long duration, often associated with nasal mucosa changes (e.g., submucosal fibrosis) at the middle meatus, but also in the inferior turbinate [23]. Atrophic rhinitis is a significant nasal pathologic condition, because it has been associated with overaggressive turbinectomy procedures, although this issue remains under debate [5, 20]. This rare condition is characterized by progressive, slow atrophy of the nasal mucosa with crusting and foul odor from the nose (ozena), typically beginning at puberty.

Deviation of the nasal septum is associated with an overgrowth of the inferior turbinate on the contralateral side. This compensatory hypertrophy involves the bone as well as the mu-

Table 49.1 Common causes of inferior turbinate hypertrophy

Allergic rhinitis
Vasomotor rhinitis (hyperreflectoric rhinitis)
Drug-induced rhinitis
Acute/chronic rhinosinusitis
Idiopathic rhinitis
NARES (chronic nonallergic rhinitis with eosinophilia syndrome)
Hormonal (e.g. pregnancy)

cosa [3]. Although the turbinate tends to adopt the new condition after septoplasty with bone absorption, this process lasts many months, even years [3, 13]. Thus, turbinate reduction at the time of septoplasty for compensatory hypertrophy (at least the bony part) is recommended.

Medical Management

Medical therapy is the first-line treatment of turbinate hypertrophy; however, the appropriate choice of therapy relies on the underlying pathology. In allergic rhinitis, treatment is directed toward the inflammatory response. Medications such as topical and systemic antihistamines along with topical steroid sprays are usually needed for better control. Systemic decongestants are occasionally used; however, these drugs are sympathomimetic and patients should be asked whether they suffer from hypertension, cardiovascular diseases, or glaucoma. Systemic steroids can also be given in selected cases. Intraturbinate injections of steroids are also used to treat inflammatory mucosal hypertrophy. Care must be taken because cases of blindness have been reported with this technique [11]. Allergy desensitization is the last treatment choice when other medical means have failed. Avoidance of allergens is counseled. Drug-induced rhinitis is treated with cessation of the etiologic factor (usually topical decongestant) with aid of a steroid spray. In case of inferior turbinate pathology being associated with acute or chronic sinusitis, treatment of sinusitis is the first step. However if medical management fails, surgical options may need to be considered.

Preoperative Evaluation

Evaluation of the nasal airway and turbinates should always include a detailed history and a proper physical exam. Important symptoms to elicit are nasal obstruction, rhinorrhea, sneezing, and nasal itchiness. History elicits the nature of turbinate dysfunction and helps to categorize it into causes. The physical exam consists of a complete examination of the dynamic and static properties of the nasal airways. Thus nasal assessment should be always performed before and after decongestion using anterior rhinoscopy or nasal endoscopy. Endoscopy offers a detailed view and localization of the obstructed areas, as the turbinate can grow toward the nasal septum, even sometimes having contact points with it, or toward the choana, obstructing it. Failure of swollen turbinate mucosa to shrink after application of decongestant suggests the possibility that the patient has bony hypertrophy of the inferior turbinate, chronic unresponsive soft-tissue hypertrophy, or drug-induced rhinitis [14]. Inferior turbinate hypertrophy can be confirmed objectively by rhinomanometry. This investigation is performed with and without decongestion and total resistance is calculated. Resistance above 0.3 Pa/ml/s is usually symptomatic [17]. A limitation of rhinomanometry is that no resistance can be measured when the nasal cavity is completely obstructed. Marked reduction in resistance with decongestion suggests mucosal disease. Decongestion causing less than a 35% decrease in resistance suggests a structural cause of nasal obstruction rather than a mucosal cause [17]. Acoustic rhinometry is another objective method of nasal airway assessment [8]. However, both methods still have poor correlation with the patients' subjective symptom ratings [23].

Computed tomography (CT) scan (see Chap. 45) is indicated in the evaluation of nasal obstruction when a cause cannot be identified on physical exam with endoscopy or when evaluating tumors or polyps. CT is not indicated in the workup of inferior turbinate hypertrophy alone. However, if a CT scan of the nose and paranasal sinuses has been obtained for other reasons, it may provide useful information, like assessment of bony versus mucosal hypertrophy. In a recent study based on CT scan images, inferior turbinate bones were classified in four groups: lamellar (the most common), compact, combined (lamellar and compact), and bullous [26]. The authors suggested that the cross-sectional area of the inferior turbinate bone is relatively larger in compact and combined types. CT scan can also reveal cases of pneumatization of the inferior turbinates. A study reported an incidence of pneumatized inferior turbinates of 1 in 250 cases [4].

Surgical Treatment

Inferior turbinate surgery can be performed under local or general anesthesia (usually with concomitant septal surgery). The patient's position is supine with the head elevated by 30°. Preparation of the nose for local anesthesia includes local application of lidocaine 4% or xylocaine 2% with vasoconstrictor on cotton pledgets. Intraturbinate injection of lidocaine 2% with 1:100.000 epinephrine is not generally recommended. Sedation of patients undergoing turbinate interventions under local anesthesia is of great help for the patient and the surgeon. A rigid 0 nasal endoscope of 4 mm is the standard instrument required in endoscopic surgical treatment. Depending on the type of surgery planned, further instruments like a Freer elevator, suction, turbinate scissors, microdebrider, diathermy, laser probes, and/or radiofrequency probes are used (see Chap. 46).

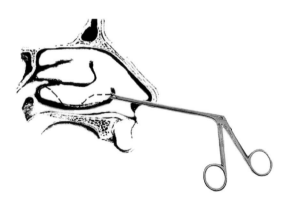

Fig. 49.1 Schematic representation of partial inferior turbinate removal when the hypertrophy affects its anterior or posterior part

Surgical Techniques

Numerous procedures are available for this purpose, and controversy exists as to which is the best [6]. In general, techniques that reduce the mucosal surface, such as cauterization or laser application, help to reduce the symptom nasal secretion, whereas measures that reduce the turbinate volume are indicated to reduce nasal obstruction. In this chapter, techniques are presented divided in two main categories: conventional and latest. Total inferior turbinectomy is not considered as an option, in this chapter, because it is believed that it results in significant nasal airflow disturbance (turbulent flow) and a sense of nasal obstruction. It is also associated with a high rate of complications (crusting, bleeding, nasal dryness), although its relationship to ozena is controversial [20].

Conventional Methods

Turbinate Displacement (Lateral Out-Fracture)

Lateral out-fracture of the inferior turbinate can be useful for anatomical bony deviations, but has no value in cases of mucosal hypertrophy. This procedure can be helpful to surgeons in order to gain space in some cases of paranasal sinuses surgery. However, this method offers only short-term results as the turbinate returns to its previous position after a period of time [10].

Submucosal Cauterization

Treatment of inferior turbinate hypertrophy using electrical cauterization can be performed with a monopolar cautery using a special electrode. A needle is inserted into a submucosal plane without contact between the electrode and the bony portion of the turbinate in order to avoid bone necrosis and osteitis. It is useful to burn the entry mucosal point on the head of the turbinate to avoid bleeding during the procedure.

The procedure can be repeated several times, but it has no value in cases where the cause of turbinate hypertrophy is the bony portion. Postoperative bleeding is uncommon and nasal packing is rarely required. Nasal packing for 24 h is usually enough in these patients. Postoperative care includes daily irrigation and weekly crust removal for 3–4 weeks. Late complications such as atrophic rhinitis may occur in cases of overcoagulated turbinates and bone necrosis [21]. The use of nasal splints is helpful to prevent adhesion formation. This method offers good short-term results but its main disadvantages remain the high intraoperative temperature, which is a risk factor for bone necrosis, and the poor long-term results [21].

Partial Inferior Turbinectomy

This method, which is performed under endoscopic view, provides a precise excision of the hypertrophied part of the turbinate, decreasing the risk of excessive or inadequate resection. All techniques involving removal of turbinate mucosa have been criticized for the potential risk of atrophic rhinitis. However, some authors believe that this method is effective and safe when performed properly [7]. The inferior turbinate is gently out-fractured medially using a Freer elevator. The inferior third of the turbinate is resected in the anterior (anterior turbinectomy), in the posterior (posterior turbinectomy), or along its anteroposterior length depending on the hypertrophy location (Fig. 49.1). The excision is performed with turbinate scissors after hemostatic clamping of the portion to be resected and cauterization of the marked sulcus. Repositioning of the turbinate and nasal packing for 24–48 h are required. Mucosal hypertrophy at the posterior end of the inferior turbinate can be effectively reduced using snares followed by coagulation to prevent bleeding.

The most common complications are crusting and bleeding. Severe bleeding may require hospital admission. Postoperative osteitis is uncommon; however, in cases of exposed bone, debridement is mandatory. Inferior turbinoplasty is a modified method of partial turbinectomy [16]. Two mucoperiosteal flaps are created and excessive mucosa from the inferior portions (mainly the lateral one) are trimmed along with the excessive bone. The remaining lateral mucoperiosteal flap is placed laterally, covering the exposed bone. This method offers less crusting because it covers the mucosal defect. Saline irrigation is required. The flap is packed in place with the aid of rubber finger stalls. This method is technically problematic, because the flap fixation is difficult, a fact that can result in inadequate flap attachment [16].

Latest Techniques

Lasers

Various laser systems have been tested for turbinate hypertrophy management. There are six basic laser systems that can be used [15]:
1. Carbon dioxide (CO_2)
2. Diode
3. Neodymium-doped yttrium aluminium garnet (Nd:YAG)
4. Potassium-titanyl-phosphate (KTP)
5. Argon:ion
6. Holmium-doped yttrium aluminium garnet (Ho:YAG)

The depth of coagulation is up to 2 mm. Diode and Nd:YAG lasers are poorly absorbed by water, tissue protein, and blood. These lasers are therefore able to transmit energy to deeper tissue layers. The CO_2 laser is strongly absorbed by water, causing surface tissue ablation. The Ho:YAG laser is likewise strongly absorbed by water, but it also provides better coagulation capabilities for improved hemostasis. All lasers except the CO_2 laser can be applied with the use of a flexible quartz fiber in a contact or noncontact mode.

Described techniques of laser application include linear, anterior-to-posterior stripes along the entire turbinate, or along

the inferior edge. An alternative technique is a crosshatched pattern on the turbinate surface. In cases of nasal valve obstruction, additional laser spots to the head of the inferior turbinate are indicated. This single-spot technique seems to be the most suitable for the CO_2 laser. Its straight beam is ideal for reducing the hyperplastic tip of the turbinate. Up to ten spots (1–2 W; 1 s; power density: 2,038 W/cm^2) are applied under endoscopic or microscopic control. Shrinkage of the turbinate can be observed during the procedure. Treatment of the turbinate disease with the Nd:YAG laser is performed with a special laser rhinoscope. The turbinate is irradiated until the mucosa becomes pale (5–10 W; 600 μm bare fiber; power density: 3,540 W/cm^2). The Nd:YAG laser initially results in reactive swelling of the turbinate and this leads to nasal obstruction in the immediate postoperative period. The clear benefit of this procedure is evident several weeks later.

A submucous laser application has also been described using the KTP laser [24]. In this technique, an 18-gauge needle is used to introduce an optical fiber into the inferior turbinate in an effort to reduce the mucosal damage. All of these methods demonstrate widely variable success rates, ranging from 50 to 100% improvement. The comparison of outcome results is difficult as the follow-up period vary. Complications include nasal crusting, epistaxis, and synechiae. Takeno et al. studied the effect of CO_2 laser partial turbinectomy in patients with allergic rhinitis with or without seasonal exacerbations [25]. The authors suggest that although the results indicate significant symptom improvement, the response to the treatment was not vigorous and immediate in seasonal allergy patients. Therefore, laser surgery can be applied during allergy exacerbations, but results may not be evident until the allergy season has ended. All patients should be advised to use decongestants for 2–3 days postoperatively and saline irrigation for 2–3 weeks to avoid crust formation.

Radiofrequency Volumetric Tissue Reduction

Low-frequency energy is delivered with a probe, which induces ionic agitation of the surrounding tissues. This causes a localized thermal lesion. The extent of injury is controlled by monitoring the increase in tissue temperature. Postoperative wound contracture and fibrosis induces tissue volume reduction. The probe, which typically has a distal active portion, is inserted submucosally into the turbinate (Fig. 49.2). The maximal tissue temperature for this technique ranges from 60 to 90 C, much lower than either electrocautery or laser techniques, where tissue temperature may reach 600 C [19].

Procedures such as electrocautery and surgical resection result in mucosal injury and are associated with crusting on the turbinate that may last for several weeks. During this period, the mucociliary function is affected. A recent study demonstrated that mucosal ciliary transport is preserved with radiofrequency volumetric tissue reduction (RFVTR), as the probe is placed submucosally and the temperatures reached are much lower [22]. Another radiofrequency device called "coblation" is a bipolar thermal-ablation device that causes molecular degeneration through a lower-heat-generating process. The probes are

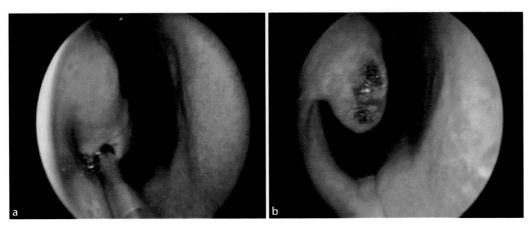

Fig. 49.2a, b Endoscopic view. **a** Insertion of the radiofrequency probe into the inferior turbinate for submucosal abla-tion with radiofrequency volumetric tissue reduction. **b** The inferior turbinate is reduced in size 9 days postoperatively and a normal healing process is visible at the entry point of the probe

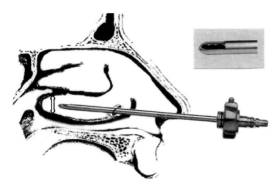

Fig. 49.3 Schematic representation of submucosal inferior turbinate reduction with the aid of a microdebrider. The *white arrow* indicates the movements of the instrument submucosally

supposed to convert a conductive medium (saline) into an ionic plasma layer that disrupts adjacent tissue with minimal thermal effect.

This method is not useful in cases where the hypertrophy in-volves the bony part of the turbinate. A light packing for 3–4 h is usually sufficient. In cases of excessive bleeding, a Merocel nasal tampon is placed for 24–48 h. Recent studies report that the RFVTR procedure was well tolerated by the patients with minimal pain intra- and postoperatively [1].

Powered Instrumentation

The microdebrider (see Chap. 47) can be used directly on the turbinate surface or, after incision, in the anterior portion of the turbinate and submucosal insertion. Gupta et al. described a technique using an endoscopic microdebrider to remove the lat-eral mucosa and part of the underlying bone, similar to Mabry's turbinoplasty [16, 12]. The authors suggested that the debrider

allowed a more precise resection. A true submucosal technique has also been described with the use of microdebrider. In sub-mucosal resection a submucous pocket is dissected from the an-terior head of the turbinate medially to the turbinate bone with the use of freer elevator. The microdebrider is inserted with an oscillatory rotation of 800–1000 rpm and removes the hypertro-phied submucosal stroma (Fig. 49.3). The use of a microdebri-der allows the appropriate management of cases with bony-part involvement where other techniques (lasers, RFVTR) are not effective. In the submucosal technique it is helpful to make the incision on the head of the turbinate by monopolar cautery for minimal bleeding.

Although the goal is to preserve the mucosa as much as pos-sible, some authors reported that 55% of patients had mucosal tears immediately following the procedure [9]. Rubber-finger stall packing for 24–48 h postoperatively is recommended. Re-moval is less painful than after packing with Merocel or gauze. Bleeding, crusting and synechiae may occur.

Conclusion

The surgical management of inferior turbinate hypertrophy tends to be more conservative as our knowledge about the long term results of our intervention in nasal function is limited. Endoscopic view for precise resection combined with a sub-mucosal technique seems to be the basis of modern treatment modalities. The use of new techniques is increasing the number of procedures into the office-based setting rather than the op-erating room. The literature regarding the efficacy of different treatment modalities suffers from a lack of controlled prospec-tive studies. There is no established gold-standard technique for inferior turbinate reduction. Thus surgeons should always individualize their cases with detailed dynamic preoperative as-sessment and use of the surgical technique that presents more advantages in each case separately.

Tips to Avoid Complications

- Overexaggerating cauterization requires coverage with antibiotic at least for a week to avoid osteitis.
- Exposed bone needs debridement and coverage with the mucoperiosteum.
- Meticulous removal of blood clots and crusts in the postoperative period is necessary for a good result and avoidance of synechiae formation. Longer packing with rubber finger stalls is a less painful alternative. Nasal splints (e.g., silicone films) for a few days postoperatively can be useful in cases where the surgeon feels that synechiae may occur.
- Daily saline irrigation is highly significant for the recovery of nasal mucosa and avoidance of crust formation.
- It is useful to burn the entry mucosal point of the probe on the head of the turbinate to avoid bleeding during the procedure.
- Patients are discouraged to blow their nose for several weeks. Sneezing is aided by the opened-mouth technique or in selected cases with antihistamines. Heavy lifting and straining is not recommended for the early postoperative period.

Take-Home Pearls

- There is no established gold-standard technique for inferior turbinate reduction. There is a need for more prospective controlled studies.
- A detailed preoperative dynamic assessment of the nose helps to individualize each case and select the appropriate surgical technique.
- The presence of bone hypertrophy is a significant factor for the treatment choice.
- Submucosal resection is always preferable when possible.
- Low-temperature techniques (e.g., RFVTR) result in less mucosal damage.
- Avoidance of overaggressive therapies and control of the underlying disease are basic in the modern disease management.
- Because no surgical procedure cures the underlying condition, further medical therapy may be necessary.
- Turbinate dysfunction should be treated as a quality-of-life issue.

References

1. Back LJ, Hytonen ML, Malmberg HO, Ylikoski JS (2002) Submucosal bipolar radiofrequency thermal ablation of inferior turbinates: a long-term follow-up with subjective and objective assessment. Laryngoscope 112:1806–1812
2. Becker W, Naumann HH, Pfaltz CR (1989) Ear, Nose and Throat diseases, 3rd edn. Thieme, Stuttgart, pp 180–185
3. Berger G, Hammel I, Berger R, Avraham S, Ophir D (2000) Histopathology of the inferior turbinate with compensatory hypertrophy in patients with deviated nasal septum. Laryngoscope 111:2100–2105
4. Braun H, Stammberger H (2003) Pneumatization of turbinates. Laryngoscope 113:668–672
5. Chang D, Ries R (2004) Surgical treatment of the inferior turbinate: new techniques. Curr Opin Otolaryngol Head Neck Surg 12:53–57
6. Clement WA, White PS (2001) Trends in turbinate surgery literature: a 35-year review. Clin Otolaryngol 26:124–128
7. Elwany S, Harrison R (1990) Inferior turbinectomy: comparison of four techniques. J Laryngol Otol 104:206–209
8. Fisher EW (1997) Acoustic rhinometry. Clin Otolaryngol Allied Sci 22:307–317
9. Friedman M, Tanyeri H, Lim J (1999) A safe alternative technique for inferior turbinate reduction. Laryngoscope 109:1834–1837
10. Goode RL (1978) Surgery of the turbinates. J Otolaryngol 7:262–268
11. Goodman LF, Goodman RS (2002) Safety of steroid injections. Am J Rhinol 16:287
12. Gupta A, Mercurio E, Bielamovitz S (2001) Endoscopic inferior turbinate reduction: an outcome analysis. Laryngoscope 111:1957–1959
13. Illum P (1997) Septoplasty and compensatory inferior turbinate hypertrophy: long term results after randomized turbinoplasty. Eur Arch Otorhinolaryngol 254:89–92
14. Jafek B (2001) Nasal obstruction. In: Bailey B, Healey GB, Johnson JT, Pillbury HC, Jackler RK, Tardy ME Jr, Calhoun KH (eds) Head and Neck Surgery – Otolaryngology, 3rd edn. Lippincott Williams and Wilkins, Philadelphia, pp 293–308
15. Janda P, Sroka R, Baumgartner R (2001) Laser treatment of hyperplastic inferior turbinates: a review. Lasers Surg Med 28:404–413
16. Mabry RL (1988) Inferior turbinoplasty: patient selection, technique and long term consequences. Otolaryngol Head Neck Surg 98:60–66
17. McCaffrey T (2001) Nasal function and evaluation. In: Bailey B, Healey GB, Johnson JT, Pillbury HC, Jackler RK, Tardy ME Jr, Calhoun KH (eds) Head and Neck Surgery – Otolaryngology, 3rd edn. Lippincott Williams and Wilkins, Philadelphia, pp 261–271
18. Merkus P, Ebbens FA, Muller B, Fokkens WJ (2006) Influence of anatomy and head position on intranasal drug deposition. Eur Arch Otorhinolaryngol 263:827–832
19. Nease C, Krempl G (2004) Radiofrequency treatment of turbinate hypertrophy: a randomised, blinded, placebo-controlled clinical trial. Otolaryngol Head Neck Surg 130:291–299

49

20. Ophir D, Shapira A, Marshak G (1985) Total inferior turbinectomy for nasal airway obstruction. Arch Otolaryngol 111:93–95

21. Quine SM, Aitken PM, Eccles R (1999) Effect of submucosal diathermy to the inferior turbinates on unilateral and total nasal airflow in patients with rhinitis. Acta Otolaryngol 119:911–915

22. Sapci T, Sahin B, Karavus A, Akbulut UG (2003) Comparison of the effects of radiofrequency tissue ablation, CO_2 laser ablation, and partial turbinectomy applications on nasal mucociliary functions. Laryngoscope 113:514–519

23. Smith T (2004) Outcomes research in rhinology: chronic rhinosinusitis. ORL 66:202–206

24. Supiyaphun P, Aramwatanapong P, Kerekhanjanarong V, Sastarasadhit V (2003) KTP laser inferior turbinoplasty: an alteration procedure to treat the nasal obstruction. Auris Nasus Larynx 30:59–64

25. Takeno S, Osada R, Ishino T, Yajin K (2003) Laser surgery of the inferior turbinate for allergic rhinitis with seasonal exacerbation: an acoustic rhinometry study. Ann Otol Rhinol Laryngol 112:455–460

26,. Uzun L, Ugur M, Savranlar A, Mhmutyazicioglu K, Ozdemir H, Beder L (2004) Classification of the inferior turbinate bones: a computed tomography study. Eur J Radiol 51:241–245

27. Wexler DB, Davidson TM (2004) The nasal valve: a review of the anatomy, imaging, and physiology. Am J Rhinol 18:143–150

Chapter 50

Endonasal Maxillary Sinus Surgery

50

Jannis Constantinidis

Core Messages

- Successful surgery to treat inflammatory diseases of the maxillary sinus as well as of the remaining paranasal sinuses is based on a sound understanding of the pathophysiology of the sinonasal mucosa.
- Indications for surgical intervention are based on thorough history-taking, careful endoscopic examination of the nose and sinuses, and excellent imaging.
- There are three different endonasal approaches to the maxillary sinus: through the middle meatus (middle meatal antrostomy), inferior meatus (inferior meatal antrostomy), and through the nasal vestibule and crista piriformis (Sturmann-Canfield operation).
- Endoscopic middle meatal antrostomy permits drainage, aeration, and excellent access to the maxillary sinus.
- The Sturmann-Canfield operation represents a good alternative to the Caldwell-Luc operation and allows excellent visualization and ample space for instrumentation.

Contents

Introduction

Already in the beginnings of classic paranasal sinus surgery, the maxillary sinus was approached by various surgeons transnasally as well as transorally. Mikulicz (1886) and Lothrop (1897) are regarded as the founders of transnasal maxillary sinus fenestration [24, 28]. The procedure to open the maxillary sinus transorally by creating a window into the nose was described independently by Caldwell (1893) [5] and Luc (1897) [25]. While the transoral opening of the maxillary sinus was frequently used to remove the maxillary mucosa almost completely, the endonasal fenestration of the maxillary sinus was intended to preserve the mucosa. Not least due to the technical limitations of endonasal surgery, the transoral Caldwell-Luc procedure was used extensively in the 20th century. It became obvious, however, that the negative sequelae of radical maxillary sinus procedures such as the Caldwell-Luc procedure occur quite frequently. Reports of such sequelae include neuralgias of the infraorbital nerve, permanent loss of sensation over the cheek, dental pain, and obliteration of the maxillary sinus with subsequent mucocele formation [10, 11, 13].

A better understanding of the ostiomeatal complex in the development of maxillary sinus disease led to the understanding that with reconstitution of physiologic drainage, the previously diseased sinus mucosa can regain its healthy physiologic function [26, 27]. Moreover, the development of improved anesthesiologic techniques as well as greatly enhanced visualization with microscopes and endoscopes have led to a renaissance of endonasal approaches to the paranasal sinuses [8, 9, 43]. Therefore, over recent years the endonasal approach has become the gold standard in the therapy of inflammatory diseases of the maxillary sinus as well as of the remaining paranasal sinuses [12, 19, 21, 23, 31, 33, 36, 41, 42, 44]. The term "functional endoscopic surgery" (FESS) has been coined and describes the surgical reconstitution of physiologic drainage and ventilation of the paranasal sinuses by means of repairing the natural drainage pathways endoscopically.

Preoperative Endoscopy and Radiographic Evaluation

All endonasal procedures of the maxillary sinus and the neighboring paranasal sinuses are planned after a thorough history has been obtained, the endonasal anatomy has been studied with an endoscope, and imaging has been obtained. Anterior rhinoscopy allows the assessment of the condition of the nasal septum and the anterior aspects of the inferior turbinates, but not of the middle meatus and the posterior middle turbinate. After topical application of local anesthetics and vasoconstrictors to the nasal mucosa, the nasal anatomy is inspected with a 0° or 30°, 4-mm rigid endoscope or a flexible endoscope. Pathologic changes of the nasal mucosa may include secretions, erythema, edema, polyps, or purulent secretions; for example in the middle meatus. The middle turbinate may be carefully medialized in order to improve the visualization of important anatomic structures such as the uncinate process, the ethmoidal bulla, and the hiatus semilunaris. The natural ostium of the maxillary sinus is in most cases not visible during endonasal endoscopy since it is obscured by the uncinate process. An accessory ostium may be visible since these are more posteriorly located. Pediatric rigid endoscopes (2.7 mm) and pediatric flexible endoscopes are very helpful to examine children or adults with narrow endonasal anatomy.

Computed tomography (CT) is of paramount importance as it provides us with important information about the individual anatomy and the extent of the pathology (see Chap. 45). In order to assess the maxillary sinus and the anterior ethmoid sinuses, coronal cuts allow excellent visualization of the anatomy of the middle nasal meatus and the anterior skull base [45, 46]. In rare cases, dental artifacts may limit the assessment of the important anatomic structures of the anterior ethmoid. A CT scan should be obtained when the patient is least symptomatic, not at the time of an acute flare of infection or inflammation. Moreover, topical application of cortical steroids and vasoconstrictors prior to obtaining the CT scan may be helpful to avoid imaging of nonpermanent mucosal reactions. One should bear in mind that there may be discrepancies between radiologic and intraoperative findings [20]. A magnetic resonance imaging scan is indicated if the orbita is involved, or when for example in unilateral pathology a suspected tumor is to be delineated from surrounding mucosal edema, inflammation, and secretions [22].

Prior to surgical procedures of the paranasal sinuses, a general or pediatric examination may be advisable in order to diagnose and treat general diseases such as hypertension. In children with chronic and recurrent signs and symptoms of rhinosinusitis, a chloride sweat test, assessment of immunoglobulins including IgG subclasses, and potentially mucosal biopsy to rule out ciliary dyskinesia should be considered [40].

Surgical Indications

Because of its anatomic relationship to the nose and the remaining paranasal sinuses, the maxillary sinus is susceptible to infections, especially if there are other predisposing factors such as an allergic rhinitis or a septal deviation. The most frequent indication for surgical therapy of the maxillary sinus is chronic rhinosinusitis that has been refractory to medical treatment. Additional indications are listed in Table 50.1. Adjunctive procedures such as septoplasty or turbinate out-fracture should be considered if pathology is identified and can be correlated with the patient's symptoms.

Endonasal Surgery of the Maxillary Sinus

Modern maxillary sinus surgery is surgery of the microanatomic space of the middle nasal meatus. Opening of stenoses allows improved ventilation and drainage of the maxillary sinus, which in turn provides an environment that may allow the mucosa to recover and mucocilliary clearance to be reconstituted [33, 36].

Middle Meatal Antrostomy

Fenestration of the maxillary sinus through the middle meatus begins if necessary with careful medialization of the middle turbinate using the Freer elevator (see Chap. 46). Care should be taken not to fracture the bony insertion of the middle turbinate. The uncinate process is identified and the hiatus semilunaris and the ethmoid bulla are visualized. The uncinate pro-

Table 50.1 Indications for endonasal surgery of the maxillary sinus

Inflammatory diseases	Acute bacterial rhinosinusitis with orbital complications
	Recurrent acute bacterial rhinosinusitis
	Chronic bacterial rhinosinusitis
	Fungal rhinosinusitis
	Sinonasal polyposis
	Antrochoanal polyp
	Mucoceles (primary, after Caldwell-Luc operation)
Neoplastic diseases	Biopsy (malignant tumors)
	Complete resection (benign tumors, inverted papillomas)
Other	Foreign bodies

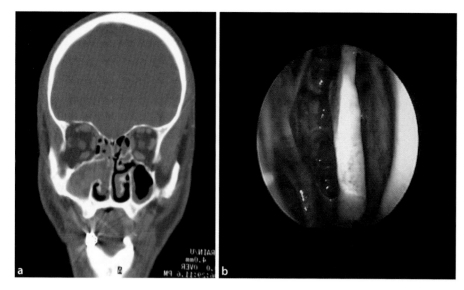

Fig. 50.1 **a** Coronal computed tomography of a patient with chronic maxillary and ethmoidal sinusitis. **b** Postoperative endoscopic view after middle meatal antrostomy and complete ethmoidectomy

cess may be medialized with the ballpoint probe, and is then incised along its insertion into the lateral nasal wall using the sickle knife or a sharp elevator. The straight Blakesley forceps is then used to mobilize the superior and inferior insertion of the uncinate process into the lateral nasal wall with a rotary motion. Care must be taken not to strip the mucosa at the superior and inferior margins. After removal of the uncinate process, the natural ostium of the maxillary sinus can be visualized and palpated with a ballpoint probe or a curved suction. The maxillary sinus ostium may then be enlarged with sharp cutting forceps inferiorly, posteriorly, and anteriorly. The upper aspect of the inferior turbinate, the ground lamella of the middle turbinate, and the nasolacrimal duct are at risk during this maneuver and must be carefully preserved (see Chap. 54). The use of the 45 endoscope or alternatively the 30 or 70 endoscope improves visualization and inspection of the maxillary sinus. If an accessory maxillary sinus ostium is present, this should be sharply enlarged posteriorly in order to unify it with the natural ostium. This maneuver prevents reentry of the nasal mucin through the accessory ostium [34, 35]. The neo-ostium should be at least 1 cm in diameter in order to reduce the risk of scarry stenosis. When performed properly, middle meatal antrostomies remain patent in up to 98% of cases [21, 36].

In rare cases the maxillary sinus infundibulum is obstructed by a large anterior ethmoid cell (Haller cell) that extends along the medial aspect of the floor of the orbit. In order to achieve a sufficient fenestration of the maxillary sinus, it is necessary to remove the Haller cell. Overall, middle meatal antrostomy is frequently combined with an anterior or total ethmoidectomy (Fig. 50.1a, b). The endonasal middle meatal antrostomy is a procedure with relatively few complications and a high success rate. Complications may include: bleeding, synechia, loss of sensation over the cheek or pain secondary to irritation to the infraorbital nerve, and restenosis. Davis et al. [7] reported on 310 patients who underwent endoscopic middle meatal an-

trostomy: Epiphora was observed in 1 patient, and synechiae in 20 patients. Stankiewicz [37] observed 2 cases of epiphora in 300 patients who underwent middle meatal antrostomy. Orbital complications such as retro-orbital hematoma, diplopia, or visual changes are rare in endonasal maxillary sinus surgery.

Inferior Meatal Antrostomy

Although the fenestration of the maxillary sinus into the inferior meatus does not necessarily follow our pathophysiologic understanding of maxillary sinusitis, this procedure remains popular among some surgeons who may perform isolated inferior meatal antrostomies or combined inferior and middle meatal antrostomies. It has been shown that inferior middle meatal antrostomies are unfavorable since the mucociliary drainage of the sinus mucosa continues to target the middle meatus [4, 15]. However, some authors report excellent clinical results with inferior middle meatal antrostomies [1, 2]. The authors feel that inferior middle meatal antrostomy is only indicated if access to the maxillary sinus through the middle meatus is not safe or not possible secondary to foreign bodies, tumors, or other pathology. In addition, for patients who do not have a functioning mucociliary clearance, as in patients with ciliary dyskinesia, an inferior window may allow passive drainage of the maxillary sinus [36, 39].

After the inferior turbinate has been carefully medialized, a nasal speculum is inserted into the inferior meatus. A trocar is used to perforate the lateral nasal wall at the transition of the anterior to the middle third of the inferior turbinate. This opening is then enlarged with straight and back-cutting forceps. A persistent ledge along the nasal floor should be avoided. The dissection should also not be carried too high in order to avoid risk of damage to the nasolacrimal duct and Hasners valve. The maxillary sinus may then be inspected with various endo-

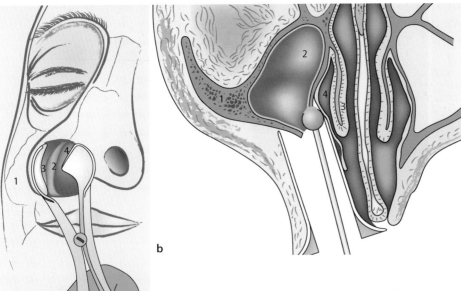

Fig. 50.2a,b Sturman-Canfield operation. **a** Through an incision in the nasal vestibule, the rim of the piriform crest and the anterior wall of the maxillary sinus are exposed. *1* Maxilla, *2* piriform crest, *3* canine fossa, *4* inferior turbinate. **b** The piriform crest is removed, after which the medial and anterior walls of the maxillary sinus can also be removed. *1* Maxilla, *2* maxillary sinus, *3* inferior turbinate, *4* inferior meatus

scopes, which allows the removal under direct vision of polyps, cysts, or other pathologies. Potential complications of inferior meatal antrostomy include: bleeding (e.g., after injury to the greater palatine artery), synechiae, or loss of sensation in the anterior teeth (see Chap. 44). Sogg [32] reported on 174 inferior meatal antrostomies performed in 87 patients. The procedure was performed under local anesthesia and no complications were reported. If this technique is performed in children, special care is to be taken to avoid the more superiorly located roots of the permanent teeth [30, 32]. Overall inferior meatal antrostomy carries a higher risk of scarry stenosis or synechiae [11, 15]. Therefore, generous enlargement of the inferior window and thorough postoperative inspection and debridement are needed.

Sturmann-Canfield Operation

Sturmann (1908) [38] and Canfield 1908 [6] described the same procedure of a maxillary sinus approach different from middle and inferior meatal antrostomy. This approach is based on opening the maxillary sinus endonasally by removing the crista piriformis and, if needed, the anterior medial wall of the maxillary sinus. This procedure is useful if a broad endonasal approach to the maxillary sinus is needed and fenestration of the middle and inferior meatus is not sufficient to remove the maxillary sinus pathology. This larger approach may be performed under microscopic or endoscopic visualization, or a combination of the two modalities. The procedure represents a good alternative to the Caldwell-Luc operation and allows excellent visualization and ample space for instrumentation. This method is similar to

the procedure described by Denker and may also be referred to as the endonasal Denker procedure, which is especially useful for removal of tumors of the maxillary sinus [3, 11, 29, 39].

The nasal vestibule is incised in a vertical, slightly curved fashion. The piriform crest is identified and the periosteum and soft-tissue envelope of the anterior wall of the maxillary sinus are dissected with an elevator. The infraorbital nerve is identified and preserved. Medially, the periosteum of the maxillary sinus wall is also dissected. The crista piriformis is removed with a rongeur or a cutting burr, after which the medial and anterior wall of the maxillary sinus may be removed if necessary (Fig. 50.2a, b). Possible complications include irritation, edema, and infection of the soft tissues of the cheek. Sensory deficits of the infraorbital nerve as well as injuries of the tooth roots have also been observed. Epiphora may be observed if the medial wall of the maxillary sinus is removed. This complication may be prevented by performing an endonasal dacryocystorhinostomy.

Postoperative Care

After endonasal surgery, raw mucosal surfaces of various degrees are present and require specific care. Hosemann et al. [16] demonstrated four stages of wound healing of the nasal mucosa and recommended postoperative therapy specific to these stages. Close follow-up with frequent endoscopic local debridements during the first 3 months after surgery is recommended. During the first 10–14 days the patient should be seen every 2–3 days. Various protocols of postoperative care have been proposed [14, 18]. The extent of the surgery and the nature of the disease will dictate individual variations to these standardized protocols. Local care of the mucosa includes debridement of crusts under local anesthesia, opening of synechiae, and suctioning of the neo-ostium.

Edema of the nasal mucosa and formation of granulation tissue may be treated with topical antibiotics and corticosteroids [14, 18, 42]. Despite the best therapy, mucosal pathology including edema may occur or persist after the procedure. Potential causes include alterations to the natural lymphatic drainage of the maxillary sinus, and persistent and recurrent disease [16]. It has been suggested that providing moisture to the healing nasal mucosa reduces edema, crusting, and inflammation of the surgical site [17]. Mildly hyperosmotic nasal flushes are used and may be started immediately after surgery or removal of packing. Peri- and postoperative administration of systemic antibiotics is not necessary for routine endonasal surgery, but may be indicated in cases of purulent infection or osteomyelitis [12, 23]. The administration of systemic corticosteroids may be indicated in cases of extensive polyposis and may be initiated a few days prior to the surgical procedure [17]. Children do not tolerate well the routine postoperative care of the operated paranasal sinuses; in some cases, sedation or even general anesthesia may be required to perform postoperative care [14].

Conclusions

The combined endoscopic and microscopic endonasal access to the maxillary sinus allows the treatment of inflammatory diseases of the maxillary sinus, to control possible complications and to remove benign tumors. The morbidity associated with endonasal procedures is minimal and less frequent than that associated with external approaches.

Tips to Avoid Complications

- Careful study of high-resolution CT scans provides crucial information regarding the individual anatomy and the extent of pathology. Thus, the risk of intraoperative complications is reduced.
- Identification of the maxillary sinus ostium with a curved ballpoint probe or suction is very helpful to avoid orbital complications.
- In middle meatal antrostomy, anterior dissection further forward than the attachment line of the uncinate process substantially increases the risk of injury of the nasolacrimal duct.
- Keep the patient's eyes uncovered in the surgical field in order to provide surgical orientation in relation to the orbit and earlier identification of possible orbital complications.
- Identification of the infraorbital nerve and subperiosteal dissection reduce the risk of sensory deficits after the Sturmann-Canfield operation.

Take-Home Pearls

- Endonasal endoscopic middle meatal antrostomy is the primary procedure for the treatment of inflammatory diseases of the maxillary sinus that are resistant to medical therapy.
- Benign tumors of the maxillary sinus can be completely removed endonasally by means of the Sturmann-Canfield procedure.
- A thorough postoperative follow-up and treatment regimen is a crucial aspect, complements the surgical therapy, and is the basis for excellent surgical results.

Acknowledgment

The author would like to thank Professor of Art Anatomy, Sourvalis Dimitrios for the medical illustrations.

References

1. Arias R, Ariza H, Correa I, Stamm A (2000) Micro-endoscopic surgery of the maxillary sinus. In: Stamm A, Draf W (eds) Micro-endoscopic Surgery of the Paranasal Sinuses and the Skull Base. Springer, Berlin, Heidelberg, pp 249–256
2. Arnes E, Anke JM, Mair IS (1985) A comparison between middle and inferior meatal antrostomy in the treatment of chronic maxillary sinus infection. Rhinology 23:65–69
3. Brors D, Draf W (1999) The treatment of inverted papilloma. Curr Opin Otolaryngol Head Neck Surg 7:33–38
4. Buiter CT, Straatman NA (1981) Endoscopic antrostomy in the nasal fontanelle. Rhinology 19:17–24
5. Caldwell GW (1893) Diseases of the accessory sinuses of the nose and an improved method of treatment for suppuration of the maxillary antrum. N Y State J Med 58:526–528
6. Canfield KB (1908) The submucous resection of the lateral nasal wall in chronic empyema of the antrum, ethmoid and sphenoid. JAMA 51:1136–1141
7. Davis WE, Templer JW, Lamear WR, Davis WE Jr, Craig SB (1991) Middle meatus antrostomy: patency rates and risk factors. Otolaryngol Head Neck Surg 104:467–472
8. Dixon H (1976) Microscopic antrostomies in children: a review of the literature in chronic sinusitis and plan of medical and surgical treatment. Laryngoscope 86:1796–1813
9. Draf W (1973) Wert der Sinuskopie für Klinik und Praxis. Laryngol Rhinol Otol 52:890–896
10. Draf W (1980) Der Gesichtsschmerz nach Caldwell-Luc-Operation. Prophylaxe und Therapie. Laryngol Rhinol Otol 59:99–107
11. Draf W (1982) Die chirurgische Behandlung entzündlicher Erkrankungen der Nasennebenhöhlen. Arch Otorhinolaryngol 235:133–205
12. Draf W, Weber R (1993) Endonasal micro-endoscopic pansinusoperation in chronic sinusitis. I. Indications and operation technique. Am J Otolaryngol 14:394–398

13. Eichel B (1973) Surgical management of chronic paranasal sinusitis. Laryngoscope 83:1195–1203

14. Gross CW, Gross WE (1994) Post-operative care for functional endoscopic sinus surgery. Ear Nose Throat J 73:476–479

15. Hosemann W, Wigand ME, Nikol J (1989) Klinische und funktionelle Aspekte der endonasalen Kieferhöhlen-Operation. HNO 37:225–230

16. Hosemann W, Wigand ME, Göde U, Langer F, Dunker I (1991) Normal wound healing of the paranasal sinuses: clinical and experimental investigations. Eur Arch Otorhinolaryngol 248:390–394

17. Jorissen M (2004) Postoperative care following endoscopic sinus surgery. Rhinology 42:114–120

18. Kennedy DW (1992) Prognostic factors, outcomes and staging in ethmoid sinus surgery. Laryngoscope 102:1–18

19. Kennedy DW, Zinreich SJ (1988) The functional endoscopic approach to inflammatory sinus disease: current perspectives and technique modifications. Am J Rhinol 2:89–96

20. Kennedy DW, Zinreich SJ, Rosenbaum AE, Johns ME (1985) Functional endoscopic sinus surgery. Theory and diagnostic evaluation. Arch Otolaryngol 111:576–582

21. Kennedy DW, Zinreich SJ, Shaalan H, Kihn F, Naclerio R, Loch E (1987) Endoscopic middle meatal antrostomy: theory, technique, and patency. Laryngoscope 97:1–9

22. Kraus DH, Lanzieri CF, Wanamaker JR, Little JR, Lavertu P (1992) Complementary use of computed tomography and magnetic resonance imaging in assessing skull base lesions. Laryngoscope 102:623–629

23. Levine HL (1993) Endoscopic Sinus Surgery. Thieme, New York

24. Lothrop HA (1897) Empyema of the antrum of Highmore. A new operation for the cure of obstinate cases. Boston Med Surg J 136:455–462

25. Luc H (1897) Une nouvelle methode operatoire pour la cure radicale et rapide de empyeme chronique du sinus maxillaire. Arch Laryngol (Paris) 10:185–207

26. Messerklinger W (1972) Nasenendoskopie: Der mittlere Nasengang und seine unspezifischen Entzündungen. HNO 20:212–215

27. Messerklinger W (1978) Endoscopy of the Nose. Urban and Schwarzenberg, Baltimore

28. Mikulicz J (1886) Zur operativen Behandlung des Empyems der Highmoreshöhle. Prager Z Heilkd 7:27

29. Minovi A, Kollert M, Draf W, Bockmühl U (2006) Inverted papilloma: feasibility of endonasal surgery and long-term results of 87 cases. Rhinology 44:205–210

30. Muntz H, Lusk R (1990) Nasal antral windows in children: a retrospective study. Laryngoscope 100:643–646

31. Rice DH, Schäfer SD (1988) Endoscopic paranasal sinus surgery. Raven, New York

32. Sogg A (1982) Intranasal antrostomy: causes of failure. Laryngoscope 92:1038–1041

33. Stammberger H (1986) Endoscopic endonasal surgery. Concepts in treatment of recurring rhinosinusitis. Part II. Surgical technique. Otolaryngol Head Neck Surg 94:143–146

34. Stammberger H (1991) Functional endoscopic sinus surgery. Decker, Philadelphia

35. Stammberger H, Hawke M (1993) Essentials of functional endoscopic sinus surgery. Mosby, St. Louis

36. Stammberger H, Posawetz W (1990) Functional endoscopic sinus surgery. Concept, indications and results of the Messeklinger technique. Eur Arch Otorhinolaryngol 247:63–76

37. Stankiewicz JA (1989) Complications in endoscopic intranasal ethmoidectomy: an update. Laryngoscope 99:686–690

38. Sturmann D (1908) Die intranasale Eröffnung der Kieferhöhle. Berl Klin Wochenschr 27:1273–1274

39. Toffel PH, Aroesty DJ, Weinmann RH (1989) Secure endoscopic sinus surgery as an adjunct to functional nasal surgery. Arch Otolaryngol Head Neck Surg 515:822–825

40. Tomenzoli D, Castelnuovo P, Pagella F, Berlucchi M, Pianta L, Delu G, Maroldi R, Nicolai P (2004) Different endoscopic surgical strategies in the management of inverted papilloma of the sinonasal tract: experience with 47 patients. Laryngoscope 114:193–200

41. Wald ER (1992) Sinusitis in children. N Engl J Med 326:319–323

42. Wigand ME (1981) Transnasale, endoskopische Chirurgie der Nasennebenhöhlen bei chronischer Sinusistis. II. Die endonasale Kieferhöhlenoperation. HNO 29:263–269

43. Wigand ME (1990) Endoscopic surgery of the paranasal sinuses and anterior skull base. Thieme, New York

44. Wigand ME, Steiner W (1977) Endonasale Kieferhöhlenoperation mit endoskopischer Kontrolle. Laryngol Rhinol Otol 56:421–425

45. Wigand ME, Buiter CT, Griffiths MV, Perko D (1988) Treatment of antral pathology – which surgical route? Rhinology 26:253–255

46. Zinreich SJ (1994) Imaging of inflammatory sinus disease. Otolaryngol Clin North Am 26:535–547

50

Chapter 51

Ethmoid Sinus Surgery

51

Alessandro Varini

Core Messages

- Chronic rhinosinusitis and nasal polyposis are the main indications for ethmoid surgery.
- The pathogenesis of these diseases remains unclear and surgery may be palliative, although effective if adequately combined with proper medical treatment.
- Computed tomography is the preoperative modality of choice in creating a road map and in showing the bony architecture and features.
- Obstruction of the ostiomeatal complex represents the crucial surgical target.
- Limited procedures are frequently successful.
- Surgical steps are tailored to individual cases.
- Preoperative and postoperative care plays an essential role in the safe and efficacious treatment of ethmoid diseases.

Contents

Aims and Objectives

Introduction

The most common diseases affecting the ethmoid that establish a need for surgery are inflammations, especially acute/intermittent rhinosinusitis, chronic rhinosinusitis (CRS), and nasal polyposis (NP) [23]. CRS is one of the most common chronic diseases [2] and shows a trend toward increasing prevalence. The usual surgical indication for rhinosinusitis is lack of response to maximal conservative medical treatment [20, 23]. Surgery is tailored to the individual patient's specific history and symptoms, general conditions, age, sex, extent of disease, anatomy, radiologic findings, and other individual characteristics [11, 16, 20, 32, 35]. The surgical technique carried out should be based on the individual patient's symptoms and on quality of life [1].

The ethmoid labyrinth, as the name indicates, represents an intricate territory. Ethmoid surgery needs above all a correct understanding of its anatomy, so as not to err. Furthermore, it requires deepening the comprehension of the underlying physiology and mechanisms that predispose to or causing the pathology. Surgery may not act as an etiopathogenetical, but as a symptomatic treatment that is unable to completely cure the underlying basic pathology (see Chap. 57). The combination of surgical and medical treatments has thus become the method of choice [31, 46, 47, 58].

Predisposing Local Anatomic Factors and Surgical Anatomy

As yet, the basic principle of CRS surgical treatment is the removal of pathological tissue and anatomic obstruction in the ethmoid, restoring ventilation and drainage of the large functionally dependent paranasal sinuses [51]. The ostiomeatal complex is a functional unit composed of the maxillary sinus ostia, anterior ethmoid cells and their ostia, ethmoid infundibulum, hiatus semilunaris, and the middle meatus [23]. Thickening of facing mucosal surfaces can lead to tissue contacts, which may result in loss of ciliary beating activity and mucociliary transport. The resulting vicious circle is hypothesized to finally result

Table 51.1 Anterior ethmoid "accessory" cells (modified from Kuhn)

Ethmoid infundibulum cells	Cells surrounding the frontal ostium	Cells behind the bulla lamella
Terminal recess	Frontal recess	Suprabullar recess
Agger nasi cell(s)	Frontal bullar cell	Retrobullar recess
Infundibular cells	Interfrontal sinus septal cell	Supraorbital ethmoid cell
Lacrimal cell	Frontal cells (types I–IV)	

Table 51.2 Main structures involved in frontal sinus obstruction. *CT* Computed tomography

Ethmoid infundibulum	The ethmoid infundibulum is a three-dimensional funnel-shaped space (V-like shape in axial CT) The superior configuration of the infundibulum depends on the anatomy of the uncinate process The uppermost uncinate attachment bends laterally attaching to the lamina papyracea, closes superiorly the infundibulum, and creates a blind end, "dome-shaped," the terminal recess
Terminal recess	It is similar to a pouch created when the superior segment of the uncinate process attaches laterally onto the lamina papyracea Part and partition of the ethmoid infundibulum, as the superior blind end Below the frontal recess or a frontal cell The terminal recess has revealed a high prevalence with a variable degree of pneumatization This recess may be found as the only, and single "cell," and its dome the only bony wall, obscuring the frontal recess
Agger nasi cell	The agger nasi cell "results when the mound or crest on the lateral wall immediately anterior and superior to the insertion of the middle turbinate undergoes pneumatization" "The most constant and anterior of the anterior ethmoid air cells"
Suprabullar and retrobullar recesses	These spaces, less correctly called the sinus lateralis, are located between the ethmoid roof superiorly (first foveola ethmoidalis), the ethmoid bulla anteriorly and inferiorly, the lamina papyracea laterally, and the basal lamella posteriorly The recesses are typically separated by a bony crest or mucosal projection from the basal lamella to the ethmoid bulla These recesses communicate medially with the middle meatus through the hiatus semilunaris superior Anteriorly, the suprabullar recess may be separated from the frontal recess by the bulla lamella, if it reaches and attaches to the skull base Thus, the two recesses do not communicate with the frontal sinus outflow tract through the frontal recess The anterior ethmoid artery is located on the roof of the suprabullar recess, running onto the skull base or, in case of more pneumatization, inside or behind a tissue bridge from the base of the skull to the ethmoid bulla, or inside a free mesentery
Supraorbital ethmoid cell	This cell extends over the orbit from the suprabullar recess, and it is essentially a pneumatization of this recess into the orbital plate of the frontal bone The cell arises anteriorly to the anterior ethmoid artery and posteriorly to the frontal recess, separated by the bulla lamella

51

in obstruction and impairment of secretions evacuation [62]. Following this theory, most diseases of the maxillary and frontal sinuses originate in the ethmoid, in the narrow clefts of the ostiomeatal complex [62]. The aim of functional surgery is to eliminate only those structures directly involved in the genesis of the obstruction.

The complexity of the ethmoid labyrinth is strictly related to the richness of different anatomic structures in a relatively small space [43, 62, 70]. Due to high variability, the ethmoid can be thought of as a fingerprint. Each single structure shows a wide range of variations due to the individual characteristics or pa-

thologies or previous surgical interventions and is able to create a site of obstruction. Variations of the curvature of the uncinate process, laterally and medially, may constrict the infundibulum at different levels. Variations like a hyperpneumatized ethmoid bulla, concha bullosa, and a paradoxically curved or variably shaped and bent middle turbinate can lead to additional obstacles.

Blockage of this inferoanterior aspect of the ethmoidal infundibulum results in the promotion of disease into the subordinate maxillary sinus. The frontal sinus drainage pathway anatomy is even more "labyrinthine" [4, 39, 40, 42, 43, 52, 70]. The so-called accessory cells of the anterior ethmoid are considered at the root of frontal sinus disease as responsible, in the majority of cases, for impeding ventilation and drainage (Tables 51.1 and 51.2) [9, 13, 27, 41]. The posterior ethmoid cells drain through the superior or supreme meatus. These cells are usually less incriminated, although they are almost always affected. The walls and the drainage of the cells in particular should be well known in order to perform "functional" surgery, respecting the physiology and following the "anatomical route predesigned by nature" [63].

Imaging

The radiological investigation is of utmost importance for evaluation of sinus disease localization, extent and complications, depiction of anatomic abnormalities, reconstruction of the anatomical architecture, and orientation [5, 6, 10, 49, 50]. Computed tomography (CT) is the radiologic examination of choice (see Chap. 45). Findings may range from minimal to extensive CT disease involvement, namely from minor mucosal thickening, partial or isolated opacification, to complete opacification of all sinuses, without air-filled cavities ("white out"). Lund-Mackay (whose system has been adopted by the Task Force on Rhinosinusitis of the American Academy of Otolaryngology-Head and Neck Surgery) and Friedman have proposed a different and useful CT scoring system that is now commonly used for CRS (Tables 51.3 and 51.4) [25, 48, 49]. Isolated sinus opacification may represent a mucocele. Unilateral sinus opacification, even without bone destruction, usually signifies neoplasm or mycosis [44] and needs to be imaged with contrast, sometimes also magnetic resonance imaging, and histological confirmation by biopsy.

It is preferable to initiate the CT examination after adequate medical treatment and during an intervening period without infections, in a quiescent phase of the disease. Mucosal swelling and polyp size will thus be minimal and so areas of persistent thickening can be identified and, at the same time, the resolution of the bony partition will be improved. A commonly used protocol trial of medication consists of 1–3 weeks of antibiotic therapy and a burst of oral and nasal steroids [25].

Important data derived from imaging the ethmoid include its height and slope (take-off angle between the cribriform plate and ethmoid roof), the course of the ethmoid arteries, demarcation of the frontal sinus outflow tract, the relationship between the posterior ethmoid and optic nerve, the presence of Onodi cells, and identification of any bony dehiscences at the lamina papyracea and along the ethmoidal roof. Magnetic resonance tomography (MRT) provides more and complementary data regarding numerous diseases like mucoceles, invasive fungal sinusitis, cerebrospinal fluid fistulas, meningoencephaloceles, and benign and malignant tumors [61, 67, 68].

Preoperative Care

The preoperative study is essentially based on a thorough history, microendoscopic clinical examination, and imaging. Nasal cavity examination should be performed before and after decongestion; this provides information about the extent and current activity of the disease, anatomical details, and abnormalities. Biopsies are reserved for monolateral or suspected lesions, but only after CT or MRT investigation. Allergy tests, rhinomanometry and acoustic rhinometry, olfactory detection, and nasal mucociliary clearance times are carried out, although not all of them routinely. Quality-of-life questionnaires and symptom scores are helpful in the assessment of disease severity, in treatment planning, and in evaluating results.

In the case of CRS, a preoperative medical therapy must be planned, as indication for surgery is based on failure of conservative treatment. The common pre- and perioperative systemic medications are basically antibiotics and corticosteroids, which improve the condition of the surgical field and thus reduce inflammation, bleeding, and complications [11]. Prophylaxis

Table 51.3 Lund-Mackay CT staging system. *0* No abnormalities, *1* partial opacification, *2* total opacification

Sinus System	Left	Right
Maxillary (0,1,2)	-	-
Anterior ethmoids (0,1,2)	-	-
Posterior ethmoids (0,1,2)	-	-
Sphenoid (0,1,2)	-	-
Frontal (0,1,2)	-	-
Ostiomeatal complex (0 or 2 only)*	-	-
Total points	-	-

0 Not occluded, *2* occluded

Table 51.4 Friedman CT staging system

Stage I	Single sinus involvement, either unilateral or bilateral
Stage II	Discontiguous or patchy areas of disease, in any sinus; clinically responsive to medication
Stage III	Contiguous disease throughout the ethmoid labyrinth (other sinuses may be involved); clinically responsive to medication
Stage IV	Contiguous mucosal thickening involving the ethmoid labyrinth with massive involvement of other sinuses (not necessarily all sinuses); clinically unresponsive to medication

should start 1–2 weeks before surgery and can continue post-operatively for some days to weeks. A short course of systemic steroids given before the operation is also recommended [19], especially for severe NP, such as in acetylsalicylic acid (ASA) triad. The commonest prescribed oral steroid is prednisolone (1 mg/kg daily for 5–15 days preoperative) [29]. Other medications like antileukotrienes are still under debate. No precise data are available with regard to the role and efficacy of systemic and topical antifungal medications [28, 56]. Previous surgery reduces the improvements obtainable with common preoperative medication, as a result of scars.

Routine laboratory studies are necessary, including bleeding and clotting assessment. Reduction of bleeding is the key point in this surgery in order to obtain the best possible surgical view. Medications that affect coagulation and prolong bleeding must be discontinued or substituted. Nonsteroidal analgesics/antirheumatics should be suspended at least 3 weeks before surgery. Hypertension must be controlled absolutely. The treatment and monitoring of hypertension is definitely required.

Principles

As for any other surgical discipline, the ethmoid surgery armamentarium undergoes continuous innovation; the "state of the art," as a unique and universally accepted technique, is constantly evolving. The nature and extent of the disease are the main factors to be considered in treatment planning and predicting outcome [32, 34, 42, 71]. In decision-making, each technique should be analyzed in terms of subjective symptomatic improvement [64], recurrence rate [66,71], impact on quality of life [1], and percentage of complications [37]. Modern surgery has moved from more extended to functional treatments. The surgical strategy varies from partial or minimal circumscribed ethmoidectomy, to complete, anterior and/or posterior, ethmoidectomy with maxillary, frontal, and sphenoid sinusotomy, the so-called pansinus operation [21, 33]. The most extensive surgery may be suggested only after failure of repetitive surgeries [66].

Mucosal Preservation

The proposed philosophies range from the functional limited removal of only the pathological tissues or structures obstructing the ostia [62,69] to extensive and subtotal extirpation of the mucosa underlying the ethmoid. However, stripping of the mucosa and leaving denuded bone modifies the mucosa to a metaplastic epithelium, damages the mucociliary transport function, and results in more granulations, osteitis, and scar formation [62].

Since the disease is probably systemic and a nasal manifestation of an underlying disorder, the basic philosophy adopted most often is to do less rather than more, sparing the structures that are not directly responsible for the obstruction. The mucosa should be left intact, unless it is directly and grossly involved in the pathogenesis. Exposure of only minimal bony areas allows

faster and better mucosal healing. Once key ethmoid areas are treated, preservation of the mucosa inside the frontal and maxillary sinuses is recommended. Maintenance of mucosal continuity prevents blockage of lymphatic drainage. The removal of mucosa from around the total circumference of the ostia should be avoided as this leads to stenosis [69].

Endonasal Ethmoid Surgery Techniques

Minor interventions are reserved for circumscribed diseases in primary cases. Limited ethmoidectomy, leaving the mucosa untouched inside the frontal, maxillary, and sphenoid sinus, seems to be as sufficient as more extended procedures in most of the cases. Resection is targeted only on the obstructing structures, preserving the key landmarks in order to reach the goal of identifying, exposing, opening, and, rarely, widening the natural ostia. This surgical concept, termed functional endoscopic sinus surgery (FESS), was introduced by Messerklinger and spread worldwide by Stammberger and Kennedy [38, 62]. FESS, more or less modified, has been accepted as the standard for the surgical management of sinus inflammations. If the entire ethmoid is affected, a complete ethmoidectomy is performed in accordance with the principles of FESS. More extended procedures are only indicated in a limited number of patients.

The correction of septal deviation may be recommended when it undoubtedly causes such a nasal obstruction that the patient would undergo surgery for septal deviation alone, when septal deviation causes mechanical obstruction on the ostiomeatal complex, or when it limits or impedes access and surgical manipulation in the ethmoid [18]. A mild or moderate degree of septal deviation is not a risk factor for CRS. Septoplasty is performed before operating the ethmoid on the narrow side, using classic or microendoscopic techniques.

The middle turbinate should be preserved as much as possible, even if it does not represent a dogma [36]. The physiologic roles of the middle turbinate in terms of humidification, heating, olfaction, and guiding the inhaled air should be preserved. The basal lamella of the second segment is usually opened and resected while performing a complete ethmoidectomy. The head and third horizontal segment remain the points of maximal stability. Turbinates originate from a common and continuous bony plate, the conchal lamina of the turbinal wall of the ethmoid, superiorly attached to the junction between the cribriform plate and the lateral lamella. As a consequence, fractures should be avoided because of the risk of skull-base injury. The middle meatus needs to be kept opened after surgery. Manipulation that causes destabilization, such as resection of the horizontal segment, are at risk of lateralization, which, it has been found, is the most common anatomic factor associated with primary surgery failure (see Chap. 55) [26, 55]. Subtotal resection may obviate this problem and has been proposed as a systematic and routine procedure in ethmoid surgery [34]. On the other hand, extended resections can cause crusts, atrophy, and uncontrolled adhesions. Stabilization is accomplished and lateralization prevented by keeping and fixing the head medially, creating a controlled synechia between the middle turbinate

51

and the septum, or by means of transseptal-transturbinate sutures [26,45]. Tail resection risks bleeding from the sphenopalatine artery branch to the middle turbinate. In revision surgery, the head of the middle turbinate is usually the most important anatomical landmark.

Partial inferior uncinectomy, achieved with the aid of back-biting forceps, gives the surgeon enough access to the natural maxillary ostium (see Chap. 50). The inferior resection is usually performed at the expense of the remaining lower part of the uncinate, which is adherent to the inferior mucosal border of the ostium and should be first luxated medially for correct identification. Simply opening the ethmoid infundibulum in this way frees the maxillary sinus of obstruction. Incomplete removal, leaving inferoposterior remnants, may cause failure to recognize and expose the natural ostium. In this case, the creation of a neo-ostium, disconnected and distant from the natural ostium, may result in recirculation ("missed ostium sequence") [17].

The aim of FESS for CRS and NP is to restore drainage and ventilation, removing the obstruction in the ethmoid with precision. FESS comprises several possible steps, the choice of which depends upon individual anatomy as well as the type and extent of disease. The steps are performed inside a sort of surgical "box" bounded by the turbinal wall medially, the skull base superiorly, and the orbital wall laterally. The operation is begun by first examining and carefully palpating the structures, trying to identify the landmarks and the location of the obstruction. Depending on the operating direction, the anterior-to-posterior and posterior-to-anterior dissection must be distinguished [33, 59]; the anterior-to-posterior procedure moves step by step from front to back and from medial to lateral (centrifugal). Typical signs of opening of a cavity are the appearance of air bubbles or secretions. Progressive opening of the main four ethmoid "doors," the uncinate process, bulla lamella, basal lamella, and anterior sphenoid wall, allows access to the main anatomical "air spaces." Safe opening is usually located at the inferomedial aspect, because the skull base and orbit are at risk superolaterally. The skull base and medial orbital wall must be identified progressively and respected as the main landmarks of dissection.

Anterior-to-Posterior FESS Dissection

The first step is commonly partial resection of the uncinate process, which opens the infundibulum (infundibulotomy). Removal of the medial wall of the infundibulum may be completed by luxating and displacing medially and resecting the uncinate from the anterior convex attachment line up to the maxilla with the middle turbinate. Removal of the uppermost attachment of the uncinate in many patients opens the frontal recess, with a view onto the frontal ostium. Less frequently, it is also necessary to remove the dome of one or more frontal cells above and behind, in order to provide a good enough view of the frontal ostium. Removal of the bulla lamella, when it reaches the skull base, exposes the suprabullar and retrobullar recesses and the anterior ethmoid artery, located on the roof [9]. After removing the anterior ethmoid cells, the last access before entering the

posterior ethmoid is the basal lamella of the middle turbinate. Once identified, the basal lamella is opened, inferomedially, in its second frontal third, to enter the posterior ethmoid. This unnatural opening does not usually create recirculation between the anterior and posterior ethmoid through the superior meatus. Interlamellar cells should be removed. One or more posterior ethmoid cells need to be cleared before identifying the anterior wall of the sphenoid or an Onodi cell. The presence of an Onodi cell puts the optic nerve at risk for damage. The bulge of the optic nerve at the lateral wall may be frequently covered only by a paper-thin bony lamina, or may be dehiscent. The third horizontal segment of the middle turbinate should not be removed, thus avoiding its lateral luxation. Moreover, the branch of the sphenopalatine artery for the middle turbinate runs along the inferomedial border of this segment. The final ethmoid cavity, when performing a complete ethmoidectomy, is bounded laterally by the lamina papyracea, medially by the lateral surface of the middle, superior and supreme turbinates, and superiorly by the ethmoid roof, the skull base.

Posterior-to-Anterior FESS Dissection

Complete ethmoidectomy can also be performed in a posterior-to-anterior direction [69]. Here, the sphenoid sinus is opened first transnasally, and then the ethmoid roof is exposed from posterior, opening the posterior ethmoid cells, followed by further opening of the anterior ethmoid cells. This approach avoids surgery directed toward the skull base from the anterior direction, which may be considered more dangerous.

Fungus Balls

Fungus balls develop as saprophytic growths inside the sinus and needs to be removed without the underlying mucosa, and with sinus lavage (washing the cavity). Maxillary fungus balls are not associated with ostiomeatal complex obstruction. In the case of eosinophilic rhinosinusitis [24, 33], the eosinophilic mucin has to be removed, also by washing the cavities.

Ethmoid Mucoceles

Ethmoidal mucoceles or pyoceles are treated by removing the obstruction, incising the cyst, draining the contained secretions, and marsupializing the wall, as wide as possible [7, 14]. Pulling the mucosa is unnecessary and risky, promoting long-lasting granulations and scarring.

Ethmoid Tumors

Ethmoid benign and malignant tumors are treated with increasing frequency using endonasal microendoscopic approaches, applying the same concepts of CRS surgery [3,8]. However, radical removal of the adjacent mucosa, bone, and dura are performed at the tumor site as necessary. The indication depends on the histology, and tumor site, size, and surrounding area of invasion. Advanced technologies and increased skills have widened the indications, allowing safe and effective endonasal removal, especially of benign tumors [3, 30, 53, 60].

Postoperative Care

Postoperative protocols vary widely among surgeons and studies [33, 54]. It should be diversified according to the nature and extent of the pathology. The usage of nasal packing is advocated by some, while not by others [22]. The packs, when inserted, are usually removed between the 1st and 7th postoperative day. In any case, packing should be minimized and, when used as hemostats, may be avoided if adequate intraoperative hemostasis has been ensured. Some apply or drip antibiotic/steroid ointments or solutions onto the walls of the cavity, or directly to the sponges. The more recently developed absorbable agents, like gels or foams, which dissolve spontaneously, have to be left covering the wound, but their efficacy remains to be clarified [12]. Splints are removed 1–2 weeks afterwards. It is essential to give patients information, instructions, and counsel regarding late complications and nasal hygiene. Blowing the nose has to be avoided immediately after the operation, and in some cases for few days thereafter, because of the risk of orbital emphysema or pneumocephalus.

Postoperative wound care is a matter of debate. The operated nasal cavities need to be cleaned daily, from the day of surgery or after removal of packing, using nasal watery and saline solutions, sprays, douches, or irrigations, for moistening until the clots and crusts subside. Patients are advised to repeat this treatment twice or more times a day for weeks. Sometimes, but infrequently, the crusts need to be gently and cautiously removed from the ethmoid. The crusts do not generally require any care and are left inside until they clear spontaneously, thus avoiding bleeding and crust reformation. Any bony debridement should be removed owing to the process of necrosis. In some cases, for example when there is a pronounced tendency toward extreme granulation formation or a risk of secondary adhesion and obstruction by scarring, mitomycin C may be applied locally [15].

Local corticosteroids are usually given for several months, even starting soon after the operation. The most commonly used topical steroids are beclomethasone diproprionate, flunisolide, fluticasone proprionate, mometasone furoate, and budesonide [57].

Purulent secretions are an indication for administrating broad-spectrum antibiotics for 7–10 days. The use of antibiotics is questionable in the absence of pus. Oral medical therapy, steroids and antibiotics, started before surgery, should be continued. Atopic patients with nasal polyps should take antihistamines for several months, although with CRS there is no evidence of benefit from this [23]. Diffuse polyposis often requires systemic steroids at intervals. In ASA triad patients, additional therapy with antileukotrienes is suggested [65]. Postoperative office endoscopic examinations are scheduled at 2 weeks, 3 and 6 months, and 1 year; thereafter once a year for long-term follow up.

Tips to Avoid Complications

- Detailed knowledge of the anatomy is mandatory.
- Preoperative medical treatment reduces inflammation and risk of bleeding.
- Correct interpretation of preoperative imaging and intraoperative findings is required.
- Bone remodeling such as thickening and thinning, dehiscences, erosion, or destruction must be recognized on CT.
- Excessive manipulation of the middle turbinate puts the lateral lamella of the cribriform plate at risk of injuries.
- Lateralization of the middle turbinate must be prevented since it is considered the most common anatomic factor associated with primary surgery failure.
- Adequate removal of the uncinate process, identification of the lamina papyracea, careful attention to orbital fat protrusion, and avoidance thereof, keeping the tip of the microdebrider in a lateral direction, contribute to the prevention of orbital complications.
- Bleeding represents the main enemy, leading to disorientation, and needs to be minimized, also by being familiar with the vascular anatomy.
- The anterior ethmoid artery may run separate from the skull base; its usual position is between the bulla and the basal lamellae in the suprabullar recess or, less frequently, in the supraorbital cell.
- Branches of the sphenopalatine artery may be damaged by resecting the tail or the horizontal segment of the middle turbinate.
- Hyperpneumatization signifies thinner bony structures and the need for careful instrumentation, especially near the lateral lamella of the cribriform plate.

Take-Home Pearls

- The most optimal and universally accepted procedure in ethmoid surgery for inflammations is still under debate, essentially owing to a lack of understanding of the underlying pathophysiology.
- Evidence-based surgery, comparative studies, and quality randomized controlled trials should be obtained.
- Conservative surgical techniques combined with medical therapy should be chosen.
- Identification of the maxillary ostium and restoration of maxillary sinus function may be achieved by inferior uncinectomy.
- More extended approaches may be required in cases of diffuse disease and recurrences, but at the price of a higher risk of complications.
- The objectives striven for by surgery should be symptom and quality of life improvement by dealing with inflammations and radical eradication of tumors.

51

References

1. Alobid I, Benitez P, Bernal-Sprekelsen M (2006) Nasal polyposis and its impact on quality of life: comparison between the effects of medical and surgical treatments. Allergy 60:452–458

2. Anand VK (2004) Epidemiology and economic impact of rhinosinusitis. Ann Otol Rhinol Laryngol Suppl 193:3–5

3. Banhiran W, Casiano RR (2005) Endoscopic sinus surgery for benign and malignant nasal and sinus neoplasm. Curr Opin Otolaryngol Head Neck Surg 13:50–54

4. Bent JP III, Cuilty-Siller C, Kuhn FA (1994) The frontal cell as a cause of frontal sinus obstruction. Am J Rhinol 8:185–191

5. Bhattacharyya N (2005) A comparison of symptom scores and radiographic staging systems in chronic rhinosinusitis. Am J Rhinol 19:175–179

6. Bhattacharyya N, Fried MP (2003) The accuracy of computed tomography in the diagnosis of chronic rhinosinusitis. Laryngoscope 113:125–129

7. Bockmuhl U, Kratzsch B, Benda K, et al (2005) Paranasal sinus mucoceles: surgical management and long term results. Laryngorhinootologie 84:892–898

8. Bockmuhl U, Minovi A, Kratzsch B, et al (2005) Endonasal micro-endoscopic tumor surgery: state of the art. Laryngorhinootologie 84:884–891

9. Bolger WE, Mawn CB (2001) Analysis of the suprabullar and retrobullar recesses for endoscopic sinus surgery. Ann Otol Rhinol Laryngol 110:3–14

10. Bolger WE, Butzin CE, Parsons DS (1991) Paranasal sinus bony anatomic variations and mucosal abnormalities: CT analysis for endoscopic sinus surgery. Laryngoscope 101:56–64

11. Castelnuovo P, De Bernardi F, Delù G, et al (2005) Rational treatment of nasal polyposis. Acta Otorhinolaryngol Ital 25:3–29

12. Chandra RK, Kern RC (2004) Advantages and disadvantages of topical packing in endoscopic sinus surgery. Curr Opin Otolaryngol Head Neck Surg 12:21–26

13. Chiu AG, Vaughan WC (2004) Using the frontal intersinus septal cell to widen the narrow frontal recess. Laryngoscope 114:1315–1317

14. Chiu AG, Vaughan WC (2004) Management of the lateral frontal sinus lesion and the supraorbital cell mucocele. Am J Rhinol 18:83–86

15. Chung JH, Cosenza MJ, Rahbar R, et al (2002) Mitomycin C for the prevention of adhesion formation after endoscopic sinus surgery: a randomized, controlled study. Otolaryngol Head Neck Surg 126:468–474

16. Clement PA, Bluestone CD, Gordts F, et al (1998) Management of rhinosinusitis in children: consensus meeting. Arch Otolaryngol Head Neck Surg 124:31–34

17. Coleman JR, Duncavage JA (1996) Extended middle meatal antrostomy: the treatment of circular flow. Laryngoscope 106:1214–1217

18. Collet S, Bertrand B, Cornu S, et al (2001) Is septal deviation a risk factor for chronic sinusitis? Review of the literature. Acta Otolaryngol Belg 55:299–304

19. Damm M, Jungehulsing M, Eckel HE, et al (1999) Effects of systemic steroid treatment in chronic polypoid rhinosinusitis evaluated with magnetic resonance imaging. Otolaryngol Head Neck Surg 120:517–523

20. Doufur X, Bedier A, Ferrie JC, et al (2004) Diffuse nasal polyposis and endonasal endoscopic surgery: long-term results, a 65-case study. Laryngoscope 114:1982–1987

21. Draf W (1991) Endonasal micro-endoscopic frontal sinus surgery: the Fulda concept. Oper Tech Otolaryngol Head Neck Surg 2:234–240

22. Eliashar R, Gross M, Wohlgelertner J, et al (2006) Packing in endoscopic sinus surgery. Is it really required? Otolaryngol Head Neck Surg 134:276–279

23. European Academy of Allergology and Clinical Immunology (2005) European position paper on rhinosinusitis and nasal polyps. Rhinology Suppl 18:1–87

24. Ferguson BJ (2004) Categorization of eosinophilic chronic rhinosinusitis. Curr Opin Otolaryngol Head Neck Surg 12:237–242

25. Friedman WH, Katsantonis GP, Bumpous JM (1995) Staging of chronic hyperplastic rhinosinusitis: treatment strategies. Otolaryngol Head Neck Surg 112:210–214

26. Friedman WH, Landsberg R, Tanyeri H (2000) Middle turbinate medialization and preservation in endoscopic sinus surgery. Otolaryngol Head Neck Surg 123:76–80

27. Gaafar H, Abdel-Monem MH, Qawas MK (2001) Frontal sinus outflow tract "anatomic study". Acta Otolaryngol 121:305–309

28. Helbling A, Baumann A, Hanni C (2006) Amphotericin B nasal spray has no effect on nasal polyps. J Laryngol Otol 11:1–3

29. Hissaria P, Smith W, Wormald PJ (2006) Short course of systemic corticosteroids in sinonasal polyposis: a double-blind, randomized, placebo-controlled trial with evaluation of outcome measures. J Allergy Clin Immunol 118:128–133

30. Hofmann T, Bernal-Sprekelsen M, Koele W, et al (2005) Endoscopic resection of juvenile angiofibromas – long term results. Rhinology 43:282–289

31. Holliday RA, Shpizner BA (1995) Avoiding complications of endoscopic sinus surgery: analysis of coronal, axial, and sagittal computed tomographic images. Oper Tech Otolaryngol Head Neck Surg 6:149–156

32. Hopkins C, Browne JP, Slack R, et al (2006) Complications of surgery for nasal polyposis and chronic rhinosinusitis: the results of a national audit in England and Wales. Laryngoscope 116:1494–1499

33. Hosemann W, Weber RK, Keerl RE, et al (2000) Minimally Invasive Endonasal Sinus Surgery. Thieme, Stuttgart

34. Jankowski R, Pigret D, Decroocq F, et al (2006) Comparison of radical (nasalisation) and functional ethmoidectomy in patients with severe sinonasal polyposis. A retrospective study. Rev Laryngol Otol Rhinol (Bord) 127:131–140

35. Kennedy DW (1992) Prognostic factors, outcomes and staging in ethmoid sinus surgery. Laryngoscope 102:1–18

36. Kennedy DW (1998) Middle turbinate resection: evaluating the issues – should we resect normal middle turbinates? Arch Otolaryngol Head Neck Surg 124:107

37. Kennedy DW, Shaman P, Han W, et al (1994) Complications of ethmoidectomy: a survey of fellows of the American Academy of Otolaryngology – Head and Neck Surgery. Otolaryngol Head Neck Surg 111:589–599

38. Kennedy DW, Zinreich SJ, Rosenbaum AE, et al (1985) Functional endoscopic sinus surgery: theory and diagnostic evaluation. Arch Otolaryngol Head Neck Surg 111:576–582

39. Kew J, Rees GL, Close D, et al (2002) Multiplanar reconstructed computed tomography images improves depiction and understanding of the anatomy of the frontal sinus and recess. Am J Rhinol 16:119–123

40. Kountakis S, Senior B, Draf W (2005) The Frontal Sinus. Springer, Berlin Heidelberg New York

41. Kuhn FA, Bolger WE, Tisdal RG (1991) The agger nasi cell in frontal recess obstruction: an anatomic, radiologic and clinical correlation. Oper Tech Otolaryngol Head Neck Surg 2:226–231

42. Landsberg R, Sergev Y, Friedman M, et al (2006) A targeted endoscopic approach to chronic isolated frontal sinusitis. Otolaryngol Head Neck Surg 134:28–32

43. Lang J (1989) Clinical anatomy of the nose, nasal cavity and paranasal sinuses. Thieme, Stuttgart New York

44. Lehnerdt G, Weber J, Dost P (2001) Unilateral opacification of the paranasal sinuses in CT or MRI: an indication of an uncommon histologic finding. Laryngorhinootologie 80:141–145

45. Lindermann J, Keck T, Rettinger G (2002) Septal-turbinate-suture in endonasal sinus surgery. Rhinology 40:92–94

46. Lund VJ (2001) Evidence-based surgery in chronic rhinosinusitis. Acta Otolaryngol 121:5–9

47. Lund VJ (2006) Surgical outcomes in chronic rhinosinusitis and nasal polyposis. Rhinology 44:97

48. Lund VJ, Kennedy DW (1997) Staging for rhinosinusitis. Otolaryngol Head Neck Surg 117:35–40

49. Lund VJ, Mackay IS (1993) Staging in rhinosinusitis. Rhinology 31:183–184

50. Lund VJ, Draf W, Friedman WH, et al (1995) Quantification for staging sinusitis. Ann Otol Rhinol Laryngol 104:17–21

51. Messerklinger W (1978) Endoscopy of the Nose. Urban and Schwarzenberg, Baltimore Munich

52. Messerklinger W (1982) The recessus frontalis and its clinical aspects. Laryngol Rhinol Otol 61:217–223

53. Minovi A, Kollert M, Draf W, et al (2006) Inverted papilloma: feasibility of endonasal surgery and long-term results of 87 cases. Rhinology 44:205–210

54. Moriyama H (1992) Postoperative care and long term results. Rhinol Suppl 14:156–161

55. Musy PY, Kountakis SE (2004) Anatomic findings in patients undergoing revision endoscopic sinus surgery. Am J Otolaryngol 25:418–422

56. Ponikau JU, Sherris DA, Weaver A, et al (2005) Treatment of chronic rhinosinusitis with intranasal amphotericin B: a randomized, placebo-controlled, double-blind pilot trial. J Allergy Clin Immunol 115:125–131

57. Rowe-Jones JM, Medcalf M, Durham SR (2005) Functional endoscopic sinus surgery: 5 year follow up and results of a prospective, randomized, stratified, double-blind, placebo controlled study of postoperative fluticasone propionate aqueous nasal spray. Rhinology 43:2–10

58. Scadding GK (2002) Comparison of medical and surgical treatment of nasal polyposis. Curr Allergy Asthma Rep 2:494–499

59. Schaefer SD, Li JC, Chan EK, et al (2006) Combined anterior-to-posterior and posterior-to-anterior approach to paranasal surgery: an update. Laryngoscope 116:509–513

60. Sciarretta V, Pasquini E, Farneti G (2006) Endoscopic sinus surgery for treatment of vascular tumors. Am J Rhinol 20:426–431

61. Shetty PG, Shroff MM, Kirtane MV, et al (1998) Evaluation of high resolution CT and MR cisternography in the diagnosis of cerebrospinal fluid fistula. Am J Neuroradiol 19:633–639

62. Stammberger H (1991) Functional Endoscopic Sinus Surgery. BC Decker, Philadelphia

63. Stammberger H (2001) FESS – "Uncapping the Egg" – The Endoscopic Approach to Frontal Recess and Sinuses. A Surgical Technique of the Graz University Medical School. Endo-Press, Tuttlingen, Germany

64. Terris MH, Davidson TM (1994) Review of published results for endoscopic sinus surgery. Ear Nose Throat J 73:574–580

65. Ulualp SO, Sterman BM, Toohill RJ (1999) Antileukotriene therapy for the relief of sinus symptoms in aspirin triad disease. Ear Nose Throat J 78:604–606

66. Videler WJ, Wreesmann VB, van der Meulen FW, et al (2006) Repetitive endoscopic sinus surgery failure: a role for radical surgery? Otolaryngol Head Neck Surg 134:586–591

67. Wani MK, Ruckenstein MJ, Parikh S (2001) Magnetic resonance imaging of the paranasal sinuses: incidental abnormalities and their relationship to patient symptoms. J Otolaryngol 30:257–262

68. Weiss F, Habermann CR, Welger J, et al (2001) MRI in the preoperative diagnosis of chronic sinusitis: comparison with CT. Rofo 173:319–324

69. Wigand ME (1990) Endoscopic Surgery of the Paranasal Sinuses and Anterior Skull Base. Thieme, Stuttgart New York

70. Wormald PJ (2005) Endoscopic Sinus Surgery. Thieme, Stuttgart New York

71. Wynn R, Har-El G (2004) Recurrence rates after endoscopic sinus surgery for massive sinus polyposis. Laryngoscope 114:811–813

51

Chapter 52

The Frontal Sinus

Bernhard Schick and Wolfgang Draf

Core Messages

- Frontal sinus surgery is indicated after failure of conservative treatment.
- In many patients an adequate drainage of the anterior ethmoid already leads to resolution of frontal sinus affection.
- To avoid postoperative closure of the frontal sinus drainage, meticulous dissection within the confines of the frontal recess with minimal mucosal injury is of utmost importance.
- The lateral mucosal linings of the frontal sinus infundibulum and frontal recess are of great importance in mucociliary clearance of the frontal sinus.
- Maximal widening of the frontal sinus drainage with sufficient resection of the upper nasal septum is demanded for successful frontal sinus type III drainage.

Contents

Introduction

Endonasal frontal sinus drainage was first reported by Schaeffer in 1890, but was not accepted by most rhinologists for a long time. Indeed it is true that external approaches toward this sinus in particular have dominated for many decades and are still not uncommon. Even though not all frontal sinus problems can be managed endonasally, it has clearly been determined that in most situations endonasal frontal sinus drainage can be achieved. Awareness of the complex anatomical relationships within the frontal recess, improved understanding of the physiology and pathophysiology of the frontal sinus, advances in endoscopic/microscopic surgery, and the availability of specialized instrumentation have contributed to the successful adoption of endonasal frontal sinus drainage. However, one should bear in mind that despite these various improvements, transnasal frontal sinus surgery still remains one of the most difficult challenges in surgical management of the paranasal sinuses. This chapter will provide an overview of endonasal surgical concepts involving the frontal sinus.

Aims and Objectives

In most situations endonasal frontal sinus surgery is performed to treat chronic sinusitis. Here, the frontal sinus function might be impaired due to narrowed mucus clearance pathways. In the case of narrowed pathways, a vicious circle of edema, decrease in mucociliary clearance, mucus stasis, pH changes, and bacterial overgrowth can develop. If conservative treatment fails to restore frontal sinus ventilation, endonasal frontal sinus surgery aims to remove frontal recess obstruction, thus enabling restoration of ventilation. In this context it is important to remember the mucociliary clearance pattern of the frontal sinus described by Messerklinger [12]. While 60% of the fontal sinus mucus that is transported from the interfrontal sinus septum, laterally across the frontal sinus roof, medially along the frontal sinus floor to the frontal ostium, recirculates, 40% of the mucus is drained down to the lateral frontal recess. Thus, the mucosa of the lateral frontal recess is most important for frontal sinus drainage and should be carefully preserved in frontal sinus surgery.

Furthermore, the patient's symptoms are most important in the decision to perform frontal sinus surgery. Pain, headaches, pressure, or purulent drainage from the frontal sinus that are refractory to medical treatment are an indication for frontal sinus surgery. In nasal polyposis, it is important to keep in mind that diagnostic radiology frequently shows opacification of the frontal sinus, with these patients quite often reporting no or only minimal symptoms related to the frontal sinus. It has been pointed out that in most of these cases surgical opening of the frontal sinus is not necessary [15]. Furthermore, in several cases of chronic sinusitis, as in nasal polyposis, a complex treatment concept has to be considered. In addition to the surgical treatment, other components like medical treatment, avoidance of allergens, and desensitization in patients with aspirin intolerance may be necessary for long-term success (see Chap. 57). In the case of allergic fungal infection of the frontal sinus, the surgeon should ensure complete suction of the thick mucus filling the sinus cavity.

Difficulties may occur in patients with symptomatic recurrent or persistent frontal sinus disease after previous endonasal frontal sinus surgery that does not respond to intensive conservative treatment. Due to distorted anatomy and possible neo-osteogenesis, endoscopic revision surgery remains a great challenge [1]. In the case of an incomplete anterior ethmoidectomy with incomplete opening of the frontal recess in previous surgery, the chances of a successful revision surgery of the frontal sinus are much better than in situations of a frontal recess that is closed by scar tissue. Previous stripping of the mucosa in the frontal recess followed by closure of the frontal sinus ostium due to scar tissue presents a difficult situation; in this situation a stable reopening of the frontal sinus is hard to achieve. Thus, it is the great responsibility of the first surgeon to dissect the frontal recess very meticulously.

Removal of frontal sinus tumors (e.g., osteoma) or repair of cerebrospinal fluid fistulas are rare indications for endonasal frontal sinus surgery. Here, adequate opening of the frontal sinus is required for sufficiently treating the specific pathology. Another rare indication for endonasal opening of the frontal sinus is a barotrauma, in terms of resolving subpressure in the sinus (Fig. 52.1).

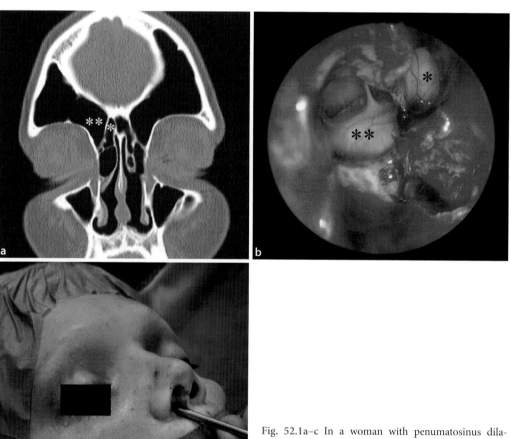

Fig. 52.1a–c In a woman with penumatosinus dilatans, the right frontal sinus (**) and a frontal cell (*) are shown on preoperative coronal computed tomography scanning (**a**), and intraoperatively (**b**) after frontal sinus opening. Positive diaphanoscopy (**c**) confirms opening of the frontal sinus

Table 52.1 Kuhn (1996) classification of frontoethmoidal cells, modified by Wormald (2005) [10, 17]

Frontal cell type 1	Single frontal recess cell above the agger nasi cell
Frontal cells type 2	Tier of cells in the frontal recess above the agger nasi cell
Frontal cell type 3	Single massive cell pneumatizing cephalad into the frontal sinus
Frontal cell type 4	A cell pneumatizing into the frontal sinus and extending >50% of the vertical height of the frontal sinus

Surgical Anatomy

A keystone in endonasal frontal sinus surgery is to understand the anatomical relationships of the frontal recess (see Chap. 44). Only precise knowledge of the frontal recess anatomy and its variations enables meticulous endonasal frontal sinus drainage by opening the frontal recess with the least possible injury to its mucosa. The frontal recess, as part of the anterior ethmoid, represents the connection between the frontal sinus and the ethmoidal infundibulum, resembling an inverted, funnel-shaped space. Thus, the frontal recess borders the frontal sinus infundibulum with its narrow end. The borders of the frontal recess are well defined as the agger nasi ventrally, the lateral lamella of the middle turbinate medially, the ethmoidal bulla posteriorly, and the lamina papyracea laterally. In close relation to the bulla lamella, the anterior ethmoid artery is located at the posterior border of the frontal recess (see Chap. 54). It is important to understand that the frontal recess can be narrowed by numerous cellular structures. Frontal recess cells are known as agger nasi cells, supraorbital ethmoid cells, frontal cells, frontal bulla cells, suprabullar cells, and interfrontal sinus septal cells [2]. Four types of frontoethmoidal cells can be distinguished (Table 52.1).

If a wider opening of the frontal sinus is necessary, it is important to consider that resection of the medial part of the frontal sinus floor has to respect the olfactory groove as its posterior border. The anterior border of the olfactory groove may protrude into the frontal sinus, here only covered by a thin bony layer. This is a situation of higher risk for anterior skull-base injury during surgery and was therefore termed a "dangerous frontal bone" by Boenninghaus in 1923 (see Chap. 44). The most anterior attachment of the middle turbinate is found about 5 mm ventral to the olfactory groove. The frontal sinus infundibulum (also termed the frontal sinus ostium) is bordered anteriorly by the nasal peak, which narrows the frontal sinus infundibulum as a thick bone.

Radiology

Diagnostic radiology in concert with detailed anamnesis and thorough endoscopic evaluation enables determination of indications for frontal sinus surgery and to define the appropriate surgical concept. Computed tomography (CT) without use of contrast medium is the radiological assessment of first choice to evaluate the frontal sinus as well as the anterior ethmoid anatomy (see Chap. 45). The great value of CT here lies in precisely defining the bony anatomy. The degree of frontal sinus aeration in chronic sinusitis, the presence of a possible bony defect at the anterior skull base in situations of cerebrospinal fluid fistulas, and delineation of the bony borders in cases of tumor diseases are additionally obtained. Since the frontal sinus recess is a particularly complex area anatomically it is of major importance to the surgeon to obtain prior to surgery a precise description of the cells narrowing the frontal recess. CT is further excellently suited for explaining the surgical concept to the patient [13]. CT can be of particular use in obtaining the information necessary for image-guided surgery (see Chap. 48). Additional magnetic resonance imaging is of benefit for the analysis of tumors or cerebrospinal fluid fistulas.

CT-scans are available in coronal, sagittal, and axial sections, which each provide specific information to the surgeon. Axial sections allow determination of the anterior–posterior diameter of the frontal sinus infundibulum and to estimate the maximal anterior–posterior diameter that can be created by performing type III frontal sinus drainage. Sagittal sections also illustrate the anterior–posterior diameter of the frontal sinus infundibulum, attachment of the ethmoidal bulla, and the possible presence of a suprabullar recess as well as other cells like agger nasi cells and suprabullar cells that might narrow the frontal recess. Coronal sections allow the position of the middle turbinate to be defined in relation to cells extending into the frontal recess, attachment of the uncinate process, and the various frontal cells. Nowadays high-quality reconstructions are available. Thus, every rhinologist should discuss with the radiologist the primary section being taken with the necessary reconstructions of the other section planes. Secondary coronal reconstructions might be of benefit compared to primary coronal sections in terms of avoiding dental artifacts that might disrupt the detailed evaluation of the individual cellular architecture.

How to Do it

Endonasal surgery as a treatment for frontal sinusitis comprises a wide range of strategies. The surgical options range from very limited opening of the anterior ethmoid to enlarged openings of the frontal sinus. Selection of the appropriate strategy is based on the individual pathophysiology that is judged preoperatively as the reason for fontal sinus affection. If the pathology is located in the anterior ethmoid and does not extend to the frontal recess, it is sufficient to open the anterior ethmoid. In these cases the secondary affection of the frontal sinus can be expected to resolve. This strategy particularly aims to keep the confines of the frontal recess untouched, as surgery in this area may cause persistent frontal sinusitis postoperatively [9].

For frontal sinus drainage, three different degrees of frontal sinus opening have been developed [3]: (1) simple drainage (type I), (2) extended drainage (type II), and (3) endonasal median drainage (type III). From type I to type III, frontal sinus drainage surgery is increasingly invasive; however, this concept gives the rhinologist the chance to resolve the vast majority of frontal sinus pathologies endonasally.

Type I: Simple Drainage

In the case where obstruction of the frontal sinus is attributed to frontal recess pathology, opening of the frontal recess is required [3, 8, 17]. Thus, it is of great importance that the surgeon, as pointed out before, observes closely the preoperatively taken CT images, focusing on the individual anatomy of all cellular structures narrowing the frontal recess. Whether the frontal sinus drains into the ethmoidal infundibulum or the middle nasal meatus needs to be determined. Two situations have to be distinguished:

1. If the uncinate process is attached to the lateral nasal wall, the lamina papyracea, or agger nasi cells, the frontal recess is reached between the uncinate process and bulla lamella. In these situations the cranial parts of the uncinate process form the terminal recess. The way toward the frontal sinus is found thus between the terminal recess and the middle turbinate.
2. If the uncinate process is attached cranially to the anterior skull base or middle turbinate, it blocks the access to the frontal recess. In this situation, the frontal recess is opened by resection of the uncinate process (Fig. 52.1).

As mucosal injury must be minimalized, it is very useful to repeatedly place decongestant pledgets. Prevention of bleeding and mucosal decongestion are very beneficial for the least traumatic dissection within the frontal recess, which is performed with angled endoscopes like a 45° endoscope. The principle of further meticulous dissection is to gain access to the frontal sinus infundibulum by opening and removal of the cellular structures that cover the frontal sinus from below. The view from below enables the surgeon to look into various opened cells within the frontal recess. Removal of the dome of these cells is necessary to obtain a view behind them. The comparison of this situation with "egg shells" reported by Stammberger [14] reflects on the surgical strategy that is needed (Fig. 52.2). With an angled spoon or angled bulb-headed probe, the thin bony borders of cells in the frontal recess are dissected and finally removed. In the case of submucosal bone removal, the adjacent mucosa is pushed aside providing a view onto the structures that had previously been hidden by the cell [13]. Frontal sinus drainage type I is achieved with exposure of the fontal sinus opening (Fig. 52.3a). Thus, the frontal recess is completely exposed with great importance placed on preserving its mucosa.

It is very important that a terminal recess, such as the cranial border of the uncinate process or frontal cells, are not misinter-

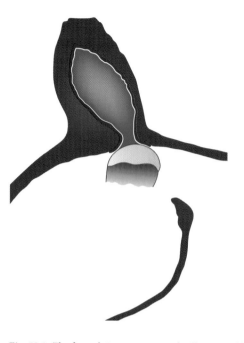

Fig. 52.2 The frontal sinus opening is finally covered by the cranial part of cells that have to be gently removed with specialized instruments like curved spoons. The mucosal trauma at the frontal sinus opening is thus minimized

preted as the frontal sinus. Comparison of a curved instrument placed into the assumed frontal sinus with the position of the same instrument beside the nose in the same direction as previously being placed in the nose gives the surgeon an impression as to whether the tip of the instrument is placed at the level of the medial canthus or clearly above it [13]. A more trustworthy technique by which to confirm opening of the frontal sinus is a positive diaphanoscopy at the forehead (Fig. 52.1).

Type II: Extended Drainage

A further widening of the frontal sinus access at one side is achieved by resection of the frontal sinus floor, a procedure that has been termed frontal sinus drainage type II. Two different forms can be distinguished. Resection of the frontal sinus floor can extend from the lamina papyracea to the middle turbinate (type IIa, Fig. 52.3b) or from the lamina papyracea to the nasal septum (type IIb, Fig. 52.3c). According to the classification of nasofrontal approach (NFA) given by May and Schaitkin [11], NFA II corresponds with type IIa and NFA III with type IIb. Indications for frontal sinus type II drainage are serious complications of acute sinusitis, medial mucopyocele, benign tumors, and situations of frontal sinus obstruction with "good-quality mucosa" [5]. The indications for type IIa or type IIb drainage depend on the frontal sinus opening that is achieved by a type IIa drainage. If type IIa drainage results in an opening less than 5×7 mm, type IIb drainage is carried out. Where a frontal sinus drainage type IIb is intended, a drill is required due to the medially increasing thickness of the bone. One should pay careful

52

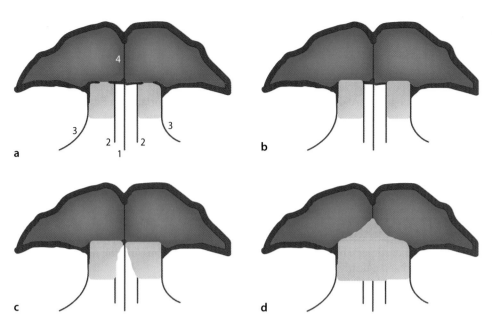

Fig. 52.3a–d Exposure of the frontal sinus opening after removal of all cells within the confines of the frontal recess is termed frontal sinus drainage type I (**a**). Resection of the frontal sinus floor can be performed from the lamina papyracea to the middle turbinate (**b**, type IIa) or from the lamina papyracea to the nasal septum (**c**, type IIb). Endonasal median drainage (**d**, type III) means resection of the frontal sinus floor from the right lamina papyracea to the left lamina papyracea with additional resection of the upper nasal septum and the inferior part of the interfrontal septum

attention to mucosa preservation, at least at the most beneficial part of the circumference, at the lateral border. This will contribute significantly to successful long-term frontal sinus drainage patency.

Type III: Endonasal Median Drainage

Maximal opening of the frontal sinus is achieved by frontal sinus type III drainage [3, 4]. Here, the frontal sinus floors on both sides of the adjacent upper nasal septum as well as most of the interfrontal septum are removed (Fig. 52.3d). There are two approaches to performing a type III frontal sinus drainage, which is also known as endonasal median drainage – the lateral and middle approaches. The lateral approach starts with identification of the frontal sinus opening on both sides after complete ethmoidectomy. This is well suited to revision surgery if the middle turbinate is preserved and the previous ethmoidectomy is found to be incomplete. Both frontal sinus openings are then connected to a maximal large drainage. In the middle approach, performance of the type III frontal sinus drainage starts with resection of the perpendicular plate of the nasal septum with identification of the first olfactory fiber [5]. The medial approach is attractive if after previous surgery landmarks are missing, and in the presence of an intersinusoidal cell that can be opened with further enlargement to both lateral sides.

Sufficient removal of the upper nasal septum (approximately 1.5 cm) is of great importance for the success of this extended frontal sinus drainage. The extended drainage is bordered dorsally by the olfactory groove. Here, identification of the first olfactory fiber clearly defines the maximal posterior resection border and allows removal of the most anterior part of the middle turbinate at a length of about 5 mm. At the end of surgery the surgeon has created the so-called "frontal-T." Its long crus is formed by the posterior border of the perpendicular ethmoid lamina resection, and the shorter wings on both sides are shaped by the posterior margins of the frontal sinus floor resection. For bone removal, especially at the nasal peak, extensive drilling is necessary; the use of a microscope can be beneficial. Curved drills nowadays offer improved possibilities for resecting bony structures within the frontal sinus, like the cranial parts of the interfrontal septum. The intention is to gain the greatest possible frontal sinus access by extended bone removal, but one always has to keep in mind that the frontal sinus opening should be bordered at the end of surgery by bone on all sides. Again, preservation of the lateral-most mucosal lining as far as possible is highly beneficial, thus avoiding circumferential loss of all mucosa. Furthermore, epithelialization of the created large nasofrontal drainage by free mucosal flaps diminishes the risk of postoperative reclosure [16].

Aspects in Revision Surgery

In revision surgery an endonasal approach for opening the frontal sinus might be very difficult due to the loss of important landmarks such as the middle turbinate, as well as thick scar layers and neo-osteogenesis. Circumscript opening of the frontal sinus via a short skin incision at the medial eye brow with illumination of the frontal sinus or application of fluorescein solution may facilitate endonasal opening following the diaphanoscopy or fluorescein signal [13]. For endonasal management of frontal sinus obstruction after middle turbinate resection, the frontal sinus rescue procedure has been recommended [2]. After removal of the frontal sinus stenosis, a small mucoperiosteal flap is placed on the denuded region of the frontal neo-ostium.

Frontal Sinus Stenting

Frontal sinus stenting has been recommended to increase long-term patency rates. However, use of this procedure remains a matter of debate, and accepted indications for postoperative stenting of the frontal sinus outflow tract are lacking. Reported indications for frontals sinus stenting include a frontal sinus neo-ostium diameter less than 5 mm, situations of extensive or circumferential exposure of bone, polyposis/allergic fungal sinusitis, flail/lateralized middle turbinate, and frontal sinus revision surgery [7].

Postoperative Care

The need for nasal packing depends on the extent of surgery. If the mucosa has almost completely been preserved and a nearly bloodless field is found at the end of surgery, nasal packing might not be necessary. Nasal packing for 2–3 days is used for hemostasis and cases of limited mucosal injury. In the case of major mucosal removal (e.g., in extended frontal sinus drainage where the drill has been used for widening), an even more prolonged nasal packing is necessary. For frontal sinus drainage type IIb and type III it is recommended to place rubber fingers into the created drainage. This nasal packing stimulates the reepithelialization of the bar bone, thereby reducing the risk of frontal sinus drainage reclosure. Nasal packing should be removed 5 days after type IIb drainage and 7 days after type III drainage.

The extent of postoperative care in terms of crust removal depends on the surgical strategy that was been selected for frontal sinus management. In this context it is important to mention that removal of crusts intends to avoid reclosure of the drainage. However, cleaning may induce new injuries, with the formation of granulation tissue and removal of new epithelium. Thus, the frequency of mechanical cleaning of the frontal sinus drainage depends on the individual situation. Nevertheless, it has become clear that daily mechanical cleanings are not as beneficial as has been thought for a long time. Indeed, a first, careful cleaning 1 week after surgery might be sufficient in cases of mainly preserved mucosa.

Similar to other paranasal sinuses, nasal irrigations by the patients as well as medical treatments determined by the pathology are indicated after frontal sinus surgery. Topical corticosteroid application has been found to have a favorable effect, with reduction of swelling and faster healing [6]. Use of systemic corticosteroids after surgery in cases of severe nasal polyposis is not uncommon, yet without general acceptance. Furthermore, there are various regimes of systemic postoperative corticosteroid medication in terms of different durations, dosages, and drugs being used. Postoperative antibiotics have been recommended after extended frontal sinus drainage with the first nasal packing. Further indications for postoperative antibiotics are based only on individual findings. Adaptive desensitization after surgery as part of a whole treatment concept in patients suffering from acetylsalicylic acid triad should also be considered (see Chap. 57).

Summary

Frontal sinus surgery is one of the most challenging topics in endonasal surgery. It requires thorough anatomical knowledge, a precise analysis of the CT findings, and a meticulous preparation technique. Due to the high variability of different cell configurations within the frontal recess, frontal sinus surgery demands an individual approach in every patient. Initial surgical interventions to resolve frontal sinus drainage problems should carefully take the physiological and pathological conditions into account, aiming to preserve as far as possible the mucosal lining of the frontal sinus drainage. If needed, extended frontal sinus drainage can be achieved endonasally with high success rates. The option of an enlarged frontal sinus opening enables today's rhinologist to approach the vast majority of frontal sinus pathologies endonasally, thus decreasing the need for external approaches.

Tips to Avoid Complications

- Have a close cooperation with the radiologist so that CT scans are available that provide the best information on the individual anatomy of the patient.
- Limit as far as possible mucosal injury within the confines of the frontal recess.
- Maximal mucosal decongestion and maximal reduction of bleeding by repeated placement of epinephrine-soaked pledgets is beneficial for the best possible intraoperative orientation.
- Ensure complete anterior ethmoidectomy following the concept of frontal recess exposure for frontal sinus drainage.
- Specialized instrumentation greatly facilitates the preparation within the frontal recess.
- Avoid destabilization of the middle turbinate to prevent middle-turbinate lateralization.
- Clear identification of the first olfactory fiber is helpful for achieving maximal frontal sinus drainage.
- Adequate removal of the upper nasal septum is mandatory for successful frontal sinus type III drainage.
- Nasal packing for 1 week and mucosal grafts to cover free bone are valuable to ensure stable opening after frontal sinus type III drainage.

Take-Home Pearls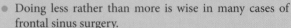

- Doing less rather than more is wise in many cases of frontal sinus surgery.
- Secondary affections of the frontal sinus frequently resolve after removal of the ethmoidal obstruction.
- Complete dissection of obstructing cells like agger nasi and frontal recess cells with wide exposure of the frontal recess may ensure frontal sinus drainage.

- Always intend to preserve as much of the natural mucosal lining as possible, as this is a keystone for successful frontal sinus drainage.
- If necessary, wide frontal sinus drainage can be achieved endonasally with high success rates, thus decreasing the number of external frontal sinus procedures.
- Frontal sinus type III drainage enables the surgeon to work transnasally at the area of the inferior posterior frontal sinus wall, medially to a sagittal plane through the lamina papyracea.

References

1. Chiu AG, Kennedy DW (2005) Revision endoscopic frontal sinus surgery. In: Kountakis S, Senior B, Draf W (eds) The Frontal Sinus. Springer, Berlin Heidelberg New York, pp 191–199
2. Citardi MJ, Batra PS, Kuhn FA (2005) Frontal sinus rescue. In: Kountakis S, Senior B, Draf W (eds) The Frontal Sinus. Springer, Berlin Heidelberg New York, pp 243–249
3. Draf W (1991) Endonasal micro-endoscopic frontal sinus surgery: the Fulda concept. Oper Tech Otolaryngol Head Neck Surg 2:234–240
4. Draf W, Weber R, Keerl R, Constantinidis J, Schick B, Saha A (2000) Endonasal and external micro-endoscopic surgery of the frontal sinus. In: Stamm AC, Draf W (eds) Micro-Endoscopic Surgery of the Paranasal Sinuses and the Skull Base. Springer, Berlin Heidelberg New York, pp 255–278
5. Draf W (2005) Endonasal frontal sinus drainage type I–III according to Draf. In: Kountakis S, Senior B, Draf W (eds) The Frontal Sinus. Springer, Berlin Heidelberg New York, pp 219–232
6. Hosemann WG, Weber RK, Keerl RE, Lund VJ (2000) Minimally Invasive Endonasal Sinus Surgery. Principles, Techniques, Results, Complications, Revision Surgery. Thieme, Stuttgart New York
7. Kanowitz SJ, Jacobs JB, Lebowitz RA (2005) Frontal sinus stenting. In: Kountakis S, Senior B, Draf W (eds) The Frontal Sinus. Springer, Berlin Heidelberg New York, pp 261–266
8. Karanfilov BI, Kuhn FA (2005) The endoscopic frontal recess approach. In: Kountakis S, Senior B, Draf W (eds) The Frontal Sinus. Springer, Berlin Heidelberg New York, pp 179–189
9. Kennedy DW (1992) Prognostic factors, outcomes and staging in ethmoid sinus surgery. Laryngoscope 102:1–18
10. Kuhn FA (1996) Chronic frontal sinusitis: the endoscopic frontal recess approach. Oper Tech Otolaryngol Head Neck Surg 7:222–229
11. May M, Schaitkin B (1995) Frontal sinus surgery: endonasal drainage instead of an external osteoplastic approach. Oper Tech Otolaryngol Head Neck Surg 6:184–192
12. Messerklinger W (1967) On the drainage of the normal frontal sinus of man. Acta Otolaryngol 63:176–181
13. Simmen D, Jones N (2005) Manual of Endoscopic Sinus Surgery and its Extended Applications. Thieme, Stuttgart New York
14. Stammberger H (2001) FESS – "Uncapping the Egg" – The Endoscopic Approach to Frontal Recess and Sinuses. A Surgical Technique of the Graz University Medical School. Endo-Press, Tuttlingen
15. Stankiewicz JA, Chow JM (2005) The fontal sinus and nasal polyps. In: Kountakis S, Senior B, Draf W (eds) The Frontal Sinus. Springer, Berlin Heidelberg New York, pp 87–93
16. Stennert E (2001) Rhino-frontal sinuseptotomy (RFS): a combined intra-extra nasal approach for the surgical treatment of severely diseased frontal sinuses. Laryngoscope 111:1237–1245
17. Wormald PJ (2005) Surgery of the frontal recess and frontal sinus. Rhinology 43:82–85

Chapter 53

The Sphenoid Sinus

Paolo Castelnuovo, Francesca De Bernardi,
Giorgio Minonzio, Giovanni Delù, and Maurizio Bignami

Core Messages

- The sphenoid sinus, known in the past as the "neglected sinus" [30], has attracted growing attention over the past 10 years due to the development of diagnostic techniques, the innovation of selective endonasal endoscopic approaches to the sinus itself and to the latest advancement in surgery, which foresees using the sphenoid sinus as the gateway to the sellar area and to the middle and posterior skull base.

- Improved diagnostic techniques. The routine use of nasal endoscopy, computed tomography scans and magnetic resonance imaging has increased the number of diagnoses of sphenoid disease [4, 7, 9, 10, 16, 19, 28]. Early diagnosis is fundamental because the presenting symptoms are both poor and non-specific, and often diagnosis is made after the arousal of a complication, due for instance to bone erosion involving the surrounding structures [9]. The possible complications can be very serious; in fact, the sphenoid sinus is strictly related to important and vulnerable structures such as the pituitary gland, the optic nerves, the cavernous sinuses, the internal carotid arteries, and cranial nerves III, IV, V and VI [16].

- Improved surgical techniques. The classic approach to this region was aggressive and disfiguring. The development of intranasal endoscopic techniques offers a practical alternative to the traditional methods; the endoscopic approach allows direct access to the sphenoid sinus while preserving other nearby anatomical structures and, furthermore, being an easier and quicker surgical manoeuvre it is able to prevent the complications that may arise with the sphenoid disease [7, 9, 10, 17–19, 22].

- Surgical access to the skull base. Endoscopic surgery on the middle and posterior skull base is becoming increasingly refined and the sphenoid sinus is the chief anatomical structure for the various approaches to the skull base [5, 6, 10, 11, 13, 14, 21, 22, 27].

Contents

Radiology

Radiological diagnosis of intrinsic lesions or those that have extended to the nearby sphenoid sinus is reached principally through computed tomography (CT) scans and magnetic resonance (MR) images, in a manner similar to that used for other sinus and skull-base structures [20,29]. The CT scan, using the basic screening method without contrast medium, should be examined first of all to assess the bone walls, differentiating normal aspects and anatomical variations from four fundamental types of pathological variation: thickening (chronic sinusitis, fibrous dysplasia); thickening with diffuse areas of reabsorption (chronic osteomyelitis); thinning with swelling (mucocele); various forms of destruction nearly always associated with a mass (tumours in general). The cavity is then examined to see if it is normally aerated, partially aerated or totally opaque, relating these aspects to those found in the walls. When suspecting the presence of tumour tissue, it is essential to investigate further by means of MR; according to whatever emerges from the images acquired, this will be either basal or, more frequently, with paramagnetic contrast.

In cases of acute inflammation in the sinus, the only radiological sign (immediately noticeable in the CT scan) is the presence of an air-fluid level (differential diagnosis with pseudolevels from cystic components or haemosinus) with no mass obstructing the ostium.

In specifically chronic inflammatory diseases (of any nature), the aforementioned signs on the bone walls are associated with mucoperiosteal thickening and often with polyps that are not distinguishable on the CT scan. In the majority of cases, the use of contrast medium in both CT scanning and MR imaging facilitates defining the profile by means of the enhanced images that emerge exclusively in the peripheral portions of the polyps.

Mucous cysts, although found most frequently in the maxillary sinus, are nevertheless also possible in the sphenoid and are easily recognisable with MR on the grounds of the type of liquid they contain.

In this area, which is the lateral or pterygoid recess of the sphenoid, differential diagnosis between a mucous cyst and a meningocele is performed using MR imaging in T2-weighted fluid-attenuated inversion-recovery (FLAIR) sequence. In this sequence, the mucous cyst maintains the hyperintense signal typical of liquids, while the meningocele shows a hypointense signal secondary to the suppression of the liquor signal typical of the FLAIR sequence (Fig. 53.1). In cases of intrasphenoid meningocele in which the site of the leakage is located in the lateral parasellar portions, the bone defect must be accurately assessed in order to consider a persistence of the lateral cranial-pharyngeal canal (Sternberg's canal). In these cases, the nature of the defect is to be considered congenital since it is situated at a point where primordial sphenoid portions fuse and where it is highly unlikely that acquired defects can arise [8].

Certain secondary aspects consent differential diagnosis between aspecific chronic forms of inflammation and fungal forms (calcifications, dehydration typically distinguishable as an "iron-like" hyperdensity on the CT or extremely hypointense – "signal-void" – on T2-weighted MR).

In the invasive fungal forms there can also be signs of a destructive process on the walls that may complicate the morphological diagnostic approach even further, and for which acquisition of fat-saturation data with the aid of contrast medium are recommended, since there is a possibility of there being extensions into the adjacent anatomical structures through the perivascular venous route (Figs. 53.2 and 53.3). The most frequent complications arising from this type of diffusion are to be found intraorbitally and intracranially in the form of: orbital abscess and/or cellulitis, optic neuritis, meningitis, subdural abscess/empyema or cerebral abscess.

The possible presence of lymphomatoid components underlying an inflammatory process, usually with high cellularity and with high uptake of the contrast medium, might make diagnosis

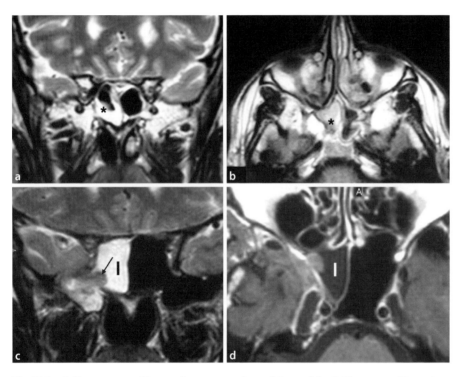

Fig. 53.1a–d The sequence of images demonstrates the usefulness of the fluid-attenuated inversion-recovery (FLAIR) sequence in magnetic resonance (MR) imaging for a differential diagnosis between a pathological lesion in the lateral sphenoidal recess and a meningocele/meningoencephalocele (with or without liquor in the sinus) originating in the Sternberg canal. a, b An inflammatory cyst in the lateral sphenoid recess with effusion and mucous hyperplasia in the sphenoid floor (*). In this case, the pathological tissue appears hyperintense both in the T2-weighted MR (a) and in the FLAIR sequence (b). c, d On the contrary, in the case of a Sternberg canal meningoencephalocele (arrow) with the sphenoid sinus filled with liquor (l), the typical hyperintensity of the T2-weighted MR (c) results seems to be diminished in the FLAIR sequence (d). Hypointensity at this point indicates the intrasphenoidal presence of cerebral tissue and liquor

53

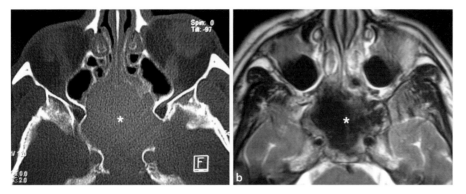

Fig. 53.2a,b Clinical case of extramucous eosinophilic mycosis (*). **a** Extensive lesion progressively destroying the skull base, with bone lysis of the superior clivus and the left lateral wall of the sinus. Slight hyperdensity is observed within the lesion. **b** T2-weighted MR scan revealing a vast area of poor signal within the lesion, typical of fungal dehydration (signal void). There is evident invasion of the lesion into the left cavernous sinus

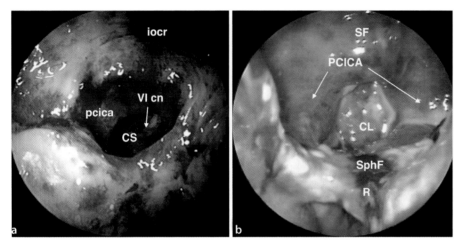

Fig. 53.3a,b Endoscopic images, 45°, 4 mm. **a** image of the sphenoid sinus during surgery after removal of the mycotic lesion, showing erosion and devascularisation of the left cavernous sinus (*CS*) and exposure of the VI cranial nerve (*VI cn*). **b** Control endoscopy 20 days after surgery. The interior of the sphenoid sinus appears free of disease. *iocr* Interoptic carotid recess, *pcica* paraclival internal carotid artery, *CL* clivus, *SF* sellar floor, *SphF* sphenoid floor, *R* sphenoid rostrum

even more difficult, but it is highly unusual to see this in the sphenoid.

The aforementioned bone signs indicating a slowly expanding mucocele are associated with MR images that vary according to a continuous spectrum that is linked with the progressive increase in the protein content (with reduced fluidity), which goes from an initial status (fluid) with hyperdensity in T1 (hyperproteinaemia) and in T2 (prevalently aqueous; Fig. 53.4) to a status of significant thickening with extreme reduction in the signal in T1 and in T2. In this latter case, the association of the two methods of investigation is very important to enable exclusion of the false-negatives – pseudonormoaeration – that may

result with MR on its own. The differential diagnosis of the mucocele can be with mixed forms or forms of allergic sinusitis or expansive polyps on the bone. Certain tumour forms can mimic a mucocele; however, a non-infected mucocele never takes up contrast medium. A CT scan can be useful for confirming what an MR has revealed, and it can show the hyperdensity corresponding to advanced forms of dehydration of the mucocele contents.

Some of the lesions that mimic the appearance of a tumour (e.g. granulomatosis, necrotising vasculitis) generally have some form of nasosinusal involvement, and in this respect it is advisable to always assess the facial mass as a whole rather than

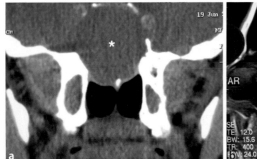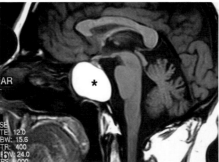

Fig. 53.4a, b Clinical case of a sphenoid mucocele (*). **a** Coronal computed tomography (CT) scan with intermediate algorithm setting showing an alteration of slow and regular expansion in the sphenoid cavity, the interior of which is slightly but homogeneously hypodense; convexity and lysis of the osseous walls of the sinus. **b** Sagittal MR image in basal T1: diagnosis of mucocele with diffuse hyperintensity (considering the protein content of a significantly fluid mucocele)

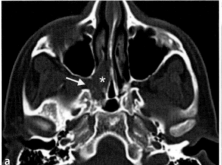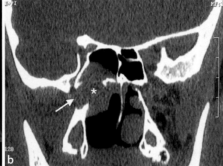

Fig. 53.5a, b Clinical case of a juvenile angiofibroma (*). **a** Axial view CT scan clearly showing the characteristic enlargement of the sphenopalatine foramen (*arrow*) caused by the angiofibroma. **b** The erosion caused by the lesion and its invasion of the sphenoid floor and the base of the pterygoid process can be seen in this coronal view

acquire images of the sphenoid selected from excessively segmental studies (e.g. sellar MR in coronal view).

In tumour investigation, the first step in imaging diagnostics is to establish the starting point of a lesion, followed by collection of information useful for classifying it as either benign or malignant.

In cases of benign tumours it must be remembered that angiofibromas extend as far as the sphenoid sinus in 60% of cases and that their diagnosis – generally well defined in the first images because of the presence of multiple "flow void" areas and due to their significant uptake of contrast medium – is angiographically typical, showing a capillary reticulum fed by the distal branches of the internal maxillary, but in the case of extension to the skull base this is fed by the Vidian artery and by the inferolateral trunk.

The origin is typically at the margin of the sphenopalatine foramen and penetration in the pterygopalatine fossa occurs early (seen in about 90% of cases at the time of diagnosis). Consequently, the progressive expansion between foramen and fossa is nearly always detected with the CT scan (Fig. 53.5). It is reported that in over half of cases, the sphenoid is reached through the nasopharyngeal roof.

The differential diagnosis of an intrasinusal haemangiopericytoma must nevertheless also take into account the protrusions of residual bone as well as typicality according to the age range.

An inverted papilloma can reach the sphenoid in 10–20% of cases and can be classified not only by the first endoscopic and imaging investigations performed, but also because of particular MR signs (T2 with cerebriform aspects, however, are more commonly seen in the maxillary area; Fig. 53.6).

Of the sinusal lesions that originate in the bone, osteomas are more rarely found in the sphenoid sinus than in the frontoethmoid area. These are easily distinguishable on a CT scan, although MR investigation can give significant results if the in-

53

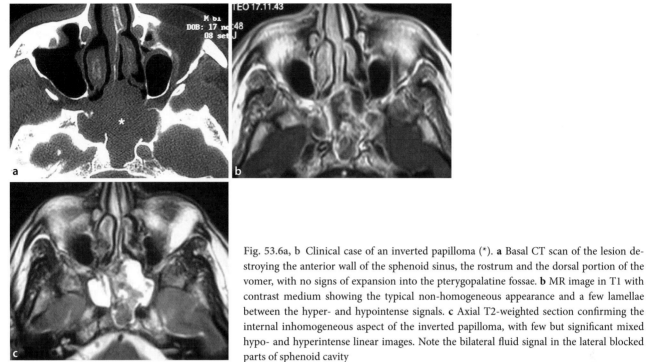

Fig. 53.6a, b Clinical case of an inverted papilloma (*). **a** Basal CT scan of the lesion destroying the anterior wall of the sphenoid sinus, the rostrum and the dorsal portion of the vomer, with no signs of expansion into the pterygopalatine fossae. **b** MR image in T1 with contrast medium showing the typical non-homogeneous appearance and a few lamellae between the hyper- and hypointense signals. **c** Axial T2-weighted section confirming the internal inhomogeneous aspect of the inverted papilloma, with few but significant mixed hypo- and hyperintense linear images. Note the bilateral fluid signal in the lateral blocked parts of sphenoid cavity

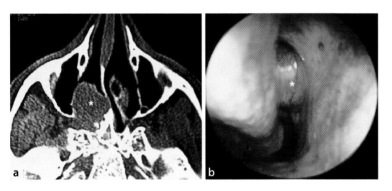

Fig. 53.7a, b Clinical case of a sphenoid chondrosarcoma (*). **a** Basal axial CT scan showing a mass situated in the basisphenoid area, similar to an angiofibroma but with signs of aggressive erosion and a few rather typical calcifications. **b** Diagnostic endoscopic image, 0°, 4 mm, revealing the tumour occupying the right sphenoid-ethmoid recess and covered with apparently undamaged mucosa

tracranial growth is sufficient for defining the meningeal planes. A differential diagnosis to exclude fibrous dysplasia does not require the use of a contrast medium and the latter is distinguished principally by its overall appearance, being more "swollen", even in the monostotic forms, and by its matrix looking like "sandpaper" (although this can vary).

The typical starting points of a chondrosarcoma are the petrous-clival fissure and the vomer–sphenoid junction; it can reach the sphenoid cavity from both of these sites. Its characteristic feature in a basal CT scan is the presence of chondroid or annular calcifications in a hypodense, lobulated and progressively osteodestructive matrix with precise borders (Fig. 53.7). The MR aspects are non-specific, either with or without contrast medium, because of the low vascularity of the lesion, and the various differential diagnoses are with not only primitive bone lesions (e.g. chordoma), but also with metastases or with lesions that have expanded to nearby structures. Squamous cell carcinomas, as well as the adenocarcinomatous and non-differentiated forms, rarely start in the sphenoid, but they must always be considered when performing differential diagnosis because of the possibility of there being an underlying lesion of another nature. In these cases, it is essential to use fat-saturation sequences to be able to discover any perineuronal extensions.

How to Do it

For many years, surgical access to the sphenoid sinus was problematic. The most popular technique was the sublabial transseptal approach; other routes were the transethmoidal and transpalatal approaches [4, 15, 16]. The external fronto-orbital approach to this region was aggressive and sometimes disfiguring, hence the ever-growing interest in endoscopic intranasal techniques,

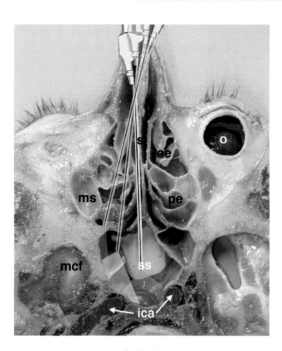

Fig. 53.8 Axial section of a fresh anatomical preparation showing how the three approaches to the sphenoid sinus allow lateral expansion of the surgical field (paraseptal – *green*, transethmoid – *yellow*, transethmoid-pterygoid – *blue*) as far as a complete view of the lateral sphenoid recess and the base of the middle cranial fossa. *mcf* Middle cranial fossa, *ae* anterior ethmoid, *pe* posterior ethmoid, *ss* sphenoid sinus, *ica* internal carotid artery, *ms* maxillary sinus, *o* orbit

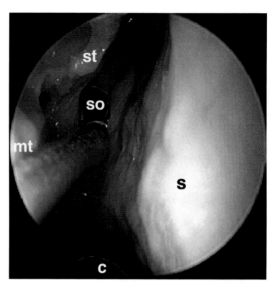

Fig. 53.9 Endoscopic image, 4 mm, 0°, anatomical dissection. The paraseptal approach to the sphenoid sinus enables the identification of its natural ostium medially to the tail of the superior turbinate (the tail of which is partially sectioned here) and widening it with sharp cutting instruments. The *dashed blue line* indicates the superior choanal margin. *c* Choana, *S* nasal septum, *mt* tail of the middle turbinate, *SO* sphenoidal ostium, *st* superior turbinate

which offer a practical alternative to the classic approaches. The endoscopic approach allows direct access to the sphenoid sinus while preserving other anatomical structures; the endoscope also permits the assessment of the lateral walls of the sphenoid sinus, given the possibility of lateral viewing (30°, 45°, 70° scopes). Moreover, in experienced hands, this surgical technique offers reduced operating time, minimal loss of blood, decrease in morbidity and shorter post-operative hospitalisation [10].

The transnasal endoscopic approaches to the sphenoid sinus are (Fig. 53.8):

1. The direct paraseptal approach.
2. The transethmoid approach.
3. The transethmoid-pterygoid-sphenoid approach [1, 2, 8, 17, 23, 26].

The choice of the type of approach depends upon the nature and the extension of the disease involving the sphenoid sinus. Isolated diseases (about 2–3% of the sinus lesions) [3,10] are preferably treated with the paraseptal approach direct to the sphenoid sinus, plurisinusal diseases with the transethmoid approach, and conditions involving the lateral wall of the sphenoid sinus require the transethmoid-pterygoid-sphenoid approach [9, 12, 25].

The Direct Paraseptal Approach

The sphenoid sinus can be reached through a direct transnasal paraseptal surgical approach; a 0° optic device 4 mm in diameter is used. In patients with a wide sphenoid-ethmoid recess and a non-pneumatised rostral sphenoid, the natural ostium of the sphenoid sinus is easily detected. A pre-surgery CT scan, performed with axial projection on the sphenoid ostia, will reveal the presence of a wide ethmoid-sphenoid recess and will show the strictly median position of the ostia themselves. The surgical access proceeds parallel to the nasal septum and to the nasal floor, with the medial margin of the inferior turbinate as the lateral landmark and the superior margin of the choana as the supradorsal landmark. When this latter point has been reached, the approach continues upwards, following the medial margins of the tails of the ethmoid turbinates (middle, superior and supreme). The sphenoid ostium is to be seen medially to the tail of the superior or supreme turbinate and is widened by centrifuging with circular clamp forceps or with Citelli forceps, or even with an intranasal drill (Fig. 53.9).

It is difficult to detect the sphenoid ostium in patients with a narrow sphenoethmoid recess and a pneumatised sphenoid rostrum. A pre-operative CT scan, performed with an axial

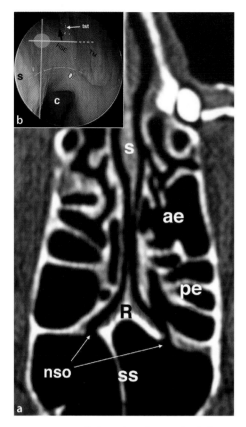

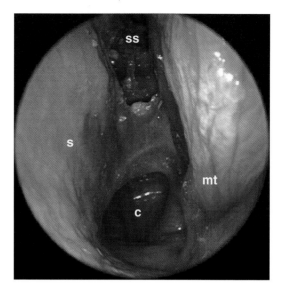

Fig. 53.11 Endoscopic image, 4 mm, 0°, anatomical dissection. In cases when the pneumatisation of the sphenoidal nostrum lateralises the lateral sphenoidal ostia, the sphenoid sinus can be accessed by milling the rostrum at the aforementioned safety point. The image shows the sphenoid sinus after its aperture. *mt* Middle turbinate, *s* nasal septum, *ss* sphenoid sinus, *c* choana

Fig. 53.10 **a** Radiological axial image (CT) showing pneumatisation of the sphenoid rostrum, with lateralisation of the natural sphenoid ostium. **b** Endoscopic image, 4 mm, 0°, left nasal fossa. The safety point for the transrostral paraseptal aperture of the sphenoid sinus (*orange area*) lies on the point where the line parallel to the medial choana margin (*green line*) joins the line parallel to the tail of the superior turbinate (*yellow line*). Projection of the septal branch of the sphenopalatine artery (*light blue broken line*). *s* Nasal septum, *ae* anterior ethmoid, *pe* posterior ethmoid, *R* sphenoidal rostrum, *ss* sphenoid sinus, *nso* natural sphenoidal ostium, *C* choana, *TM* tail of the middle turbinate, *tst* tail of the superior turbinate, *RSE* sphenoethmoidal recess

projection on the sphenoid ostia, will show the presence of a lateral protrusion of the sphenoid rostrum with a cleft-shaped sphenoethmoid recess and the ostia themselves in a very lateral position (Fig. 53.10a). In this case, to access the sphenoid sinus it will be useful to drill the rostrum at the safety point where two lines unite: the vertical one parallel to the interchoanal septum and the horizontal one parallel to the tail of the superior turbinate. In this manner, the sinus can be penetrated in a median position farthest away from the cavernous and paraclival internal carotid artery and the optic nerve, which are vital structures. Furthermore, the use of this intersection of the two lines as the point of access will avoid damaging the septal branch of the sphenopalatine artery, which, after emerging from the tail of the superior turbinate, runs through the sphenoethmoid recess and reaches the septum, following a curved line (see Chap. 44), parallel to the superior choanal margin (Fig. 53.10b). In this

case, the natural ostium of the sphenoid sinus is lateral to the sagittal portion of the basal lamina of the superior turbinate, although it still remains medial to the point where the superior turbinate inserts.

CT scanning thus allows an analysis of the degree of lateral shifting of the ostia and consequently of the difficulties that may be encountered with direct access to them. The type of approach can be then decided upon, conserving the integrity of the posterior ethmoid and the olfactory neuroepithelium (Fig. 53.11).

If the disease is seen to involve both sphenoid sinuses, the same type of approach can be performed contralaterally and the procedure can be continued using both nasal fossae. From this moment on, it will be useful to have the collaboration of a second operator who can irrigate and aspirate simultaneously in order to keep the surgical field as free as possible of blood, and perhaps assist the first operator by holding the endoscope so that he can use both hands (thus the "four-hands" technique; Fig. 53.12). The technique involves removing the anterior wall of the sphenoid sinus completely, uniting the two sinusal ostia and removing the intersphenoid septum. The same surgical procedure is used for accessing the sellar region [10].

Indications

1. Isolated sphenoid sinus diseases (chronic rhinosinusitis, mycosis, mucocele, benign tumours, liquoral fistula of the sella floor or of the median clivus).
2. Expansive lesions invading the sellar region.

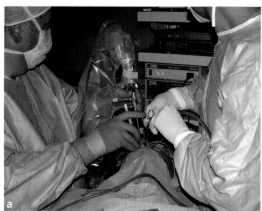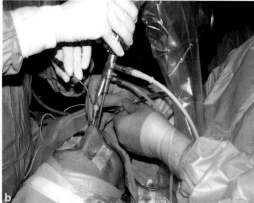

Fig. 53.12a,b These external images illustrate the versatility of the four-hands technique, during which the first operator can hold the endoscope by himself (**a**) or use two surgical instruments at the same time (**b**) and leave the endoscope to be held by the second operator

Risks

1. CSF-leak caused by interruption of the skull base at the posterior third of the olfactory cleft.
2. Hyposmia caused by damage to the olfactory neuroepithelium.
3. Damage to the optic nerve.
4. Damage to the paraclival or cavernous internal carotid artery.

Tips to Avoid Complications

- Identification of the surgical landmarks prevents losing one's bearings and reduces the risk of complications. The landmarks for this approach are: the choanal margin, protrusion of the sphenoid rostrum, the tail of the superior turbinate and the sphenoid ostium.
- The use of appropriate instruments allows greater surgical precision. Circular clamp forceps permit centrifugal widening of the sphenoidotomy. Instruments capable of removing greater quantities of bone should be used, such as Citelli forceps or an intranasal drill with sharp mills for removing the sphenoid rostrum.
- Bleeding from the septal branch of the sphenopalatine artery can be avoided by electrocoagulating the area under the tail of the superior turbinate with bipolar forceps.

53

The Transethmoidal Approach

This approach involves entering the middle meatus, laterally to the middle turbinate, and removing the second portion of the middle turbinate (frontal portion). In the case of plurisinusal dis-

ease, the patency of all sinusal ostia has to be obtained. Complete uncinectomy, removal of the ethmoid bulla and aperture of both the frontal recess and the natural ostium are also performed.

In conditions that do not involve the anterior ethmoid, it is possible to preserve the uncinate process and either partially or completely the ethmoid bulla. When removing the second portion of the middle turbinate, care should be taken to avoid injuring the first and third portions, to maintain stability in the turbinate. The next step is detection of the free inferior margin of the superior turbinate. The turbinate is gently lateralised, allowing visualisation of the sphenoid ostium. After cutting the caudal portion of the superior turbinate, the sinusal ostium is widened with circular clamp forceps. The anterior wall of the sphenoid sinus is then completely removed (Fig. 53.13a, b) [9, 10].

If a four-handed procedure in the sphenoid sinus is required, a direct paraseptal approach is performed contralaterally. The contralateral insertion of instruments allows wider movements with the endoscope, a better view of the surgical field, a three-dimensional orientation of the field and a broader view of the sphenoid-ethmoid region. The use of a 45° angled optic device permits visualisation and checking the instruments that have been inserted, even on the contralateral side, and in this manner the endoscope can be used even through the paraseptum (Fig. 53.14) [10].

Indications

1. Chronic ethmosphenoid rhinosinusitis (bacterial and mycotic).
2. Plurisinusal polyposis.
3. Optic nerve decompression [24].
4. Benign ethmosphenoid tumours.
5. Malignant tumours that do not infiltrate the lateral or posterior walls of the sphenoid sinus.
6. The centripetal multilayer technique is used when removing the lesions [7].

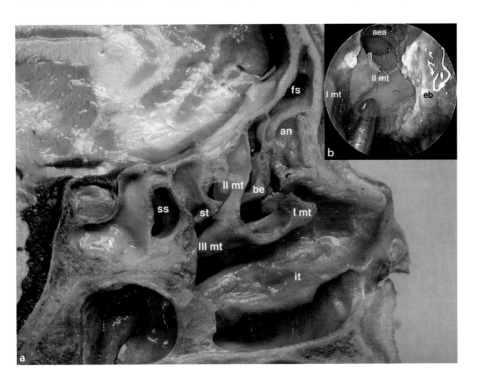

Fig. 53.13a,b Sagittal section of a fresh anatomical preparation showing the anatomy of the left lateral nasal wall. **a** The *blue line* indicates the second portion of the middle turbinate (which enters the lamina papyracea laterally, and which separates the anterior ethmoid from the posterior ethmoid) that must be removed to be able to reach the posterior ethmoid endoscopically via the transethmoidal route. **b** endoscopic image, 0°, 4 mm. After uncinotomy and aperture of the ethmoidal bulla, it is possible to see the second portion of the middle turbinate (*blue area*), which has to be removed to reach the posterior ethmoid. The safety point for this aperture is situated inferomedially, where the three portions of the middle turbinate meet. *fs* Frontal sinus; *an* agger nasi; *eb* ethmoidal bulla; *it* inferior turbinate; *I mt, II mt, III mt* first, second and third portions of the middle turbinate, respectively; *st* superior turbinate; *ss* sphenoid sinus; *aea* anterior ethmoidal artery; *be* residue of the ethmoidal bulla

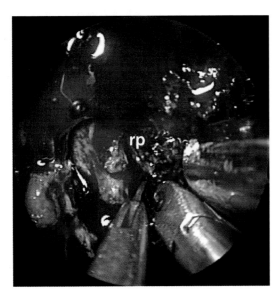

Fig. 53.14 Endoscopic image, 4 mm, 0°. During the debulking of a lesion in the rhinopharynx (*rp*), the endoscope, an aspirator, Veil forceps and a sharp cutting instrument can be seen in use simultaneously. The four-hands technique enables a clean surgical field to be maintained and allows complex surgical manoeuvres to be carried out, even within a small space

Risks

1. CSF-leak caused by interruption of the skull base at the posterior third of the olfactory cleft.
2. Hyposmia due to damage in the olfactory neuroepithelium.
3. Damage to the optic nerve.
4. Damage to the internal carotid artery.
5. Damage to the orbit causing diplopia, proptosis or amaurosis.

Tips to Avoid Complications

- The safe point for accessing the posterior ethmoid is the medial inferior angle that links the three portions of the middle turbinate.
- The safe points for accessing the sphenoid sinus are:
  1. The superior turbinate and its caudal portion, which should be cut with sharp instruments to avoid injuries.
  2. The natural ostium of the sphenoid sinus, which should be widened in a centrifugal manner.
- Pre-operative investigations carried out with CT scans and, in selected cases, with MR, allow the detection of any Onodi cells. This ethmoidal cell is recognisable in the successive axial scans observed in the caudal–cranial direction. The gradual reduction in pneumatisation in the sphenoid can then be seen, as well as the increased pneumatisation of the last cell of the posterior ethmoid (the Onodi cell) that goes beyond the sphenoid in a lateral and/or cranial direction. The following coronal projections should be observed in an anteroposterior direction to achieve a better view of the lateral or superior progression of the last ethmoid cell. In the coronal projection, the presence of either vertical or horizontal partitioning of the sphenoid can be seen. This is not to be confused with an intersphenoid septum; it is the lateral or superior wall of the sphenoid that separates it from the Onodi cell, which goes beyond it in a lateral or cranial direction (Fig. 53.15). A second important radiological investigation performed prior to surgery should distinguish the different forms of the sphenoid sinus: sellar, pre-sellar or conchal. These three types have different anatomical, endoscopic and radiological landmarks (Fig. 53.16). Morphological analysis will reveal the different position of the vital structures in the lateral wall of the sinus: optic nerve, and cavernous and paraclival internal carotid artery.

53

The Transethmoid-Pterygoid-Sphenoidal Approach

This approach is a lateral extension of the transethmoidal approach. A 0° optic telescope is used and both anteroposterior ethmosphenoidotomy and middle-meatus antrostomy are per-

formed in order to expose the posterior wall of the maxillary sinus, the anterior wall of the sphenoid sinus, the orbital apex area and the base of the pterygoid.

The site where both the nasal branch and the septal branch of the sphenopalatine artery emerge is identified and then electrocoagulated with bipolar forceps. The sphenopalatine foramen is then identified (see Chap. 44) and the pterygomaxillary fossa is opened, widening its foramen with Citelli forceps. The medial portion of the posterior wall of the maxillary sinus is then removed. Good lateral vision may be obtained with a 45° optic device. By lateralising the contents of the pterygomaxillary fossa, the Vidian foramen and the foramen rotundum can be seen. After electrocoagulation of the Vidian artery, the base of the pterygoid and the base of the sphenoid are drilled, especially at the bony margin that links the two ostia (Vidian and rotundum). In this manner it is possible to have a complete view of the pterygoid recess of the sphenoid, even if it is greatly pneumatised, and wide access to the floor of the middle cranial fossa (Fig. 53.17) [3, 8, 18].

In the four-handed technique, a direct paraseptal approach is performed contralaterally, milling the intersphenoid septum and sphenoid nostrum. Thereafter, a portion of the vomer, large enough to allow reaching the floor of the contralateral middle cranial fossa, is removed [10].

Indications

1. CSF-leak and encephalocele of the middle cranial fossa floor (persistence of the embryonal Sternberg canal; Fig. 53.18).
2. Diseases of the lateral recess of the sphenoid sinus.

Risks

1. CSF-leak due to interruption of the skull base at the olfactory cleft.
2. Hyposmia caused by damage to the olfactory neuroepithelium.
3. Damage to the optic nerve.
4. Damage to the internal carotid artery.
5. Damage to the rectus medialis muscle.

Tips to Avoid Complications

- The landmarks to look for are the posterior wall of the maxillary sinus, the Vidian foramen and the foramen rotundum, which should be identified to avoid damaging the optic nerve and the carotid artery.
- Preservation of the first portion of the middle turbinate and the cranial part of the basal lamina.

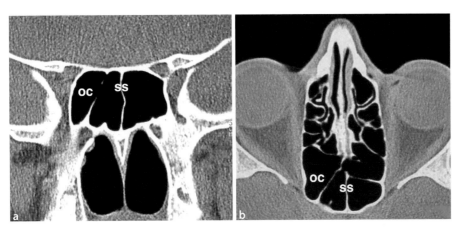

Fig. 53.15a,b Radiological image (CT) in coronal (a) and axial (b) views of the sphenoid sinus showing the presence of an Onodi cell on the right, which goes beyond the right sphenoid sinus laterally. *ss* Sphenoid sinus, *oc* Onodi cell

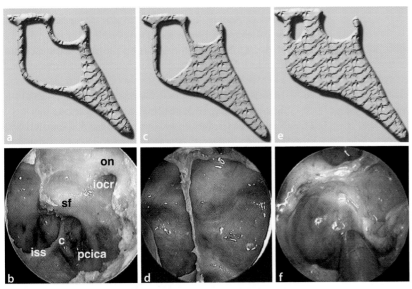

Fig. 53.16a–f The illustrations show sagittal sections of the different degrees of pneumatisation in sellar- (a), pre-sellar- (c) and conchal-type (e) sphenoid sinuses. The endoscopic images show the corresponding endoscopic areas in which the anatomical landmarks on the posterior sphenoid wall are always less visible (b, d, f). *sf* Sella floor, *on* optic nerve, *iocr* interoptic-carotid recess, *c* clivus, *iss* intersphenoidal septum, *pcica* paraclival internal carotid artery

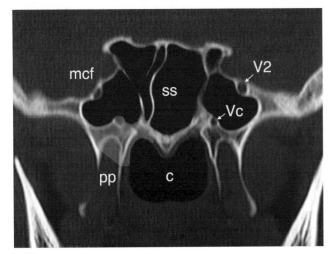

Fig. 53.17 Coronal view radiological image (CT) of the sphenoid sinus. This image demonstrates particularly pneumatised lateral sphenoidal recesses; in this case, the transethmoid-pterygoid endoscopic access to the lateral portion of the sphenoid sinus (*ss*) requires removal of the sphenoid floor an the base of the pterygoid process (*pp*); that is, the area highlighted in *blue*. *c* Choana, *Vc* Vidian canal, *V2* canal of the second branch of the fifth cranial nerve, *mcf* middle cranial fossa

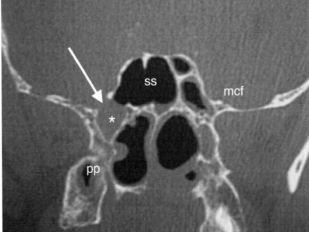

Fig. 53.18 Coronal view radiological image (CT) of the sphenoid sinus. This image shows, in the right lateral sphenoid recess area, a bone defect (indicated by the *arrow*) in the middle cranial fossa (*mcf*), with herniation of cerebral tissue inside the sphenoid sinus. This is the typical site of a meningoencephalocele in the Sternberg canal. *pp* Pterygoid process

Take-Home Pearls

- MR imaging, depending on how it is weighted (T1, T2, FLAIR, fat saturation), permits the differentiation of the various different diseases of the sphenoid sinus.
- Knowledge of radiological anatomy (CT and MR) is of fundamental importance for reducing the risks of iatrogenic damage during surgery.
- The different endoscopic endonasal approaches to the sphenoid sinus have revolutionised treatment for these diseases, guaranteeing reliable results and a significant reduction in morbidity.

References

1. Al-Nashar IS, Ismail S, Carrau RL, Herrera A, Snyderman CH (2004) Endoscopic transnasal transpterygopalatine fossa approach to the lateral recess of the sphenoid sinus. Laryngoscope 114:528–532
2. Bolger WE (2005) Endoscopic transpterygoid approach to the lateral sphenoid recess: surgical approach and clinical experience. Otolaryngol Head Neck Surg 133:20–26
3. Bolger WE, Osenbach R (1999) Endoscopic transpterygoid approach to the lateral sphenoid recess. Ear Nose Throat J 78:36–46
4. Cakmak O, Shohet MR, Kern EB (2000) Isolated sphenoid sinus lesions. Am J Rhinol 14:13–9
5. Cappabianca P, Cavallo LM, de Divitiis E (2004) Endoscopic endonasal transsphenoidal surgery. Neurosurgery 55:933–940; discussion 940–941
6. Carrau RL, Jho HD, Ko Y (1996) Transnasal-transsphenoidal endoscopic surgery of the pituitary. Laryngoscope 106:914–8
7. Castelnuovo P, Battaglia P, Locatelli D, Delù G, Sberze F, Bignami M (2006) Endonasal micro-endoscopic treatment of malignant tumors of the paranasal sinuses and anterior skull base. Oper Tech Otolaryngol Head Neck Surg 17:152–167
8. Castelnuovo P, Dallan I, Pistochini A, Battaglia P, Locatelli D, Bignami M (2007) Endonasal endoscopic repair of Sternberg's canal cerebrospinal fluid leaks. Laryngoscope 117:345–349
9. Castelnuovo P, Pagella F, Semino L, De Bernardi F, Delu G (2005) Endoscopic treatment of the isolated sphenoid sinus lesions. Eur Arch Otorhinolaryngol 262:142–147
10. Castelnuovo P, Pistochini A, Locatelli D (2006) Different surgical approaches to the sellar region: focus on the "two nostrils four hands technique". Rhinology 44:2–7
11. Cavallo LM, Messina A, Gardner P, Esposito F, Kassam AB, Cappabianca P, de Divitiis E, Tschabitscher M (2005) Endoscopic endonasal surgery of the midline skull base: anatomical study and clinical considerations. Neurosurg Focus 19:E2
12. Cheung DK, Martin GF, Rees J (1992) Surgical approaches to the sphenoid sinus. J Otolaryngol 21:1–8
13. Cohen NA, Kennedy DW (2005) Endoscopic sinus surgery: where we are – and where we're going. Curr Opin Otolaryngol Head Neck Surg 13:32–38
14. de Divitiis E (2006) Endoscopic transsphenoidal surgery: stone-in-the-pond effect. Neurosurgery 59:512–20; discussion 512–20
15. Doglietto F, Prevedello DM, Jane JA Jr, Han JA, Laws ER Jr (2005) A brief history of endoscopic transsphenoidal surgery – from Philipp Bozzini to the First World Congress of Endoscopic Skull Base Surgery. Neurosurg Focus 19:E3
16. Elwany S, Elsaeid I, Thabet H (1999) Endoscopic anatomy of the sphenoid sinus. J Laryngol Otol 113:122–126
17. Frank G, Pasquini E, Doglietto F, Mazzatenta D, Sciarretta V, Farneti G, Calbucci F (2006) The endoscopic extended transsphenoidal approach for craniopharyngiomas. Neurosurgery 59:ONS75–83; discussion ONS75–83
18. Frank G, Pasquini E, Mazzatenta D (2001) Extended transsphenoidal approach. J Neurosurg 95:917–918
19. Hadar T, Yaniv E, Shvero J (1996) Isolated sphenoid sinus changes – history, CT and endoscopic finding. J Laryngol Otol 110:850–853
20. Harnsberger HR, Hudgins P, Wiggins R, Davidson C (2004) Diagnostic Imaging Head and Neck. Amirsys, Salt Lake City
21. Kassam AB, Gardner P, Snyderman C, Mintz A, Carrau R (2005) Expanded endonasal approach: fully endoscopic, completely transnasal approach to the middle third of the clivus, petrous bone, middle cranial fossa, and infratemporal fossa. Neurosurg Focus 19:E6
22. Locatelli D, Castelnuovo P, Santi L, Cerniglia M, Maghnie M, Infuso L (2000) Endoscopic approaches to the cranial base: perspectives and realities. Childs Nerv Syst 16:686–691
23. Locatelli D, Rampa F, Acchiardi I, Bignami M, De Bernardi F, Castelnuovo P (2006) Endoscopic endonasal approaches for repair of CSF leaks: nine-year experience. Oper Neurosurg 58:246–257
24. Luxenberger W, Stammberger H, Jebeles JA, Walch C (1998) Endoscopic optic nerve decompression: the Graz experience. Laryngoscope 108:873–882
25. Metson R, Gliklich RE (1996) Endoscopic treatment of sphenoid sinusitis. Otolaryngol Head Neck Surg 114:736–744
26. Pasquini E, Sciarretta V, Farneti G, Mazzatenta D, Modugno GC, Frank G (2004) Endoscopic treatment of encephaloceles of the lateral wall of the sphenoid sinus. Minim Invasive Neurosurg 47:209–213
27. Rosen MR, Saigala K, Evans J, Keanea WM (2006) A review of the endoscopic approach to the pituitary through the sphenoid sinus. Curr Opin Otolaryngol Head Neck Surg 14:6–13
28. Sethi DS (1999) Isolated sphenoid lesions: diagnosis and management. Otolaryngol Head Neck Surg 120:730–736
29. Som PM, Curtin HD (2003) Head and Neck Imaging. Mosby, St. Louis
30. Van Alyea OE (1941) Sphenoid sinus: anatomic study, with consideration of the clinical significance of the structural characteristics of the sphenoid sinus. Arch Otolaryngol 34:225–253

Chapter 54

Complications of Endonasal Endoscopic Sinus Surgery

54

Amir Minovi, Bernhard Schick and Wolfgang Draf

Core Messages

- Every surgeon – even with long-term experience – should bear in mind that there is no simple sinus operation.
- A learning curve is observed for each individual sinus surgeon.
- For safe endonasal sinus surgery, careful preoperative analysis of radiological imaging is mandatory.
- Identification of defined anatomical landmarks during surgery is most important to prevent complications.
- Loss of landmarks in revision surgery increases surgical risk.
- Orbital haematoma with rapid loss of vision needs immediate orbital decompression (transnasal decompression, lateral canthotomy).
- If a cerebrospinal fluid fistula is discovered during the surgery it should be repaired immediately.
- Internal carotid artery and intracranial vessel injuries need interdisciplinary treatment (neurosurgeon, neuroradiologist).

Contents

Introduction

Endonasal surgery of the paranasal sinuses began near the beginning of the 20th century [6, 28]. However, catastrophic complications during endonasal surgery at this time, like skull-base injuries followed by meningitis, brain abscess and/or encephalitis, were life threatening in this preantibiotic area. Early in the 20th century, Mosher described, therefore endonasal ethmoid surgery as the most dangerous operation in all of surgery [21]. Thus, for many decades most surgeons favoured the external approach for paranasal sinus surgery, considering them to be associated with a lower risk for life-threatening complications. Better understanding of the landscape of the surgical area and the pathophysiology of the paranasal sinus mucosa played an important role in the renaissance of endonasal sinus surgery in the 1970s, with the development of new optical aids; namely, endoscopes and operating microscopes [3, 7, 20]. Nowadays, the principles of endonasal sinus surgery have been well established and the specific risks of endonasal surgery are well defined.

According to May et al. [18] minor and major complications can be distinguished in endonasal paranasal sinus surgery. Minor complications (incidence about 3%) are associated with little morbidity and are not followed by any significant sequelae for the patient. On the contrary, major complications (incidence about 0.5%) present significant morbidity, require in most situations urgent treatment and may be associated with catastrophic outcome for the patient (Table 54.1).

The paranasal sinuses present a complex anatomy surrounded by important structures, a situation that might be further complicated by severe paranasal pathologies. Therefore, even in the case of extensive surgical experience, complications may still occur. Several studies have been undertaken to measure the complication rates of sinus surgery, like the incidence of skull-base defects among large populations of patients. Weber et al. [34] analysed the complication rates in 1,178 patients who underwent endonasal ethmoidectomy. A dural lesion with cerebrospinal fluid (CSF) leak occurred in 2.5% of the patients. Findings from a later study [11], in which complications were analysed in 1,000 patients operated by 5 surgeons, revealed that a CSF leak occurred in 0.5% of the patients. The incidence of a specific complication may range in different series, and so ev-

Table 54.1 Classification of complications of endonasal sinus surgery, modified after May [18, 19]

Minor complications	Major complications
Periorbital emphysema	Epiphora requiring surgery
Bleeding into the lids	Loss of intact sense of smell
Bronchospasm	Haemorrhage requiring transfusion
Epistaxis requiring nasal packing	Cerebrospinal fluid leak
Dental or lip pain/numbness	Postoperative meningitis
Adhesions requiring treatment	Orbital haematoma
Postoperative atrophic rhinitis	Diplopia persistent for weeks/permanent
	Impairment or loss of vision
	Brain haemorrhage, cerebral abscess
	Injury to the carotid artery

ery surgeon should bear in mind that there is no simple sinus operation.

Complications may occur in every stage of experience in endonasal sinus surgery. However, a learning curve has to be considered in this respect. Three stages in the learning curve of sinus surgery have been hereby defined:

1. Stage I (surgeries 1–30): greatest risk of complication, with dural injury.
2. Stage II (surgeries 30–100): slighter risk of complication, with frequent periorbital injuries.
3. Stage III (surgery 100 onwards): least risk, corresponding to an experienced surgeon [10].

Nevertheless, it has been pointed out that serious complications occur most frequently among experienced surgeons [11].

Fortunately, major complications are rare. But with regard to the possible severity of complications, sinus surgery remains one of the most dangerous surgical treatments in otorhinolaryngology. Strategies to avoid complications and to deal with them properly in case of occurrence are highly warranted. This chapter will focus in detail on selected complications in endonasal sinus surgery.

Synechiae and Adhesions

The formation of synechiae is the most common sinus surgery complication and can be expected in 6–22% of cases despite adequate local aftercare. In most cases adhesion develops between the middle turbinate and the lateral nasal wall. Excessive removal of mucosa and manipulation in the area of frontal recess often results in adhesions, causing postoperative frontal sinusitis (see

Chap. 52). Approximately 15% of patients with synechiae need revision surgery [30]. If correction of a significant septal deviation was not performed in combination with the sinus surgery, a septoplasty should be done in revision surgery. For adhesions between the nasal septum and the turbinates, one can insert a silicone stent and leave it in place for 2 weeks. Postoperative care, with removal of crusts and frequent irrigation with a saline solution, reduces the chances of scar-tissue formation.

Nasolacrimal Duct

The bony cover of the nasolacrimal duct by the lacrimal bone can vary widely; it can be thick, thin or may be absent in single individuals. The least bony protection of the nasolacrimal duct is usually found superior to the inferior nasal turbinate. Injury to the nasolacrimal duct is mainly caused by extensive widening of the middle meatal antrostomy in the anterior direction (see Chap. 50). One should keep in mind that the attachment of the uncinate process indicates the nasolacrimal duct. Thus, middle meatus antrostomy should respect the attachment of the uncinate process. Injury of the nasolacrimal duct/sac may also occur during intended removal of agger nasi cells. In difficult situations it is advisable to expose the nasolacrimal sac, as this clear landmark allows definition of the anterior border of the ethmoidectomy. This strategy allows both avoidance of nasolacrimal duct injury and complete opening of the anterior ethmoid. Most injuries to the nasolacrimal duct resolve spontaneously; hence, it is possible to observe patients with epiphora initially in most situations (Fig. 54.1) [1, 26]. The treatment of choice in cases of extended permanent epiphora is endonasal dacryocystorhinostomy (see Chap. 58) [24, 29].

54

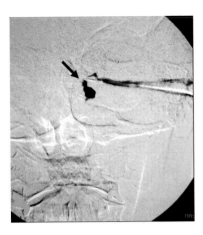

Fig. 54.1 Nasolacrimal duct injury leading to stenosis of the lacrimal sac. Dacryocystogram in anteroposterior projection after irrigation of the inferior lacrimal canaliculus with contrast medium: note the dacryocele and postsaccal stenosis (*arrow*) at Krause's valve

Orbital Complications

The close anatomical position of the orbit to the nose and paranasal sinuses makes it susceptible to surgical injury; injuries to the lamina papyracea, orbital haematoma, diplopia, and blindness have to be considered. In order to detect the possibility of serious orbital complication, the eyes should remain uncovered throughout the surgery and checked by the surgeon at the end of the operation. The assisting nurse should be instructed to observe the bulb when the surgeon is working close to the orbit. Observations by the assisting nurse like eye movements can indicate early manipulations at the lamina papyracea or periorbita.

Fracture or Perforation of the Lamina Papyracea

Fracture or perforation of the lamina papyracea during sinus surgery can lead to periorbital emphysema and ecchymosis. Periorbit emphysema usually occurs when the patient is awakened coughing and blowing the nose, permitting air to enter the soft tissues surrounding the orbit. The typical clinical sign of emphysema is a rustling of the soft tissue in the infraorbital region with a soft eye bulb and no decrease in vision. The emphysema is treated by simple observation and instructing patients not to blow their nose. The emphysema usually reabsorbs within 7–10 days [31].

In difficult anatomical situations the risk of injury to the lamina papyracea increases. In revision surgery and massive polyposis in particular, the lamina papyracea may be thinned out or partially dehiscent. One should further keep in mind that for a right-handed surgeon standing on the right side of the patient, there is a higher risk of perforating the lamina papyracea on the left side of the patient. Localised injury of the lamina papyracea is not a serious event. If perforation of the lamina papyracea has occurred, patients should be informed not to blow their nose in order to avoid postoperative emphysema. Furthermore, ointments containing petrolatum should not be used for nasal packing in these situations, as this could lead to microspherulocytosis/paraffingranuloma [10].

In cases of laceration of the periorbita, periorbital fat usually bulges out and can be identified by its yellow appearance. Performing the bulb-pressing test, which was developed by Draf and Stankiewicz [4, 31], can be helpful when there is suspicion of injury to the lamina papyracea and/or periorbita. Gentle application of pressure to the bulb leads to a corresponding movement of the periorbita if only the lamina papyracea is injured, or to protrusion of fat if the periorbita has been opened. It is important not to resect any herniated fat. If only a slight fat herniation is observed, this needs no further treatment. If orbital fat herniates extensively into the ethmoid, gentle replacement of the fat is performed and the large periorbital laceration sealed with connective tissue transplants. Postoperative antibiotic treatment has been recommended in these situations.

Orbital Haematoma

Orbital haematoma is caused mainly by penetration of the lamina papyracea and can occur whether or not the periorbita is injured. Orbital haemorrhage is caused most frequently by laceration of the orbital veins lining the lamina papyracea, and rarely by injury to the ethmoid arteries [32]. Lateral laceration of one of the ethmoid arteries, however, is a serious complication. The vessel may retract into the orbit, leading quickly to clinical signs and symptoms of retrobulbar haematoma. One should keep in mind that the location of the anterior ethmoid artery can vary markedly (see Chap. 44). This vessel may be placed in the skull base or below the skull base, a situation that is found when the ethmoid sinuses are more pneumatised. The degree of anterior ethmoid sinus pneumatisation, as an indicator of the risk of injury to the anterior ethmoidal artery, can be determined on preoperative computed tomography (CT) scans [27]. In the case of more pneumatised ethmoid sinuses in particular, the course of the ethmoid artery is even more directly evident below the skull base on the CT scans. If the course of the anterior ethmoidal artery is unclear during preparation at the frontal recess, it may be beneficial not to work along the border to the orbit. If the anterior ethmoidal artery is injured at this border the vessel may retract immediately into the orbit, not allowing the surgeon coagulation time. If the anterior ethmoidal artery is injured at some distance from the orbital border, more time is available to coagulate the artery, thus avoiding severe complications.

Rapid onset of an orbital haematoma develops, however, when a lacerated anterior ethmoid artery retracts into the orbit, becoming obvious as proptosis. Untreated orbital haematoma causes an increase in orbital pressure, which may lead to

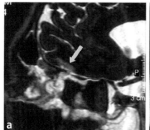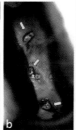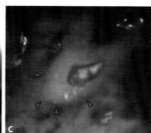

Fig. 54.2a–c Condition after laser polypectomy (elsewhere) with multiple cerebrospinal fluid leaks at the left posterior ethmoidal roof. **a** Magnetic resonance imaging in sagittal view showing a skull-base defect with liquor fistula (*yellow arrow*). **b** Intraoperative view: multiple defects along the skull base (*yellow arrows*). **c** Positive fluorescein test (*red arrows*) after injection of intrathecal sodium fluorescein

at least temporary visual impairment or blindness [22]. This is caused by a reduction in the vascular supply to the optic nerve, which is very sensitive to ischaemia. Therefore, an orbital haematoma has to be treated immediately to prevent permanent visual impairment or blindness. In this case, it is necessary to decrease immediately the intraorbital pressure. Removal of nasal packing, upraising of the upper body, medical treatment (azetazolamide, mannitol and cortisone) and surgical treatment are recommended. As a highly valuable surgical option, lateral canthotomy with inferior cantholysis and possible superior cantholysis allows immediate orbital decompression. Furthermore, transnasal orbital decompression with removal of the lamina papyracea and incision of the orbital periosteum should be considered. In addition, the patient should be examined by an ophthalmologist as part of his/her interdisciplinary treatment.

Diplopia

This is a major complication of sinus surgery that can be caused by injury to the ocular muscles that are located close to the sinuses, the medial rectus and superior oblique muscles. Most commonly the injury is caused to the medial rectus muscle, which runs just lateral to the periorbita at the centre of the lamina papyracea. It is important to know that the layer of intraorbital fat becomes thinner as one moves posteriorly, which means less protection of the medial rectus muscle. Damage to the medial rectus muscle frequently results in complicated strabismus and disturbing diplopia. The injury can be caused by direct laceration of either the muscle or its surrounding nervous and vascular supply. Spontaneous healing of mechanically injured muscles is rarely seen. Permanent diplopia is a very rare complication that needs neuro-ophthalmologic consultation and possible strabismus surgery [5, 23, 33].

Damage to the Optic Nerve

Direct damage to the optic nerve is less common than indirect injury via a retrobulbar haematoma. Typical high-risk areas for direct damage of the optic nerve are the sphenoid sinus and the posterior ethmoid (see Chap. 44), especially when there is extended pneumatisation in these areas [8]. Fortunately, direct optic nerve injury is extremely rare and only a few individual cases have been reported [2, 14, 15].

CSF Leak

CSF leak may occur by iatrogenic perforation of the skull base, especially in the area of the anterior ethmoid roof in the region of the lateral lamella of the cribriform plate (Fig. 54.2) or at the junction of the posterior ethmoid roof and the sphenoidal plane. Indeed, if the olfactory groove is very deep in relation to the ethmoidal roof (type III according to Keros) [13] there might be only a very thin bony border separating the olfactory groove from the ethmoidal cavity (see Chap. 44). The anterior half of the middle turbinate is an excellent landmark when performing dissection in the ethmoid region. One should always stay lateral to the middle turbinate, since further medial dissection may lead to a perforation of the cribriform plate, resulting in a CSF fistula. For a right-handed surgeon being placed on the right side of the patient, there is an increased risk of perforating the olfactory groove on the right side.

CSF leaks recognised intraoperatively should be closed immediately because of the risk of developing potentially fatal late meningitis. Endonasal duraplasty with the underlay or onlay technique can be used to close the fistula. The long-term results of immediate duraplasty are excellent [25]. Postoperative CT is strongly recommended to evaluate any possible intracranial injury that may need interdisciplinary cooperation with neurosurgery. If a CSF fistula first recognised after endonasal sinus surgery, CT is indicated before surgical exploration. Frontobasal skull base injuries should not generally be managed conservatively. A tight dura repair is required in most circumstances. A skull-base defect resulting from endonasal sinus surgery can almost always be closed using the endonasal approach.

Major Vessel Injury and Brain Haemorrhage

Injury to the major blood vessels, namely the internal carotid artery, and brain are extremely rare during sinus surgery. Injury to the internal carotid artery occurs most frequently during sphenoid sinus surgery. In 20% of the sphenoid sinuses the bony carotid canal may be dehiscent (see Chap. 44). Before opening the sphenoid sinus one must study the axial CT to look for a protruding internal carotid artery. The anterior wall of the sphenoid sinus is removed by working medially with downbiting and upbiting forceps. If it is possible to visualise the natural opening of the sphenoid sinus, this can be widened (see Chap. 53). Another very safe technique for opening the sphenoid sinus is us-

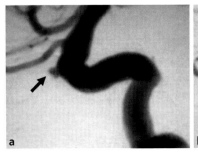
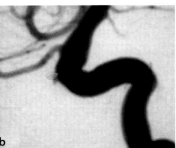

Fig. 54.3a, b Laceration of the internal carotid artery (ICA) in revision sinus surgery (elsewhere) after sphenoidotomy. **a** Angiography showing a false aneurysm (*arrow*) of the ICA. **b** Condition after successful embolisation

ing a drill. Close to the septum, the inferior part of the anterior sphenoid sinus wall can be opened with the drill approximately 1.5 cm above the choanal bridge. One should be very careful with surgical manipulations at the intersphenoidal septum. The septum sinuum sphenoidalium may be attached posteriorly to a thin carotid artery canal, hence removal of the septum requires cutting instruments or a diamond drill. One should not fracture the septum. This manoeuvre can lead to partial laceration of the carotid artery and development of false aneurysm, often occurring weeks or even months later [16].

Injury to the carotid artery is one of the least common, but one of the most catastrophic complications during sinus surgery and requires immediate treatment. In this case, the surgery has to be stopped immediately and the sphenoid sinus packed. Even if the bleeding can be controlled, it is necessary to consider the development of a false aneurysm likely. Further management needs interdisciplinary cooperation with the neuroradiologist and neurosurgeon (Fig. 54.3).

Take-Home Pearls

- The learning curve in endonasal sinus surgery is triphasic.
- Sinus surgery should be taught by supervised surgery and practiced on cadavers.
- The most serious complications occur during operations performed by experienced surgeon.
- Detailed study of the preoperative CT scan is key to avoiding complications.
- Retrobulbar haematoma should be treated intraoperatively through endonasal orbital decompression. Consider lateral canthotomy as a quick treatment of retrobulbar haematoma in the anaesthetic recovery room or the ward.
- In cases of serious complications inform the family of the patient immediately.

Tips to Avoid Complications

- Early identification of the middle turbinate and attachment of the uncinate process, as these are important anatomic landmarks.
- Control of the eye bulb during surgery by the surgeon and the operating nurse.
- Bulb-pressing test after Draf and Stankiewicz can be helpful when there is suspicion of injury to the lamina papyracea/periorbita.
- Always dissect laterally to the middle turbinate, never medially.
- The middle meatal antrostomy should be performed just above the inferior turbinate and should not go further anteriorly than the attachment of the uncinate process.
- The septum sinuum sphenoidalium may be attached posteriorly to a thin carotid artery canal, hence removal of the septum with cutting instruments or a diamond drill is recommended. Do not fracture the septum!

Acknowledgement

The authors would like to thank Mo Motamedi, PhD, Department of Cell Biology, Harvard Medical School for his kind cooperation.

References

1. Bolger WE, Parsons DS, Mair SA, et al (1992) Lacrimal drainage system injury in FESS. Incidence, analysis, and prevention. Arch Otolaryngol Head Neck Surg 118:1179–1184
2. Buus DR, Tse DT, Farris BK (1990) Ophthalmic complications of sinus surgery. Ophthalmology 97:612–619
3. Draf W (1983) Endoscopy of the Paranasal Sinuses. Springer, Berlin Heidelberg New York (German edition 1978: Die Endoskopie der Nasennebenhöhlen)
4. Draf W (1986) Course of Advanced Endonasal Micro-endoscopic Sinus Surgery. Academic Teaching Hospital, Fulda
5. Dutton JJ (1986) Orbital complications of paranasal sinus surgery. Ophthalmic Plast Reconstr Surg 2:119–127
6. Halle M (1906) Externe und interne Operation der Nasennebenhoehleneiterungen. Berl Klein Wschr 43:1369–1372

7. Heermann H (1958) Ueber endonasale Chirurgie unter Verwendung des binokularen Mikroskops. Arch Ohr-Nas-Kehlk-Heilk 171:295–297

8. Hosemann WG, Weber RK, Keerl RE, Lund VJ (2000) Minimally Invasive Endonasal Sinus Surgery. Thieme, Stuttgart New York

9. Hudgins PA (1993) Complications of endoscopic sinus surgery. The role of the radiologist in prevention. Radiol Clin North Am 31:21–32

10. Keerl R, Weber R, Draf W, Kind M, Saha A (1996) Periorbital paraffingranuloma following paranasal sinus surgery. Am J Otolarnygol 17:264–268

11. Keerl R, Stankiewicz JA, Weber R, et al (1999) Surgical experience and complications during endonasal sinus surgery. Laryngoscope 109:546–550

12. Keerl R, Weber R, Draf W (2000) Teaching and learning in endonasal sinus surgery. In: Stamm AC, Draf W (eds) Micro-endoscopic Surgery of the Paranasal Sinuses and the Skull Base. Springer, Berlin Heidelberg New York, pp 153–160

13. Keros P (1965) Über die praktische Bedeutung der Niveauunterschiede der Lamina cribrosa des Ethmoids. Z Laryngol Rhinol 41:808–838

14. Kennedy DW, Shanan P, Han W, et al (1994) Complications of ethmoidectomy: a survey of fellows of the American Academy of Otolaryngology-Head Neck Surgery. Otolaryngol Head Neck Surg 111:589–599

15. Kim JY, Kim HJ, Kim CH, Lee JG, Yoon JH (2005) Optic nerve injury secondary to endoscopic sinus surgery: an analysis of three cases. Yonsei Med J 46:300–304

16. Lister JR, Syper GW (1979) Traumatic false aneurysm and carotid-cavernous fistula: a complication of sphenoidotomy. Neurosurgery 5:473–475

17. Maniglia AJ (1991) Fatal and other major complications of endoscopic sinus surgery. Laryngoscope 101:349–354

18. May M, Levine HL, Schaitkin B, et al (1993) Complications of endoscopic sinus surgery. In: Levine HL, May M (eds) Endoscopic Sinus Surgery. Thieme, New York, pp 193–243

19. May M, Levine HL, Mester SJ, et al (1994) Complications of endoscopic sinus surgery: an analysis of 2108 patients – incidence and prevention. Laryngoscope 104:1080–1083

20. Messerklinger J (1970) Die Endoskopie der Nase. Monatsschr Ohrenheilk 104:451–456

21. Mosher H (1929) The surgical anatomy of the ethmoid labyrinth. Ann Otol Rhinol Laryngol 38:869–901

22. Oeken J, Bootz F (2004) Severe complications after endonasal nasal sinus surgery. An unresolved problem. HNO 52:549–553

23. Penne RB, Flanagan JC, Stefanyszyn MA, et al (1993) Ocular motility disorders secondary to sinus surgery. Ophthal Plast Reconstr Surg 9:53–61

24. Schauss F, Weber R, Draf W, et al (1996) Surgery of the lacrimal system. Acta Otorhinolaryngol Belg 50:143–146

25. Schick B, Weber R, Mosler P, et al (1997) Long-term follow-up of fronto-basal dura-plasty. HNO 45:117–122

26. Serdahl C, Berris C, Chole R (1990) Nasolacrimal duct obstruction after endoscopic sinus surgery. Arch Ophthalmol 108:391–392

27. Simmen D, Raghavan U, Briner HR, et al (2006) The surgeon's view of the anterior ethmoid artery. Clin Otolaryngol 31:187–191

28. Spiess G (1899) Die endonasale Chirurgie des Sinus frontalis. Arch Laryngol 9:285–291

29. Sprekelsen MB, Barberan MT (1996) Endoscopic dacryocystorhinostomy: surgical technique and results. Laryngoscope 106:187–189

30. Stammberger H, Posawetz W (1990) Functional endoscopic sinus surgery. Concept, indications and results of the Messerklinger technique. Eur Arch Otorhinolaryngol 247:63–76

31. Stankiewicz JA (1989) Complications of endoscopic sinus surgery. Otolaryngol Clin North Am 22:749–758

32. Stankiewicz JA, Chow JM (1999) Two faces of orbital hematoma in intranasal (endoscopic) sinus surgery. Otolaryngol Head Neck Surg 120:841–847

33. Thacker NM, Velez FG, Demer JL, et al (2005) Extraocular muscle damage associated with endoscopic sinus surgery: an ophthalmology perspective. Am J Rhinol 19:400–405

34. Weber R, Keerl R, Draf W, et al (1996) Management of dural lesions occurring during endonasal sinus surgery. Arch Otolaryngol Head Neck Surg 122:732–736

54

Chapter 55

Endoscopic Sinus Surgery for Nasal Polyposis

55

Philippe Gevaert, Sofie Claeys, and Claus Bachert

Core Messages

■ Nasal polyposis is a chronic disorder; patients must be prepared for long treatment periods and follow-up.

■ Co-morbidity with lower airway disease is important in the treatment decision.

■ Pre-operative medical treatment facilitates the surgical procedure.

■ Careful post-operative follow-up is necessary to increase the success of surgery.

■ In recurrent cases of nasal polyps it is preferable to keep the period between two operations as long as possible.

Contents

Introduction

The management of patients with nasal polyps is one of the major problems otorhinolaryngologists have to face in daily practice. Nasal polyposis (NP) is a chronic disease with a high recurrence rate; even with careful medical and surgical treatment a definite cure cannot be assured. Hippocrates removed polyps with a snare and this remained the only treatment available until recently [1]. However, there have been two remarkable therapeutic innovations in the last two decades: first, the introduction of topically active corticosteroids, and second, endoscopic sinus surgery [2].

When reviewing different studies on endoscopic sinus surgery in NP there is an absolute paucity of "double-blind placebo-controlled studies", and the lack of an overall accepted classification makes comparisons between studies very difficult. The European Position Paper on Rhinosinusitis and Nasal Polyps (EPOS) document tries to close that gap, but differences in aetiology, disease severity or the extent of the polyp disease already influence the outcome of surgery [3, 4]. It is widely known that concomitant conditions such as asthma and aspirin intolerance are risk factors for recurrences of NP (see Chap. 57). Another confounding factor is that the majority of patients receive additional topical or systemic medication such as steroids or antibiotics. Finally, the outcome measures are not standardised (e.g. symptoms, olfaction, recurrences, complications) and the length of the follow-up ranges from a few months up to 10 years. All of this makes comparison between different surgical approaches and pre-, peri-, and post-operative medical treatments difficult.

Indications for Endoscopic Sinus Surgery in NP

The primary goal of treatment is the relief of symptoms, the primary symptoms being nasal blockage, congestion, hypo- or anosmia and secretion. Other symptoms include post-nasal drainage, facial pain, headache, sleep disturbance and decreased quality of life [5]. A decrease in the frequency of infections and disease recurrences, the improvement of associated lower airway symptoms, and the prevention of complications such as mucoceles and orbital involvement [5] are indications for thorough and careful medical and/or surgical intervention.

Planning of endoscopic sinus surgery in patients with NP depends on several factors. It is recommended to try medical therapy first and see how the primary symptoms of the patient improve. Patients failing medical treatment should be considered for surgical intervention. In general the decision for surgery will be based on the extent of polyp disease and control of symptoms and lower airways diseases. Several staging systems for polyps have been proposed [3, 4]: The absence of NP is graded as 0. Grade 1 polyps are visible in the middle meatus only, whereas grade 2 polyps extend beyond the middle meatus without completely blocking the nose. Grade 3 polyps are massive and obstruct the nose completely. For grade 1 and 2 polyps, a medical treatment with topical glucocorticoids and eventually antibiotics (long-term clarithromycin or doxycyclin) should be considered before surgery is indicated (Fig. 55.1). In grade 3, additional systemic glucocorticoids can be added (Fig. 55.1). Although long-term oral glucocorticoids and antibiotics will improve the symptoms, one has to consider whether some long-term treatment schemes are not more harmful than surgery. Endoscopic sinus surgery offers to a vast percentage of patients a solution with long-term symptom improvement and even a possible total cure of NP. Therefore, in massive NP or if your patient was never operated before, the threshold to operate might be lower than in recurrent NP. In the latter group one should prefer to keep the period between two operations as long as possible supposing that previous surgery was appropriate (see Chap. 57).

Polypectomy Versus Extended Endoscopic Sinus Surgery in NP

The extent of surgery varies according to the extent of the disease and the surgeon's individual practice, and ranges from removal of polyps within the middle meatus, perhaps combined with uncinectomy, middle meatal antrostomy and opening of the bulla, to a complete "nasalisation" of all sinuses. However, exenteration of all sinus mucosa must be avoided.

Intranasal Snare Polypectomy or Endoscopic Polypectomy

Over the last two millennia, intranasal snare polypectomy was the golden standard for treating patients with NP. Although this proposition is attractive at a first glance and is commonly done, there is little to substantiate it in the literature.

The endoscope now offers the possibility to delicately remove polyps with the nasal forceps. This can be done under local anaesthesia as an outpatient procedure. Since the removal of nasal polyps is essentially confined to the nasal cavity, however, the results are less favourable in the longer term than with more extended procedures and it does not offer the chance of a long-term problem solution. This approach may be attractive for patients when general anaesthesia is not allowed, when small recurrences occur or in between consecutive endoscopic sinus surgeries.

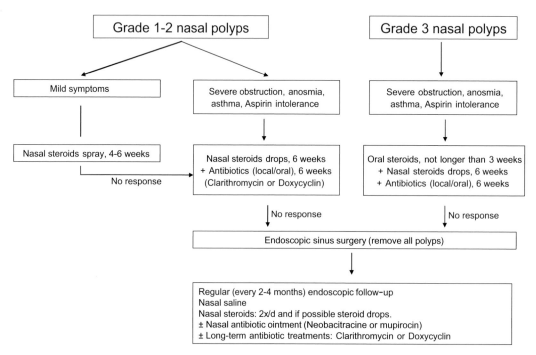

Fig. 55.1 Treatment algorithm for nasal polyposis

55

Endoscopic Sinus Surgery for NP

Functional endoscopic sinus surgery (FESS) is applied to any sinus surgery undertaken with endoscopic control. The aim is to restore sinus ventilation and drainage by opening the key areas while preserving sinus mucosa, which has the potential to regenerate. Removing the disease out of all sinuses is essential. Nasal polyps should not only be removed from the maxillary sinus and the ethmoids, but also from the frontal and sphenoid sinuses. Based on histopathological studies, one could argue that all follicle-like and lymphoid accumulations that are characteristic of NP should be removed [6]. These contain memory cells (T- and B-cells) that are responsible for a reactive hyperglobulinaemia to many allergens and *Staphylococcus aureus* enterotoxins and so maintain the disease. In daily practice, however, we understand that complete exenteration of all sinus mucosa is not possible and can cause many post-operative problems such as "empty nose syndrome" and long-term crusting.

Recent epidemiological data and scientific arguments favour extensive endoscopic sinus surgery over polypectomy. In a systematic review of endoscopic sinus surgery for nasal polyps, 33 studies were evaluated, 3 randomised controlled trials (RCTs), 3 non-RCTs and 27 case series studies [7, 8]. The RCTs and controlled trials reported overall symptomatic improvement that ranged from 78 to 88% for endoscopic sinus surgery compared with 43–84% for comparative techniques (including polypectomy, Caldwell-Luc and intranasal ethmoidectomy) [7, 8]. Disease recurrence was 28% for endoscopic ethmoidectomy, compared with 35% for polypectomy. The percentage of overall complications was reported in only one comparative study and was 1.4% for FESS compared with 0.8% for conventional procedures [7, 8]. Total complications in the case series studies ranged from 0.3 to 22.4% (median 6%).

Microdebriders Versus Classical Instruments in Endoscopic Sinus Surgery in NP

The success of powered instruments such as "microdebriders" or "shavers" in endoscopic sinus surgery is for a great part due to the ease of use in NP. Numerous advantages of microdebriders over standard instruments have been suggested, including reduced operation time, decreased intra-operative and post-operative bleeding, improved visualisation and precision for tissue removal, decreased tissue laceration with mucosal preservation, decreased crusting and synechia formation, reduced ostial reocclusion and overall faster wound healing. In case of NP, the issue is complete removal without complete exenteration of the mucosa or trimming a polypoid middle turbinate without turbinectomy. Without a microdebrider this may be difficult or impossible to achieve. However, to date little information in the literature supports these advantages of microdebriders over standard instruments. In addition, most studies are underpowered, resulting in a series of non-significant results.

Some studies compared the outcome of endoscopic sinus surgery when using the microdebrider on one side of the nose and standard (Blakesley) instruments on the other side. Both instruments resulted in symptom improvement and in endoscopically visible healing over time, but no significant difference was found between the two techniques. In endoscopic evaluation, the total score at 3 weeks after surgery was significantly better in the microdebrider group. Synechia formation, patency of middle meatal antrostomy and open access to the ethmoid were the same in both groups [9].

Nowadays, you have an extended choice of blades ranging from a straight blade to 40° degree bended blades and with or without a turning head of the blade. The 40° degree bended blade has the advantage that one sees what it is cutting away and that the blade can access the maxillary sinus and the frontal recess. As a consequence, one only needs a single blade for the whole procedure. On the other hand, more experience is needed to use a 40° degree bended blade and debrided tissue causes blockage more frequently than with straight blades, because of the reduced suction power. Microdebriders (see Chap. 47) will continue to advance the field of endoscopic surgery, providing clearer operative fields and causing less tissue trauma in experienced hands. However, the severity of complications, including the potential for rapidly aspirating orbital and cerebral contents when laminae are violated, septal defects and even endoscope damage if handed wrongly, must be taken into account. To date, no studies have been reported that test the clinical safety of these instruments, but the risk of complication appears to be dependent on the surgeon's experience [7, 8].

Post-operative Follow-up and Treatment

The goal of pre-, peri- and post-operative medical treatment should be symptom relief, but also control of complications (e.g. infection, asthma exacerbation) and prevention of recurrences. Given the high recurrence rate (even under optimal medical treatment) and the paucity of controlled studies, some surgeons prefer to give absolutely no treatment, whereas others give a maximal treatment with long-term local and systemic glucocorticoids, antibiotics and antifungal medications. Nowadays, with the combination of adequate surgery and medical treatment, good long-term results can be achieved in the majority of cases.

Control of Asthma

NP is frequently associated with late-onset (severe) asthma and aspirin intolerance. During the first 4 weeks post-operatively in particular, the risk for exacerbations is increased and the asthma is often difficult to treat. The increased incidence of post-nasal drip, crusting and aspiration that occur during the wound-healing period should be considered. Therefore, optimal pulmonary treatment with inhaled and systemic glucocorticoids and long-term antibiotics has to be considered pre-, peri- and post-operatively. In patients at risk, a pre-operative consultation with a pulmonary physician is mandatory.

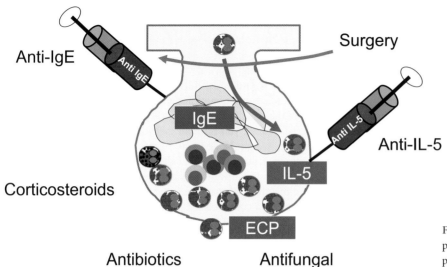

Fig. 55.2 Therapeutic options for nasal polyposis. *IL-5* Interleukin-5, *ECP* eosinophilic cationic protein

Medical Treatment for NP

A diagrammatic summary of the medical treatments for NP is shown in Fig. 55.2.

Nasal Glucocorticosteroids

The symptomatic efficacy of intranasal corticosteroids in patients with nasal polyps is well documented (Fig. 55.3) [10]. In an extensive review of the literature on treatment modalities in NP, the European Position Paper on Rhinosinusitis and Nasal Polyps proposes an evidence-based treatment strategy for NP [3, 4]. Steroids are the cornerstone for treating NP. Symptoms such as nasal blockage, rhinorrhoea and occasionally hyposmia are reduced during the period of treatment, especially in obstructive polyposis [11, 12]. After surgery, topical corticosteroids may also reduce the incidence of polyp recurrences or prolong the symptom-free time interval (EPOS evidence level is Ib). Only one study describes the effect after FESS in a group of patients who underwent this procedure after an inadequate response to at least 3 months of local corticosteroid treatment. It did not show a positive effect of local corticosteroids over placebo. Topical application of corticosteroids significantly reduces symptoms, but does not impact polyps within the sinuses. In fact, the distribution of the drug within the nasal cavity, partially or completely obstructed by polyp tissue, already presents a notable problem to treatment success [5]. In this respect the use of nasal glucocorticoid drops might partially overcome this problem [13]. In a direct comparison of steroid sprays and droplets, 50% of the patients who did not respond to nasal spray did respond to the same medication when applied as a droplet [13]. Most likely, the "lying head back position" allows the steroid drop to reach the nasal polyps better than the common spray [13].

Systemic Glucocorticosteroids

Systemic oral glucocorticosteroids are indicated to start off or enforce conservative local treatment. Furthermore, pre-operative oral glucocorticoid treatment increases visibility during surgery. Oral glucocorticosteroids induce a significant effect for some months, with an improvement of symptoms in 72% of the patients and a reduction of polyp size and of sinus opacification in the computed tomography (CT) scan in 52% [14]. Recurrences occurred within 5 month in almost all subjects. Thus, oral glucocorticosteroids may be indicated to delay or facilitate surgery. However, so far there is no evidence that the natural course of the disease might be influenced by short- or long-term low-dose treatment regimes.

Antibiotics

Bacteria are frequently encountered pathogens in the mucus of NP patients. Van Zele et al. reported that *S. aureus* colonisation of the middle nasal meatus is higher in patients with NP (64%) compared to patients with chronic rhinosinusitis (CRS; 27%) and healthy controls (33%) [6, 15]. In patients with atopic dermatitis, the eradication of *S. aureus* has been shown to significantly improve symptomatology, although temporarily. This potential therapeutic effect of *S. aureus* eradication has not yet been studied in NP. Possible treatment schemes are: long-term antibiotics (doxycyclin, erythromcyin or clarithromycin) and regular application of mupirocin ointment.

In a clinical study, roxithromycin (150 mg/day) was administered for at least 8 weeks to 20 patients with nasal polyps associated with chronic sinusitis; the authors observed an improvement in 52%. The combination of roxithromycin with azelastine (1 mg twice/day), an antihistamine that also inhibits the release of leucotrienes, was examined in another 20 polyp patients,

55

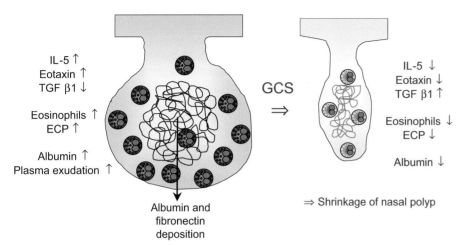

IL-5 ↑
Eotaxin ↑
TGF β1 ↓

Eosinophils ↑
ECP ↑

Albumin ↑
Plasma exudation ↑

GCS ⇒

IL-5 ↓
Eotaxin ↓
TGF β1 ↑

Eosinophils ↓
ECP ↓

Albumin ↓

Albumin and
fibronectin
deposition

⇒ Shrinkage of nasal polyp

Fig. 55.3 Effect of glucocorticos-teroids (*GCS*) on nasal polyposis. *TGF* Transforming growth factor

with further increase of improvement to 68% [16]. However, in a placebo-controlled study to determine the effects of another macrolide, clarithromycin (500 mg twice a day for 6 weeks), in patients with asthma, sinus CT revealed no relevant changes related to the treatment [17]. Further large-scale placebo-controlled studies with macrolides in NP are required before final conclusions on the role of macrolides in the management of this disease can be drawn.

Antifungals

Ponikau et al. demonstrated the presence of fungi in 96% of 210 consecutive patients with CRS [18]. Two double-blind, placebo-controlled, randomised trials were performed to test the effectiveness of topical antifungal treatment in CRS with NP [13]. Both an antifungal spray and antifungal nasal lavages, when administered over a period of 2–3 months, were ineffective in reducing patient symptoms and nasal endoscopy scores. Furthermore, a 6-week course of orally administered terbinafine also failed to bring about any improvements in patient symptom scores or CT scores [19]. Therefore, antifungals are only indicated nowadays in invasive forms of sinus mycosis or in immunocompromised hosts.

Antileukotrienes

It has been suggested that changes in the arachidonic acid metabolism are involved in the pathomechanism underlying NP, especially in aspirin-sensitive subjects. Theoretically, the use of antileucotrienes, especially in aspirin-sensitive nasal polyp patients, could be appropriate [20]. Montelukast, a leucotriene D4 receptor antagonist, was studied as an add-on therapy to topical and inhaled corticosteroids in patients with or without aspirin sensitivity, with both NP and asthma [21]. Clinical subjective improvement in NP occurred in 64% of aspirin-tolerant and 50% of aspirin-sensitive patients; asthma improved in 87% and 61% of these patients, respectively. However, acoustic rhinometry, nasal inspiratory peak flow and nitric oxide levels did not change significantly in any group, and improvement following montelukast therapy was not associated with aspirin sensitivity.

Antihistamines

Antihistamines may be indicated in subjects with NP and allergic rhinitis complaints. In a clinical study including 45 patients with residual or recurrent NP after ethmoidectomy, patients were treated with either cetirizine at twice the recommended daily dose (20 mg) or placebo for 3 months [22]. Although the size of polyps remained unchanged during the study period, the active treatment reduced sneezing and rhinorrhoea effectively, and also had a late effect on nasal obstruction.

Anti-interleukin-5

In a double-blind, placebo-controlled, randomised, 2-centre, safety, and pharmacokinetic study, 24 subjects with bilateral NP were randomised to receive a single intravenous infusion of Reslizumab, a humanised anti-human interleukin (IL)-5 monoclonal antibody, at a dose of either 3 mg/kg or 1 mg/kg, or placebo [23]. Individual nasal polyp scores improved in half of the verum-treated patients for up to 4 weeks. When carefully analysing responders and non-responders, only those nasal polyps with increased levels of IL-5 in nasal secretions before treatment seemed to benefit from anti-IL-5 treatment. Indeed, repeated injections need to be evaluated. Given the cost of antibody treatments, if commercialised, they will probably only be restricted for severe recurrent NP with difficult-to-control asthma.

Anti-IgE

Considering the marked local production of IgE-antibodies in nasal polyps and its relation to severity of disease, it appears that local IgE is functional and involved in the regulation of chronic inflammation [6]. Thus, strategies to antagonise IgE antibodies could be of relevance. No studies in NP have yet been performed to answer the question as to whether high concentrations of IgE-antibodies within the NP tissue can be targeted with success.

Symptom Control and Recurrences

In a 20-year follow-up study of 41 patients with nasal polyps, 85% of patients still suffered from the disease, with anosmia present in 61% [24]; 8 subjects, including 7 with aspirin sensitivity, had undergone 11 or more surgical operations during the 20-year period. Although the recurrence rates in long-term studies are often high (disease present or not), the symptom control of is much better. The overall symptomatic improvement reported in three randomised controlled and five controlled trials (reported in five studies) ranged from 78 to 88% for FESS. Polyp recurrences range from 28% to 35% for endoscopic sinus surgery (depending on the length of observation).

The case series studies reported overall symptomatic improvement for patients with nasal polyps that ranged from 37 to 99% (median 89%). Improved sense of smell decreased rapidly after 6 months in the ethmoidectomy group compared with nasalisation in one comparative study. Overall improvement compared with pre-operative scores ranged from 13 to 91%, with a median of 31% (six studies). Improvement in nasal obstruction post-operatively (compared with pre-operative scores) ranged from 29 to 100%, with a median of 72% (six studies). Overall post-operative patency ranged from 57 to 100%, with a median of 93% (seven studies).

The medical or surgical treatment of NP may have an impact on the control of asthma. A study involving 205 patients with asthma and aspirin sensitivity indicated that surgery improves asthma for relatively long periods of time [25]. However, there are no data concerning the evolution of asymptomatic bronchial hyperreactivity in patients with NP, and individual patients may develop asthma symptoms after surgery. This development may represent the natural course of the disease rather than a true shift from upper- to lower-airway disease.

Long-Term Management of Recurrent NP

First of all, it is wise to inform your patient about the state of his disease and the long-term consequences. Some symptoms (such as nasal obstruction) are easy to manage, whereas other symptoms (such as loss of smell and taste) are difficult to control. The patient should know what you really can or cannot offer them. Therefore, all of the therapeutic options and limitations should be discussed and the management should based on the patient's desire, rather than on the itch in the surgeons fingers when he sees big polyps.

One should generally keep the period between two operations as long as possible, for the comfort of the patient. The decision to perform surgery will generally be based on the extent of polyp disease, the control of symptoms, the presence of lower-airways diseases, and the quality of previous surgery. In this respect, a good dialogue with the pulmonary physician is mandatory.

In recurrent NP grade 1 or 2 it is recommended that your patient undergo a long-term medical treatment scheme (Table 55.1), whereas in the case of difficult-to-control asthma or massive polyposis (grade 3), revision endoscopic surgery might be preferred.

Summary

The treatment of nasal polyps will depend very much upon the individual experience and philosophy. No medical or surgical treatment guarantees a cure; however, endoscopic sinus surgery at least gives the patient a chance of total cure of NP.

Management of recurrent NP is still unsatisfactory and long-term medical treatment should be maintained to control symptoms and concomitant lower-airway problems in between revision surgeries.

Table 55.1 Extending the period between two endoscopic sinus surgeries in recurrent nasal polyposis

Essential	• Regular (every 2–4 months) endoscopic follow-up: evaluation of the polyp status and infection, eventual suction cleaning of infected crusts and mucus. • Nasal saline: minimum twice a day to remove crust and decrease chronic colonisation. • Nasal glucocorticoids: preferably twice a day and if possible glucocorticoid drops.
Consider	• Nasal antibiotic ointment (Neobacitracine or mupirocin). • Long-term antibiotic treatment: clarithromycin (500 mg/day) or doxycyclin (100 mg/day) for 6 weeks. • Occasional oral glucocorticoid burst (rescue medication, only if necessary). • Repeated endoscopic polypectomies under local anaesthesia (microdebrider) in the outpatient clinic can relieve your patient of nasal blockage.

55

Tips to Avoid Complications

- Pre-operative oral glucocorticoid treatment increases visibility during surgery.
- Microdebrider provides a clearer operative field and causes less tissue trauma.
- Microdebriders should only be used in experienced hands.
- Patients should stop smoking for optimal wound healing after surgery.
- Avoid asthma exacerbations by pre-treating patients at risk.

References

1. Mygind N, Lildholdt T (1997) Nasal Polyposis: An Inflammatory Disease and its Treatment. Munksgaard, Copenhagen
2. Mygind N, Lildholdt T (1996) Nasal polyps treatment: medical management. Allergy Asthma Proc 17:275–282
3. Fokkens W (2005) Evidence based diagnosis and treatment of rhinosinusitis and nasal polyps. Rhinology 43:1
4. Fokkens W, Lund V, Bachert C, Clement P, Helllings P, et al (2005) EAACI position paper on rhinosinusitis and nasal polyps executive summary. Allergy 60:583–601
5. Bachert C, van Cauwenberge P (2003) Nasal Polyps and Sinusitis. In: Adkinson NF, Yunginger JW, Busse WW, Bochner BS, Simons FER, Holgate ST (eds) Middleton's Allergy: Principles and Practice. Mosby, Philadelphia, pp 1421–1436
6. Gevaert P, Holtappels G, Johansson SG, Cuvelier C, Cauwenberge P, Bachert C (2005) Organization of secondary lymphoid tissue and local IgE formation to Staphylococcus aureus enterotoxins in nasal polyp tissue. Allergy 60:71–79
7. Dalziel K, Stein K, Round A, Garside R, Royle P (2006) Endoscopic sinus surgery for the excision of nasal polyps: A systematic review of safety and effectiveness. Am J Rhinol 20:506–519
8. Dalziel K, Stein K, Round A, Garside R, Royle P (2003) Systematic review of endoscopic sinus surgery for nasal polyps. Health Technol Assess 7:iii, 1–iii159
9. Sauer M, Lemmens W, Vauterin T, Jorissen M (2007) Comparing the microdebrider and standard instruments in endoscopic sinus surgery: a double-blind randomised study. B-ENT 3:1–7
10. Badia L, Lund V (2001) Topical corticosteroids in nasal polyposis. Drugs 61:573–578
11. Lund VJ, Flood J, Sykes AP, Richards DH (1998) Effect of fluticasone in severe polyposis. Arch Otolaryngol Head Neck Surg 124:513–518
12. Tos M, Svendstrup F, Arndal H, Orntoft S, Jakobsen J, et al (1998) Efficacy of an aqueous and a powder formulation of nasal budesonide compared in patients with nasal polyps. Am J Rhinol 12:183–189
13. Ebbens FA, Scadding GK, Badia L, Hellings PW, Jorissen M, et al (2006) Amphotericin B nasal lavages: not a solution for patients with chronic rhinosinusitis. J Allergy Clin Immunol 118:1149–1156
14. van Camp C, Clement PA (1994) Results of oral steroid treatment in nasal polyposis. Rhinology 32:5–9
15. van ZT, Gevaert P, Watelet JB, Claeys G, Holtappels G, et al (2004) Staphylococcus aureus colonization and IgE antibody formation to enterotoxins is increased in nasal polyposis. J Allergy Clin Immunol 114:981–983
16. Ichimura K, Shimazaki Y, Ishibashi T, Higo R (1996) Effect of new macrolide roxithromycin upon nasal polyps associated with chronic sinusitis. Auris Nasus Larynx 23:48–56
17. Kraft M, Cassell GH, Pak J, Martin RJ (2002) Mycoplasma pneumoniae and Chlamydia pneumoniae in asthma: effect of clarithromycin. Chest 121:1782–1788
18. Ponikau JU, Sherris DA, Kita H (2007) The role of ubiquitous airborne fungi in chronic rhinosinusitis. Clin Allergy Immunol 20:177–184
19. Kennedy DW, Kuhn FA, Hamilos DL, Zinreich SJ, Butler D, et al (2005) Treatment of chronic rhinosinusitis with high-dose oral terbinafine: a double blind, placebo-controlled study. Laryngoscope 115:1793–1799
20. Parnes SM (2002) The role of leukotriene inhibitors in allergic rhinitis and paranasal sinusitis. Curr Allergy Asthma Rep 2:239–244
21. Ragab S, Parikh A, Darby YC, Scadding GK (2001) An open audit of montelukast, a leukotriene receptor antagonist, in nasal polyposis associated with asthma. Clin Exp Allergy 31:1385–1391
22. Haye R, Aanesen JP, Burtin B, Donnelly F, Duby C (1998) The effect of cetirizine on symptoms and signs of nasal polyposis. J Laryngol Otol 112:1042–1046
23. Gevaert P, Lang-Loidolt D, Lackner A, Stammberger H, Staudinger H, et al (2006) Nasal IL-5 levels determine the response to anti-IL-5 treatment in patients with nasal polyps. J Allergy Clin Immunol 118:1133–1141
24. Vento SI, Ertama LO, Hytonen ML, Wolff CH, Malmberg CH (2000) Nasal polyposis: clinical course during 20 years. Ann Allergy Asthma Immunol 85:209–214
25. English GM (1986) Nasal polypectomy and sinus surgery in patients with asthma and aspirin idiosyncrasy. Laryngoscope 96:374–380

Chapter 56

Endoscopic Sinus Surgery on the Patient Without the Usual Landmarks

56

Rainer Weber

Core Messages

- Surgery in patients with no landmarks needs proper pre-operative imaging (at least CT in axial and coronal planes) and strict indications.
- Optimal instrumentation is necessary, like specific instruments for frontal and maxillary sinus surgery.
- Revision sinus surgery should be performed only by very experienced sinus surgeons.
- Always use identifiable landmarks:
  - For the sphenoid sinus these are the choana and the nasal septum.
  - For the ethmoid it is the sphenoid sinus.
  - For the maxillary sinus they are the inferior turbinate, the nasal bottom, and the nasolacrimal duct.
  - For the frontal sinus they are the frontal prozess of maxilla, the ethmoidal

Contents

Introduction

Endonasal sinus surgery is usually carried out in a stepwise manner [5]. The surgeon becomes orientated with the aid of certain landmarks. In revision surgery or in special cases with severe pathology (Fig. 56.1), after trauma or in tumor patients, some of these landmarks are missing, for example the middle and superior turbinate or different cell groups of ethmoidal cells. It is assumed that the complication rate in these patients is (much) higher than in normal patients, although there are no data to support this assumption. This chapter provides an overview of how to deal with the difficult situation where the normal landmarks for sinus surgery are missing. This is a combination of personal experience and review of the literature. Evidence-based strategies are not available.

Preoperative Evaluation and Radiology

In considering patients with no landmarks for endonasal sinus revision surgery it is of utmost importance to check that there is an indication to do this type of surgery and to carefully weigh up the benefits and risks for the individual patient. To this end, the surgeon should collect a detailed history, precise imaging (see Chap. 45), and careful preoperative endoscopy. It has to be clearly established which symptoms can be addressed by revision sinus surgery in conjunction with conservative treatment options (see Chap. 57) so that the patient can be given realistic goals. To help achieve this, a high-resolution CT in axial and coronal planes should be performed to outline the following structures (see Chap. 45):

1. Internal carotid artery.
2. Optic nerve.
3. Depth of the olfactory cleft.
4. Remnants of the middle and superior turbinate.
5. Lateral and anterior–posterior diameter of the frontal sinus.
6. Anterior ethmoidal artery.
7. Extent of the pathology.
8. Irregular scarring or ossification of the ethmoidal cells.

Precise radiological evaluation and endoscopic examination allows determination of the presence or loss of important landmarks. In most cases the absence of landmarks is the result of resection of the middle turbinate and in some situations resection of the superior turbinate. This may be combined with major scarring inside the ethmoid or the nasal cavities, or with a major recurrent polyposis (see Chap. 55). In combination with missing structures of the ethmoid, like the uncinate process, agger nasi cells, and the bulla ethmoidalis, orientation may be extremely difficult. As such, this surgery should be performed only by an experienced surgeon, as he or she may be faced with various difficult situations of altered anatomy and increased intraoperative bleeding.

It is assumed, without supportive data, that intraoperative bleeding is increased in revision sinus surgery, and indeed this is my experience. This may be attributable to the ongoing inflammatory disease or by a better vascularization of fibrous tissue following previous surgery in comparison to the normal tissue in a healthy sinus system. So, an optimal preparation of the operative field should be done, including local infiltration with xylocain/epinephrine, topical application of xylometazolin, and additional topical application of epinephrine. The anesthetist should run a deep anesthesia, maintaining a mean blood pressure of 60 mmHg with a heart rate of 60 beats/min [2, 6].

Proper instrumentation and optimal visualization of the operative field is a precondition for endonasal sinus surgery, but it is much more relevant in surgery in patients with no landmarks. The author recommends performing this surgery primarily endoscopically to be able to deal with *all* problems of *all* sinuses. In addition, in some cases it may be beneficial to use the microscope if a more detailed view is necessary, for instance inside the sphenoid sinus.

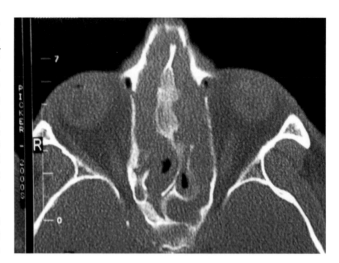

Fig. 56.1 Severe recurrent polyposis with complete opacification of all sinuses and sclerosis of the surrounding bone after multiple previous surgeries (axial computed tomography, CT scan)

How to Do it – Ethmoid and Sphenoid Sinus

The fundamental aim in sinus surgery is removal of the pathology (major polyps, tumor) with creation and maintenance of a sufficient drainage. The normal way of preparing the ethmoid is the step-by-step removal of ethmoidal cells and pathology from anterior to posterior. In revision ethmoid surgery with loss of the typical landmarks (see Chap. 51) there is an increased risk of damage to the orbit (penetration of the lamina papyracea or periorbit) and to the skull base (ethmoidal roof, cribriform plate). In such situations it is safer to use the posterior–anterior approach [5], starting from the sphenoid sinus and the sphenoid sinus roof and going backwards along the ethmoidal roof.

A clear and consistent landmark by which to locate and open the sphenoid sinus is the choana and the natural opening of the sphenoid sinus, which is consistently found 10–15 mm upwards of the choana, medial to the attachment of the superior turbinate, and paramedian to the nasal septum (Fig. 56.2) [3]; the precise individual anatomy should be checked by CT in axial and coronal planes.

The anterior wall of the sphenoid sinus can be nearly completely resected. In this way the posterior skull base and the posterior lamina papyracea might be exposed and further prepara-

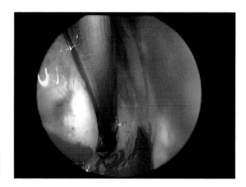

Fig. 56.2 Endoscopic view (achieved with a 45° telescope and the AIDA documentation system; Karl Storz, Tuttlingen, Germany) of the entrance of the sphenoid sinus on the right side, 10–15 mm upwards from the choana, medial to the attachment of the medial turbinate

tion can be performed in a safe way from posterior to anterior. The author uses the 130° angled Kerrison punch to do this work (Fig. 56.2). The skull base and the lamina papyracea run in a soft plane with no breaks. Thus, preparation can be performed safely by moving anteriorly in a tangential manner from the clearly posterior visible plane of the sphenoid sinus/exposed ethmoid roof and the lamina papyracea.

It should be borne in mind in revision sinus surgery lacking usual landmarks that the landmark for ethmoid is the sphenoid sinus, with the chance of posterior-to-anterior exposure of the ethmoidal roof, and those for the sphenoid are the choana and the nasal septum.

56

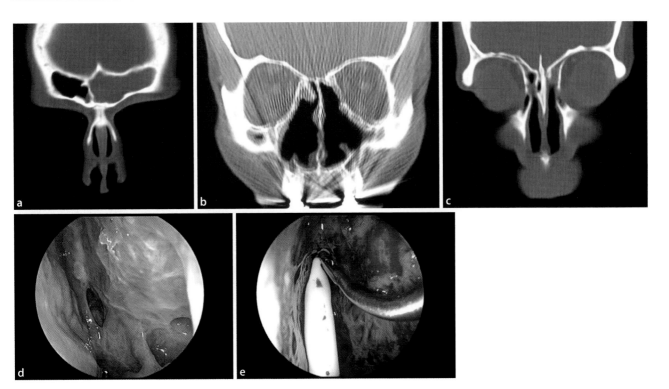

Fig. 56.3a–e Mucocele of the frontal sinus after previous surgery. **a** Coronal CT showing complete opacification of the left frontal sinus. **b** Coronal CT showing nearly complete resection of all turbinates, with wide access to both the maxillary and ethmoid sinuses. **c** Coronal CT showing the beginning of the supraorbital recessus with scarring. **d** Corresponding endoscopic view to **c** (with a 45° telescope and the AIDA documentation system; Karl Storz) showing the empty nose with a wide opening to the maxillary sinus (opening of the sphenoid sinus) and purulent secretion at the skull base. **e** Insertion of a Rains frontal sinus stent into the left frontal sinus using a Giraffe forceps (Karl Storz)

How to Do it – Maxillary Sinus

Depending on the anatomy and the previous operation(s), an approach via the obstructed or scarred middle nasal meatus is frequently possible. This can be done using a bended suction, which is introduced behind the nasolacrimal duct and directly above the insertion of the inferior turbinate to penetrate the scar. It is directed in a lateral and inferior direction. Before doing this, however, a coronal CT plane of the anatomy should be viewed to check that there is enough space between the upper border of the inferior turbinate and the inferior border of the lamina papyracea so as avoid penetrating the orbit. The first opening should be enlarged stepwise with through-cutting punches and forceps to create a larger and sufficient opening.

If there is not enough space in the middle meatus (e.g., in cases of mucoceles of the maxillary sinus after Caldwell-Luc operation) [11], the opening should be made in the inferior nasal meatus after medialization of the inferior turbinate (see Chap. 50). As described previously, the exact localization of a mucocele relative to the inferior turbinate should be checked by CT, and the first opening could be made with a bended suction. The enlargement should also be performed in the same way as

described earlier. In very difficult cases it may be necessary to cut the inferior turbinate behind the orifice of the nasolacrimal duct - temporarily (!) - to provide sufficient access to a lateral localized mucocele. After creation of a sufficient opening, the inferior turbinate should be reinserted at the transection area with two resorbable sutures.

The inferior turbinate is a very important structure for the climatizing function of the nose. In the author's experience it is advisable for a better healing of the reattached turbinate to perform an occlusive aftercare for 2–3 weeks, which permits a moist wound healing and prevents necrosis. The blood supply for the inferior nasal turbinate is ensured from posterior. If the inferior turbinate is missing, the marsupialization of a mucocele of the maxillary sinus is carried out in the same way, starting with the bended suction or a comparable instrument, using the nasolacrimal duct and the nasal bottom as landmarks. The opening is enlarged downwards to create a smooth transition from the nasal cavity into the maxillary sinus.

It should be borne in mind in revision sinus surgery lacking usual landmarks that the landmarks for the maxillary sinus are the nasal floor, the inferior nasal turbinate, and the nasal lacrimal duct.

How to Do it – Frontal Sinus

The most difficult approach is that to the frontal sinus [1, 4, 7–10, 12]. Again it is of utmost importance to analyze the individual preoperative CT to look for the best way to enter the frontal sinus (Fig. 56.3). Depending on the anatomy and the lateral and anterior–posterior dimensions of the frontal sinus outflow tract, the size of the spina nasalis interna, and the underlining pathology, it may be:

1. possible to achieve a sufficient drainage (e.g., type IIa or type IIb drainage according to Draf) by removing some remnant ethmoidal cells [1, 9];
2. sufficient to resect scars or some new bone formation;
3. necessary to make a much larger opening like a type III drainage (synonyms: median drainage, or frontal drill-out procedure, or modified Lothrop procedure) [1, 7, 9].

For enlargement of the frontal sinus drainage, one should create an opening to the frontal sinus of at least 5 mm (Type IIa) [4], as otherwise the risk of reclosure is high.

There are at least four endonasal ways to enter an obstructed frontal sinus in revision sinus surgery:

1. If the ethmoidal roof is exposed intraoperatively, it is first recommended to go along the ethmoidal roof and the anterior ethmoidal artery to the posterior frontal sinus wall. The anterior ethmoidal artery runs a few millimeters *posteriorly* to the posterior frontal sinus wall across the ethmoidal roof (see Chap. 44).
2. Preparing along the frontal process of the maxilla leads *anteriorly* to the frontal sinus floor.
3. In preparing a type III drainage, which means the complete bilateral resection of the frontal sinus floor, the upper part of the nasal septum, and the lower part of the septum of the frontal sinus (see Chap. 52), it is necessary to resect parts of the adjacent nasal septum. Thus, in cases of difficult orientation without landmarks one can perform resection of the nasal septum as a first step to expose the frontal sinus floor and enter it from *inferiorly* in front of the cribriform plate. Identification of the first olfactory fiber has been recommended by Draf [1]. Anterior to this first olfactory fiber, one can enter the frontal sinus and perform a type III drainage by a stepwise enlargement with punches or with a burr creates. This enlargement depends on the individual anatomy and pathology.
4. An additional way to enter the frontal sinus in patients without landmarks and difficult orientation, or in patients with major scarring and osteogenesis in the frontal sinus outflow tract, is via the contralateral normal frontal sinus. The first step is to prepare a type IIa drainage (see Chap. 52); like uncapping the egg – removal of anterior superior ethmoidal cells and exposing the normal drainage pathway of the healthy frontal sinus. Then one can proceed stepwise medially to the other side in front of the posterior sinus wall. In doing this one has to resect the anterior attachment of the middle turbinate and the adjacent part of the nasal septum and the frontal sinus floor. This is also a very safe way to enter a completely obstructed frontal sinus of one side.

It should be borne in mind in revision sinus surgery lacking usual landmarks that Landmarks for the maxillary sinus are:

1. the frontal process of the maxilla;
2. the nasal septum;
3. the ethmoidal roof and anterior ethmoidal artery;
4. the first olfactory fiber;
5. the contralateral frontal sinus.

How I Do it? Frontal Sinus Additional Procedures

In cases with a narrow entrance to the frontal sinus despite enlarging with a burr and performing a type III drainage, a special frontal sinus stent could be inserted (Fig. 56.3). The author uses a Rains frontal sinus stent (Gyrus Medical). It should be left inside for 3–6 months [10, 12]. Careful attention should be paid to the development of edema or infection as a result of stenting. In this case it should be removed earlier.

In some cases an external approach will be necessary by performing an osteoplastic frontal sinus operation with fat obliteration [8, 9].

Navigation System

The author has performed all of the types of surgery described herein without a navigation system (see Chap. 48); this is possible without increased risk. Despite this personal experience, the use of navigation systems might be of help in difficult cases and it could be used to reduce the operation time.

Pre- and Postoperative Care

A chronic polypoid sinusitis or acute superinfection of a mucocele is managed in the usual way using systemic and topical steroids or antibiotics. After the operation, the author recommends in cases of severe polyposis the following anti-inflammatory medications:

1. Prednisolone 100 mg/day for 3 days.
2. Prednisolone 50 mg/day for 7–10 days.
3. Topical steroid.
4. Cefuroxime 2×500 mg/day or Cotrum forte 2×1 for 14 days.
5. Additionally, a nasal douche with Ems salt.

In cases of a mucopyocele, antibiotic treatment for 14 days with cefuroxime without steroids is performed. In cases with major granulation tissue, particularly after type III drainage, intensive endoscopically guided aftercare is important. Fibrin and granulations should be removed to prevent the development of scarring via the granulation tissue. This should be done once or twice a week in the first 2 weeks, and weekly thereafter. There is no proof that the application of mitomycin C prevents the development of postoperative scarring after frontal sinus surgery; however, it may be of help in difficult revision cases if it can be applied on granulation tissue in the frontal sinus outflow tract and not on the bare bone. Further studies on this topic are necessary.

Take-Home Pearls

- Check carefully by preoperative endoscopic and radiological evaluation which landmarks used in primary surgery still exist.
- It is possible to perform revision surgery in patients lacking the usual landmarks by considering other specific landmarks (the nasal septum, nasal floor, inferior nasal turbinate, choana, and nasal lacrimal duct).
- Ethmoid sinus surgery in revision surgery can be performed after identification of the sphenoidal plane along the ethmoidal roof in a posterior-to-anterior direction.
- The insertions of the inferior nasal turbinate and the nasolacrimal duct are important landmarks for access to the maxillary sinus in revision sinus surgery.
- The most difficult sinus to approach in revision sinus surgery is the frontal sinus, which necessitates a very careful analysis of radiological imaging. Access to the frontal sinus may be reached along the frontal process of the maxilla, the ethmoidal roof together with the anterior ethmoidal artery, remnants of agger nasi cells, the first olfactory fiber, or the contralateral normal frontal sinus.
- A careful endoscopic aftercare and control is necessary.

References

1. Draf W (2006) Endonasal frontal sinus drainage type I–III according to Draf. In: Kountakis S, Senior B, Draf W (eds) The Frontal Sinus. Springer New York, pp 219–32
2. Eberhart LH, Folz BJ, Wulf H, Geidner G (2003) Intravenous anesthesia provides optimal surgical conditions during microscopic and endoscopic sinus surgery. Laryngoscope 113:1369–1373
3. Hosemann W, Groß R, Göde U, Kühnel T, Röckelein G (1995) The anterior sphenoid wall: relative anatomy for sphenoidotomy. Am J Rhinol 9:137–144
4. Hosemann W, Kühnel T, Held P, Wagner W, Felderhoff A (1997) Endonasal fenestration of the frontal sinus in surgical management of chronic sinusitis – a critical evaluation. Am J Rhinol 11:1–11
5. Hosemann W, Weber R, Keerl R, Lund V (2000) Minimally invasive endonasal sinus surgery. Thieme, Stuttgart New York
6. Rathjen T, Bockmühl U, Greim C-A (2006) Modern anaesthesiology concepts supporting paranasal sinus surgery. Laryngorhinootologie 85:20–23
7. Weber R, Kratzsch B (2001) Endonasal median drainage: indications and surgical technique. HNO 49:1047–60
8. Weber R, Draf W, Keerl R, Kahle G, Schinzel S, Thomann S, Lawson W (2000) Osteoplastic frontal sinus surgery with fat obliteration. Technique and long-term results using magnetic resonance imaging in 82 operations. Laryngoscope 110:1037–1044
9. Weber R, Draf W, Kratzsch B, Hosemann W, Schaefer SD (2001) Modern concepts of frontal sinus surgery. Laryngoscope 111:137–46
10. Weber R, Hochapfel F, Draf W (2000) Packing and stents in endonasal surgery. Rhinology 38:49–62
11. Weber R, Keerl R, Draf W (2000) Endonasal endoscopic surgery of maxillary sinus mucoceles after Caldwell-Luc operation. Laryngorhinootologie 79:532–535
12. Weber R, Mai R, Hosemann W, Draf W, Toffel PH (2000) The success of 6-month stenting in endonasal frontal sinus surgery. Ear Nose Throat J 79:930–941

Chapter 57

Role of Aetiology in Revision Endoscopic Sinus Surgery

57

Susanne Mayr and Bernhard Schick

Core Messages

■ All available diagnostic measures are to be used to define the pathology of recurrent sinus disease to the best possible extent.

■ Optimised conservative treatment comes before, parallel to and after revision sinus surgery.

■ Revision surgery should be embedded in a concept of conservative and surgical treatment.

■ The strategy of revision sinus surgery depends on the individual pathology.

Contents

Introduction

Functional endoscopic sinus surgery is performed worldwide and improves the symptoms caused by chronic rhinosinusitis (CRS) in 75–95% of cases. However, it is a well-known experience that there are patients responding less well to surgical therapy; after endoscopic sinus surgery, 5–15% of all patients need to be considered for revision sinus surgery. When focussing on subgroups of patients, such as those with aspirin-exacerbated respiratory disease (AERD), even higher rates of disease recurrence are noted.

Due to the nature of the disease, it should be noted that sinus surgery is unable to provide a cure for many forms of inflammatory sinus disease. Sinus surgery contributes to the relief of symptoms in these situations, but needs to be combined with additional treatment options that target the underlying pathology. It is therefore of utmost importance that the underlying pathological condition is investigated, as this could benefit from additional conservative treatment. Improved understanding of the aetiology enables the physician to select further post-operative conservative treatment options that could contribute to the success of revision sinus surgery.

In this chapter, conservative treatment options before, parallel and after revision sinus surgery will be discussed as part of a combined conservative/surgical treatment concept.

Aims and Objectives

The term CRS with or without nasal polyps is used as a generalised term for various inflammatory sinus affections and symptoms caused by different underlying aetiologies and pathomechanisms. As identification of new pathomechanisms is an ongoing process, it is important to check carefully over the years if the individual pathology can be defined more precisely when following patients with chronic sinus disease. Since known that certain patients are specifically prone to recurrences, depending on the aetiology, it will be of interest if further therapeutic options arise as a result of improved understanding of the individual pathology.

57

Thus the first aim in dealing with the situation of revision sinus surgery is to work out to what extent the reason for surgical failure is linked to the pathology itself. The second important point is to analyse the surgical strategy being used in primary surgery and the result of the healing process after that primary surgery. Based on these two important aspects it should be possible to establish an individually tailored strategy composed of optimised conservative treatment and a surgical concept that is dependent upon the extent of sinus disease and the anatomical situation.

Preoperative Assessment

General Assessment

Medical History

The first step to workup recurrent sinus disease is a detailed assessment of the patient's symptoms. The presence of major local symptoms such as nasal blockage, congestion or stuffiness, nasal discharge or post-nasal drip, facial pain or pressure, headache and reduction/loss of smell should be queried, as well as distant symptoms such as sore throat, dysphonia and coughing (Table 57.1) [27]. The severity of each symptom should be graded for follow-up purposes. A four-grade scale (severe, moderate, slight and no symptom/normal) is recommended, or alternatively the use of visual analogue scales [11]. Other more general complaints to mention are malaise, drowsiness and fever in acute boosts of disease. Note that patients may either present with the same range of symptoms as they did prior to their initial surgery, or with a more detailed knowledge of their disease, describing their major and minor symptoms very specifically.

Table 57.1 Major and minor symptoms in chronic rhinosinusitis (CRS)

Symptom
Nasal blockage/congestion/stuffiness
Mucopurulent drainage
Post-nasal drainage
Loss of smell/taste
Facial pain or pressure
Coughing/sore throat/dysphonia
Headaches
Ear pressure
Epiphora
Dryness/crusting
Sneezing

Table 57.2 Endoscopic appearances. Additionally evaluated: nasal septum, lower turbinate

Polyps[a]	Right	
	Left	
Oedema[b]	Right	
	Left	
Discharge[c]	Right	
	Left	
Scarring[b]	Right	
	Left	
Crusting[b]	Right	
	Left	
Total points		

[a]Scoring for polyps: 0=absence of polyps; 1=polyps in the middle meatus only; 2=polyps beyond the middle meatus
[b]Scoring for oedema, scarring and crusting: 0=absent; 1=mild; 2=severe
[c]Scoring for discharge: 0=no discharge; 1=clear, thin discharge; 2=thick, purulent discharge

Sinus symptoms have an enormous impact on the quality of life (QoL) [11, 22]. In that context the use of standardised questionnaires is very helpful for measuring QoL, and in a practical way these questionnaires help to make the need of therapeutic interventions more understandable for patients. However, should be pointed out that the severity of local symptoms does not always correlate with QoL scales [39]. The most frequently used QoL instruments today are the 16-Item Sino-Nasal Outcome Test [37], the Chronic Sinusitis Survey [12], the Rhinosinusitis Disability Index [5] and the Rhinoconjunctivitis QoL questionnaire. The Medical Outcomes Study Short Form 36 is the most commonly used generic instrument for general health in addition to those mentioned above [41, 51].

Clinical Examination

Correct understanding of the individual anatomy requires detailed rhinoscopic and endoscopic inspection of the inner nose using endoscopes of different angles. It is crucial to examine before and after decongestion. One should be reminded when making the diagnosis that the severity of nasal symptoms and the results of nasal endoscopy often do not correlate. It should also be borne in mind that with the "headache" symptom in particular, the underlying cause might be of non-sinus aetiology.

Endoscopic examination has to answer the question of possible closure of the sinus drainage pathways. Incomplete removal

Table 57.3 Radiological grading of sinus systems proposed by Lund and Mackay

Sinus system	Right	Left
Maxillary sinus[a]		
Anterior ethmoidal[a]		
Posterior ethmoidal[a]		
Sphenoidal[a]		
Frontal[a]		
Ostiomeatal complex[b]		
Total points for each side		

[a]Scoring: 0=no abnormalities; 1=partial opacification; 2=total opacification
[b]Scoring: 0=not occluded, 2=occluded

of the uncinate process and incomplete anterior ethmoidectomy may be involved in recurrent sinusitis. Scarring or lateralisation of the middle turbinate can further block the ethmoid drainage (see Chap. 56). A missed natural ostium of the maxillary sinus in primary surgery with creation of a neo-ostium may prevent physiological drainage of the sinus with recirculation, also termed "missed ostium sequence". The presence of residual bone fragments should be confirmed as a possible continuous source for inflammation, chronic osteiitis or osteomyelitis. Furthermore, nasal congestion has to be considered due to turbinate pathology, septal deviations and valve problems.

Accurate documentation of the diseased areas and documenting results using semi-quantitative scores for polyps, oedema, nasal discharge, crusting and scarring are beneficial for further planning of revision sinus surgery (Table 57.2) [21, 24, 28].

Imaging

Computed tomography (CT) is essential for determining the extent of the pathologic condition (see Chap. 45). CT findings are analysed with reference to the surgical strategy selected for primary surgery and to define the possible crucial narrowings of the sinus drainage pathways. The bony borders of the sinuses are checked carefully in order to obtain information regarding the extent of primary surgery and possible bony lacerations at the anterior skull base or lamina papyracea. Recognition of such alterations is the key to preventing complications. We recommend the use of one of the numerous and proven evaluation systems for pre-surgical evaluation. The authors use the Lund-Mackay system, which has facilitated the highest level of both interobserver and intraobserver agreement (Table 57.3) [28, 34, 50, 55–58]. Magnetic resonance imaging is generally relevant for the assessment of intracranial or orbital complications [9].

Laboratory Studies

Due to the fact that there is a higher prevalence of atopy in patients with CRS, we check for atopic disposition with a skin-prick test including the common aeroallergens (e.g. trees, grasses, moulds, house dust mites, and dog and cat dander) and test for total IgE in serum.

Aetiology-Specific Assessments

The reason that primary surgery fails to improve symptoms is frequently related to the aetiology of the disease, and patients with certain aetiologies are specifically prone to recurrences. Therefore, a detailed understanding of the relevant pathomechanisms is needed at the time of presentation. The most important reasons are: mechanical obstruction, atopic disposition, bronchial asthma, AERD, bacterial and viral infections, inflammation induced by bacterial superantigens, colonisation and immunological reaction to fungi. Other causes include gastro-oesophageal reflux (GERD), immunodeficiencies, and rare diseases such as primary ciliary dyskinesia, cystic fibrosis (CF) and Churg-Strauss-Syndrome. In general, patients initially presenting with nasal polyps have a higher rate of recurrent disease despite the most aggressive surgeries than patients initially presenting without nasal polyps.

Signs and Symptoms that Should Prompt Aetiology-Specific Assessments

Certain signs, symptoms or laboratory results found during the general workup suggest a potentially treatable pathology. The most common signs that call for a more detailed workup are shown in Table 57.4.

Specific Aetiological Aspects

Mechanical Obstruction

Endoscopy and imaging (CT scan) play a key role in revealing relevant anatomical dispositions that are responsible for mechanical obstructions. A narrowed or blocked drainage can be an anatomical situation that has not been addressed by the primary surgery, or also might be the result of the post-surgical healing process.

Bacteria

Acute Rhinosinusitis

Mucopurulent discharge seen by rhinoscopy/endoscopy, especially in combination with generalised malaise and signs of inflammation in blood tests, suggests acute exacerbation [11]. Microbiology culture and resistance pattern should be assessed in immunocompromised patients. One has to bear in mind that

Table 57.4 Signs/symptoms for a specific aetiology. *GERD* Gastrointestinal reflux, *AERD* aspirin-exacerbated respiratory disease, *CF* cystic fibrosis, *ASA* acetylsalicylic acid, *NSAIDs* non-steroidal anti-inflammatory drugs

Sign/symptom	Search for
"Allergic" symptoms: runny nose, congestion, itching, sneezing, loss of smell, epiphora	Allergy
Mucopurulent discharge	Bacteria, fungi, immunodeficiency, ciliary dyskinesia
Coughing	Bronchial hyperactivity, bronchial asthma
Heartburn	GERD
Massive recurrent nasal polyps	AERD, fungi, ciliary dyskinesia
Young age	Immunodeficiency, CF
Unwanted reactions to ASA, NSAIDs	AERD
Positive skin test	Allergy
Elevated total IgE and/or specific IgE	Allergy

patients who have already had sinus surgery might misinterpret their secretions as purulent, although it may be simply loosened granulocyte-rich crustings from areas of scarred mucosa.

Superantigens

Of patients with CRS with nasal polyps, 60% were found to have *Staphylococcus aureus* in their nose, together with strong eosinophilic inflammation and local IgE production causing persistent inflammation and formation of nasal polyps. The pathophysiological aspect is thought to be toxins produced by the bacteria acting as superantigens [2, 53]. The suspicion for this aetiology is based mainly on clinical aspects, with recurrent nasal polyps and persistent mucopurulent drainage. There is currently no validated test available to reliably identify this subgroup of patients.

Allergy

Further skin-prick testing is only indicated when certain allergens are suspected and are available in standardised solutions. It should be carried out in cases with clinical suspicion of allergy underlying the recurrent disease. Testing for specific IgEs (SX1, Phadiatop) in serum is recommended. A possible allergy to dust mites and moulds should be tested intracutaneously.

The next step to determining the clinical relevance of specific allergens is a specific intranasal allergen challenge. A specific amount of the allergen is applied intranasally as a drop or spray. The reaction is monitored by rhinometric methods and symptom scores. There is no clear evidence that food allergy or its testing is of relevance for recurrent sinus disease. Epicutaneous skin testing helps to assess atopic disposition; however, due to

the substances tested it has no relevance as diagnostic tool for CRS.

Bronchial asthma has previously been reported to have a negative effect on surgical outcome and an increased need for revision sinus surgery. In patients presenting with lower-airway involvement, bronchial hyper-reactivity and bronchial asthma, more extensive sinus disease is generally suspected. The basic evaluations to rule out bronchial hyper-reactivity are spirometry and broncholysis testing. When patients primarily complain about chronic cough we need to be aware that post-nasal drip might be the cause.

Aspirin-Exacerbated Respiratory Disease

Sensitivity to acetylsalicylic acid (ASA) and other non-steroidal anti-inflammatory drugs (NSAIDs) is a major prognostic factor for recurrent disease. These patients often return with clinically massive nasal polyps after primary surgery, as well as with prolonged episodes of recurrent rhinosinusitis [1]. Detailed questioning regarding unwanted reactions to NSAIDs after oral, intramuscular or other application is essential. The typical feature patients will report is an onset of rhinorrhoea, conjunctival irritation, nasal congestion, a sense of tightness in the throat and chest, and scarlet flush of the head and neck immediately or within a couple of hours following the ingestion. This might lead up to the point of exacerbation of bronchial asthma or even anaphylactic reaction. The full clinical picture of AERD is the combination of CRS with nasal polyps, bronchial asthma and sensitivity to NSAIDs [13, 33, 47, 48]. The special feature of these patients is an extensive eosinophilic infiltration in tissues and lavages of the upper and lower airways.

However, it is essential, especially in otolaryngology, to identify those individuals who do not yet present the complete clinical picture. If AERD is suspected on the basis of medical history, further specific challenges with ASA and other NSAIDs should be applied next. Oral challenges should be done in a specialised medical centre with close (inpatient!) monitoring, because of the high risk of anaphylactoid reactions. The oral route is the best-validated and most frequently used provocation scheme. The bronchial and intravenous route is less advisable. The intra-nasal challenge presents a valuable alternative for an outpatient setting due to its low-risk potential and short duration; however, once dissolved in water, the test substance (lysine-ASA) is only stable for 1 day.

The current pathogenic hypothesis for AERD suggests an imbalance of prostaglandin E_2 (PGE_2) and cysteinyl-leukotrienes (cys-LTs) due to a metabolic shift towards the lipoxygenase pathway and reduced formation of prostanoids by inhibiting cyclo-oxygenase isozymes [7, 47]. An in vitro assay has recently been established that is valuable in diagnosing AERD. For this assay a mixed leukocyte culture is used to analyse the eicosanoid release of cys-LTs and PGE_2 using competitive enzyme immunoassays [3, 4, 43]. A positive test result is defined as elevated cys-LT release and lowered PGE_2 release (LiPiDoC-AIT). Alternatively the cellular allergy stimulation test (CAST 2000-ELISA) to measure only the leukotrienes (LTC_4, LTD_4, LTE_4) can be used [29].

Various

Signs of GERD may be symptoms such as heartburn, acid regurgitation or other gastrointestinal diseases. The airways might be involved, with sore throat, coughing and dysphonia. Refer these patients to internal medicine for diagnosis and treatment before surgery [10, 20].

Fungi may cause a range of pathologies, ranging from non-invasive fungus balls to invasive debilitating disease. They may also induce an altered local immune (non-allergic) response in nasal/sinus secretions resulting in chronic eosinophilic rhinosinusitis or nasal polyps. While the invasive forms are diagnosed by clinical examination and radiological assessment, the last has no specific symptoms other than simply recurrent disease, nasal polyps and mucopurulent discharge. In order to uncover this aetiology, specific handling is required to culture fungi from the nasal discharge.

Timing of Surgery and Conservative Treatment

Surgery and conservative treatment methods should always be combined in a concept that is suitable for the underlying aetiologies and symptoms. The aim of surgery is mainly to remove the specific focus for the disease and to recover proper drainage. Hence, to a certain degree, relief from various symptoms is achieved, at least in the short-term. The aims of additional medical treatment are to achieve stable relief from rhinitis symptoms, such as nasal obstruction, loss of smell and recurrence of disease. This concept includes pre-surgical, surgical and post-surgical treatment. The aim of combined conserva-

tive/surgical treatment is to achieve the best long-term symptom improvement (see Chap. 55).

A critical question is whether surgery and conservative treatment is done in parallel or sequentially. This decision has to be made individually for each patient. In general, however, acute, and especially inflammatory conditions benefit from conservative treatment at least 2 days before surgery. When a specific treatment for allergy or GERD has been started it is reasonable to wait for some time before a decision about surgery and the extent of surgery is made.

On the other hand, all conditions that show an anatomically unfavourable situation that is unlikely to respond to medical treatment, such as scarring, or an obstruction that may even prevent topical treatment from working should be treated by surgery first. Even if a condition is expected to benefit from conservative treatment, the severity and subjective impairment of the patient may call for surgery before medical treatment (e.g. patients with massive nasal polyps).

Pre-surgical Conservative/Medical Management

Allergy

If allergy is a major factor for complaints, patients should be treated according to individual symptoms. Second-generation antihistamines are considered first-choice treatment, as well as topical corticosteroids with their strong effect on nasal blockage and long-lasting anti-inflammatory properties. Treat with topical corticosteroids such as budesonide, flunisolide, triamcinolon acetonide, fluticasone-17-propionate and mometasone furoate with high receptor affinity and low bioavailability. Topical antihistamines are considered an "on demand" treatment in addition to a continuous medication. Specific immunotherapy is indicated in specific IgE-mediated disease when pharmacotherapy and avoidance measures are insufficient. If surgery still needs to be considered for other reasons, it needs to be performed outside allergy season and all treatments for allergic rhinitis can be continued independently from surgery.

Antileukotrienes, antagonists of cys-LT_1 receptors (montelukast) and 5-lipoxygenase inhibitors (zileuton) have shown a benefit in mild asthmatics. A few trials indicate that antileukotriene treatment may have a beneficial effect on nasal symptoms and decrease polyp regrowth in patients with CRS, and especially in those with AERD [15, 40]. However, ASA desensitisation is significantly more effective against polyp regrowth.

Various

In patients with recurrent boosts of acute rhinosinusitis and exacerbations of CRS we have to deal with drug-resistant organisms more often than in sporadic bacterial rhinosinusitis. The antimicrobial agents to use are amoxicillin clavulanate, cefuroxime axetils, chinolones (ciprofloxacin, levofloxacin, moxifloxacin). In selected cases it is advisable to set up a culture and adjust the treatment accordingly [46]. Topical steroids have recently been proven to be beneficial in combination with antibi-

57

otics [30]. Decongestants and nasal douches have an alleviating effect on symptoms.

If all other causes have been ruled out and superantigens are suspected, long-term, low-dose macrolide treatment with 150 mg roxithromycin daily for 3 months can be considered (see Chap. 55) [46]. A benefit is also seen in combination with surgery [14].

The administration of antifungal agents was considered a potential treatment in the past; however, recent data question amphotericin B nasal lavages (25 ml amphotericin B; 100 μg/ml) to each nostril twice daily for 3 months) to be effective in the treatment of CRS. Further studies on this topic are needed [38, 42, 52].

has frequently been implicated in recurrent sinus disease; however, indisputable evidence is rare. Much of the support for a link between reflux disease and several extra-oesophageal complications is based on the observation that reflux disease frequently coexists with other disorders. Long-term treatment with a proton pump inhibitor, independent of the time point and extent of surgery, in cooperation with an internal medicine specialist is advised [10, 20].

Patients with immunodeficiencies or CF benefit from pre-surgical topical corticosteroids in combination with nasal douches. Short-term clinical trials have shown that nebulised hypertonic saline improves mucociliary clearance, and new systems (e.g. Pari Sinus) have been developed recently [49].

Systemic corticosteroids (e.g. prednisolone, prednisone) are a last resort for medical treatment in the case of severe symptoms of CRS with nasal polyps refractory to first-choice treatment. Short courses of oral steroid therapy can be prescribed (<3 weeks) starting with 80 mg prednisone/100 mg prednisolone and successive decrease. One has to be aware of the strong rebound effect, however, especially in patients with AERD. Steroids may also be given orally several days before surgery in order to reduce swelling and facilitate surgery [9, 16, 17, 23, 25, 26, 32].

Alternative Ways

Many other types of preparations have been investigated, but the evidence of their benefit is poor. Phytopreparations claim an effect on CRS. Different immunomodulators or immunostimulants such as bacterial lysates have been tested for acute and CRS, as an altered immune response may be responsible for frequent recurrences and the antibiotic courses could be reduced significantly [44]. Certain groups of antibiotics may be regarded as immunomodulators, such as quinolones and macrolides [8]. The topical application of capsaicin, the active substance from red-hot chilli peppers, is discussed as an option to stop recurrent nasal polyps [54]; it may act as a long-lasting desensitiser on nasal mucosa when applied due to depletion of substance P and neurokinins in unmyelinated axons. Very recently, furosemide came into discussion as a treatment option, but its value has yet to be proved [35].

Surgical Management

Extent of Surgery

Anatomical problems need localised intervention. The relevance of surgery in diseases that can not be cured by surgery must be considered. The main anatomical problems specific to revision sinus surgery are:

1. Scarring in the area of the frontal recess and the frontal sinus ostia.
2. Lateralisation of the middle turbinate and scarring on the lateral nasal wall.
3. Persistent lateral cells in the area of the lamina papyracea and/or agger nasi cells.

Patients with general disease of the sinus mucosa need restoration of drainage from all sinuses, but as much unaffected mucosa as possible should be spared. Disturbance of lymphatic drainage and scarring may be the consequence of extended mucosa resection.

Concomitant Medical Treatment

Patients with problems in the frontal sinus benefit from concomitant medical treatment during surgery (e.g. application of steroid-containing ointments). Application can be repeated after surgery, but should be considered on an individual basis depending on wound healing. Use of mitomycin C has been suggested in situations of pronounced tendency towards extreme granulation formation (see Chap. 51). Instillation or lavage with antimicrobial agents (e.g. tobramycin) is discussed for patients with CF; however, evidence-based data is inconclusive and therefore this treatment is reserved for interdisciplinary, individualised treatment concepts.

Post-surgical Conservative/Medical Management

General Aspects

For all patients undergoing revision sinus surgery, mechanical care is advised, whereas the amount of treatment should be dependent on the extent of surgery. As an example, intensified mechanical care is certainly needed in complicated frontal sinus disease. The further use of nasal douches with isotonic or slightly hypertonic saline is recommended. Initially, after surgery a topical decongestant or preferably decongesting drops in solutions with other soothing ingredients are advised.

Topical corticosteroids with the least systemic effect are recommended, because they reduce oedema and facilitate the drainage of secretions. During the period of granulation tissue forming it prevents adhesions that might later lead to unpleasant scarring [18, 19]. The addition of antibiotics is advised in patients with signs of acute bacterial infection and mucopurulent drainage.

Oral corticosteroids are considered in patients with nasal polyps attributable to different aetiologies as a post-surgical

Table 57.5 Treatment plan for AERD

	Plan for AERD	Time point
1.	History	Initial office visit
	Whole blood test (LiPiDoC-AIT)	Initial office visit
2.	Surgery	
3.	Healing period, steroids oral/nasal	4 weeks
4.	Oral ASA provocation	6–8 weeks post-surgery
5.	Oral ASA desensitisation (300 mg)	6–8 weeks post-surgery
6.	Continue ASA plus topical steroids	Lifelong
7.	Patient follow-up	Every 6 months
8.	Additional treatment	Topical steroids, montelucast
9.	Individual suggestion	Change in ASA dosage, increase/decrease

Table 57.6 Protocol for ASA desensitisation

ASA desensitisation	Dose (ASA mg)
Day 1	15 mg
	30 mg
	60 mg
Day 2	60 mg
	150 mg
Day 3	150 mg
	150 mg
Day 4	300 mg
	Demission

short course of 1–4 weeks. However, the dose of oral corticosteroid should be under the Cushing level in less than 2 weeks. Hence, the duration of treatment should take into account possible side effects due to the systemic effect, and also with respect to the different phases of wound healing after surgery.

Post-surgical treatment with oral antihistamines in combination with topical corticosteroids is beneficial in patients with known allergies. It helps to reduce the influx of proinflammatory mediators that might complicate the wound-healing process.

If no ASA desensitisation is planned or about to be performed, treatment with antileukotrienes (montelucast) can be considered in patients with heavy nasal polyps due to proven or suspected AERD [15, 31]. The medication should start overlapping the oral corticosteroid course and be continued at least until after wound healing is completed.

Aspirin-Exacerbated Respiratory Disease

In patients with AERD a further anti-inflammatory treatment is absolutely necessary otherwise polyps reoccur in 90% of the cases after weeks or months [1]. Patients with AERD have a decreased risk of recurrent nasal polyps if desensitisation to ASA or topical lysine-ASA treatment is performed. The combined treatment of topical corticosteroids and desensitisation to ASA is effective in 65% of patients, improving the symptoms of rhinorrhoea and nasal blockage, while 73% show reduced regrowth of nasal polyps and improvement of smell [6].

A plan for treatment needs to be set up for standardisation (Table 57.5). Desensitisation to ASA consists of daily administration of increasing doses of ASA (Table 57.6). The airway resistance (e.g. by peak flow or forced expiratory volume in 1 s) needs to be monitored closely during the induction period. As soon as patient reports any clinical symptoms related to AERD, further ASA administration is stopped for the day and on the next day it is started with the same dosage. A coated tablet of 300 mg is the long-term maintenance dose used by the authors. Only long-term treatment can secure a beneficial outcome over time [6, 13, 45]. Alternative options are nasal desensitisation with lysine-ASA [36].

Summary

Treatment of recurrent sinus disease is a challenging task due to the variability in underlying pathophysiology. It has been demonstrated that a combination of sinus surgery, careful pre-surgical, surgical and post-surgical treatment with an appropriate conservative and medical therapy can have a favourable long-term effect on clinical symptoms. Revision surgery is a highly individualised type of procedure, and a precise knowledge of all aspects of the disease is very important to implement a combined medical and surgical approach with maximum benefit for the patient.

57

Tips to Avoid Complications

- Do everything to understand the underlying pathology and analyse carefully the possible reasons for surgical failure.
- Previous to revision surgery, search for so far unknown aetiologic factors like atopic diseases, AERD, immunodeficiency and GERD.
- Treat allergies according to guidelines; try not to operate during allergy season.
- Safety features in revision sinus surgery are even more important due to altered anatomy.

Take-Home Pearls

- Preoperative diagnostics are important to define the aetiology of recurrent sinus pathology in order to create an optimised treatment plan.
- Surgery is indicated when having symptoms despite optimal conservative treatment.
- Surgical management follows individual anatomy and pathology in terms of a specific tailored operative strategy.

References

1. Amar YG, Frenkiel S, Sobol SE (2000) Outcome analysis of endoscopic sinus surgery for chronic sinusitis in patients having Samter's triad. J Otolaryngol 29:7–12

2. Bachert C, Gevaert P, Holtappels G, van Cauwenberge P (2002) Mediators in nasal polyposis. Curr Allergy Asthma Rep 2:481–487

3. Baenkler HW, Schafer D, Hosemann W (1996) Eicosanoids from biopsy of normal and polypous nasal mucosa. Rhinology 34:166–170

4. Baenkler HW, Zeus J, Schenk J, Schafer D (2004) Abnormal eicosanoid pattern by blood leukocytes in gastroduodenal ulcer. Med Sci Monit 10:CR557–562

5. Benninger MS and Senior BA (1997) The development of the Rhinosinusitis Disability Index. Arch Otolaryngol Head Neck Surg 123:1175–1179

6. Berges-Gimeno MP, Simon RA, Stevenson DD (2003) Long-term treatment with aspirin desensitization in asthmatic patients with aspirin-exacerbated respiratory disease. J Allergy Clin Immunol 111:180–186

7. Bochenek G, Banska K, Szabo Z, Nizankowska E, Szczeklik A (2002) Diagnosis, prevention and treatment of aspirin-induced asthma and rhinitis. Curr Drug Targets Inflamm Allergy 1:1–11

8. Dalhoff A, Shalit I (2003) Immunomodulatory effects of quinolones. Lancet Infect Dis 3:359–371

9. Damm M, Jungehulsing M, Eckel HE, Schmidt M, Theissen P (1999) Effects of systemic steroid treatment in chronic polypoid rhinosinusitis evaluated with magnetic resonance imaging. Otolaryngol Head Neck Surg 120:517–523

10. Dibaise JK, Sharma VK (2006) Does gastroesophageal reflux contribute to the development of chronic sinusitis? A review of the evidence. Dis Esophagus 19:419–424

11. Fokkens W (2005) Evidence based diagnosis and treatment of rhinosinusitis and nasal polyps. Rhinology 43:1

12. Gliklich RE, Hilinski JM (1995) Longitudinal sensitivity of generic and specific health measures in chronic sinusitis. Qual Life Res 4:27–32

13. Gosepath J, Hoffmann F, Schafer D, Amedee RG, Mann WJ (1999) Aspirin intolerance in patients with chronic sinusitis. ORL J Otorhinolaryngol Relat Spec 61:146–150

14. Gotfried MH (2004) Macrolides for the treatment of chronic sinusitis, asthma, and COPD. Chest 125:52S–60S; quiz 60S–61S

15. Grundmann T, Topfner M (2001) Treatment of ASS-Associated Polyposis (ASSAP) with a cysteinyl leukotriene receptor antagonist – a prospective drug study on its antiinflammatory effects. Laryngorhinootologie 80:576–582

16. Henriksson G, Norlander T, Forsgren J, Stierna P (2001) Effects of topical budesonide treatment on glucocorticoid receptor mRNA down-regulation and cytokine patterns in nasal polyps. Am J Rhinol 15:1–8

17. Hosemann W, Michelson A, Weindler J, Mang H, Wigand ME (1990) The effect of endonasal paranasal sinus surgery on lung function of patients with bronchial asthma. Laryngorhinootologie 69:521–526

18. Hosemann W, Gode U, Langer F, Rockelein G, Wigand ME (1991) Experimental studies of wound healing in the paranasal sinuses. I. A model of respiratory wounds in the rabbit maxillary sinus. HNO 39:8–12

19. Hosemann W, Gode U, Langer F, Wigand ME (1991) Experimental studies of wound healing in the paranasal sinuses. II. Spontaneous wound healing and drug effects in a standardized wound model. HNO 39:48–54

20. Jecker P, Orloff LA, Wohlfeil M, Mann WJ (2006) Gastroesophageal reflux disease (GERD), extraesophageal reflux (EER) and recurrent chronic rhinosinusitis. Eur Arch Otorhinolaryngol 263:664–667

21. Johansson L, Akerlund A, Holmberg K, Melen I, Stierna P, Bende M (2000) Evaluation of methods for endoscopic staging of nasal polyposis. Acta Otolaryngol 120:72–76

22. Khalid AN, Quraishi SA, Kennedy DW (2004) Long-term quality of life measures after functional endoscopic sinus surgery. Am J Rhinol 18:131–136

23. Larsen K, Tos M (1997) A long-term follow-up study of nasal polyp patients after simple polypectomies. Eur Arch Otorhinolaryngol 254:S85–88

24. Lildholdt T, Rundcrantz H, Lindqvist N (1995) Efficacy of topical corticosteroid powder for nasal polyps: a double-blind, placebo-controlled study of budesonide. Clin Otolaryngol Allied Sci 20:26–30

25. Lildholdt T, Rundcrantz H, Bende M, Larsen K (1997) Glucocorticoid treatment for nasal polyps. The use of topical budesonide powder, intramuscular betamethasone, and surgical treatment. Arch Otolaryngol Head Neck Surg 123:595–600

26. Llorente JL, Martinez-Farreras A, Rodrigo JP, Perez P, Munoz C, Baragano L, Suarez C (2002) Nasal polyposis: postoperative long term results (5 years) after endoscopic sinus surgery. Acta Otorrinolaringol Esp 53:102–109

27. Lund VJ, Kennedy DW (1995) Quantification for staging sinusitis. The Staging and Therapy Group. Ann Otol Rhinol Laryngol Suppl 167:17–21

28. Lund VJ, Mackay IS (1993) Staging in rhinosinusitis. Rhinology 31:183–184

29. May A, Weber A, Gall H, Kaufmann R, Zollner TM (1999) Means of increasing sensitivity of an in vitro diagnostic test for aspirin intolerance. Clin Exp Allergy 29:1402–1411

30. Meltzer EO, Orgel HA, Backhaus JW, Busse WW, Druce HM, Metzger WJ, Mitchell DQ, Selner JC, Shapiro GG, Van Bavel JH, et al (1993) Intranasal flunisolide spray as an adjunct to oral antibiotic therapy for sinusitis. J Allergy Clin Immunol 92:812–823

31. Micheletto C, Tognella S, Visconti M, Pomari C, Trevisan F, Dal Negro RW (2004) Montelukast 10 mg improves nasal function and nasal response to aspirin in ASA-sensitive asthmatics: a controlled study vs placebo. Allergy 59:289–294

32. Mygind N (1999) Advances in the medical treatment of nasal polyps. Allergy 54:12–16

33. Namazy JA, Simon RA (2002) Sensitivity to nonsteroidal anti-inflammatory drugs. Ann Allergy Asthma Immunol 89:542–550; quiz 550, 605

34. Oluwole M, Russell N, Tan L, Gardiner Q, White P (1996) A comparison of computerized tomographic staging systems in chronic sinusitis. Clin Otolaryngol Allied Sci 21:91–95

35. Passali D, Mezzedimi C, Passali GC, Bellussi L (2000) Efficacy of inhalation form of furosemide to prevent postsurgical relapses of rhinosinusal polyposis. ORL J Otorhinolaryngol Relat Spec 62:307–310

36. Patriarca G, Bellioni P, Nucera E, Schiavino D, Papa G, Schinco G, Fais G, Pirotta LR (1991) Intranasal treatment with lysine acetylsalicylate in patients with nasal polyposis. Ann Allergy 67:588–592

37. Piccirillo JF, Merritt MG Jr, Richards ML (2002) Psychometric and clinimetric validity of the 20-Item Sino-Nasal Outcome Test (SNOT-20) Otolaryngol Head Neck Surg 126:41–47

38. Ponikau JU, Sherris DA, Weaver A, Kita H (2005) Treatment of chronic rhinosinusitis with intranasal amphotericin B: a randomized, placebo-controlled, double-blind pilot trial. J Allergy Clin Immunol 115:125–131

39. Radenne F, Lamblin C, Vandezande LM, Tillie-Leblond I, Darras J, Tonnel AB, Wallaert B (1999) Quality of life in nasal polyposis. J Allergy Clin Immunol 104:79–84

40. Ragab S, Parikh A, Darby YC, Scadding GK (2001) An open audit of montelukast, a leukotriene receptor antagonist, in nasal polyposis associated with asthma. Clin Exp Allergy 31:1385–1391

41. Ragab SM, Lund VJ, Scadding G (2004) Evaluation of the medical and surgical treatment of chronic rhinosinusitis: a prospective, randomised, controlled trial. Laryngoscope 114:923–930

42. Ricchetti A, Landis BN, Maffioli A, Giger R, Zeng C, Lacroix JS (2002) Effect of anti-fungal nasal lavage with amphotericin B on nasal polyposis. J Laryngol Otol 116:261–263

43. Schafer D, Schmid M, Gode UC, Baenkler HW (1999) Dynamics of eicosanoids in peripheral blood cells during bronchial provocation in aspirin-intolerant asthmatics. Eur Respir J 13:638–646

44. Serrano E, Demanez JP, Morgon A, Chastang C, Van Cauwenberge P (1997) Effectiveness of ribosomal fractions of *Klebsiella pneumoniae*, *Streptococcus pneumoniae*, *Streptococcus pyogenes*, *Haemophilus influenzae* and the membrane fraction of Kp (Ribomunyl) in the prevention of clinical recurrences of infectious rhinitis. Results of a multicenter double-blind placebo-controlled study. Eur Arch Otorhinolaryngol 254:372–375

45. Stevenson DD, Hankammer MA, Mathison DA, Christiansen SC, Simon RA (1996) Aspirin desensitization treatment of aspirin-sensitive patients with rhinosinusitis-asthma: long-term outcomes. J Allergy Clin Immunol 98:751–758

46. Suzuki H, Shimomura A, Ikeda K, Oshima T, Takasaka T (1997) Effects of long-term low-dose macrolide administration on neutrophil recruitment and IL-8 in the nasal discharge of chronic sinusitis patients. Tohoku J Exp Med 182:115–124

47. Szczeklik A, Stevenson DD (2003) Aspirin-induced asthma: advances in pathogenesis, diagnosis, and management. J Allergy Clin Immunol 111:913–921; quiz 922

48. Szczeklik A, Nizankowska E, Duplaga M (2000) Natural history of aspirin-induced asthma. AIANE Investigators. European Network on Aspirin-Induced Asthma. Eur Respir J 16:432–436

49. Talbot AR, Herr TM, Parsons DS (1997) Mucociliary clearance and buffered hypertonic saline solution. Laryngoscope 107:500–503

50. Van Camp C, Clement PA (1994) Results of oral steroid treatment in nasal polyposis. Rhinology 32:5–9

51. Ware JE Jr, Sherbourne CD (1992) The MOS 36-item short-form health survey (SF-36) I. Conceptual framework and item selection. Med Care 30:473–483

52. Weschta M, Rimek D, Formanek M, Polzehl D, Podbielski A, Riechelmann H (2004) Topical antifungal treatment of chronic rhinosinusitis with nasal polyps: a randomized, double-blind clinical trial. J Allergy Clin Immunol 113:1122–1128

53. Zhang N, Gevaert P, van Zele T, Perez-Novo C, Patou J, Holtappels G, van Cauwenberge P, Bachert C (2005) An update on the impact of *Staphylococcus aureus* enterotoxins in chronic sinusitis with nasal polyposis. Rhinology 43:162–168

54. Zheng C, Wang Z, Lacroix JS (2000) Effect of intranasal treatment with capsaicin on the recurrence of polyps after polypectomy and ethmoidectomy. Acta Otolaryngol 120:62–66

55. Zinreich J (1993) Imaging of inflammatory sinus disease. Otolaryngol Clin North Am 26:535–547

56. Zinreich SJ, Mattox DE, Kennedy DW, Chisholm HL, Diffley DM, Rosenbaum AE (1988) Concha bullosa: CT evaluation. J Comput Assist Tomogr 12:778–784

57. Zinreich SJ, Kennedy DW, Kumar AJ, Rosenbaum AE, Arrington JA, Johns ME (1988) MR imaging of normal nasal cycle: comparison with sinus pathology. J Comput Assist Tomogr 12:1014–1019

58. Zinreich SJ, Kennedy DW, Malat J, Curtin HD, Epstein JI, Huff LC, Kumar AJ, Johns ME, Rosenbaum AE (1988) Fungal sinusitis: diagnosis with CT and MR imaging. Radiology 169:439–44

Chapter 58

Endoscopic Surgery on the Lacrimal Apparatus

58

Gert Jeunen and Mark Jorissen

Core Messages

- Dacryocystorhinostomy (DCR) is indicated in distal outflow obstruction of the lacrimal system.
- The fluorescein dye retention test and lacrimal irrigation and probing are used to detect the presence and site of obstruction.
- Dacryocystography is used to determine the site of stenosis or obstruction.
- Computed tomography can be used to define the diameter of the bony lacrimal canal, and identifies concurrent nasal or paranasal disease.
- Lacrimal scintillography is a more functional assessment.
- Endoscopic DCR can easily be performed by an otolaryngologist who is experienced in endonasal endoscopic surgery.
- New endoscopic techniques have been developed involving wide bony removal and creation of epithelium-lined mucosal anastomosis, resulting in improved surgical results.
- Postoperative care consists of topical steroid and antibiotic eye drops, nasal douching with saline, nasendoscopic removal of crusting and blood clots, and removal of silicone tubes.

Contents

Introduction

Obstruction of the lacrimal pathways is a common problem that can be corrected with dacryocystorhinostomy (DCR), which involves diverting the lacrimal flow into the nasal fossa through an artificial opening made at the level of the lacrimal bone [1]. This procedure can be carried out by an external or endonasal surgical approach [2]. The external approach, described by Toti in 1904 [3] became very popular and is still the mainstay of treatment for most ophthalmologists, with modifications in the 1920s including the addition of flaps, and in 1962 with Silastic tube intubation by Jones [4–6]. The original intranasal technique was described in 1893 by Caldwell but was largely abandoned as a result of problems with visualization. However, since the development of the endonasal microsurgical techniques and the now-thorough knowledge of paranasal and orbital anatomy, endonasal DCR presents itself as an alternative choice to the conventional external approach.

58

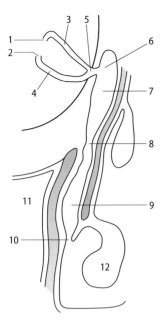

Fig. 58.1 Anatomy of the lacrimal system. *1* Punctum superius, *2* punctum inferius, *3* canaliculus superior, *4* canaliculus inferior, *5* canaliculus communis or Maier's sinus, *6* Rosenmüller's valve, *7* lacrimal sac, *8* Krause's valve, *9* nasolacrimal duct, *10* Hasner's valve, *11* maxillary sinus, *12* concha inferior

Anatomy/Physiology of the Lacrimal System

The function of tears is to keep the ocular surface moist and clear of debris and bacteria. Tears are produced by the lacrimal and accessory lacrimal glands and drain through the lacrimal drainage system, which begins at the punctum, a small opening on the medial surface of each eyelid (Fig. 58.1). The punctum is the opening of the canaliculus, which drains into the common canaliculus and then into the lacrimal sac. Tears that collect in the lacrimal sac drain through the nasolacrimal duct and into the nose through the inferior meatus, which is located below the inferior turbinate. The valve of Hasner, a mucosal fold at the distal end of the nasolacrimal duct, prevents air from entering the lacrimal sac when the nose is blown. Tears are swallowed after they pass from the nose into the nasopharynx.

The drainage of tears is both passive and active. Gravity is responsible for passive drainage, and blinking facilitates active drainage by activating the pump mechanism (orbicularis oculi muscles) and creating a negative pressure in the canaliculus and lacrimal sac, resulting in drawing of tears into the drainage system.

Pathology of the Lacrimal System

Epiphora is defined as the overflow of tears and is caused by a disruption in the balance between tear production and drainage. In the absence of conditions that increase tear production,

abnormality in tear drainage is the most likely cause of epiphora. Abnormalities of tear drainage can be subdivided further into functional and anatomical. Functional failure is related to poor lacrimal pump function, which may be due to a displaced punctum, eyelid laxity, weak orbicularis, or cranial nerve VII palsy. Anatomical obstruction may occur at any point along the lacrimal drainage pathway and may be congenital or acquired. Acquired nasolacrimal duct obstruction can be further subdivided into primary and secondary [7].

Acute and chronic dacryocystitis are clinical entities that are mostly caused by an underlying lacrimal system obstruction.

Primary Acquired Nasolacrimal Duct Obstruction

Primary acquired nasolacrimal duct obstruction (PANDO) is a mostly idiopathic "shrinking process" of the lacrimal sac and nasolacrimal duct and affects adults, progressively resulting in significant stenosis of the lacrimal drainage system, often at the preexisting most narrow locations (e.g., Rosenmüller's, Krause's, and Hasner's valves; Fig. 58.1).

There is no evidence of a bacterial or other precipitating cause of PANDO. Linberg and McCormick reported the histopathological changes in PANDO [8]. An initial lumen obstruction by mucosal edema is followed by progressive fibrosis due to chronic inflammation, resulting in further ductal narrowing. Stasis of cellular debris and mucus in the ductal lumen results not only in aggravation of the inflammation, but also in rebound hypersecretion of tears and thus increasing epiphora [8]. PANDO is more common in middle-aged and elderly females. Using CT scans, Groessl et al. demonstrated that women have significantly smaller dimensions in the lower nasolacrimal fossa and middle nasolacrimal duct [9]. They noted that changes in the anteroposterior dimensions of the bony nasolacrimal canal coincide with osteoporotic changes throughout the body. These quantitative measurements may help explain the higher incidence of PANDO among women. Others have suggested menstrual and hormonal fluctuations and a heightened immune status as factors that may contribute to the disease process.

Secondary Acquired Lacrimal Drainage Obstruction

The general categories of causes of secondary acquired lacrimal drainage obstruction include infectious, inflammatory, neoplastic, traumatic, and mechanical. These subjects will not be discussed in detail in this chapter.

Acute Dacryocystitis

Acute infection is mostly associated with preexisting nasolacrimal duct obstruction, which facilitates inflammation and impedes the distal evacuation of pus. In addition, cranial clearance can be hampered by obstruction of the common canaliculus, due to vigorous swelling of the lacrimal sac. In a review of 54 children with dacryocystitis, two-thirds of the cases were chronic and one-third were acute. The most common organisms isolated from children with acute dacryocystitis were *alpha-hemolytic Streptococci*, *Staphylococcus epidermidis*, and *Staphylococcus aureus* [10].

Chronic Dacryocystitis

This chronic disease is also associated with underlying nasolacrimal duct obstruction. The organisms most commonly isolated from the lacrimal sac in one study of 47 young children with nasolacrimal duct obstruction included *Streptococcus pneumoniae* (35%), *Haemophilus influenzae* (20%), *Pseudomonas aeruginosa* (11%) and *Streptococcus viridans* (11%) [11].

Diagnosis and Evaluation

Clinical Evaluation

Patients present with epiphora and mucoid or purulent discharge, with or without signs of acute or chronic infection, such as pain and skin edema/erythema in the region of the medial canthus. Acute dacryocystitis can be complicated by spread of infection in the orbital region, with preseptal or orbital cellulitis and orbital abscess. Sepsis and meningitis have also been described in the literature as a rare complication of acute dacryocystitis [12].

All patients should be subjected to an ophthalmologic and ear, nose, and throat examination. In order to attain good postoperative results, the patient's assessment should be focused on making sure the pathology is caused by distal outflow obstruction of the lacrimal system. The following relevant investigations are highlighted.

Nasal Endoscopy

To assess the anatomical accessibility of the operative site, particular attention is paid to the presence of significant deviations of the nasal septum at the level of the middle meatus or at the anterior end of the inferior turbinate. The presence of coexistent paranasal sinus disease such as nasal polyposis or inflammatory conditions forewarns the surgeon of the potential need for endoscopic ethmoidal or middle-meatal surgery [13].

Fluorescein Dye Retention Test

The fluorescein dye retention test is a semiquantitative test of delayed or obstructed tear outflow [14]. Instill one drop of fluorescein 2% into the unanesthetized conjunctival sac; the amount of residual color after 3 and 5 minutes in one or both eyes is noted and the intensity of residual fluorescein dye is graded on a scale of 0–4 (where 0 = no dye, 4 = all of the dye). The test is positive if residual fluorescein is present. The dye normally drains down the system in this time. A strongly positive test is found if obstruction is present. False negative findings may occur due to

a large lacrimal sac or mucocoele, or a distal nasolacrimal duct block, where the dye can pool in the sac or duct.

Penetration of the dye thus confirms patency of the nasolacrimal system. However, drawbacks are the high false negative rate and the fact that the test does not identify patients with a partial obstruction of the nasolacrimal system. According to Wormald and Tsirbas, this test has been largely superseded by dacryocystography (DCG) and lacrimal scintillography [15, 16].

Lacrimal Irrigation and Probing

Probing and syringing the proximal lacrimal drainage system can detect both the presence and site of partial or complete lacrimal outflow [16]. Firstly, topical anesthetic drops are placed in the eye. The upper and lower puncta are gently dilated with a blunt Bowman's "00" probe (Martin, Tuttlingen, Germany), rotating it for the first 1 mm with the lid margin taut. Following dilatation, the probe is angled medially. As the probe enters the common canaliculus, slight resistance may be felt – the "soft stop" – and then as it touches the medial wall of the sac, there is a "hard stop." At this point the probe is angled vertically down to feel whether there is any sac pathology or distal obstruction.

Distal obstruction is diagnosed by probing and then syringing to see whether the fluid can initially be passed through the canaliculi into the nose. If it refluxes through the other punctum, this indicates that there is distal obstruction. If there is reflux through the same punctum, then there is canalicular or common canalicular stenosis, and this can be confirmed be gentle probing [17]. Irrigation is at a higher hydrostatic pressure than the normal tear outflow. Therefore, patients with functional epiphora from dacryostenosis may have apparently normal findings on irrigation, and scintillography should be done [16].

Jones Tests

Jones I and II tests, which in short involve instilling copious amounts of fluorescein into the eye with the suspected blockage and checking the recovery of fluorescein after blowing the nostril on the same side only into a tissue, are only performed to confirm and localize functional epiphora and are not done if there is a complete obstruction on syringing [16].

Imaging Studies

Ancillary radiological investigations help to confirm the site of stenosis or obstruction, to assess functional tear drainage delay, and demonstrate paranasal pathology. Tests are complementary and more then one test may be necessary.

Dacryocystography

This involves injection of a radio-opaque fluid (e.g., Ultravist 300; Schering, Berlin, Germany) into the lower or upper canaliculus and taking magnified X-rays (Fig. 58.2). DCG enables an

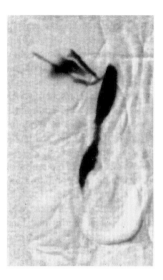

Fig. 58.2 Digital subtraction dacryocystography of the right lacrimal system

accurate assessment of the anatomy of the canaliculi, sac, and nasolacrimal duct. It is good for determining the site of stenosis or obstruction, and is particularly useful in distinguishing between post-sac and pre-sac stenosis. It outlines diverticula and fistulae, and shows intra-sac pathology (dacryoliths or tumors), and sac size. It also helps to define the cause of failed lacrimal surgery. DCG may be useful in determining whether individual patients are good candidates for endonasal surgery. Mannor and Millman found that endonasal DCR was successful in 82% of patients with normal or large lacrimal sacs on DCG, but the success rate was only 29% in individuals with small lacrimal sacs [18]. However, one must be aware that intubation and the pressure generated by the injection of contrast may alter the normal physiology by causing dilatation, which may mask a mild obstruction [15, 16, 19]. The DCG proves open tearways until the point the contrast medium is reaching. If, for example, contrast medium is not going into the sac, this may be due to detritus or stones in the sac; it is not proof of a canalis communis stenosis.

Nuclear Lacrimal Scintillography

A more physiological and functional assessment is provided by lacrimal scintillography, in which a radioisotope (technetium-99m pertechnetate) is placed in the lower fornix of the eye and assessments are made at regular time intervals as to whether the radioisotope reaches the nasal cavity [19]. Lack of sac filling will often indicate a presaccal obstruction, while delay in sac emptying may indicate a postsaccal obstruction [15].

The combination of a dacryocystogram and lacrimal scintillography allows both the anatomical detail and the function of the system to be assessed.

Computed Tomography

Computed Tomography can be used to define the diameter of the bony lacrimal canal. Zinreich et al. described the combination of CT with DCG, making it a more functional examination [20]. This examination is indicated in posttraumatic or postoperative nasolacrimal duct obstruction and as preoperative exam when performing an endoscopic DCR procedure. It also allows identification of nasal or paranasal sinus abnormalities that might require concomitant correction, and permits preoperative visualization of the thickness of the bone surrounding the lacrimal sac as well as the presence of an agger nasi cell, which may require surgical removal [21].

Magnetic Resonance Imaging

Magnetic resonance imaging is superior to CT in imaging soft tissues. In selected cases of complex pathology, such as tumors, it could add valuable information, but is not routinely used.

How to Do it

Endoscopic DCR can be performed under local or general anesthesia. It is possible to open the lacrimal sac endonasally with either conventional instruments with or without powered instrumentarium, or a laser. The laser procedure has the advantage that it can be done more readily as a day-stay procedure, as there is a minimal amount of bleeding. The disadvantages of the laser are its expense, the precautions that need to be taken, and the fact that the results are not as good as with conventional instruments, with success rates ranging from 64% to 85% [17, 22–25].

There are a variety of surgical techniques for endoscopic DCR, all with the aim of producing an opening of the lacrimal sac. However, it is not always easy to identify the lacrimal duct or sac via the endonasal route. In view of that, it is important to understand the anatomy of the lacrimal bone at the lateral wall of the nose and the relevance to endoscopic surgery.

Surgical Anatomy

The lacrimal sac (12–15 mm long) is housed in the lacrimal fossa between the anterior and posterior lacrimal crests (Fig. 58.3). The anterior lacrimal crest is formed by the frontal process of the maxillary bone and the posterior crest by the lacrimal bone. The fossa measures up to 8 mm anteroposteriorly, 16 mm vertically, and 2–4 mm deep. Its vertical axis is slightly posterior, inferior, and lateral. The nasolacrimal duct (18-mm long) leads from the sac into the lateral wall of the nose, where it opens in the inferior meatus. The bony canal for the duct is formed by the maxilla, lacrimal bone, and the inferior nasal concha. The bony canal starts as a near-spherical opening in the inferoanterior orbital floor, approximately 3–5 mm from the rim. It becomes slightly oval as it descends, with the longer dimension anteroposterior. The interosseous part is approximately 12 mm

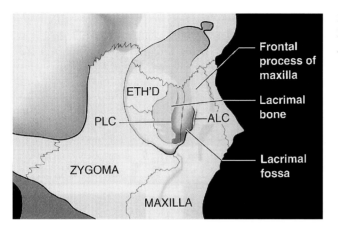

Fig. 58.3 Lateral view of the right lacrimal fossa. *PLC* Posterior lacrimal crest, *ALC* anterior lacrimal crest, *ETH'D* ethmoid

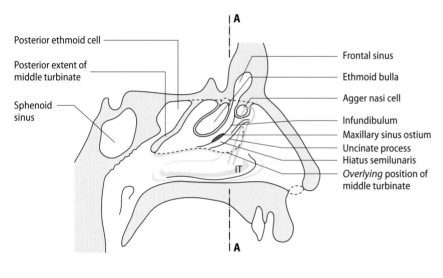

IT   Inferior turbinate

⬤   Yellow outline indicates *underlying* position of lacrimal sac and nasolacrimal duct.

Fig. 58.4 Left lateral nasal wall of the middle turbinate removed to reveal the structures in the middle meatus. The uncinate process, hiatus semilunaris and infundibulum are to be avoided (posterior to line A–A). The *yellow outline* indicates the underlying position of the lacrimal sac and nasolacrimal duct. *IT* Inferior turbinate

long and inclines posteriorly (approximately 15°) and laterally, toward the first molar (Fig. 58.4). The width of the bony canal is wider in men than in women [16].

Viewed intranasally, the lacrimal ridge, starting at the highest point of the inferior turbinate, extending vertically and ending immediately in front of the middle turbinate's attachment, corresponds to the frontal process of the maxilla immediately anterior to its junction with the lacrimal bone. The lacrimal bone is paper thin, making identification of this junction with the hard frontal process easy. This vertical junction lies approximately 3 mm behind the ridge and extends upwards under the anterior attachment of the middle turbinate and above the ethmoid crest for approximately 5 mm. The nasolacrimal duct and sac lie immediately lateral to this junction in a vertical plane. Posterior to the ridge there is a slight concave depression in front of the uncinate process. This process is attached to the lacrimal

bone and the inferior turbinate by a series of delicate footpieces. The anterior footpieces are at the junction of the lacrimal fossa and the orbital plate of the lacrimal bone, and should therefore be regarded as the extreme posterior limit of safety [26]. In a cadaver study, Yung and Logan showed that the uncinate process is a better landmark in endoscopic DCR, compared with the middle turbinate, the appearance of which is known to be highly variable [27].

Surgical Procedure

While numerous authors have described various techniques for endonasal DCR, the basic steps in this procedure are summarized below. Whatever technique is used, the main objectives are to:

58

1. Create a rhinostomy from the sac through the lateral nasal wall.
2. Minimize trauma to the lacrimal system and sac.
3. Minimize damage to the mucosa around the rhinostomy site.
4. Avoid a high rhinostomy, as this can produce a sump syndrome.
5. Avoid collateral mucosal damage in the nose, to minimize the formation of adhesions.

Important in endoscopic DCR is nasal mucosa decongestion, by applying topical vasoconstrictors followed by a submucosal injections of lidocaine containing epinephrine. In cases performed under local anesthesia, topical ocular anesthetic is instilled in the operative eye, after which a local anesthetic solution is infiltrated in the medial portion of the eyelids and medial canthal region [21].

Abnormalities that may potentially interfere with the creation of the intranasal ostium or comprise its patency, such as nasal septal deviation or nasal polyposis, are addressed surgically as required. Nussbaumer et al. pointed out that 55 out of 256 patients (21.5%) who underwent endoscopic DCR required additional endonasal procedures to improve access to the lacrimal area, with overall DCR success rates of almost 90% [28].

To help to identify the location of the lacrimal sac endonasally, a 20-gauge endoilluminator probe (used in vitreoretinal surgery) may be introduced through the canaliculus and advanced into the lacrimal sac. The location of the lacrimal sac can be visualized endonasally by transillumination [21].

The next step is to incise the nasal mucosa overlying the lacrimal sac. Although various modifications of incisions and mucosal flap creation are described, most authors choose to make an incision in the region of the lacrimal ridge and create an elevated posterior-based mucoperiostal flap, in this way exposing the maxilla and lacrimal bone. Some of the redundant mucosa may be excised.

The bone overlying the lacrimal sac is now removed. Firstly, the thin lacrimal bone is identified by moving the inserted light pipe around or inserting a periost elevator and feeling the bone suture. The thin lacrimal bone is very flexible and is removed using a Freer's elevator and Blakesley forceps. Be careful to remove all of the small pieces of lacrimal bone, because remnants could later occlude the rhinostomy. At this point the thicker bone of the maxilla, overlying the superior part of the sac can be removed by using either hammer and chisel, forceps, rongeurs, or a diamond burr. There is some controversy in literature about the rhinostomy ostium size and location.

After the removal of the bone of the lateral nasal wall, the lacrimal sac mucosa can be incised. It is useful to identify the sac by moving the light pipe around and to "tent up" the mucosa in order to incise its anterior surface. This is preferentially done in a vertical direction, from inferior to superior, anterior to the light beacon. Be careful not to damage the inside of the sac by pushing the blade in too deep, and do not leave any excess of mucosa flapping, as it could obstruct the common opening. A too-posterior-orientated sac incision could lead to inadvertent orbital penetration, resulting in orbital fat prolapse.

Since postoperative scarring with granulation and fibrosis at the rhinostomy site is the most common cause of DCR failure, most authors prefer to create a mucosal-lined fistula by apposing the lacrimal and nasal mucosal flaps at the end of the procedure.

A silicone tube is routinely placed through the upper and lower canaliculi into the nasal cavity, where it is fixed with a hemoclip. There are some authors who use tubing of the stenosis only in more complicated cases, avoiding this trauma to the pathways epithelium in straight-forward postsaccal stenosis.

Pre- and Postoperative Care

Preoperative Care

As stated earlier, the most important preoperative measure is to decongest the nasal mucosa, in order to prevent excessive hemorrhage, which can significantly impair surgical visualization and safety.

When surgery is performed under general anesthesia, vasoconstriction is achieved by nasal fossa packing with neurosurgical pads soaked in cocaine 10% solution, or infiltration of the nasal mucosa with 0.001% adrenalin/xylocaine in the region of the lacrimal sac and head of middle turbinate.

When surgery is performed under local anesthesia, nasal decongestion is complemented by anesthetizing the following tissues [16]:
1. Ocular surface with topical guttae amethocaine.
2. Medial upper and lower eyelids, anterior lacrimal crest, and lacrimal fossa with lidocaine 2% and epinephrine 1:200,000

Postoperative Care

The following guidelines should be noted [16, 29]:
1. Unless associated nasal procedures are performed, nasal packing is not routinely used.
2. Topical steroid and antibiotic eye drops are given for about 4 weeks.
3. There is usually no need for a nasal steroid spray.
4. Patients are told not to blow their nose for 1 week.
5. Nasal douching with saline solution has to be carried out four times a day at home.
6. Patients are initially followed up at the outpatient clinic at weeks 1 and 2, for nasendoscopic suction cleaning of crusting and blood clots.
7. If silicone intubation is performed, patients are seen after 6 weeks for stent removal.
8. At 6 months, the surgical result is evaluated.

In 1999 the Royal College of Ophthalmologists published guidelines for clinical governance suggesting that freedom from epiphora for 3 months after surgery is the marker for a satisfactory procedure [30].

Results

External DCR has a 90–95% success rate and this technique has therefore been generally accepted as the gold standard in lacrimal surgery for distal nasolacrimal duct obstruction. Woog et al. published an overview of surgical results of the endonasal DCR technique (Table 58.1), with success rates ranging from 59% to 100%. Follow-up information provided in these studies is highly variable and the results should be interpreted accordingly [21]. However, the endoscopic DCR technique has several advantages compared with the external approach [21, 24]:

1. Avoidance of a cutaneous incision and scar, resulting in less disruption of medial canthal anatomy and lacrimal pump function.
2. Decreased operative time.
3. Decreased intraoperative hemorrhage.
4. Decreased postoperative morbidity and enhanced recovery.
5. Direct access to the lacrimal system through the lacrimal bone, avoiding double-sided dissection of the sac.
6. The ability to concurrently address nasal and/or paranasal sinus abnormalities through the same surgical approach.
7. The ability to treat acute dacryocystitis with empyema.
8. The procedure may be performed on an outpatient basis and/ or under local anesthesia.
9. No nasal packing is required unless associated nasal procedures are performed.

The higher primary success rates reported with external DCR are probably due to the creation of a controlled epithelium-lined mucosal anastomosis, instead of the common removal of the mucosal wall of the lacrimal sac and nose in the endonasal approach [31].

A prospective study comparing endoscopic to external DCR was performed by Hartikainen et al. [31]. These authors looked at 64 patients and followed up at 1 year. They found a patency rate of 75% in the endoscopic cases versus 91% in externally operated cases. The difference was not, however, statistically significant. It should be noted that after revision procedures, there was a 97% success rate in both groups [31].

Throughout the years several modifications of the classically performed endoscopic DCR technique have been described in literature, and these have resulted in improvements of the surgical success rates.

The endoscopic DCR technique reported by Yung and Hardman-Lea involved wide bone removal and marsupialization of the inferior three-quarters of the lacrimal sac and superior nasolacrimal duct into the nose [32]. The level of obstruction was assessed preoperatively and confirmed peroperatively. In cases with lacrimal sac/duct obstruction, a success rate of 93% was yielded.

In a prospective, nonrandomized cohort study, Wormald described a new powered endoscopic DCR technique, with full

Table 58.1 Results of primary endonasal dacryocystorhinostomy. *CO₂* Carbon dioxide, *DCR* dacryocystorhinostomy, *endosc* patent ostium on nasal endoscopy, *FESS* functional endoscopic sinus surgery, *Ho:YAG* holmium:yttrium-aluminium-garnet, *instr* instruments, *irrig* patency to lacrimal irrigation, *KTP* potassium titanyl phosphate, *MMC* mitomycin C, *NS* not specified, *RF* radio frequency, *Sx* symptomatic relief

First author (year)	N	Follow-up (months)	Outcome measures	Success rate (%)	Comments
Jokinen (1974) [35]	126	NS	Sx, irrig	83	Direct vision, microscope, chisel, drill
Woog (1993) [36]	40	1,5–23	endosc, irrig	83	Ho:Yag laser
Reifler (1993) [37]	19	10–16	Sx, endosc	68	KTP laser
Whittet (1993) [13]	18	9–15	Sx, endosc	94	Chisel, drill; postoperative endoscopy
Metson (1994) [22]	34	7–23	endosc, irrig	82	including 27 primary/7 revision DCR; Ho:YAG laser
Seppa (1994) [38]	12	11–17	Sx	83	CO₂/Nd:YAG laser
Weidenbecher (1994) [39]	56	12	Sx, endosc	86	FESS instr, chisel, drill
Eloy (1995) [2]	28	6–39	Sx	82	Microscope/endoscope, flaps
Java (1995) [40]	50	9	Sx, irrig	90	External DCR controls; RF, rongeurs, curette, MMC
Sprekelsen (1996) [1]	152	NS	Sx, endosc	86	FESS instr, drill
Shun-Shin (1998) [41]	40	NS	Sx	86	Chisel
Hartikain (1998) [24]	32	12	Sx, irrig	75	randomized controlled nonmask study; external DCR
Yung (1998) [42]	81	6–12	Sx	92	Endoscope, inferior location of ostium, stent removal 3 months, weekly endoscopy

lacrimal sac exposure and primary mucosal anastomosis, yielding a success rate of 95.7% [25].

In a prospective, nonrandomized interventional comparative case series, these high success rates of endoscopic DCR were confirmed by Tsirbas. Surgical success was defined as relief from symptoms and by anatomic patency. The same technique of full lacrimal sac exposure and primary mucosal anastomosis was used in a series of 31 consecutive patients with anatomic nasolacrimal duct obstruction, and compared with 24 external DCR procedures. There was no statistical difference between the success rates of endoscopic DCR (93.5%) and external DCR (95.8%) [33].

The high success rates with these new endoscopic DCR techniques are comparable with those reported with the external technique. This is explained by the authors by the full lacrimal sac exposure and the creation of a large ostium, which is similar in size to that made with external DCR. Others have suggested that the initial size of the ostium is not related to eventual success [34], but a larger ostium allows an approximation between nasal and sac mucosa. Traditionally, this was only achieved via the external approach, but in this new endoscopic DCR technique, the lacrimal sac mucosa and significant amounts of nasal mucosa are preserved [33].

Conclusion

Nasolacrimal duct obstruction is a common disorder that can be treated surgically by the DCR procedure. Since its early description, the external approach has been accepted by most ophthalmologists as the gold standard of treatment. Recent developments of modern endoscopic sinus surgery and modifications of the various described endoscopic techniques have resulted in higher success rates that are comparable with those achieved with the external technique. Together with the various advantages of an endoscopic approach, this promotes the role of the ENT surgeon in the treatment of this pathology. Future prospective randomized trials are needed to prove the equivalence in long-term efficiency of the endoscopic DCR technique.

> ### Tips to Avoid Complications
>
> - Master a perfect knowledge of surgical anatomy.
> - Ensure good mucosal decongestion to increase visualization and decrease bleeding.
> - Avoid collateral mucosal damage in the nose to minimize crusting and formation of adhesions.
> - Make sure of wide bony removal to avoid rhinostomy stenosis.
> - The extreme posterior limit of safety of bony removal is the anterior attachment of the uncinate process.
> - Try to create an epithelium-lined mucosal anastomosis.
> - Avoid a high rhinostomy, as this can produce a sump syndrome.
> - Do not tie the intubation tubes too tightly intranasally, to prevent punctal cheesewiring.

> ### Take-Home Pearls
>
> - Use clinical examination and imaging studies to detect and confirm distal lacrimal outflow obstruction.
> - A thorough knowledge of endonasal surgical anatomy and experience in endoscopic nasal surgery are imperative.
> - Endoscopic DCR has several important advantages in comparison with the classical external approach.
> - Recently described endoscopic DCR technique modifications yield success rates comparable to those achieved with external DCR.

References

1. Sprekelsen MB, Barberan MT (1996) Endoscopic dacryocystorhinostomy: surgical technique and results. Laryngoscope 106:187–189
2. Eloy P, Bertrand B, Martinez M, et al (1995) Endonasal dacryocystorhinostomy: indications, technique and results. Rhinology 33:229–233
3. Toti A (1904) Nuovo Metodo conservatore dicura radicale delle suppurazione croniche del sacco lacrimale. Clin Moderna (Firenza) 10:385
4. Dupuy-Dutemp L, Bouguet M (1921) Note preliminaire sur en procede de dacryocystorhinostomie. Ann Ocul 158:241
5. Jones LT (1962) The cure of epiphora due to canalicular disorders, trauma and surgical failures on the lacrimal passages. Trans Am Acad Ophthalmol Otolaryngol 66:506
6. Tsirbas A, Wormald PJ (2003) Mechanical endonasal dacryocystorhinostomy with mucosal flaps. Br J Ophthalmol 87:43–47
7. Camara JG, Bengzon AU (2006) Nasolacrimal duct obstruction. eMedicine http://www.emedicine.com/oph/TOPIC465.HTM
8. Linberg JV, McCormick SA (1986) Primary acquired nasolacrimal duct obstruction. A clinicopathologic report and biopsy technique. Ophthalmology 93:1055–1063
9. Groessl SA, Sires BS, Lemke BN (1997) An anatomical basis for primary acquired nasolacrimal duct obstruction. Ophthalmology 115:71–4
10. Campolattaro BN, Lueder GT, Tychsen L (1997) Spectrum of pediatric dacryocystitis: medical and surgical management of 54 cases. J Pediatr Ophthalmol Strabismus 34:143–153
11. Kuchar A, Lukas J, Steinkogler FJ (2000) Bacteriology and antibiotic therapy in congenital nasolacrimal duct obstruction. Acta Ophthalmol Scand 78:694–698
12. Janssen AG, Brenkman CJ (2002) Beeldvormende diagnostiek en röntgenologische interventie procedures van de traanwegen. In: Brenkman CJ, de Vries N (eds) Neusbijholte Chirurgie, Goedaardige Aandoeningen. Kugler, The Hague, pp 333–359
13. Whittet HB, Shun-Shin GA, Awdry P (1993) Functional endoscopic transnasal dacryocystorhinostomy. Eye 7:545–549
14. Newell FW (1986) The lacrimal apparatus. In: Newell FW (ed) Ophthalmology Principles and Concepts, 6th edn. Mosby, St. Louis, p 254

15. Wormald PJ, Tsirbas A (2004) Investigation and endoscopic treatment for functional and anatomic obstruction of the nasolacrimal duct system. Clin Otolaryngol 29:352–356

16. Olver J (2002) Colour Atlas of Lacrimal Surgery. Butterworth-Heinemann, Oxford

17. Simmen D, Jones N (2005) Manual of Endoscopic Sinus Surgery. Thieme, New York Stuttgart

18. Mannor GE, Millman AL (1992) The prognostic value of preoperative dacryocystogram in endoscopic intranasal DCR. Am J Ophthalmol 113:134–137

19. Wearne MJ, Pitts J, Frank J (1999) Comparison of dacryocystography and lacrimal scintigraphy in the diagnosis of functional nasolacrimal duct obstruction. Br J Ophthalmol 83:1032–1035

20. Zinreich SJ, Miller NR, Freeman LN, et al (1990) Computed tomographic dacryocystography using topical contrast media for lacrimal system visualisation. Orbit 9:79–87

21. Woog JJ, Kennedy RH, Custer PL, et al (2001) Endonasal dacryocystorhinostomy: a report by the American Academy of Ophthalmology. Ophthalmology 108:2369–2377

22. Metson R, Woog JJ, Puliafito CA (1994) Endoscopic laser dacryocystorhinostomy. Laryngoscope 104:269–274

23. Hehar SS, Jones NS, Sadiq A (1997) Endoscopic holmium:Yag laser dacryocystorhinostomy – safe and effective as day-case procedure. J Laryngol Otol 111:1056–1059

24. Hartikainen J, Grenman R, Puukka P, et al (1998) Prospective randomized comparison of external dacryocystorhinostomy and endonasal laser dacryocystorhinostomy. Ophthalmology 105:1106–1113

25. Wormald PJ (2002) Powered endoscopic dacryocystorhinostomy. Laryngoscope 112:69–72

26. McDonogh M, Meiring JH (1989) Endoscopic transnasal dacryocystorhinostomy. J Laryngol Otol 103:585–587

27. Yung MW, Logan BM (1999) The anatomy of the lacrimal bone at the lateral wall of the nose: its significance to the lacrimal surgeon. Clin Otolaryngol 24:262–265

28. Nussbaumer M, Schreiber S, Yung MW (2004) Concomitant nasal procedures in endoscopic dacryocystorhinostomy. J Laryngol Otol 118:267–269

29. Yuen KSC, Lam LYM, Tse MWY, et al (2004) Modified endoscopic dacryocystorhinostomy with posterior lacrimal sac flap for nasolacrimal duct obstruction. Hong Kong Med J 10:395–400

30. Royal College of Ophthalmologists (1999) Guideline for Clinical Governance in Ophthalmology. RCO, London

31. Hartikainen J, Antila J, Varpula M, et al (1998) Prospective randomized comparison of endonasal endoscopic dacryocystorhinostomy and external dacryocystorhinostomy. Laryngoscope 108:1861–66

32. Yung MW, Hardman-Lea S (2002) Analysis of the results of surgical endoscopic dacryocystorhinostomy: effect of the level of obstruction. Br J Ophthalmol 86:792–794

33. Tsirbas A, Davis G, Wormald P (2004) Mechanical endonasal dacryocystorhinostomy versus external dacryocystorhinostomy. Ophthal Plast Reconstr Surg 20:50–56

34. Linberg JV, Anderson RL, Busted RM (1982) Study of intranasal ostium external dacryocystorhinostomy. Arch Ophthalmol 100:1758–1762

35. Jokinen K, Karja J (1974) Endonasal dacryocystorhinostomy. Arch Otolaryngol 100:41–44

36. Woog JJ, Metson R, Puliafito CA (1993) Holmium:YAG endonasal laser dacryocystorhinostomy. Am J Ophthalmol 116:1–10

37. Reifler DM (1993) Results of endoscopic KTP laser-assisted dacryocystorhinostomy. Ophthal Plast Reconstr Surg 9:231–236

38. Seppa H, Grenman R, Hartikainen J (1994) Endonasal CO_2-Nd:YAG laser dacryocystorhinostomy. Acta Ophthalmol (Copenh) 72:703–706

39. Weidenbecher M, Hosemann W, Buhr W (1994) Endoscopic endonasal dacryocystorhinostomy: results in 56 patients. Ann Otol Rhinol Laryngol 103:363–367

40. Javate RM, Campomanes BS, Co ND, et al (1995) The endoscope and the radiofrequency unit in DCR surgery. Ophthal Plast Reconstr Surg 11:54–58

41. Shun-Shin GA (1998) Endoscopic dacryocystorhinostomy: a personal technique. Eye 12:467–470

42. Yung MW, Hardman-Lea S (1998) Endoscopic inferior dacryocystorhinostomy. Clin Otolaryngol 23:152–157

Chapter 59

Epistaxis: Diagnosis, Evaluation, and Treatment

59

Piero Nicolai, Davide Tomenzoli, Johnny Cappiello, and Cesare Piazza

Core Messages

- The vast majority of epistaxis episodes are self-limiting events.
- When anterior epistaxis takes origin from Kiesselbach's plexus, cauterization with the aid of a headlight or loupes under local anesthesia can be easily performed.
- In anterior epistaxis from the anterior ethmoid artery (AEA) and posterior epistaxis from the posterior ethmoidal artery (PEA) or the sphenopalatine artery (SPA), nasal packing should be used only as a temporary measure in order to appropriately plan the next therapeutic step.
- An endoscopic approach under general anesthesia is always warranted as first-line surgical treatment. Arterial embolization and open-field ligation should be reserved only for cases of failure of appropriate endoscopic attempts or for patients with contraindications to an endoscopic approach.
- In posterior epistaxis, SPA should be addressed first and, only in case of inadequate bleeding control, the AEA and PEA should be subsequently coagulated.
- In anterior epistaxis, the first surgical step should be AEA coagulation, followed by SPA and PEA cauterization only in where there is insufficient control of epistaxis.
- In hereditary hemorrhagic teleangiectasia (HHT) syndrome (Rendu-Osler-Weber syndrome), aggressive nasal packing should be always avoided in order to minimize mucosal trauma.
- In HHT, endoscopic photocoagulation with different types of laser under local or general anesthesia is a cost-effective therapeutic tool that is associated with minimal morbidity.

Contents

Introduction

Nasal bleeding is an event experienced by virtually all individuals during some point in their life. Nevertheless, as nearly all episodes of epistaxis are self-limiting, its actual incidence remains undetermined and is undoubtedly underestimated. In a retrospective 10-year study period of a total of 973,900,000 visits to emergency departments in the United States, patients with epistaxis accounted for 0.46%; however, only 6% of them required hospitalization [1]. The need for surgical intervention is reported to be 9.5% among hospitalized patients [2].

The term "epistaxis" can be used to describe a variety of situations ranging from self-limiting mild nasal bleeding to life-threatening nasal hemorrhage. Apart from posttraumatic nasal bleeding caused by mucosal injuries or severe bony fractures, and epistaxis due to sinonasal neoplasms, coagulative disorders, or vascular congenital diseases, the etiology of the condition remains uncertain. Predisposing factors that may lead to nasal hemorrhage include environmental irritants, mucosal drying, infectious and granulomatous diseases, anticoagulation and nonsteroidal anti-inflammatory drugs, and hypertension [3–5].

Epistaxis is usually subdivided into anterior and posterior. The former originates from Kiesselbach's plexus (also called Little's or Valsalva's area), which is located in the anterior portion of the nasal septum, while the latter arises from Woodruff's nasopharyngeal plexus. Treatment of epistaxis is strongly dependent on the site (anterior or posterior nasal fossa), visibility of the bleeding source, and amount/duration of blood loss. When bleeding arises from Little's area, cauterization with silver nitrate or bipolar forceps may be easily performed with the aid of a headlight and following application of adequate topical anesthesia (usually with cottonoid pledgets soaked in 4% lidocaine). Using a rigid nasal endoscope, the source of bleeding can be visualized and treated even when located in the middle or posterior part of the nasal fossa. However, when the origin of bleeding is not readily visible or the hemorrhage is overwhelming the nasal fossa, packing with hemostatic gauzes, a Foley catheter, or other devices specifically designed for the nasal cavity is temporarily indicated before planning ligation/cauterization of the involved vessel or selective arterial embolization.

Blood Supply of the Nose and Paranasal Sinuses

The nasal fossae and paranasal sinuses are vascularized by the terminal vessels of collaterals from the external and internal carotid arteries (see Chap. 44). The external carotid artery branches into the superficial temporal and maxillary arteries (MAs). The latter vessel, arising behind the condyle of the mandible and giving rise to several branches, passes through the pterygomaxillary junction and enters the pterygopalatine fossa. From this point, before reaching the nasal fossa, it gives rise to five branches, in caudal–cranial order, the posterior superior alveolar artery, the inferior orbital artery, the vidian artery, the descending palatine artery, and the sphenopalatine artery (SPA). The latter exits the pterygopalatine fossa through the sphenopalatine foramen.

In 1991, Morton and Khan [6], in a study on 30 cadaver heads, described the variability of the course of the MA in the pterygopalatine fossa. According to that study, it is possible to distinguish five different MA branching types: the Y type (180° between the two arteries), intermediate type (90°), T type (>90°), M type (0°), and a fifth type, those that can not be classified into one of the previous four categories. The intermediate type was the most frequently encountered (33.3%) by the authors in their dissection study.

The SPA enters the nasal fossa through the sphenopalatine foramen, which lies between the basal lamellae of the middle and superior turbinates. It is bordered anteriorly by a constant, triangular bony landmark, called the crista ethmoidalis of the palatine bone (Fig. 59.1). Different descriptions concerning the branching pattern of the SPA distal to the pterygopalatine fossa have been reported. According to Simmen et al. [7], the SPA enters the nasal fossa as a single arterial trunk in only 2.6% of cases, while in the majority of cadaver head sides it divides into 2–10 branches before exiting the sphenopalatine foramen. Babin et al. [8] observed a single trunk in 20% of cases, with 2–5 branches crossing the sphenopalatine foramen in the remaining cases. In contrast, Holzmann et al. [3] found a single trunk in 52.1% of patients treated for epistaxis, and two or three branches in 43.5% and 4.4% of individuals, respectively. One interesting aspect of SPA branching is that the posterior nasal artery, also called the septal artery, enters the lateral wall of the nasal fossa through a separate foramen (posterior to the sphenopalatine foramen) in 12% of cases [9]. This vessel exits its foramen and then runs over the anterior wall of the sphenoid sinus, reaching the posterior nasal septum. According to Babin

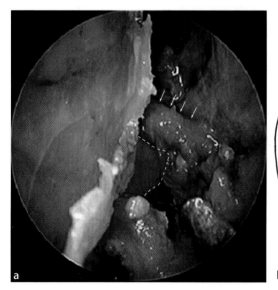
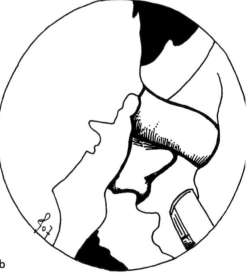

a   b

Fig. 59.1 **a** Endoscopic view with a 0° rigid endoscope of the right nasal fossa in a cadaver head (a diagrammatic version is shown in **b**). The *dotted line* outlines the ethmoid process of the palatine bone (crista ethmoidalis), which is used as a "pointer" for identification of the sphenopalatine artery (SPA) foramen. *White arrows* indicate the SPA. *PWMS*, posterior wall of the maxillary sinus (courtesy of Professor P. Castelnuovo and Professor P. Palma, Insubria University, Varese, Italy)

et al. [8], from this point the septal artery moves forward and branches into three different vessels: the superior branch supplies Kiesselbach's plexus and anastomoses with a branch of the facial artery and with collaterals of the anterior ethmoid artery, while the two inferior branches vascularize the inferior septal area. Furthermore, the lowest one passes through the incisive canal and anastomoses with a branch of the descending palatine artery, the greater palatine artery (Fig. 59.2).

The second vessel coming from the external carotid artery and contributing to the blood supply of the nasal fossa is the facial artery with one of its collateral vessels, the superior labial artery, which anastomoses to branches of the anterior ethmoid and septal arteries at the level of Kiesselbach's plexus [10].

The anterior ethmoid artery (AEA) and posterior ethmoid artery (PEA) are feeding vessels of the sinonasal tract that arise from the ophthalmic artery, an intracranial collateral of the internal carotid artery. After its origin in the orbital cavity, the AEA enters the anterior ethmoid through the anterior ethmoid foramen (Fig. 59.3). In 1961, Kirchner et al. [11] published a surgical anatomy study of the ethmoid arteries: they studied 150 orbits and found the AEA within the frontoethmoid suture line in 68% of cases, and 1–4 mm above it in the remaining 32%. The distance from the anterior lacrimal crest to the anterior ethmoid foramen ranged from 14 to 18 mm in 64% of the specimens. Inside the anterior ethmoid, the AEA is surrounded by a thin bony wall, termed the ethmoid canal, which is embedded in the roof of the anterior skull base (Fig 59.4). The anterior ethmoid canal runs from the orbit to the lateral lamella of the cribriform plate, taking an oblique direction from posterior-lateral to anterior-medial, and in the majority of cases is located between the

second (bullar lamella) and the third (ground lamella) of the middle turbinates [12]. The AEA canal generally lies close to the skull base, but less frequently it is enveloped in a bony mesentery at a mean distance of 3–5 mm from the rhinobasis [12,13]. This anatomic variation seems to be a consequence of extensive pneumatization of the ethmoid sinus, particularly in the presence of a supraorbital cell [7]. A partially dehiscent AEA canal has been reported to be present in 16–40% of cases (Fig 59.5) [14]. The AEA leaves the ethmoid sinus by piercing the lateral lamella of the cribriform plate, reaching the anterior cranial fossa. After branching off the anterior meningeal artery, it turns downward and enters the nasal fossa, giving rise to several vessels that feed the anterior portion of the roof of the nasal fossa, anterior nasal septum, and anterior ethmoid sinus.

The PEA branches from the ophthalmic artery and leaves the orbit through the posterior ethmoid foramen, which is located at the level of the frontoethmoid suture line in 87% of cases. It lies about 10 mm behind the anterior ethmoid foramen, while its distance from the optic canal ranges between 4 and 7 mm in 84% of orbits [11]. The PEA traverses the posterior ethmoid sinus in the posterior ethmoid canal, enters the anterior cranial fossa giving off a meningeal branch, and then descends between the cribriform plate and the fovea ethmoidalis. In the nasal fossa, the PEA divides into medial and lateral branches, feeding the roof of the nose down to the superior turbinate and corresponding portion of the septum [15].

The venous drainage of the nasal cavities generally follows the course of the arteries. The anterior and posterior ethmoid veins mainly drain into the cavernous sinus through the superior ophthalmic vein, even though connections with the supe-

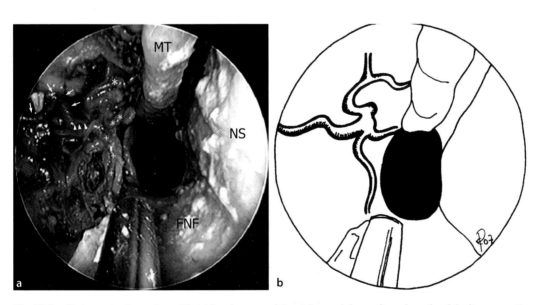

Fig. 59.2 a Endoscopic view using a 0° rigid endoscope of the right nasal fossa of a cadaver head (a diagrammatic version is shown in **b**). The posterior wall of the maxillary sinus and a wide portion of the palatine bone have been removed, exposing the arterial network of the infratemporal and pterygopalatine fossae. *White arrows* indicate the maxillary artery and *white arrowheads* point to the SPA. The *single white asterisk* indicates the septal branch of the SPA, *double white asterisk* shows the branch of the SPA for the middle turbinate, and *white crosses* indicate the descending palatine artery. *MT* middle turbinate, *NS* nasal septum, *FNF* floor of the nasal fossa. (Courtesy of Professor P. Castelnuovo and Professor P. Palma, Insubria University, Varese, Italy)

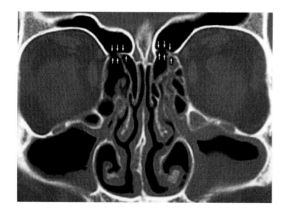

Fig. 59.3 Coronal computed tomography scan of the paranasal sinuses. *White arrows*, which appear bilaterally on the micrograph, show the course of the anterior ethmoidal arteries (AEAs) from the medial wall of the orbit to the perpendicular lamella of the cribriform plate

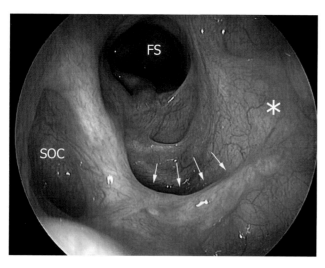

Fig. 59.4 Endoscopic view, taken with a 45° rigid endoscope, of a right nasal fossa previously operated for chronic rhinosinusitis. *White arrows* delineate the AEA bony canal running from the orbit (*left*) to the perpendicular lamella of the cribriform plate (*right, asterisk*). *SOC* Supraorbital cell, *FS* frontal sinus

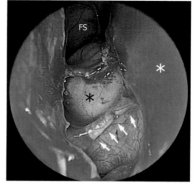

Fig. 59.5 Endoscopic view, taken with a 70° rigid endoscope, of a right nasal fossa previously operated for nasal polyposis. *White arrows* indicate the AEA crossing the anterior skull base outside its usual bony canal, here completely dehiscent. The *white asterisk* indicates the vertical lamella of the cribriform plate, while the *black asterisk* shows the roof of the first ethmoid cell

rior sagittal sinus and veins of the dura mater of the anterior cranial fossa have also been described [16]. The sphenopalatine veins drain into the maxillary vein or cavernous sinus through a system of emissary vessels, the greater palatine veins into the maxillary and posterior facial veins or cavernous sinus, and the septal veins into the anterior facial vein. The pterygoid venous plexus is located between the temporalis and the pterygoid muscles and receives venous drainage from the sphenopalatine vein, making an inferior anastomosis with the posterior facial vein through the deep facial vein and superiorly with the cavernous sinus through several emissary vessels.

Therapeutic Strategy

When the bleeding source is not readily visible even with adequate topical vasoconstriction and local anesthesia and is not controlled by anterior nasal packing, more invasive therapeu-

tic maneuvers are warranted. In this regard, posterior nasal packing should not be considered as a definitive therapeutic approach, but rather a temporary measure in order to reduce blood loss while stabilizing the patient. The option is then available to choose between several treatment strategies, ranging from endoscopic or traditional techniques for cauterization/ligation of nasal vessels to selective arterial embolization under angiographic control.

Open-field ligation of arterial vessels was the first invasive technique described in the international literature to treat otherwise uncontrollable epistaxis. In 1925, Hyde [17] first used external carotid artery ligation for management of massive nasal bleeding. In subsequent years, Seiffert [18] and Chandler and Serrins [19] described MA ligation in the pterygopalatine fossa through a transmaxillary approach. Specific drawbacks of this technique were related to difficulties in ready identification of the MA and its branches [20], with possible complications and sequelae such as dental trauma, maxillary sinusitis, infraorbital nerve lesion, oral-antral fistula, blindness, and ophthalmoplegia [21]. If the bleeding source was located in the upper and lateral portion of the nasal cavity, even the AEA and PEA were addressed by an open-field approach via a skin incision similar to that utilized for external ethmoidectomy.

An endonasal approach for SPA cauterization was first used at the end of the 1970s. In 1976, Prades [22] described a transnasal approach to the pterygopalatine fossa for surgical division of the vidian nerve through the middle meatus using an operating microscope. In this procedure, the author always ligated the SPA before addressing the vidian nerve. Stamm et al. [23] first described a series of 145 patients treated for posterior epistaxis by transnasal microsurgical ligation of the SPA.

During the last 20 years the advent and wide popularization of endoscopes has offered an additional tool for management of otherwise uncontrollable nasal bleedings. Growing evidence has demonstrated comparable success rates of endoscopic and microsurgical techniques in the management of epistaxis originating from the SPA and its branches. Moreover, the endoscopic approach presents significant advantages in the treatment of AEA and PEA bleeding. In fact, 45° and 70° angled endoscopes, coupled to angled and thin instruments specifically designed for frontal sinus surgery allow magnified exposure of the anterior skull base.

Surgical management of nasal bleeding using an endoscopic approach is usually performed under general anesthesia, with the patient in the anti-Trendelenburg position and the surgical bed inclined to about 30°. After removal of nasal packings and aspiration of clots, cottonoid pledgets with oxymetazoline are positioned in the middle meatus and nasal fossa. In the case of suboptimal endoscopic visualization of the nasal fossa due to septal spur or deviation, the surgical procedure begins with a standard or endoscopic septoplasty, according to the complexity of the anatomic situation. Subsequent submucosal injections of xylocaine and 1:100,000 epinephrine at the level of the uncinate process and the axilla of the middle turbinate leads to adequate decongestion of the mucosa. Identification of landmarks such as the uncinate process laterally, the vertical lamella of the middle turbinate medially, the bulla ethmoidalis superiorly, and the second and third portions of the middle turbinate posteriorly allows safe access to the middle meatus area. Some authors [24, 25] propose inferior uncinectomy and middle meatus antrostomy with removal of the bulla ethmoidalis to gain more space for subsequent isolation and cauterization of the SPA and its branches. Holzmann et al. [3] suggested resecting the horizontal portion of the middle turbinate, which can add further space for the adequate identification of the sphenopalatine foramen. However, we concur with others [23, 26–28] that these surgical steps are not always required and the sphenopalatine foramen can be identified even with an intact middle meatus. Palpatory maneuvers in the region between the posterior fontanella and the anterior margin of the palatine bone should be performed carefully in order to assess precisely the point of entry of the SPA in the nasal cavity. We usually start the procedure with a vertical mucosal incision placed 1 cm in front of the insertion of the third portion of the middle turbinate, on the lateral wall of the nasal fossa. Blunt dissection of a mucoperiosteal flap with a Freer suction elevator in the pos-

terior direction exposes the ethmoid crest of the palatine bone. This triangular bony "pointer" constitutes the anterior margin of the sphenopalatine foramen and represents its main surgical landmark. Its careful removal with a small rongeur allows visualization of the neurovascular bundle entering the nasal fossa through the sphenopalatine foramen. Complete exposure of this area is obtained by circumferential blunt dissection until the SPA and its branches are clearly visible. It is worth mentioning that the SPA runs through its foramen as a single vessel in only 2.6–20% of cases, while branches in its terminal rami at the level of the pterygopalatine fossa or inside the sphenopalatine foramen itself in the vast majority of patients [7, 8]. Two hemostatic clips are placed on the SPA, while the other branches are usually coagulated with bipolar forceps. We always accomplish submucosal blunt dissection medial to the sphenopalatine foramen up to the anterior wall of the sphenoid sinus. This is justified by the entry of the septal branch of SPA in the nasal cavity as a separate vessel through a foramen located posteriorly to the sphenopalatine foramen in 12% of cases. Holzmann et al. [3] strongly suggest sphenoidotomy and identification of the septal artery at the level of the anterior wall of the sphenoid sinus whenever no active bleeding is encountered during isolation of the main trunk of the SPA.

In the event of no active bleeding during surgical identification and ligation of the SPA in a patient with a history of massive epistaxis that is uncontrollable by anterior and posterior packings, we also address both the ethmoid arteries. According to Stammberger [13], the surgical landmark for AEA identification is the anterior wall of the bulla ethmoidalis, which marks the junction between the posterior boundary of the frontal recess and the roof of the first ethmoid cell. Usually, the AEA is located 1–2 mm posterior to this landmark. Computed tomography (CT) scan could provide the surgeon with information on the specific anatomy of the frontal recess, with special reference to the pattern of the uncinate process superior insertion [29], the presence of a hyperpneumatized agger nasi cell or a supraorbital cell (possibly indicating an anterior ethmoid foramen outside and inferior to the skull base) [30], and the precise morphology and position of the lateral lamina of the cribriform plate. All of these variants should be anticipated by the radiologist to reduce the possibility of an accidental AEA lesion with the risk of intraorbital hemorrhage or creation of a cerebrospinal fluid leak (see Chap. 54). Surgical steps for AEA identification and cauterization are the same as those for a Draf type II frontal sinusotomy (see Chap. 52) [31]. It begins with complete removal of the uncinate process and bulla ethmoidalis (and of the aforementioned anatomical variants if present, and limiting the surgical approach to the frontal sinus) to fully expose the frontal recess and identify the AEA canal. In the case of a bony canal fully encircling the AEA, a diamond burr aids in exposing the artery as much as possible, which is then safely coagulated with bipolar forceps. After perforation of the ground lamella of the middle turbinate and complete removal of the posterior ethmoid cells, identification of the PEA is usually accomplished about 1 cm posterior to the AEA, at the level of the skull base. Its bony canal should be approached with a diamond burr to fully expose and coagulate the artery.

Management of Epistaxis in Rendu-Osler-Weber Syndrome

Rendu-Osler-Weber syndrome, or hereditary hemorrhagic telangiectasia (HHT), is a systemic vasculopathy that is inherited as an autosomal dominant trait in 80% of cases and is without any known family history of disease in the remaining 20% (interpreted as the occurrence of spontaneous mutations or incomplete penetrance of the responsible gene in asymptomatic relatives) [32]. A multitude of mutations have been found in at least two gene loci on chromosomes 9 and 12 [33–35]. The prevalence of HHT is estimated to be between 1:3,500 and 1:8,000, with no differences between Japan, Europe, and North America [36]. Vascular dysplasias encountered in HHT can also encompass arteriovenous malformations and aneurysms, but the most frequent hallmark is represented by mucocutaneous and visceral teleangiectasias. These are fragile pathologic dilatations arising from capillaries and postcapillary venules that lack elastic tissue and a muscular layer, which are therefore prone to easy bleeding and have no vasoconstrictive potential [32].

The single most common clinical sign of HHT is recurrent epistaxis, occurring sooner or later in more than 90% of patients, depending on the clinical definition of the disease. Nose bleedings sometimes begin in childhood, but more frequently between the third and fourth decade of life, becoming increasingly frequent and heavier with aging. Associated clinical manifestations are cutaneous, gastrointestinal, genitourinary, pulmonary, intracranial, and intraocular hemorrhage.

Epistaxis in HHT invariably tends to recur despite sophisticated therapeutic approaches that include surgical ligation of the MA [37], endoscopic photocoagulation by neodymium-doped yttrium aluminium garnet, potassium titanyl phosphate, argon, flashlamp-pulsed dye, or diode lasers [38–42], septal dermoplasty [43–45], Young's closure of the nostrils by skin flaps [46], microvascular free flaps [47], arterial embolization [48], and hormonal therapy with estrogens [49, 50]. Temporary nasal packings should be inserted with great caution to reduce further mucosal trauma and should be held in place for the shortest time possible [51] prior to carrying out appropriate therapeutic procedures. These should never include cauterization of telangiectasias, which is responsible for both exacerbation of immediate bleeding and delayed nasal crusting with possible septal perforation [32, 51].

Neoformation of telangiectasias in previously uninvolved areas of nasal mucosa is the most likely explanation for the frustrating long-term results usually achieved in the treatment of HHT, as recently demonstrated by in vivo observation of these lesions with contact endoscopy by Folz and Werner [52]. This phenomenon explains the palliative nature of the majority of the therapeutic armamentarium developed to date and, together with the intrinsic rarity of HHT, justifies the absence of a commonly shared management algorithm.

At our Institution, between June 2001 and December 2006, we treated 52 HHT patients using photocoagulation with diode laser under general anesthesia. During the procedure great care was made to photocoagulate only the ectasic and more prominent vascular dilatations, addressing them in a noncontact manner,

holding the laser fiber 3–4 mm from the mucosal surface and firing until whitening of the blood vessels and surrounding tissue occurs. Gentle application of local vasoconstrictors and meticulous attention in not touching the ectasias with the endoscope, fiber, or other instruments are essential in obtaining hemostasis without excessive intraoperative bleeding. Among these patients, 7 familial clusters, accounting for 26 (50%) patients of our series, were identified. Twenty (38%) patients were submitted to a 2nd endoscopic procedure, 15 (29%) to a 3rd operation, 11 (21%) to a 4th, 6 (11%) to a 5th, and 5 (10%) to a sixth. Two patients (4%) have been treated 11 times and 1 (2%) has needed 13 procedures.

Arterial Embolization for Epistaxis

Sokoloff et al. [53] first described arterial embolization for otherwise uncontrollable nasal bleedings. Since then, several authors have reported their experience in elective management of recurrent posterior epistaxis using this technique [5, 21, 54–58]. This procedure is usually performed under local anesthesia, is well-tolerated, and normally lasts no more than 15–20 min in experienced hands. Access is obtained by percutaneous catheterization of the right femoral artery. The pre-embolization angiogram, performed through the same catheter used for the therapeutic maneuvers, allows the viewing of an initial panoramic view of the entire common carotid artery territory to assess all possible sources of nasal bleeding. Moreover, vascular anomalies can be adequately anticipated in this pre-embolization phase. In the absence of signs of radiopaque contrast extravasation at the level of the internal carotid artery branches, selective catheterization of the external carotid artery is performed. A subsequent superselective catheterization of the internal maxillary artery is needed to exclude possible anastomosis with the internal carotid or vertebral artery systems, the presence of reflux, or the rare occurrence of an ophthalmic artery arising from the external carotid artery system. When the bleeding source has been localized, its embolization is accomplished under fluoroscopic control using particles of polyvinyl alcohol, dextran microspheres, absorbable gelatin sponge, or detachable balloons until the contrast extravasation from the identified vessel has stopped. Superselective angiographic embolization offers some advantages compared to surgical management of epistaxis: these include accurate evaluation of the precise source of bleeding, the identification of possible vascular anomalies, and the possibility of repeating the therapeutic procedure in case of bleeding recurrence. It is strongly recommended for patients who are unsuitable for general anesthesia due to compromised medical conditions, while it is contraindicated in patients with hemorrhage from the AEA or PEA, in presence of severe atherosclerotic disease of the carotid arteries, and in patients with a suspect history of allergy to contrast medium [59, 60]. The success rate reported in the literature ranges from 75% to 97%, with a complication rate between 6% and 27% [5, 21, 54–58]. It is noteworthy that complications encompass facial pain and paresthesia, nasal ala necrosis, trismus, ophthalmoplegia, temporary and permanent amaurosis, hemiplegia, and ataxia.

Summary

Our proposed algorithm for the management of nose bleeding is as follows: anterior and posterior nasal packings should be always considered as temporary measures to gain time while preparing the patient for the most appropriate therapeutic approach. Moreover, especially in patients with HHT, nasal packing should never be attempted aggressively for the intrinsic risk of worsening diffuse nasal mucosa bleedings due to further trauma. If the bleeding source is readily visible with a headlight or loupes in the anterior portion of the nasal cavity, cauterization of the responsible vessels is usually performed under local anesthesia. If the bleeding originates from the posterior part of the nasal fossa and the involved vessel may be clearly identified, cauterization with endoscopic magnification under local anesthesia can be attempted in compliant patients without major epistaxis and favorable nasal anatomy. In all other cases and whenever the source of bleeding is not clearly identifiable or remains uncertain even after adequate endoscopic examination, it should be addressed under general anesthesia. SPA should be always endoscopically clipped in posterior bleedings, while the AEA should be addressed in the anterior ones. In case of uncertain origin or insufficient control of the epistaxis, after cauterization of one of these two vessels the other should be coagulated at the same time together with PEA, although it is rarely the main cause of bleeding. Open-field ligation of the AEA, PEA, and SPA as a first-step surgical approach should be considered an obsolete procedure. Nonetheless, it may still play a role after failure of an endoscopic approach or when endoscopic instrumentation is not available, when the clinician has limited experience in endoscopic procedures, or in some specific situations (i.e., major craniofacial traumas). Photocoagulation with different types of laser is useful for the management of recurrent epistaxis in HHT. Even though not able to get definitive results (as most of the other therapeutic approaches described), it is relatively less time-consuming, associated with minimal surgical and postoperative morbidity, and can be repeated as often as needed. For both HHT and epistaxis of other origins, arterial embolization should be considered as a last resort in the management of otherwise intractable nose bleedings.

Tips to Avoid Complications

- Perform a septoplasty before any attempt of surgery on the SPA, AEA, or PEA whenever, in spite of adequate mucosal decongestion, a septal spur or deviation impairs endoscopic visualization of the nasal fossa and ethmoidal complex.
- For SPA cauterization, identify the uncinate process, the bulla ethmoidalis, and the second and third portions of the middle turbinate; then identify the ethmoid crest of the palatine bone and expose the SPA foramen by removing it; coagulate the main trunk of the SPA and its septal branch in front of the anterior wall of the sphenoid sinus.

- In epistaxis requiring AEA coagulation, a CT scan may help the inexperienced surgeon to gain precise information on the specific anatomy of the patient, with special reference to those details that can guide the identification of the AEA with minimal risks (i.e., pattern of uncinate process superior insertion, configuration of the lateral lamina of the cribriform plate, presence of a hyperpneumatized agger nasi or supraorbital cell).
- Whenever the AEA and PEA are running in a bony canal, use a diamond burr to expose and coagulate them.
- During photocoagulation of vascular ectasias in HTT, address only the more prominent lesions, using a noncontact mode, with the laser tip maintained 3–4 mm from the mucosal surface.

Take-Home Pearls

- In general, nasal packing should be used as a temporary measure while planning the definitive treatment. This concept has to be strictly applied, especially to the management of HHT patients.
- In case of profuse anterior epistaxis, CT scan can be useful in order to provide the surgeon with a better understanding of the anatomic area surrounding the AEA and therefore in preventing serious complications during the endoscopic procedure.
- When an endoscopic approach is elected, address the SPA first in posterior epistaxis and the AEA first in the anterior epistaxis, but maintain a low threshold of suspicion in case of insufficient bleeding control in order to shift your attention to the other vessel during the same surgical procedure.
- Leave arterial embolization and open-field ligation as the last resource in case of repeated endoscopic failures.
- In case of HHT, apply a minimally invasive approach by laser photocoagulation in a noncontact mode.

References

1. Pallin DJ, Chng Y-M, McKay MP, Emond JA, Pelletier AJ, Camargo CA (2005) Epidemiology of epistaxis in US emergency departments, 1992 to 2001. Ann Emerg Med 46:77–81
2. Goddard JC, Reiter ER (2005) Inpatient management of epistaxis: outcomes and cost. Otolaryngol Head Neck Surg 132:707–712
3. Holzmann D, Kaufmann T, Pedrini P, Valavanis A (2003) Posterior epistaxis: endonasal exposure and occlusion of the branches of the sphenopalatine artery. Eur Arch Otorhinolaryngol 260:425–428
4. Umapathy N, Quadri A, Skinner DW (2005) Persistent epistaxis: what is the best practice? Rhinology 43:305–308

5. Viehweg TL, Roberson JB, Hudson JW (2006) Epistaxis: diagnosis and treatment. J Oral Maxillofac Surg 64:511–518

6. Morton AL, Khan A (1991) Internal maxillary artery variability in the pterygopalatine fossa. Otolaryngol Head Neck Surg 104:204–209

7. Simmen DB, Raghavan U, Briner HR, Manestar M, Groscurth P, Jones NS (2006) The anatomy of the sphenopalatine artery for the endoscopic sinus surgery. Am J Rhinol 20:502–505

8. Babin E, Moreau S, Goullet de Rugy M, Delmas P, Valdazo A, Bequignon A (2003) Anatomic variations of the arteries of the nasal fossa. Otolaryngol Head Neck Surg 128:236–239

9. Schwartzbauer HR, Shete M, Tami TA (2003) Endoscopic anatomy of the sphenopalatine and posterior nasal arteries: implications for the endoscopic management of epistaxis. Am J Rhinol 17:63–66

10. Chiu T, Dunn JS (2006) An anatomical study of the arteries of the anterior nasal septum. Otolaryngol Head Neck Surg 134:33–36

11. Kirchner JA, Yanagisawa E, Crelin ES (1961) Surgical anatomy of the ethmoidal arteries. Arch Otolaryngol 74:382–386

12. Moon H-J, Kim H-U, Lee J-G, Chung IH, Yoon JH (2001) Surgical anatomy of the anterior ethmoidal canal in ethmoid roof. Laryngoscope 111:900–904

13. Stammberger H (1991) Special endoscopic anatomy of the lateral nasal wall and ethmoidal sinuses. In: Stammberger H (ed) Functional Endoscopic Sinus Surgery. BC Decker, Philadelphia, pp 49–87

14. Floreani SR, Nair SB, Switajewski MC, Wormald P-J (2006) Endoscopic anterior ethmoidal artery ligation: a cadaver study. Laryngoscope 116:1263–1267

15. Gluckman JL, de Vries EJ (1995) Epistaxis. In: Donald PJ, Gluckman JL, Rice DH (eds) The Sinuses. Raven, New York, pp 623–640

16. Lang J (1989) Vessels of the nasal cavity and paranasal sinuses. In: Lang J (ed) Clinical Anatomy of the Nose, Nasal Cavity and Paranasal Sinuses. Georg Thieme, New York, pp 106–111

17. Hyde FT (1925) Ligation of the external carotid artery for control of idiopathic nasal hemorrhage. Laryngoscope 35:899–904

18. Seiffert A (1928) Unterbindung der Arteria maxillaris interna. Z Hals Nasen Ohrenheilk 22:323–325

19. Chandler JR, Serrins AJ (1965) Transantral ligation of the internal maxillary artery for epistaxis. Laryngoscope 75:1151–1159

20. Metson R, Lane R (1988) Internal maxillary artery ligation for epistaxis: an analysis of failures. Laryngoscope 98:760–764

21. Strong EB, Bell DA, Johnson LP, Jacobs JM (1995) Intractable epistaxis: transantral ligation vs. embolization. Efficacy review and cost analysis. Otolaryngol Head Neck Surg 113:674–678

22. Prades J (1976) Abord endonasal de la fosse pterygo-maxillaire. LXXIII Cong Franc Compt Rendus des Seanc pp 290–296

23. Stamm AC, Pinto JA, Neto AF, Menon AD (1985) Microsurgery in severe posterior epistaxis. Rhinology 23:321–325

24. Ram B, White PS, Saleh HA, Odutoye T, Cain A (2000) Endoscopic endonasal ligation of the sphenopalatine artery. Rhinology 38:147–149

25. Pothier DD, MacKeith S, Youngs R (2005) Sphenopalatine artery ligation: technical note. J Laryngol Otol 119:810–812

26. Wormald PJ, Wee DTH, van Hasselt CA (2000) Endoscopic ligation of the sphenopalatine artery for refractory posterior epistaxis. Am J Rhinol 14:261–264

27. Voegels RL, Curti Thomè D, Vasquez Iturralde PP (2001) Endoscopic ligature of the sphenopalatine artery for severe posterior epistaxis. Otolaryngol Head Neck Surg 124:464–467

28. Rockey JG, Anand R (2002) A critical audit of the surgical management of intractable epistaxis using sphenopalatine artery ligation/diathermy. Rhinology 40:147–149

29. Landsberg R, Friedman M (2001) A computer-assisted anatomical study of the nasofrontal region. Laryngoscope 111:2125–2130

30. Simmen DB, Raghavan U, Briner HR, Manestar M, Schuknecht B, Groscurth P, Jones NS (2006) The surgeon's view of the anterior ethmoid artery. Clin Otolaryngol 31:187–191

31. Draf W (1991) Endonasal micro-endoscopic frontal sinus surgery, the Fulda concept. Oper Tech Otolaryngol Head Neck Surg 2:234–240

32. Peery WH (1987) Clinical spectrum of hereditary hemorrhagic telangiectasia (Osler-Weber-Rendu disease) Am J Med 82:989–997

33. McAllister KA, Grogg KM, Johnson DW, Gallione CJ, Baldwin MA, Jackson CE, Helmbold EA, Markel DS, McKinnon WC, Murrell J, et al (1994) Endoglin, a TGF-ß binding protein of endothelial cells, is the gene of hereditary haemorrhagic telangiectasia type 1. Nat Genet 8:345–351

34. Johnson DW, Berg JN, Baldwin MA, Gallione CJ, Marondel I, Yoon SJ, Stenzel TT, Speer M, Pericak-Vance MA, Diamond A, Guttmacher AE, Jackson CE, Attisano L, Kucherlapati R, Porteous ME, Marchuk DA (1996) Mutations in the activin receptor-like kinase 1 gene in hereditary hemorrhagic telangiectasia type 2. Nat Genet 13:189–195

35. Gallione CJ, Repetto GM, Legius E, Rustgi AK, Schelley SL, Tejpar S, Mitchell G, Drouin E, Westermann CJ, Marchuk DA (2004) A combined syndrome of juvenile polyposis and hereditary haemorrhagic telangiectasia associated with mutations in MADH4 (SMAD4) Lancet 363:852–859

36. Dakeishi M, Shioya T, Wada Y, Shindo T, Otaka K, Manabe M, Nozaki J, Inoue S, Koizumi A (2002) Genetic epidemiology hereditary hemorrhagic telangiectasia in a local community in the northern part of Japan. Hum Mutat 19:140–148

37. Golding-Wood PH (1983) The role of arterial ligation in intractable epistaxis. J Laryngol Otol 8:120–122

38. Siegel MB, Keane WM, Atkins JF Jr, Rosen MR (1991) Control of epistaxis in patients with hereditary hemorrhagic telangiectasia. Otolaryngol Head Neck Surg 105:675–679

39. Ducic Y, Brownrigg P, Laughlin S (1995) Treatment of haemorrhagic telangiectasia with the flashlamp-pulsed dye laser. J Otolaryngol 24:299–302

40. Lennox PA, Harries M, Lund VJ, Howard DJ (1997) A retrospective study of the role of the argon laser in the management of epistaxis secondary to hereditary haemorrhagic telangiectasia. J Laryngol Otol 111:34–37

41. Lund VJ, Howard DJ (1999) A treatment algorithm for the management of epistaxis in hereditary hemorrhagic telangiectasia. Am J Rhinol 13:319–322

42. Shah RK, Dhingra JK, Shapshay SM (2002) Hereditary hemorrhagic telangiectasia: a review of 76 cases. Laryngoscope 112:767–773

43. Saunders W (1964) Hereditary hemorrhagic telangiectasia: effective treatment of epistaxis by septal dermoplasty. Acta Otolaryngol 58:497–502

44. Ross DA, Nguyen DB (2004) Inferior turbinectomy in conjunction with septodermoplasty for patients with hereditary hemorrhagic telangiectasia. Laryngoscope 114:779–781

45. Fiorella ML, Ross DA, Henderson KJ, White Jr RI (2005) Outcome of septal dermoplasty in patients with hereditary hemorrhagic telangiectasia. Laryngoscope 115:301–305

46. Young A (1967) Closure of the nostrils in atrophic rhinitis. J Laryngol Otol 81:515–524

47. Bridger GP, Baldwin M (1990) Microvascular free flap in hereditary hemorrhagic telangiectasia. Arch Otolaryngol Head Neck Surg 116:85–87

48. Weissman JL, Jungreis CA, Johnson JT (1995) Therapeutic embolization for control of epistaxis in a patient with hereditary hemorrhagic teleangiectasia. Am J Otolaryngol 16:138–140

49. Pau H, Carney AS, Walker R, Murty GE (2000) Is oestrogen therapy justified in the treatment of hereditary haemorrhagic telangiectasia? A biochemical evaluation. Clin Otolaryngol 25:547–550

50. Sadick H, Ramin N, Oulmi J, Karl H, Bergler W (2003) Plasma surgery and topical estriol: effects on the nasal mucosa and long-term results in patients with Osler's disease. Otolaryngol Head Neck Surg 129:233–238

51. Abelson TI (1991) Epistaxis. In: Paparella MM, Shumrick DA, Gluckman JL, Meyerhoff WL (eds) Otolaryngology. Saunders, Philadelphia, PA, pp 1831–1841

52. Folz BJ, Werner JA (2007) Contact endoscopy of the nose in patients with Rendu-Osler-Weber syndrome. Auris Nasus Larynx 34:45–48

53. Sokoloff J, Wickbom J, McDonald D, Brahme F, Goergen TG, Goldberger LE (1974) Therapeutic percutaneous embolization in intractable epistaxis. Radiology 111:285–287

54. Vitek JJ (1991) Idiopathic intractable epistaxis: endovascular therapy. Radiology 181:113–116

55. Sinilnuoto TM, Leinonen AS, Karttunen AI, Karjalainen HK, Jokinen KE (1993) Embolization for the treatment of posterior epistaxis. An analysis of 31 cases. Arch Otolaryngol Head Neck Surg 119:837–841

56. Tseng EY, Narducci CA, Willing SJ, Sillers MJ (1998) Angiographic embolization for epistaxis: a review of 114 cases. Laryngoscope 108:615–619

57. Klotz DA, Winkle MR, Richmon J, Hengerer AS (2002) Surgical management of posterior epistaxis: a changing paradigm. Laryngoscope 112:1577–1582

58. Sadri M, Midwinter K, Ahmed A, Parker A (2006) Assessment of safety and efficacy of arterial embolisation in the management of intractable epistaxis. Eur Arch Otorhinolaryngol 263:560–566

59. Romagnoli M, Marina R, Sordo L, Gaini RM (2000) Indications for selective arterial embolization in the treatment of epistaxis. Acta Otorhinolaryngol Ital 20:330–335

60. Andersen PJ, Kjeldsen AD, Nepper-Rasmussen J (2005) Selective embolization in the treatment of intractable epistaxis. Acta Otolaryngol 125:293–297

Chapter 60

Endoscopic Surgery of the Orbit

60

Olaf Michel

Core Messages

- The medial and inferomedial part of the orbit as well as the orbital apex with the optic nerve are easily accessible transnasally.
- Good results have been obtained using endonasal orbital decompression for inhomogeneous space-occupying intraorbital lesions like malignant endocrine orbitopathy and bleedings.
- In indicated cases, fractures of the medial orbital wall and medial orbital floor might be managed transnasally.
- In reachable primary and secondary malignant lesions, including pseudotumors, transnasal biopsy is an attractive diagnostic option.
- Transnasal removal of a foreign body and selected tumors should be considered.

Contents

Aims and Objectives

In rhinology, the external approaches to the paranasal sinuses have been abandoned in favor of the endonasal endoscopically controlled techniques [7, 29]. With increasing experience these techniques were used to approach also adjacent structures like the pituitary gland, the nasolacrimal duct and sac, the anterior skull base, and – last but not least – the orbit. Due to anatomical and instrumental restrictions, the orbit can be approached transnasally by its medial part (lamina orbitalis) and the inferomedial part (orbital floor). Tumors and lesions in the following areas are accessible via this transnasal approach:

1. Those involving the bony structures of the orbit in extension of the paranasal sinuses.
2. Those in the compartments between the lamina orbitalis and the periorbit.
3. Those in the periorbit itself.
4. Those in the compartment between the periorbit and the extraocular muscles.
5. To some extent, those in the intraconal compartment, mainly the medial and inferomedial part with the limit of the optic nerve (ON) and the eyeball.

Surgical Anatomy

It goes without saying that it is necessary for the surgeon to have a clear-cut anatomical concept of the orbital and adjacent structures. They can be studied in relevant anatomical textbooks and publications [21, 26, 28]. Only the essential anatomical facts will be mentioned hereafter.

Vascular Supply

The human orbit contains within it a highly organized connective tissue system that contains the orbital blood vessels: the ophthalmic (OA), anterior and posterior ethmoidal (AEA and PEA, respectively), and infraorbital arteries, as well as the orbital venous system.

The OA is the main source of arterial blood for the orbit and every caution should be taken to ensure its conservation; damage to this vessel causes blindness. The infraorbital artery also contributes to the eye, but to a far lesser degree. The OA usually arises from the internal carotid artery and generally passes the optic foramen at the inferolateral aspect of the ON (see Chap. 61). After its entry into the orbit, the OA proceeds to cross over or under the ON and subsequently follows a medial direction [14]. The course of the OA varies considerably! Nevertheless, the approach to the orbit from the nose has the advantage that the OA is lateral to the medial rectus muscle and therefore less endangered than in other approaches.

The AEA most often arises from the third part of the OA, between the superior oblique and medial rectus muscles [14]. After its origin, the AEA proceeds via the anterior ethmoidal foramen to the anterior cranial fossa, where it gives off an anterior meningeal artery. Intracranial bleeding can occur from this artery if it is injured in the case of anterior skull-base fistula during surgery. Next, the AEA runs to the anterior and medial ethmoid cells and continues into the anterior part of the nasal cavity. Intraorbitally, it may contribute to the vascularization by branches to the medial rectus and inferior oblique muscles.

The PEA is usually smaller in diameter than the AEA and less constant. The vessel takes origin mostly from the "bend" of the OA. It then usually runs between the superior levator palpebrae muscle and the superior oblique muscle, thus above the OA. The PEA occasionally supplies branches to the orbital periosteum and fat tissue. It should not be underestimated as source of bleeding.

The infraorbital artery contributes to the vascularization of the lower orbital parts. It arises from the maxillary artery in the pterygopalatine fossa and enters the orbit through the posterior end of the inferior orbital fissure. It then runs along the inferior orbital sulcus and canal to emerge on the face via the infraorbital foramen. The vessel supplies branches to the orbital adipose tissue, the inferior rectus and inferior oblique muscles, the lacrimal gland, and the lacrimal sac. This artery can cause severe intraorbital bleeding, requiring immediate orbital decompression when injured (e.g., during repair of the orbital floor).

The orbital venous system drains directly or indirectly, via the superior ophthalmic vein in the cavernous sinus. Another posterior communication is presented by the ophthalmomeningeal vein and the vein that travels through the inferior orbital fissure and connects the inferior ophthalmic vein with the pterygoid plexus. The ophthalmofacial vein also takes up branches from the mucosal membranes of the maxillary sinus.

Compartments

All extraocular muscles insert into the apex of the orbit, forming a muscle cone with insertion in the annulus of Zini, where the periorbit is also contacted. This muscle cone maintains a grip on the ON. In case of muscle swelling, the ON becomes subject to pressure precisely in this area (see Chap. 61).

Each extraocular muscle is surrounded by a thin fascial sheath, which is attached to thin fascial septa. Tenon's capsule

and the fascia around the extraocular muscles separate the intra- from the extraconal compartment. A connective tissue network connects Tenon's capsule to the anterior periorbit. The periorbit forms the periost of bony surroundings of the orbit. It exhibits a certain resistance, but also easily tears, when manipulated.

All muscle and orbital structures are embedded in orbital fat. The fat consists of relatively large fat cells, which are connected by thin septa. One should not try to extract fat tissue because it is coupled to other tissues behind. It may cause a chain reaction that may result in damage to other structures (e.g., avulsion of capillaries).

Radiology

In native computed tomography (CT) all orbital tumors exhibit a higher density compared to the orbital fat tissue, with the exception of lipomas and dermoid cysts. The outline of the lesion and its relationship to other structures may provide hints as to their histopathologic nature.

Magnetic resonance tomography (MRT) provides the best information in combination with surface coils and T1-weighted spin echo sequences for the delineation of muscles, nerves, blood vessels, and connective tissue [11]. T2-weighted spin echo sequences allow the differentiation between different tissues. MRT can give first clues as to the vascularization of the tumor.

Digital subtraction angiography is indicated for the diagnosis of vascular changes (mainly carotid-cavernous fistulae, aneurysms, angiomas). Angiography is usually performed to ascertain the possibility of an interventional procedure (e.g., embolization of pathologic vessels) [10]. In such a case, the surgical procedure should be planned and previewed within the next 3 days (e.g., embolization on Tuesday – possible intervention on Wednesday, Thursday, or Friday). Going beyond this period causes weakening of the effect.

A single photon emission CT scan can be useful to quantify an inflammatory process (e.g., malignant orbitopathy with activated lymphocytes) and the clinical differentiation between active and inactive disease. This can ease the decision making between surgical intervention and conservative therapy with immunosuppressive drugs [20].

Indications for a Transnasal Approach to the Orbit

Trauma

Fractures of the Medial Orbital Wall and Floor

Every orbital trauma should prompt investigation for evidence of entrapment of the inferior or medial rectus muscle if a fracture of the orbital floor or of the medial wall of the orbit is suspected. In a large number of cases, the latter goes unrecognized. The typical clinical sign for entrapment is diplopia (Fig. 60.1a). Horizontal double vision is noticed by the patient if the medial rectus muscle is involved, and vertical double vision if the infe-

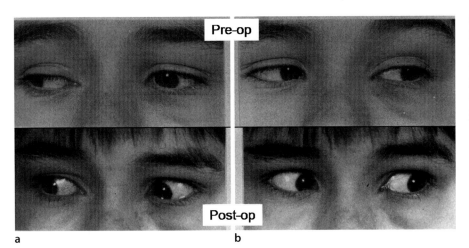

Fig. 60.1a,b Preoperative (a *Pre-op*) horizontal diplopia caused by entrapment of medial rectus muscle on right side following orbital trauma and same patient (b *Post-op*) after transnasal repair of the orbital lamina binocular fusion is restored

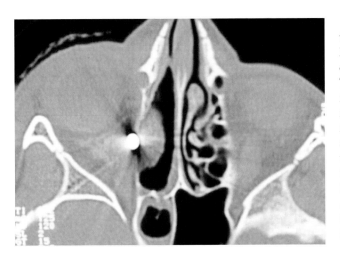

Fig. 60.2 Foreign metal-dense body within the orbit

In the case of an orbital floor fracture (classic blow-out), transnasal repair has proven to be useful only in selected cases. Even by creating a large antral window, the usual instruments do not allow unrestricted handling within the maxillary sinus. The lateral region (lateral from the impression of the infraorbital nerve) is particularly difficult to reach. A transnasal attempt to reset a dislocated orbital floor can be attempted when the fragment is located medially and consists of one part. Nevertheless, a proper support must be archived (e.g., by an antral balloon, which is left in place for about 5 days). The balloon should be filled up with water-soluble contrast medium in order to assess its proper unfolding and its postoperative placement by X-ray. Another disadvantage of the procedure is the inability to control the orbital rim, which is often involved in this kind of orbital fracture.

rior rectus muscle is involved. Entrapment may cause effusion into the muscle sheath, or intramuscular hemorrhage, subsequent cicatrization, and a delayed impaired function. Reposition of the soft tissue and removal of the fragments is recommended.

In case of an ethmoidal blow-out fracture with entrapment, an ethmoidectomy has to be performed to reach the medial orbital wall. After removal of remnant bony parts, the orbital contents have to be brought back in place and sealed in order to restore binocular vision (Fig. 60.1b). In smaller lesions the gap can be covered solely by a thin silicone sheet and reinforced temporarily by a selfexpanding package, which is left in situ for about 5 days. A larger dehiscence of the medial orbital wall should be closed by fascia using an underlay technique, covered by a thin silicone sheet, and stabilized for 5 days with a package. The use of a blue-dyed silicone sheet is meaningful for better recognition and the prevention of accidental removal of the fascia. This method was first described by us in 1993 [23] and has been successfully adopted by several surgeons [6, 16].

Penetrating Lesions

Penetrating lesions of the orbit with or without the inclusion of foreign bodies may be amenable to a transnasal procedure, when the ethmoid cells are involved or when there is suspicion of a foreign body in the area of the ethmoid, the medial, or the intraconal parts of the orbit (Fig. 60.2).

The risks of imminent surgical intervention (with regard to unwanted side effects) must be weighed against the risk of a wait-and-see policy. Foreign bodies may lead to later problems in form of loss of vision, lasting motility disturbances or swelling, purulent sinusitis, or mucocele. For intraoperative localization of metallic foreign bodies, an X-ray image converter (C-arch) is useful. More precisely, foreign bodies can be detected with the help of modern three-dimensional navigation systems (see Chap. 48).

One must be aware that many types of plastic material, glass splinters, and wood particles are difficult to detect by any type of imaging. Wood splinters cause a strong tissue reaction as foreign bodies or due to infection, and should therefore never be left in place. Nevertheless, the intraoperative difficulties of localizing a foreign body embedded in the orbital fat should not be underestimated because of its possible unpredictable evasive action [4].

60

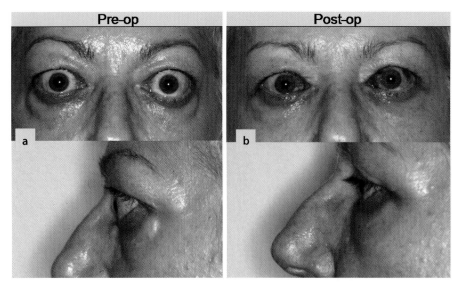

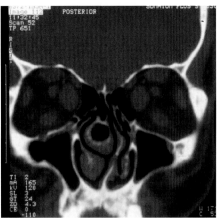

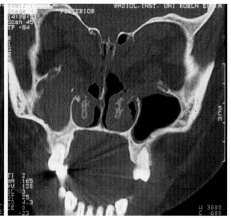

Fig. 60.3 **a** Female patient with malignant endocrine orbitopathy, proptosis, staring glance, diplopia, and visual loss. **b** 1 day postoperatively. Note the reduction of proptosis, restored binocular fusion after simultaneous squint surgery (recession of the medial rectus muscle), no visible scars

Fig. 60.4 Coronal scan of the affected orbit with enlarged extraocular muscles, preoperatively and after transnasal orbital decompression

Compressive Optic Neuropathy

Compressive optic neuropathy (CON) with visual loss is the most serious clinical sign encountered in Graves' ophthalmopathy (GO), space-occupying lesions, and intraorbital bleeding – in all cases of an increase in volume of the orbital contents. Presenting signs may include loss of visual acuity, visual field defects, dyschromatopsia, and exposure keratopathy due to proptosis (Fig.60.3a).

The pathophysiology of Graves' disease has not yet been clarified. Autoimmunity against eye muscle and orbital fat antigens has been proposed as the underlying pathomechanism of GO [17]. At the onset of the disease, the inflammatory response of the extraocular muscles may be diminished by corticosteroids, radiotherapy, or immunosuppressive drugs. Later, when fibrosis has set in, medical treatment fails and the swelling of the extraocular muscles becomes out of control. If treatment fails or is contraindicated, surgical decompression is indicated to relieve CON. In particular, the muscle cone in the apex of the orbit has to be decompressed to release the pressure upon the ON.

The bilateral transnasal approach has been proven [22, 24] a safe and reliable method, particularly when combined with squint surgery (Fig. 60.3b) in the same session [25]. Our own experience is based on nearly 300 decompressed eyes. Transnasal orbital decompression (TOD) is nowadays a commonly performed operation (Fig. 60.4).

Resection of prolapsing orbital fat neither improves exposure nor provides greater decompression. Injection of cortisone into the orbital fat is risky because of the possible induction of fat necrosis.

Common Orbital Diseases

Inflammation

Orbital infections develop from the direct spread of sinusitis, most commonly ethmoidal, but also from preseptal space, particularly from preseptal (or periorbital) cellulitis in children. Infectious material can be inoculated directly into the orbital soft tissue secondary to trauma, surgery, or orbital foreign bodies.

Table 60.1 Affection table for relevant diseases involving the orbit

Disease	Affected area			
	Sinus	Periorbit	Extraconal	Intraconal
Malignant ophthalmopathy	No	No	Frequent	Frequent, compressive
Cellulitis	Yes	Frequent	Frequent	No
Phlegmona	Yes	Yes	Rare	No
Subperiosteal abscess	Yes	Yes	Yes	No
Intraorbital abscess	Yes	Yes	Yes	Yes or no
Mucocele	No	Yes	Yes, compressive	No
Pyocele	No	Yes	Yes	No
Lacrimal duct and sac	No	Yes	Yes	No

Subperiosteal Abscess

This is a collection of purulent material between the lamina papyracea and the periosteum. This infection may develop from orbital cellulitis or from spread of an adjacent infection. The diagnosis is made on CT scan or magnetic resonance imaging (MRI; Fig. 60.5), but can be suspected on physical examination or clinical signs (Table 60.1). The abscess can be drained by ethmoidectomy and transnasal ablation of part of the lamina orbitalis.

Intraorbital Abscess

This is a collection of pus within the orbital soft tissue and a serious complication of sinusitis, with the danger of permanent loss of vision. The modern recommended surgical procedure for drainage of an intraorbital abscess is the transnasal approach, particularly in children. The main advantages of this approach are the simultaneous treatment of causative disorders with surgery following the pathogenic route of the abscess formation, and lack of trauma to further structures. The field of vision is more favorable as compared with the external approach when the abscess is located right in the axis of vision and one does not have to cut through healthy tissue and the intact skin, which, especially in children, can lead to long-lasting visible scarring [30, 12].

The abscess will be drained by ethmoidectomy, transnasal ablation of part of the lamina papyracea, and incision of the periorbit. There is no rule as to how to incise the periorbit. A complete removal is unnecessary.

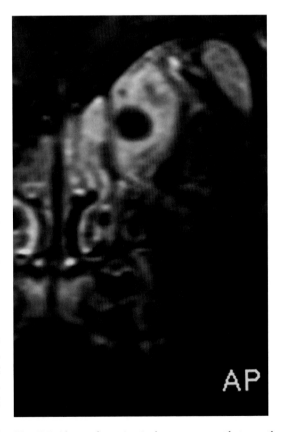

Fig. 60.5 Abscess formation in the compartment between the periorbit and the extraocular muscles as a complication of ethmoiditis

Benign Tumors

Muco- and Pyoceles

In general, mucoceles have a history of prior sinus surgery or trauma. A large proportion develops spontaneously; rarely, they derive from a nondraining concha bullosa. They grow as a result of the inner retention of mucus displacing the adjacent structures like the orbit (Fig. 60.6) and are considered to be pseudotumors. If they become infected, they become pyoceles. The obvious symptoms are displacement of the globe, diplopia, and exophthalmos. Today, most mucoceles are operated transnasally. The mucocele is delineated by removing ethmoidal structures. It is opened, evacuated, and than left with a wide drainage to the nasal cavity. Because the inner lining of a mucocele consists of mucosa, no further surgical measure is required. The mucosa will contact the mucosa of the nasal cavity (marsupialization) and becomes part of it by forming a "neosinus." It will only lead to revision when the opening is not wide or stable enough. Exophthalmos, double vision, and displacement of the eyeball generally resolve without further therapeutic measures [3].

Osteomas

These benign tumors originate mostly in the area of the ethmoid and the frontal recess and may therefore grow into the orbit. They become apparent by chance (e.g., an X-ray undertaken for headache) or by indirect symptoms like a frontal sinusitis due to blockage of the aperture. More rarely, meningitis due to a thinned out dura is the first symptom. The literature is full of case reports describing their successful transnasal removal, mostly using a piecemeal technique. When invading the orbit or when being attached only to the orbital lamina, manipulation should be done with utmost caution to avoid uncontrolled movements into the orbit. Large tumors of the frontal sinus still demand an osteoplastic frontal sinus operation.

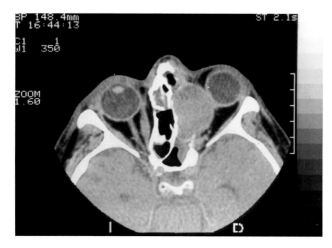

Fig. 60.6 Mucocele invading the orbit. Note the displacement of the medial rectus muscle and the globe

Vascularized Tumors

Angiofibroma

Angiofibroma is a rare fibrovascular tumor that occurs predominantly in male adolescents. By local growth it can erode into the orbit. Preoperative angiography helps to define the tumor and should be followed by embolization, which is highly recommended to avoid massive bleeding during transnasal surgery. The removal usually starts from visible parts within the nasal cavity and then follows the tumor to its extensions, thus also including the orbit.

Cavernous Hemangiomas

Cavernous hemangiomas, or lymphangiomas, may be situated within the orbit, mostly intraconally, and may affect the apex of the orbit. They do not usually reach the apex orbitae and are characterized by a pseudocapsule. Endoscopic removal is rarely recommended if the position is next to the lamina orbitalis between the medial and the inferior rectus muscles.

Other Benign Tumors

Benign tumors that are located in the orbital apex include schwannoma, neurofibroma, meningioma, and fibrous tumors. They frequently present with slow progression of exophthalmos and visual loss caused by CON. TOD may be indicated [19]. The best therapy is usually complete excision. The approach chosen depends upon the tumor size and position.

Malignant Tumors

Rhabdomyosarcoma

The preferred localizations of rhabdomyosarcoma (RMS) are the orbit and the paranasal sinuses. The prognosis of RMS, which used to be poor in former times, has been improved clearly since definitive multimodality therapy was established in the 1970s (for example the Intergroup Rhabdomyosarcoma Study in 1972, the International Society of Pediatric Oncology in 1975, or the German "Cooperative soft tissue study," or CWS, in 1981). The leading therapy of RMS, according to the CWS, is chemotherapy and radiotherapy, because orbital tumors have an excellent prognosis after this treatment. The main role of surgery is to obtain specimens for histological diagnosis. Severe mutilation by radical surgery, especially in children, should be avoided in favor of multidrug chemotherapy and radiation for a better quality of life [15].

Carcinomas

In the management of sinusoidal cancer, orbital exenteration is no longer considered to be necessary for treatment when the tu-

Table 60.2 Affection table of benign and malign tumors

Tumor type	Affected area			
	Sinus	Periorbit	Extraconal	Intraconal
Hemangioma, capillary				Rare (children)
Hemangioma, capillary				Frequent (adults)
Lymphangioma	Yes	Yes	Rarely	Adolescents
Rhabdomyosarcoma			Rarely	Rarely
Lymphoma				Frequently
Carcinoma (paranasal sinuses)	Yes	Yes	Frequently	Rarely
Metastasis	Yes	Yes	Yes	Rarely
Neuroblastoma			Rarely	No

mor is only abutting or eroding the orbital walls. The increased sensitivity of the high resolution CT scanner and MRT allows a more accurate evaluation of the extent of the tumor and determination of whether the tumor has invaded or just approached the periorbit. The actual involvement of the periorbit, however, cannot be determined until transnasal surgical exploration (Table 60.2). It is generally accepted that if the neoplasm does not penetrate the bony orbital walls or the periorbit, complete excision can also be performed transnasally. During surgery, small areas of periorbit may be locally resected with frozen-section control [13].

Sinonasal Undifferentiated Carcinoma

Sinonasal undifferentiated carcinoma is an uncommon aggressive malignancy of the nasal cavity and paranasal sinuses that is associated with a dismal outcome; the mean survival time is still less than 1 year. It has a tendency to spread from the paranasal sinuses to the orbit and anterior cranial fossa. With the exception of biopsy, it is rarely recommendable to treat this aggressive tumor by transnasal resection.

Melanomas

Malignant melanomas of the nasal cavity, and maxillary and ethmoidal sinus may invade the orbit. It should be noted that pigmented melanocytes can occur within the sinus, nasal, and oral epithelium, just as in the conjunctival epithelium.

Lymphomas

The clinical sign of a lymphoma is frequently exophthalmos. The manifestation of a lymphoma within the orbit may proceed later systemic spread. Therefore, the histopathologic classifica-

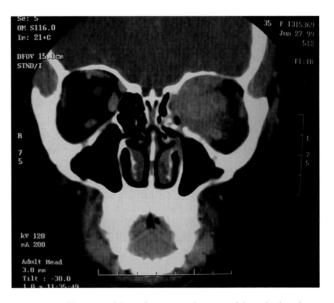

Fig. 60.7 Infiltration of the soft tissue in the apex of the orbit by a lymphoma

tion of this entity is of great importance. Transnasal biopsy is possible when the tumor is situated more inferomedial to the ON (Fig. 60.7).

Metastatic Tumors

Perhaps more than other orbital tumors, metastatic tumors may result in an infiltrative syndrome, thus presenting with motility disturbance, frozen globe, palpably firm orbit, and indurated periorbital skin (Table 60.2). Enophthalmus may be present with scirrhous tumors such as metastatic breast carcinoma. An infiltrative pattern in the CT scans may be a clue to the metastatic nature of the orbital tumor (Fig. 60.8a). In up to 25% of the patients the orbital metastasis may be the initial manifestation of a

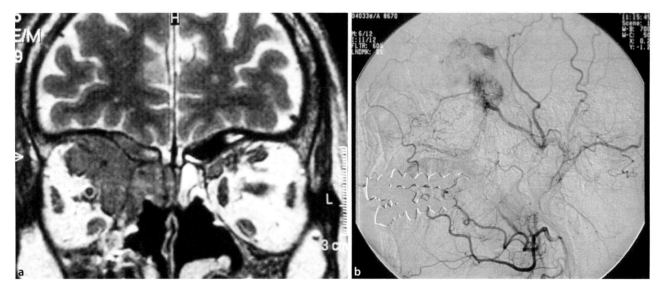

Fig. 60.8 **a** Infiltrating metastasis of a hypernephroma. **b** This metastasis of hypernephroma had a marked vascularization, as shown by angiography

primary tumor elsewhere. Some tumors (e.g., hypernephroma) tend to bleed extensively (Fig. 60.8b).

Although the prognosis is poor for patients with metastatic cancer, modern treatment methods continue to improve and long-term palliation is often possible. The limiting factor is always the primary tumor, therefore treatment of orbital metastasis is usually palliative [8, 9]. In cases of infiltrative spread of a tumor into the orbit, transnasal exenteration using a powered instrument has already been tried [2].

Complications

It is a mistake to think that transnasal endoscopically controlled orbital surgery is free of complications just because it is seemingly less invasive than other procedures. Unwanted effects and disastrous events can be minimized, however, by good preoperative evaluation, choice of the appropriate surgical approach, adequate exposure, careful manipulation of tissues, and immediate and meticulous cauterization of bleeding sources using only bipolar forceps.

Blindness might result from excessive traction or application of pressure on the eye or the ON. The blood vessels supplying the ON, or the nerve itself might be injured. Central retinal artery or vein occlusion might occur as a result of increased extraocular pressure (e.g., using a speculum or a close package).

Intraorbital hemorrhage might cause proptosis and corneal exposure, as well as posing a threat of compressive visual loss. This complication is minimized by a transnasal approach because the orbital bleeding can drain to the nasal cavity.

Extraocular muscle injury may occur during orbital surgery. Edema and hemorrhage within the muscle can cause transient motility impairment or ptosis, which usually resolves within a few weeks. Temporary or permanent paresis of extraocular muscles is a cause of diplopia.

Tips to Avoid Complications

- An ophthalmologic examination (visual acuity, ocular motility, pupillary function, ocular tensions, anterior segment, fundus) should be done prior to any decision making.
- Radiological examinations (CT with protocol for later navigation, MRI, angiography) should provide the best possible information.
- Close cooperation with ophthalmologists and discussion in a multidisciplinary conference is helpful to determine the best treatment strategy.
- The surgical equipment in the operating theater should consist of a microscope, endoscopes with different viewing angles, bipolar forceps, standard instruments for endonasal sinus surgery, and smaller-sized instruments for the orbital content. Powered instruments and lasers are not recommended as a first-line treatment choice. Fibrin glue, fascia, and silicone sheets can be helpful.

Pre- and Postoperative Care

After surgical opening of the orbit, the exposed surface of the orbital contents epithelize, usually spontaneously within some days. Surprisingly, in spite of the free contact to the nose, inflammation of the orbital contents is extremely rare. This may be due to the regular healthy mucosa before the operation. Thus, a long-time antibiotic "shield" is not necessary, although a "single-shot" perioperative application of an antibiotic (e.g., amoxicillin-clavulanate) is recommended, if only for medicolegal reasons.

The cleaning of the cavities by instruments under endoscopic control seems of some importance to the final surgical result, particularly for the prevention of synechiae. There are also surgeons who advocate a no-touch policy. A middle course could be the application of a self-resolving packing, but solid experience is not yet approved [5].

Rinsing by the patient with brine or other salt solutions has proven to have a positive effect upon wound healing in controlled studies [1]. Anyway, the use of packing soaked with ointments that contain mineral oil derivatives (e.g., Vaseline) should be strictly avoided because of the striking danger of causing paraffinomas (myospherulosis) in the tissues [18].

The results of follow-up studies corroborate the thinking that the advantages of the endoscopic transnasal orbital surgery lie in the absence of any scars, the absence of bony defects in the maxilla, and the avoidance of later complications and morbidity, such as lasting postoperative hypesthesia of the infraorbital nerve, oroantral fistula, tooth problems, nasolacrimal drainage system obstruction [27], and facial swelling.

Conclusion

Endonasal surgery can be used in orbital surgery. From this transnasal approach, the anterior skull base, the medial and inferomedial orbits, the orbital apex with the ON, and the inferomedial intraconal compartment of the orbit are within reach.

In all primary and secondary malignant lesions with extension into the orbit, the transnasal biopsy is of importance for diagnosis, particularly in metastasis to the orbit and pseudotumors. Benign lesions like mucoceles and osteomas are accessible and fully removable. Good results have been obtained with endonasal orbital decompression and inhomogeneous space-occupying intraorbital lesions like bleedings. Among the orbital traumas, this procedure is suitable for treating restricted fractures of the medial orbital wall and medial orbital floor, and removal of foreign bodies.

The transnasal approach is not indicated in all diseases that are situated mostly intraconal, supraorbital, and lateral of the eyeball, or for tumors with intracranial extension.

In summary, the transnasal orbital approach has its place as a helpful addition to the transfacial and transcranial techniques, and can even replace them in certain selected indications.

Take-Home Pearls

- Manipulation of the external eye muscles, particularly the medial rectus muscle, can trigger the oculocardiac reflex (OCR), which is a trigeminovagal reflex. The occurrence of OCR is unpredictable and may manifest as bradycardia, bigeminy, ectopic beats, nodal rhythm, atrioventricular block, and cardiac arrest, which is the most serious complication. Warn the anesthetist prior to the operation!

- Intranasal surgical opening of the orbit (e.g., in case of orbital decompression) should leave enough space for the drainage of the frontal sinus and the maxillary sinus, otherwise later revision surgery for a mucocele is programmed. The maxillary sinus can also be drained by an inferomedial antrostomy. The frontal recess (see Chap. 52) should be carefully exposed to establish a reasonable drainage. A too-extended decompression with a resulting bulky fat prolapse has to be avoided for this reason.

- In the case of surgical orbital decompression, an occluding postoperative package should be avoided in order to keep the effect of reducing the pressure on the ON; best is no package. If inevitable, customized and individualsized, self-expanding material should be used, with the pressure-giving part in the region of the posterior nasal orifice (choanae) and nasopharynx, leaving space next to the orbit by placing the package onto the nasal floor.

- The inferomedial approach between the medial and the inferior rectus muscle is safest for intraconally situated lesions, because blood vessels or nerve structures are rarely found in this quadrant of the orbit. But be aware: the anatomical situation is variant!

References

1. Bachmann G, Hommel G, Michel O (2000) Effect of irrigation of the nose with isotonic salt solution on adult patients with chronic paranasal sinus disease. Eur Arch Otorhinolaryngol 257:537–541
2. Batra PS, Lanza DC (2005) Endoscopic power-assisted orbital exenteration. Am J Rhinol 19:297–301
3. Bockmühl U, Kratzsch B, Benda K, Draf W (2006) Surgery for paranasal sinus mucoceles: efficacy of endonasal micro-endoscopic management and long-term results of 185 patients. Rhinology 44:62–67
4. Cartwright MJ, Kurumety UR, Frueh BR (1995) Intraorbital wood foreign body. Ophthal Plast Reconstr Surg 11:44–48
5. Chandra RK, Conley DB, Haines GK III, Kern RC (2005) Longterm effects of FloSeal packing after endoscopic sinus surgery. Am J Rhinol 19:240–243
6. Chen CT, Chen YR, Tung TC, Lai JP, Rohrich RJ (1999) endoscopically assisted reconstruction of orbital medial wall fractures. Plast Reconstr Surg 103:714–720
7. Draf W (1982) Die chirurgische Behandlung entzündlicher Erkrankungen der Nasennebenhöhlen. Indikation, Operationsverfahren, Gefahren, Fehler und Komplikationen, Revisionschirurgie. Arch Otorhinolaryngol 235:133–305
8. Draf W, Berghaus A (1993) Tumoren und Pseudotumoren ("tumorähnliche Läsionen") der frontalen Schädelbasis, ausgehend von der Nase, den Nasennebenhöhlen und dem Nasenrachenraum (einschliesslich der operativen Zugänge) Rhinochirurgisches Referat. Eur Arch Otorhinolaryngol 1:105–186

60

9. Draf W, Samii M (1989) Chirurgische Behandlung von bösartigen Tumoren der Nasennebenhöhlen mit Schädelbasisbeteiligung. Strahlenther Onkol 165:474–477

10. Duvoisin B, Zanella FE, Sievers KW (1998) Imaging of the normal and pathological orbit. Eur Radiol 8:175–188

11. Ettl A, Salomonowitz E, Koornneef L, Zonneveld FW (1998) High-resolution MR imaging anatomy of the orbit. Correlation with comparative cryosectional anatomy. Radiol Clin North Am 36:1021–1045, ix

12. Fakhri S, Pereira K (2006) Endoscopic management of orbital abscesses. Otolaryngol Clin North Am 39:1037–1047

13. Goffart Y, Jorissen M, Daele J, Vander Poorten V, Born J, Deneufbourg JM, Zicot AF, Remacle JM (2000) Minimally invasive endoscopic management of malignant sinonasal tumours. Acta Otorhinolaryngol Belg 54:221–232

14. Hayreh SS (2006) Orbital vascular anatomy. Eye 20:1130–1144

15. Hess A, Schroder U, Schroder R, Michel O (1998) Das Rhabdomyosarkom im Kopf-Hals-Gebiet. Eine Zusammenstellung einiger Kasuistiken, Therapiemoglichkeiten und Prognosen. Laryngorhinootologie 77:557–563

16. Jeon SY, Kim C, Ma Y, Hwang E (1996) Microsurgical intranasal reconstruction of isolated blowout fractures of the medial orbital wall. Laryngoscope 106:910–913

17. Kazim M, Goldberg RA, Smith TJ (2002) Insights into the pathogenesis of thyroid-associated orbitopathy: evolving rationale for therapy. Arch Ophthalmol 120:380–386

18. Keefe MA, Bloom DC, Keefe KS, Killian PJ (2002) Orbital paraffinoma as a complication of endoscopic sinus surgery. Otolaryngol Head Neck Surg 127:575–577

19. Kloek CE, Bilyk JR, Pribitkin EA, Rubin PA (2006) Orbital decompression as an alternative management strategy for patients with benign tumors located at the orbital apex. Ophthalmology 113:1214–1219

20. Krassas GE, Kahaly GJ (1999) The role of octreoscan in thyroid eye disease. Eur J Endocrinol 140:373–375

21. Lang J (1982) Neue Ergebnisse zur Anatomie der Orbita. Fortschr Ophthalmol 79:3–10

22. Michel O (1993) Die endonasale Optikusdekompression bei endokriner Orbitopathie. Z Prakt Augenheilk 14:316–320

23. Michel O (1993) Isolierte mediale Orbitawandfrakturen: Ergebnisse einer minimal invasiven endoskopisch – kontrollierten endonasalen Operationstechnik. Laryngorhinootologie 72:450–454

24. Michel O, Oberlander N, Neugebauer P, Neugebauer A, Russmann W (2001) Follow-up of transnasal orbital decompression in severe Graves' ophthalmopathy. Ophthalmology 108:400–404

25. Neugebauer A, Nishino K, Neugebauer P, Konen W, Michel O (1996) effects of bilateral orbital decompression by an endoscopic endonasal approach in dysthyroid orbitopathy. Br J Ophthalmol 80:58–62

26. Rontal E, Rontal M, Guilford FT (1979) surgical anatomy of the orbit. Ann Otol Rhinol Laryngol 88:382–386

27. Seiff SR, Shorr N (1988) Nasolacrimal drainage system obstruction after orbital decompression. Am J Ophthalmol 106:204–209

28. Weisman RA (1988) surgical anatomy of the orbit. Otolaryngol Clin North Am 21:1–12

29. Wigand ME (1981) Transnasale, endoskopische Chirurgie der Nasennebenhöhlen bei chronischer Sinusitis. III: Die endonasale Siebbeinausräumung. HNO 29:287–293

30. Wolf SR, Gode U, Hosemann W (1996) Endonasal endoscopic surgery for rhinogen intraorbital abscess: a report of six cases. Laryngoscope 106:105–110

Chapter 61

Endoscopic Optic Nerve Decompression

61

Bernhard Schick

Core Messages

- Medial decompression of the optic nerve at the orbital apex and along the optic canal can be performed endoscopically with excellent visualization.
- In contrast to orbital decompression, the role of optic nerve decompression remains controversial.
- Whereas in the past acute traumatic optic nerve compression was the primary focus for decompressing procedures, nowadays numerous pathological conditions that cause chronic optic nerve compression, like tumours, endocrine orbitopathy and idiopathic intracranial hypertension, are at the centre of interest for endoscopic optic nerve decompression.
- Indications for endoscopic optic nerve decompression are based on an individual patient's situation.

Contents

Introduction

Surgical optic nerve decompression has been performed primarily for the treatment of traumatic optic neuropathy. Optic nerve compression due to reactive oedema, haemorrhage and minimal bone displacements along the intracanalicular course of the optic nerve are the focus of interest, as they can cause reversible visual impairment. However, one should be aware that in practice it is a difficult task to define the reason for traumatic optic nerve affection. These difficulties contribute to the problem of defining the proper indications for optic nerve decompression in traumatic situations, especially as only very few recommendations can be derived from the literature. It is noteworthy that a meta-analysis found evidence for benefit of treatment compared to expectant management [2], while an international optic nerve trauma study described no clear benefit for either corticosteroid treatment or optic canal decompression compared to observation alone [9].

The indications for surgical optic nerve decompression in traumatic situations are usually based on an individual patient's situation. This procedure is in fact judged to be of only limited use in the management of traumatic optic neuropathy [1]. Nowadays other non-traumatic indications have gained increasing interest with regard to surgical optic nerve decompression. Space-occupying lesions like mucoceles, optic nerve meningioma or fibrous dysplasia, endocrine orbitopathy, osteopetrosis, acute optic neuropathy associated with acute retinal necrosis, inflammatory optic neuropathy, osteopetrosis and idiopathic intracranial hypertension leading to visual disturbance have been mentioned as indications for optic nerve decompression [6, 8, 10].

For surgical decompression, various approaches like the craniotomy approach, lateral orbitotomy, extranasal transethmoidal approach, transantral ethmoid access, transorbital approach and transnasal procedures are available. Not least because of the controversy surrounding the benefit of surgical optic nerve decompression and possible numerous problems in patients with multisystem trauma, the least traumatic surgical techniques are of specific interest. Endoscopic transnasal optic nerve decompression is a highly attractive option in this regard due to the reduced morbidity (no need for external incisions, preservation of olfaction) and excellent visualization afforded by this procedure. This chapter will focus on the strategy for endoscopic optic nerve decompression.

Anatomy

It is the intracanalicular segment of the optic nerve that is addressed in endoscopic optic nerve decompression. Thus, precise knowledge of its anatomy is necessary. The optic nerve and ophthalmic artery run along the optic canal and enter the orbit through the optic foramen. At the orbital apex the optic nerve is surrounded by the fibrous annulus of Zinn. This fibrous tissue fixes the optic nerve in place, which results in the optic nerve being most vulnerable at its intracanalicular segment [5]. The endoscopic sinus surgeon frequently notices the route of the optic nerve in the superior portion of the lateral sphenoid sinus wall, due to its prominence in front of the internal carotid artery. However, one has to bear in mind that this prominence is missing in up to 25% of all cases [4]. If an Onodi cell is present, the optic nerve may form a prominence at the lateral wall thereof. While the diameter of the distal part of the optic canal diameter measures only 4–6 mm, that of the proximal part ranges from 5 to 9.5 mm [7]. The medial bony border of the optic canal is thin, ranging from 0.2 to 0.6 mm, and is found to be dehiscent in up to 4% [4], necessitating great care in endoscopic optic nerve decompression. A thicker bony bulge, the optic nerve tubercle, is found at the medial conjunction of the orbit apex and the optic canal (see Chap. 44).

The ophthalmic artery enters the optic canal mostly inferior and lateral to the optic nerve. This artery can also be localized inferomedial of the optic nerve, however, a situation that needs to be considered in endoscopic optic nerve decompression. It is important to note that within the optic canal and orbit, the optic nerve, as part of the central nervous system, is surrounded by the pia mater, arachnoid, and dura [3]. The dural covering consists of two layers. Cerebrospinal fluid leakage occurs if its inner portion is opened.

Pathophysiological Aspects

One has always to consider that in acute situations of optic nerve and ophthalmic artery compression, decompression is needed within a critical period of time. Already after 1–3 h of retinal ischaemia, persistent visual impairments can be expected [14]. Based on animal studies with standardized optic nerve injury, decompression of the injured optic nerve was found to be beneficial within the first 6 h after injury [12].

In acute traumatic aetiologies, secondary optic nerve lesions like oedema, haemorrhage and minimal bone displacements are the focus of interest for indications of optic nerve decompression. It is thus important to consider that in traumas, temporary deformation of the optic canal can occur without any evidence of a fracture on computed tomography [13]. In such situations, the optic nerve is especially at risk for injury at its intracanalicu-

lar part, due to fixation of the dural optic nerve sheath at the annulus of Zinn. Besides impairment of the microcirculation, axonal damage (conduction block, demyelination, degeneration) may also result. As surgical decompression has been considered to be an additional trauma, it is noteworthy that no evidence for an additional optic nerve injury was found in an animal model as a result of the additional trauma induced by surgical decompression of the optic nerve [5]. In practice, however, it has been shown that the trauma induced by surgical decompression of the optic nerve may arise first, the actual trauma being delayed by up to 7 days after the causative event, for example in situations of failed high-dose corticoid therapy.

A different situation is found in pathologies causing chronic progressive compression of the optic nerve. Tumour lesions, like mucocele or fibrous dysplasia, as well as idiopathic intracranial hypertension are possible examples. The timing of decompression in these cases has an effect on the progress of visual impairment.

Preoperative Diagnostics

It is of utmost importance to check after trauma for visual impairment. Important findings in cases of traumatic optic nerve injury are visual loss and absence of reaction to direct light in the ipsilateral pupil. Where there is any evidence of acute visual impairments, the ophthalmologist needs to evaluate the eye bulb to rule out pathologies of ocular motility, papillary function, ocular tension, and the anterior segment and fundus. Corneal subluxation, vitreous haemorrhage, retinal detachment or orbital haematoma are possible findings that explain visual disturbance rather than intracanalicular optic nerve compression. In situations of longer-lasting pressure on the optic nerve, like idiopathic intracranial hypertension, papilloedema might be the first finding.

Computed tomography is warranted to visualize the fractures and displaced bone that may cause optic nerve compression (see Chap. 45). In addition, it provides necessary information regarding possible intracranial haematoma, intraorbital haematoma, further fractures, especially those that may affect the carotid artery [15], and of the individual anatomy. Furthermore, computed tomography may be used for image-guided surgery (see Chap. 48).

How to Do it

Surgery starts with sphenoethmoidectomy. The intention of ethmoidectomy is to expose the medial orbital wall and, in the presence of an Onodi cell, the optic nerve. Opening of the sphenoid sinus is performed paraseptally or transethmoidally like in sphenoid sinus surgery performed for other reasons. After sufficient opening of the sphenoid sinus, the course of the carotid artery and the optic nerve in the superolateral part of the sphenoid sinus are identified in case of prominence. The mucosa is then gently removed from the lateral sphenoid sinus wall, with

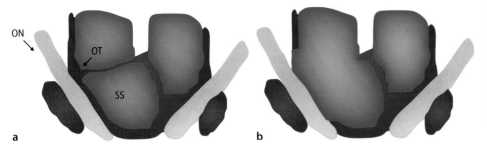

Fig. 61.1a,b Optic nerve decompression before (**a**) and after (**b**) bone removal with exposure of the posterior part of the periorbita, removal of the optic tubercle (*OT*) and medial exposure of the optic nerve (*ON*) in the sphenoid sinus (*SS*)

exposure of the optic canal. Attention has to be paid to possible bony dehiscences. Following the optic canal in the anterior direction, the optic tubercle is identified. Anterior to the optic tubercle, the lamina papyracea is removed exposing the posterior part of the periorbita. Opening of the periorbita must be avoided at this time as protruding orbital fat diminishes visualization during further surgery. This is followed by removing the bone over the optic tubercle and the optic canal from anterior to posterior. The bone is thinned out using a diamond burr. Sufficient irrigation is necessary to avoid thermal injury. The last shell of bone is removed with elongated fine dissectors. One should not start to remove the last shells of bone until the bone is thinned along the whole way, as it is this last shell of bone that provides the best protection for the optic nerve. Finally, the optic nerve is exposed medially (Fig. 61.1). Optic nerve decompression can be performed with or without optic nerve sheath incision, a procedure that remains controversial [11]. If a dural optic nerve sheath incision is intended, this is carried out with a sickle knife or, more atraumatically, with a small diamond knife, from posterior to anterior at the upper edge of the exposed optic nerve (superomedial quadrant) to avoid damaging the ophthalmic artery. The annulus of Zinn should be incised as part of the dural nerve sheath incision to achieve adequate decompression [10]. In special situations, optic nerve decompression is combined with orbital decompression (see Chap. 60). Coagulation should be avoided along the course of the optic nerve, and nasal packing is not placed in the posterior ethmoid and sphenoid sinus in order to prevent nerve injury.

Postoperative Care

Postoperative eye function is documented carefully, especially for changes in visual activity. The presence of a cerebrospinal fluid fistula, which may result in meningitis, is checked carefully. The patient is requested not to blow her or his nose in order to circumvent orbital emphysema. Otherwise, postoperative care is not very different than in other cases of paranasal sinus surgery.

Tips to Avoid Complications

- Decision-making regarding indications and performance of optic nerve decompression should be an interdisciplinary process.
- Be aware of the varying bone thicknesses along the optic canal and the possible presence of bony dehiscences.
- Where an optic nerve sheath incision is intended, this should only be performed in the exposed superomedial quadrant of the optic nerve in order to avoid injury to the ophthalmic artery, which might run along the inferomedial quadrant.
- Include incision of the annulus of Zinn in the optic nerve sheath incision.
- Placement of fibrin glue over the site of the optic nerve sheath incision may prevent a cerebrospinal fluid fistula.
- During drilling, pay careful attention to the carotid artery, which is located inferior–posterior to the course of the optic nerve.

Take-Home Pearls

- Endoscopic optic nerve decompression is a highly attractive, less invasive alternative to external approaches.
- While the indications for optic nerve decompression after traumas remains controversial, endoscopic optic nerve decompression should be borne in mind for non-traumatic pathologies like tumours (mucocele, fibrous dysplasia, meningioma), endocrine orbitopathy and idiopathic intracranial hypertension causing chronic optic nerve compression.
- Delineation of the precise aetiology of traumatic optic nerve lesions may be a difficult task that compounds the problems of determining the proper indications for endoscopic optic nerve decompression.
- So far there are no well-established, proven guidelines for indications for surgical optic nerve decompression, especially in trauma situations.

61

References

1. Acheson JF (2004) Optic nerve disorders: role of canal and nerve sheath decompression surgery. Eye 18:1169–1174
2. Chen C, Selva D, Floreani S, Wormald PJ (2006) Endoscopic optic nerve decompression for traumatic optic neuropathy: an alternative. Otolaryngol Head Neck Surg 135:155–157
3. Cook MW, Levin LA, Joseph MP, Pinczower EF (1996) Traumatic optic neuropathy. A meta-analysis. Arch Otolaryngol Head Neck Surg 122:389–392
4. Duque LAP (2000) Endoscopic optic-nerve decompression in traumatic optic neuropathy. In: Stamm AC, Draf W (eds) Micro-Endoscopic Surgery of the Paranasal Sinuses and the Skull Base. Springer, Berlin Heidelberg New York, pp 441–449
5. Fujii K, Chambers SM, Rhoton AL (1979) Neurovascular relationships of the sphenoid sinus: a microsurgical study. J Neurosurg 50:31–39
6. Gellrich NC, Kankan J, Maier W, Aschendorff A, Klenzner T, Schipper J (2006) Single and temporally displaced second nerve lesions in an animal model and their clinical significance. HNO 54:761–767
7. Gupta AK, Ganth MG, Gupta A (2003) Modified endoscopic optic nerve decompression in idiopathic intracranial hypertension. J Laryngol Otol 117:501–502
8. Habal M, Maniscalco J, Rhoton A (1977) Microsurgical anatomy of the optic canal: correlates to optic nerve exposure. J Surg Res 22:527–533
9. Haller D, Gosepath J, Mann WJ (2006) The management of acute visual loss after sinus surgery – two cases of rhinogenic optic neuropathy. Rhinology 44:216–218
10. Levin LA, Beck RW, Joseph MP, Seiff S, Kraker R (1999) The treatment of traumatic optic neuropathy. The International Optic Nerve Trauma Study. Ophthalmology 106:1268–1277
11. Luxenberger W, Stammberger H, Jeveles JA, Walch C (1998) Endoscopic optic nerve decompression: the Graz experience. Laryngoscope 108:873–882
12. Metson R, Pletcher SD (2006) Endoscopic orbital and optic nerve decompression. Otolaryngol Clin North Am 39:551–561
13. Ohlsson M, Svensson M (2006) Early decompression of the injured optic nerve reduces axonal degeneration and improves functional outcome in the adult rat. Exp Brain Res 179:121–130
14. Rochels R (1990) Holographic deformation analysis of the optic canal in blunt cranial trauma. Fortschr Ophthalmol 87:182–185
15. Rochels R, Rudert H (1995) Emergency therapy of traumatic orbital hematoma with acute visual impairment. Laryngorhinootologie 74:325–327
16. Steigerwald C, Draf W, Hofmann E, Minovi A, Behr R, Bockmuhl U (2005) Angiography of the carotid artery in centro-lateral skull base fractures? Laryngorhinootologie 84:910–914

Endoscopic Surgery of the Skull Base

Chapter 62

Endoscopic Management of Rhinobasal Cerebrospinal Fluid Fistulae

62

Andrew C. Swift

Core Messages

- A dural fistula may present with cerebrospinal fluid (CSF) rhinorrhoea, a pneumoencephalocele or recurrent bacterial meningitis.
- A dural fistula carries a cumulative risk of meningitis of about 10% per year, even if a CSF leak has stopped.
- Anterior skull-base dural fistulae should be explored and closed, even if the leak ceases spontaneously.
- Intrathecal fluorescein is an excellent method for locating a dural defect, even if it is not actively leaking at the time of endoscopic exploration.
- Many dural fistulae can be located and closed by endoscopic surgical techniques.
- Frontal sinus leaks are not easily accessible endoscopically and present with their own unique problems.
- Meticulous technique rather than the type of graft is the key to success.

Contents

Introduction

The presence of cerebrospinal fluid (CSF) rhinorrhoea implies that there must be a dural fistula in the skull base. However, since about 70% will stop leaking within 3 weeks, it has been acceptable practice to await spontaneous cessation and repair only those patients in whom the leak persists. This approach was balanced with the fact that most leaks used to be repaired via an anterior craniotomy, with its inherent risks of anosmia and significant morbidity (10.3%) and mortality (2.6%) [12]. Endoscopic surgery has revolutionised CSF repair [20, 42]. The precise location and repair of dural defects with minimal morbidity, and preservation of the sense of smell is now possible in most patients [31].

CSF leaks are inherently dangerous and meningitis has been reported in 20–30% of cases prior to surgery [14, 16, 22]. More importantly, there is a cumulative risk of meningitis of approximately 10% per year, and 85% of patients will have had at least one episode over a 20-year period. There is therefore a powerful argument for recommending active intervention, location and repair once the diagnosis has been confirmed. The management of acute traumatic CSF leak remains controversial, and conservative therapy for 4–6 weeks is still recommended by some even though the morbidity of endoscopic exploration and repair is low and the risk of meningitis after a leak is cumulative [22].

In patients in whom the diagnosis remains uncertain, it becomes a matter of clinical judgement based on the likelihood of a true dural fistula as to whether endoscopic exploration is indicated. Beta-2 transferrin and fluorescein studies can be particularly useful in this group of patients [4].

Pathogenesis

The most practical way of classifying CSF leaks is by the cause. Defects in the skull base can be considered as either traumatic or non-traumatic.

Traumatic Causes

A fracture of the skull base after head injury is a common cause of CSF rhinorrhoea either directly into the nose or via the Eustachian tube. However, such a fracture may also cause a residual defect with subsequent herniation of the weakened dura to form a meningocele or meningoencephalocele that subsequently presents with meningitis or a delayed CSF leak many years later. Once a meningocele has formed, for whatever reason, even a minor head injury may induce a leak.

CSF rhinorrhoea is a recognised complication after pituitary surgery or following craniotomy for intracranial tumours. The incidence of CSF leak after endoscopic sinus surgery was estimated to be 0.5% in the UK in 1994 [9]. However, endonasal surgery accounts for a significant proportion of leaks in some series of repairs [17, 32, 39].

Non-Traumatic Causes

Non-traumatic leaks are often referred to as "spontaneous" leaks, but the term lacks precision and encompasses various causes and pathologies [18]. Endoscopic techniques have facilitated the recognition and accurate diagnosis of non-traumatic CSF leaks, and a small meningocele or meningoencephalocele can often be identified at the site of the leak.

Elevation of CSF pressure can predispose to a spontaneous CSF leak. Such elevation is classified as either communicating or non-communicating, the latter leading to hydrocephalus. There has been an observation that spontaneous CSF leaks are more likely to occur in obese women, probably due to elevation of CSF pressure [2, 11, 16, 25]. Interestingly, in a series of 32 patients with spontaneous CSF rhinorrhoea and intrasellar arachnoidocele (empty sellar), 90% had altered CSF dynamics and elevated pressure [29].

Skull-base defects also occur with benign/malignant tumours or granulomatous conditions that erode bone. Invasive prolactinomas may cause a particular problem of multiple defects in the sphenoid sinus.

Clinical Features

Typically, a patient with CSF rhinorrhoea will present with clear watery fluid running from the nose, particularly when the head is placed in a dependent position. Patients may also present with meningitis and watery rhinorrhoea: any patient with recurrent meningitis should be considered to have a skull-base defect that must be found. Occasionally, confusion can arise with a watery nasal discharge on exercise or with acute emotion, due to an altered autonomic response often following a previous head injury [10]. Enquiry should be made about symptoms relating to sinus disease since this may not only confuse the diagnosis, but may also need to be managed at the time of dealing with the leak.

Nasal examination, including rigid/flexible endoscopy, should assess access to the nasal cavities and the nasal septum so that corrective surgery can be planned and other pathology dealt with.

Investigation

Fluid Analysis

Traditionally, a glucose oxidase stick test was performed to detect glucose within the nasal fluid to confirm the presence of CSF, but this has a poor predictive value and lacks sensitivity and specificity [8]. It has recently been suggested that the specificity can be improved be ensuring that the nasal fluid is not blood-stained, the blood glucose is normal and the patient does not have an upper respiratory tract infection [3].

Detection of beta-2 transferrin, a polypeptide found within CSF, is a specific test for a leaking dural fistula [36]. A sample of 0.3–0.5 ml is required, and if not collected in clinic it can be collected at home and kept refrigerated until there is sufficient volume for analysis. The test is qualitative and not always easy to interpret. The sensitivity may occasionally be affected by liver disease and rare genetic transferrin anomalies, and these should be sought by analysing serum simultaneously.

A recent alternative to beta-2 transferrin is beta-trace protein (prostaglandin-D synthase), the concentration of which is second to albumin in CSF. Analysis is fast, sensitive, inexpensive and quantitative, and requires only 0.3 ml of fluid [34, 37].

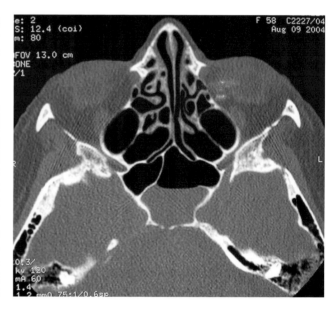

Fig. 62.1 Axial high-resolution computed tomography (CT) scan in a patient with a spontaneous cerebrospinal fluid (CSF) leak. Note the fluid level and small bony defect in posterior wall of the sphenoid sinus

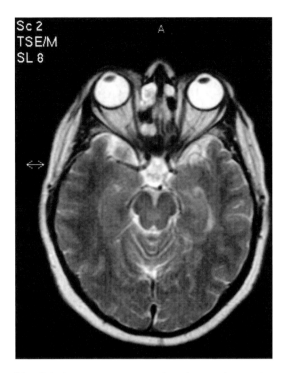

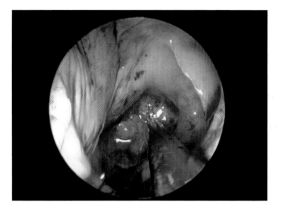

Fig. 62.3 A small meningocele in the posterior wall of the sphenoid sinus shown after intrathecal injection of fluorescein (CT shown in Fig. 62.1)

Fig. 62.2 A magnetic resonance imaging scan in a patient with three right-sided meningoencephaloceles, one in each of the anterior ethmoid, the posterior ethmoid and the sphenoid sinus. The left anterior ethmoid had previously been repaired

Imaging

Both computed tomography (CT) and magnetic resonance (MR) scans give complementary information when assessing patients with CSF leaks [40]. High-resolution CT (HRCT) scans that include the frontal and sphenoid sinuses with window settings to show fine bony detail in coronal and axial planes are required. The site of a leak may be shown as a bony defect, but other important features include localised sinus opacity or a fluid level (Fig. 62.1). An MR scan with T2-weighted images may localise the site of an active leak as a high signal return, but may also provide details of a tumour, meningocele or encephalocele if present (Fig. 62.2) [28]. However, for post-traumatic CSF leaks, a CT is essential but an MR scan may not be required.

CT-cisternography is reported as an accurate way of localising an actively leaking defect, but requires intrathecal injection of contrast such as iohexol or metrizamide via a lumbar puncture [28]. MR-cisternography with gadolinium-containing contrast medium has been described but is not approved in most countries [1]. Since scanning techniques are now much more sensitive, intrathecal injection with radioisotopes seems to have been superseded by MR/HRCT (see Chap. 45).

Surgical Location and Repair

Intrathecal Fluorescein

Endoscopic techniques combined with intrathecal fluorescein greatly enhance the ability to localise a CSF leak, although the technique is not used by all surgeons. Fluorescein stains CSF a fluorescent green that can reveal a minimal leak or defects that are not actively leaking (Fig. 62.3). Use of a blue filter will enhance the fluorescence of the fluorescein for very subtle leaks.

Purified fluorescein without preservatives (e.g. Alcon 10% solution for injection, Alcon Pharma, Freiburg, Germany) is injected into the intrathecal space via a lumbar puncture by the anaesthetist a couple of hours before endoscopic exploration. The patient remains supine during this period, ideally in a head-down Trendelenberg position, to aid circulation of fluorescein to the head. However, this is not practical in children when the lumbar puncture needs to be done under general anaesthesia just prior to skull-base exploration.

The author currently uses 50 mg as a maximal dose in adults (0.5 ml of 10% solution/1 ml of 5% solution), but doses vary amongst different surgeons, with some using much lower doses of 10–20 mg [16, 28, 45]. The fluorescein should be injected into the intrathecal space slowly, after dilution with 10 ml of CSF, using a fine 25-Fr-gauge needle.

The risks associated with intrathecal fluorescein are minimal, but patients should nevertheless be appropriately consented [21]. They should also be advised that their urine will be a strong colour for 3–4 days. There is a low incidence of seizures after fluorescein, but temporary weakness and numbness of the legs, cranial nerve deficits and opisthotonus have been described [35]. Tests of fluorescein sensitivity have been recommended and include a skin test and/or an intravenous injection of 25 mg of fluorescein prior to intrathecal injection [16, 28].

62

Recently, identification of CSF both in clinic and during surgery by applying topical fluorescein with cotton dressings has been described [38].

Endoscopic Exploration

Following intrathecal fluorescein, the nasal cavities are inspected endoscopically after suitable vasoconstriction to identify the presence of a leak. If there is an active leak, fluorescein will collect in the nasopharynx, but key places to inspect include the cribriform plate, sphenoethmoidal recess, Eustachian tube orifice and middle meatus. It is important to avoid mucosal trauma and bleeding during this process since this will make detection of a minimal leak much more difficult. The tympanic membranes should be examined for staining if there is any doubt about CSF leaking from the Eustachian tube. Minimal leaks may take patience to identify, and placing the patient head down or asking the anaesthetist to temporarily increase intracranial pressure may induce a CSF to leak through a small defect.

If fluorescein is not seen at this point, the surgeon must decide whether to proceed with further dissection and exploration. Information about the clinical facts and investigation findings will need to be considered in this decision. The surgeon should be prepared to exenterate all of the ethmoid air cells, explore the sphenoid sinus and to display the frontal recess and frontal os.

Principles of Endoscopic Repair

Prior to commencing surgery the surgeon should check that the correct instruments are available (Table 62.1). Once identified, the dural defect is prepared by removing the surrounding mucosa to encourage fibrosis and adherence of the graft. Herniation of the meninges should be mobilised and reduced, taking care not to cause a massive leak or damage to underlying intracranial structures. Bipolar diathermy may be helpful in dealing with a large prolapsed encephalocele. The possibility of multiple dural defects should always be considered, particularly after trauma.

Various grafts have been used with success and it is the attention to detail during the repair rather than specific graft material that is most important (Table. 62.2). Both underlay and overlay techniques have been described [19, 45]. Potential graft sites include the thigh, abdominal wall, temporalis muscle and intranasal tissues. The author generally uses fascia with fat for sphenoid leaks and muscle for ethmoid or cribriform plate leaks. The graft is stabilised with fibrin glue and ethmoid grafts are supported from below by a nasal pack. Fluorescein provides excellent information about the integrity of the repair.

Decisions regarding the investigation and operative intervention in patients with CSF rhinorrhoea are often quite complex and need to be tailored to individual patients. Management algorithms have been described [30, 33]. A suspected or proven dural fistula after head trauma and skull fracture presents a particularly difficult management problem for which there is no simple answer. Decisions have to be balanced between the potential risks of meningitis and operative morbidity. A leak from the nose is much more likely to require surgery compared to those from the ear [46]. Endoscopic exploration for CSF rhinorrhoea within days of a skull-base injury will be associated with mucosal inflammation and be more prone to bleeding. Elective repair within 2–4 weeks of diagnosis is therefore a reasonable plan of management. The Glasgow coma score and associated traumatic brain lesions are strong predictors of prognosis for CSF leakage from any site complicating skull-base fracture [46].

Techniques for Site-Specific Dural Defects

Frontal Sinus Leaks

Frontal sinus leaks may affect the frontal recess, frontal os or the sinus above the os. Leaks in the recess or the os may be accessible endoscopically, but consideration should always be given to both external repair and maintaining the long-term patency of the frontal os to prevent complications of the secondary effects of frontal sinusitis and mucocele formation [44].

Table 62.1 Instrument and equipment check list

- 0°, 2.7-mm- and 4-mm-diameter endoscope
- 45 or 70 degree, 4-mm-diameter endoscope
- Blue filter
- Straight and upturned fine paediatric Wild-Blakesley forceps
- Paediatric dissector
- Hajek's sphenoid punches with narrow shaft
- Straight mushroom punch for sphenoid
- Fibrin glue (Tiseel, Immuno, Vienna. Austria)

Table 62.2 Graft materials

Autograft	Nasal mucosa/mucoperiosteum
	Nasal septal cartilage/bone
	Fascia lata
	Muscle (temporalis, vastus lateralis, rectus abdominis)
	Fat (leg or abdomen)
Allograft	Lyophilised fascia lata
Xenograft	Small intestine submucosal biomaterial (Surgisis: Cook SIS, Cook Biotech, West Lafayette, Indiana, USA)

Ethmoid Sinus and Cribriform Plate Leaks

Leaks in the cribriform plate are often the quickest to find, but access is very limited. Small paediatric instruments and a 2.7-mm-diameter endoscope are required. In addition, the middle turbinate may need to be partially resected to obtain sufficient access for optimal graft placement.

Defects in the ethmoid sinus are generally easier to access but are not always easy to control. This applies particularly to large defects that may require composite grafts that include cartilage or bone [41]. Mucoperiosteum from the inferior turbinate has been reported to give a more secure seal than mucosa alone [17].

If a CSF leak occurs during endoscopic sinus surgery, a free mucosal/mucoperiosteal graft from either the septum or a turbinate should be harvested and placed over the defect. However, a leak may present several days after surgery and the patient may develop a pneumoencephalocele or an intracranial complication. Endoscopic repair should be performed as soon as the patent is well enough; intrathecal fluorescein is recommended in this situation.

Sphenoid Sinus Leaks

Sphenoid sinus leaks can be very challenging problems. For small defects in the midline, the author plugs the defect with fascia lata and then occludes the sinus with fat and tissue glue. It is sufficient to remove mucosa from around the defect only; stripping the mucosa from the whole sinus is unnecessary and potentially dangerous.

Patients with invasive prolactinomas form a very challenging group [25]. The tumour usually erodes the sphenoid walls to create multiple defects that often open and start leaking as the tumour shrinks following medication with bromocriptine [24]. Repair of such leaks requires co-ordination with an endocrinologist so that the tumour is stable throughout the period of repair.

Spontaneous leaks from defects in the lateral sphenoid wall pose a challenging problem, particularly in a well-pneumatised sinus [26]. Such cases are best dealt with by maximising the exposure to the sphenoid and the defect, and this may include extending the exposure laterally through the pterygopalatine fissure after removing the posterior wall of the maxillary sinus.

Perioperative Management

Antibiotic prophylaxis prior to surgery may induce infection with resistant micro-organisms, but overall they are considered to have a positive protective effect [6, 13]. Post-operative antibiotics are generally used in most reported series [19].

During the immediate post-operative period, sudden increases in CSF pressure should be minimised. Patients should be nursed semi-prone, stool softeners should be prescribed, and they should avoid coughing, sneezing and straining.

Packing the nose after surgery may be advantageous to supporting a graft from below, but meta-analysis has shown that packing does not influence the overall success rates of closure [19].

A lumbar drain should be considered for 4–5 days in profuse leaks that are difficult to control, particularly if intracranial pressure is raised. Their reported use is variable and meta-analysis showed no influence in the overall success rate [19]. Insertion of a temporary lumbar drain or a permanent ventriculoperitoneal shunt has even been described as a means of treating CSF rhinorrhoea and limiting the need for surgery, but it is difficult to see how this would prevent the inherent long-term risk of meningitis [29].

Complications and Outcome

Complications following endonasal repair of a CSF leak are rare, but potential complications include the standard risks of endoscopic sinus surgery as well as pneumoencephalus, meningitis, intracranial bleeding and cerebral abscess.

The most important criteria for outcomes measures are the number of successful repairs and the long-term incidence of meningitis after repair. There are no prospective randomised studies, but there are now several extensive case series of endoscopic repair of CSF fistulae.

Successful Closure

Excellent results have been reported and most quote figures for successful closure in excess of 85–90% [19, 22, 27, 32, 39]. Successful closure has been reported with multilayered free grafts [32, 41]. In the author's series of 70 patients, 10% developed a recurrent leak within weeks of endoscopic repair and 12% had a recurrent leak from 9 months to 12 years later.

Computer-assisted endoscopic surgery does not appear to improve fistula closure rates [43]. No differences in closure rates have been identified between overlay and underlay techniques or between different types of graft [19, 23]. Use of fibrin glue has not been demonstrated to improve the outcome [15].

Local mucosal advancement flaps have been associated with a high delayed failure rate due to graft retraction and are not recommended [15]. Closure failures may be due to high CSF pressure but do not seem to be influenced by the graft material, although details are often omitted [7, 39].

Meningitis

The long-term outcome of meningitis is crucial to judging the effects of surgical repair of CSF fistulae, but little is reported on this outcome measure. Within the author's series, only 2 out of 70 patients have suffered a further episode of meningitis due to recurrent defects. This compares with 24/70 (34%) who had meningitis prior to repair, in whom 10 had recurrent episodes. In a series of 39 patients with a preoperative incidence of meningitis of 38%, none have had meningitis during a review period of 22–120 months (mean 65 months) [5].

62

Conclusions

Endoscopic location and repair of CSF fistulae in the anterior skull base is a low-morbidity technique with a high degree of success. The procedure is greatly enhanced when combined with intrathecal fluorescein. Endoscopic repair can easily be repeated in patients with recurrent leaks and offers a preferable alternative to craniotomy. The risks of meningitis are greatly reduced following endoscopic repair.

Tips to Avoid Complications

- For a unilateral leak, always check if the side is correct prior to surgery.
- Ensure good vasoconstriction and nasal mucosal preparation.
- Ensure that all scans are available for review in theatre at the time of surgery.
- Intrathecal fluorescein should always be given slowly.
- Avoid profuse loss of CSF during surgery.

Take-Home Pearls

- Management decisions may be complex and are best performed jointly with a neurosurgical colleague.
- Locating a subclinical leak may take time and patience.
- Achieve optimum access to facilitate preparation of the graft site.
- Graft technique and materials are best decided by the size and location of the defect.
- Dural defects may be multiple, particularly after skull fracture, but also in malformations.
- Not all CSF leaks will be amenable to endoscopic repair – be prepared to accept defeat and revise the approach.
- Remember to inspect the graft site on the abdomen or leg.

References

1. Aydin K, Guven K, Sencer S, Jinkins JR, Minareci O (2004) MRI cisternography with gadolinium-containing contrast medium: its role, advantages and limitations in the investigation of rhinorrhoea. Neuroradiology 46:75–80
2. Badia L, Loughran S, Lund V (2001) Primary spontaneous cerebrospinal fluid rhinorrhea and obesity. Am J Rhinol 15:117–119
3. Baker EH, Wood DM, Brennan AL, Baines DL, Philips BJ (2005) New insights into the glucose oxidase stick test for cerebrospinal fluid rhinorrhoea. Emerg Med J 22:556–557
4. Bateman N, Jones NS (2000) Rhinorrhoea feigning cerebrospinal fluid leak: nine illustrative cases. J Laryngol Otol 114:462–464
5. Bernal-Sprekelsen M, Alobid I, Mullol J, Trobat F, Tomas-Barberan M (2005) Closure of cerebrospinal fluid leaks prevents ascending bacterial meningitis. Rhinology 43:277–281
6. Brodie H (1997) Prophylactic antibiotics for posttraumatic cerebrospinal fluid fistulae: a meta-analysis. Arch Otolaryngol Head Neck Surg 123:749–752
7. Castelnuovo P, Mauri S, Locatelli D, Emanuelli E, Delù G, Giulio GD (2001) Endoscopic repair of cerebrospinal fluid rhinorrhea: learning from our failures. Am J Rhinol 15:333–342
8. Chan DT, Poon WS, Ip CP, Chui PW, Goh KY (2004) How useful is glucose detection in diagnosing cerebrospinal fluid leak? The rational use of CT and beta-2 transferrin assay in detection of cerebrospinal fluid fistula. Asian J Surg 27:39–42
9. Cumberworth VL, Sudderick RM, Mackay IS (1994) Major complications of functional endoscopic sinus surgery. Clin Otolaryngol 19:248–253
10. Cusimano MD, Sekhar L (1994) Pseudocerebro-spinal fluid rhinorrhoea. J Neurosurg 80:26–30
11. Dunn CJ, Alaani A, Johnson AP (2005) Study on spontaneous cerebrospinal fluid rhinorrhoea: its aetiology and management. J Laryngol Otol 119:12–15
12. Eljamel MS (1991) The role of surgery and B₂-transferrin in the management of cerebrospinal fluid fistulae. MD Thesis, University of Liverpool
13. Eljamel MS (1993) Antibiotic prophylaxis for unrepaired CSF fistulae. Br J Neurosurg 7:501–506
14. Eljamel MS, Foy PM (1990) Acute traumatic CSF fistulae: the risk of intracranial infection. Br J Neurosurg 4:369–371
15. Gassner HG, Ponikau JU, Sherris DA, Kern EB (1999) CSF rhinorrhea: 95 consecutive surgical cases with long term follow-up at the Mayo Clinic. Am J Rhinol 13:439–447
16. Gendeh BS, Mazita A, Selladurai BM, Jegan T, Jeevanan J, Misiran K (2005) Endonasal endoscopic repair of anterior skull-base fistulas: the Kuala Lumpur experience. J Laryngol Otol 119:866–874
17. Gjuric M, Goede U, Keimer H, Wigand ME (1996) Endonasal endoscopic closures of cerebrospinal fistulas at the anterior cranial base. Ann Otol Rhinol Laryngol 105:620–623
18. Har El G (1999) Editorial: what is "spontaneous" cerebrospinal fluid rhinorrhoea? Classification of cerebrospinal fluid leaks. Ann Otol Rhinol Laryngol 108:323–326
19. Hegazy HM, Carrau RL, Snyderman CH, Kassam A, Zweig J (2000) Transnasal endoscopic repair of cerebrospinal fluid rhinorrhea: a meta-analysis. Laryngoscope 110:1166–1172
20. Jones NS, Becker DG (2001) Editorial: advances in the management of CSF leaks. BMJ 322:122–123
21. Keerl R, Weber RK, Draf W, Wienke A, Schaefer SD (2004) Use of sodium fluorescein solution for detection of cerebrospinal fluid fistulas: an analysis of 420 administrations and reported complications in Europe and the United States. Laryngoscope 114:266–272
22. Kirtane MV, Gautham K, Upadhyaya SR (2005) Endoscopic CSF rhinorrhea closure: our experience in 267 cases. Otolaryngol Head Neck Surg 132:208–212
23. Lee TJ, Huang CC, Chuang CC, Huang SF (2004) Transnasal endoscopic repair of cerebrospinal fluid rhinorrhea and skull base defect: ten-year experience. Laryngoscope 114:1475–1481

24. Leong KS, Foy PM, Swift AC, Atkin SI, Hadden DR, MacFarlane IA (2000) CSF rhinorrhoea following treatment with dopamine agonists for massive invasive prolactinomas (review). Clin Endocrinol 52:43–49

25. Lindstrom D R, Toohill RJ, Loehrl TA, Smith TL (2004) Management of cerebrospinal fluid rhinorrhea: the Medical College of Wisconsin experience. Laryngoscope 114:969–974

26. Lopatin AS, Kapitanov DN, Potapov AA (2003) Endonasal endoscopic repair of spontaneous cerebrospinal fluid leaks. Arch Otolaryngol Head Neck Surg 129:859–863

27. Lund VJ (2002) Endoscopic management of cerebrospinal fluid leaks. Am J Rhinol 16:17–23

28. Lund VJ, Savy L, Lloyd G, Howard D (2000) Optimum imaging and diagnosis of cerebrospinal fluid rhinorrhoea. J Laryngol Otol 114:988–992

29. Mangiola A, Anile C, Chirico AD, Maria G (2003) Cerebrospinal fluid rhinorrhea: pathophysiological aspects and treatment. Neurol Res. 25:708–712

30. Marshall AH, Jones NS, Robertson IJ (1999) An algorithm for the management of CSF rhinorrhoea illustrated by 36 cases. Rhinology 37:182–185

31. Marshall AH, Jones NS, Robertson IJ (2001) CSF rhinorrhoea: the place of endoscopic sinus surgery B J Neurosurg 15:8–12

32. McMains KC, Gross CW, Kountakis SE (2004) Endoscopic management of cerebrospinal fluid rhinorrhea. Laryngoscope 114:1833–1837

33. Meco C, Oberascher G (2004) Comprehensive algorithm for skull base dural lesion and cerebrospinal fluid fistula diagnosis. Laryngoscope 114:991–999

34. Meco C, Oberascher G, Arrer E, Moser G, Albegger K (2003) Beta-trace protein test: new guidelines for the reliable diagnosis of cerebrospinal fluid fistula. Otolaryngol Head Neck Surg 129:508–517

35. Moseley JI, Carton CA, Stern WE (1978) Spectrum of complications in the use of intrathecal fluorescein. J Neurosurg 48:765–767

36. Nandapalan V, Watson ID, Swift AC (1996) Beta-2-transferrin and cerebrospinal fluid rhinorrhoea Clin Otolaryngol 21:259–264

37. Reiber H, Walther K, Althaus H (2003) Beta-trace protein as sensitive marker for CSF rhinorhea and CSF otorhea. Acta Neurol Scand 108:359–362

38. Saafan ME, Ragab SM, Albirmawy OA (2006) Topical intranasal fluorescein. the missing partner in algorithms of cerebrospinal fluid fistula detection. Laryngoscope 116:1158–1161

39. Schick B, Ibing R, Brors D, Draf W (2001) Long-term study of endonasal duraplasty and review of the literature. Ann Otol Rhinol Laryngol 110:142–147

40. Shetty P, Shroff MM, Sahani DV, Kirtane MV (1998) Evaluation of high-resolution CT and MR cisternography in the diagnosis of cerebrospinal fluid fistula. Am J Neuroradiol 19:633–639

41. Silva LRF, Santos RP, Zymberg ST (2006) Endoscopic endonasal approach for cerebrospinal fluid fistulae. Minim Invasive Neurosurg 49:88–92

42. Swift AC, Foy PM (2002) Advances in the management of CSF rhinorrhoea. Hosp Med 63:28–32

43. Tabaee A, Kassenoff TL, Kacker A, Anand VK (2005) The efficacy of computer assisted surgery in the endoscopic management of cerebrospinal fluid rhinorrhoea. Otolaryngol Head Neck Surg 133:936–943

44. Woodworth BA, Schloser RJ, Palmer JN (2005) Endoscopic repair of frontal sinus cerebrospinal fluid leaks. J Laryngol Otol 119:709–713

45. Wormald PJ, McDonough M (1997) "Bath-plug" technique for the endoscopic management of cerebrospinal fluid leaks. J Laryngol Otol 111:1042–1046

46. Yilmazlar S, Arslan E, Kocaeli H, Dogan S, Aksoy K, Korfali E, Doygun M (2006) Cerebrospinal fluid leakage complicating skull base fractures: analysis of 81 cases. Neurosurg Rev 29:64–71

Chapter 63

Endonasal Microendoscopic Tumor Surgery at the Anterior Skull Base

63

Ulrike Bockmühl

Core Messages

- Sinonasal malignancies with their histological variety and their propensity to recur and cause local injury present unique challenges to the otolaryngologist.
- Tumors that in the past required open approaches may now be managed successfully with the endonasal approach alone or with combined approaches, lowering the overall morbidity while not sacrificing outcome.
- Cases must be assessed individually in order to determine the appropriate management approach.
- For most sinonasal malignancies, surgical resection followed by postoperative radiation results in superior local control and survival rates compared with single-modality therapy alone.

Contents

Introduction

While the frequency of benign tumors of the nose, the paranasal sinuses, and the anterior skull base is not known, malignant sinonasal tumors account for approximately 3–6% of all head and neck malignancies [16, 28, 36, 44]. Local extension of the malignancies often results in invasion of the skull base, the brain, and/or the orbit. The commonly used techniques in surgical resection of anterior skull-base neoplasms are craniofacial [3, 4, 9, 12, 16, 18, 19, 24, 27, 36] and transcranial procedures [10]. Craniofacial resection needs a bifrontal craniotomy and a transfacial approach usually includes a disfiguring facial incision, midfacial degloving, lateral rhinotomy, and/or extensive facial osteotomies, which result in a cosmetic defect. Transcranial resection is not popular because of the difficulties associated with tumor removal in the nasal cavity. Last but not least, because of the osteotomies that are required in all these external approaches, latency until adjuvant irradiation can start is extended, being prognostically unfavorable.

The success and experience with endonasal endoscopic and/or microscopic techniques together with the development of related surgical instruments have led to expanded endonasal surgery beyond inflammatory diseases to complete resection of sinonasal tumors and lesions at the anterior and central skull base [2, 14, 23, 26, 31, 41]. Meanwhile, several studies have been published describing endonasal surgery to be an effective treatment option for the resection of benign tumors, especially for inverted papilloma and juvenile angiofibroma [5, 25, 26, 29, 30, 40, 41, 43, 45, 46, 48–50]. Concerning malignant tumors, so far there are only few reports on small numbers of patients or single lesions treated, which were mostly esthesioneuroblastomas [2, 6, 8, 47, 51]. When properly indicated and planned, endonasal procedures are superior to the traditional external techniques for the majority of benign, but also malignant tumors [2, 14, 25, 26, 29, 35, 41].

In this chapter, our experience with the endonasal endoscopic and/or microscopic approach to anterior skull-base lesions is described.

General Principles of Endonasal Tumor Surgery

The following preconditions should be realized for successful removal of the pathology and regarding functional and aesthetic aspects:

1. The surgeon must have an extensive and reliable knowledge of the anatomy (see Chap. 44).

2. The surgeon must have vast experience in the endonasal surgery of inflammatory diseases, traumatology, and endonasal duraplasty (see Chap. 62), and last but not least, must be very familiar with the surgical technique of type III frontal sinus drainage according to Draf (see Chap. 52) [13].

3. The surgeon must be familiar with the prevention and management of possible complications (intraorbital hematoma, damage to the lacrimal system, cerebrospinal fluid – CSF – leaks, and major bleeding; see Chap. 54).

4. Since both the microscope and endoscope have advantages and disadvantages, the surgeon should be able to use both in order to optimize his work.

5. Navigation is highly recommended (see Chap. 48).

6. The surgeon should also have expertise in head and neck surgery, including the different external approaches in this area (i.e., he must be able to switch intraoperatively from an endonasal to an external approach and to perform an appropriate reconstruction of soft tissue or bone).

7. Intracranial extension by itself is not a contraindication for the endonasal approach. Rather, it depends on the degree of the extension and the experience of the surgeon. However, those cases should be discussed carefully with the neuroradiologist and the neurosurgeon.

8. If the surgeon lacks neurosurgical training himself, close cooperation with neurosurgeons not only in major intraextracranial cases is mandatory.

9. The surgical procedures should be performed under general anesthesia.

10. In general, we achieve vasoconstriction by placing cotton swabs soaked in naphazoline hydrochloride in the nasal cavity for 10 min followed by subsequent injection of lidocaine with 1:200.000 epinephrine at the lateral nasal wall as well as the septum.

11. Frozen sections should be obtained intraoperatively to ensure complete tumor removal.

Preoperative Management

Before surgery, diagnostic investigation should always include endoscopy and imaging studies, such as computed tomography (CT) and magnetic resonance (MR) imaging (MRI). These are important for evaluation of the location and extent of the lesion, surgical planning, and postoperative follow-up. To obtain the optimum information we recommend performing both CT *and* MRI. The vascularity of a lesion can be evaluated with digital subtraction angiography. If the tumor has reached or involved the internal carotid artery, a balloon occlusion test should be performed together with a perfusion scintigraphy of the brain. In cases with a suspected CSF leak, a CT- or MR-cisternography might be a helpful investigation (see Chap. 45).

Surgical Procedure

Our philosophy is to dissect around the tumor body from all sides along normal anatomical structures. In many cases this means beginning anteriorly with a frontal sinus drainage type III according to Draf [13], then resecting the upper nasal septum and exploring the anterior skull base, dissecting the tumor down to the sphenoid sinus. In many cases this includes the removal of the cribriform plate, the crista galli, and the surrounding dura. Laterally, the margin of dissection is the periorbit, medially it is usually the nasal septum or the opposite nasal cavity, and in large lesions the opposite periorbit. In case of periorbital infiltration, the periorbit can be removed and reconstructed with Tutoplast Fascia Lata (Tutogen Medical, Alachua, FL, USA). If the anterior skull base including the dura needs to be removed, we prefer to dissect from lateral to medial, but it is also possible going the other way around [21]. Duraplasty is generally performed as described by Schick et al. [34].

A criticism of the endonasal approach is the "impossibility" of achieving en bloc resection. Certainly, en bloc removal of tumors is the ideal choice and it is often achieved in smaller lesions. If it is not possible, we perform a piecemeal resection, since as yet there is no evidence that supports a risk of tumor spread because of debulking. Radical extirpation of the disease does not depend on en bloc resection, as shown by our long-term results of inverted papilloma and malignant tumors [2, 29]. Instead, the primary purpose is to identify and widely remove the tumor origin as well as the infiltrated structures (i.e., anterior skull base, dura, or lamina papyracea). It is acceptable, therefore, to resect larger tumors segmentally [2, 25, 26, 30, 43, 47, 50]. One typical example of an endonasal microendoscopic resection of an adenocarcinoma is presented in Fig. 63.1.

In some circumstances it will be necessary to combine the endonasal approach with an external procedure (i.e., a midfacial degloving [7] or a subcranial approach according to Raveh [33]) to achieve clear margins. Then, the surgeon must have the expertise to proceed. Under circumstances whereby incomplete tumor removal is expected (e.g., tumor abutting the internal carotid artery, the optic nerve, or the cavernous sinus; i.e., in adenoid cystic carcinoma or chordoma, or in metastases) endonasal palliative surgery may be indicated, not for the purpose of cure but as an attempt to achieve considerable improvement in quality of life. Finally, it is important to recognize when endonasal resection is not in the patient's interest (e.g., tumor infiltration of the frontal lobe, the cavernous sinus, or the orbit). While more recently, endonasal endoscopic techniques [21, 22] have extended what can be resected, thus far there is no evidence that these increase life expectancy or reduce morbidity, and inexperienced surgeons should be very careful of adopting advanced procedures [20].

The tumor locations in which endonasal surgery is indicated are shown in Fig 63.2. In general, stage T1 and T2 malignancies of the nasal cavity and the ethmoid sinus can be safely resected

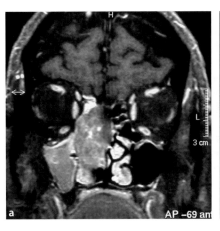
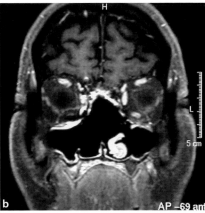
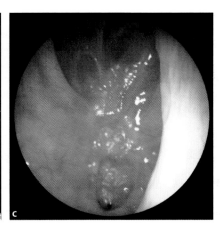

Fig. 63.1a–c Adenocarcinoma of the right ethmoid sinus extending into the nasal cavity as well as infiltrating the nasal septum. a Preoperative T1-weighted coronal image with contrast medium showing the space-occupying lesion. b Postoperative T1-weighted coronal magnetic resonance image 1 year after primary endonasal surgery. c Postoperative endoscopic control 1 year after surgery showing that wound healing is still not complete

via endonasal procedures; T3 tumors might also be removable by the endonasal approach if they only superficially infiltrate the lamina papyracea and periorbit or the cribriform plate, respectively. This also applies to T4a tumors if they have grown only marginally into the frontal sinus or have infiltrated the sphenoid sinus without major bony destruction.

In our experience there are the following major limitations to the use of the endonasal microendoscopic approach:
1. Extensive involvement of the frontal sinus, because it is difficult to remove the diseased mucosa in the supraorbital region and to even drill the underlying bone (Fig. 63.2) [25, 43, 50].
2. Extensive intracranial infiltration.
3. Intraorbital infiltration.
4. If a tumor originates from the posterolateral, anterior or inferior wall of the maxillary sinus.
5. Recurrent lesions associated with massive scar tissue.

Cases with those limitations should be managed primarily by external procedures such as the subcranial approach according to Raveh [33] or midfacial degloving [7].

Postoperative Management

Postoperative Course

In all cases with anterior skull-base resection (both ethmoid roofs, cribriform plates, and crista galli) and duraplasty or dura strengthening as well as in all cases with a large common nasal cavity it will be packed by a continuous ointment tamponade on a silicon sheet that is placed directly on the duraplasty. The silicon film helps re-epithelization, creating a moist chamber. If the tumor could be resected by a unilateral paranasal sinus operation, the nose will be packed with rubber finger stalls (Rhinotamp, Vostra, Aachen, Germany). These will be removed 3–7 days postoperatively. In all expanded endonasal resections, the silicon film and the ointment tamponade will be taken out after 7 days. Patients are usually hospitalized for 3 days (simple cases) up to 10 days (severe cases). During the time of nasal package the patients receive antibiotics (usually second-generation cephalosporin).

After removal of the nasal package the patients have to care for their noses (i.e., using greasy ointment several times a day

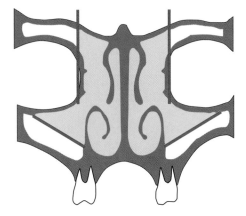

Fig. 63.2 Tumor locations in which endonasal surgery is generally indicated (*yellow area*): Lesions not exceeding more laterally than a vertical plane through the lamina papyracea (*red line*) and those that do not originate from the posterolateral, anterior, or inferior walls of the maxillary sinus

63

and if necessary have gentle debridement at an outpatient visit). In all cases without duraplasty we recommend ample douching with a physiological salt solution at least twice a day. In this regard, the patients have to know that if there was full-thickness mucosal excision it may take up to 1 year for normalization and a possible restart of cilia function [37]. With superficial mucosal damage it may take only several weeks [37].

Follow-up

Generally, follow-up consists of endoscopic examination of the nasal cavity and MRI. In all malignant tumors we perform regular clinical controls quarterly in the 1st and 2nd year after operation, in the 3rd year semiannually and thereafter only annually. Three months after surgery we usually take MRI of the paranasal sinuses and the skull base, as well as of the neck to exclude lymph node metastases. Thereafter, MRI will be repeated annually. Importantly, preoperative staging includes thoracic CT, which will also be repeated yearly postoperatively, since solitary metastases are resectable. We also recommend this regime for inverted papilloma and juvenile angiofibroma, except neck and thoracic imaging. In fibrous dysplasia, ossifying fibroma, paraganglioma, and mucoceles we follow our patients quarterly only in the 1st year and then simply annually. Patients with other benign tumors will have the first postoperative control 3 months after surgery, including a CT (in osteomas) or MRI, thereafter they will have only an endoscopic examination annually.

Outcome

Generally, 5-year disease-specific survival rates of sinonasal malignant tumors that were treated by a combination of sur-

gery (craniofacial resection) and radiotherapy are reported to be between 40% and 70% [16, 36, 39, 42]. Histology, T stage (especially brain, orbital, and deep soft-tissue involvement, and involvement of the sphenoid sinus), positive surgical margins, previous treatment, and lymph node spread have been reported to be predictive factors for poor prognosis [1, 36, 39, 42]. Survival rates vary widely even among tumors of the same histology. Table 63.1 presents the results of some selected recently published follow-up studies that evaluated more than 100 patients each. Esthesioneuroblastoma and adenoid cystic carcinoma have the most favorable prognosis, with possible 5-year disease-specific survival rates of up to 100%. However, the latter prognosis is determined mainly by distant metastases and slow perineural spread, which diminish disease-specific survival to around 40% after 15 years [15]. The two most common histologic types, adenocarcinoma and squamous cell carcinoma, have been reported to have similar outcomes for overall survival [16]. It appears that patients with adenocarcinomas seem to have better prognosis than those with squamous cell carcinomas [2, 3, 16, 36]. Only Suarez et al. [42] have found the reverse proportion in their patient cohort. Malignant melanomas have, along with undifferentiated carcinomas, the worst prognosis [16, 36, 42]. Although tumor histologic findings play an important role in treatment outcome, the prognostic effect of the histologic type is difficult to establish because of the high number of different pathologic conditions and the small number of most of the histologic types. This is also a limitation of all other predictive factors.

Concerning the outcome of patients whose sinonasal malignancies have been removed exclusively endonasally, the series reported so far are few and limited, but they have not shown an increase in local recurrence rates or poorer prognosis [2, 8, 11, 17, 32, 38]. An evaluation of our own patients with endonasally resected adenocarcinomas, squamous cell carcinomas, and esthesioneuroblastomas (n=29) showed a 5-year disease-

Table 63.1 Most common malignant sinonasal tumor histologies (descending order of frequency) including their reported 5-year disease-specific survival rates after multimodality treatment of surgery and postoperative radiotherapy. The most prevalent tumor entities of the author's patient series are marked *bold italic*. The right column includes survival rates of the author's endonasally resected tumor group

Histologic tumor type	Five-year disease-specific survival				
	Shah et al. [36]	Suarez et al. [42]	Ganly et al. [16]	Bockmühl et al. [2]	
					Endonasal resection
Squamous cell carcinoma	51%	65%	43.6%	57%	53%
Adenocarcinoma	57%	30%	52%	65%	78%
Adenoidcystic carcinoma	46%	100%	-	100%	100%
Mucosal melanoma	33%	0	0	-	-
Esthesioneuroblastoma	100%	70%		78%	100%
Undifferentiated carcinoma	-	18%	26.3%	-	-
Sarcoma	58%	-	-	22%	-
All	58%	71%	53.3%	60%	71%

specific survival rate of 78.4%, compared to 66.4% of the patients who underwent conventional external approaches (n=51) [2]. The particular survival rates of these three entities are listed in Table 63.1. Thus, especially for the resection of T2-staged squamous cell and adenocarcinomas of the nasal cavity and the ethmoid sinus, we advocate the endonasal approach. As mentioned earlier, T3 tumors may also be removable endonasally if they only superficially infiltrate lamina papyracea and periorbit or the cribriform plate and dura. This also applies to T4a tumors if they have grown only marginally into the frontal sinus or have infiltrated the sphenoid sinus without major bony destruction. In contrast, maxillary sinus tumors should be removed invariably via a transantral approach, if necessary with maxillectomy [3, 28, 36]. In cases of esthesioneuroblastomas we recommend endonasal resection for tumors of Morita/Kadish stage A or B (no evidence of intracranial extension). Interestingly, compared to squamous cell carcinomas, many esthesioneuroblastomas also infiltrate the dura, but less frequently the brain, resulting in a much higher resectability and finally better outcome.

Tips to Avoid Complications

- Never be tempted to operate without the CT and/or MRI scans.
- Take your time. Being in a hurry may mean that you forget something, that you do not pay enough attention to anatomical landmarks, thus loosing orientation, and finally this may result in complications. In the long term, any of these will slow you down.
- Operate with the body 20° head-up to reduce venous engorgement in the nasal mucosa.
- Do not tape the eyes, so that they can be examined regularly while you are operating. Also, regularly ballotte the eyes with the lids closed to check whether there is any dehiscence of the lamina papyracea.
- This is not "smash and grab" surgery. Rather, it requires good preparation, analysis of CT scans, and a thorough knowledge of the anatomy and attention to detail in surgical technique.
- Navigation should always complement the intraoperative technical setting to double-check anatomical landmarks.
- Fore most operating it is easier to use a 0° endoscope than an angled endoscope.
- If at all possible use the four-hand-technique, whereby one surgeon holds the endoscope and suction and the other prepares with both hands.
- Do not remove or grab anything that you cannot see clearly.
- Stop if visibility is poor. Place cotton swabs soaked with naphazoline hydrochloride or epinephrine (1:10.000). If bleeding is excessive, curtail the procedure or switch to an open approach.

Take-Home Pearls

- The concept of endonasal microendoscopic surgery is no longer an alternative, but a highly valid treatment modality in surgery of sinonasal and anterior, as well as central skull-base tumors. Therefore, it is always essential to check whether the endonasal approach is possible. In principle, surgery in this field should be as extensive as necessary, but as minimally traumatic as possible, which requires a lot of experience. In our hands, following a stepladder of four surgical techniques has proved to be very efficient: (1) endonasal, (2) midfacial deglov-ing [7], (3) osteoplastic frontal sinus approach, and (4) subcranial approach according to Raveh [33]. The lateral rhinotomy is generally reserved for conditions whereby exenteration of the orbit is needed simultaneously [13]. However, individual anatomy and pathology and the personal experience of the surgeon ultimately lead to the choice of approach and operative treatment. In general, oncologic principles should not be compromised in order to minimize morbidity to the patient. The key to success in endonasal microendoscopic surgery is locating the origin of the tumor, defining its extent, and completely removing all diseased tissue including the surrounding normal mucosa. So far, results achieved by this approach are comparable to those of external procedures.

Acknowledgment

To Professor W. Draf for teaching in skull-base surgery.

References

1. Blanch JL, Ruiz AM, Alos L, Traserra-Coderch J, Bernal-Sprekelsen M (2004) Treatment of 125 sinonasal tumors: prognostic factors, outcome, and follow-up. Otolaryngol Head Neck Surg 131:973–976

2. Bockmühl U, Minovi A, Kratzsch B, Hendus J, Draf W (2005) Stellenwert der endonasalen mikro-endoskopischen Tumorchirurgie. Laryngol Rhinol Otol 84:884–891

3. Bridger GP, Kwok B, Baldwin M, Williams JR, Smee RI (2000) Craniofacial resection for paranasal sinus cancers. Head Neck 22:772–780

4. Cantu G, Solero CL, Mariani L, Salvatori P, Mattavelli F, Pizzi N, Riggio E (1999) Anterior craniofacial resection for malignant ethmoid tumors – a series of 91 patients. Head Neck 21:185–191

5. Carrau RL, Snyderman CH, Kassam AB, Jungreis CA (2001) Endoscopic and endoscopic-assisted surgery for juvenile angiofibroma. Laryngoscope 111:483–487

6. Casiano RR, Numa WA, Falquez AM (2000) Endoscopic resection of olfactory neuroblastoma. Am J Rhinol 15:271–279

63

7. Casson PR, Bonnano PC, Converse JM (1974) The midfacial degloving procedure. Plast Reconstr Surg 53:102–113

8. Castelnuovo P, Delù G, Sberze F, Pistochini A, Cambria C, Battaglia P, Bignami M (2006) Esthesioneuoblastoma: endonasal endoscopic treatment. Skull Base 16:25–30

9. Cheesman AD, Lund VJ, Howard DJ (1986) Craniofacial resection for tumors of the nasal cavity and paranasal sinuses. Head Neck Surg 8:429–435

10. Clifford P (1977) Transcranial approach for cancer of the antro-ethmoidal area. Clin Otolaryngol 2:115–130

11. Colclasure JC, Gross CW, Kountakis SE (2004) Endoscopic sinus surgery in patients older than sixty. Otolaryngol Head Neck Surg 131:946–949

12. Delfini R, Iannetti G, Belli E, Santoro A, Ciappetta P, Cantore G (1993) Cranio-facial approaches for tumours involving the anterior half of the skull base. Acta Neurochir (Wien) 124:53–60

13. Draf W (2005) Endonasal frontal sinus drainage type I–III according to Draf. In: Draf W (ed) The Frontal Sinus. Springer, Berlin Heidelberg New York, pp 219–232

14. Draf W, Schick B, Weber R, Keerl R, Saha A (2000) Endonasal micro-endoscopic surgery of nasal and paranasal sinus tumors. In: Stamm A, Draf W (eds) Micro-Endoscopic Surgery of the Paranasal Sinuses and the Skull Base. Springer, Berlin Heidelberg New York, pp 481–488

15. Fordice J, Kershaw C, El-Naggar AK, Goepfert H (1999) Adenoid cystic carcinoma of the head and neck: prediction of morbidity and mortality. Arch Otolaryngol Head Neck Surg 125:149–152

16. Ganly I, Patel SG, Singh B, Kraus DH, Bridger PG, Cantu G, Cheesman A, De Sa G, Donald P, Fliss DM, Gullane P, Janecka I, Kamata SE, Kowalski LP, Levine PA, Medina Dos Santos LR, Pradhan S, Schramm V, Snyderman C, Wei WI, Shah JP (2005) Craniofacial resection for malignant paranasal sinus tumors: report of an International Collaborative Study. Head Neck 27:575–584

17. Goffart Y, Jorissen M, Daele J, Vander Poorten V, Born J, Deneufbourg JM, Zicot AF, Remacle JM (2000) Minimally invasive endoscopic management of malignant sinonasal tumours. Acta Otorhinolaryngol Belg 54:221–232

18. Howard D, Lund VJ (1993) Surgical options in the management of nose and sinus neoplasia. In: Lund VJ (eds) Tumours of the Upper Jaw. Churchill Livingstone, Edinburgh, pp 329–336

19. Janecka IP, Sen C, Sekhar L, Curtin H (1994) Treatment of paranasal sinus cancer with cranial base surgery: results. Laryngoscope 104:553–555

20. Janecka IP, Sen C, Sekhar LN, Ramasastry S, Curtin HD, Barnes EL, D'Amico F (1994) Cranial base surgery: results in 183 patients. Otolaryngol Head Neck Surg 110:539–546

21. Kassam A, Snyderman CH, Mintz A, Gardner P, Carrau RL (2005) Expanded endonasal approach: the rostrocaudal axis. Part I. Crista galli to the sella turcica. Neurosurg Focus 19:E3

22. Kassam A, Snyderman CH, Mintz A, Gardner P, Carrau RL (2005) Expanded endonasal approach: the rostrocaudal axis. Part II. Posterior clinoids to the foramen magnum. Neurosurg Focus 19:E4

23. Kassam AB, Snyderman C, Gardner P, Carrau R, Spiro R (2005) The expanded endonasal approach: a fully endoscopic transnasal approach and resection of the odontoid process: technical case report. Neurosurgery 57:E213; discussion E213

24. Ketcham AS, Wilkins RH, Vanburen JM, Smith RR (1963) A combined intracranial facial approach to the paranasal sinuses. Am J Surg 106:698–703

25. Kraft M, Simmen D, Kaufmann T, Holzmann D (2003) Long-term results of endonasal sinus surgery in sinonasal papillomas. Laryngoscope 113:1541–1547

26. London SD, Schlosser RJ, Gross CW (2002) Endoscopic management of benign sinonasal tumors: a decade of experience. Am J Rhinol 16:221–227

27. Lund VJ, Howard DJ, Wei WI, Cheesman AD (1998) Craniofacial resection for tumors of the nasal cavity and paranasal sinuses – a 17-year experience. Head Neck 20:97–105

28. Maghami E, Kraus DH (2004) Cancer of the nasal cavity and paranasal sinuses. Expert Rev Anticancer Ther 4:411–424

29. Minovi A, Kollert M, Draf W, Bockmühl U (2006) Inverted papilloma: feasibility of endonasal surgery and long-term results of 87 cases. Rhinology 44:205–210

30. Nicolai P, Berlucchi M, Tomenzoli D, Cappiello J, Trimarchi M, Maroldi R, Battaglia G, Antonelli AR (2003) Endoscopic surgery for juvenile angiofibroma: when and how. Laryngoscope 113:775–782

31. Pasquini E, Sciarretta V, Frank G, Cantaroni C, Modugno GC, Mazzatenta D, Farneti G (2004) Endoscopic treatment of benign tumors of the nose and paranasal sinuses. Otolaryngol Head Neck Surg 131:180–186

32. Poetker DM, Toohill RJ, Loehrl TA, Smith TL (2005) Endoscopic management of sinonasal tumors: a preliminary report. Am J Rhinol 19:307–315

33. Raveh J, Turk JB, Laedrach K, Seiler R, Godoy N, Chen J, Paladino J, Virag M, Leibinger K (1995) Extended anterior subcranial approach for skull base tumors: long-term results. J Neurosurg 82:1002–1010

34. Schick B, Ibing R, Brors D, Draf W (2001) Long-term study of endonasal duraplasty and review of the literature. Ann Otol Rhinol Laryngol 110:142–147

35. Schick B, Steigerwald C, El Tahan AER, Draf W (2001) The role of endonasal surgery in the management of frontoethmoidal osteomas. Rhinology 39:66–70

36. Shah JP, Kraus DH, Bilsky MH, Gutin PH, Harrison LH, Strong EW (1997) Craniofacial resection for malignant tumors involving the anterior skull base. Arch Otolaryngol Head Neck Surg 123:1312–1317

37. Shaw CK, Cowin A, Wormald PJ (2001) A study of the normal temporal healing pattern and the mucociliary transport after endoscopic partial and full-thickness removal of nasal mucosa in sheep. Immunol Cell Biol 79:145–148

38. Shipchandler TZ, Batra PS, Citardi MJ, Bolger WE, Lanza DC (2005) Outcomes for endoscopic resection of sinonasal squamous cell carcinoma. Laryngoscope 115:1983–1987

39. Spiro JD, Soo KC, Spiro RH (1989) Squamous cell carcinoma of the nasal cavity and paranasal sinuses. Am J Surg 158:328–332

40. Stamm AC, Watashi CH, Malheiros PF, Harker LA, Pignatari SSN (2000) Micro-endoscopic surgery of benign sino-nasal tumors. In: Stamm A, Draf W (eds) Micro-Endoscopic Surgery of the Paranasal Sinuses and the Skull Base. Springer, Berlin Heidelberg New York, pp 489–514

41. Stammberger H, Anderhuber W, Walch C, Papaefthymiou G (1999) Possibilities and limitations of endoscopic management of nasal and paranasal sinus malignancies. Acta Otorhinolaryngol Belg 53:199–205

42. Suarez C, Llorente JL, Fernandez De Leon R, Maseda E, Lopez A (2004) Prognostic factors in sinonasal tumors involving the anterior skull base. Head Neck 26:136–144

43. Tomenzoli D, Castelnuovo P, Pagella F, Berlucchi M, Pianta L, Delù G, Maroldi R, Nicolai P (2004) Different endoscopic surgical strategies in the management of inverted papilloma of the sinonasal tract: experience with 47 patients. Laryngoscope 114:193–200

44. Tufano RP, Mokadam NA, Montone KT, Weinstein GS, Chalian AA, Wolf PF, Weber RS (1999) Malignant tumors of the nose and paranasal sinuses: hospital of the University of Pennsylvania experience 1990–1997. Am J Rhinol 13:117–123

45. Tufano RP, Thaler ER, Lanza DC, Goldberg AN, Kennedy DW (1999) Endoscopic management of sinonasal inverted papilloma. Am J Rhinol 13:423–426

46. Von Buchwald C, Larsen AS (2005) Endoscopic surgery of inverted papillomas under image guidance – a prospective study of 42 consecutive cases at a Danish university clinic. Otolaryngol Head Neck Surg 132:602–607

47. Walch C, Stammberger H, Anderhuber W, Unger F, Kole W, Feichtinger K (2000) The minimally invasive approach to olfactory neuroblastoma: combined endoscopic and stereotactic treatment. Laryngoscope 110:635–640

48. Winter M, Rauer RA, Gode U, Waitz G, Wigand ME (2000) Invertierte Papillome der Nase und der Nasennebenhöhlen. Langzeitergebnisse nach endoskopischer endonasaler Resektion. HNO 48:568–572

49. Wolfe SG, Schlosser RJ, Bolger WE, Lanza DC, Kennedy DW (2004) Endoscopic and endoscope–assisted resections of inverted sinonasal papillomas. Otolaryngol Head Neck Surg 131:174–179

50. Wormald PJ, Ooi E, van Hasselt CA, Nair S (2003) Endoscopic removal of sinonasal inverted papilloma including endoscopic medial maxillectomy. Laryngoscope 113:867–873

51. Yuen AP, Fan YW, Fung CF, Hung KN (2005) Endoscopic-assisted cranionasal resection of olfactory neuroblastoma. Head Neck 27:488–493

Chapter 64

Beyond the Sphenoid Sinus

64

Paolo Castelnuovo, Andrea Pistochini, Giorgio Minonzio, and Davide Locatelli

Core Messages

- Endonasal endoscopic surgery, which was originally developed to treating sinus conditions, has allowed us to reach deeper and deeper into the intracranial and intradural structures without demolishing the facial skeleton. Nowadays, this endoscopy enables visualisation of the entire ventral skull base, from the crista galli to the odontoid process [12, 15, 28, 31].
- The sphenoid sinus is an important anatomical gateway for surgery on those intracranial structures that would otherwise be accessed traditionally by destructive transcranial or transfacial approaches.
- The development of neuroendoscopy, which has attracted much attention in recent years because of the great possibilities it offers, is linked with the improvement in surgical skills using "four-hands" endonasal techniques and with the improvement in appropriately designed surgical instruments. These new tools are: rigid optics with angled vision, double-angled instruments and powered instruments such as intranasal drills, shavers, lavage systems, surgical Doppler probes and neuronavigation.

Contents

Objectives

The use of an endonasal surgical approach to reach the rhinobase and the sellar as well as parasellar areas has greatly advanced over the past years as the result of a search for less invasive surgical accesses. In fact, experience gained in otorhinolaryngology with endoscopic instruments [3, 40] has offered neurosurgeons a minimally invasive access to intracranial pathologies. Thus, "four-handed" endonasal endoscopy has become an important alternative to the traditional approaches (transcranial and transseptal), firstly allowing the treatment of sellar and parasellar conditions [1, 20, 22, 32], then lesions in the petrous bone apex, and finally those in the posterior fossa (Fig. 64.1) [31].

Intracranial lesions are reached through an "upside-down cone-shaped tunnel" created by the nasal-sphenoid tract. This

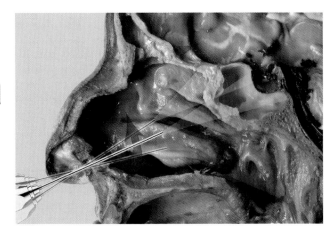

Fig. 64.1 Sagittal section of a fresh anatomical preparation showing the lateral wall of the right nasal fossa and the rhinobase. Using the transsphenoid route, the different inclination of the endoscope and surgical instruments, together with removal of the nasosinusal structures located in the foreground, permits reaching the skull base at the ethmoid-sphenoid planum (*yellow*), the sella and the lateral parasellar regions (*green*) and the clivus and petrous-occipital clival areas (*blue*)

64

avoids both anterior and lateral destruction of the facial skeleton and in selected cases allows the preservation of vitally important vascular-nervous structures along the surgical route.

The experience of certain schools of surgery [2, 4, 5, 9, 10, 14, 17, 19, 29, 33–39] during recent years has demonstrated, in a selected population of patients, the great possibilities of neuroendoscopic techniques in improving surgical results while simultaneously guaranteeing lower morbidity [7, 11, 13, 16, 21, 25, 26]. The common denominator in all of these schools is a continuous collaboration between neurosurgeons and otorhinolaryngologists.

Radiology

Imaging of the Sellar Region

Imaging of the sellar region is of major importance both in the preoperative evaluation and in follow-up of all of the lesions to be treated or cured via the endoscopic route. Before endoscopic surgery, diagnostic imaging capabilities are focused on description of the variations of normal anatomy (particularly the intraoperatively dangerous ones), lesion detection and description of its anatomic relationships and – when possible – to report about the radiological semeiotics specific for a presumptive diagnosis based on pathological nature.

Sella Turcica/Sphenoid Sinus Variability

Sphenoid bone variations are easily detected with non-enhanced computed tomography (CT), which remains mandatory preoperatively. Moreover, multislice units are now free from artefact and positional limitations (see Chap. 45). Multiplanar image reformatting is recommended in the three orthogonal planes, as the adjunct of sagittal plane views is of significant importance and can be obtained with no radiation dose increase. Reports should include not only a description of the classical sinus pneumatisation types (conchal, presellar and sellar), but also underlying focal airy space variations (clinoid, hypertrophied recess, accessory compartments), and should focus on carotid and optic canals dehiscence/transsphenoid course aspects, conjoined septa and on the sphenoid body/clivus inner bone structure (see Chap. 44).

Intrasellar Lesions

For pituitary and other, rarer intrasellar lesions, plain magnetic resonance (MR) imaging (MRI) (sagittal/coronal T1-weighted, T2-weighted, T1 contrast enhanced, specifically optimised thickness, field of view and signal-to-noise ratio) is still a sound diagnostic imaging tool that can be used for any case. Thanks to the evolution of MRI technology, MR examinations can now be customised by adjunctive sequences according to the needs of each individual diseased patient. So, in cases of suspected pituitary intraparenchymal lesion, a dynamic-contrast-enhanced sequence is almost always performed due to its capability of differentiating between delayed (and displaced portal system "tuft") enhancement in pathologic areas and regular enhancement-in-time of normal glandular parenchyma. Fluid-attenuated inversion recovery and gradient echo are at times added in cases of cystic or haemorrhagic lesions.

In cases of suspected sellar bony-wall dehiscence, sequences optimised to obtain an MR cisternography effect are of great importance due to their ability to demonstrate cerebrospinal fluid (CSF) leakages in a non-invasive, simple radiological way.

Suprasellar Lesions

Many of the radiological guidelines described previously for the intrasellar compartment can be applied to the suprasellar region. In these cases, a panoramic brain MRI view is more useful to search for associated lesions. MR angiography (MRA) is more frequently needed in order to disclose the relationships between the lesion mass and the supraclinoid arteries, and in some instances to exclude an aneurysmatic nature of the mass itself.

Vessel Variations

MRA is suitable for the detection of carotid, anterior cerebral artery and posterior communicating artery variations when endoscopy or MRI reveals a course suspected to originate in an area associated with increased risk. Persistence of the trigeminal artery (Fig. 64.2), particularly dangerous when it lies its medial to cranial nerve VI, is easily depicted and graded. The angles typical of the carotid siphon and other region (interfaces) and

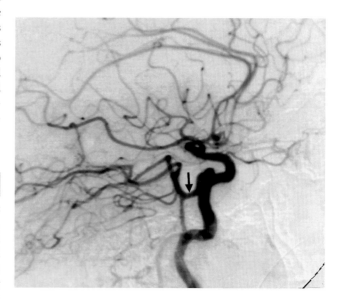

Fig. 64.2 Angiographic image showing the presence of a persistence of the trigeminal artery (associated with an embolised anterior cerebral artery – ACA – aneurysm) identifiable as Salzman type 2 (*arrow*)

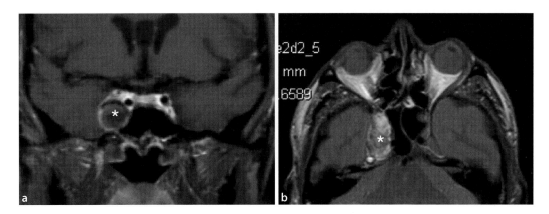

Fig. 64.3a,b Clinical case of epidermoid cyst. **a** Magnetic resonance imaging (MRI) with contrast medium in axial view demonstrating the right cavernous sinus expanded on the whole, but with a roundish area of reduced uptake. **b** Coronal image with the same technique: the area of reduced uptake is more clearly visible

method-related artefacts can at times reduce the MRA image quality. CT angiography also suffers from some (different) technical limitations in this region, but the qualities and drawbacks of the two methods are often complimentary and acquisition of both is recommended when exclusion criteria are needed in doubtful vascular aspects. Digital subtraction angiography (DSA) can be reserved for selected cases in which the flow dynamics are more relevant than simple vessel depiction (e.g. fistulas and collaterals).

Follow-up Studies

Surgical procedures may give rise to heterogeneous signals due to homologous or heterologous tissues, procedure-related devices, and blood, for example, which can mimic or even mask residual or recurrent lesions. An accurate retrospective evaluation of the surgical procedure and of the preoperative imaging is the key to a better study sensibility in these cases. Contrast enhancement is mandatory, even in preoperatively non-enhancing lesions.

Parasellar Imaging

Parasellar structures are complex both in structure and in space arrangement. For general CT and MRI characteristics, one can refer to the earlier sellar-sphenoid section. Each parasellar anatomic region should then be discussed with regard to its imaging-specific characteristics.

Cavernous Sinus

In the last few years, MR has progressively improved the in-vivo detection of intracavernous structures, as it allows acquisition of high-definition thin-slice images with excellent depiction of border zones and of the intracavernous course of the cranial

nerves; the exit foramina and paracavernous dural and CSF boundaries are also clearly visible. This allows radiology grading of cavernous invasion and identification of tiny intracavernous lesions of both expansile and inflammatory origin (Figs. 64.3 and 64.4).

Petrous Apex–Middle Cranial Fossa Boundary Lesions

Most important in this region is determination of the vascular relationships of the lesions, both arterial and venous. MRA and CT angiography should therefore be widely employed and compared with plain panoramic images. Due to the relevance

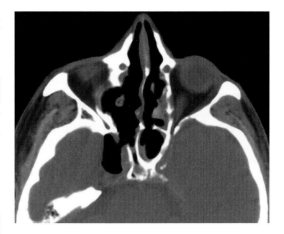

Fig. 64.4 Basal axial view computed tomography (CT) scan of the previous clinical case taken in the post-operative period showing the results of the ethmoid-sphenoidotomy and endonasal removal of the lesion, the breach, and the presence of air in the treated cavity

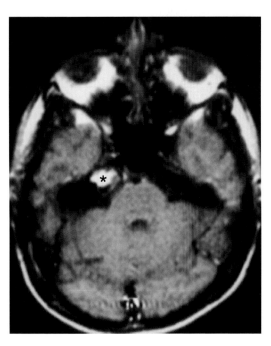

Fig. 64.5 MRI showing a cholesterol granuloma at the apex of the right petrous apex in basal T1-weighted image (differential diagnosis of fatty tissue in an abnormal site)

of bone reaction/destruction, the combined CT and MRI approach is very often , if not always, used (Fig. 64.5).

Posterior Fossa Invasion

Many of the previous general guidelines can be employed in cases of posterior fossa invasion, as these are often included in the parasellar study due to contiguous invasion of lesions arising in both regions. The most relevant use of MR is MR cisternography for posterior CSF spaces; its importance is emphasised by the need to determine the course of the cranial nerves at the root entry zone and cisternal-cavernous side.

Differential Diagnosis of Retroclival Masses

Chordoma

Chordomas from notochordal remnants are often spheno-occipital-fissure related. Imaging findings vary depending on its mixed bony, myxoid and haemorrhagic content, as follows:
1. CT: midline bone-destructive mass with multiple intratumoural hyperdense bone fragments.
2. MR: typically hyperintense on T2-weighted images and mixed intensity (hypointense and hyperintense haemorrhage/myxoid) on T1-weighted images,
3. Contrast enhancement "reticular" or "honeycomb" due to hypointense bony foci.

4. MRA/DSA: avascular, vessel encasement with infrequent stenosis.

Chondrosarcoma

Chondroid calcifications are observed typically on CT, but are not always visible, and MR signal features can mimic chordomas (hyaline and myxoid matrix); the tumour base is not in a midline location (petro-occipital fissure).

Pituitary Macroadenoma with Clival Invasion

1. CT: benign, well-defined margins.
2. MR: origin and continuity with the intrasellar region; signal and enhancement heterogeneity is possible, but not as frequent and diffuse as in chordomas. Concomitant suprasellar and cavernous extension is observed.

Meningioma

1. CT: hyperostosis, hyperdensity, calcifications.
2. MR: often with "en-plaque" disposition and dural tail borders; hyperenhancement in the majority of cases.
3. DSA: typical external carotid artery feeders, pial feeders peripherally, rather homogeneous, slow lesion staining.

Metastasis and Plasmacytoma

Destructive and obvious when multiple in patients with known primitive disease. In single midline lesions, the T2-weighted signal is intermediate in comparison to the chordomatous hyperintensity. Nasopharyngeal carcinoma may erode the contiguous clivus from below.

How to Do it

Approaches

The approach to the sphenoid sinus and its complete exposure are the first surgical steps for treating the anatomical structures surrounding it (Fig. 64.6). This can vary from a paraseptal approach to a transethmoid-pterygoidal one, depending upon how necessary it is to proceed laterally to reach the site (Table 64.1). In any case, it is advisable to expose the entire sinus, creating a single cavity that is open anteriorly. The "beyond the sphenoid" access, described further on, is another factor that is dependent on the size of the lesion. The extra- or intradural dissection of a mass via endoscopy foresees an initial debulking of the lesion. These debulking techniques depend on the consistency of the lesions and can be performed with an aspirator or with cutting instruments or powered aspirators (shaver, ultrasonic surgical aspirator). The next steps are identification and mobilisation of the tumour capsule, dissection and protec-

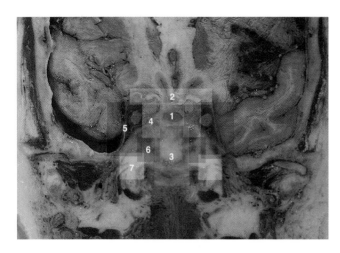

Fig. 64.6 Coronal section of a fresh anatomical preparation at the level of the sellar cavity. Different colours define the anatomical areas that can be reached by the transsphenoid route: *1* sellar (*green*), *2* superior parasellar (*yellow*), *3* clival (*blue*), *4* medial parasellar (*orange*), *5* lateral parasellar (*purple*), *6* apex of the petrous rocca and the petrous-clival fissure (*red*), *7* petrous-occipital (*white*) (picture taken at the Department of Anatomy, University of Vienna, M. Tschabitcher, MD)

Table 64.1 Anatomical areas that can be reached via an endoscopic endonasal approach, and the relative routes of access to the sphenoid [10]

Four-handed transsphenoid approach	Anatomical areas reached
Bilateral direct paraseptal	Sellar and inferior parasellar area
Bilateral transethmoidal	Superior and medial parasellar area
Transethmoid-pterygoidal	Lateral parasellar, middle cranial fossa, petrous bone apex

tion of the adjacent neurovascular structures, then removal of the capsule, taking care not to cause damage with the heat of the electrocoagulator.

Sellar Area – via a Direct Transsphenoidal Approach

The direct bilateral paraseptal approach allows good exposure of the sellar area and permits the treatment of intrasellar conditions [24].

With removal of the sellar floor, which allows access to the sellar clivus, anatomical landmarks such as the internal carotid artery (ICA) and the optic nerve can be recognised (see Chap. 44) and are useful for avoiding damage to important structures. These intrasphenoid landmarks (interoptic-carotid recess, cavernous carotid and paraclival protrusion) appear differently depending on whether the pneumatisation of the sinus is presellar, sellar or conchal, and they surround the sellar floor, around a central area that can be removed surgically without the risk of iatrogenic damage (Fig. 64.7).

Once the central bony portion of the sellar floor has been removed, the periosteal layer of the dura mater is cut to start extracting the tumour. Intrasellar navigation (hydroscopy; Fig. 64.8) [34] is the technique of choice for completing sellar evacuation: it enables both detachment of the tumour using water and continuous cleansing of the sellar cavity, as well as achieving better control over bleeding. Another important manoeuvre is raising the suprasellar cistern, which very often

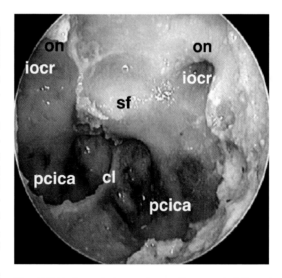

Fig. 64.7 Endoscopic image, 4 mm, 0°, anatomical dissection. The interior of the sphenoid sinus (sellar type) is visible after opening the left of its anterior wall and removing the intersphenoid septum. The following are noticeable on the posterior sphenoid wall: sellar floor (*sf*), clival bone depression (*cl*), bone protrusion in the paraclival portions of the internal carotid artery (ICA; *pcica*) and of the optic nerves (*on*), depression in the inter-optic-carotid recesses (*iocr*)

protrudes downwards, blocking the visual field and making it difficult to see if there are any residual parts of the tumour. The use of 45° optics permits a 360° view of the sellar cavity recesses.

Risks

Damage to the optic nerve, the internal cavernous carotid and the meningopituitary branch, and dural lesion of the ethmoid-sphenoid planum.

Tips to Avoid Complications

- To open the sellar floor, the surgeon must have adequate knowledge of the anatomical and radiological (MR) landmarks and the ability to relate them to each other:
  a. in the upper part, the line connecting the interoptic carotid recesses; detection of the Onodi cell and detection of the superior intercavernous sinus;
  b. laterally, the cavernous ICA protrusion;
  c. in the lower part, detection of the sellar floor and the inferior intercavernous sinus.
- In the conchal-type sphenoid sinuses it is useful to use the midline indicated by the rostrum as a landmark, at a point near the sphenoid floor.
- Use of surgical Doppler in the intrasellar step for indicating the position of the ICA; use of hydrodissection.

Superior Parasellar Region – via the Transtuberculum/Transplanum Approach

The technique of opening of the ethmoid-sphenoid planum is an extension of the previous approach in the rostral direction. This allows access to the anterior skull base and the suprasellar cistern without passing through the sella turcica.

In this case, the transsphenoid access is accompanied by selective opening of the posterior ethmoid in order to reveal the posterior ethmoid arteries, which are considered to be the anterior margins of this approach, to avoid damaging olfaction (Fig. 64.9). This is followed by extraction of the portion of bone between the interoptic-carotid recesses, which corresponds to removal of the tuberculum sellae area on the intracranial side. After accurate coagulation, the opening of the dura mater here enables control over the optic chiasm, and thereafter, the pituitary peduncle and the hypophysis. At this point, exposure of the superior intercavernous sinus and its aperture after vascular clipping will allow the surgeon to see if there is any suprasellar extension of the tumour in the prechiasmatic cistern. After identifying the neurovascular structures that must be preserved, removal of the tumour involves its systematic devascularisation and extracapsular dissection according to the principles of endoscopic intradural dissection.

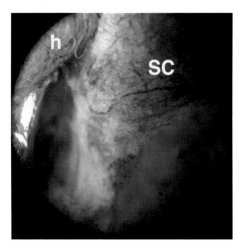

Fig. 64.8 Endoscopic image, 4 mm, 45°. Using the optic device on continuous lavage, it is possible to obtain an immersion view (hydroscopy) of the interstellar area; in this case, immersion curettage of the paracavernous recess can be seen. *h* Residual hypophysis after removal of the tumour, *SC* medial wall of the left cavernous sinus

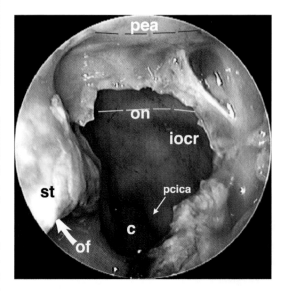

Fig. 64.9 Access to the skull base through the ethmoid-sphenoid planum requires the identification of the posterior ethmoid artery, which represents the anterior boundary of this approach. Endoscopic image, 0°, 4 mm, anatomical dissection. Once the posterior ethmoidectomy at the ethmoid roof has been performed, it is possible to see the posterior ethmoid artery (*pea*). After cutting the tail of the superior turbinate (*st* – the landmark for identifying the natural sphenoid ostium) then removing the anterior sphenoid wall, the intrasphenoid structures can be distinguished. The ethmoid-sphenoid planum may be opened in the area situated between the optic nerve and the posterior ethmoid artery. *on* Optic nerve, *iocr* inter-optic-carotid recess, *c* clivus, *pcica* paraclival internal carotid artery, *c* clivus, *of* olfactory fissure

Risks

1. Damage to the olfactory neuroepithelium.
2. Damage to the optic nerves.
3. Damage to the intracranial nerves.

Tips to Avoid Complications

- Not extending the dissection of the planum anteriorly to the posterior ethmoid arteries preserves olfaction.
- Abundant irrigation, especially during drilling manoeuvres in the tuberculum sellae area, protects the optic nerve from damage produced by heat.
- Inferior parasellar region (via the rostrocaudal approach).
- When proceeding along the median line in the rostrocaudal direction, the extension of the tumour may be such that an approach exposing the retroclival spaces is required.

Superior Third of the Clivus

The approach to the superior portion of the clivus, corresponding to the sellar dorsum, involves transsellar exposure. If the tumour does not involve the gland, this should be positioned with a view to opening the diaphragm, as in the case of access to the planum. This placement will allow access to the retrosellar spaces after drilling the dorsum. This surgical route offers access to the basilar and interpeduncular cisterns. Intradural dissection of the tumour should always be performed according to the techniques described previously.

Middle and Inferior Thirds of the Clivus

An inferior extension of the previous approach leads to a view of the lower retroclival spaces, of the craniovertebral junction and of the anterior portion of the foramen magnum. The paraclival tracts of the ICA are the lateral limits of the clival fenestration. The technique, which is similar to the previous ones, regards the approach to the sphenoid sinus, involving drilling the floor of the sphenoid sinus itself instead of opening the planum or the sellar floor. This manoeuvre, together with resection of the posterior third of the vomer, enables identification of the fundamental landmarks, which are: (1) cranially and laterally the carotid canals, the medial pterygoidal laminae and the pterygoid canals; (2) caudally the Rosenmuller fossae, the Eustachian tubes, the laryngobasilar fascia and the nasopharyngeal mucosa.

Exposure of the clivus is achieved by creating an inferior hinged mucofascial flap from the rhinopharyngeal mucosa and pharyngobasilar fascia. We utilise the diode laser to create this flap because of the consistency and adherence to deeper planes (Fig. 64.10). During this surgical approach, the Vidian canal becomes an important landmark for safety during this manoeuvre, since the Vidian nerve and Vidian artery, which join the ICA at its anterior genu, run through it. Furthermore, the Vidian canal is an important landmark if there is a need to move inferiolaterally to the ICA genu in order to proceed towards the petrous bone (Fig. 64.11a). Opening of the dura mater at the anterior genu of the paraclival ICA requires particular care due to the presence of cranial nerve VI in this area, and necessitates identification of the vertebral artery and the vertebral-basilar junction with the aid of surgical Doppler. Finally, the basilar artery and the structures that are rostral to it can be identified (Figs. 64.11b, c and 64.12). Through this approach it is also possible to decompress the medulla at the cervicomedullary junction, removing the odontoid process after posterior vertebral clamping at C3 (Figs. 64.13 and 64.14) [27].

Risks

1. Damage to the ICA and to cranial nerve VI.
2. Abundant bleeding coming from the venous plexus of the clival periosteum.
3. Persistence of a dural defect with significant liquoral fistula.

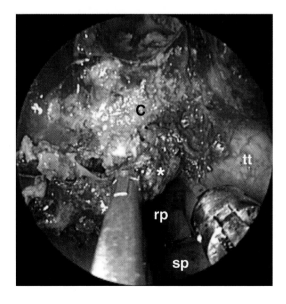

Fig. 64.10 Endoscopic image, 0°, 4 mm. The diode laser proves to be extremely useful for creating a pedunculated flap (*) in the rhinopharyngeal area (*rp*). This permits performing accurate incisions of the mucosa and the basilar-pharyngeal fascia, which in this area adhere firmly to the anterior bone wall of the clivus (*C*). *sp* Soft palate, *tt* torus tubaricus

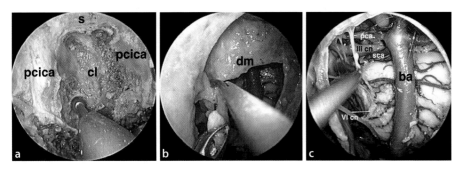

64

Fig. 64.11a–c Endoscopic images, 0°, 4 mm, anatomical dissection. **a** The lateral boundaries for milling the clivus in its inferomedial segment are the paraclival areas of the ICA. *s* Sella, *pcica* paraclival portions of the ICA, cl clivus. **b** Opening of the dura mater (*dm*) allows a view of the intracranial retroclival structures. **c** Cranial nerve III (*III cn*), which passes through the posterior cerebral artery (*pca*) and the superior cerebellar artery (*sca*), is immediately visible rostral to the basilar artery (*ba*); laterally, cranial nerve VI (*VI cn*) can be seen running towards the Dorello canal

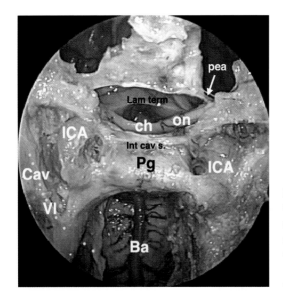

Fig. 64.12 Endoscopic image, 0°, 4 mm, anatomical dissection. The image shows the anatomical structures exposed after opening the ethmoid-sphenoid planum, the sellar floor, the cavernous sinuses and the clivus. *pea* Posterior ethmoid artery, *Lam term* lamina terminalis, *ch* chiasm, *on* optic nerve, *Pg* pituitary gland, *Int cav s.* intercavernous sinus, *ICA* internal carotid artery, *Ba* basilar artery, *Cav* cavernous sinus, *VI cn* cranial nerve VI (its course from where it exits the Dorello canal to inside the cavernous sinus is indicated by the *yellow dotted line*)

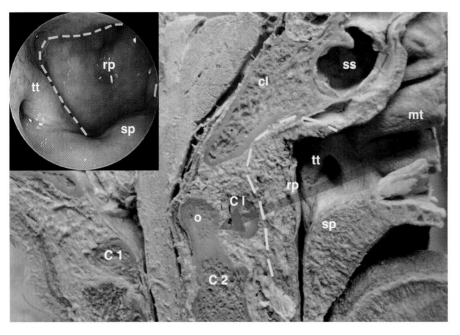

Fig. 64.13 Sagittal section of an anatomical preparation fixed in formalin showing the rhinopharyngeal area, the clivus and the articulation between the first and second cervical vertebrae (C1 and C2, respectively). *ss* Sphenoid sinus, *mt* tail of the middle turbinate, *Cl* clivus, *tt* torus tubaricus, *rp* rhinopharynx, *sp* soft palate, *C1* first cervical vertebra, *C2* second cervical vertebra, *o* odontoid process. The *yellow dashed line* indicates the section required for creating the inferiorly pedunculated mucous flap necessary for endoscopic exposure of the articulation between C1 and C2. *Inset:* Endoscopic image, 0°, 4 mm, showing the supralateral margins of the pedunculated flap in the rhinopharyngeal region

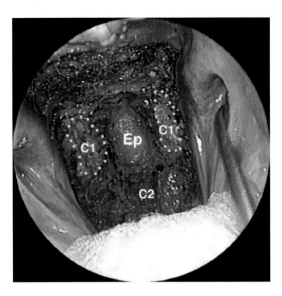

Fig. 64.14 Endoscopic image, 0°, 4 mm, anatomical dissection. The anterior arches of C1 and C2 can be accessed after freeing the inferior portion of the rhinopharyngeal flap and retracting the soft palate. The image shows the odontoid process (*Ep*) after the removal of the C1 anterior arch

Tips to Avoid Complications

- During drilling of the clivus, use the Vidian canal as landmark, keeping to the medial side of it.
- The use of an electromagnetic neuronavigator and surgical Doppler is important.
- Use pedunculated flaps for the duraplasty.
- The use of fibrillar collagen or fibrin cement allows the management of venous bleeding during surgery.
- Avoiding opening the Liliequist membrane reduces the risk of persistent liquoral fistula.

Medial Parasellar Region – via the Transethmoid-Sphenoidal Approach

This route is used for the removal of lesions involving the sellar region with extension into the medial parasellar area, to the lateral recess of the sphenoid and to the posterolateral portion of the ethmoid, and for decompressing the optic nerve. In fact, the posterior ethmoid, the apex of the orbit, the lateral wall of the sphenoid (pterygoid recess) and the medial component of the cavernous sinus can all be seen without difficulty. The inclination of the surgical tools, which is different to that used in the paraseptal route, facilitates management of these structures.

On the other hand, complete exposure of the medial portion of the cavernous sinus requires removal of the bony wall that covers the internal cavernous carotid and thereafter the lateral wall of the sphenoid as far as the orbital apex (Fig. 64.15). In

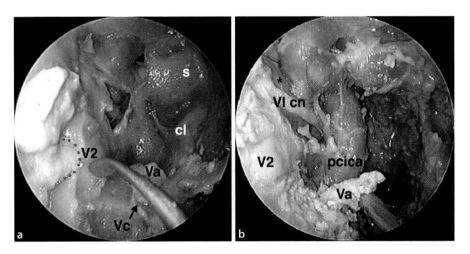

Fig. 64.15a, b Endoscopic image, 0°, 4 mm, anatomical dissection. Removal of the anterior sphenoid wall and drilling the sphenoid floor and the pterygoid allows exposure of the lateral recess of the sphenoid sinus (medial wall of the cavernous sinus). **a** In this image, the right Vidian canal (*Vc*), with the Vidian artery (*Va*), and the canal of the second branch of cranial nerve V (*V2*) have been reached laterally and the medial wall of the cavernous sinus has been incised. *s* Sella, *cl* clivus. **b** Opening of the right cavernous sinus is now complete and the ICA and cranial nerve VI (*VI cn*) can be seen. *Persistent trigeminal artery. *pcica* Paraclival portion of the ICA, *V2* second branch of cranial nerve V, *Va* Vidian artery (picture taken at the Department of Anatomy, University of Vienna, M. Tschabitcher, MD)

particularly pneumatised sphenoids, removal may involve the medial portion of the great wing of the sphenoid. When the cavernous sinus is affected by an expansive process, venous bleeding is nearly always absent due to the devascularisation produced by the tumour, and this makes it possible to treat expanded lesions in this area.

Lateral Parasellar Region – via the Transethmoid-Sphenoid-Pterygoidal Approach

Indications for using this surgical approach include the need to view the lateral structures of the anterior and middle skull base, like the lateral portion of the cavernous sinus, the base of the middle cranial fossa – particularly in cases of very pneumatised pterygoid-sphenoid recesses – and the infratemporal fossa (Fig. 64.16). After removal of the medial portion of the posterior wall of the maxillary sinus and lateralisation of the contents of the pterygoid-maxillary fossa, the Vidian canal is exposed (with cauterisation of the Vidian artery), as well as the foramen rotundum. At this point in the dissection, drilling the pterygoid and sphenoid bases enables the view to be extended to the lateral portion of the cavernous sinus and to the floor of the middle cranial fossa.

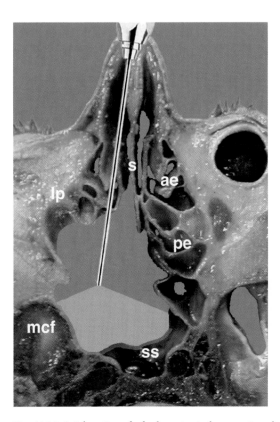

Fig. 64.16 Axial section of a fresh anatomical preparation showing the structures removed in a transethmoid-pterygoid-sphenoid approach towards the parasellar region. This approach allows the view to be widened laterally in order to see the base of the middle cranial fossa (*mcf*). *s* Nasal septum, *ae* anterior ethmoid, *pe* posterior ethmoid, *lp* lamina papyracea, *ss* sphenoid sinus

Risks

1. Damage to the ICA, cranial nerve VII and the optic nerve.
2. Damage to cranial nerve VI.
3. A persistent CSF leak.

Tips to Avoid Complications

- It is important to use an electromagnetic neuronavigator and surgical Doppler.
- During opening of the lateral sphenoidal wall, the anatomical landmarks that are useful during sellar floor removal must be recognised.
- Cranial nerve VI runs through the cavernous sinus in a midlateral direction.
- The use of fibrillar collagen and fibrin cement permits the control of venous bleeding during surgery.

Petrous Bone

Access to the petrous apex may be facilitated if it is medialised and pushed forward by the tumour. If this is not the case, the difficulty of this approach lies in the need to lateralise the ICA. The approach starts with the creation of a pedunculated septal [18] or pharyngeal-basilar flap. Exposure of the posterior wall of the maxillary sinus, bipolar electrocoagulation of the nasal branches of the sphenopalatine artery and dissection of its septal branch afferent to the pedunculated flap allow dislocation of the flap itself inside the maxillary sinus until the reconstructive step. By dissecting the medial portion of the pterygoid and identifying the Vidian foramen, the safety surgical landmarks can be maintained. Drilling of the sphenoidal floor is then performed, identifying the middle pterygoid lamina, which is also an essential landmark.

In fact, if this lamina is drilled perpendicularly to the clivus it is possible to reach the ICA at its anterior genu, where its petrous tract becomes vertical. Once identified, the ICA can be skeletalised, first by thinning it down and removing the bone that covers it, then lateralising it to allow access to the petrous apex (Fig. 64.17). Furthermore, along this route it is also possible to reach the petrous-clival region, the exposure of which requires removal of part of the petrous bone. At this point, the drilling, which proceeds medially to the ICA genu, results in removal of the petrous-clival junction until the underlying dura mater is exposed. The superior and lateral margins of the dissection are the cavernous sinus and the middle cranial fossa, respectively.

Closure Techniques

In the majority of sellar surgical procedures, there is no need to reconstruct the sellar floor once the tumour has been removed, applying only fibrin cement at the sellar aperture. On the other

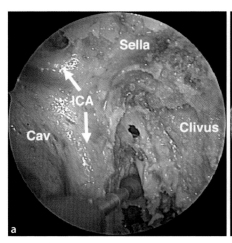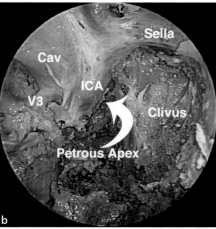

Fig. 64.17 Endoscopic images, 0°, 4 mm, anatomical dissection. **a** Drilling the clivus near the paraclival portion of the ICA, underneath the Vidian canal, allows access to the petrous apex. *Cav* Cavernous sinus. **b** The ICA can be shifted delicately to the side to provide a better view of the petrous-clival and petrous-occipital areas. *V3* Third branch of cranial nerve V

hand, sellar plastic surgery is required in all the cases in which there is liquorrhoea at the conclusion of the sellar evacuation.

The technique involves reconstructing the sellar floor with several layers of different materials (see Chap. 62). We prefer using autologous materials such as the temporal (or abdominal) fascia, the septal or turbinal mucoperiosteum, the quadrangular cartilage or the turbinal bone. Heterologous materials may also be used, like synthetic dural substitutes or collagen matrix. The material to be used is chosen according to the type of surgical approach employed (the site and degree of the defect) and the anatomy of each individual patient. For instance, if the patient presents a concha bullosa, the lateral portion of this structure will be used and is obtained by means of conchal plastic surgery. The tissue obtained is fragmented to achieve a free graft of turbinal bone and turbinal mucoperiosteum. All of this takes place without demolishing any anatomical structures, but results in improvement of nasal function. If the middle turbinate is sacrificed during surgery (for example, in a transethmoid-pterygoid-sphenoid procedure), this will become a donor of turbinal bone and mucoperiosteum, both of which can be used as free grafts. The reconstruction technique generally involves placing the grafts in a multilayer manner (one intradural intracranial layer, an extradural intracranial layer then an extracranial layer), to guarantee greater stability of the plasty [6, 8].

In the sellar region, an intrasellar layer of fascia or collagen matrix is generally applied, followed by a second layer of bone or cartilage, then a third of extracranial mucoperiosteum (overlay) on the sellar floor. The layers may be reduced to two (an underlay and an overlay), and fascia alone may be used. As already mentioned, the various combinations will be applied differently in each individual patient. In our experience, in the anterior cranial fossa an intradural fascia is more easily applied, whereas from the sellar tuberculum backwards, both cerebral pulsation and the force of gravity would shift the intradural flap. In this latter site, it is important to stabilise the flap by placing it in an extradural position and pushing it intradurally and centrally with the filling material (e.g. abdominal fat, cartilage; Fig. 64.18).

Approaches that are more extensive require more complex reconstructive procedures because of the larger defect that they produce [23]. First of all, it is advisable to fill the intracranial defect caused by removal of the tumour (for example with collagen matrix); here, it is more difficult to apply an intradural layer for efficacious closure of the defect because of its size. Therefore, an overlay of fascia (or acellular dermis) is applied and can be stabilised with autologous fat or simply with reabsorbent material. The use of a pedunculated mucous flap that is vascularised at the base of the sphenopalatine artery is particularly useful (Fig. 64.19) [18].

Fibrin glue should be applied at the end of the procedure, over the flaps and not between them to avoid creating empty spaces and consequently the possible recurrence of liquorrhoea once it has been absorbed. The use of a balloon stent in the sphenoid sinus as a support for the graft is at times recommended. Tem-

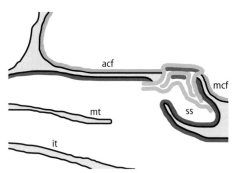

Fig. 64.18 Illustration showing the stabilisation of a multilayer plasty of a large defect in the skull base at risk of implant extrusion due to liquor pressure. Implants of greater consistency, such as cartilage and autologous bone (*purple layers*), are placed between implants of minor consistency, such as fascia lata (*blue coloured layer*), to provide better stability and firmness in the intracranial area. *Green* indicates the intracranial dura mater and *red* the nasosinusal mucosa. *acf* Anterior cranial fossa, *mcf* middle cranial fossa, *ss* sphenoid sinus, *mt* middle turbinate, *it* inferior turbinate

64

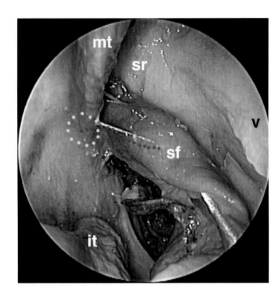

Fig. 64.19 Endoscopic image, 0°, 4 mm, anatomical dissection. The image shows the creation of a pedunculated septal flap on the septal branch of the sphenopalatine artery. The *yellow dots* indicate the position of the sphenopalatine foramen, the *red spots* indicate the course of the septal branch above the choanal margin. *sf* Septal flap, *mt* tail of the middle turbinate, *sr* sphenoethmoidal recess, *it* tail of the inferior turbinate, *v* vomer

porary lumbar drainage in the post-operative period does not appear to decrease the probability of recurrences, which occur more frequently in cases of very large defects [23]. Other factors that can lead to recurrences are: wrong evaluation of the size of the defect and the use of flaps that are insufficient in size, failure to apply the flap to the skull base without first exposing the bone and levelling the margins of the defect, and lack of compliance by the patient who does not heed the recommendations given concerning the post-operative period [30].

Indications and Contraindications

The indications for these types of approach depend upon the site, type and consistency of the lesion (Table 64.2). They are generally indicated when, because of the lesion's features, a surgical approach with a lateral-middle direction is considered best and when the neurovascular structures are peripheral to the lesion. Once the lesion has been reached, the surgeon can decide either on a biopsy or on its immediate removal.

This possibility of a minimally invasive approach for bioptic procedures is particularly advantageous in the case of diseases that respond better to medical treatment (such as lymphomas). Moreover, it must be remembered that these approaches are useful when treating CSF fistulas at the ventral skull base. The contraindications for removal of the tumour are obviously the proximal position of vital structures with respect to the lesion and where it is impossible to drain the lesion through the nasosphenoid tunnel because of arachnoid adherences or adherences with the vessel structures. Furthermore, these approaches are contraindicated in cases when a major vessel has to be either

Table 64.2 Choice of approach according to the disease. CSF Cerebrospinal fluid

Sellar approaches	Sellar lesions (e.g. pituitary adenomas, craniopharyngiomas)
Transplanum approaches	• Anterior skull-base lesions (e.g. suprasellar meningiomas) • CSF leaks of the ethmoid-sphenoidal planum
Transsellar and subsellar/transclival rostrocaudal approaches	• Retroinfundibular/retrosellar region tumours (e.g. petroclival meningiomas) • Clival/retroclival lesions (e.g. chordomas, lipomas) • Removal of the pannus behind the odontoid process affected by rheumatoid arthritis with cervicomedullary junction compression
Transpterygoidal approach to the cavernous sinus and middle cranial base	Selected cases of tumours: • Pituitary macroadenomas or meningiomas refractory to radiotherapy or with pre-existing cranial nerve deficits. • Tumours of cranial nerves V and VI (e.g. Schwannomas). • CSF leaks of the anterior middle cranial fossa (e.g. Sternberg's canal)
Transpterygoidal-sphenoidal approach to the medial petrous apex	• Lesion that has expanded the petrous apex towards the clivus and the lateral recess of the sphenoid sinus (e.g. extradural cholesterol granulomas, cholesteatomas, dermoid tumours)
Transpterygoidal-sphenoidal approach to the petroclival region	• Intradural or extradural lesions situated along the medial portion of the petroclival junction (e.g. chondrosarcomas, chordomas, lesions arising in the sinonasal region) • CSF leaks of the petroclival junction

sacrificed or reconstructed, and they do not offer substantial advantages if an exenteratio orbitae or the removal of the anterior facial skeleton tissue is deemed necessary.

Nevertheless, the most important contraindication when choosing the type of approach remains the surgeon's lack of experience in the endoscopic management of these anatomical regions and in the handling of complications.

Pre- and Post-operative Care

The presurgical evaluation of a patient includes an overall assessment of his respiratory and cardiocirculatory system, in addition to the routine blood tests. In order to avoid excessive bleeding during surgery, the patient should be made to suspend all anti-coagulant drugs (to be substituted with anti-aggregates) and nonsteroidal anti-inflammatory drugs (NSAIDs; to be substituted with drugs containing paracetamol and codeine). Any rhinosinusal conditions should be resolved prior to surgery.

The patient must be informed about the risks involved in removal of the tumour, about the possibility of duraplasty becoming necessary and that the endoscopic approach employed might have to be converted into an external one. In patients with endocranial hypertension, a lumbar drainage is inserted in the post-operative period. Moreover, during the post-operative period, the patients should not take NSAIDs for at least 20 days and should perform nasal lavage (or medicated nasal douches) to keep the nasal cavities clean. A CT scan or nuclear MR is usually carried out 24 h after surgery to check for any haemorrhage, ischaemia or pneumocephalus. In addition, the patients should be submitted to a strict follow-up programme of endoscopic examinations (once a month for the first 6 months, then every 6 months thereafter until 2 years after surgery, then once a year thereafter, if there are no complications). Furthermore, MR investigations should be performed at 6, 12 and 24 months after surgery.

General Tips to Avoid Complications

- Before proceeding with the removal of the lesion, it is important to presume its histological features by considering its radiological characteristics, then confirming this by means of histological analysis; it is also important to determine its relationship with vascular-nervous structures and the presence of any adherences in order to avoid iatrogenic damage or pointless surgical removal.

▼

- The ability to find and keep one's bearings is essential for undertaking this type of surgery. The fundamental nasosinusal, intra- and extracranial anatomical landmarks must be checked continuously during surgery in order to guarantee safe access to the structures, even when they are in deep positions. In the case of access to the sphenoid sinus, the choanal border and the sphenoid rostrum must be detected. For removal of the sellar floor, the interoptic-carotid recesses and the paraclival carotid bulges must be recognised. The cavernous sinus must be opened after exposure of the Vidian canal and the foramen rotundum, while the medial pterygoid lamina, the Vidian canal and the anterior and inferior genu of the paraclival ICA have to be recognised in the case of access to the petrous apex.

- If the principal requisite for the surgeon is that he must always know the exact position he is in, the continuous comparison between the two views – the macroscopic and the endoscopic one – is what permits him to achieve this result. Essential to a surgeon's training is, therefore, the anatomical dissection of cadavers.

- The surgeon must be able to embrace the three spatial planes, creating a three-dimensional view, a mental picture that blends endoscopy with radiology. In this respect, neuronavigation offers fundamental support, but should never be used regardless of the surgeon's knowledge of anatomy and surgery. Another essential aspect of training in endoscopic surgery is the acquisition of knowledge regarding radiological anatomy (CT) and a continuous comparison with the relative endoscopic and macroscopic images acquired during dissection.

- Finally, performance of this type of surgery should always imply the use of appropriately devised instruments. The industries that specialise in this field have produced numerous innovations over recent years, such as neuronavigation, the high degree of definition that has been reached in imaging systems and the synthetic materials that facilitate haemostasis or the reconstruction of defects caused by surgery. The great availability of appropriately devised instruments, together with the increasing need for efficacious endoscopic handling of the anatomical structures, has contributed to the development of the "four-handed" intranasal technique. This technique has offered otorhinolaryngologists and neurosurgeons the possibility of interdisciplinary surgical training, leading to an important and profitable exchange of technical know-how.

Take-Home Pearls

- It is extremely important to work in a team comprising otorhinolaryngologists, neurosurgeons, neuroradiologists, the intensive care unit staff, neuroendocrinologists and neuro-oncologists, in a department for head and neck surgery where skull-base surgery is performed.
- A further essential feature is accurate presurgical evaluation of the lesion that has to be treated, whether it is a fistula or a benign or malignant lesion, in order to know beforehand the advantage and feasibility of using an endoscopic approach.
- It must be stressed that each and every time an endonasal microendoscopic surgical approach is contemplated, profound knowledge of the anatomy of the area, whether macroscopic, endoscopic or radiological, is the primary requisite. It takes time to accomplish these techniques, but every step taken when learning them must be followed meticulously, and the surgeon must have a thorough knowledge of the traditional external approaches to be able to be able to handle any complications that may arise.

References

1. Alfieri, Jho HD (2001) Endoscopic endonasal approaches to the cavernous sinus: surgical approaches. Neurosurgery 49:354–360; discussion 360–362
2. Bockmuhl U, Khalil HS, Draf W (2005) Clinicoradiological and surgical considerations in the treatment of cholesterol granuloma of the petrous pyramid. Skull Base 15:263–267
3. Bockmuhl U, Minovi A, Kratzsch B, Hendus J, Draf W (2005) Endonasal micro-endoscopic tumor surgery: state of the art. Laryngorhinootologie 84:884–891
4. Cappabianca P, Buonamassa S, Cavallo LM, Mariniello G, de Divitiis O (2004) Neuroendoscopy: present and future applications. Clin Neurosurg 51:186–190
5. Carrau RL, Jho H, Ko Y (1996) Transnasal-transsphenoidal endoscopic surgery of the pituitary gland. Laryngoscope 106:914–918
6. Castelnuovo P, Mauri S, Locatelli D, Emanuelli E, Delu G, Giulio GD (2001) Endoscopic repair of cerebrospinal fluid rhinorrhea: learning from our failures. Am J Rhinol 15:333–342
7. Castelnuovo P, Locatelli D, Mauri S, De Bernardi F (2003) Extended endoscopic approaches to the skull base, anterior cranial base CSF leaks. In: de Divitiis E, Cappabianca P (eds) Endoscopic Endonasal Trans-sphenoidal Surgery. Springer, New York, Wien, pp 137–138
8. Castelnuovo PG, Delu G, Locatelli D, Padoan G, Bernardi FD, Pistochini A, Bignami M (2006) Endonasal endoscopic duraplasty: our experience Skull Base 16:19–24
9. Castelnuovo P, Battaglia P, Locatelli D, Delù G, Sberze F, Bignami M (2006) Endonasal micro-endoscopic treatment of malignant tumors of the paranasal sinuses and anterior skull base. Oper Tech Otolaryngol Head Neck Surg 17:152–167
10. Castelnuovo P, Pistochini A, Locatelli D (2006) Different surgical approaches to the sellar region: focusing on the "two nostrils four hands technique". Rhinology 44:2–7
11. Cavallo LM, Messina A, Cappabianca P, Esposito F, de Divitiis E, Gardner P, Tschabitscher M (2005) Endoscopic endonasal surgery of the midline skull base: anatomical study and clinical considerations. Neurosurg Focus 19:E2
12. Cohen NA, Kennedy DW (2005) Endoscopic sinus surgery: where we are – and where we're going. Curr Opin Otolaryngol Head Neck Surg 13:32–38
13. de Divitiis E, Cappabianca P, Cavallo LM (2002) Endoscopic transsphenoidal approach: adaptability of the procedure to different sellar lesions. Neurosurgery 51:699–705; discussion 705–707
14. de Divitiis E, Cavallo LM, Cappabianca P, Esposito F (2007) Extended endoscopic endonasal transsphenoidal approach for the removal of suprasellar tumors: part 2. Neurosurgery 60:46–45
15. Doglietto F, Prevedello DM, Jane JA Jr, Han JA, Laws ER Jr (2005) A brief history of endoscopic transsphenoidal surgery – from Philipp Bozzini to the First World Congress of Endoscopic Skull Base Surgery. Neurosurg Focus 19:E3
16. Frank G, Sciarretta V, Mazzatenta D, Farneti G, Modugno GC, Pasquini E (2005) Transsphenoidal endoscopic approach in the treatment of Rathke's cleft cyst. Neurosurgery 56:124–128; discussion 129
17. Frank G, Sciarretta V, Calbucci F, Farneti G, Mazzatenta D, Pasquini E (2006) The endoscopic transnasal transsphenoidal approach for the treatment of cranial base chordomas and chondrosarcomas. Neurosurgery 59:ONS50–7
18. Hadad G, Bassagasteguy L, Carrau RL, Mataza JC, Kassam A, Snyderman CH, Mintz A (2006) A novel reconstructive technique after endoscopic expanded endonasal approaches: vascular pedicle nasoseptal flap. Laryngoscope 116:1882–1886
19. Hofmann T, Bernal-Sprekelsen M, Koele W, Reittner P, Klein E, Stammberger H (2005) Endoscopic resection of juvenile angiofibromas – long term results. Rhinology 43:282–289
20. Jane JA Jr, Han J, Prevedello DM, Jagannathan J, Dumont AS, Laws ER Jr (2005) Perspectives on endoscopic transsphenoidal surgery. Neurosurg Focus 19:E2
21. Jho HD (2001) Endoscopic transsphenoidal surgery. J Neurooncol 54:187–195
22. Jho HD, Carrau RL (1997) Endoscopic endonasal transsphenoidal surgery: experience with 50 patients. J Neurosurg 87:44–51
23. Kassam A, Carrau RL, Snyderman CH, Gardner P, Mintz A (2005) Evolution of reconstructive techniques following endoscopic expanded endonasal approaches. Neurosurg Focus 19:E8
24. Kassam A, Snyderman CH, Carrau RL, Gardner P, Mintz A (2005) Endoneurosurgical hemostasis techniques: lessons learned from 400 cases. Neurosurg Focus 19:E7
25. Kassam A, Snyderman CH, Mintz A, Gardner P, Carrau RL (2005) Expanded endonasal approach: the rostrocaudal axis. Part II. Posterior clinoids to the foramen magnum. Neurosurg Focus 19:E4

26. Kassam AB, Gardner P, Snyderman C, Mintz A, Carrau R (2005) Expanded endonasal approach: fully endoscopic, completely transnasal approach to the middle third of the clivus, petrous bone, middle cranial fossa, and infratemporal fossa. Neurosurg Focus 19:E6

27. Kassam AB, Snyderman C, Gardner P, Carrau R, Spiro R (2005) The expanded endonasal approach: a fully endoscopic transnasal approach and resection of the odontoid process: technical case report. Neurosurgery 57L:E213

28. Locatelli D, Castelnuovo P, Santi L, Cerniglia M, Maghnie M, Infuso L (2000) Endoscopic approaches to the cranial base: perspectives and realities. Childs Nerv Syst 16:686–691

29. Locatelli D, Levi D, Rampa F, Pezzotta S, Castelnuovo P (2004) Endoscopic approach for treatment of relapses in cystic craniopharyngiomas. Childs Nerv Syst 20:863–867

30. Locatelli D, Rampa F, Acchiardi I, Bignami M, De Bernardi F, Castelnuovo P (2006) Endoscopic endonasal approaches for repair of cerebrospinal fluid leaks: nine-year experience. Neurosurgery 58:ONS246–256

31. Maroon JC (2005) Skull base surgery: past, present, and future trends. Neurosurg Focus 19:E1

32. Mattox DE (2004) Endoscopy-assisted surgery of the petrous apex. Otolaryngol Head Neck Surg 130:229–241

33. May M, Hoffmann DF, Sobol SM (1990) Video endoscopic sinus surgery: a two-handed technique. Laryngoscope 100:430–432

34. Schick B, Ibing R, Brors D, Draf W (2001) Long-term study of endonasal duraplasty and review of the literature. Ann Otol Rhinol Laryngol 110:142–147

35. Senior BA, Dubin MG, Sonnenburg RE, Melroy CT, Ewend MG (2005) Increased role of the otolaryngologist in endoscopic pituitary surgery: endoscopic hydroscopy of the sella. Am J Rhinol 19:181–184

36. Snyderman CH, Kassam AB (2006) Endoscopic techniques for pathology of the anterior cranial fossa and ventral skull base. J Am Coll Surg 202:563

37. Stamm AM (2006) Transnasal endoscopy-assisted skull base surgery. Ann Otol Rhinol Laryngol Suppl 196:45–53

38. Stammberger H, Anderhuber W, Walch C, Papaefthymiou G (1999) Possibilities and limitations of endoscopic management of nasal and paranasal sinus malignancies. Acta Otorhinolaryngol Belg 53:199–205

39. Unger F, Haselsberger K, Walch C, Stammberger H, Papaefthymiou G (2005) Combined endoscopic surgery and radiosurgery as treatment modality for olfactory neuroblastoma (esthesioneuroblastoma). Acta Neurochir (Wien) 147:595–601

40. Walch C, Stammberger H, Unger F, Anderhuber W (2000) A new therapy concept in esthesioneuroblastoma. Laryngorhinootologie 79:743–748

Chapter 65

Congenital Choanal Atresia

65

Cristina Molina-Martínez, José-María Guilemany-Toste,
Javier Cervera-Escario, and Manuel Bernal-Sprekelsen

Core Messages

- In more than 75% of bilateral choanal atresia cases, further associated anomalies have to be considered.
- Computed tomography allows definition of the bony/membranous nature of a choanal atresia with precise definition of the bony situation due to thickening and displacement of the bony surroundings.
- While bilateral choanal atresia needs an immediate response, treatment of unilateral choanal atresia may be postponed.
- The endonasal approach is nowadays widely accepted as the treatment option of first choice for choanal atresia.
- There is no consensus regarding the efficacy of stents in the treatment of choanal atresia.

Contents

Introduction

Congenital choanal atresia (CCA) was first reported in 1830. Its incidence is estimated to be about 1:5,000 to 1:8,000 births [19–21]. CCA is two times more prevalent in females and on the right side. CCA is unilateral in 65–75% of cases and bilateral in the rest. Harris et al. [14] showed that CCA has the same incidence in all races.

More than 75% of bilateral cases of CCA have other associated anomalies, such as CHARGE (coloboma and cranial nerves, heart defects, choanal atresia, retardation of growth and development, genital and urinary abnormalities, and ear abnormalities and/or hearing loss) [5,11,14,26]. Other anomalies associated with CCA include polydactyly, nasal-auricular and palatal deformities, Crouzon's syndrome, craniosynostosis, microencephaly, meningocele, meningoencephalocele, facial asymmetry, orbital-midfacial hypoplasia, cleft palate, and hypertelorism [5].

About 30% of atresias are pure bony; 70% are mixed bony-membranous [9]. The four aspects of the deformity include a narrow nasal cavity, lateral bony obstruction by the lateral pterygoid plate, medial obstruction caused by thickening of the vomer, and membranous/bony obstruction. Histopathologic studies have revealed that the lateral pterygoid plate and the posterior vomer are expanded by endochondral bone formation and are associated with a delicate fibroepithelial membrane that obstructs the choanae [26].

Nasal Embryology

Nasal placodes have an ectodermal origin appearing at the 3rd week of gestation. The nasal cavities extend posteriorly during development under the influence of the posteriorly directed fusion of the palatal processes. Thinning of the membrane occurs, which separates the nasal cavities from the oral cavity. By the 38th day of development, the two-layer membrane consisting of nasal and oral epithelia ruptures and forms the choanae.

The epithelium around the forebrain increases to become specialized olfactory sensory cells. The maxillary process fuses anteriorly with the lateral and medial nasal processes, forming the nasolacrimal groove. This groove invaginates, and the epithelium within is reabsorbed to form the nasolacrimal duct. The nasal septum and premaxilla are formed from the frontonasal process. The maxillar palatal shelves grow medially, fusing with each other and the septum, forming the secondary palate. The nostrils are occluded with an epithelial plug by the 24th week of gestation. Development failure at any point during these processes results in a nasal abnormality.

Etiology

Etiologic and hereditary aspects of choanal atresia remain unclear. A slightly increased risk exists in twins [9,24], with no relation to maternal age [16]. CCA is usually sporadic, but CCA affecting siblings and successive generations has been reported. This malformation can be transmitted as recessive autosomal inheritance [9,18, 24]. It has been suggested that methimazole intake during pregnancy is responsible for specific embryopathies, including choanal atresia [2,3,8, 12].

Several theories have been proposed to explain the pathogenesis of CCA [15]:
1. Persistence of the buccopharyngeal membrane.
2. Persistence of the oronasal membrane (Hochstetter's bucconasal membrane).
3. Abnormal persistence and location of mesenchyme in the choana.
4. Abnormal growth of bony structures surrounding the choana: vomer, sphenoid, pterygoid and palatal bones.
5. Misdirected mesenchyme flow during embryogenesis.

The most likely explanation of the genesis of CCA seems to be the persistence of the bucconasal membrane. Between the 3rd and 4th weeks of gestation, the nasal placodes, which are ectodermal thickenings on each side of the midline, invaginate to form the nasal pits. These enlarged nasal pits burrow into the mesoderm of the developing face, and the primitive nasal pouches are formed. These pouches lie immediately above the buccal cavity, and its floor thins out to become a nasal and oral cavity separated by a thin bucconasal membrane. This membrane ruptures between the 5th and 6th weeks of gestation to produce the choanae. Failure of this membrane to rupture may cause CCA [19].

Diagnosis

Classically, the simplest diagnostic procedure, performed right after the birth, is to press air through the nose with a Politzer balloon or try to introduce a small catheter through the nose till the nasopharynx. The conclusive diagnosis is based on a complete nasal and nasopharyngeal examination using a rigid or flexible fiber-optic endoscope after decongestion to assess the malformation (Fig. 65.1). Instilling contrast material into the nasal cavity and performing an X-ray with the patient in a supine position is no longer used.

Radiology

Computed tomography (CT) scan is the method of choice to assess CCA, revealing the nature and thickness of the obstructing segment [1,8,10,11] and allowing the surgical procedure and its extent to be planned. Thin axial sections (1.5 mm) with bone and soft-tissue windows can give detailed information about the imperforate membranes and bony overgrowth. Images can also be reconstructed in the sagittal plane. In addition, CT scans may detect a skull-base defect being associated with a meningocele/meningoencephalocele (see Chap. 45). Before performing the CT scan, the nose should be aspirated to eliminate any retained

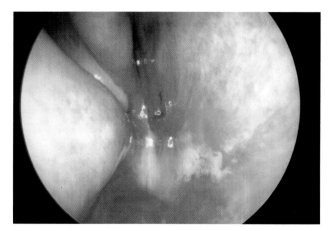

Fig. 65.1 Endoscopic view of a choanal atresia in an infant aged 5 months. The middle and inferior turbinates can be seen fusing posteriorly with the nasal septum in a "cul de sac"

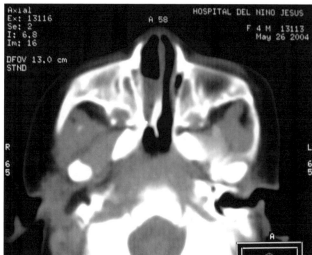

Fig. 65.2 Computed tomography (CT) image of a unilateral mixed (osseous – membranous) choanal atresia. Note the hypertrophy of the pterygoid lamina and atresia of the posterior aspect of the nasal fossa

secretions that may impede the correct assessment of the true thickness of the soft tissue.

Under normal conditions the choanal orifices measure more than 0.37 cm in children under 2 years old, and the vomer doesn't exceed 0.34 cm in children less than 8 years of age. In children with bony choanal atresia, CT demonstrates medial bowing and thickening of the lateral walls of the nasal cavity, which are fused with the enlarged vomer. Some degree of bone narrowing and vomer thickening is usually also present in just membranous CCA (Figs. 65.2–65.4)[11].

Clinical Diagnosis

The newborn epiglottis is near the soft palate and the tongue has a close contact with both the soft and hard palates. These anatomical factors are the reason why newborns breathe nasally, a bilateral CCA is thus an important respiratory emergency in the newborn [4] with an immediate respiratory distress, as infants are obligate nasal breathers. Bilateral CCA produces an immediate respiratory distress that can lead to severe asphyxia and death after birth [13]. Normal newborns are able to breathe through the nose and to swallow almost simultaneously. The adoption of oral breathing happens between hours and 2 weeks after the birth.

A history of respiratory distress and cyanosis are mostly associated with oral intake and sleeping, and is relieved by crying. The respiratory obstruction is cyclic: when the child falls asleep the mouth closes, starting a progressive obstruction with stridor followed by increased respiratory effort and cyanosis. Either the observer opens the child's mouth or the child cries, thus clearing the obstruction. Occasionally, bilateral CCA is de-tected later, when newborns compensate nasal obstruction with constant mouth breathing. Clinically, bilateral nasal mucous discharge, absence of taste and smell, undernourishment, defective speech, chronic rhinosinusitis, and conductive hearing loss may be observed. Excoriation of the nares and upper lip may also be noted.

Unilateral CCA rarely causes any acute respiratory distress. Most common finding is a unilateral nasal mucous discharge on the same side of the atresia. Thick and solid secretions occlude the nasal cavity [7]. Unilateral CCA does not require immediate surgical attention. Conservative management is recommended, sometimes with the use of a McGovern nipple for feeding. A large nipple can be modified by having its end cut off and then ties are attached to the nipple and placed around the head. This provides an airway through which the baby can breathe while its mouth is closed. Alternatively, a surgeon's mask may be fixed around the head to secure the oral airway. In an emergency, the infant can be stimulated to cry; if this is unsuccessful, a finger can be inserted into the mouth until the airway is patent. With this management, the infant can be fed and the airway is protected while definitive therapy is delayed to allow time for a complete workup with the chance to rule out other anomalies.

Surgical Treatment

Unilateral atresia is rarely an emergency. Definitive repair can be planned later, when pneumatization of the paranasal sinuses and growth of the midface are more advanced, facilitating treatment. The management of bilateral atresia requires an immediate response by experienced surgeons.

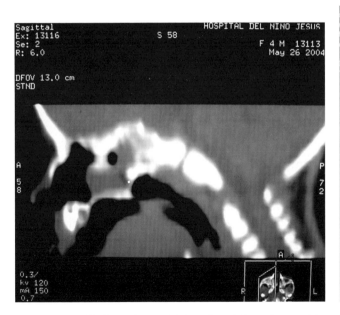

Fig. 65.3 Lateral high-resolution CT of a unilateral choanal atresia. The extent of the atresia can be observed

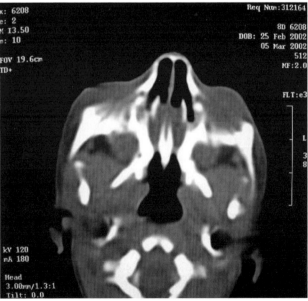

Fig. 65.4 CT of a bilateral bony atresia in a newborn indicating thickening of the vomer and hypertrophy of the lateral pterygoid plates

The stenotic area is found in the palatomaxillary joint, at the posterior margin of the vomer and the palatal process. The atresia plate has a variable size from 1 to 12 mm, representing the posterior margin of a funnel deformation. Additional changes can be an accentuated arch of the hard palate, a sweeping inward of the lateral and posterior nasal walls, and a narrowing of the nasopharynx by the posterior and lateral pharyngeal walls. In cases with a bony atresia, a thin fibrous layer in the inferomedial portion of the wall often exists.

Preoperative Planning

1. Preoperative assessment of choanal atresia: uni-/bilateral; bony, mixed or membranous, symmetric/asymmetric narrowing, additional changes (see above).
2. Accurate assessment of the skull and midface anatomy before determining the therapeutic strategy, including recognition of potential associated malformations. Flexible and/or rigid endoscopic evaluation will be completed with CT.
3. The mucous layer should be reconstructed, preferably with flaps, to avoid restenosis and granulomas. Different lasers may be helpful to create and to enlarge the new opening.
4. There is no consensus about the position and duration of stenting.

Indications

Surgical time and technique selection is based on:
1. Age.
2. Uni-/bilateral atresia.
3. Bony or membranous atresia.
4. Associated anomalies.
5. Potential side effects and complications of each surgical technique.
6. Previous surgical failure.

Methods

Transnasal Approaches

Simple Perforation

The atretic plate is perforated and a calibrated sound is placed on this perforation. This kind of intranasal approach is recommended only as an emergency procedure. The main disadvantages or complications are the increased risk of a "via falsa" and the persistence of respiratory insufficiency.

Endonasal Resection

Endonasal resection involves cleaning and aspiration of the nasal fossa with epinephrine injection into the mucosa overlying the bony atresia, and identification of anatomical landmarks in the nasal fossa (mainly the nasal floor and turbinates). The en-

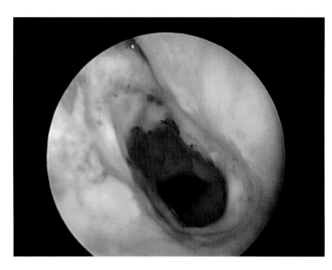

Fig. 65.5 Endoscopic view of an operated choana 10 days postoperatively. The procedure was carried out with a CO_2 laser and topical application of mitomycin C

doscopic procedure starts with incisions of the nasal mucous layer overlying the bony atretic plate. Mucosal flaps are thus created; these will be used at the end of the procedure to cover the borders of the new choanal opening. Opening of the choanal atresia is commenced inferomedially in order to avoid complications like skull-base injuries. CT data-based navigation has been reported as an additional tool for removal of the atresia plate (see Chap. 48). The perforation can be achieved with different instruments: punches, diamond burrs mounted on a long, angled handpiece, or a CO_2-laser beam (the latter may be indicated for thinner atretic bony plates or for membranous atresia). An important step might be the resection of the posterior part of the vomer, which is performed to further widen the choanal opening. If mucosal flaps have been used they are replaced at the end of the procedure for covering the wound surfaces and are kept in place with a packing (Fig. 65.5).

Transpalatine Approach

A mucosal incision is made, beginning just behind the maxillary tuberosity on one side, continued medial to the alveolar ridge up to the canine region, and then angled back to the nasopalatine foramen. A likewise incision is made on the opposite side and the mucosal flaps are elevated, taking care not to damage the greater palatine arteries. The mucosa of the nasopharynx and nose is elevated and preserved. The palatine bones posterior to the greater palatine foramina, the atresia plates, and the posterior vomer are then carefully drilled away using a diamond burr. The preserved mucosa is then used to cover the superior and inferior surfaces of the newly formed choana, and then sutured in place to cover the bone. To avoid alterations in palatal growth, this approach must be performed after the age of 18 months. It is still recommended by some authors for use in cases of bilateral CCA and in revision cases.

Transseptal Approach

This approach is recommended for unilateral CCA. A submucosal septal hemitransfixion incision is made, followed by submucosal dissection of the vomer and bony atresia plate. After the atresia plate is resected, a lateral- and medial-based door-like flap is created by appropriate transnasal mucosal incisions. The flaps are used to cover the medial and lateral surfaces of the newly formed choana. It has been suggested that the flaps should be fixed with fibrin glue and nasal tamponade for 2 days with no insertion of a stent [23].

Discussion

The transpalatine approach to the nasal choana has largely been abandoned in favor of endonasal approaches. The transnasal endoscopic method is the most widely accepted repair technique [22]. The endonasal approach has a lower morbidity compared to the transpalatine approach. The blood loss is minimal; there are no risks of postoperative palatal fistulas, and reduced postoperative pain and discomfort [19]. However, in newborns and little children, the sphenoid sinus is not yet pneumatized and therefore the skull base lies much lower. Drilling the atretic plate could lead to exposure of dura and ultimately to a cerebrospinal fluid leak. To avoid the exposure of the superiorly located skull base, perforation of the atresia has to commence inferiorly along the floor of the nasal fossa.

Unfortunately, the problem of restenosis (9–36%) is significant. Revision surgery may be a recurring theme in some children. McLeod and Brooks [19] described a successful revision using a microdebrider with straight and 120 telescopes, image-guided surgery, and topical mitomycin C to keep the choana patent without stenting. Mitomycin C is an antimitotic drug that inhibits in vitro fibroblastic proliferation and may prevent fibrosis and scar-tissue formation in humans [17,22].

Postoperative Care

There is no consensus regarding the efficacy of stents and their duration of use to maintain the patency of the choana after CCA surgery. The stent is used to prevent obliterative scarring based on fibrosis and granulation tissue. The use of all kinds of packing has been described, such as endotracheal tubes, soft silicone, self-inflating silastic tube, silicone suction tubes, and metal-reinforced rubber silicone tubes. They are usually left in place for about 2–3 months, depending upon the author. In revision cases the duration of stenting described is even longer. However, prolonged mucosal trauma from stenting [6,22,25], plus the heat produced by burrs despite irrigation with saline may lead to obliterative scarring. Our personal experience shows that, similar to what has been observed after drilling and stenting the frontal sinus ostium, the scarring surrounds the stents and then later, when it is removed, collapses, closing the choana. Recently, studies have shown transnasal endoscopic repair of choanal atresia, both unilateral and bilateral, to be effective without stenting [6,22,23,25].

Tips to Avoid Complications

- Precise delineation of the bony components involved in choanal atresia is recommended.
- Pay careful attention to possible skull-base defects in order to be prepared to treat, in addition, a possible meningocele/meningoencephalocele.
- With regard to the high incidence of additional anomalies in bilateral choanal atresia, the best possible cooperation with the anesthesiological team is necessary.
- Begin with inferomedial endonasal opening of the choanal atresia, using the nasal floor and the turbinates as important landmarks.

References

1. Ayari S, Abedipour D, Bossard D, Froehlich P (2004) CT-assisted surgery in choanal atresia. Acta Otolaryngol 124:502–504
2. Barbero P, Ricagni C, Mercado G, Bronberg R, Torrado M (2004) Choanal atresia associated with prenatal methimazole exposure: three new patients. Am J Med Genet A 129:83–86
3. Barwell J, Fox GF, Round J, Berg J (2002) Choanal atresia: the result of maternal thyrotoxicosis or fetal carbimazole? Am J Med Genet 111:55–56
4. Bergonse G, Carneiro AF, Vassoler TM (2005) Choanal atresia, analysis of 16 cases – the experience of HRAC–USP from 2000 to 2004. Rev Bras Otorrinolaringol (Engl Ed) 71:730–733
5. Bonafos G, Capon-Degardin N, Fayoux P, Pellerin P (2004) Choanal atresia and rare craniofacial clefts: report of three cases with a review of the literature. Cleft Palate Craniofac J 41:78–83
6. Cedin AC, Fujita R, Cruz OL (2006) Endoscopic transseptal surgery for choanal atresia with a stentless folded-over-flap technique. Otolaryngol Head Neck Surg 135:693–698
7. Cenjor Español JR, Montserrat J, Cervera Escario T (2000) Figueroa imperforación de coanas. In: Tomás Barberan M, Bernal Sprekelsen M (eds) Tratado de Otorrinolaringología Pediátrica. Gráficas Alzamora, Gerona, pp 339–346
8. Chabrolle JP, Bruel H, El Khoury E, Poinsot J, Amusini P, Benouada A, Marie JP. (2003) Methimazol and choanal atresia. Arch Pediatr 10:463–464
9. Chia SH, Carvalho DS, Jaffe DM, Pransky SM (2002) Unilateral choanal atresia in identical twins: case report and literature review. Int J Pediatr Otorhinolaryngol 62:249–252
10. Crockett DM, Healy GB, McGill TJ, Friedman EM (1987) Computed tomography in the evaluation of choanal atresia in infants and children. Laryngoscope 97:174–183
11. Cummings CW, Frederickson JM, Harker LA, Krause CH, Richardson M, Schuller DE (1998) Choanal atresia. In: Cummings CW, Frederickson JM, Harker LA, Krause CH, Richardson M, Schuller DE (eds) Otolaryngology – Head and Neck Surgery, 3rd edn. Mosby, St. Louis, pp 93–95

12. Ferraris S, Valenzise M, Lerone M, Divizia MT, Rosaia L, Blaid D, Nemelka O, Ferrero GB, Silengo M (2003) Malformations following methimazole exposure in utero: an open issue. Birth Defects Res A Clin Mol Teratol 67:989–992

13. Gujrathi CS, Daniel SJ, James AL, Forte V (2004) Management of bilateral choanal atresia in the neonate: an institutional review. Int J Pediatr Otorhinolaryngol 68:399–407C

14. Harris J, Robert E, Kallen B (1997) Epidemiology of choanal atresia with special reference to the CHARGE association. Pediatrics 99:363–367

15. Hengerer AS, Strome M (1982) Choanal atresia: a new embryologic theory and its influence on surgical management. Laryngoscope 92:913–921

16. Jones JE, Young E, Heier L (1998) Congenital bony nasal cavity deformities. Am J Rhinol 12:81–86

17. Kubba H, Bennet A, Balley CM (2004) An update on choanal atresia surgery at Great Ormond Street Hospital for Children: preliminary results with Mitomycin C and the KTP laser. Int J Pediatr Otorhinolaryngol 68:939–945

18. Lin S, Kirk EP, McKenzie C, Shalhoub C, Turner AM (2004) De novo interstitial duplication 4 (q28.1q35) associated with choanal atresia. J Paediatr Child Health 40:401–403

19. McLeod IK, Brooks DB, Mair EA (2003) Revision choanal atresia repair. Int J Pediatr Otorhinolaryngol 67:517–527

20. Pagon RA, Graham JM Jr, Zonana J, Yong SL (1981) Coloboma, congenital heart disease and choanal atresia with multiple anomalies: the CHARGE association. J Pediatr 99:223–227

21. Pasquini E, Sciarretta V, Saggese D, Cantaroni C, Macri G, Farneti G (2003) Endoscopic treatment of congenital choanal atresia. Int J Pediatr Otorhinolaryngol 67:271–276

22. Rombaux P (2003) Transnasal repair of unilateral choanal atresia. Rhinology 41:31–36

23. Rudert H (1999) Combined transseptal-transnasal surgery of unilateral choanal atresia without using stents. Laryngorhinootologie 78:697–702

24. Schroederer JW Jr, Watson JD, Walner DL, Silvestri JM (2006) Premature monozygotic twins with bilateral choanal atresia: a case report. Laryngoscope 116:149–150

25. Schoem SR (2004) Transnasal endoscopic repair of choanal atresia: why stent? Otolaryngol Head Neck Surg 131:362–366

26. White DR, Giambra BK, Hopkin RJ, Daines CL, Rutter MJ (2005) Aspiration in children with CHARGE syndrome. Int J Pediatr Otorhinolaryngol 69:1205–1209

65

Rhinoplasty

Chapter 66

Surgical Anatomy of the External Nose 66

Fred J. Stucker, Jack W. Pou, and Trang Vo-Nguyen

Core Messages

- When describing the relationship of one anatomical structure to the other in the nose, use the cephalic–caudal and anterior–posterior orientation.
- Nasal subunits should be taken into consideration when performing nasal reconstruction. Reconstruction of the entire subunit is preferred.
- The anterior, middle, and posterior septal angles lend shape to the nasal tip.
- An L-strut of at least 1.5 cm should be left in septoplasty to maintain nasal support.

Contents

Introduction

An in-depth understanding of the anatomy of the nose is essential in rhinoplasty. Careful analysis of the anatomy of the nose and an understanding of the anatomical variances will assist the surgeon in planning and executing a successful rhinoplasty. This chapter will describe the surgical anatomy of the nose.

The nose is a complex, three-dimensional structure which gives character to the face. The external nose consists of discreet aesthetic subunits including the dorsum, the sidewalls, the ala, the soft-tissue triangles, and the tip (Fig. 66.1).

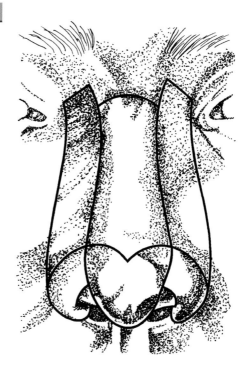

Fig. 66.1 Subunits of the nose. (1) Nasal dorsum (2) Nasal sidewall (3) Nasal alar (4) Nasal tip

Aesthetic Nasal Proportions

On the frontal view, important landmarks of the surface anatomy of the nose include the forehead, the nasion, the tip-defining points, the alar-sidewall, the supra-alar crease, and the philtrum. There should be a gentle and smooth curve from the brows to the nasal dorsum. The width of the nose should be the same as the intercanthal distance. The length of the nose should be approximately one-third of the distance from the hairline to the chin (Fig. 66.2).

From the basal view, the relative proportion of the columella and the infratip lobule can be clearly visualized. The relative ratio between the columella and the infratip lobule is approximately 2:1. The soft tissue triangles are seen with smooth margins. The nasal sills curve gently as the alae merge to form the ala-facial grooves (Fig. 66.3).

On the lateral view, the nose is seen extending from the nasofrontal angle to the subnasale. The nasion corresponds to the nasofrontal suture line. The rhinion corresponds to the soft tissue at the osseocartilaginous junction of the nasal dorsum. The supratip is seen with a slight depression cephalic to the tip defining point. The infratip lobule curves gently as it merges with the columella. The columella has a subtle double break and is slightly visible. The nasofrontal angle is approximately 115–135°. The nasolabial angle is approximately 90–105° (Fig. 66.4). The nasal projection is best appreciated using the 3-4-5 triangle (Fig. 66.5).

Nasal Anatomy (Framework)

The complex contour of the nose is the result of harmonious blending of nasal framework and the soft tissue covering it. The nasal framework includes the nasal bone, the ascending process of the maxilla, the upper and lower lateral cartilages, and the nasal septum. The caudal septum has an important function in maintaining nasal support. A 1.5-cm dorsal and caudal struts are prudently preserved in septal surgery in order to maintain

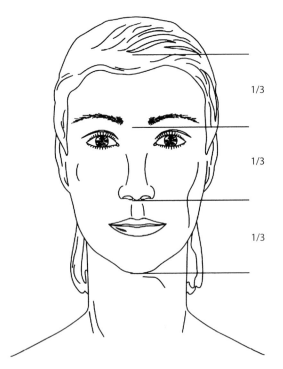

Fig. 66.2 Facial aesthetic propositions

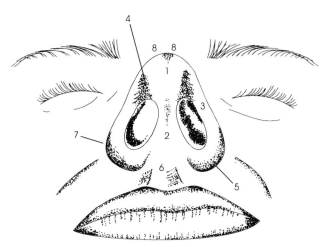

Fig. 66.3 Surface anatomy of a nasal base. (1) Infratip lobule (2) Columella (3) Nasal alar sidewall (4) Soft tissue triangle (5) Nasal sill (6) Columella—labial angle (7) Alar—facial angle (8) Nasal tip

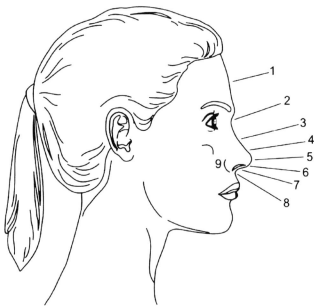

Fig. 66.4 Surface anatomy of the lateral nose. (1) Glabella (2) Nasofrontal angle (3) Rhinion (4) Supratip (5) Nasal tip (6) Infratip lobule (7) Columella (8) Nasolabial angle (9) Alar—facial angle

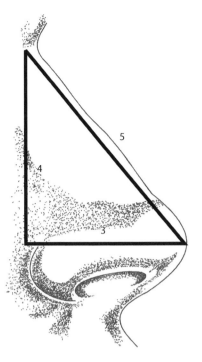

Fig. 66.5 Aesthetic propositions of the lateral nose

the nasal profile. The anterior, middle, and posterior septal angles must be maintained so that nasal contour is preserved. Nasal tip support depends upon the upper and lower lateral cartilages, the attachment of the lower lateral cartilages to the piriform aperture, the caudal septum, the interdomal ligament, the maxillary crest, the nasal spine, and the attachment of the caudal septum to the medial crura (Fig. 66.6).

The tripod concept explains tip dynamics and the various surgical procedures used to alter tip rotation and projection. The two medial crura of the lower lateral cartilages act as one leg of the tripod. The other legs are formed by the two lateral crura. By changing the pivot point of the tripod, tip rotation and tip projection can also be changed.

The paired nasal bones form the upper third or the bony vault of the nose. The nasal bones articulate with the frontal bone as well as the ascending process of the maxilla. The upper lateral cartilage forms the middle third of the nose or the midvault, and fuses with the undersurface of the nasal bone at its cephalic border. The cephalic edge of the lower lateral cartilage overlaps the caudal edge of the upper lateral cartilage in the scroll area (Fig. 66.7).

Soft Tissue Support

Skin thickness is an important consideration in rhinoplasty. It is difficult to achieve a sculpted appearance in thick-skinned patients. However, thin-skinned patients will reveal all irregularities and asymmetries in the contour of the nose following rhi-

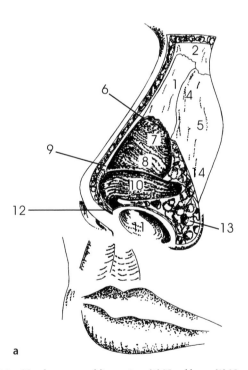

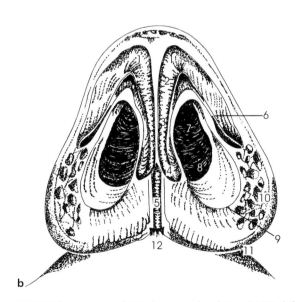

Fig. 66.6 **a** Nasal anatomy oblique view. (1) Nasal bone (2) Nasofrontal suture line (3) Internasal suture line (4) Naso-maxillary suture line (5) Ascending process of maxilla (6) Rhinion (7) Upper lateral cartilage (8) Caudal edge of upper lateral cartilage (9) Septal angle (10) Lower lateral cartilage (11) Medial crus (12) Intermediate crus (13) Sesamoid aper-

ture (14) Pyriform aperture. **b** Nasal anatomy, basal view. (1) Tip defining point (2) Intermediate crus (3) Medial crus (4) Medial crural footplate (5) Caudal septum (6) Lateral crus (7) Naris (8) Nostril floor (9) Nostril sill (10) Alar lobule (11) Alar—facial groove (12) Nasal spine

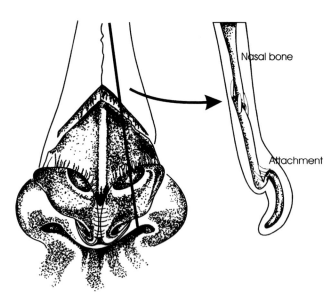

Fig. 66.7 Relationships between the nasal bone and the upper and lower lateral cartilages

66

There are three major groups of nasal musculature. The elevator muscles include the procerus and the levator labii alaeque nasi. The depressor muscles include ala nasalis and depressor septi nasi. The compressor muscles include the transverse nasalis and the compressor narium minor. The dilator muscle includes the dilator naris anterior. Important adjacent muscles include the corrugator and the orbicularis oculi (Fig. 66.8).

Vascular supply and lymphatic drainage are found superficial to the nasal musculature. Major vessels of nasal vasculature include the lateral dorsal artery, the lateral nasal artery, the angular artery, and the columella artery (Fig. 66.9). The lymphatic drainage of the nose converges in the submandibular nodes. Of noted, there is minimal lymphatic drainage in the columella (Fig. 66.10). Therefore, the columella incision in open rhinoplasty causes minimal edema.

noplasty. Generally speaking, the skin is thicker at the nasion, thinner over the rhinion, and then thicker in the supratip.

The superficial musculoaponeurotic system (SMAS) of the nose is similar to the SMAS of the face. The SMAS should be preserved in rhinoplasty to camouflage any bony or cartilaginous irregularities.

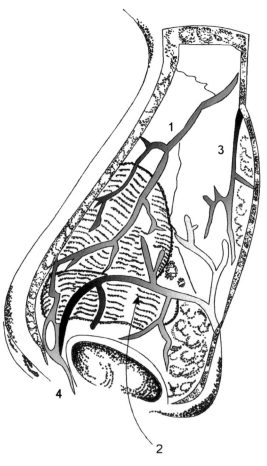

Fig. 66.9 Nasal vasculature (1) Dorsal nasal artery (2) Lateral nasal artery (3) Angular artery (4) Columella artery

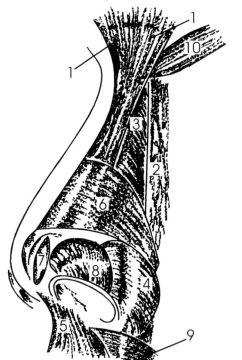

Fig. 66.8 Nasal musculature **A**. Elevator muscles (1) Procerus (2) Levator labii alaeque nasi (3) Anomalous nasi **B**. Depressor muscles (4) Alar nasalis (5) Depressor septi nasi **C**. Compressor muscles (6) Transverse nasalis (7) Compressor narium minor **D**. Minor dilator muscles (8) Dilator naris anterior **E**. Other muscles (9) Orbicularis oris (10) Corrugator

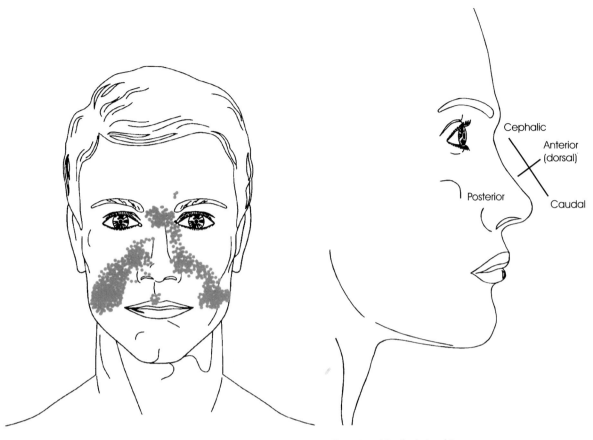

Fig. 66.10 Lymphatic drainage of the nose

Fig. 66.11 Nasal relationships

Take-Home Pearls

- When describing the relationship of one anatomical structure to the other in the nose, use the cephalic/caudal and anterior/posterior orientation (Fig. 66.11).
- Nasal subunits should be taken into consideration when performing nasal reconstruction. Reconstruction of the entire subunit is preferred.
- The anterior, middle, and posterior septal angles lend shape to the nasal tip.
- L-strut of at least 1.5 cm should be left in septoplasty to maintain nasal support.

References

1. Anderson JR (1984) A reasoned approach to nasal base surgery. Arch Otolaryngol 110:349–358
2. Burget GC, Menick FJ (1985) The subunit principles in nasal reconstruction. Plast Reconstr Surg 76:239–247
3. Crumley RJ, Lancer M (1988) Quantitative analysis of nasal tip projection. Laryngoscope 98:202–208
4. Larrabee WF, Makielski KH, Henderson JL (2004) Surgical anatomy of the face. Lippincott Williams & Wilkins, Philadelphia
5. Powell N, Humphreys B (1984) Proportions of the aesthetic face. Thieme-Stratton, New York
6. Tardy ME, Brown R (1990) Surgical anatomy of the nose. Raven Press, New York
7. Toriumi DM, Becker DG (1999) Rhinoplasty dissection manual. Lippincott Williams & Wilkins, Philadelphia

Chapter 67

Septorhinoplasty: Management of the Nasal Vault and Septum

67

Randolph B. Capone and Ira D. Papel

Core Messages

- Thorough understanding of nasal anatomy, facial analysis, and the duality of nasal form and function is essential for rhinoplasty surgeons.
- Crumley's method for determination of tip projection is also useful to determine dorsal projection at any point along the dorsum.
- Septal, auricular, and/or costal cartilage grafts are routinely required to correct middle vault deformities.
- Successful correction of iatrogenic, traumatic, and congenital nasal deformities requires careful consideration of the interplay between the bony vault, cartilaginous vault, and septum.

Contents

Introduction

Of all the aesthetic facial units, the nose plays perhaps the most important role in facial proportion and harmony. A single unpaired structure occupying the midface, it serves to balance the facial thirds and fifths as well as those aesthetic units surrounding it. Seemingly small changes after rhinoplasty or traumatic injury frequently affect dramatic changes in nasal appearance. The nose is not, however, only an aesthetic structure, but also a respiratory and olfactory organ. This duality of nasal form and function mandates that rhinoplasty must enhance nasal appearance and optimize the nasal airway. It is essential, therefore, that the nasal surgeons have a detailed understanding of nasal anatomy and physiology, and a thorough grasp of the many interventions available in rhinoplasty. In this chapter, the editors have asked us to discuss these issues with regard to management of the nasal vault and septal deformity.

Anatomy of the Upper Two Thirds of the Nose

The upper two thirds of the nose contains the dorsum and sidewall aesthetic subunits while the tip, columella, soft tissue triangles, and alae constitute the lower third of the nose (Fig. 67.1) [1]. Topographically, the upper two thirds of the nose is that portion from the *nasion* to the level of the alar crease (Fig. 67.2), where the nasion is defined as the most posterior point along the curve from the glabella to the nasal dorsum. The *radix* is the region of the nasal dorsum that defines the contour of the paired nasal bones from the glabella towards the nasal tip.

Skin and Subcutaneous Tissue

The skin overlying the upper nasal two thirds has variable thickness. Relatively thick at the nasion (2–5 mm), it becomes thin and mobile over the dorsum (3.2 mm), thinnest at the rhinion (2–2.2 mm), and gradually thickens again, becoming sebaceous towards the tip (5 mm) [2]. This variability is important in planning the dorsal profile because creation of a straight skeletal profile will not likely create a straight postoperative profile.

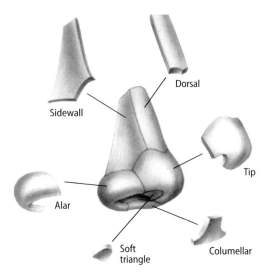

Fig. 67.1 Nasal subunits. (Modified from [1])

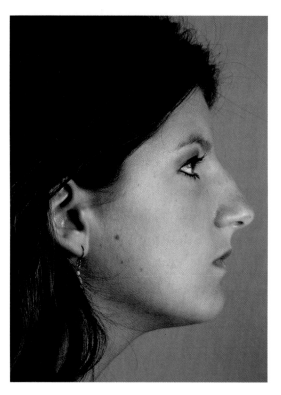

Fig. 67.2 Upper nasal two thirds: nasion to alar crease

67

When edema diminishes, the surgeon may find that the rhinion has been overresected if no allowance for skin thickness was considered during surgery.

Beneath the skin is a thin fibrous layer designated the nasal superficial musculo-aponeurotic system (SMAS) [3]. Analogous to the facial SMAS, the nasal SMAS encompasses the nasal musculature and is located immediately superficial to the periosteum and perichondrium. Dissection just below the nasal SMAS provides a less traumatic and easier dissection plane during rhinoplasty, with preservation of nasal vasculature, nerves, and lymphatics that lie within the skin-soft tissue envelope [4].

Nasal Bones and Upper Lateral Cartilages

Deep to the nasal SMAS are the paired nasal bones and upper lateral cartilages. The nasal bones fuse with the frontal bone approximately 11 mm superior to the intercanthal line, and are on average 2.5 cm in length [5]. This length can be quite variable and represents a significant risk factor for airway compromise after rhinoplasty [6]. The caudal margin of the nasal bones overlaps the cephalic margin of the upper lateral cartilages, which in turn interlock with the paired lower lateral cartilages at the *scroll* (Fig. 67.3). Each of these connections is an important structural component that contributes to nasal integrity and support.

Laterally, the caudal margin of the nasal bones and the anterior margin of the ascending processes of the maxilla form the pyriform aperture. The lateral margin of the upper lateral cartilages fuses with dense connective tissue, and the medial margin fuses with the septum superiorly, but separates and is mobile inferiorly. Mucosa is tightly adherent to the internal surface of the cartilages and is continuous with the lining of the septum and lateral nasal wall.

The caudal margin of the upper lateral cartilage, the anterior head of the inferior turbinate, the proximate septum, and floor of the nose define the borders of the internal nasal valve. The angle between the upper lateral cartilages and the septum is the nasal valve angle, normally 10-20°. The nasal valve typically has a cross-sectional area of 55–83 mm [2] and represents the site of greatest nasal resistance and primary airflow limiting segment of the nasal cavity [7].

The Bony and Cartilaginous Vaults

The upper nasal two thirds can be thought of as two contiguous arches, or vaults—a superior bony vault and an inferior cartilaginous vault. The nasal bones and the paired ascending processes of the maxilla comprise the bony vault, while the cartilaginous vault is composed of the upper lateral cartilages and the cartilaginous dorsal septum. The region of transition of the bony vault to the cartilaginous vault is known as the rhinion. The soft tissue linkage that occurs at the rhinion is comprised of upper lateral cartilage perichondrium that inserts upon the undersurface of the paired nasal bones. This union allows for motion of the inferior vault relative to the superior vault.

As the name implies, nasal vaults are critical for support, distribution of forces, maintenance of dorsal height, and maintenance of nasal projection. As with any arch, the most essential support element occurs at the keystone. The nasal keystone area

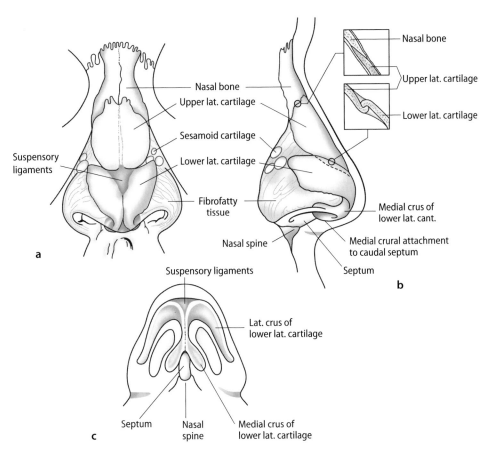

Fig. 67.3 **a–c** Anatomic relationships of the nasal bones, upper lateral cartilages, and lower lateral cartilages. (Modified from [7])

is the convergence of the caudal margin of the nasal bones, the perpendicular plate of the ethmoid bone, the cephalic margin of the upper lateral cartilages, and cartilaginous septum. Understanding this area is critical during planning and execution of osteotomies so as to effect a change without disruption of important support mechanisms.

Nasal Analysis

The face is a complex set of surfaces with tremendous variability. The goal of facial analysis is to provide a consistent framework to compare pre- and postoperative results in spite of this variability. Nowhere is this more important than in rhinoplasty. Every rhinoplasty candidate should have high-quality six-view photography to facilitate analysis. In addition, an additional chin-down view is especially useful in evaluation of patients with nasal vault deformity (Fig. 67.4).

Aesthetic Angles

Of the five facial aesthetic angles, three are determined using the geometry of the nasal dorsum: the nasofacial, the nasofrontal, and the nasomental angles. The *nasofacial angle* is the

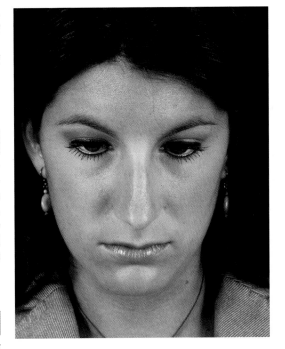

Fig. 67.4 Chin down view of nasal dorsum

angle prescribed by the intersection of the facial plane (glabella to pogonion) and a line tangent to the nasal dorsum. Ideally, it is 36–40°. The *nasofrontal angle* is determined by the intersection of the line connecting the nasion and glabella and the nasal dorsum tangent, and is ideally 115–130°. Lastly, the *nasomental angle* is determined by the intersection of the line connecting the tip-defining point to the pogonion and the nasal dorsum tangent. The ideal nasomental angle is 120–132°. Each of these angles should be carefully considered during the examination and in photographic evaluation of the rhinoplasty candidate.

Nasal Length

Leonardo da Vinci introduced the practice of dividing the face into equal vertical thirds and horizontal fifths for the purpose of facial analysis. Later modified by Powell and Humphreys, this serves as the basis for modern-day facial analysis [8]. A method more specific to nasal analysis, however, divides the lower face into two parts using the nasion, subnasale, and menton as landmarks [9]. Using this method, nasal length (nasion-subnasale) should be three fourths the distance from the subnasale to the menton (Fig. 67.5).

Nasal Width and Radix Contours

On frontal view, nasal width should increase along its length, with the narrowest part occurring at the intercanthal line. Maximal nasal width occurs at the alae and should equal one fifth the width of the face. The upper nasal contour should follow a gentle curve from the medial eyebrow to the ipsilateral tip-defining point. Any irregularities in this contour will quickly be noted as different from the contralateral side, thereby contributing to asymmetry and an unsightly appearance. The pair of these curves, known as *radix contours*, is highlighted by the nasal light reflex and should be symmetric (Fig. 67.6).

Dorsal Projection

The nose projects anteriorly from the face, with its forward thrust orthogonal to the facial plane and parallel to the midsagittal plane. Quantification of nasal projection is a critical component of the rhinoplastic evaluation, yet of the many methods previously described, none specifically address dorsal projection (i.e., dorsal height) [10–12]. Determination of proper tip projection using Crumley's method, however, simultaneously yields the upper limit of ideal dorsal projection along the entire nasal length, since the proportions of a 3:4:5 triangle do not change (Fig. 67.7). If dorsal projection exceeds this limit, it is indicative of the presence of an unsightly dorsal hump. Since a slight dorsal concavity can be attractive, dorsal projection slightly less than this limit is allowable, but a significantly lower measurement would be indicative of a saddle nose deformity.

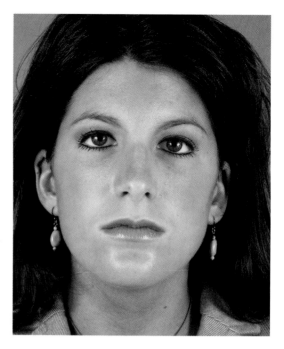

Fig. 67.5 Determination of nasal length using the nasion, subnasale, and menton: a = ¾ b

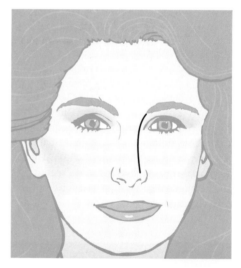

Fig. 67.6 Radix lines. (Modified from [38])

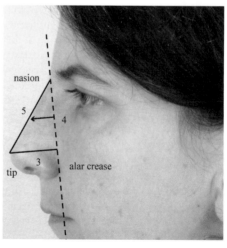

Fig. 67.7 Determination of ideal dorsal projection using tip projection analysis

Defects of the Nasal Vaults

Bony Vault Defects

Most deformities involving the bony vault arise from blunt trauma (Table 67.1). Fractured nasal bones can be comminuted and/or displaced, often resulting in an unsightly twist, depression, spur, or hump. Frequently, the skin overlying the bony dorsum is lacerated causing additional deformity by the presence of cicatrix and adherence of the dermis to the nasal bone periosteum. Severe fractures such as naso-orbital ethmoid fractures are often quite disfiguring due to retrodisplacement of the nasal bones, deprojection and flattening of the nasal dorsum, and shortening of the nose. The resultant telescopic defect is often associated with traumatic telecanthus due to the disruption of the medial canthal tendon insertion upon the nasal bones. Trauma involving the bony vault does not typically cause functional defect, unless the keystone area, the septum, or the middle vault is also affected. Less common causes of upper vault deformity include prior rhinoplasty, neoplasia, and congenital anomalies [13, 14].

Cartilaginous Vault Defects

Deformity of the middle nasal vault can be more complex than that of the bony vault since it is frequently accompanied by internal nasal deformity contributing to airway compromise. The internal nasal valve occurs near the junction of the upper and lower lateral cartilages and is often weakened or narrowed subsequent to trauma affecting the middle vault. Furthermore, the soft tissue nature of the middle vault makes it susceptible to deformity caused by other etiologies, including unrecognized birth trauma, infections, inflammatory diseases, or autoimmune processes [15–17].

Treatment of the middle vault in rhinoplasty was for many years considered little more than removal of a hump deformity. In the 1980s, however, surgeons began to describe numerous long-term complications of this limited approach, including the inverted-v deformity, nasal valve collapse, open roof deformity,

Table 67.1 Nasal vault defects

Dorsal hump	Twists
Deep nasion	Curvatures
Saddle nose	Pollybeak
Asymmetric nasal bones	Bony prominences
Short/long nasal bones	Rocker deformity
Wide/narrow bony pyramid	Open roof deformity
Depressions	Inverted v deformity
Partial/total rhinectomy (nasal cancer, gunshot wound)	

and pollybeak deformity. As a result, rhinoplasty techniques were modified to avoid these problems [18, 19].

Management of the Cartilaginous Vault

Surgical correction of the middle vault involves correction of existing deformities, while ever mindful of additional deformity prevention. When certain risk factors are present, such as short nasal bones, weak upper lateral cartilages, thin skin, narrow bony pyramid, or previous trauma or surgery, preventative action may be required utilizing cartilage grafting, precise structural realignment, and fixation of nasal valve structures.

Correction of middle vault starts with septoplasty. The old saying "as the septum goes, so goes the nose" indicates the importance of straightening the central strut of the nose. With the goal of making the dorsal septum as straight as possible, the open approach is often utilized. Accessing the septum from above via the separation of the lower lateral cartilages allows better exposure than the traditional endonasal approach [20]. The deviated portions of the quadrangular cartilage and perpendicular plate of the ethmoid bone are removed, making sure that 1-cm dorsal and caudal struts are maintained. Wide mucoperichondrial elevation, weakening incisions, wedge excisions, and sutured struts are adjuncts useful in straightening the deviated septum.

Spreader grafts are probably the next most common corrective modality used for middle vault rehabilitation. First described by Sheen and Sheen, these rectangular cartilage grafts are placed between the junctions of the upper lateral cartilages and septum to widen and stabilize the nasal valve [21]. Spreader grafts not only lateralize the upper lateral cartilages but also strengthen the middle vault to resist the inward motion on inspiration associated with Bernoulli's principle. They can be placed either through open or closed rhinoplasty techniques, but are easier to stabilize with direct sutures via the open approach. Septal cartilage is the most frequently used grafting material, but costal cartilage and auricular cartilage may be used if septum is not available. Spreader grafts can also be used for aesthetic purposes. For patients with unilateral middle vault depressions, a single spreader graft can elevate and lateralize the upper lateral cartilage to restore symmetry.

In many revision rhinoplasty cases involving middle vault pathology, separation of the septum and upper lateral cartilages has occurred due to prior hump removal. There is usually fibrous connective tissue present instead of the native cartilaginous junction. Therefore, preservation of the mucoperichondrium and creation of a pocket for graft placement through the open approach is usually preferred. If the upper lateral cartilages are fused with the septum in the internal nasal valve area, sharp dissection with an elevator will preserve the mucoperichondrium and maintain stability. In cases where the upper lateral cartilages have been almost completely resected, conchal cartilage onlay grafts may be needed in addition to spreader grafts to augment lateral support or camouflage depressions. The grafts are carved, aligned, and fixed into position with 5-0 PDS (Polydiaxonone, Ethicon, Sommerville, NJ) mattress sutures. Most spreader grafts are 1.5–2.5 cm in length and 1–3 mm in width. In general, the grafts should run along the dorsal septum from below the bony-cartilaginous junction to the anterior septal angle. In severe cases, the grafts may be layered to provide additional bulk. Grafts of unequal width may also be used to correct asymmetries in the middle vault. Spreader grafts can also be used as internal splints to help straighten a caudal septal deflection. The technique of spreader graft placement and fixation is demonstrated in Fig. 67.8–11. Placement of spreader grafts is greatly facilitated by placement of a 30-gauge needle through the cartilage complex while suturing.

A corollary to spreader grafting that deserves mention is reverse spreader grafting. This technique can be useful in patients with an overly broad middle vault, minimal nasal obstruction,

and no nasal valve collapse. In these cases, patients can benefit from reduction of the horizontal width of the cartilaginous dorsum, which can be thought of as the reverse of spreader grafts [22].

Patients with saddle-nose deformity frequently have middle vault collapse without soft tissue support, commonly due to a large septal perforation. Fixation of a dorsal graft helps to enhance dorsal projection, support the soft tissues, and restore the integrity of the nasal valve. Calvarial bone secured with a lag screw or rib cartilage secured with sutures have been very useful in these patients [23, 24]. In addition, dorsal calvarial grafts can serve as anchors for other reconstructive grafts [25]. In some

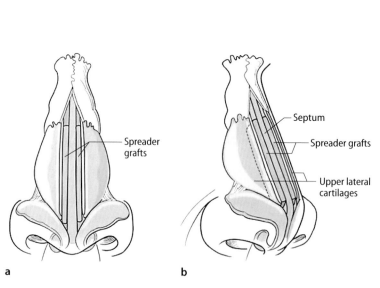

a   b

Fig. 67.8 **a,b** Ideal placement of spreader grafts between septum and upper lateral cartilages. (Modified from [7])

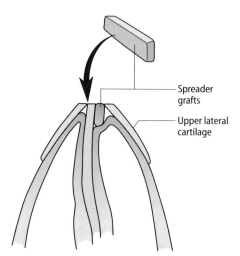

Fig. 67.9 Placement of spreader graft lateralizes and elevates the upper lateral cartilage, widening the middle vault. (Modified from [7])

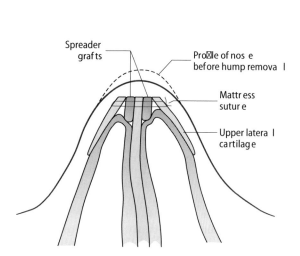

Fig. 67.10 Spreader grafts in place and fixed with mattress sutures. The original dorsal height is identified. (Modified from [7])

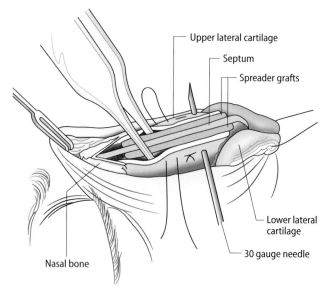

Fig. 67.11 Demonstration of mattress suture fixation and use of 30-gauge needle for stabilization. (Modified from [7])

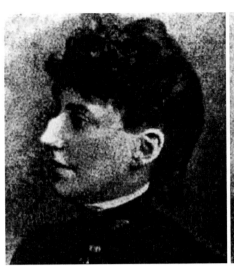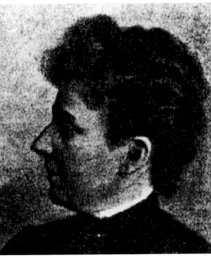

Fig. 67.12 John Orlando Roe patient: before and after dorsal hump removal. (From [27])

cases, the use of crushed cartilage or Alloderm (LifeCell Corp., Branchburg, NJ) over the dorsum and graft material can help smooth an irregular profile.

While pollybeak deformity appears to be a caudal cartilaginous vault problem, it actually represents a lack of tip projection relative to middle vault projection. Therefore, pollybeak deformity is not a true cartilaginous vault defect. As such, its correction requires augmentation of tip support, not deprojection of the middle vault.

Additional methods to augment the function of the nasal valve involve the placement of alar batten grafts, butterfly grafts, and various suture methods. Schlosser and Park described the use of 5-0 clear nylon flaring sutures that span the upper lateral cartilages and septum horizontally [26]. Tightening the suture theoretically increases the angle of the internal nasal valve and therefore improves nasal airflow. Their study indicated that flaring sutures used concomitantly with spreader grafts increase airflow more than the use of spreader grafts alone. Other suture techniques such as tip-lifting sutures, or valve maneuvers like internal valve M-Plasty or lateral crural j-flap, can also be useful adjuncts but are outside the scope of this chapter.

Management of the Bony Vault

Deformity of the upper nasal vault represents a challenge to the rhinoplasty surgeon, requiring thorough preoperative evaluation and careful surgical technique to manage. Improper or incomplete treatment of the bony vault may lead to suboptimal results, including persistence of existing defects or the creation of new ones. The presence of iatrogenic deformities listed in Table 67.1 bear witness to this. Surgical treatment of the bony vault should aim to accomplish the following: (1) establishment of appropriate dorsal projection, (2) creation of a smooth dorsal contour free of bony irregularity, (3) correction of nasal width, and (4) straightening of the crooked nose.

Techniques used to accomplish these aims include hump reduction, osteotomies, and grafting.

Hump Reduction

John Orland Roe (1848–1915) provided the modern age with the first account of correction of a dorsal defect in 1891 (Fig. 67.12) [27]. Regional dorsal overprojection is managed with wide soft tissue envelope elevation and the removal of portions of the nasal bones. This can be done either through an open or closed approach. Adequate exposure must be balanced with the maintenance of soft tissue support, and it must be remembered that the upper lateral cartilages insert deep to the caudal margin of the nasal bones. Care must be taken not to disarticulate this union. The best way to avoid this is to elevate the nasal bone periosteum using a Joseph elevator 1–2 mm superior to the rhinion [28]. Bone removal is subsequently accomplished with a double-guarded osteotome or a carbide tungsten pull rasp, depending on the amount of bone to be removed. After sharp incision of the cartilaginous component, large humps typically require removal with the osteotome. Care should be taken to follow the planned trajectory and not make an oblique cut by straying laterally or canting the osteotome (Fig. 67.13). Refinements can then be performed by rasping just off midline in a slightly oblique manner so as not to avulse the upper lateral cartilages [29].

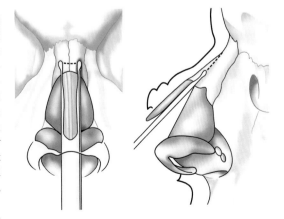

Fig. 67.13 Removal of dorsal excess. (Modified from [29])

Osteotomies

Osteotomies have evolved greatly since the time of Jacques Joseph (1865–1934), one of the rhinoplasty pioneers who touted their importance [30]. Early techniques were fraught with nasal airway compromise largely due to a trajectory that caused wide disruption of periosteum and release of lower lateral cartilage lateral suspensory ligaments. Modifications have led to the emergence of modern techniques that place equal importance upon preservation of the nasal airway and aesthetic improvement, in accord with the dual tenet of the rhinoplasty operation [31, 32].

Osteotomies can be performed laterally, medially, or intermediately. Lateral osteotomies should be limited to the thin bone of the pyriform aperture, lateral to the anterior margin of the ascending maxillary processes. If too far lateral, the thick bone at the nasofacial transition will be encountered, rather than the average 2.5 mm thickness typically encountered along the osteotomy path [33].

Lateral osteotomies can be linear or perforating, internal or external. The ideal trajectory is described as "high–low–high," which indicates the antero-posterior position on the nasal pyramid. A standard lateral osteotomy is a linear, internal cut that is initiated with a mucosal stab incision made just lateral to the anterior face of the inferior turbinate. The curved, guarded 4-mm osteotome is placed into the incision on the margin of the pyriform aperture, at about a 45° angle to the facial plane, or roughly perpendicular to the face of the aperture (Fig. 67.14). Preservation of the inferior segment of the pyriform maintains the lateral suspensory ligaments and width important for the nasal airway. Soon after the initial cut, the osteotome should be transitioned roughly parallel to the facial plane and directed toward the medial canthal area. The osteotomy should then curve anteriorly and superiorly to terminate at the level of the medial canthus, midway between the dorsal line and the medial canthus. The tell-tale sound of the osteotome meeting the thicker frontal bone is indicative of the proper stopping point. If the osteotomy extends superior to the medial canthus, there is greater risk of creating a rocker deformity, which occurs when the nasal

bone inferior to the osteotomy sinks relative to the bone superior to the cut. The osteotomy is completed with pronation and medialization of the osteotome, causing back-fracture across the superior aspect of the nasal bone. Elevation of the periosteum in this vicinity liberates the nasal bones from the soft tissue envelope, allowing the osteotomized bone to heal free of the influence of soft tissue contracture. If the back-fracture is incomplete or inadequate, it can be augmented percutaneously using a 2-mm osteotome. Alternatively, the entire back-fracture can be completed percutaneously.

Perforating lateral osteotomies can be performed either internally (transnasally) or externally (percutaneously). The perforating technique is the ideal method to complete an exact osteotomy with minimal trauma. It is preferred when maintenance of support is critical, such as in revision rhinoplasty or short nasal bones, since there is far less disruption of periosteal support and the intact periosteum stabilizes and splints the mobilized segments, enhancing precise healing [34, 35]. A series of perforations are made at fixed intervals along the desired fracture trajectory and then completed with minimal manual manipulation. The intranasal perforating osteotomy is useful to widen the pyriform aperture by displacing the bones laterally [36].

Medial and intermediate osteotomies should be used judiciously; however, they can be essential when the pyriform is very thick, the nose is significantly deviated, or a very large nose needs to be reduced. Both medial and intermediate osteotomies are usually performed transnasally with a 3-mm osteotome. Medial osteotomies are initiated on the medial aspect of the caudal margin of the nasal bones near the septum. This is very near the keystone area of the nasal vaults so considerable care must be taken. The percutaneous perforation technique can be used to perform medial osteotomies to further ensure preservation of the keystone. The trajectory of the fracture is superolateral, meeting with the back fracture of the previously performed lateral osteotomy. If further correction is needed, intermediate osteotomies can also be performed. The intermediate osteotomy is also initiated on the caudal margin of the nasal bones, intermediate to the medial and lateral osteotomies. The trajectory should parallel the lateral osteotomy and meet with the superior back fracture. Since intermediate osteotomies are difficult to execute if the lateral bone has already been mobilized, they are best performed prior to lateral osteotomies.

Grafts

Contemporary grafts useful in treatment of the bony vault include radix grafts, onlay grafts, and anchored bone grafts. Radix grafts serve to increase the projection of the nasofrontal trough,

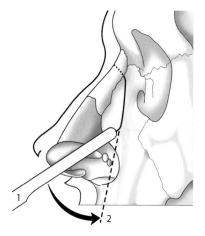

Fig. 67.14 The lateral osteotomy is initiated at the anterior face of the inferior turbinate, initially perpendicular to the plane of the pyriform aperture (position 1). The osteotomy is then transitioned (position 2), and carried to the medial canthal area. (Modified from [29])

correcting the excessively deep nasion. If septal or auricular cartilage is readily accessible, it can be used either as a single morsellized piece or multiple fragments sutured together as a plumping graft [37]. The graft is placed either superficial or deep to the nasal bone periosteum and held in place by the overlying skin envelope. Although Alloderm can also be used as a radix graft, it is perhaps more useful as a dorsal onlay graft to camouflage small irregularities as well as add height. When significant bony defects are present, as after cancer resection or NOE telescoping nasal deformity, calvarial bone grafts may be required to reconstruct the upper vault. These grafts are cantilevered off the frontal bone and anchored precisely with titanium screws.

Septum

The nasal septum is often injured by seemingly minor trauma. Starting with birth canal trauma, the nose is frequently struck during childhood and adolescence. In essence, our noses represent a collection of injuries from birth into adulthood. Therefore it is not unusual to find significant septal deviations, many of which are symptomatic.

Evaluation of the deviated septum is typically by physical exam. Deviations in the anterior one third of the nose tend to be more obstructive, especially if impinging upon the nasal valve. Low deviations tend to be more symptomatic than high deviations if away from the internal valve. Of course, concomitant factors such as chronic inflammatory disease, turbinate hypertrophy, and nasal valve deficiency must be considered as additional causes of nasal obstruction.

Anatomy

The surgical anatomy of the septum involves the soft tissue of the columella and mucosa, in addition to the cartilage and bone

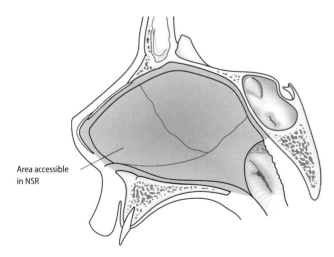

Area accessible in NSR

Fig. 67.15 Sagital view of septum showing areas involved with septal reconstruction. (Modified from [39])

of the septum, premaxilla, and maxillary crest. The cartilaginous septum sits in a groove defined by the maxillary crest and its nasal spine extension. Deviations can exist in any or all of these components, and must be addressed individually. In addition to the premaxilla/maxillary crest the major components of the septum include the quadrangular cartilage, vomer, and perpendicular plate of the ethmoid (Fig. 67.15).

Technique

The authors prefer to utilize techniques which preserve nasal support and normal anatomic conformation. Resection of septal structure should be conservative, correcting only the deviated portions and maintaining strong dorsal and caudal struts. This can be accomplished via a hemitransfixion, or Killian incision, depending upon the segment of septum needing repair. Often the septum is utilized for cartilage grafts to repair other parts of the nose. Caudal septal deviations will require a hemitransfixion or full transfixion incision, but a more posterior defect may benefit from a limited dissection via a Killian incision. On some occasions the septum can be approached and repaired by splitting the medial crura exposing the caudal septum. This may be indicated for severe caudal septal deviations, or correction of alar columellar disproportions.

Dissection should be limited to the submucoperichondrial plane, which facilitates easy elevation, less bleeding, and a stronger mucosal flap. Not observing this important plane of dissection will result in more bleeding, edema, and difficulty obtaining the desired results. There is also a higher incident of septal perforation and other complications such as postoperative bleeding (Fig. 67.16).

After elevation of an anterior tunnel, the bony-cartilaginous junction is separated and posterior tunnels elevated on the bone. At this point the inferior tunnels can be elevated by dissecting from posterior to anterior along the maxillary crest. This exposes most of the septal contents and makes selective resection much easier with good exposure (Fig. 67.17).

At this point the deviated portion of the quadrangular cartilage is resected leaving caudal and dorsal struts of at least one centimeter. This exposes the bony septum, which is also resected after dividing the superior connection with the cribiform plate sharply to avoid a superior fracture into the skull base. The maxillary crest can be trimmed with an osteotome or scissors if it projects into the airway. We try to avoid removal of the maxillary crest or nasal spine to maintain support and prevent damage to the nasopalotine nerve. Damage to this nerve may result in significant hypesthesia of the anterior hard palate.

Caudal Deviations

Caudal septal deviations can be challenging. This type of septal deformity may require fixation of the caudal septum to the nasal spine with permanent sutures. If the caudal deflection is high in the septum, extended spreader grafts may be necessary to splint the dorsal edge and achieve straightening (Fig. 67.18).

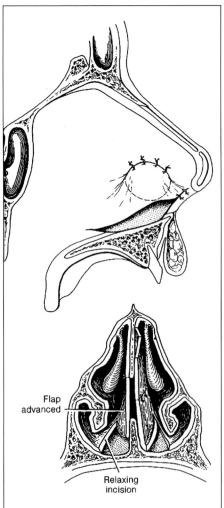

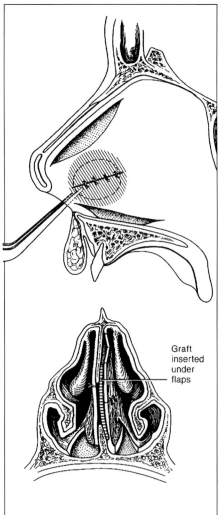

Fig. 67.16 Technique for repair of septal perforation. (From [40])

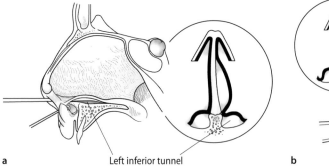

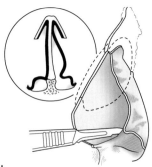

Fig. 67.17 **a,b** Inferior and anterior tunnel technique for septoplasty (Modified from [39])

After all segments of the septum are realigned, crushed cartilage (if available) is used to fill the septal envelope. Closure may utilize chromic sutures in addition to a running 4-0 plain gut mattress suture. Silastic splints are often used when an extensive dissection has been necessary. Both methods result in adequate fixation and prevention of fluid in the septal envelope. The Silastic splints are typically left in place 5–7 days.

When approaching a septorhinoplasty which involves deviations of the septum and nasal vaults, the authors prefer to perform the septoplasty first. This often releases any internal tension in the nose, and may help straighten the lower one third of the nose. The use of septal cartilage as grafting material also facilitates repairing depressions and deviations in other areas.

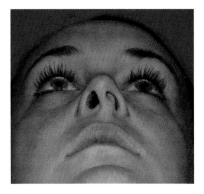

Fig. 67.18 Significant caudal septal deviation

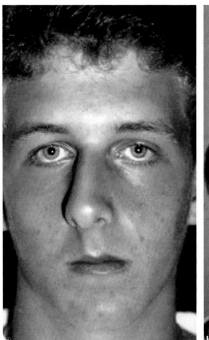

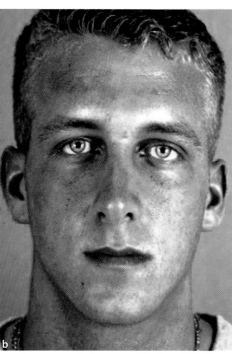

Fig. 67.19 **a** Patient #1 prior to septorhinoplasty for crooked nose. **b** One year postoperative result

Conclusion

Facial aesthetics and attractiveness rely in large part on the appearance of the nose. Deformities affecting the nasal vaults are distinct and independent from those affecting the nasal tip, and contribute not only to unsightly appearance, but also improper nasal function. Building on the past experience of prior rhinoplasty surgeons, surgical techniques dealing with nasal vault deformities have evolved, ever mindful that restoration of proper anatomic vault relations significantly enhances the appearance of the nose and nasal function (Figs. 67.19, 20).

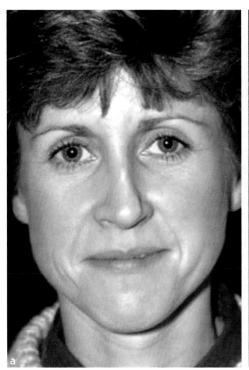

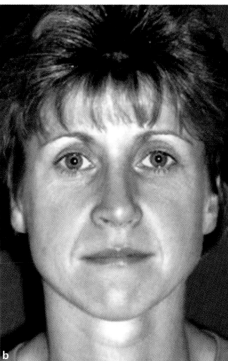

Fig. 67.20 **a** Patient #2 prior to septorhinoplasty for revision rhinoplasty. **b** One year postoperative result

The nasal septum plays a large role in nasal function, and is often involved in traumatic nasal deviations. It is essential to repair septal pathology in a timely manner, in coordination with the other nasal components.

The contemporary rhinoplasty surgeon must be facile with analysis and management of the bony and cartilaginous nasal vaults that comprise the upper two thirds of the nose, and be able to integrate this into management of the nasal tip and septum for successful performance of the septorhinoplasty operation.

67

References

1. Burget GC, Menick FJ (1994) Aesthetic reconstruction of the Nose. Mosby, St. Louis

2. Behrbohm H (2004) Preoperative Management. In: Behrbohm H, Tardy ME Jr, (eds) Essentials of septorhinoplasty: Philosophy, approaches, techniques. Thieme, Stuttgart, pp 89–106

3. Mitz V, Peyronie M (1976) The superficial musculo-aponeurotic system in the parotid and cheek area. Plast Reconstr Surg 58:80–88

4. Tardy ME, Brown RJ (1995) Surgical anatomy of the nose. Raven Press, New York

5. Oneal RM, Beil RJ Jr, Schlesinger J (1999) Surgical anatomy of the nose. Otolaryngol Clin North Am 32(1):145–181

6. Guryon B (1998) Nasal osteotomy and airway changes. Plast Reconstr Surg 102(3):856–860

7. Papel ID (2002) Management of the middle vault. In: Papel ID (ed) Facial plastic and reconstructive surgery, 2nd edn. Thieme, Stuttgart, pp 407–413

8. Powell N, Humprheys B (1984) Proportions of the aesthetic face. Thieme, New York

9. Papel ID, Capone RB (2004) Facial proportions and esthetic ideals. In: Behrbohm H, Tardy ME Jr (eds) Essentials of septorhinoplasty: Philosophy, approaches, techniques. Thieme, Stuttgart, pp 65–74

10. Simons R (1982) Nasal tip projection, ptosis, and supratip thickening. Ear Nose Throat J 61:452–457

11. Crumley R (1988) Quantitative analysis of nasal tip projection. Laryngoscope 98:202–208

12. Baum S (1982) Introduction. Ear Nose Throat J 61:426–428

13. Dingman RO, Natvig P (1977) The deviated nose. Clin Plast Surg 4:145–152

14. Vuyk HD (2000) A review of practical guidelines for correction of the deviated, asymmetric nose. Rhinology 38(2):72–78

15. Verwoerd CDA, Verwoerd-Verhoef HL (1989) Developmental aspects of the deviated nose. Facial Plast Surg 6:95–100

16. Fernandez-Vozmediano JM, Armario Hita JC et al (2004) Rhinoscleroma in three siblings. Pediatr Dermatol 21(2):134–138

17. Pirsig W, Pentz S, Lenders H (1993) Repair of saddle nose deformity in Wegener's granulomatosis and ectodermal dysplasia. Rhinology 31(2):69–72

18. Sheen JH (1984) Spreader graft: A method of reconstructing the roof of the middle nasal vault following rhinoplasty. Plast Reconstr Surg 73:230–237

19. Toriumi DM, Johnson CM (1993) Open structure rhinoplasty: Featured technical points and long-term follow-up. Facial Plast Surg Clin North Am 1:1–22

20. TerKonda RP, Sykes JM (1999) Repairing the twisted nose. Otolaryngol Clin North Am 32(1):53–64

21. Sheen JH, Sheen AP (1987) Aesthetic rhinoplasty. Mosby, St. Louis

22. Thomas JR, Prendiville S (2004) Overly wide cartilaginous middle vault. Facial Plast Surg Clin North Am 12(1):107–110

23. Frodel JL, Marentette LJ, Quatela VC, Weinstein GS (1993) Calvarial bone graft harvest: Techniques, considerations, and morbidity. Arch Otolaryngol Head Neck Surg 119:17–23

24. Quatela VC, Jacono AA (2002) Structural grafting in rhinoplasty. Arch Facial Plast Surg 18(4):223–232

25. Papel ID (1991) Augmentation rhinoplasty utilizing cranial bone grafts. Md Med J 40:479–483

26. Schlosser RJ, Park SS (1999) Surgery for the dysfunctional nasal valve. Arch Facial Plast Surg 1:105–110

27. Lam SM, (2002) John Orlando Roe: Father of aesthetic rhinoplasty. Arch Facial Plast Surg 4:122–123

28. Larrabee WF Jr (1993) Open rhinoplasty and the upper third of the nose. Facial Plast Surg Clin North Am 1(1):23–38

29. Mostafour SP, Murakami CS, Larrabee WF Jr (2002) Management of the bony nasal vault. In: Papel ID (ed) Facial plastic and reconstructive surgery, 2nd edn. Thieme, Stuttgart, pp 402–406

30. Aufricht G (1971) Joseph's rhinoplasty with some modifications. Surg Clin North Am 51:299–316

31. Webster RC, Davidson RC, Smith RC (1977) Curved lateral osteotomy for airway protection in rhinoplasty. Arch Otolaryngol 103:454–458

32. Thomas JR, Griner NR, Remmler DJ (1987) Steps for a safer method of osteotomies in rhinoplasty. Laryngoscope 97:746–747

33. Larrabee WF Jr, Murakami CS (2000) Osteotomy techniques to correct posttraumatic deviation of the nasal pyramid: A technical note. J Craniomaxillofac Trauma 6(1):43–47

34. Tardy ME Jr (2004) Contemporary rhinoplasty: Principles and philosophy. In: Behrbohm H, Tardy ME Jr (eds) Essentials of septorhinoplasty: Philosophy, approaches, techniques. Thieme, Stuttgart, pp 37–63

35. Rohrich RJ, Minoli JJ, Adams WP, Hollier LH (1997) The lateral nasal osteotomy in rhinoplasty: An anatomic endoscopic comparison of the external versus internal approach. Plast Reconstr Surg 99:1309–1313

36. Byrne PJ, Walsh WE, Hilger PA (2003) The use of inside-out lateral osteotomy to improve outcome in rhinoplasty. Arch Facial Plast Surg 5(3):251–255

37. Daniel RK, Calvert JW (2004) Diced cartilage grafts in rhinoplasty surgery. Plast Reconstr Surg 113(7):2156–2171

38. Orten SS, Hilger PA (2002) Facial analysis of the rhinoplasty patient. In: Papel ID (ed) Facial plastic and reconstructive surgery, 2nd edn. Thieme, Stuttgart, p 361

39. Kasperbauer JL, Facer GW, Kern EB (2002) Reconstructive surgery of the nasal septum. In: Papel ID (ed) Facial plastic and reconstructive surgery, 2nd edn. Thieme, Stuttgart, p 461

40. Kridel RW (2002) Nasal septal perforation: Prevention, management, and repair. In: Papel ID (ed) Facial plastic and reconstructive surgery, 2nd edn. Thieme, Stuttgart, p 478

Chapter 68

The Endonasal Approach to Rhinoplasty

68

Robert L. Simons and Lisa D. Grunebaum

Core Messages

■ The ultimate success in rhinoplasty depends more upon the initial consultation and analysis of the patient than it does upon the technical approach to the nose. In the author's experience, the endonasal approach affords the opportunity to satisfy the patient's needs in the overwhelming majority of cases.

Contents

Introduction

Times have changed. Thirty years ago most rhinoplasties were performed through endonasal incisions. Today, the more prevalent technique is with external or transcolumellar (open) approach. Why the change? Are better rhinoplasty results today directly related to the increasing use of the external approach?

To answer those questions we must first recognize that surgeons are justifiably influenced by their training. Today, most residency programs emphasize the external approach almost to exclusion. Therefore, for many of the newer rhinoplasty surgeons the endonasal approach is foreign, distant, if not antiquated.

From our standpoint, no well-trained rhinoplasty surgeon should feel limited by either approach. The answer to good rhinoplasty results rests not with the approach or technique, but rather with underlying diagnosis. Favorable outcomes with this operation emanate from the initial consultation and the physician/surgeon's ability to make the right diagnosis to satisfy the patient's individual needs.

The senior author was trained at the Mt. Sinai Hospital in New York City over 40 years ago. His primary mentoring influence was Dr. Irving Goldman who required that all rhinoplasties employ the endonasal approach and the Goldman technique. Today Dr. Simons continues to utilize the endonasal approach in over 90% of his primary and secondary procedures, though the Goldman tip procedures are used in just 13% of the cases.

The Importance of the Initial Patient Consultation

As noted above, the initial consultation is crucial to a successful outcome in rhinoplasty. Listening carefully to the patient's medical, social, and occupational background allows for an understanding of the individual's personality. Take the time to learn who the person is before inquiring about concerns regarding his/her nose. It is worthwhile to note in reference to the patients own words, major complaints, or desire for change. Your goals are twofold with their surgery; first to satisfy the patient's desire for change, but secondarily to do it in a manner which does not draw attention to the surgery.

68

The history should include complete understanding of any previous nasal trauma or functional disabilities that the patient experiences with nasal breathing or associated concerns of epistaxis or sinusitis. The physical examination includes a thorough head and neck exam in order to assess any cranial or facial abnormalities especially those that could affect the outcome.

Significant differences between what the doctor and patient sees, unrealistic expectations, and overly demanding or perfectionist behavior are infrequent but easily detectable "warning signs" by the interested listener. The bottom line is one of comfort. If the patient or procedure makes the surgeon uncomfortable, it is wise to pass on this opportunity to operate.

Nasal Analysis and Preoperative Planning for the Endonasal Approach

How surgeons analyze the nose depends greatly on the information provided. Accurate photographic documentation is critical. We employ two light sources, a blue background and take photographs from a defined and consistent distance from the patient. Frontal, right and left lateral unsmiling, oblique and right lateral smiling views allow the surgeon to assess nasal width, height, dorsal alignment, tip position, and dorsal highlights. The importance of the base view cannot be overstated. Tip projection, ratio of structural support to skin thickness, and functional breathing problems related to the external valve can all be evaluated from this view.

In order to assess an individual's degree of nasal tip projection, a lateral view and base view are examined. Adequate tip projection will have a 1:1 ratio between the length of the base of the nose and the upper lip (Fig. 68.1). The base view will reveal an equilateral triangle with strong medial and lateral support. The medial crura should have a 2:1 relationship of the columella to lobule (Fig. 68.2).

Every rhinoplasty deserves at least five operations! (Fig. 68.3) The photographic analysis following the initial consultation is the second time the specific procedure is planned. The third takes place on the return office visit or just before surgery. The fourth is in the operating room (OR) and the fifths occurs sometime during one of the postoperative visits. This type of attention to detail and deliberative "game planning" allows the patient and the surgeon to arrive in the OR with the calming assurance that they know what to expect and how the problem will be approached. It is not acceptable to say, "we'll wait until we get into the OR and open up the nose to decide what we will do."

Rhinoplasty is an elegant, yet difficult operation even in the most experienced hands. Preoperative preparation allows the surgeon to consider the entire range of any problems associated with each patient's nasal anatomy and plan accordingly to address each issue in an appropriate and stepwise fashion. The "game plan" approach, as well as presence of preoperative pho-

TIP PROJECTION

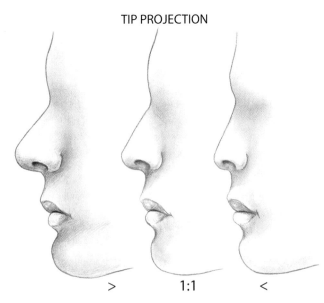

>   1:1   <

Fig. 68.1 Adequate tip projection will have a 1:1 ratio between the length of the base of the nose and the upper lip, as demonstrated in the *center* figure

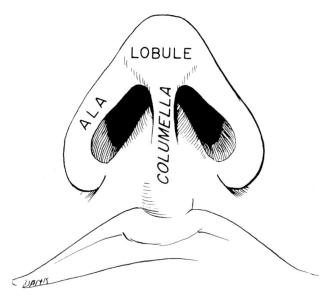

Fig. 68.2 The length of the columella should be two times that of the lobule. The base view should reveal an equilateral triangle

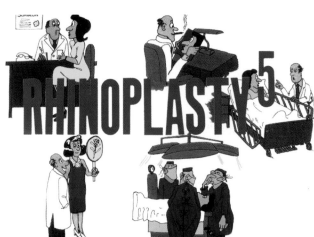

Fig. 68.3 Every rhinoplasty deserves at least five operations!

tographs in the operating room is further necessitated by the fact that with the patient supine on the OR table and following the injection of local anesthetics the preoperative nasal appearance can change dramatically. Allowing 5–10 min for the vasoconstrictive effects of the local anesthetic to occur is important, as is the opportunity to again revisit the "game plan."

In well over 90% of the time both primary and revisional cases are approached by the senior author with an endonasal technique.

With complete transfixion and marginal incisions, the endonasal approach affords excellent visualization of all areas except the lateral osteotomy site. It allows variation of technique, with delicate "touch" evaluation, small pocket size for grafts, and avoids any external scar. For this surgeon, a real advantage of the endonasal approach over the external approach is that a final profile adjustment and the appropriate relationship of tip to dorsum are made easier with the skin envelope intact.

The external approach is employed in unique situations of extreme scarring, tissue deficiency, or marked curvature of the dorsum. Usually the placement of spreader grafts or the need for high septal repositioning is more easily approached and controlled from above.

We continue to see a disadvantage in differentiating the endonasal and external approach in terms of "closed" and "open." The endonasal approach hardly limits the surgeon's ability to evaluate or correct the patient's problem, yet "closed" is a term that suggests less capability to observe or maneuver. The beauty and delicate nature of rhinoplasty demands more intelligent and precise descriptive terminology.

Intraoperative Details for the Endonasal Approach

Transfixion

With the endonasal approach, the complete transfixion incision becomes full when there is the need for shortening or straight-ening the caudal septum. Through this extended incision the depressor septi muscle is cut when the dependent and ptotic nature of the tip is accentuated in the preoperative smiling view. In a retrograde manner soft tissue can be removed from between the medial crura to narrow a widened columella.

Preliminary Dorsal Work

Following the transfixion the senior author will normally perform the preliminary lowering of the nasal dorsum. This reduction of excess projection is carried out in a staged manner. First the cartilaginous dorsum in the area of the septal angle and upper lateral cartilage is lowered with a right angle scissors or knife. Following the preliminary lowering of the septal angle a line between the caudal end of the remaining bony projection and the desired nasal frontal angle is easily discerned. The shaving of the access bone is usually carried out with a sharp osteotome or occasionally a dorsal rasp may be utilized (Fig. 68.4).

Two points are to be made about this preliminary dorsal reduction at the beginning of the procedure. Since septal surgery is frequently necessitated with the rhinoplasty, assurance for preserving a good L-shaped dorsal and caudal septal support is more readily achieved by carrying out the septal work after the dorsum has been lowered.

Cartilaginous Reduction

The cartilaginous reduction on a high, wide nose is often facilitated by separating the upper lateral cartilages from the septum. Transmucosal incisions parallel to the septum allow for accurate, segmental sliver reduction of the septal angle. Waiting until after lateral osteotomies to determine the need for trimming the upper laterals lessens the tendency for excess upper lateral cartilage excision and consequently, the potential for later upper valve collapse or midvault pinching.

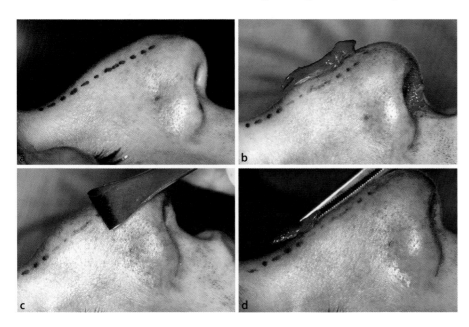

Fig. 68.4 Intraoperative photo showing the planned dorsal resection with osteotome. Staged dorsal reduction with first cartilage and then bone removed

Tip Modification and the Endonasal Approach

Regarding tip surgery, a marginal incision is preferred for visualization and modification of the alar cartilages. We begin the marginal incision behind the infradomal soft tissue facet and continue the incision anteriorly, approximately half way down the columella (Fig. 68.5).

The lateral extension of the incision along the caudal margin of the lateral crus rarely parallels the marginal rim. A lateral and medial release of the soft tissue with scissors allows an easy delivery of the chondrocutaneous bipedicle flap. Extraction of that flap with the right angle hook will mark the lobular apex and identify the anatomic high point of the dome (Fig. 68.6).

This is an important landmark in deciding whether one is to increase, decrease, or maintain the present tip projection.

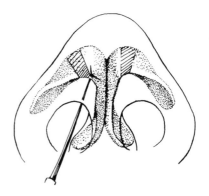

Fig. 68.6 Drawing of right-angled hook at dome. Notice the figuratively planned vertical dome division (as shown by *diagonal lines*) borrowing no more than 2–3 mm along the caudal border

Vertical Dome Division

In more than 80% of the cases the senior author uses some form of vertical dome division. The rationale behind the vertical dome division is the ability to change projection directly and to narrow and rotate the lobule with minimum cartilage excision. Inherent in this philosophy is the preservation of surrounding tissues (i.e., the septal angle and caudal septum), which further decrease the risk of postoperative appearance of an overoperated nose.

Today's trends in tip surgeries are for improved visualization with preservation of the cartilage as well as better medial stabilization and support. These tenets are inherent in vertical dome

division techniques. It is important to remember that vertical dome division (VDD) is an incisional technique that allows for repositioning of nasal tissue and should not be combined with excisional techniques. "One should always leave behind more than one takes." Preservation of at least 6–8 mm of lateral crus will help prevent alar collapse and stabilize the nasal base as well as allow for a strong natural-appearing tip.

Vertical dome division (VDD), a generic description of tip procedures first employed by the senior author in the late 1970s, allows for narrowing, rotation, and change in tip projection by repositioning rather than excision of any sizable amount of cartilage.

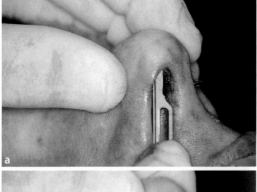

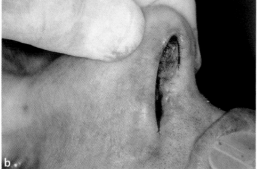

Fig. 68.5a,b As seen here, the marginal incision is begun behind the facet and extended 50% along the anterior columella

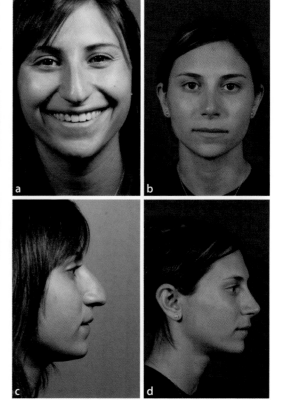

Fig. 68.7 **a,b** Preoperative and views of young woman with dorsal hump and underprojected tip. **c,d** 2-year postoperative views of same woman after rhinoplasty with Goldman technique

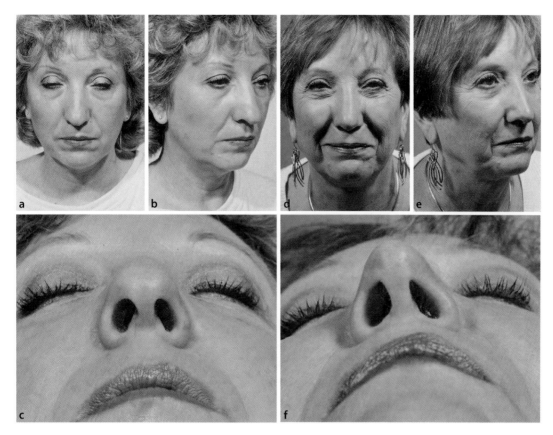

Fig. 68.8 **a–c** Preoperative views of woman with underrotated tip. **d–f** 17-year postoperative views of same woman after rhinoplasty with Goldman technique. The change in tip direction is maintained long term

The prototype of VDD was the Goldman tip technique first described by Dr. Irving Goldman in 1957. The Goldman tip technique employs the use of the vertical cut through cartilage and mucosa lateral to the apex of the dome (not more than 2–3 mm) (Fig. 68.6) which allows the creation of a chondrocutaneous strut of medial crura, increasing the tip projection. As previously stated, this technique should not be combined with excisional techniques. The Goldman technique is used in cases that require increase in tip projection or change in direction, such as in the downwardly displaced ptotic ageing nose (Figs. 68.7a–d, 8a–f).

The other forms of vertical dome division utilized are the Hockey stick excision and the Simons' modification. The Hockey stick excision was initially attributed to Brown and McDowell and then modified by Smith. The domal area is excised keeping intact the underlying mucosa. This procedure can help correct an overly projected or rotated nasal tip (Figs. 68.9a–f, 10a–f).

Most commonly employed by the senior author is the Simons' modification of vertical dome division, which allows for moderate change in tip projection, as well as narrowing and increased tip rotation. In the Simons' modification the anatomic apex and lobular dome is marked by the right angle hook as the bipedicle flap is delivered through the marginal incision. The infradomal space is defatted following delivery of both domes. The lobular domes are vertically incised individually. No effort is made to deliver both domes at the same time. Symmetry and

control of tip projection demand bilateral cuts equidistant from the right angle marker.

Vertically cutting the dome allows direct inward and upward movement of the medial lobular portion. As with the classic Goldman maneuver, limiting the lateral distance of the cut to 3 mm from the lobular apex at the caudal margin of the cartilage prevents notching (Fig. 68.11a).

Maintenance of symmetry and further influence of lobular projection depend on proper placement of the lobular suture. Initially, both lobular domes are delivered into the right nostril. The medial edge of the vertical cut on the left side is grasped with Brown-Adson forceps and a 5-0 clear nylon suture used in a horizontal mattress fashion. The first pass with the needle is closer to the superior edge than the more medial inferior exit with no attempt made to pass through the interior perichondrium. A mirror image of that needle passage is performed in the right side with the knot buried between the medial crura superiorly (Fig. 68.11b, c).

Careful attention to accurate placement of the suture assists symmetric healing. The direction of the pull influences supralobular narrowing and tip rotation. This medialization of the lobule without significant cephalic excision affects the desired long-term pyramidal appearance of the nasal base (Figs. 68.12a–f, 13a–f).

When the cut medial edge gently leads the lateral, nature does a wonderful job of reconstituting the dome. The senior

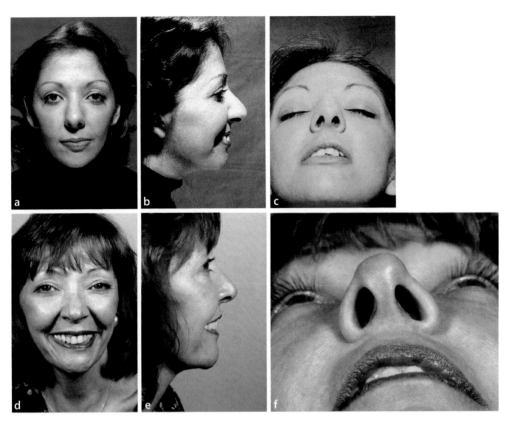

Fig. 68.9 **a–c** Preoperative views of woman with overprojected and broad tip. **d–f** 25-year postoperative views of same woman after rhinoplasty with hockey stick approach to tip. The decrease in projection and tip refinement is well-maintained long term

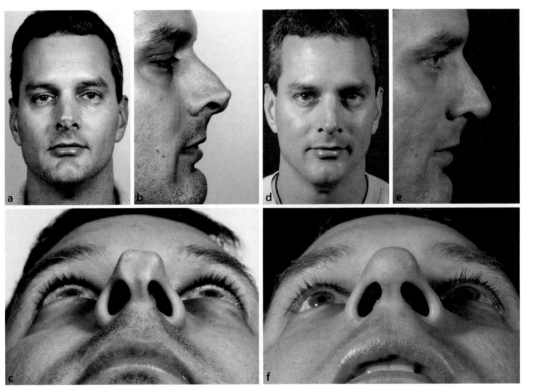

Fig. 68.10 **a–c** Preoperative view of patient with pre-existing natural bossae and overrotated as well as over-projected tip. **d–f** 1-year postoperative view of same patient. Tip is deprojected and bossae are effaced with hockey stick excision and crushed cartilage in infradomal area

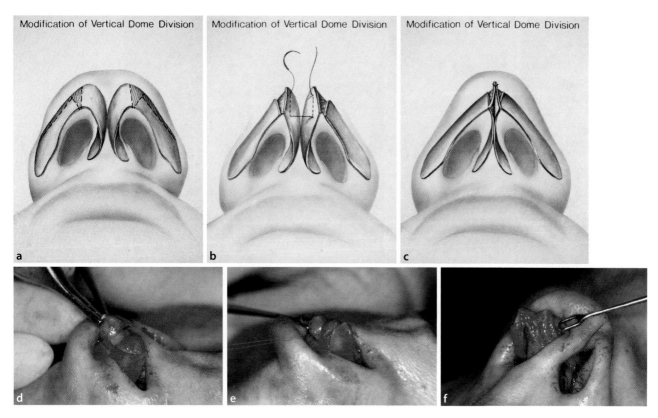

Fig. 68.11 **a** The excision for Simons' modification is shown by the first figure. The lateral distance of the cut is limited to 3 mm from the lobular apex. **b** The suture is placed in a horizontal mattress fashion with the needle closer to the superior edge than the more medial inferior exit. **c** Result of Simons modification after suture placement. The alar cartilages are returned to the natural position. The pyramidal appearance of the base is achieved. **d–f** Intraoperative photos of Simons' modification as shown in previous diagrams

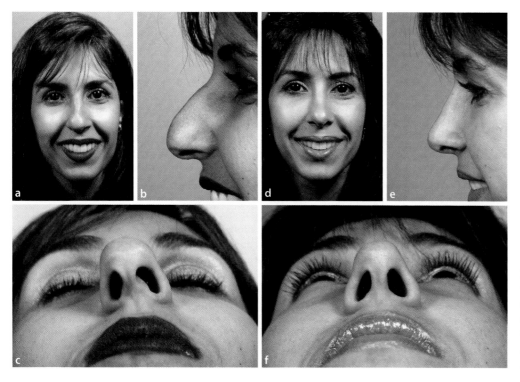

Fig. 68.12 **a–c** Preoperative views of young woman with asymmetric and broad tip. **d–f** 2-year postoperative views of same woman after rhinoplasty with Simons' tip modification

68

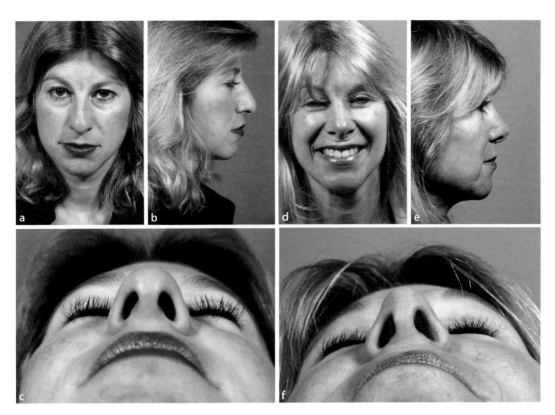

Fig. 68.13 **a–c** Preoperative views of patient with broad, underrotated tip. **d–f** 23-year postoperative views of same woman following Simons' tip modification

author's use of sutures in the tip is limited to stabilizing medial components. Attempting to reconstruct the dome by suturing the cut medial crura to the lateral crus is unnecessary and might lead to asymmetries. Moreover, suturing medial-to-lateral or lateral-to-lateral crural components defeats the purpose of vertical dome division and might result in an unnatural narrowing of the lobular apices.

The Use of Crushed Cartilage in the Endonasal Approach

Over the past decade, the senior author has been using crushed cartilage in the infralobular space. The cartilage is placed in the infratip through the medial right marginal incision (Fig. 68.14). This only can help hide irregularities and it can also act as an adjunctive measure to increase tip projection or lengthen the nose. Additionally, a cartilaginous columellar batten may be placed anterior to the medial crura to increase columella show and decrease the appearance of a retracted columella.

Marginal incisions and the lower transfixion incision are closed with two or three interrupted sutures of 4-0 chromic catgut. These sutures at the marginal incisions are placed obliquely to encourage medial movement of the bipedicle chondrocutaneous flap. It is important not to cause notching by placing the medial exit too close to the alar rim.

Osteotomies

Following the tip and dorsum work the lateral osteotomies are performed. Whether performed through an endonasal or external approach the osteotomies are hidden from view and thus subject to less control than other parts of the operation. The generally preferred osteotomy line is a curved high (preserving a bony triangle at the pyriform base) to low (in the nasofacial groove) to high (into the nasion). The senior author uses the straight Parkes chisel with its initial placement in the downward and outward direction at the pyriform aperture, advancing towards the inner canthus, where the chisel turns inward then upward towards the nasion with palpable direction. A complete osteotomy is preferred to a partial or greenstick fracture.

Intermediate osteotomies are useful with asymmetrically wide or broad convex nasal bones and precede the lateral osteotomy. Occasionally the medial osteotomy is used as an outfracture procedure to fully complete the bony infracture and at times to ensure a straighter break in a twisted nose.

Following the osteotomies, a rise in the cartilaginous dorsum often occurs from the medial movement of the attached upper lateral cartilage. It is at this time, usually near the end of the procedure, that the excess upper lateral cartilage can be trimmed judicially.

A good taping job cannot fix a poorly executed rhinoplasty; however, a bad taping job can ruin a good rhinoplasty. A "cinch

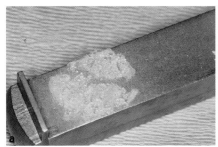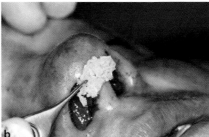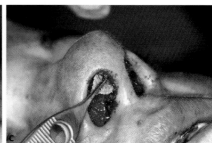

Fig. 68.14 **a** The appearance of the cartilage after crushing. **b,c** The cartilage is moistened and placed through the marginal incision on the right

dressing" of clear tape is placed around the lobular tissues with tape and plaster cast applied as an external splint. Telfa pads are used as an intranasal splint for approximately 2 days. The external splint remains in place for approximately 1 week.

Postoperative Care and Instructions

Before surgery every patient is counseled about the postoperative period. Most patients return to work and normal activity within 1 to 2 weeks following surgery. All patients must be reassured that full recovery and the desired refinement generally takes months, not days or weeks to occur. With the expected natural resolution of swelling and its concomitant subtle changes, it is generally best to resist the desires for revision for at least 1 year.

To improve the quality of your work there is no better teacher than long-term follow-up of one's own patients. When well performed the subtle nature of the operation provides long-lasting rejuvenation of facial features almost unparalleled in other facial plastic procedures. Remembering that the diagnosis is more important than technique and that in rhinoplasty, "we do a little to

achieve a lot" will enable us to enjoy greater success in rhinoplasty whether our preferred approach is external or endonasal.

References

1. Simons RL (1987) Vertical dome division in rhinoplasty. Otolaryngol Clin North Am 20(4):785–796
2. Simons RL (2004) A personal report: Emphasizing the endonasal approach. Facial Plast Surg Clin North Am 12:15–34
3. Simons RL (1999) Nasal tip bossae in rhinoplasty. Arch Facial Plast Surg 1:83–89
4. Brown JB, McDowell F (1951) Plastic surgery of the nose. Mosby, St Louis
5. Goldman IB (1957) The importance of the medial crura in nasal tip reconstruction. AMA Arch Otolaryngol 65:143–147
6. Gillman GS, Simons RL, Lee DJ (1999) Nasal tip bossae in rhinoplasty: Etiology, predisposing factors and management techniques. Arch Facial Plast Surg 1:83–89
7. Simons RL, Adelson R (2005) Rhinoplasty in male patients. Facial Plast Surg 21:240–249

Chapter 69

Nasal Tip Management Utilizing the Open Approach

69

Russell W. H. Kridel and Peyman Soliemanzadeh

Core Messages

- As experience with tissue shrinkage and scar contracture has increased, many surgeons have moved away from more aggressive cartilage resection and scoring techniques toward the use of more conservative suture techniques for restructuring the tip cartilages.
- Combining knowledge of the three dimensional nasal anatomy with a clear aesthetic understanding enables the surgeon to develop a clear surgical plan.
- The surgeon can follow an algorithm for nasal tip management which allows for proper tip analysis and the determination of the techniques he/she can utilize to achieve the needed aesthetic goals.
- In examining tip projection, the surgeon must understand the critical importance of examining tip projection in relation to the height of the radix.
- Binding the medial crura together, to a columella strut, or to the caudal septum will ensure a solid foundation for the nasal tip and helps to avoid postoperative loss of nasal tip projection, which could eliminate any supratip break and may result in supratip fullness (pollybeak deformity).
- If more tip projection is required than is provided by simple stabilization of the nasal base via the medial crura, the surgeon can look to additionally increase projection via either the Double Dome technique for minor increases or through the Lateral Crural Steal for greater projection.
- In classic nasal tripod theory, a standard way to retrodisplace the tip is to shorten one or both of the legs of the tripod. When one shortens only the lateral crura or only the medial crura, a change in rotation will ensue. One can take advantage of this principle to accomplish both retrodisplacement as well as a change in rotation by selecting the proper technique.

Contents

Introduction

Nasal tip management has always been the key component of successful rhinoplasty. And in most cases this has meant an emphasis on projecting or deprojecting, narrowing, and refinement of the nasal tip structure. As experience with scar contracture has increased, many surgeons have moved away from more aggressive cartilage resection and scoring techniques toward the use of more conservative suture techniques for restructuring the cartilage. These new techniques rely on precise suture placement and tension control to create a natural-appearing nasal tip contour.

In approaching the nasal tip, the rhinoplastic surgeon must be able to seamlessly connect and integrate the underlying anatomic form with the individualized "ideal" nasal aesthetics. In other words, the variable surface features of the patient's nose must be correlated to the underlying internal structural components and compared to an aesthetic "ideal" for that patient. Combining knowledge of the three dimensional anatomy with a clear aesthetic understanding then enables the surgeon to develop a precise surgical plan.

There are many nasal tip techniques which modify the nasal tip cartilages by suturing cartilages, dividing cartilages, or a combination of both. However, with time certain techniques result in excessive narrowing or asymmetries of the nasal tip with or without attendant nasal dysfunction. This chapter will first briefly review surgically relevant nasal tip aesthetic analysis. The remainder of the chapter will be dedicated to elucidat-

69

ing a clear surgical algorithm for management of the nasal tip. Specifically, the tongue in groove (TIG) technique, double dome suture (DDS) technique, the lateral crural steal (LCS), the lateral crural overlay (LCO), the medial crural overlay (MCO), and dome truncation (DT) will each be detailed as part of an overall surgical algorithm for tip management [1–8].

Nasal Analysis

In order to reliably address the nasal tip, the surgeon must understand the correlation between the external nasal contour and the shape of the underlying tip cartilages. Once this relationship between the external tip shape and the underlying structure is understood, the surgeon can simplify nasal tip surgery to the techniques required in order to create a sound tip structure that will tolerate the forces of scar contracture over time. Knowledge of the many formulas, specific angles, and anatomic proportions that have been described is important but cannot accomplish the surgical goal alone. What is more, many of these general "ideal" aesthetic parameters are used to evaluate the nasal tip from the lateral or base view rather than the frontal view, which is what the patient sees.

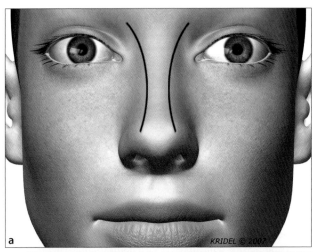

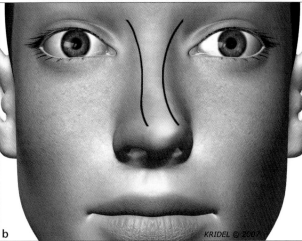

Ideally, on front view the nose should have a subtle hourglass appearance with two divergent concave lines. These gently curving lines, referred to as the brow-tip aesthetic line by Tardy, extend from the infraorbital rim to the nasofrontal angle and then into a slightly narrower middle nasal vault (Fig. 69.1a). These lines then continue in the transition from the middle nasal vault to the nasal tip with a slight divergence at the nasal tip, especially as they approach the alar margins. When these lines diverge or converge irregularly, the nose appears crooked either at the tip or middle vault depending on the irregularity (Fig. 69.1b).

On frontal view, the most common deformity in the dome is generally a lack of dome definition. This is due to rounded dome cartilages, a lack of defined transition between the intermediate and lateral crura, or to an excessive degree of divergence between the intermediate crura, i.e., a wide interdomal distance. Moreover, Daniel noted that the most aesthetically pleasing nasal tips have a dome structure defined with a convex domal segment and a concave lateral crus [9]. Thus many of the commonly described tip-refining techniques act to convert a convex lateral crus into one that is concave. However, the over-accentuation of such a concavity in the lateral crus can pinch the nasal tip and create an unnatural demarcation between the tip and the alar lobule [9], and therefore, these authors (Russell Kridel and Peyman Soliemanzadeh) would prefer to say the lower laterals should be made flat rather than concave.

In the supratip region, excessive fullness creates an unfavorable shadow. This supratip fullness is most commonly caused by either excessive prominence of the cephalad portion of the lateral crus (producing a "bulbous" appearance) or lateral alar convexities located lateral to the dome which produce a "boxy" tip configuration [10]. A high anterior septal angle and a cartilaginous fullness in the nasal dorsal septum may be the source of any supratip fullness. This fullness in the supratip region should be eliminated to create a supratip shadow and to enhance the resultant attractive nasal tip.

On profile, the nasal tip should have a curvilinear shape with no sharp contours. Ideally on profile, when examining the line that extends from the base of the columella to the tip there is a subtle bend which occurs at the columellar–lobular junction, which corresponds to the junction of the medial crura and intermediate crura and differentiates the tip lobule from the columella. This columellar–lobular angle or double break should be preserved by avoiding blunting the normal divergence of the intermediate crura.

The nasal tip analysis on profile can then be divided into an evaluation of projection and rotation. With regard to tip projection, one can begin by referring to the excellent review of

Fig. 69.1 a On frontal view the nose should have a subtle hourglass appearance with two divergent concave lines. These gently curving lines, referred to as the brow-tip aesthetic line by Tardy, extend from the infraorbital rim to the nasofrontal angle and then into a slightly narrower middle nasal vault. **b** When these lines diverge or converge irregularly, the nose appears crooked either at the tip or middle vault depending on the irregularity (© 2007 Russell W.H. Kridel, used with permission)

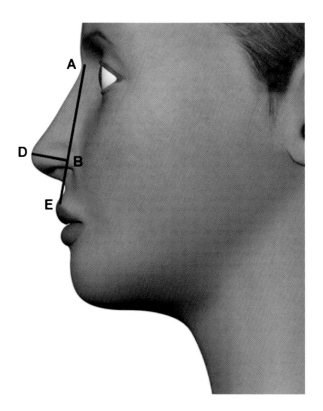

Fig. 69.2 Crumley's analysis derived from a combination of the Powell and Simons methods found a ratio of BD/AE equal to .2833 to most closely achieve the ideal nasal projection. The vertical vector (AE) combines nasal length and upper lip length. (© 2005 Russell W.H. Kridel, used with permission)

the topic done by Crumley [12] (Fig. 69.2). We would add that in examining tip projection, the surgeon must understand the critical importance of examining the tip projection in relation to the height of the radix. The radix should be considered not as a separate unit but as a "key part of a dynamic form" [13] (Fig. 69.3). In other words, the tip is only projected in relation to the projection of dorsal height at the nasion. As such, one needs to consider not only the height and position of the tip but also the height and depth of the radix, as well as the nasofacial angle produced in its relation to the nasal tip [13, 14].

If true overprojection is determined, the surgeon can then do an objective analysis as to the underlying cause for overprojection. Components of the nasal anatomy that lead to tip overprojection can include (1) over-elongated alar cartilages—including lateral crura, medial crura, intermediate crura, or combinations therein; (2) a tension nose with overdeveloped quadrangular cartilage; (3) combinations of the above; and (4) trauma or iatrogenic injury causing dorsal saddling [15].

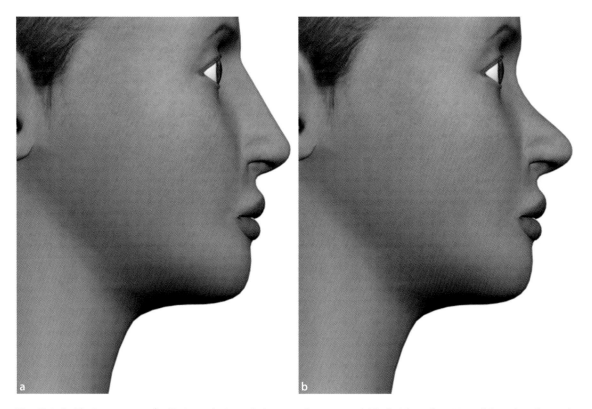

Fig. 69.3a,b The importance of radix in aesthetic analysis cannot be overstated. The height and position of the radix affect each other, define the nasofacial angle, and serve as the counterpoise of the nasal base. While projection is the same in both figures, the change in radix positioning causes the illusion of overprojection in **b** (© 2005 Russell W.H. Kridel, used with permission)

Having completed analysis of nasal projection, the next step is to determine whether rotation is adequate or will need to be addressed as many tip techniques can or will alter rotation. A nasolabial angle of 95–100° in males, and 100–115° in females, is generally regarded as ideal. Nasolabial angles more acute than these accepted standards are generally found to be aesthetically unattractive. If a nasal tip is found to be ptotic, the surgeon may consider that (1) most commonly, the lower lateral cartilages are excessively long and push down the medial crura; (2) the lateral crura are vertically oriented; (3) there are weakened tip support mechanisms (secondary to previous surgery or as part of normal aging); (4) there may be atrophy of bone or premaxillary subcutaneous tissue at the nasolabial angle.

Finally, the nose is further examined for tip asymmetries, skin thickness, dorsal humps or irregularities, as well as nasal valve competence and other functional components. With analysis of the patient's external nasal contour and underlying cartilaginous structure complete, a comparison is made to the set "idealized" end point of a natural appearing 3-dimensional nasal tip contour. The surgeon then proceeds to our algorithm to determine how to accomplish the surgical goal (Fig. 69.4 Algorithm).

The first tier to be determined in our nasal tip algorithm is whether the nose is under- or overprojected. If the nose is underprojected, the surgeon can look to achieve increased projection via a number of techniques including (1) binding together the medial crura if they are splayed apart; (2) double dome technique; (3) the lateral crural steal (LCS); (4) the use of a columellar strut with or without a premaxillary plumping graft; (5) a tip graft, or (6) setting the medial crura onto the caudal septum in

a more projected position and then suturing them in place in a tongue-in-groove maneuver.

Prior to working on the domal region of the nasal tip, one must examine and stabilize the medial crura since they act as a base to support the tip and its projection. Generally, noses with strong medial crura that extend down toward the nasal spine have excellent support and will tend not to lose projection postoperatively. Conversely, noses with short medial crura that do not reach the posterior septal angle/nasal spine are more likely to lose projection postoperatively [9]. Occasionally, the surgeon will find the medial crura are buckled due to their natural shape or trauma and need to be sutured together with or without an intervening columellar strut. Stabilizing the nasal base will ensure that tip projection is maintained postoperatively, or in cases where the medial crura are buckled, will actually increase projection.

Binding the medial crura together, to a columella strut, or to the caudal septum will ensure a solid foundation for the nasal tip and helps to avoid postoperative loss of nasal tip projection, which could eliminate any supratip break and may result in supratip fullness (pollybeak deformity).

If more tip projection is required than is provided by simple stabilization of the nasal base via the medial crura, the surgeon can look to additionally increase projection via either the double dome technique for minor increases or through the Lateral Crural Steal [3] for greater projection. The double-dome unit procedure is predominantly effective in narrowing the wide or bulbous lobule but can also be utilized for an incremental increase in tip projection. However, when more significant tip

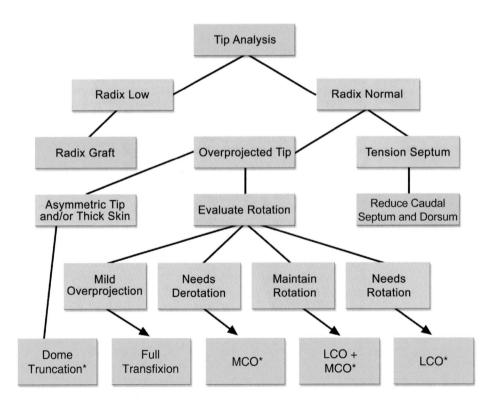

Fig. 69.4 Algorithm developed to help simplify the approach to deprojection. Note that analysis begins with evaluation of the radix. Also note that *asterisk* is utilized to show that a Full Transfixion Incision can be added to said procedures to allow further retro-displacement (© 2005 Russell W.H. Kridel, used with permission)

projection is necessary, the surgeon can utilize the LCS. The LCS is a horizontal mattress suture that spans the nasal dome anterior to the vestibular lining. With its lateral placement, the medial crura are lengthened at the expense of the lateral crura. In other words, the lateral crus is recruited medially into the dome. And the result is increased tip projection, increased rotation and tip narrowing.

When, on the other hand, the nasal tip is found to be over-projected, our algorithm begins with an evaluation of the radix (Fig. 69.4 Algorithm). Oftentimes what is needed to bring the nasal tip back into proper balance with the remainder of the patience profile is a radix graft and not deprojection. For that reason we stress the importance of the radix by placing it at the top of the evaluation. In these cases, overprojection is not the problem and a simple radix graft will restore balance.

Once the radix has been evaluated, and the nose has been defined as truly overprojected, attention can then be turned toward the next ladder. If minimal deprojection is needed the surgeon can do a simple full transfixion incision in order to effect the desired retrodisplacement. This method works by lysing the supporting fibrous connections between the septum and the medial crura. However, when more pronounced deprojection is necessary, other methods that may also affect rotation are considered.

In classic nasal tripod theory, a standard way to retrodisplace the tip is to shorten one or both of the legs of the tripod (Fig. 69.5). However, if one shortens only the medial crura or only the lateral crura, a change in rotation will ensue. One can take advantage of this principle to accomplish both retrodisplacement as well as a change in rotation by selecting the proper technique. Kridel and Konior showed that when overprojection is accompanied by tip ptosis, the LCO (which shortens the lower lateral crural leg) permits incremental retrodisplacement with increased rotation [4]. On the other hand, the medial crural overlay (MCO), which shortens the medial crural leg of the tripod, leads to controlled deprojection and decreased rotation [6]. When used together at the same surgical intervention (to shorten both tripod legs), the MCO and the LCO can effect large amounts of retrodisplacement with little effect on rotation. These two techniques, alone or in combination, accomplish the needed retrodisplacement in the vast majority of patients. It is relatively uncommon to need further deprojection than can be accomplished with either the MCO or LCO alone or together. Large increments of retrodisplacement can be achieved with these techniques, and therefore the surgeon needs to consider

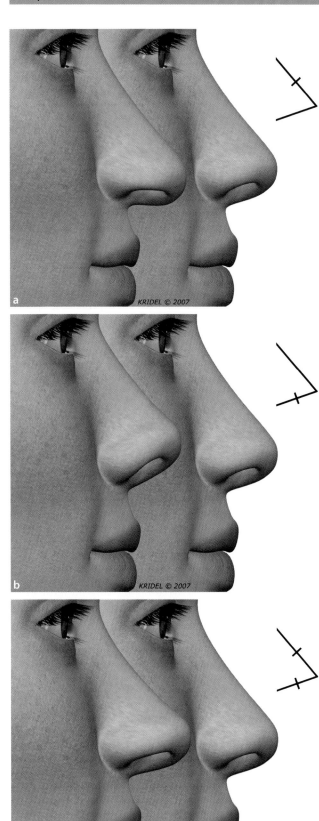

Fig. 69.5a–c Anderson Tripod Theory. Analysis of the nose must allow for the subtleties. **a** The increased rotation effect of shortening of the lateral crura. Note that there is an increase in rotation as well as subtle deprojection. **b** Shortening of the medial crura results in a decreased nasolabial angle and subtle retrodisplacement. **c** If both the medial and lateral crura are shortened equally, there is a resultant retrodisplacement without change in rotation (© 2007 Russell W.H. Kridel, used with permission)

that the skin soft tissue envelope must be able to contract down to the newly deprojected cartilaginous support structure or one will risk losing refinement in tip definition. Alternatively, tip deprojection can be accomplished by removing an equal amount of lateral crura and medial crura in a technique called dome truncation (DT), which we will discuss later.

In those patients with a tension nose deformity, we recommend that attention first be directed toward lowering the overdeveloped cartilaginous dorsum, which often tents up the tip artificially. Thereafter the surgeon can follow the same algorithm for deprojection. In our experience most of these patients require increased rotation and were found to have excellent results when treated with the LCO after dorsal reduction.

In the situations when further deprojection is called for than can be accomplished with either the LCO or MCO, the surgeon can choose one of two separate options. In order to effect retrodisplacement while maintaining rotation, the MCO can be combined with the LCO. On the other hand, as indicated in the last arm of our algorithm, it has been our experience that when significant tip asymmetry is present or when the patient has thick skin, DT [7] can be used to accomplish much of the same deprojection in a slightly easier one-step maneuver. Finally, any one of the procedures can again be combined with a full transfixion incision in order to cause another incremental decrease in projection.

Surgical Technique

Bilateral alar marginal incisions and an inverted V-shaped midcolumellar incision are made. The nasal skin is elevated from the alar cartilages in the supraperichondrial avascular plane up unto the radix. Wide undermining is necessary to allow a favorable redraping advantage for the skin-soft tissue envelope. Dorsal profile adjustments, if any are needed, precede tip work finalization in order to minimize disruption of the reconstructed nasal tip.

Prior to contouring the nasal tip, the surgeon must stabilize the base of the nose. If tip support is found to be lacking, a sutured-in-place columellar strut can effectively stabilize the base (Fig. 69.6). This graft is placed into a pocket dissected between the medial crura. When it is necessary to alter tip projection, the alar columellar relationship, and the nasolabial angle, the Tongue-in-Groove technique [1] can be utilized to stabilize the base (Fig. 69.7). Specifically, if the patient has a hanging columella and prominent caudal septum that would otherwise require trimming, the surgeon can set the medial crura back on the midline caudal septum (Fig. 69.8). Dissection generally begins in a retrograde fashion via a previously accomplished transfixion incision. If no previous septoplasty has been done, dissection is accomplished between the medial crura utilizing fine tenotomy scissors to create a potential pocket, and bilateral mucoperichondrial flaps are developed for about 1 cm over the caudal septum for exposure. The medial crura are then advanced cephaloposteriorly, placing the denuded caudal septum into the space created between them. The medial crura can then be sutured to the caudal septum utilizing 3 or 4 chromic sutures. Bilateral membranous septum excision is almost

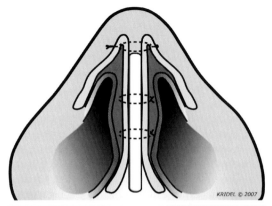

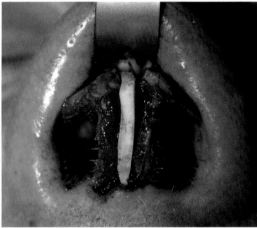

Fig. 69.6 Example of columella strut in space created between the medial crura. The strut not only provides increased support but can also increase the length of the nose or the nasolabial angle (Upper drawing © 2007 Russell W.H. Kridel, used with permission)

always necessary to remove excess tissue which results from the TIG technique. The membrane excision should always be done posterior to the transfixion incision so that only the septal mucous membrane is excised and not the vestibular columellar skin, thereby reducing the possibility of persistently weeping nose. Prior to suturing, one must be sure that the caudal septum is in the midline; otherwise, the tip will be deviated. After initial fixation, careful assessment of tip projection, nasolabial angle, alar columellar relationship, and tip rotation is critical to avoid deformity.

The TIG can also be varied in order to enhance rotation and or to increase projection (Fig. 69.9). In order to allow for increased rotation, the depth of the medial crural pocket and the amount of denuded corresponding caudal septum should be greatest at the dorsal or anterior aspect. On the other hand, to counter rotate the nasal tip or to correct excess columellar show in the posterior region, the deepest portion of the pocket and greatest corresponding advancement should be accomplished posteriorly. Finally, once the septum is placed into the space, the medial crura may be advanced anteriorly and fixed in this position in order to increase and maintain projection.

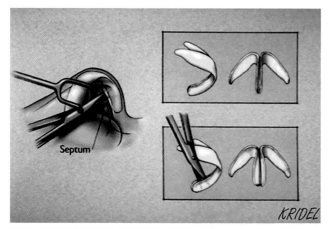

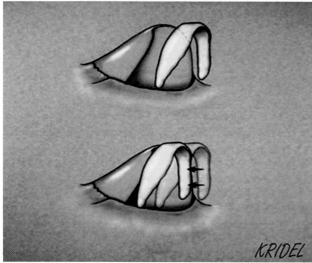

Fig. 69.7 The Tongue in Groove technique (TIG) provides a method for stabilizing the nasal base while also correcting excess columellar show or caudal septal deflections. To counter rotate the nasal tip or to correct excess columellar show, the deepest portion of the pocket and greatest corresponding advancement should be accomplished posteriorly (© 1999 Russell W.H. Kridel, used with permission)

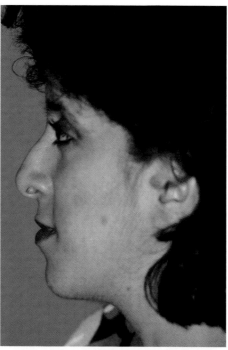

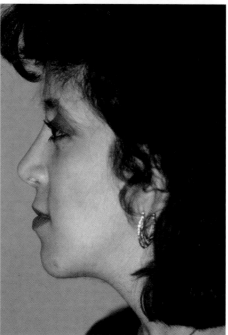

Fig. 69.8 Preoperative and 2-month postoperative profile view of patient with tongue-in-groove technique to decrease columellar show

If the nasal tip is broad, bulbous, or poorly defined, changes in contour begin with a conservative cephalic trim of the lateral crura followed by reorientation of the existing tip structures (Fig. 69.10). A conservative trim of the cephalic margin of the lateral crura will decrease supratip fullness. If the dorsal septum at the supratip and tip area is higher than the domes, it too will need to be trimmed. The extent of the cephalic trim of the lower lateral cartilages depends on the intrinsic cartilaginous strength, shape, and configuration and care is generally taken to maintain a maximal amount or at least 6 mm of lateral crus in order to prevent future valve collapse. Essentially, the cephalic trim is performed to increase tip definition and decrease convexity but sometimes is only done minimally in order to release the cephalic portion of the lateral crus from the scroll

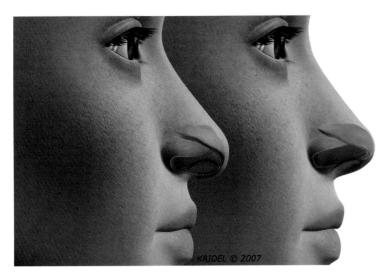

Fig. 69.9 The profile view shows how the TIG can be used to both increase projection and increase rotation by advancing the medial crura anteriorly and more cephalically prior to fixation onto the caudal septum (© 2007 Russell W.H. Kridel, used with permission)

region, thereby allowing manipulation by suture techniques. If the domes are narrow, it is best not to perform medial cartilage excision near the domes. The cephalic trim of the lateral crura is often performed primarily medially and is tapered as it extends into the lateral third of the lateral crus to avoid excessive supra-alar pinching and lateral wall collapse.

Having stabilized the nasal base and accomplished the cephalic trim, attention is then turned toward the dome. When the cartilaginous framework in the tip of the nose fails to provide adequate definition, the rhinoplastic surgeon must create refinement while maintaining strength. To achieve these results, we advocate the utilization of the double dome (Fig. 69.11). This sequence of dome binding sutures effects a stronger, more triangular lobule in those patients with wide, bulbous, or bifid tips. While the double-dome unit procedure is effective in narrowing the wide or bulbous lobule it generally only minimally increases nasal tip projection.

Dome binding sutures are a good way to narrow the bulbous nasal tip contour in the primary rhinoplasty patient and are also an effective means of decreasing supratip fullness. The vestibular skin is undermined from the undersurface of the alar cartilage, starting at the junction of the medial and lateral crura (intermediate crura), then proceeding both laterally and medially for a few millimeters to each side to allow free lateral crura mobilization without restriction by the underlying skin attachments. Following independent creation and fixation of the right and left domes, additional narrowing and refinement are accomplished using a transdomal mattress suture placed through the entire tip complex. In this way, the dome sutures act to variably narrow the dome angle, depending on the stiffness of the lateral crura and on how tightly the sutures are tied. A secondary objective is to create flat lateral crura with the dome sutures (Fig. 69.11).

In patients with soft cartilage, the dome sutures can tend to pinch and deform the dome and leave convexity of the lateral crus laterally. Placement of dome sutures can also deform the lateral crura and displace the caudal margin of the lateral crura well below the cephalic margin. This can result in a pinched na-

sal tip with a characteristic demarcation between the tip and the alar lobule [10]. The thickness of the skin of the tip will modify how tight the domes should be bound: thicker skin allows tighter binding; thinner skin will show sharp edges if the domes are bound too tightly. In these cases crushed cartilage may need to be placed over the domes to camouflage edges.

If increased projection is necessary, a Lateral Crural Steal is accomplished (Fig. 69.12). The vestibular skin is undermined from the undersurface of the alar cartilage, starting at the junction of the medial and lateral crura (intermediate crura), then proceeding both laterally and medially for about 5 mm to each side to allow free lateral crura mobilization without restriction by the underlying skin attachments. First find the anatomical dome. Then, pick a point *lateral* to the dome where the new dome will be created; make sure the vestibular skin underneath has been adequately undermined *in both directions* to allow for suture placement. The lateral crus is advanced medially in a curvilinear fashion onto the medial crus and fixed in its new position using 6-0 permanent mattress sutures just below the newly established dome. Following independent creation and fixation of the right and left domes, additional narrowing and refinement are accomplished using a transdomal mattress suture placed through the entire tip complex. To create a favorable nasal tip contour, it is preferable to have the caudal margin of the dome positioned above the cephalic margin of the dome; otherwise the tip gives a boxy appearance on profile.

To provide additional tip projection and definition or to camouflage sharp edges in thin skin, a soft, gently crushed cartilage graft can be sutured horizontally across both domes with 6-0 permanent suture. It is important to gently crush the cartilage by compressing it with Brown-Adson forceps or by gently crushing the cartilage in a block-type morcellizer; otherwise, the graft may become visible postoperatively. The graft should be sutured to the caudal margin of the domes to ensure that the caudal margin of the dome structure lies above the cephalic margin. The cartilage excised during the cephalic trim of the lateral crura is ideal for this graft because it is pli-

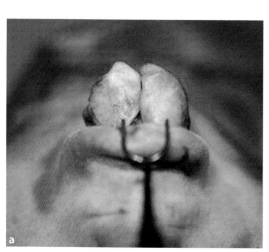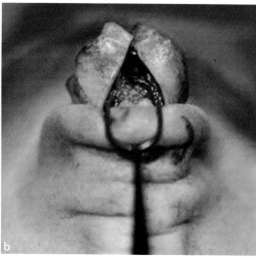

Fig. 69.10a,b The extent of the cephalic trim of the lower lateral cartilages depends on the intrinsic cartilaginous strength, and care is generally taken to maintain a maximal amount or at least 6 mm of lateral crus in order to prevent future valve collapse. If the domes are narrow, it is best not to perform medial cartilage excision near the domes

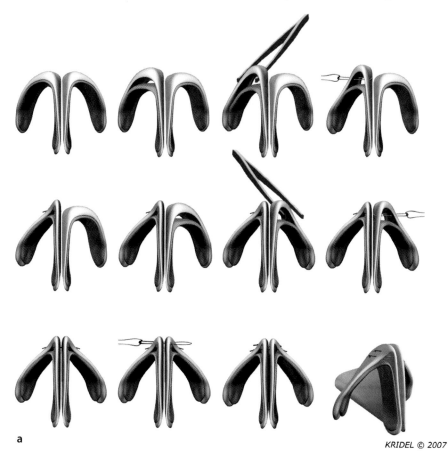

KRIDEL © 2007

Fig. 69.11a–e This illustrative sequence shows how dome binding sutures effect a stronger, more triangular lobule in those patients with wide, bulbous, or bifid tips. Following independent creation and fixation of the right and left domes, additional narrowing and refinement are accomplished using a transdomal mattress suture placed through the entire tip complex. In this way, the dome sutures act to variably narrow the dome angle, depending on the stiffness of the lateral crura and on how tightly the sutures are tied. **a** Result of the double dome technique. **b–e** *see next page* (© 2007 Russell W.H. Kridel, used with permission)

able and has soft tissue attached to it for easy fixation to the domes.

Shield tip grafts are often not necessary in patients undergoing primary rhinoplasty when the surgeon can work with the patient's existing domes with suture techniques, except when the tip skin is very thick, such as in some male patients (Fig. 69.13). Shield tip grafts are used primarily in secondary rhinoplasty, augmentation rhinoplasty, or in primary rhinoplasty patients who have an underprojected tip with thick skin and a deficient

tip lobule, which is common in some ethnic patients. In such patients needing tip projection, the lower lateral cartilages are very weak or diminutive and will not provide adequate projection with suturing methods alone. In these patients and in the revision patient with scarring, sutured-in-place shield tip grafts can be used to help give increased projection and tip definition. If one does use a shield tip graft, it must be properly carved and camouflaged to avoid visibility of the graft, since the skin tends to thin and contract over time. All shield tip grafts are at risk of

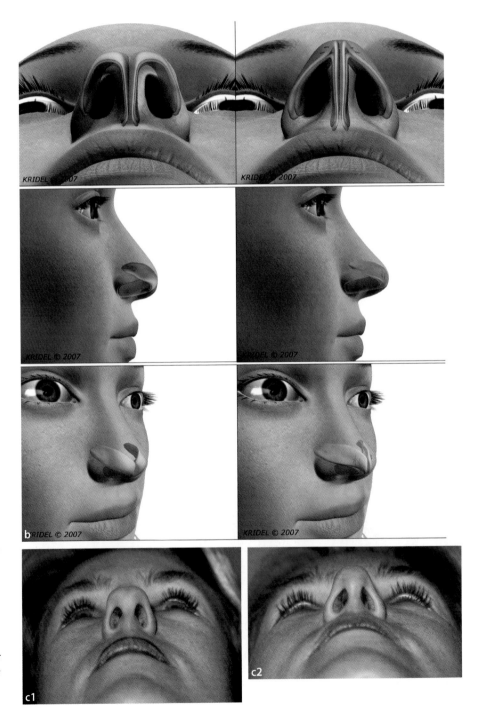

Fig. 69.11a–e (continued) This illustrative sequence shows how dome binding sutures effect a stronger, more triangular lobule in those patients with wide, bulbous, or bifid tips. Following independent creation and fixation of the right and left domes, additional narrowing and refinement are accomplished using a transdomal mattress suture placed through the entire tip complex. In this way, the dome sutures act to variably narrow the dome angle, depending on the stiffness of the lateral crura and on how tightly the sutures are tied. a,b Result of the double dome technique. c The preoperative base view and 11-months postoperative view of a patient who underwent double dome suturing after a cephalic trim. d,e see next page (© 2007 Russell W.H. Kridel, used with permission)

becoming visible regardless of skin thickness with time. As such we recommend that tip projection can be controlled in most primary rhinoplasty patients by placement of dome sutures, stabilization of the base (columellar strut graft, TIG), and *soft* cartilage grafts positioned over the domes to project and further *refine* the tip.

If deprojection is necessary, the technique utilized will depend on what if any change in rotation is necessary. *When increased rotation is desired, a lateral crural overlay (LCO) is per-* *formed* (Fig. 69.14) allowing the nasal tip to be repositioned to an aesthetically pleasing position. The incisions in the lateral crura are planned so as to cross the central-lateral portion of each lateral crus. The cartilage cut extends in a straight line from the cephalic to the caudal crural margin, taking care to stay at least 1 cm away from the dome. Before making the cartilage cut, the vestibular skin is elevated from the overlying lateral crus for approximately 5 mm on each side of the planned rotation point. Release of the vestibular skin releases tethering forces that could

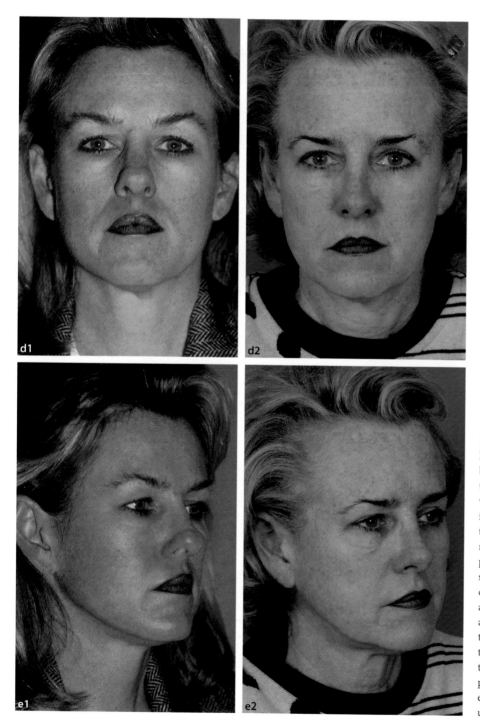

d1   d2
e1   e2

Fig. 69.11a–e (*continued*) This illustrative sequence shows how dome binding sutures effect a stronger, more triangular lobule in those patients with wide, bulbous, or bifid tips. Following independent creation and fixation of the right and left domes, additional narrowing and refinement are accomplished using a transdomal mattress suture placed through the entire tip complex. In this way, the dome sutures act to variably narrow the dome angle, depending on the stiffness of the lateral crura and on how tightly the sutures are tied. **d,e** Frontal and three quarter views of the same patient preoperatively and 12-years postoperatively (© 2007 Russell W.H. Kridel, used with permission)

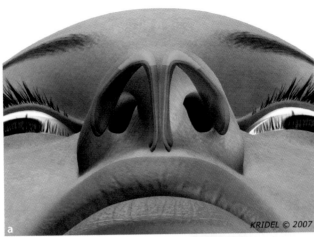

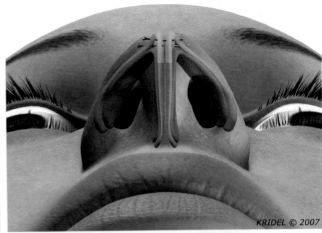

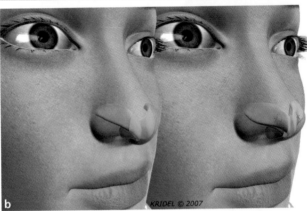

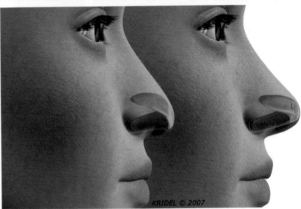

Lateral Crural Steal

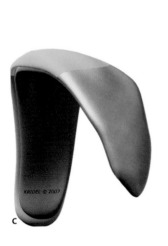

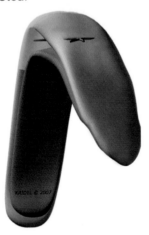

Fig. 69.12a–f The LCS is a horizontal mattress suture that spans the nasal dome anterior to the vestibular lining. With its placement, the medial crura are lengthened at the expense of the lateral crura. And the result is increased tip projection, increased rotation and tip narrowing. **a–c** Result of the lateral crural steal technique in Base, Three Quarter, and Profile view. **d–f** *see next page* (© 2007 Russell W.H. Kridel, used with permission)

restrict tip rotation, and it allows for safe transcartilaginous suture placement. In patients who have overprojection and tip ptosis, the free anterior segment of the lateral crus is both rotated and retrodisplaced over the stationary, posteriorly based lateral crural flap. Rotation of the tip superiorly functionally shortens the lateral crura. The integrity of the divided lateral crus is then re-established with 6-0 permanent transcartilaginous, horizontal mattress sutures. One can judge the resultant rotation and make adjustments in the amount of overlay and placement of the sutures as needed. Following tip rotation, the inferior corner of the lateral crural transection margin may extend below the existing caudal alar cartilage margin and may be excised with a blade to create a smooth inferior alar cartilage border. This technique is in turn followed up with dome binding sutures since the LCO will laterally distract the domes.

If on the other hand, the nose is noted to be overrotated or the reason for increased projection is secondary to overelongated medial crura, the decision is made to proceed with the MCO

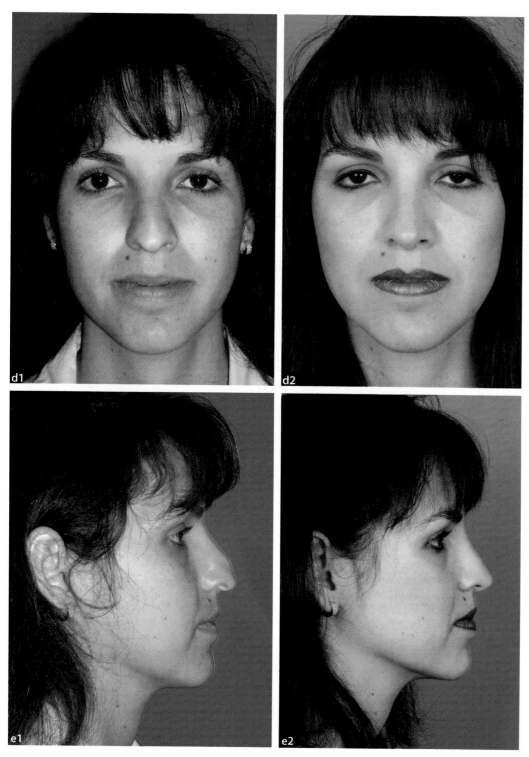

Fig. 69.12a–f (*continued*) The LCS is a horizontal mattress suture that spans the nasal dome anterior to the vestibular lining. With its placement, the medial crura are lengthened at the expense of the lateral crura. And the result is increased tip projection, increased rotation and tip narrowing. **d–e** The preoperative and 4-month postoperative Frontal, Profile, and Three Quarter view of a patient who had rhinoplasty utilizing the LCS technique for tip correction as well as a columellar strut and premaxillary plumping graft **f** *see next page* (© 2007 Russell W.H. Kridel, used with permission)

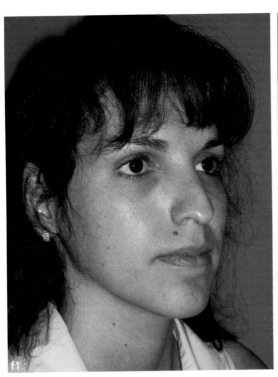
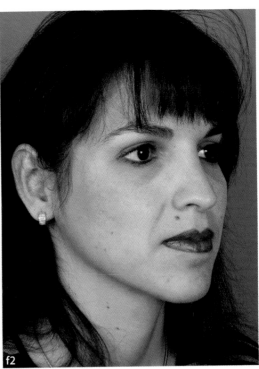

Fig. 69.12a–f (*continued*) The LCS is a horizontal mattress suture that spans the nasal dome anterior to the vestibular lining. With its placement, the medial crura are lengthened at the expense of the lateral crura. And the result is increased tip projection, increased rotation and tip narrowing. **a–c** Result of the lateral crural steal technique in Base, Three Quarter, and Profile view. **d–f** The preoperative and 4-month postoperative Frontal, Profile, and Three Quarter view of a patient who had rhinoplasty utilizing the LCS technique for tip correction as well as a columellar strut and premaxillary plumping graft. When increased rotation is desired, a lateral crural overlay (LCO) allows the nasal tip to be repositioned to be repositioned to an aesthetically pleasing position (© 2007 Russell W.H. Kridel, used with permission)

69

(Fig. 69.15). Incisions cross the central portion of each medial crus. Unlike other Lipsett-like transection techniques, the MCO requires no cartilage to be excised. As such, there is no need to predetermine which portion of the medial crus needs to be removed. As with the LCO, before making the cartilage cut, the vestibular skin is elevated from the overlying medial crus thereby permitting safe transcartilaginous permanent suture placement. After rechecking the ideal tip projection, the integrity of the medial crus is re-established by overlapping and stabilizing the cartilage with 6-0 permanent transcartilaginous, horizontal mattress stitches. The two-point fixation obtained with this suturing technique gives excellent long-term stability while allowing deprojection of the nasal tip into proper position. Moreover, the overlapping of the medial crural segments adds structural strength to the medial crura.

On those occasions when more deprojection is required than can be effected by either the LCO or MCO, a combination of both techniques can be used to retrodisplace the nasal tip without significant changes in tip rotation (Fig. 69.16). In these cases the LCO precedes the MCO. This order allows for control over

not only the extent of deprojection but also allows the surgeon to exactly determine what if any changes are desired in tip rotation.

In those patients who are found to have overprojection and have pre-existing tip asymmetries or overtly thick skin, the decision may be made to proceed with DT, as described by Kridel and Konior [7] (Fig. 69.17, DT patient and illustration). With DT, after conservative cephalic trim is completed, the vestibular skin underlying the angle of the domes is elevated for approximately 1 cm. Blunt forceps are then introduced between the vestibular skin and the dome cartilages. The alar cartilages are then elevated behind the existing domes to delineate the precise location of the tip defining point. With the alar cartilages tented up, the overprojected distance is subtracted from the most forward projecting point of the domes and is marked. *The measurement is critical as it marks the new tip defining point, which in turn will define the ultimate tip projection.*

A 6-0 permanent mattress stitch is placed transdomally through both lateral and medial crus; care being taken to bury the suture within the vestibular pockets. This stitch is placed im-

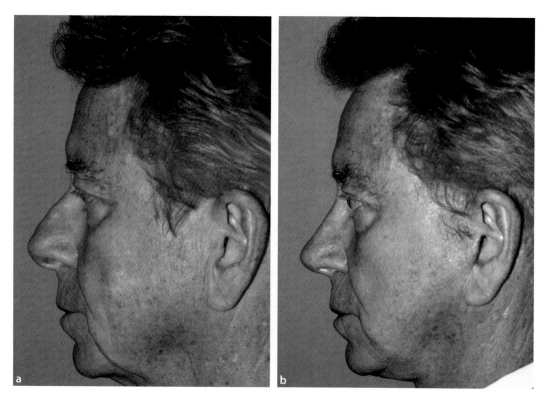

Fig. 69.13 **a** Patient after nasal trauma. **b** Patient after tip graft, columellar strut and double dome suturing to achieve tip definition (© 2007 Russell W.H. Kridel, used with permission)

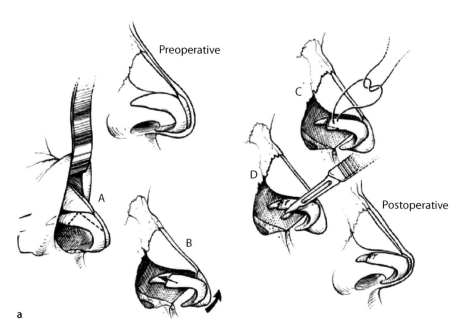

Fig. 69.14a–e Lateral Crural Overlay (LCO) allows for controlled retrodisplacement along with increased rotation. **a** Result of the lateral crural overlay technique. **b–e** *see next page* (**a** is taken from [18], **b–e** © 2007 Russell W.H. Kridel, used with permission)

69

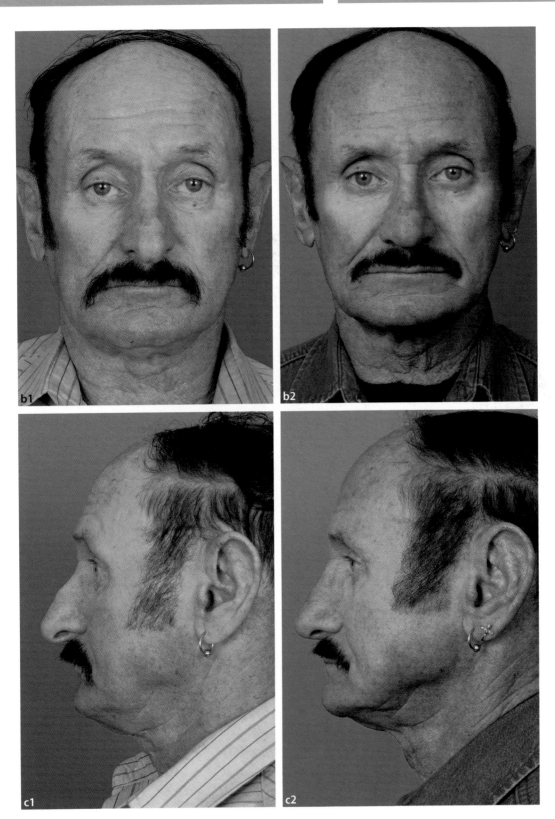

Fig. 69.14a–e (*continued*) Lateral Crural Overlay (LCO) allows for controlled retrodisplacement along with increased rotation. **b–e** Preoperative and 18-month postoperative Frontal, Profile, Base, and Three Quarter views of patient who underwent LCO, cephalic trim, full transfixion incision, and double dome suture. **d,e** *see next page* (**a** is taken from [18], **b–e** © 2007 Russell W.H. Kridel, used with permission)

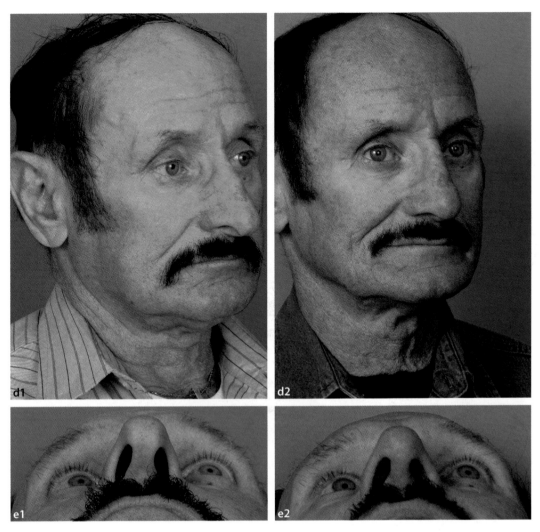

Fig. 69.14a–e (*continued*) Lateral Crural Overlay (LCO) allows for controlled retrodisplacement along with increased rotation. **b–e** Preoperative and 18-month postoperative Frontal, Profile, Base, and Three Quarter views of patient who underwent LCO, cephalic trim, full transfixion incision, and double dome suture (**a** is taken from [18], **b–e** © 2007 Russell W.H. Kridel, used with permission)

mediately posterior to the desired tip defining point and must be oriented parallel to the intended dome plane of dome truncation. By placing this transdomal suture just below the proposed truncation, the relationship between the lower lateral crura and the medial crura are maintained so that rotation will remain unchanged. The overprojected alar domes are then excised by transecting the lobular cartilages along the previously marked projection line, just anterior to the stabilizing sutures. This cut should be oriented just above and slightly oblique to the dorsal profile line, so that the inferior margin of the recreated crural junction lies slightly anterior to the cephalad margin. This arrangement achieves maximal lobular refinement and produces a supratip break along the new profile line. A stable and well-tailored lobular cartilage complex minimizes the chance for notching, valve collapse, or tip asymmetry. As with the combination of overlay LCO with MCO wherein both the medial and lateral crura are shortened by the overlay, dome truncation allows for equivalent amounts of the medial and lateral crura to be excised, and therefore nasal rotation remains unchanged (as predicted by the tripod theory) while achieving deprojection.

The nasal skin is then redraped and the tip is re-evaluated for position and definition. As greater tip refinement is generally desired, a 6-0 permanent suture is routinely placed in a double dome fashion. If any concerns exist regarding loss of tip support after completion of the alar alterations herein described, the medial crura should be reapproximated with buried 6-0 permanent or semipermanent mattress sutures. Should even further deprojection be needed, the hemitransfixion incision is converted to a full transfixion. The incision is made at the junction of the septal cartilage and membranous septum, and causes tip

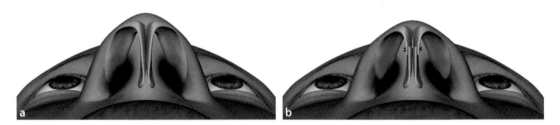

Fig. 69.15a,b Medial Crural Overlay (MCO) allows for controlled retrodisplacement along with a decreased nasolabial angle (© 2005 Russell W.H. Kridel, used with permission)

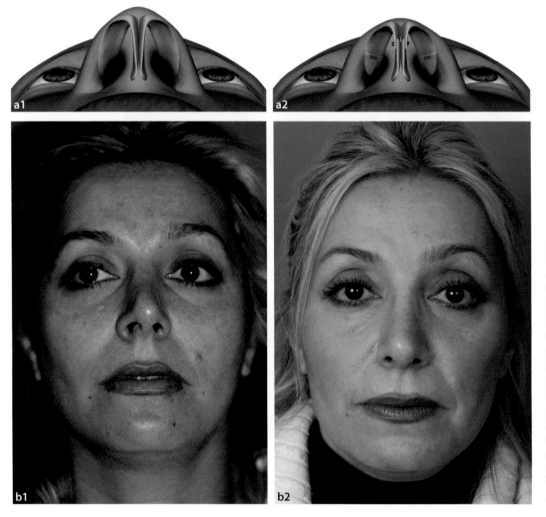

Fig. 69.16a–e The LCO and MCO can be combined when more significant deprojection is needed. **a** After LCO and MCO are combined. **b–e** Preoperative and 1-year postoperative Frontal, Profile, Three Quarter, and Base views of patient who underwent MCO, cephalic trim, and double dome suture. **c–e** *see next page* (© 2005 Russell W.H. Kridel, used with permission)

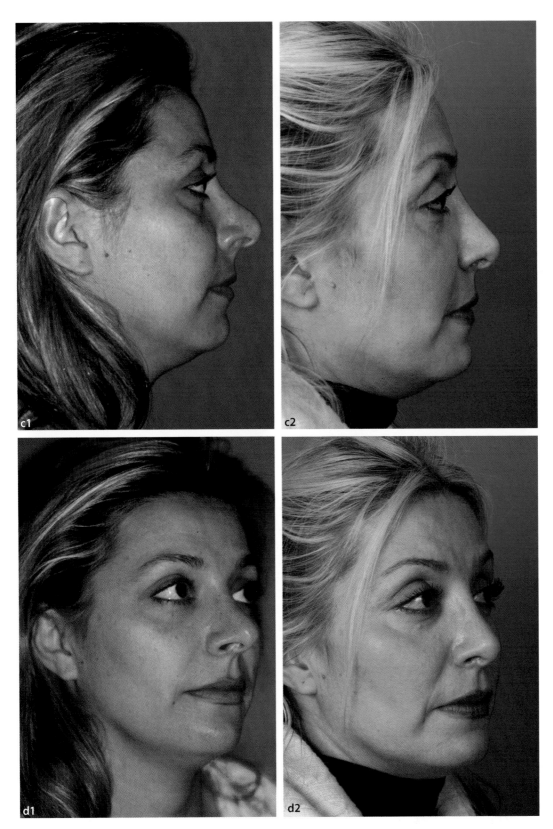

Fig. 69.16a–e (*continued*) The LCO and MCO can be combined when more significant deprojection is needed. **b–e** Preoperative and 1-year postoperative Frontal, Profile, Three Quarter, and Base views of patient who underwent MCO, cephalic trim, and double dome suture (© 2005 Russell W.H. Kridel, used with permission)

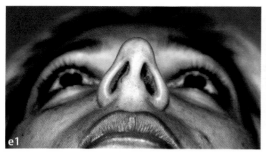
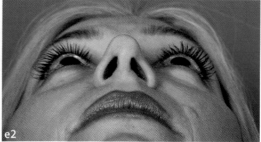

Fig. 69.16a–e (*continued*) The LCO and MCO can be combined when more significant deprojection is needed. **b–e** Pre-operative and 1-year postoperative Frontal, Profile, Three Quarter, and Base views of patient who underwent MCO, cephalic trim, and double dome suture (© 2005 Russell W.H. Kridel, used with permission)

retrodisplacement by releasing the attachments from the medial crural footplates to the caudal septum. The nasal incisions are then carefully closed. *The alar base should then be carefully evaluated to ensure that alar flaring has not occurred due to the retrodisplacement.* Occasionally, alar wedge excisions may be required to decrease the excess alar length and flare [8]. The nose is then taped to provide nasal tip support and a splint is placed over the dorsum. The splint is removed after 1 week, and the nose is again retaped for approximately 5 days to help support the tip during the early postoperative period.

The elegance of both the LCO and the MCO lies in the fact that no bridges are burned. Because no cartilage is excised, the surgeon is left with the flexibility to modify the result on the table. If too much deprojection is seen, the overlapping sutures can be released and reapproximated with less overlay. Furthermore, some have argued that excision of portions of the lateral crura results in a high risk of tip contour irregularities (notching and/or bossae) as a result of displacement and distortion of the transected, weakened cartilage. Webster encountered this difficulty with his lateral crural flap technique [19]. With

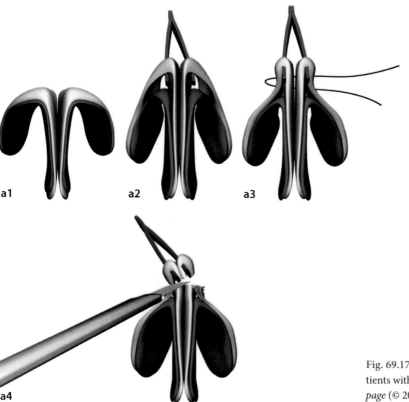

Fig. 69.17a–d Dome Truncation can be used in those patients with tip asymmetry. **a** Dome truncation. **b–d** *see next page* (© 2005 Russell W.H. Kridel, used with permission)

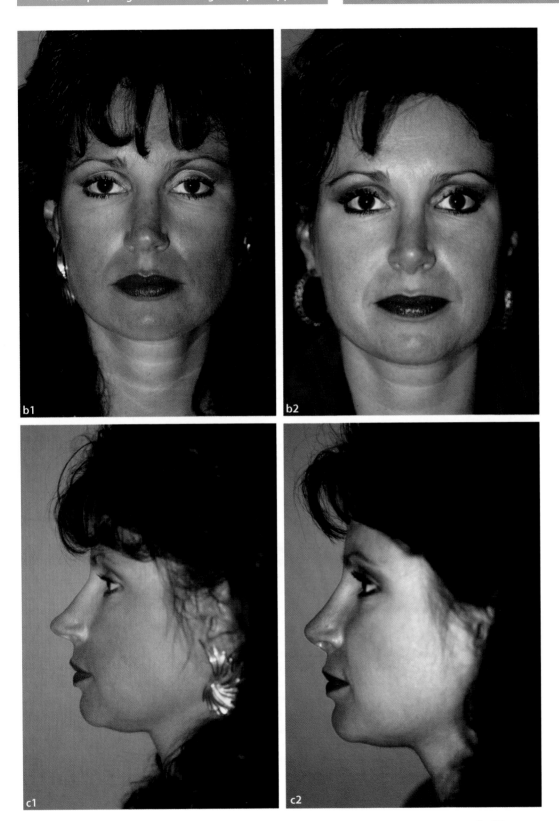

Fig. 69.17a–d Dome Truncation can be used in those patients with tip asymmetry. **a** Dome truncation. **b–d** Preoperative and 18-month postoperative Frontal, Profile, and Three Quarter views of patient who underwent dome truncation and cephalic trim (© 2005 Russell W.H. Kridel, used with permission)

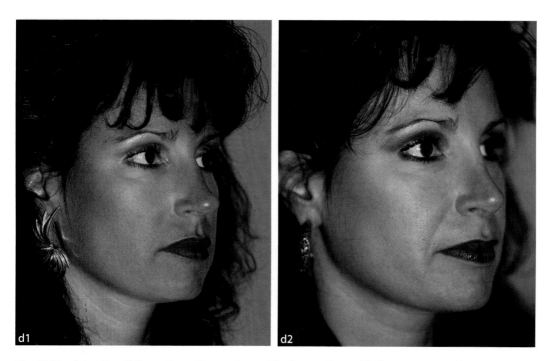

Fig. 69.17a–d (*continued*) Dome Truncation can be used in those patients with tip asymmetry. **a** Dome truncation. **b–d** Preoperative and 18-month postoperative Frontal, Profile, and Three Quarter views of patient who underwent dome truncation and cephalic trim (© 2005 Russell W.H. Kridel, used with permission)

both the LCO and the MCO, since no cartilage is excised and since sutures are used to control and maintain the correction, the overlapped crura maintain their integrity over years without buckling or any of the other associated complications. Moreover, with overlapping of cut cartilage segments, more strength is imparted to the correction. On the other hand, when cartilage segments are excised and sewn end-to-end as other authors advocate, the edges migrate with time and afford little stability. Our experience has shown that with the MCO and the overlap suturing of the cut ends, tip support can be maintained or obtained without the need for a columella strut. Because the edges are overlapped, we are not relying on a simple fibrous union and so there is much less likelihood of developing notching or collapse. In fact, the only case of MCO that needed revision in our experience was secondary to partial resorption of a piece of cartilage for an unrelated reason and not due to any tip irregularity arising from the MCO.

Of interest, numerous authors have pointed to the tripod theory and suggested that when the medial crura are shortened in relation to the lateral crura, there would be high tendency for alar flaring. That has not been our finding when the MCO is used. In fact, there were no cases were the MCO used alone ne-

cessitated alar base reduction. And even more surprising was our finding that in our entire deprojection experience only 7% of the patients needed alar base reduction, and that many of these patients desired this reduction prior to deprojection [8].

Conclusion

In all, we have found that this algorithm for nasal tip management allows the surgeon to follow a simple step-by-step plan to do proper tip analysis and to determine the techniques he/she can utilize to achieve the needed aesthetic goals. Most importantly, our long-term experience with these procedures has shown that when properly utilized, the algorithm can be used to accomplish projection or retrodisplacement of the tip with the desired changes required in tip rotation in a safe, functionally appropriate way. As with any rhinoplasty, tip asymmetries can arise. However, our tip revision rate of 4% and our finding that no patients had postoperative functional complaints allows us to feel confident that this algorithmic paradigm can be used to accomplish proper tip management in almost any circumstance.

Take-Home Pearls

- In order to reliably address the nasal tip, the surgeon must understand the correlation between the external nasal contour and the shape of the underlying tip cartilages. Once this relationship between the external tip shape and the underlying structure is understood, the surgeon can simplify nasal tip surgery to the techniques required in order to create a sound tip structure that will tolerate the forces of scar contracture over time.
- The most aesthetically pleasing nasal tips have an angle of dome defined with a convex domal segment and a flat lateral crus.
- The surgeon should be aware that a high dorsal septum and/or convex dome cartilages may be the source of supratip fullness.
- Prior to contouring the nasal tip, the surgeon must stabilize the columella and base of the nose.
- In those patients with a tension nose deformity, we recommend that attention first be directed toward lowering the overdeveloped cartilaginous dorsum, which often tents up the tip artificially.
- When overprojection is accompanied by tip ptosis, the LCO (which shortens the lower lateral crural leg) permits incremental retrodisplacement with increased rotation.
- The medial crural overlay (MCO), which shortens the medial crural leg of the tripod, leads to controlled deprojection and decreased rotation.
- When used together at the same surgical intervention (to shorten both tripod legs), the MCO and the LCO can effect large amounts of retrodisplacement with little effect on rotation.
- In those patients who are found to have overprojection and have pre-existing tip asymmetries or overtly thick skin, the decision may be made to proceed with dome truncation.
- If more tip projection is required than is provided by simple stabilization of the nasal base via the medial crura, the surgeon can look to additionally increase projection via a columellar strut, the double dome technique for minor increases or through the Lateral Crural Steal for greater projection. On those occasions when due to thick skin or weak cartilage sufficient projection is not possible via suture techniques, a shield tip graft can be utilized.

References

1. Kridel RWH, Scott B, Foda H (1999) The tongue-in-groove technique in septorhinoplasty. Arch Facial Plast Surg 1(4):246–256
2. McCollough EG, English JL (1985) A new twist in nasal tip surgery. An alternative to the Goldman tip for the wide or bulbous lobule. Arch Otolaryngol 111(8):524–529
3. Kridel RWH, Konior R, Shumrick K, Wright W (1991) Advances in nasal tip surgery. The lateral crural steal. In: Barton F (ed) Selected Readings in Plastic Surgery, vol 6. Dallas
4. Kridel RWH, Konior RJ (1991) Controlled nasal tip rotation via the lateral crural overlay technique. Arch Otolaryngol Head Neck Surg 117(4):411–415
5. Konior RJ, Kridel RWH (1993) Controlled nasal tip positioning via the open rhinoplasty approach. Facial Plast Surg Clin North Am 1(1):53–62
6. Soliemanzadeh P, Kridel RWH (2005) Nasal tip overprojection: Algorithm of surgical deprojection techniques and introduction of medial crural overlay. Arch Facial Plast Surg 7(6):374–380
7. Kridel RWH, Konior RJ (1990) Dome truncation for management of the overprojected nasal tip. Ann Plast Surg 24(5):385–396
8. Kridel RWH, Castellano R (2005) A simplified approach to alar base reduction: A review of 124 Patients over 20 years. Arch Facial Plast Surg 7(2)81–93
9. Daniel RK (1992) The nasal tip: Anatomy and aesthetics. Plast Reconstr Surg 89:216–224
10. Toriumi DM (2006) New concepts in nasal tip contouring. Arch Facial Plast Surg 8(3):156–185
11. Tebbets JB (1996) Rethinking the logic and techniques of primary tip rhinoplasty. A perspective of the evolution of surgery of the nasal tip. Clin Plast Surg 23:245–253
12. Crumley RM, Lanser M (1988) Quantitative analysis of nasal tip projection. Laryngoscope 98(2):202–208
13. Sheen JH, Sheen AP (1987) Aesthetic rhinoplasty, 2nd edn. Mosby, St. Louis, pp 70–74
14. Byrd HS, Hobar PC (1993) Rhinoplasty: A practical guide for surgical planning. Plast Reconstr Surg 91(4):642–654
15. McKinney P, Sweiss I (2002) A clinical definition of an ideal nasal radix. Plast Reconstr Surg 109(4):1416–1418
16. Tardy ME, Walter MA, Patt BS (1993) The overprojecting nose: Anatomic component, analysis and repair. Facial Plast Surg 9(4):306–317
17. Kridel RWH, Soliemanzadeh P (2006) Tip grafts in revision rhinoplasty. Facial Plast Surg Clin North Am 4:331–341
18. Kridel RWH, Konior RJ (1991) Controlled nasal tip rotation via the lateral cural overlay technique. Arch Otolaryngol Head Neck Surg 117:412
19. Webster RC, Smith RC. Lateral crural retrodisplacement for superior rotation of the tip in rhinoplasty. Aesthetic Plast Surg. 1979;3 65–78

Chapter 70

Revision Septorhinoplasty

70

Scott B. Roofe, Bryan T. Ambro, and Wayne F. Larrabee, Jr.

Core Messages

- Careful analysis and clear communication are of utmost importance in developing a surgical plan for revision rhinoplasty.
- The surgeon should emphasize maintenance of structural support and avoidance of destabilizing maneuvers.
- Osteotomies can be performed in a variety of ways to and should be precisely placed to avoid functional disruption.
- Camouflage techniques are a useful adjunct to restore cosmesis and avoid more disruptive techniques.

Contents

Introduction

Revision rhinoplasty is one of the most challenging tasks in facial plastic surgery. Even in experienced hands, revision may be necessary in 8–15% of cases [1]. Therefore, the possibility of additional surgery should be broached with all patients at the time of initial consultation. In addition to the patient's cosmetic and functional concerns, consultation for revision rhinoplasty may be complicated by frustration with their previous surgery. Open and direct communication should be used to convey realistic expectations after assessing the patient's desires and concerns. This consultation, along with a careful and systematic nasal and facial analysis, will help ensure a successful outcome.

As with the initial rhinoplasty, a detailed history and physical are essential. The history should address any previous trauma, cosmetic and functional concerns, allergies, medication and drug use. The physical exam should include anterior rhinoscopy, with and without topical decongestion. The septum, turbinates, external and internal nasal valves should be examined, and the nasal cavities inspected for nasal polyps. The external nasal exam, via inspection and palpation, allows for evaluation of the nasal skin as well as underlying structural support. Precise placement of a small elevator intranasally during nasal inspection will help isolate and define any areas of intranasal or external obstruction. Preoperative photographs are an essential component of the consultation. They serve to document any pre-existing naso-facial deformities and assist in presurgical planning. Reviewing these photographs with the patient will help them convey their concerns and discuss irregularities. Computer imaging can supplement the consultation. At times, further surgery may not improve the appearance and/or function of the nose and this should be conveyed clearly to the patient. It may be appropriate to refer the patient to a colleague for a second opinion.

Surgical Approach

Correction of deformities in revision cases may be approached externally or endonasally. The external approach provides excellent exposure to the middle and lower third of the nose for the precise placement of cartilaginous grafts. This approach involves raising the skin soft tissue envelope via a combination of transcolumellar and marginal incisions to expose the underlying bony and cartilaginous framework.

The endonasal approach provides less exposure and visualization, although it facilitates the creation of precise subcutaneous pockets for placement of grafts thus reducing the need for suturing. The endonasal approach offers minimal disruption of the nasal tip support structures decreasing the likelihood of postoperative tip ptosis. This approach can be more challenging especially in the presence of significant postsurgical scarring.

Surgical Anatomy

For purposes of analysis, the nose may be divided into horizontal upper, middle, and lower third segments. An understanding of the anatomic composition of each segment will help with the correction of associated anomalies.

Upper Third Deformities

70

Etiologies of upper third deformities after a prior rhinoplasty include over- or underreduction of the nasal dorsum, open roof deformities, asymmetries or incomplete osteotomies, and persistent septal deviation [2–4]. Collapsed nasal bones and overresection may lead to narrowing of the nasal airway and compromise breathing [3].

Surgical Management of the Upper Third Deformities

The management of postrhinoplasty deformities of the upper third of the nose can be quite variable and may require minimally invasive rasping or camouflage techniques, revision osteotomies, or major structural grafting.

Osteotomies

Osteotomies are commonly performed in both primary and revision rhinoplasty to reposition the nasal bones. Osteotomies are performed primarily to close an open nasal vault, straighten a deviated nasal septum, or narrow widened nasal sidewalls. Their use should be individualized based on the anatomical deformity one is trying to repair. Osteotomies may not be necessary in all cases of postrhinoplasty deformity and should be avoided if they may further destabilize the nose. In many instances, camouflage alone may suffice, avoiding any destabilization maneuvers that could compromise the nasal airway or cosmesis [3].

Osteotomies are generally classified as lateral, medial, and intermediate, referencing their course along the bony pyramid relative to midline. These may be modified according to the deformities being addressed. Lateral osteotomies are the most commonly performed in a "high-low-high" fashion, preserving a small triangle of bone at the piriform aperture to avoid airway compromise (Fig. 70.1). The "low-low" and "low-high" osteotomies are much less commonly used. When employing these techniques care must be taken to avoid postoperative nasal valve collapse. Osteotomies may be performed directly and linearly, or via a percutaneous perforating "postage-stamp" pattern. The percutaneous osteotomy is performed through a single stab incision on the skin of the nasal sidewall. Next, a series of small perforations are made in the bone along the lateral osteotomy path. This helps to better preserve the overlying periosteum while allowing the mobilization of the nasal bones [5]. A "push out" perforating osteotomy can lateralize n bones that are too medialized. A series of perforations are created intranly along a high-low-high lateral osteotomy path and the n bone is lateralized using an elevator (Fig. 70.2) [7]. Care should be taken to preserve as much of the overlying periosteum as possible in order to retain soft tissue support of the n bones after osteotomies. In some difficult cases, the nasal bones may collapse inward. This can be remedied by lightly packing the nose to support the bone until it heals in a favorable position. Another useful technique in this situation is to place a suture intranasally through the fractured segment and tie the two ends either over a bolster or through the perforations in the aquaplast dressing.

Medial osteotomies are performed to correct most twisted noses and ensure that fracture lines occur as desired by the surgeon. The nasal skin is thin and unforgiving in the region of the medial osteotomy thus irregularities can occur. Care must be taken to prevent overmobilization and collapse. The medial oblique osteotomy is performed by placing the osteotome between the nasal bone and the septum, and guiding it curvilinearly cephalad.

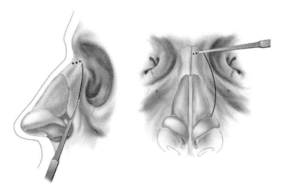

Fig. 70.1 The high-low-high osteotomy helps to preserve the airway after a lateral osteotomy. A transcutaneous perforating osteotomy may be added superiorly as necessary to complete the infracture

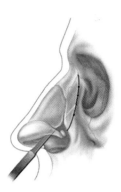

Fig. 70.2 "Push Out" perforating osteotomy is performed by creating a small number of perforations, directing the osteotome from Intranasally to outwards

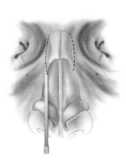

Fig. 70.3 The intermediate osteotomy is used in specific situations. These include reducing a marked nasal bone convexity or shortening an extremely long asymmetric nasal bone

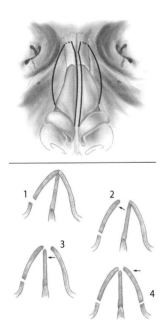

Fig. 70.4 Sequential osteotomies. The nose deviated significantly to one side can best be approached with a series of osteotomies, performed as if opening a book. In this example, a space for the deviated left nasal bone to move is created by moving the septum and right nasal bone first

Intermediate osteotomies are used less frequently but are indicated when the nasal sidewalls are of unequal height, in cases of a marked irregularity, convexity of the nasal bones or in the very wide nose. The intermediate osteotomy should be performed prior to the medial or lateral osteotomy, in order to provide stability during the maneuver. An intercartilaginous incision with a 3-mm osteotome at the midpoint or point of maximum convexity of the nasal bone (Fig. 70.3). Sequential osteotomies are indicated in the case of the extremely deviated nose. These osteotomies are performed sequentially beginning laterally contralateral to the direction of the deviation, creating a space in which to move the lateralized nasal bone. The technique is similar to turning the pages of an open book, where the nasal walls and septum represent the pages of the book (Fig. 70.4).

Osteotomies are not risk free and can result in worsening of nasal obstruction. Incomplete or greenstick fractures may fail to move the bony pyramid and correct the deformity [6]. Carrying lateral osteotomies too far cephalad may result in a rocker deformity, as the osteotomies extends into the thicker nasofrontal bone [5]. In order to correct this deformity, a 2-mm osteotome may be employed percutaneous to create an appropriate superior fracture line.

Camouflage

To avoid further destabilization it is important to preserve as much of the structural integrity of the nose as possible. Osteotomies can be potentially disruptive. Alternatively, camouflaging techniques can address nasal asymmetries and irregularities without further disrupting the structural integrity of the nose. Prior to placement of camouflaging agents described below, rasping of the bony irregularities and the bony dorsum may be necessary to optimize results.

Multiple techniques and materials have been advocated to camouflage with variable results. Autologous materials are favored over alloplasts because they are less likely to cause inflammation, fibrosis, or become infected. Septal cartilage is our first choice if there is sufficient material to repair the defect. In many revision cases due to the lack of septal cartilage, it may be necessary to harvest cartilage from one or both ears to obtain sufficient material. Harvested septal or auricular cartilage may be contoured to the desired size and shape, and morselized prior to placement. Dissection of precise pockets in the overlying soft tissues of the nose will allow for better stabilization of the graft. 5-0 or 6-0 permanent or resorbable sutures can be utilized to further stabilize these grafts.

If the appropriate amounts of septal and/or auricular cartilage are not available, other sources, such as costal cartilage, or alloplastic materials may be considered. Autologous costal cartilage is more desirable than radiated cadaveric rib cartilage, which has a higher incidence of warping and resorption [9]. Expanded polytetrafluoroethylene (e-PTFE), and polyglactin (Vicryl) mesh are commonly used synthetic materials. Processed acellular human dermis (Alloderm), porcine intestinal collagen (Surgisis), and collagen implant (EnduraGen) are useful for camouflage and minor augmentation. Hyaluronic acid (Restylane), human or bovine collagen, micronized acellular human dermis (Cymetra), and hydroxyapetite (Radiesse) have been advocated as camouflaging agents for injection in the dermal, subdermal, or subcutaneous plane. The injectable substances are temporary and thus require repeat treatments [10].

Cartilage and Bone Grafts

Cartilage and bone are used for structural support and major augmentation. Cartilage grafts are more easily carved, less metabolically demanding, and have a lower incidence of resorption than bone [8]. Costal cartilage is an option when septal and auricular cartilage are lacking, or where more support or a large volume is needed. Radiated rib cartilage is an option, particularly in the older patient where costal cartilage is ossified and difficult to harvest or carve. In some cases, bone grafting may be a suitable alternative, particularly if maximal structural support is needed. Portions of the perpendicular plate of the ethmoid or vomer may be utilized if only minimal support is needed; however, most cases requiring bony support need larger, more substantial quantities, harvested from calvarium or iliac bone. Iliac, rib, or calverial bone grafts may be considered in cases requiring structural support [9], keeping in mind that endochondral iliac bone is less likely to resorb [2]. The bony graft may be cantilevered with a percutaneously placed screw at the nasion for support, and the graft must often extend as far inferiorly as the nasal tip to provide the necessary support and to provide an aesthetic, uninterrupted dorsum.

Middle Third Anatomy and Associated Deformities

Postrhinoplasty deformities of the middle third of the nose often occur with deformities that affect the upper third as well. The "inverted V" deformity is often the result of overaggressive resection of the nasal dorsum, affecting both the upper and middle thirds of the nose. Soft tissue scarring can result in irregularities, whereas soft tissue contraction can make any prior nasal grafts more conspicuous [12, 13].

Deviation of the middle third may result in functional airway compromise as well as cosmetic concerns. Unilateral or bilateral collapse of an osteotomized nasal bone can result in an asymmetric middle third as well as obstruction [3].

Certain predisposing factors of the middle third of the nose, including a narrow middle vault and short nasal bones, create an increased risk for middle vault collapse following rhinoplasty. Constantian defines a narrow middle vault as any upper cartilaginous vault at least 25% narrower than either the upper or lower nasal thirds. He stresses the importance of recognizing such a narrowing to avoid postoperative deformities [11].

Surgical Management of the Middle Third Deformities

As with upper third deformities, surgeons can choose from a variety of techniques to address deformities of the middle third of the nose. Camouflaging, cartilage grafts, suturing techniques, and steroid injections are often utilized in this area. The patient should be evaluated for nasal obstruction and techniques selected to address the specific anatomical deformity.

Minor asymmetries of the middle third may be managed with camouflage techniques alone. Often onlay grafts of crushed or intact cartilage will be sufficient. They are placed in precise subcutaneous pockets, or directly sutured to the underlying soft tissue via an external approach. In the absence of nasal obstruction, injections of corticosteroids alone may be enough to address scarring from prior rhinoplasties.

Often, deformities of the middle third are due to overresection of the ULC, or failure to appropriately reapproximate the ULC to the nasal septum [14]. In the absence of nasal obstruction, this malposition may be corrected by simply reapproximating the ULC to the nasal septum using permanent or resorbable mattress sutures. In many cases however—particularly when there is functional compromise due to overresection and collapse of ULC—placement of spreader grafts may be necessary [15]. Although there is some disagreement as to the benefit of spreader grafts on nasal obstruction, their placement will often correct cosmetic asymmetries. Spreader grafts may be placed bilaterally if the deformity is symmetric, or unilaterally in selected asymmetric cases. More often, for asymmetry, it is best to place spreader grafts that have been fashioned asymmetrically in their thickness, rather than unilateral grafts [3]. In cases of saddle nose deformity, an onlay spreader graft may improve both middle third narrowing, as well as dorsal deformities described below [16].

Profile Deformities of the Middle and Upper Third of the Nose

Dorsal deformities, by definition, involve the middle and upper third of the nose. The most common major deformities of the dorsum are pollybeak deformities and saddle nose deformities.

The pollybeak deformity is a manifestation of supratip fullness, resulting from inadequate resection of the ULC, or septal angle [4]. Overresection in the lower one third can result in poor tip support and a relative pollybeak deformity. Addressing poor nasal tip support and projection may alleviate the appearance of the pollybeak, without the need to manipulate the dorsum [20]. In selected cases where soft tissue scarring creates supratip fullness, subdermal corticosteroid injections may improve this deformity.

The saddle deformity is a result of excessive removal of dorsal bone or cartilage. Correction requires augmentation with septal or auricular cartilage grafts, costal cartilage grafts, autogenous bone, irradiated cadaver rib, or alloplasts. A number of alloplastic materials exist such as Mersilene mesh (Ethicon Corporation, Somerville, NJ), Medpore, e-PTFE, and silicone. Of these, e-PTFE (Gore-Tex, WL Gore and Associates, Flagstaff, AZ) is least likely to cause persistent inflammation and rejection [8)].

Lower Third Deformities

The lower third complications are most commonly associated with overresection of the lower lateral cartilages or disruption of the major or minor tip support mechanisms. Most commonly there is overresection of the lateral crura. Conceptually one should approach these deformities with the goal of reconstituting the tip support mechanisms as best possible using autogenous cartilage. More minor asymmetries of the lower third can be corrected using camouflage techniques.

Surgical Management of Lower Third Deformities

Tip deformities may be approached via an endonasal, or external approach. Reconstruction of the lower third must be individualized to the anatomical deficits in each situation. Typical revision cases are provided as examples (cases 1, 2, and 4) to describe grafts frequently used. Grafts we commonly use in nasal lower one third reconstruction and are demonstrated in the cases (1–4) and include struts, shield tip grafts, CAP grafts, lateral crural replacement grafts, lateral crural strut grafts, alar batten grafts, and extended tip batten grafts. Every attempt is made preoperatively to evaluate the nose and determine which grafts are most appropriate but the actual decisions are made at the time of surgery by evaluating the anatomy and determining which grafts will override better results.

Alar retraction presents a specific problem. Alar retraction often results from lateral crura overresection, but may also follow excision of vestibular skin. Retraction of the ala results from overlying soft tissue scar contraction with little inherent support remaining in the weakened, overresected cartilage. Correction of alar retraction typically involves cartilage-grafting techniques. Mild cases may be improved by placement of cartilage grafts along the inferior margin LLC, while more severe cases often require auricular composite grafts to restore both cartilaginous support and vestibular lining.

Nasal Septal Revision

Persistent deviation of the caudal septum is a common cause of lower nasal third asymmetry. Mobilizing the quadrangular cartilage along the inferior and posterior margins and realigning the septum in the midline usually corrects dislocations of the septum from the maxillary crest. Treatment of more severe caudal septal deformities may require resection, scoring, or splinting of a portion of the caudal septum. Caudal septal extension grafts are commonly used. In extreme cases, extracorporeal septoplasty may be necessary. This involves resection, extracorporeal straightening, and reimplantation of the nasal septum [23].

In addition to its role as support mechanism for the nasal dorsum and tip, its relationship to the ULC in forming the nasal valve plays a significant role in the nasal airway. Untreated nasal septal deviation may contribute to persistent deflection of the nose as well as to obstruction. The most common septal deviations affecting nasal symmetry are those involving the dorsal and caudal parts of the quadrangular cartilage.

To assist in straightening the middle third, the ULC may be released from the nasal septum and then reapproximated in the appropriate position. Violation of the nasal mucosa should be avoided to prevent scarring in the area of the nasal valve, and to maintain soft tissue support of the ULC. Combinations of maneuvers including scoring of the cartilage, suturing to periosteum, and resection of cartilage may be used to straighten the nasal septum [20]. Batten grafts compromised of bone, cartilage, or alloplastic materials may be used as supporting mechanisms for the caudal septum or the middle third. Unilateral or bilateral spreader grafts may be placed between the upper lateral cartilage and the nasal septum. One of the grafts may be made thicker to correct asymmetry if bilateral grafts are placed [6]. Septal deviation should be addressed carefully in the revision case. Further resection, particularly in the patient who has undergone submucous resection, may result in loss of dorsal or tip support. It is imperative that an appropriate amount of cartilage be maintained. The patient is at increased risk of septal perforation in these revision cases.

Cases

The following four cases are recent ones from our practice demonstrating typical approaches to these complex problems. The accompanying diagrams demonstrate the multiple grafts utilized.

Case One

Patient is a 48-year-old woman who had had two previous rhinoplasties. She presented with aesthetic and functional concerns. On physical examination she had septal deviation, internal and external valve collapse, minimal tip support, minimal cartilage present in the tip to palpation, and a relative pollybeak deformity. She was reconstructed with auricular and septal cartilage grafts. Structural grafts used include a strut, bilateral alar batten grafts, bilateral spreader grafts, and a shield graft (Fig. 70.5a–i).

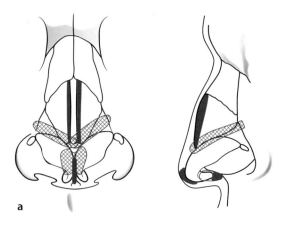

a

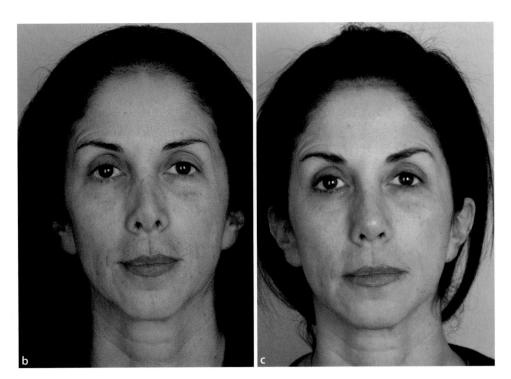

Fig. 70.5a–i Case 1 (*continuing next page*)

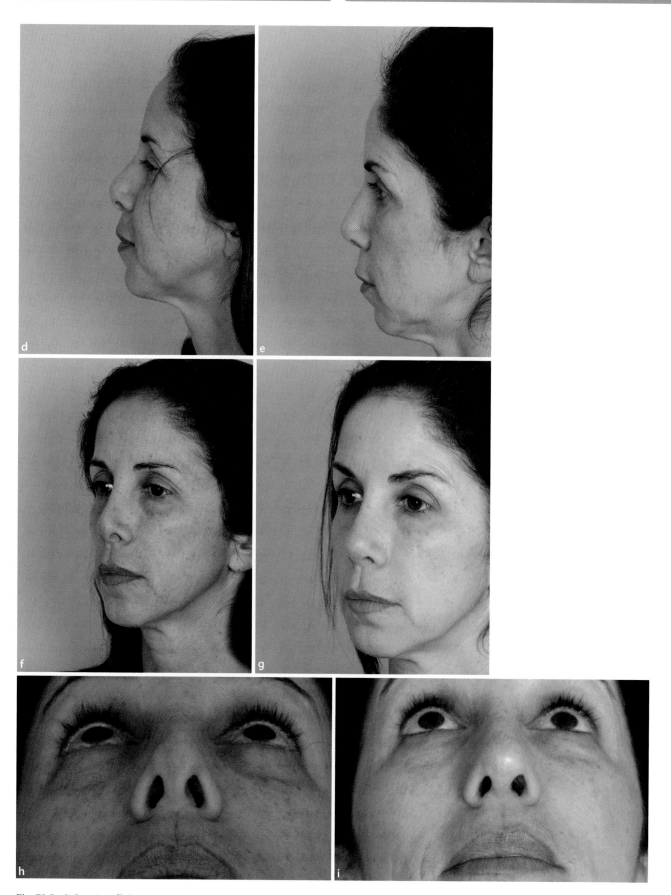

Fig. 70.5a–i *(continued)* Case 1

Case Two

This patient is a 45-year-old woman who presented with a complex history of previous rhinoplasty. She had had her first rhinoplasty at age nineteen. She subsequently had two procedures performed by other surgeons, and finally at approximately age twenty-five had a reconstruction using auricular cartilage grafts. On examination she presented with an inverted "V" deformity, internal and external valve collapse, dorsal irregularities, and poor tip symmetry. She underwent an open nasal reconstruction with auricular and septal cartilage grafts, to include bilateral spreader grafts, shield tip graft, strut, and bilateral lateral crural strut grafts (Fig. 70.6a–i).

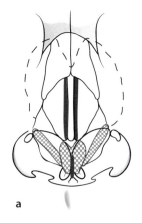
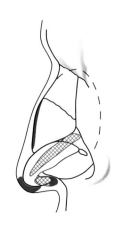

a

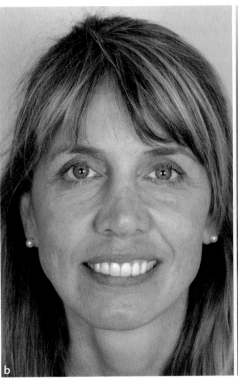
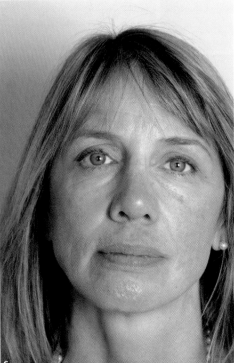

b   c

Fig. 70.6a–i Case 2 *(continuing next page)*

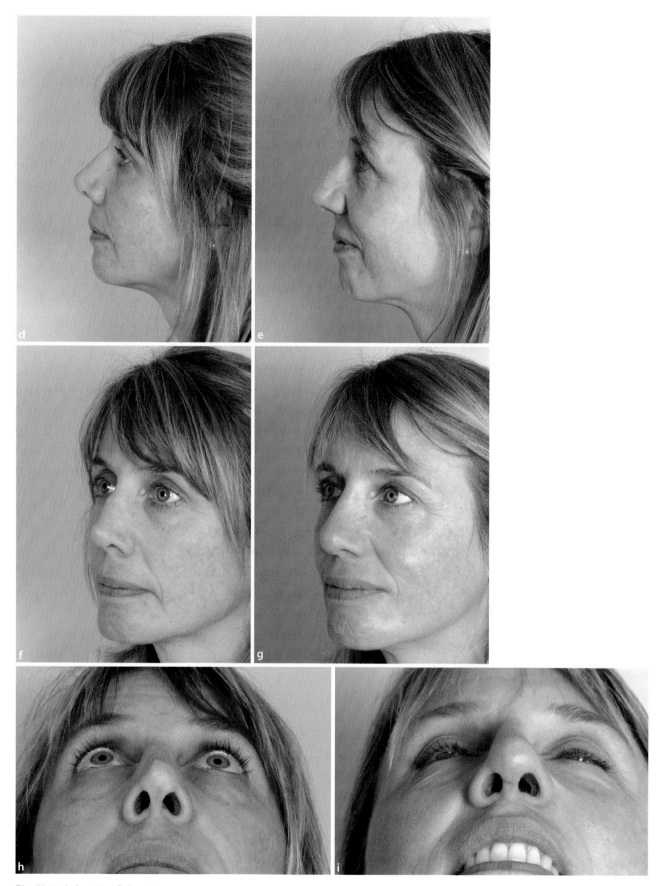

Fig. 70.6a–i *(continued)* Case 2

Case Three

This patient is a 29-year-old man who approximately 7 years ago had an auto accident, and his nose was repaired, in another state with a series of operations. The second surgeon utilized a rib graft. The patient developed a postoperative deformity with warping and partial resorption of the rib graft resulting in a saddle nose deformity. He did not wish to undergo another rib graft procedure. His breathing was unremarkable with no significant functional problems. The nose was repaired through an open approach by reshaping the underlying rib graft and augmenting it with a Gortex dorsal nasal implant (Fig. 70.7a–i).

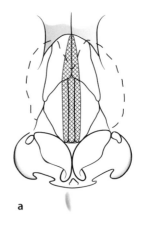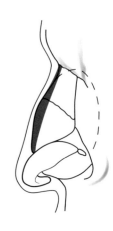

a

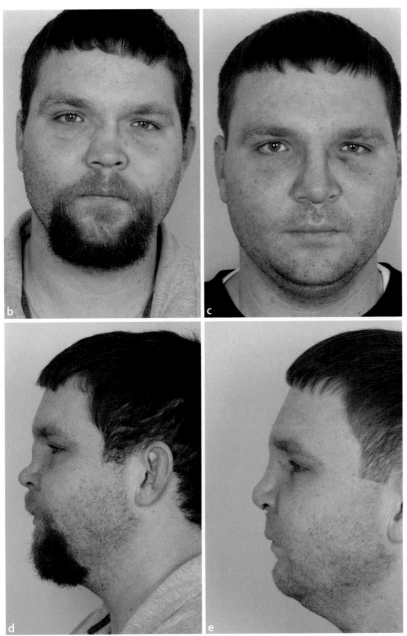

b

c

d

e

Fig. 70.7a–e   Case 3

Case Four

This 84-year-old woman presented with nasal obstruction. She had had a rhinoplasty many years ago and presented with collapse of the tip, and external and internal valve collapse. She underwent an open nasal reconstruction with septal and auricular cartilage grafts including an extended tip columellar batten graft, bilateral lateral alar replacement grafts, and a dorsal graft. She additionally underwent a lip lift procedure to shorten her long upper lip (Fig. 70.8a–i).

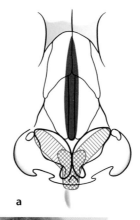
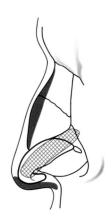

a

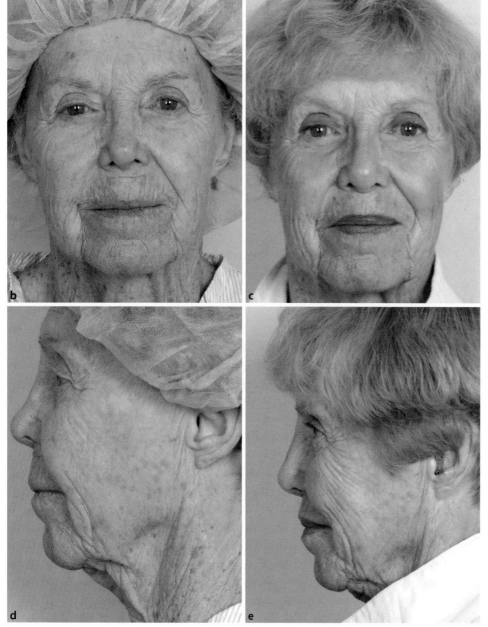

b   c

d   e

Fig. 70.8a–i Case 4

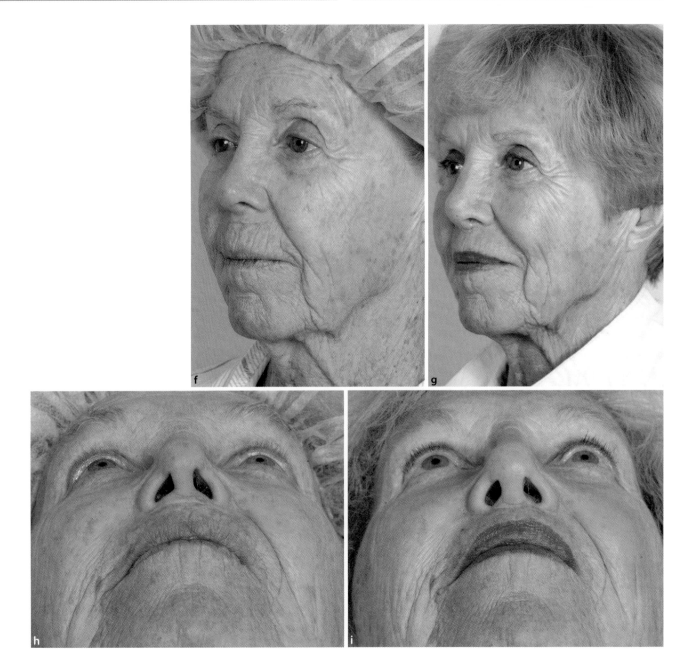

Fig. 70.8a–i Case 4 *(continued)*

Conclusion

Although revision rhinoplasty surgery can be challenging, successful revision surgery may be a source of satisfaction for both the patient and the surgeon. Careful analysis and clear and constant communication with the patient are imperative. A systematic approach, dividing the nose into thirds, facilitates surgical planning.

References

1. Quatela VC, Wayne I (2000) Challenges of secondary rhinoplasty. Facial Plast Surg Clin North Am 8:515–537
2. Bagal AA, Adamson PA (2002) Revision rhinoplasty. Facial Plast Surg 18(4):233–243
3. Murakami CS, Younger RL (1995) Management of the post-rhinoplasty crooked nose. Facial Plast Clin North Am 3(4):1–27
4. Simons RL, Gallo IF (1994) Rhinoplasty complications. Facial Plast Surg Clin North Am 2:521–529
5. Murakami CS, Larrabee WF (1992) Comparison of osteotomy techniques in the treatment of nasal fractures. Facial Plast Surg 8(4):209–219
6. Porter JP, Toriumi DM (2002) Surgical techniques for management of the crooked nose. Aesthetic Plast Surg 26 (Suppl)1:18
7. Byrne PJ, Walsh WE, Hilger PA (2003 The use of the "inside-out" lateral osteotomies to improve outcome in rhinoplasty. Arch Facial Plast Surg 5:251–255
8. Khurana D, Sherris DA (1999) Grafting materials for augmentation septorhinoplasty. Facial Plast Surg 7(4):210–216
9. Quatela VC, Jacono AA (2002) Structural grafting in rhinoplasty. Facial Plast Surg 18(4):223–232
10. Sclafani AP, Romo T, Barnett JG, Barnett CR (2003) Adjustments of subtle postoperative nasal defects: Managing the "near-miss" rhinoplasty. Facial Plast Surg 19(4):349–361
11. Constantian MB (2000) Four common anatomic variants that predispose to unfavorable rhinoplasty results: A study based on 150 consecutive secondary rhinoplasties. Plast Reconstr Surg 105(1):316–331
12. Kamer FM, McQuown SA (1988) Revision rhinoplasty: Analysis and treatment. Arch Otolaryngol Head Neck Surg 114:257–266
13. Rohrich RJ (1999) Treatment of the nasal hump with preservation of the cartilaginous framework. Plast Reconstr Surg 103(6):1734–1735
14. Toriumi DM (1995) Management of the middle nasal vault in rhinoplasty: Operative techniques. Plast Reconstr Surg 2:16–30
15. Sheen JN (1984) Spreader graft: A method of reconstructing the roof of the middle nasal vault following rhinoplasty. Plast Reconstr Surg 73:230–237
16. Murakami CS (2004) Nasal valve collapse. Ear Nose Throat J 83(3):163–164
17. Paniello RC (1996) Nasal valve suspension. An effective treatment for nasal valve collapse. Arch Otolaryngol Head Neck Surg 122(12):1342–1346
18. Clark JM, Cook TA (2002) The 'butterfly' graft in functional secondary rhinoplasty. Laryngoscope 112(11):1917–1925
19. Park SS (1998) The flaring suture to augment the repair of the dysfunctional nasal valve. Plast Reconstr Surg 101:1120–1122
20. Foda HM (2005) Rhinoplasty for the multiply revised nose. Am J Otolaryngol 26:28–34
21. Johnson CM, Toriumi DM, Friedman CD (1990) Revision rhinoplasty. In: Johnson CM, Toriumi DM (eds) Open Structure Rhinoplasty. Saunders, Philadelphia, pp 411–511
22. Becker DG (2002) Complications of rhinoplasty. In: Papel ID, Nachlas NE (eds) Facial plastic and reconstructive surgery. Thieme, New York, pp 452–460
23. Gubisch (2005) Extracorporeal septoplasty. Arch Facial Plast Surg 7(4):218–226

Chapter 71

Aesthetic Reconstruction of the Platyrrhine Nose

71

Thomas Romo and Paul Presti

Core Messages

- Porous polyethylene implants provide a reliable option in augmentation of the platyrrhine nose.
- Understanding and implementing appropriate aesthetic norms is mandatory in this type of rhinoplasty.
- Meticulous placement of multiple implants is faciliated through the open surgical approach.

Contents

Introduction

Increasing demand for facial plastic surgery especially within the African American and Asian American population has lead to further investigation of these ethnic aesthetics and anatomic stereotypes. In turn the challenges of dealing with the "ethnic nose" are on the forefront of rhinoplasty advancement as patient's expectations are not easily addressed with classic operative techniques.

Added to the complexity of the subject is the difficultly with which we define and address the African American and Asian nose. Many (including the author) argue that these patients should not be treated as a homogenous cohort [1, 2, 33]. A paradigm shift in nomenclature is necessary when discussing the Negroid or Asiatic nose since these are misnomers— as the anatomic variability within each respective community abounds [19, 24] It is more appropriate, rather, to discuss the surgical refinement of the *Platyrrhine* nose which is commonly found within the Asian-American and African-American community. This nomenclature is used to invoke concepts of nasal anatomy subtypes rather than erroneously stereotyped ethnic "nasal structure."

Rhinoplasty of the platyrrhine should not intend to anglicize the nose. Patients with a platyrrhine nose looking to transform them into a leptorrhine nose or that in line with the Caucasian aesthetic do not have reasonable expectations. More importantly, such an endpoint is incongruous with their respective ethnic features. The majority of ethnic patients seeking surgery are not looking to appear more Caucasian [6, 11] For most patients the endpoint of surgery is the improvements of aesthetics without losing their ethnic identity. The objective of the facial plastic surgeon is to restore harmony of facial features and provide symmetry to asymmetric anatomy.

Nasal Structural Anatomy

Several common elements define the platyrrhine nose. In contrast to the leptorrhine nose, with sharp well-demarcated anatomy, the platyrrhine nose does not reveal the structure beneath its skin envelope [25]. This is related to the thick sebaceous in-elastic skin overlying the wide, low dorsum and nasal tip. Under the skin lies a 2- to 4-mm thick fibrofatty layer of connective tissue. Surprisingly, the alar cartilages are always present (contrary to common thought) and similar in size to the leptorrhine nose [18, 24]. The piriform aperture and nares are oval in shape and the alae flare out laterally [21]. An acute naso-labial angle is combined with a shorter, more rounded columella, and a short nasal spine that does not project the tip [25]. In sum, the platyrrhine nose lacks internal support, has a thick unrevealing skin envelope and, projects poorly (Fig. 71.1).

Given the flaccid nature of the structural components in the platyrrhine nose, aesthetic reconstruction requires implementation of architectural support. Autologous and homologous graft material and alloplast implants have all been considered for this purpose. Nasal septal cartilage is considered the ideal graft material in rhinoplasty because it does not require a separate operative site to harvest, and it is usually straight and carves easily. Moreover, septal cartilage has proven to maintain its shape over time without the tendency to warp or resorb. However, sufficient septal cartilage is often not available for use. In addition to those cases with a history of prior surgery or trauma, it has been our experience that septal cartilage is often lacking in the platyrrhine nose. Excessive resection of septal support can cause saddle nose deformity and worsen the structural integrity of the platyrrhine nose.

Auricular cartilage may be harvested, but its utility is often restricted due to the innate curvature of conchal cartilage and the difficulty in carving the appropriate shape. Ortiz-Monasterio and Michelena described the use of rib cartilage for the correction of the platyrrhine nose, but long term warping of the graft has posed a significant problem [20]. Split calvarium, iliac, olecranon, and other bony graft material have also been proposed for use in reconstructive ethnic rhinoplasty, but these options entail significant additional morbidity not acceptable to the aesthetic patient. Rohrich and Muzaffar reported their use of acellular dermis (AlloDerm) in platyrrhine noses requiring 2- to 5-mm dorsal augmentation [24]. Almost all homologous graft material and many autologous grafts are prone to resorption or fracture. All autologous graft materials, excluding nasal septal cartilage, are saddled with the inherent and potentially significant morbidity of a second operative donor site and additional operative time.

Synthetic materials offer ease of availability and may be easily carved. For these reasons, a number of synthetic materials have been introduced for use in nasal reconstruction: silicone rubber [Silastic], polyamide mesh [Supramid], polytetrafluoroethylene carbon [Proplast, Teflon], polypropylene mesh [Prolene], polyethylene terephthalate [Mersilene mesh], and expanded polytetrafluoroethylene [e-PTFE, Gore-Tex]. However, high rates of infection and extrusion, in addition to the excessive fibrosis and contracture due to chronic foreign body response have left many surgeons dissatisfied with most synthetic materials. Most of these implant materials are not rigid enough to provide structural support, and have been used primarily for augmentation purposes. L-shaped silicone struts do provide some structural support and have been used in platyrrhine rhinoplasty, especially Asians [10, 11]. It has been proposed that the implant is offered better protection by the thicker overlying skin. Deva et al. reviewed their experience with silicone nasal implants in 422 patients, the majority (98%) of which were South-East Asian women [5]. The study highlighted a 9.7% complication rate (due to hemorrhage, displacement, extrusion, overprominence, supratip deformity, and excessive pressure) requiring removal of the graft, and a 15.8% patient dissatisfaction rate. Tham et al. reported a 16% total complication rate with 8% being categorized as being major complications (e.g., implant removal) in a group of 355 consecutive patients, using silicone augmentation [31].

There have been several reports of nasal augmentation using Gore-Tex. Godin et al. presented their results using Gore-Tex for augmentation in 309 patients during a 10-year period [8]. Their overall complication rate (cases necessitating implant removal) was 3.2%, with a significantly greater proportion of complications in cases of revision rhinoplasty. Mendelsohn and Dunlop reported a 20% complication rate (6 of 30 patients) in using Gore-Tex augmentation in rhinoplasty with a minimum 18-month follow-up. Three cases (10%) required removal of the implant [15]. However, there have been case series with long-term follow-up that have not had any complications using Gore-Tex for rhinoplastic augmentation [12].

In our opinion, PHDPE implants offer all of the benefits of alloplasts without any of the significant disadvantages found with the other implant materials. Medpor implants are rigid and provide excellent structural support. Carving is easy and takes

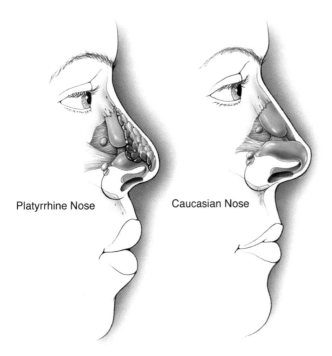

Fig. 71.1 Lateral view comparing the structure of the leptorrhine nose (*left*) with the platyrrhine nose (*right*). Note the reduced dorsal bony and cartilaginous support and the prominent subcutaneous fibrofatty tissue pad, resulting in less tip projection and definition in the platyrrhine nose

Platyrrhine Nose

Caucasian Nose

71

minimal time. If necessary, the implant can be molded to the desired contour by heating with hot water or saline in the operating theater, but after implantation, the material permanently holds its shape. Medpor's large pore size (average 150 μm) allows fibrovascular ingrowth, promoting stability and resistance to infection. In 1998, Romo et al. published a retrospective review of 187 patients who had undergone nasal reconstruction with Medpor implants (66 patients for non-Caucasian rhinoplasty, and 121 patients for revision surgery) [26]. Postoperative follow-up ranged from 6 months to 3.5 years, with an average of 26 months. Complications were limited to five patients (2.6%), all of whom had impaired healing secondary to heavy smoking, cocaine abuse, collagen vascular disease, or multiple previous surgeries. Of these, three patients had early infection and two patients had delayed infection necessitating implant removal. Implants were easily removed, without damage to the overlying soft tissue and skin envelope.

Porous high-density polyethylene implants are well tolerated in the platyrrhine nose, and provide a suitable alloplast material for augmentation rhinoplasty.

Porous High Density Polyethylene Implants in Aesthetic Reconstruction of the Platyrrhine Nose

The authors experience with PHDPE implants is extensive and the success derived from its implementation is reflective of its utility.

From January 1993 to January 2004, a total of 243 patients underwent aesthetic reconstruction of the platyrrhine nose using multiple PHDPE implants.

During the preoperative evaluation of this patient population, meticulous rhinoplasty analysis was performed, with special attention to platyrrhine features amenable to correction with PHDPE implants. The lack of bony and cartilaginous nasal support; the shape, relative weakness, and pliability of the upper and lower lateral cartilages; the lack of tip projection, rotation, and definition; and the width of the alae and any deficiency in the premaxillary area were all evaluated in this regard. The skin and soft tissue envelope were examined carefully to determine if there was sufficient subcutaneous padding to provide adequate coverage of the alloplast implants. Patients who were heavy smokers or who had dermatologic, collagen vascular, or other systemic disease that could compromise flap viability were screened out. Similarly, patients who had poorly controlled diabetes or active HIV disease, those on immuno-suppressive therapy, or those who were in any way immuno-compromised, were excluded. All patients were informed and accepted the risks and potential complications of using an alloplast implant.

Two different types of prefabricated PHDPE implants were used (Medpor surgical implants, Porex Surgical, Inc., College Park, GA): the 1.1-mm thick sheet and the large nasal dorsum implant, 8-mm height × 66-mm length (Fig. 71.2). The 1.1-mm sheet was cut and fashioned into a columella strut and multiple small premaxillary plumper implants. The dorsum implant was used with or without the tip component, depending on the type of augmentation desired. The optimal size, shape, and placement of the implants were customized based on the preoperative structural analysis of the platyrrhine features of the nose and the individual aesthetic needs of each patient. An autogenous septal cartilage graft was used to contour the infratip lobule.

The external decortication approach was used in all patients. This facilitated raising the skin flap in the appropriate subcutaneous plane above the prominent fibrofatty pad found typically in the platyrrhine nose, and also helped with the accurate placement of the PHDPE implants (Fig. 71.3a, b). The small particle plumper grafts were inserted at the base of the nasal spine via the inferior transcolumella incision (Fig. 71.4). The columella strut was positioned between the medial crura, cut to appropriate size, and secured with through-and-through 5-0 Monocryl sutures at the base and subdome region of the medial crura. A 5-0 Prolene dome binding stitch was then placed at the domal angle. Osteotomies and alar base reduction were performed in each patient as deemed necessary. The large dorsum-tip implant was carved to the appropriate shape using a #10 scalpel blade, and inset precisely into the preformed pocket along the nasal bridge. An autogenous carved septal cartilage shield graft was then secured anterior and inferior to the tip component of the implant with 6-0 Prolene sutures, rounding and correctly contouring the infratip lobule. The skin envelope was then redraped, and the columella incision was closed with two 6-0 nylon vertical mat-

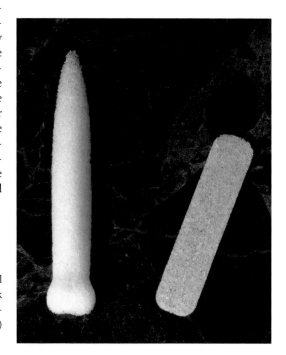

Fig. 71.2 PHDPE implants shown prior to carving (Medpor surgical implants, Porex Surgical, Inc., College Park, GA). The 1.1-mm thick sheet is used to create a columella strut and premaxillary plumper implants. The large nasal dorsum implant (8-mm height × 66-mm length) is carved appropriately and used for dorsum and tip augmentation

Fig. 71.3a,b Three quarter view and submental view of
PHDPE implant placement in the platyrrhine nose. The
nasal dorsal-tip implant, columella strut, and premaxillary plumper implants are shown. The autogenous
cartilage shield graft is depicted as transparent. Note
suture placement in the submental view. *Inset*: Preoperative platyrrhine nose

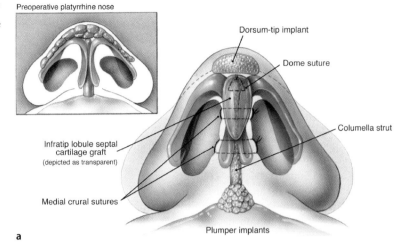

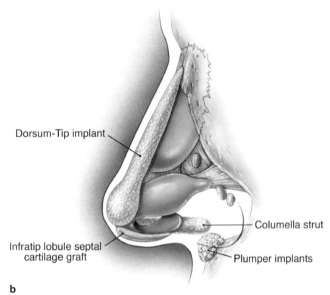

Fig. 71.4 Placement of
small particle premaxil-
lary plumper implants,
columella strut implant,
dorsal tip implant, and
infratip lobule septal
cartilage graft, all inset
precisely through an
external rhinoplasty
approach

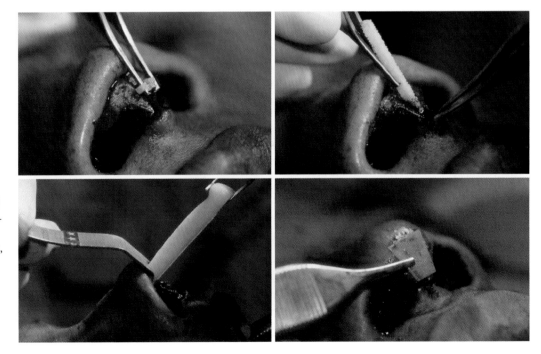

tress sutures alternating with multiple simple sutures to relieve the tension along the incision line. The marginal incisions were closed with simple 5-0 chromic stitches.

All implants were soaked in gentamycin solution prior to placement, and stringent sterile technique was observed throughout. Patients received one dose of perioperative intravenous antibiotic. An Aquaplast splint was placed on the nasal dorsum to stabilize the dorsal implant, regardless of osteotomies being performed. The sutures and splints were removed by the fifth to seventh postoperative day.

Results

Overall patient satisfaction was excellent (Fig. 71.5a, b). Minor complications occurred in five of the 243 patients (1.5%).

Early in our experience, one patient had lateral exposure of the columella strut, which was addressed by resection of the area of exposed implant, and primary closure of the columella soft tissue. With the addition of two vertical mattress sutures to close the columella incision and help relieve tension along the suture line, there have been no further problems with wound healing.

Four patients had slightly asymmetric placement or healing of the dorsal-tip implant (Fig. 71.6). This was rectified in each case by a simple touch-up procedure involving removal and re-

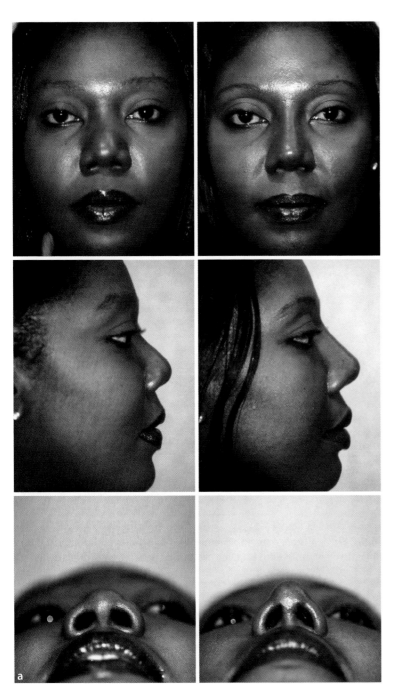

Fig. 71.5a–c Preoperative (*left*) and 1-year postoperative (*right*) views of representative African American and Asian patients after aesthetic platyrrhine rhinoplasty using multiple PHDPE implants as described in the text

Fig. 71.5a–c (*continued*) Preoperative (*left*) and 1-year postoperative (*right*) views of representative African American and Asian patients after aesthetic platyrrhine rhinoplasty using multiple PHDPE implants as described in the text

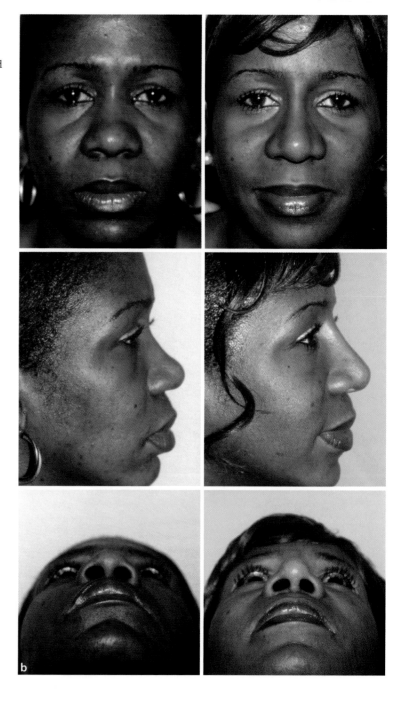

71

placement of the dorsum implant in the correct position. Despite tissue ingrowth and fixation of the implant, no difficulty was encountered in dissecting and freeing the implant, and no damage was evident to the overlying skin flap. In order to precisely inset and secure the dorsum implant during the first few days when the implant is most likely to shift, the authors currently mark the exact position of the implant and use a temporary 4-0 prolene stitch to guide placement of the implant and fix the implant in position.

There were no other major or minor complications associated with PHDPE implant use in this patient population, including no instance of implant infection or late extrusion.

Conclusion

There are certain features that define the platyrrhine nose. Bone and cartilage support is deficient, resulting in a wide dorsum

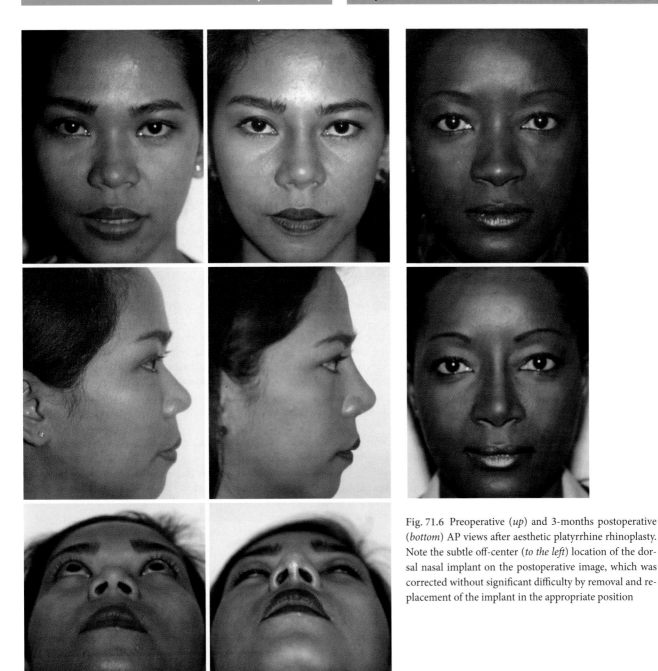

Fig. 71.6 Preoperative (*up*) and 3-months postoperative (*bottom*) AP views after aesthetic platyrrhine rhinoplasty. Note the subtle off-center (*to the left*) location of the dorsal nasal implant on the postoperative image, which was corrected without significant difficulty by removal and replacement of the implant in the appropriate position

Fig. 71.5a–c (*continued*) Preoperative (*left*) and 1-year postoperative (*right*) views of representative African American and Asian patients after aesthetic platyrrhine rhinoplasty using multiple PHDPE implants as described in the text

with poor anterior projection. The lack of skeletal support, in addition to thick skin and a prominent subcutaneous fibrofatty pad, contribute to a poorly projected tip that is amorphous and lacks definition. This is compounded by the smaller nasal spine in the platyrrhine nose with the resulting retracted columella [2]. The nasal alae tend to be wide and flared, and the premaxillary area hypoplastic.

Autologous cartilage and bone are considered optimal grafting material to provide aesthetic augmentation of the platyrrhine nose, but their supply is often limited and harvesting entails additional morbidity. Many synthetic materials have been introduced in nasal reconstruction, but high infection and extrusion rates have limited their use. Porous high-density polyethylene (PHDPE) implants present an alternative to autologous material as they allow for fibrovascular ingrowth, leading to stability of the implant and decreased infection rates.

References

1. Aung SC, Foo CL, Lee ST (2000) Three dimensional laser scan assessment of the oriental nose with a new classification of oriental nasal types. Br J Plast Surg 53:109–116
2. Baker HL, Krause CJ (1984) Update on the Negroid nose: An anatomic and anthropometric analysis. In: Ward PH, Berman WE (eds) Plastic and Reconstructive Surgery of the Head and Neck. Mosby, St. Louis
3. Burres SA (1999) Acoustic rhinometry of the oriental nose. Am J Rhinol 13:407–410
4. Canbay EI, Bhatia SN (1997) A comparison of nasal resistance in white Caucasians and blacks. Am J Rhinol 11:73–75
5. Deva AK, Merten S, Chang L (1998) Silicone in nasal augmentation rhinoplasty: A decade of clinical experience. Plast Reconstr Surg 102:1230–1237
6. Falces E, Wesser D, Gorney M (1970) Cosmetic surgery of the non-Caucasian nose. Plast Reconstr Surg 45:317–325
7. Fanous N, Yoskovitch A (2000) Premaxillary augmentation: Adjunct to rhinoplasty. Plast Reconstr Surg 106:707–712
8. Godin MS, Waldman R, Johnson CM (1999) Nasal augmentation using Gore-Tex: A 10-year experience. Arch Facial Plast Surg 1:118–121
9. Hubbard TJ (1998) Bridge narrowing in ethnic noses. Ann Plast Surg 40:214–218
10. Khoo BC (1964) Augmentation rhinoplasty in the Orientals. Plast Reconstr Surg 34:81–88
11. Larrabee WF Jr, Nishioka GL (1998) Surgery of the non-Caucasian nose. In: Bailey BJ, Tardy ME Jr (eds) Head & Neck Surgery—Otolaryngology. Lippincott, New York, pp 2648-2655
12. Lohuis PJ, Watts SJ, Vuyk HD (2001) Augmentation of the nasal dorsum using Gore-Tex: Intermediate results of a retrospective analysis of experience in 66 patients. Clin Otolaryngol Allied Sci 26:214–217
13. Malory WE Jr, Falces E (1986) Non-Caucasian rhinoplasty: 16 year experience. Plast Reconstr Surg 77:239–251
14. McKinney PW, Mossie RD, Bailey MH (1988) Calibrated alar base excision: A 20-year experience. Aesthetic Plast Surg 12:71–75
15. Mendelsohn M, Dunlop G (1998) Gore-Tex augmentation grafting in rhinoplasty—is it safe? J Otolaryngol 27:337–341
16. Neu BR (2000) Segmental bone and cartilage reconstruction of major nasal dorsal defects. Plast Reconstr Surg 106:160–170
17. Odofile FA (1994) Nasal bones and pyriform apertures in blacks. Ann Plast Surg 32:21–26
18. Ofodile FA, James EA (1997) Anatomy of alar cartilages in blacks. Plast Reconstr Surg 100:699–703
19. Ofodile FA, Bokhari FJ, Ellis C (1993) The Black American nose. Ann Plast Surg 31:209–219
20. Ortiz-Monasterio F, Michelena J (1988) The use of augmentation rhinoplasty techniques for the correction of the non-Caucasian nose. Clin Plast Surg 15:57–72
21. Pitanguy I (1972) The Negroid nose. In: Conley J, Dickinson J (eds) First international symposium on plastic and reconstructive surgery of the face and neck. Grune & Stratton, New York, pp 147–152
22. Porter JP, Tardy ME Jr, Cheng J (1999) The contoured auricular projection graft for nasal tip projection. Arch Facial Plast Surg 1:312–315
23. Rohrich RJ (1993) Rhinoplasty in the black patient. In: Daniel RK (ed) Rhinoplasty. Little Brown, Boston, pp 659–676
24. Rohrich R, Muzaffar A (2003) Rhinoplasty in the African American patient. Plast Reconstr Surg 111(3) 1322–1339
25. Romo T III, Shapiro AL (1992) Aesthetic reconstruction of the platyrrhine nose. Arch Otolaryngol Head Neck Surg 118:837–41
26. Romo T III, Sclafani AP, Sabini P (1998) Use of porous high-density polyethylene in revision rhinoplasty and in the platyrrhine nose. Aesthetic Plast Surg 22:211–221
27. Schultz AH (1913) Relation of the external nose to the bony nose and nasal cartilages in whites and Negroes. Am J Phys Anthropol 1:329–339
28. Snyder GB (1971) Rhinoplasty in the Negro. Plast Reconstr Surg 47:572–575
29. Stucker FJ (1976) Non-Caucasian rhinoplasty. Trans Am Acad Ophthalmol Otolaryngol 82:417–422
30. Stucker FJ (1987) Non-Caucasian rhinoplasty and adjunctive reduction cheiloplasty. Otolaryngol Clin North Am 20:877–894
31. Tham C, Lai YL, Weng CJ, Chen YR (2005) Silicone augmentation rhinoplasty in an Oriental population. Ann Plast Surg 54:1–5
32. Uhm KI, Hwang SH, Choi BG (2000) Cleft lip nose correction with onlay calvarial bone graft and suture suspension in oriental patients. Plast Reconstr Surg 105:499–503
33. Wang D, Qian G, Zhang M, Farkas LG (1997) Differences in horizontal, neoclassical facial canons in Chinese (Han) and North American Caucasian populations. Aesthetic Plast Surg 21:265–269
34. Yellin SA (1997) Aesthetics for the next millennium. Facial Plast Surg 13:231–239

Chapter 72

Management of the Crooked Nose Deformity

72

Philip A. Young and Fred J. Stucker

Core Messages

- Nasal trauma produces predictable anatomical changes.
- Malaligned fractured bones, once healed, hold cartilages in their malpositions.
- A geometric model aids in understanding the pathology and its correction.
- Cartilage heals in a predictable manner. It is preferable to incise completely through cartilage and align the segments rather than bending to achieve the desired shape.

Contents

Introduction

The many different approaches to the crooked nose attest to the difficulty that a surgeon faces to find a solution. Timing is crucial, in regards to treatment of an acute situation. The decision to fix the deviation closed or open and whether to use local or general anesthesia are among the options. An accurate history and exam is paramount. It can direct the surgeon down many algorithms of treatment, ultimately concentrating on what the patient deems the most important. With a chronic deformity, differing schools of thought approach the crooked nose either through (1) camouflage techniques [1, 2], (2) complete reconstruction of the anatomic deformities [3–7], (3) altering existing deformities but supporting the resulting weakened structures to rearrange the memory inherent in the tissue [8–11], (4) or a combination of each. Based on which approach a surgeon takes and what was discovered on the history and physical, the accurate execution of the different surgical techniques can lead to optimized results. Some seasoned surgeons have commented on the observation that some of their best results have occurred in the noses which they have done the least. Other surgeons take on a more radical approach, increasing variables, only to hope the tissues heal in a favorable way. In the end, what seems to matter the most is the experience of the surgeon and their technical expertise in carrying out particular maneuvers which ensure the best outcomes. Based on over 7,000 rhinoplasties, Dr. Stucker has adhered to his particular approach that has given him excellent results. It entails mostly an endonasal approach, fracture of the anterior ethmoidal septum, septoplasty with a unilateral mucoperichondrial flap and an inferior, horizontal "controlled" incision incorporating carving, scoring, planing, a "caudal septal sandwich" maneuver, and asymmetric osteotomies to effect the crooked nose to midline; in the end a septal "whip stitch" which Dr. Stucker first introduced is used to keep the septum straight [12] and has been employed by others [5]. We advocate this approach based on his greater than 25 years of experience with over 7,000 rhinoplasties and on his recent previous study of 119 patients which resulted in a 93% success rate.

The Crooked Nose in the Acute Setting

History

After clavicular and wrist fractures, a nasal fracture is one of the most common fractures in the human body [13]. It requires less force than any other facial bone. Its central and prominent location also places it at a higher risk of fracturing. When presented with an acute injury, many issues arise in caring for a patient with a nasal fracture. One must decide the severity of the injury, which can dictate the type of approach a surgeon takes to fix the problem. Minor deviations can oftentimes tolerate closed reduction under local anesthesia and can have excellent results. Others have shown that not all fractures are adequately treated, showing success rates from 14–50% [18]. These minor injuries are quite different from a nasoethmoidal fracture where fixation could require a combination of coronal, transconjunctival, sublabial, and nasal incisions along with metal plates and screws. To add to the complexity, one must address the problems with the medial canthal tendon and its fixation [14]. Thus an accurate history and physical is paramount.

With any significant trauma, one should always proceed through the ABCs. On secondary survey, the timing of the incident is vital. If within 3 h, a crooked nose has been found by some to be most easily reduced. As edema markedly increases to a peak of 6–8 h, the distortion of the deviation makes judging the fixation much more difficult [15]. Many authors then agree that the fracture should be reduced in 3–7 days, although others suggest that there is little harm allowing the swelling to resolve [16]. Beyond 2 weeks, the fractures begin to heal and solidify making a closed reduction difficult and painful, and with children this time period is shortened to 1 week.

The mechanism and whether injury was due to a high velocity impact as associated with motor vehicle accidents or due to a closed fist is crucial. Low energy impacts have a lesser chance of a telescoping injury as in a nasoethmoidal fracture. As little as 25 to 75 pounds per square inch is required to fracture the nose. With lower energies the thinner caudal portion of the nasal bones are more susceptible. As energy increases the thicker portion of the nasal bones near the nasal processes of the frontal bone are involved [17]. With higher impact energies, the frontal process of the maxilla and the nasal process of the frontal bones become involved; this can eventually include the medial canthal tendons. Progressing from a closed fist to increasingly harder, heavier objects with more force, results in a greater severity of the fracture.

Severe pain can sometimes point to a septal hematoma. Anosmia can rarely indicate a cribiform fracture, and possibly a subsequent CSF leak. Epistaxis usually indicates mucosal violation and a high incidence of an open fracture [17]. Nasal obstruction can be due to hematoma, clots, septal deviation, generalized mucosal swelling, dislocation of the upper or lower lateral cartilages, or altered tip rotation (Fig. 72.1). Orbital complaints are somewhat beyond the scope of this discussion. However, binocular diplopia can indicate possible extraocular muscle entrapment, where horizontal diplopia may indicate entrapment of the lateral or medial recti, and vertical diplopia may indicate entrapment of the superior or inferior recti. Diplopia can also be from a dislocated medial canthal tendon. Visual blurring can possibly be due to optic nerve canal swelling and entrapment of the nerve. Numbness of the medial cheek, upper lip and nasal sidewall or central teeth can indicate that the nasal fracture may be related to a maxillary wall component.

The direction of the blow dictates the appearance of the deviation. A lateral blow can fracture the ipsilateral nasal bone with lower energies. As the energy increases, the dorsum followed by the contralateral bone becomes involved. When there is any translation of the energy in a dorsal-to-ventral, caudal-to-cephalic direction, more energy is driven through the septum (Fig. 72.2). Septal fractures anteriorly have been noted to be more vertical than horizontal when located more posteriorly [17]. One group emphasized that a caudal to cephalic force tends to dislocated the caudal quadrangular cartilage off the maxillary crest, leading to shortening and possible impingement of one particular airway [16], which may be responsible for the septal tilt deformity present in nearly 40% of septonasal deviations described previously [9].

Age is an important dimension to consider. In the elderly, the nasal bones increasingly become more brittle and are more apt to become comminuted. Dislocations are more common in

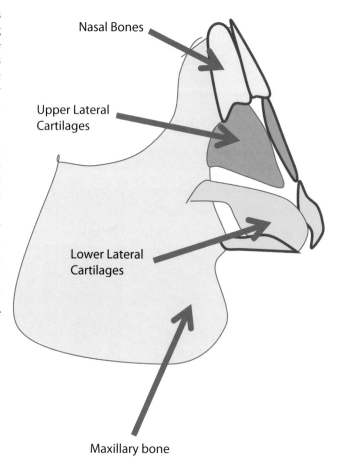

Fig. 72.1 Basic anatomical elements within the nose. The major structures within the external nose include the nasal bones, and upper and lower lateral cartilages

Nasal Bones

Upper Lateral Cartilages

Lower Lateral Cartilages

Maxillary bone

72

the young. A child's nose being more underdeveloped is composed mostly of cartilage and takes on less prominence relative to the face. Coupled with the decreased ability of the cartilage to withstand force, the facial bones become more exposed. Thus, other facial fractures are more likely. Because the cartilage is more apt to buckle and twist with an increase in the mucoperichondrium separating from the septum, the experience in some has indicated that septal hematomas are more common in children [17]. The cartilaginous structures are more apt to dislocate from the surrounding bony structures. Nasal and septal bones are more likely to greenstick fracture. Stucker et al. [19] have noted that children tend to require general anesthesia for their reduction. They re-examine children 2–3 days later and repeat the exam until the swelling decreases enough for a thorough exam to be carried out. The decreased edema also allows better judgment in the operating room. Intervention should be undertaken earlier in children versus adults. The fractures are believed to heal within 2–4 days. Closed reduction is often sufficient and a minimal invasive approach is advocated to avoid disrupting growth centers. Most surgeons advocate a conservative approach to avoid damaging growth centers and the usually sufficient management of this age group is done through closed techniques [17, 19]. Septal surgery when needed to improve airway and gross deformities is supported in the literature [17]. Crockett has proposed a more aggressive approach to avoid further growth problems and to correct airway and cosmetic issues [25].

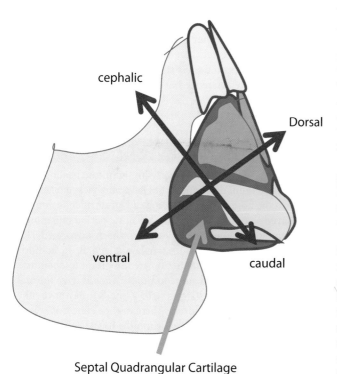

Fig. 72.2 Orientation of the nose: caudal to cephalic, and dorsal to ventral. The septal quadrangular cartilage is identified

Physical Exam

Understanding the anatomy of the nose is key. Only with this knowledge will a thorough exam be of any substance. Edema and blood often obscures an adequate exam. Repeating the exam may be necessary. Half of all patients with nasal fractures do not receive an adequate intranasal exam. Inspection should be carried out externally and internally. An accurate eye exam is a must. Testing the medial canthal tendon employing the bowstring test, measuring intercanthal distance and blunting of the canthus can indicate disruption of the central fragment and a more serious injury requiring a facial CT scan. Periorbital ecchymosis, especially with subconjunctival hemorrhage, indicates violation of periosteum and bone. This should lead the surgeon to consider an orbital fracture as well as a nasal fracture.

Lacerations with external debris should be irrigated to decrease significant bacterial load and substances that could leave a "tattoo" in the future should be removed. Gross deviations, crepitus, mobility of bone fragments are noted. Conveniently, the nose can be broken up into thirds. The upper third consists of the nasal bones, with thin and mobile skin. The middle third consists of the upper lateral cartilages (ULC) and the adjacent cartilaginous dorsum. The lower third is comprised of the lower lateral cartilages (LLC), caudal septum, and the thick, nonmobile skin of the lobule. Deviation of the upper third entails mainly a bony deviation with a variable component of septal cartilage that can maintain the bony elements in a deviated state. Hence, an internal exam with endoscopes can reveal a septal deviation that can dramatically increase the difficulty of the repair. A crooked middle third is predominated by cartilaginous tissue. Fractures, dislocations, and telescoping elements complicate the fixation. Often when these states are present, closed reduction techniques become less reliable. Caudal septal tilts and deviations almost always require some open approach to fixate the septum to the anterior nasal spine. As will be shown later, some authors advocate total caudal septal reconstruction to fix this type of deviation [3, 5–7]. Epistaxis must be handled accordingly but will not be fully addressed.

Radiographs have almost completely fallen out of the surgeon's armamentarium. A high false negative rate of up to 47% has been found [20]. The impact on the surgical approach of x-rays is insignificant to many [18, 19]. CT scans have been advocated by others from an insurance and medico-legal standpoint [21]. It can document a septonasal deformity and demonstrate impingement on the airway, while facilitating third-party payments. Photographic documentation can also help with consultation and intraoperative analysis of the fracture and are essential to any facial plastic surgeon. With cartilage memory that becomes more pertinent as the healing progresses, certain areas of deviation consisting of the cartilaginous portion of the nose can persist unless augmented in some way. Deviated ULC and LLC may persist unless weakened and resupported or completely replaced if beyond repair.

Other areas to concentrate on include involvement of the surrounding facial structures. A depressed glabella can indicate a frontal sinus fracture requiring CT evaluation. Anesthesia in the V2 components can point to maxillary fractures. Impingement of the optic nerve with attendant visual symptoms can point to a severe zygomatic component with fracture involving the optic canal. Examination of dentoalveolar structures can entail involvement of the oral maxilofacial services.

Photographic documentation of the injury is essential from a medico-legal standpoint. It can document a preinjury deformity that may not resolve with closed reduction and may require more extensive open techniques to resist the memory of the structures. Up to 30% of people have a history of a previous nasal deformity [24].

Classifications

Rohrich and Adams classified nasal fractures into 5 classes [8, 18]. Comminuted fractures, complex nasoseptal defects to nasoethmoidal fractures required greater attention on physical exam. They advocated using a 30° telescope to exam all parts of the septum and its contribution to airway and maintenance of a crooked nose. They preferred general anesthesia with closed techniques. Irreversible and posteriorly displaced septal fractures and deviations required total anatomic septal reduction or reconstruction.

Treatment

Options for fixation include using closed or open techniques, local or general anesthesia. Many others have recommended closed reduction for unilateral or bilateral deformities of the nasoseptal defects that are deviated less than one half the width of the nasal bones. They employ open reduction for extensive fracture dislocations of septonasal complex, deviations or the nasal pyramid exceeding greater than one half the width of the nasal bridge. Others add that the open approach should be used with septal hematomas, inadequate bony reduction, combined septal and alar deformities, displaced anterior nasal spine, or history of recent intranasal surgery [22].

With closed reduction, local anesthesia using lidocaine 1% with epinephrine 1/200,000, cocaine or EMLA cream separately or in some sort of combination have been employed. Others have shown that reduction under local anesthesia is just as effective as general anesthesia [23]. A newer study showed that the rate for the need for subsequent definitive rhinoplasty, septoplasty, or both was greater in the local anesthesia group (17.2%) than in the general anesthesia group (3.2%), p<0.0001. Although retrospective, the study had 324 patients and a follow-up averaging 3 years compared to other studies reviewed which had a maximum of 12 weeks follow-up. Unfortunately, given that changes to a repaired nasal fracture can sometimes take up to 2 years to fully reveal surgical changes, most of the studies with short follow-up time are repeatedly referenced in the literature.

The technique includes anesthetizing bilaterally the dorsum 5 mm from the midline at the nasal bone/ULC junction (anterior ethmoidal), sidewall including 5 mm medial to the canthus (dorsal nasal nerve), septum, and infraorbital nerve. At times, injecting the septum high and dorsally intranasally allows less painful manipulation when using the Boise elevator for nasal bone manipulation. Marking the distance between the canthal tendon horizontal height to the nostril entrance and then reducing this distance by 0.5–1.0 cm will avoid the skull base. The Boise elevator is then used to reduce the nasal bones to midline. Occasionally, a deviated dorsal septum will prevent the bones from being reduced. Asch or Walsham forceps are then applied to reduce the septum. If the septum is not reduced the nasal bones may remain deviated, requiring a possible open approach. Fractures should be reduced prior to closure if bony fragments are exposed. If tissue is healthy and not devitalized, bone fragments can be replaced. Reduced septal fractures can be stabilized through packing or silastic splints.

Others have employed traditional closed techniques and compared them with a more complete nasal fracture protocol. In a more complete approach, others have used a septoplasty, osteotomies, release of the ULCs, fracture of the anterior extension of the ethmoid perpendicular plate, followed by camouflage grafts in that order depending on reassessment between maneuvers. Compared with the more extensive approach to classical closed techniques, some have found that the more complete protocol yielded a significantly straighter nose than with traditional closed techniques (71% vs. 40%).

Most of the dominant past literature has stated that closed techniques under local anesthesia achieve equivalent results with general anesthesia [23, 26]. However, some authors are now advocating more aggressive approaches through general anesthesia [18, 27]. Courtney et al. have recently shown in a retrospective review that out of 324 patients, a general anesthesia group (194 patients) versus a local group (134 patients) required a subsequent rhinoplasty, septorhinoplasty, or septoplasty a significantly less percentage of the time (3.2 vs. 17.2%, p<0.0001). In contrast with the other highly referenced articles, their follow-up time was greater than 4–12 weeks versus an average of 3 years. They supported their study through a larger study size than other highly referenced articles (324 patients vs. 29–100 patients).

Delayed Management of the Crooked Nose

After 2 weeks, the surgeon is faced with significant healing at this point. Closed reduction approaches have much less efficacy secondary to the fibrosis. Most surgeons advocate open techniques in a delayed setting. Traditionally, a waiting period of 6 months before employing open techniques has been advocated [17]. Focusing on a patient's main complaints is vital. In addition, preinjury appearance and function are important to document, although an experienced surgeon may or should have the ability to alter this original state as well. A subject may have other issues that they wish to address. There may be concerns regarding a ptotic or bulbous tip, a wide middle third (Fig. 72.3), or a prominent nasal dorsal hump that may need addressing under a general anesthetic in one sitting [45]. An accurate history is paramount to determine the functional concerns, as well as to address any concomitant disease processes that might require new initial treatment. If the primary concern of the patient is nasal obstruction, the surgeon must determine where the obstruction is most likely located and what the cause of it is. One needs to rule out contributions from the various causes of rhinitis. Ultimately, recalling that near 50% of the resistance of the whole respiratory tract resides in the internal nasal valve area (Fig. 72.4) can be crucial [21, 28, 29]. Hence an accurate physical exam allows the surgeon to approach the causes of the patients' complaints specifically and effectively.

History

Most patients with a crooked nose will complain of their external nasal deformity. However, oftentimes they become more concerned with nasal obstruction. Duration and frequency can point a surgeon to suspect specific causes. A fixed unilateral nasal obstruction points to the nasoseptal deformity causing the obstruction.

Alternating sides of obstruction can point to the nasal cycle as a cause or possibly a dominant cause. Posturing with obstruction on the dependent side is normal. Daytime obstruction can point to allergies and occupational exposures as possible etiologies. Seasonal (weeds, trees, pollens, molds) or perennial symptoms (cockroach, dog, cat, dust mites, molds) can indicate an

IgE-mediated disease. Avoidance, pharmacologic intervention, skin testing, and immunotherapy are vital aspects to treatment. Food allergies can be a component to the rhinitis as the "shock organ" and can be diagnosed through thoughtful food elimination and reintroduction [31]. Importantly before operating one must elucidate the etiologies of obstruction and determine if any causes of rhinitis complicate the picture. Sinusitis; allergic, vasomotor, atrophic, hypertrophic rhinitis; rhinitis medicamentosa, or contributions from chemical exposures, contraceptives, pregnancy, smoking, antihypertensives, antidepressants, hypothyroidism, diabetes, Wegener's, syphilis, or sarcoidosis should be discovered prior to definitive correction of septal, turbinate, or external deformities. Prior knowledge allows surgeons to seek or apply more medical therapy, or properly counsel patients regarding less than optimal results after surgery to alleviate obstruction. Other causes include the use of continuous positive airway pressure, a prominent horizontal inferior turbinate anomaly or other congenital anomalies. A fixed unilateral obstruction since birth often indicates a correctable anatomic obstruction. Irreversible hypertrophic rhinitis of the septum and turbinates can also contribute to a problem amenable to repair and can be revealed through an accurate exam [30, 32]. (An extensive account of the physical exam needed to diagnosis and treat rhinitis is beyond the scope of this chapter; please refer to Chap. 30–32).

A history of prior rhinoplasty could have a tremendous impact on the planned revision. An operative report from the previous surgeon can prepare one to anticipate the lack of cartilaginous tissue available for augmentation and allow the surgeon to approach other sources of cartilage or bone. It can also help the surgeon to anticipate previously placed grafts and their contribution to the current state. Previous surgical maneuvers can

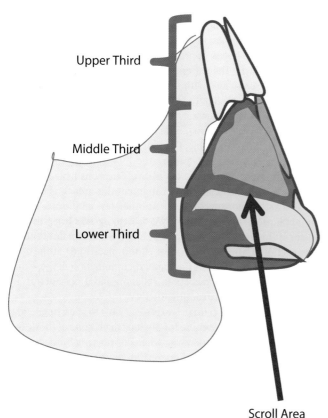

Fig. 72.3 Nasal anatomy broken up into thirds: the upper third consists of the nasal bones, the middle third consists of the upper lateral cartilages, and the lower third consists of the lower lateral cartilages. The scroll area is the attachment of the ULC with the LLC, which supports the competency of the internal nasal valve area

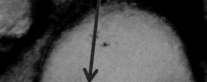
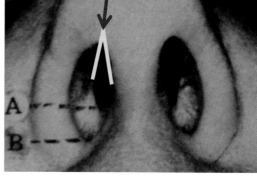

Fig. 72.4 Internal Nasal Valves (INV) at point *A*. The external nasal valves are located at point *B*. The Critical angle between the septum and the upper lateral cartilage should be between 10 and 15°

also be the cause of the new nasal obstruction. This would most likely be some narrowing found in the INV area. Past surgical approaches can impinge on the airway. Intercartilaginous incisions that were not approximated accurately can leave scarring at the internal nasal valve INV area. This approach also entails release of the scroll area (Fig. 72.3) between the LLC and ULC, which may not have been reconstituted by the previous surgeon. The aponeurosis between these two elements helps to translate the nasal dilator muscles action on the LLC to the ULC through this fibrous connection. Of the intrinsic nasal muscles, the pars transversa can dilate but mainly supports the lateral nasal wall. The pars alaris serves as the main dilator. Of the extrinsic muscles, the levator labii superioris alaeque nasi is the most important dilator, while the zyomaticus minor and orbicularis oris provide secondary lateral wall stability. Resection of the caudal aspect of the ULC can remove vital support for the INV. Overreduction during cephalic trim can weaken the alae and also disrupt the ULC connection with the LLC leading to INV impingement. Alar weir or other reduction exercises can narrow the ENV.

Physical Exam

When examining a septonasal deformity, it is convenient to break the nose up into thirds [11], the lower third being comprised of the caudal septum, lobule, LLC, columella, and alae. The skin at this region is thicker, more adherent to the underlying structures and more sebaceous. The middle third is composed of ULCs, the dorsal septum, and progressively thinner skin. The upper third is made up of the nasal bones and less adherent and thinner skin with less sebaceous quality (Fig. 72.3). Beginning caudally, a ptotic tip can be a source of both functional and aesthetic complaints. Raising the tip manually can improve a patient's breathing instantly, simulating the surgical maneuvers to rotate the tip and its likely success. A worm's eye view can allow the surgeon to examine the external and internal nasal valves (Fig. 72.4). Through the literature [21, 28, 29, 35] it is shown that approximately 30% of the respiratory tract's resistance to airflow occurs at the external nasal valves (ENV). Fifty percent of that obstruction is believed to be at the internal nasal valves (INV). Hence an accurate exam at these two anterior nasal cavity points is crucial. The external nasal slit deformity is classically used to describe an ENV source of obstruction. Deformities of the alae, lower lateral cartilages, lobule, columella; weakening or dislocation of the scroll; caudal septal deformities, tilts, or dislocations; or soft tissue defects (i.e., scars, webs) of the vestibule can contribute to narrowing.

In comparison to a deviation residing in the anterior nasal cavities (i.e., INV, ENV) versus the posterior portion (septum, turbinates), the literature contains an abundance of data illustrating the greater effect that narrowing in the prior has much greater impact than the latter [28, 29, 35–38]. One millimeter of narrowing of the ENV or INV can be critical, whereas up to 5 mm of deviation posterior to the valves can have no effect [29]. Poiseuille's law states that for laminar flow of a gas through a tube, resistance is inversely proportional to the radius to the fourth power. Thus, a decrease in radius by one half will increase

resistance by 16 fold. Bridger found that out of 144 patients through rhinomanometry less than <0.75 L/s of airflow was symptomatic [35]. Warren (using rhinomanometry) showed that a minimal cross-sectional area (MCA) of less than 16 mm2 can lead to oral breathing [36]. Bridger found that the average area at the INV was 64 mm2. Warren went on to show that at the INV area in subjects who underwent septoplasty, patients with a MCA at the INV of 54.76 mm2 were satisfied with their nasal breathing versus patients who were unsatisfied who had 20.25 mm2 (averages, p<0.000, see [36]). Constantian showed the positive effects of surgical maneuvers on the INV and ENV on airflows pre- and postoperatively [38] (Fig. 72.4).

Examining the INV entails viewing the valve from the caudal view and noting any narrowing secondary to septal deviations, septal thickening, scars, webs, granulation tissues, or contributions from the ULC or LLC. The INV is composed of the caudal ends of the ULC, the adjacent septum, and the floor of the nasal cavity. Usually, the angle formed by the septum and ULC dorsal and superiorly should be between 10 and 15° (Fig. 72.4). Less than 10° can cause subjective nasal obstructive symptoms. Deviation of the tip can impinge on one side of the airway greater than the other. This can signify a rather difficult correction. Tip deviation can indicate caudal septal deformities. When doing submucosal resection of the septum, traditionally, 8–10 mm of an "L strut" of dorsal and caudal septum are left for anterior nasal support. When one of the portions of the L strut is involved, the fixation becomes much more difficult. Oftentimes, these deformities are better approached through an open transcolumellar approach. The superior and nasal extension of the alar-facial crease coincides with the INV from an external perspective. Seen from a frontal view, the classic picture of a pinched middle third can indicate an impingement of the airway at this location. The well-known Cottle maneuver, where the examiner places pressure on a subject's medial cheek area near the alar-facial crease is used to lateralize the INV area to improve the airway. If improved the test is positive. Surgeons have used this to simulate results of surgery to augment this area. It is thought to be a rather nonspecific test. Another test employs a cotton tip applicator applied to the INV area to again open this area to see if this relieves the patient's subjective complaint of nasal obstruction. Others use a ball of cotton placed just at the apex of the INV to accomplish the same. A combination of these maneuvers can indicate success in relieving nasal obstruction by augmenting or reconstructing the INV.

Moving from the caudal, worm's eye view to the frontal view, the surgeon should examine for obvious deviations of the dorsal septum and ULCs. Importantly, when considering the approach, some surgeons advocate an open rhinoplasty approach for significant dorsal deviations [8, 10]. A dislocation of the ULC from the underside of the nasal bones is a possible sequelae of nasal trauma. Deformities of the ULC are often not addressed and spoken little of in the literature except for mentioning placement of camouflage grafts. Treatment of the ULC can markedly improve the appearance of the middle third. Ignoring its contribution can result in a persistent deformity postoperatively. In the operating room the subtleties of the ULCs' contribution are often difficult to ascertain with the swelling that results from a combination of injection, edema, and manipulation for exposure. One should utilize preoperative photos to guide their treatment of the ULCs through battens, scoring, and weakening of ULCs, or suture modifications (Fig. 72.5). Well-placed battens can be used to camouflage depressions and deviations while not actually correcting the abnormality. Scoring the cartilage can relieve tension in the perpendicular direction and help the cartilage bow towards the side of scoring. Oftentimes scoring weakens the cartilage and will need a batten to give it support. Accurate suture placement can correct unwanted bends within the cartilage to correct deviations without batten placement. However, prudent scoring combined with suture placement is needed on occasion based on the surgeon's experience. Using a 0 or 30° scope, a surgeon can identify high dorsal deviations of the quadrangular cartilage or ethmoid perpendicular plate which may need to be addressed usually from an open rhinoplasty approach. Often what is needed is complete release of the ULCs from the septum and correction of each element individually and then reconstitution of the connection between the septum and the ULCs.

Next, the upper third of the nose is examined mostly from the frontal view. Gross deviations should be noted along with identifying a unilateral or bilateral contribution. The presence of a dorsal hump can also be addressed if the patient wishes. One should note the length of the nasal bones and its relative contribution to the deviation separately from the ULC and cartilaginous dorsum. With deviations, it has been noted in the past that straight dorsal reduction can lead to asymmetric treatment of the nasal bones. The result can be one nasal bone being more shortened than the other side. Usually when this is done it is the concave nasal bone that is more reduced [8]. Further examination into the nasal cavity should be conducted with a combination of the nasal speculum and the 0 or 30° nasal endoscope before and after vasoconstriction. Response to the vasoconstriction on exam and based on patients' subjective feelings indicates a reversible component to the nasal obstruction and possible benefit from pharmacotherapy. A more diligent search for the contributing rhinitis should be conducted. Non-reversible changes indicate a fixed obstruction when the physical exam also shows no change and thus indicates that a patient has an anatomical narrowing that can be surgically improved. A trial of medication should always be used to document no improvement over the course of 1–3 months to indicate a surgical condition. The appearance of the mucosa can lead a surgeon to think allergies with pale, edematous mucosa. Erythematous mucosa can direct one to consider rhinitis medicamentosa, chemical exposure, or infection.

Other ancillary tests include allergy skin end point titration testing to rule out allergic rhinitis. Nasal cytology aids in diagnosing allergy with the presence of eosinophils or infection when large numbers of polymorphonucleocytes are found. CT scans can be used to document a septal deviation for medicolegal purposes and for insurance claims. It can also be used to diagnose sinusitis. Rhinomanometry can document the current airflow as well as the pressure of the nasal passage and resistance can be calculated. Mentioned previously, airflows <0.75 L/s were found to be symptomatic [35]. Acoustic rhinometry can aid the surgeon in finding the minimal cross sectional area. This information can direct the surgeon to the likely cause and to also attempt to reach the MCA that will lead to a satisfied patient (54.76 mm2, see above.)

Based on the completed exam, the surgeon can consider ancillary procedures to improve the airway and to augment the correction of the nasal deviation. Most of these ancillary procedures concentrate on the turbinates and their contribution to nasal obstruction and persistent septal deviation. When the physical exam demonstrates irreversible mucosal changes, and significant narrowing attributed to the area of the turbinates on visual inspection or acoustic rhinometry, multiple turbinate procedures can be utilized to ultimately reduce their size.

Avoidance of atrophic rhinitis to some surgeons represents the "bottom-line" condition to avoid. Through an analysis of the literature, Marks and Loechel showed the incidence of this is 0% for nonresection techniques (laser, chemical cautery, electrocautery, steroid injection, outfracture, radiofrequency), and 5% for total inferior turbinectomy procedures. Partial turbinectomy was found to be in between those percentages. They advocated inferior turbinoplasty to preserve the functioning medial mucosa. The advantages were that this effected a longer-lasting effect over nonresection techniques but avoided a higher chance of atrophic rhinitis by preserving the functioning mucosal side.

With regard to treating the inferior or middle turbinate, there are a few other issues to consider. When undergoing a septoplasty, the turbinates can prevent the septum from being placed in the midline. Turbinectomy or lateral outfracturing can alleviate the deviating force. Turbinate procedures to improve the airway have been beneficial in the short term but not in long-term studies [21].

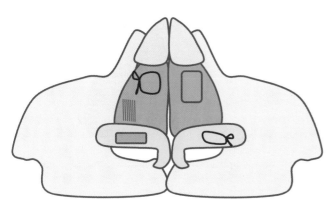

Fig. 72.5 Well-placed battens (*green*) can camouflage depressions and deviations. Scoring (*red*) in a linear manner can relieve cartilaginous stress and can increase the distance on the side of scoring and in a direction perpendicular to the scoring. Accurate suture placement (*dark brown*) can bend cartilage in a directed fashion to alter unwanted bends in the upper and lower lateral cartilages

Treatment

There are several schools of thought that can be used to guide the surgeon to treat the external components of the deviated or crooked nose: (1) predominately camouflaging techniques to affect correction of the deformity while preserving dorsal and caudal supporting forces at the expense of persistent airway issues [1, 2]; (2) a more aggressive approach via augmentation of existing structures through sutures and various maneuvers to weaken the elements but supporting the structures through a combination of sutures, grafts, and battens [8–11, 39, 40]; (3) total reconstruction by removal of deformed elements, straightening followed by replacement and reconstitution of supports [3–7]; (4) or a combination of the approaches. On a basic level, well-placed battens can be used to camouflage depressions and deviations while not actually correcting the abnormality. Scoring the cartilage can relieve tension in the perpendicular direction and help the cartilage bow towards the side of scoring. Oftentimes scoring weakens the cartilage and will need a batten to give it support. Accurate suture placement can correct unwanted bends within the cartilage to correct deviations without batten placement. However, prudent scoring combined with suture placement is needed on occasion based on the surgeon's experience. Often times many surgeons believe that what is needed is complete release of the ULCs from the septum and correction of each element individually and then reconstitution of the connection between the septum and the ULCs as discussed below (Fig. 72.5).

Sheen and Constantian have often been quoted as proponents of the camouflage technique. Sheen introduced the spreader graft [41] and popularized tip and alar batten grafts. Constantian (1989) introduced his form of camouflaging the asymmetric nose through: (1) dorsal resection of the external deviation until sufficiently close to midline; (2) submucosal resection of the septum; (3) augmentation through cartilage grafts of the upper, middle, and lower third to achieve balance; and (4) further camouflage techniques through spreader grafts and tip grafts.

Rohrich, Byrd, and Guyuron have taken a more aggressive approach in their treatment of the deviated nasal deformity. Rohrich [8] advocated an open rhinoplasty approach; wide mucoperichondrial undermining; release of the ULC, LLC, and septum from one another (Fig. 72.6); preserving the L-strut

and resecting deviated posterior elements; employing scoring, rarely morselization, and if severe 50% inferior full thickness cuts with persistent high dorsal deviations (Fig. 72.7); caudal septal swinging door, wedge resections, and caudal septal batten grafts; spreader grafts to support a weakened dorsal strut or asymmetric placement to camouflage deviation; and percutaneous osteotomies. Byrd [10] introduced Mustarde sutures to correct L-Strut deviations and septal extension grafts in a spreader or caudal batten graft orientation. He also introduced the supratip stitch to eliminate dead space to achieve "predictability of definition between the dorsum and tip." This can also avoid graft absorption (Stucker F, Buchalter G, 2004, work in progress) and eliminate a pollybeak deformity. Guyuron [9] introduced a classification system for septal deformities through which they utilized scoring of the concave side to affect asymmetric bending perpendicular to the direction of the scoring. All three groups mention the asymmetric suturing of the ULC to the septum to effect additional straightening. These types of approaches have been tried in the past, Wexler (1977) discussed elevating unilateral submucoperichondrial planes, release of ULC, use of intercartilaginous incisions (IC) (Fig. 72.6), and specifically vertical 1- to 2-mm strips of cartilage to help mobilize the caudal L strut (Fig. 72.7). More recently, a septal crossbar graft placed through full thickness cuts has recently been introduced [42]. Other techniques adhering to this type of approach include a sidewall-spreading suture, clocking sutures, triangular form of a spreader graft, an extended columellar graft, and excision of a "Burow Triangle" at the junction of the dorsal and caudal septum [11].

At times when the deviated portion of the nose extends to involve the L strut and is not amenable to correction with techniques described above, other surgeons exercise more radical

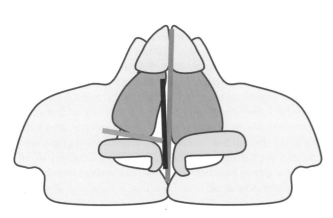

Fig. 72.6 Releasing the individual elements within the nasal anatomy can allow the surgeon to modify each element and correct the asymmetry in a more definitive manner. Releasing the ULC and LLC from the septum (*red*) and releasing the ULC from the LLC (*green*) can eliminate forces that keep the nose in an asymmetric state

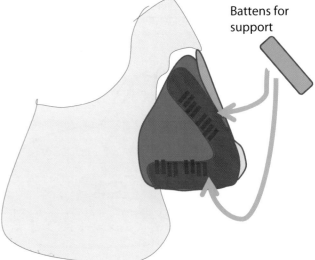

Fig. 72.7 Straightening the dorsum can entail inferior cuts to release the deviation in the dorsal segment of the L strut. A batten can support either segment of the L strut most advantageously placed on the concave side of the deviation. Well-placed cuts in the caudal segment can also be judiciously used

approaches. Rees advocated total or near total removal of the septum, reshaping then replacement with thru and thru sutures [5]. Both Peer and Maliniac advocated removal of the anterior septum and placement as a graft in the bed of the columella [6, 7]. For the tip and lower third, Menick has advocated total removal of aspects of the lower lateral cartilages to reconstruct tip deformities secondary to previous rhinoplasty and for postcancer surgeries [4]. Although most crooked nasal deformities likely contain sufficient nasal cartilage, severe crooked tips often remain resistant to surgical straightening maneuvers. Oftentimes, however, these structures in the lower third can be manipulated through alar rim grafts, alar spreader grafts, alar battens, columellar strut grafts, multiple tip suturing techniques, and lateral crural strut grafts. More recently, Persig advocated the back-to-back autogenous ear cartilage graft for irreparable caudal septal deformities to straighten the nose.

Fred J. Stucker's Approach

Dr. Stucker's approach is based on his experience with over 6,000 rhinoplasties, many consisting of the crooked nasal deformity. The approach is through a recent study of a series of 132 rhinoplasties, 39 where the patient's subjective success rate was 93% and the surgeon's was 89%. Most patients were done under general anesthesia with topical and local anesthesia to enhance hemostasis. Preoperatively, the patient received nasal decongestion. Four percent cocaine pledgets placed topically was then followed with infiltration with 1% lidocaine with 1:100,000 epinephrine.

The vital initial maneuver entails an eggshell fracture of the anterior ethmoid perpendicular plate and quadrangular cartilage with a Sayer elevator. The elevator is placed in one nostril into the apical junction between the perpendicular plate and nasal bone. The Sayer is rocked back and forth in a lateral and medial fashion to fracture the bony ethmoid septum. The elevator is then moved more inferior to mobilize the vomer with the same movements. The goal is to achieve mobilization of the septum to decrease preoperative elements holding the dorsum in a deviated position. Dr. Stucker has done this in over 6,000 rhinoplasties without a cerebrospinal fluid leak.

Endonasal or open, external approaches are both used. Elevation is begun over the cartilaginous and bony dorsal elements with blunt scissors and finished with a #15 scalpel blade. With significant scarring, the #15 blade takes a more predominant role in elevation.

The cartilaginous septum is then approached with a unilateral submucoperichondrial flap from the transfixion incision. We employ bilateral flaps especially when needed with a significantly thickened septum secondary to congenital or traumatic reasons. With septal dislocations, experience over the years has shown that overlapped, telescoped fragments tend to fibrose and lead to thickened segments of the septum. Appropriate shaving and carving, while leaving 2 mm of thickness, can markedly straighten the septum. Strip excisions can further allow midline positioning. With bilateral elevation, caution must be exercised with the increased instability. For further visualization, Dr. Stucker has advocated for quite some time an inferior,

horizontal control incision. This incision is carried from the transfixion incision along the junction between the quadrangular cartilage and the maxillary crest. The decussation of the perichondral and periosteal layers serves to hold the cartilage to the bony trough for stability but acts as a hindrance to the surgeon to elevate past. The time spent to elevate anterior and inferior tunnels is an excessive expenditure of time and effort. This incision provides access but avoids an uncontrolled tear with the attendant risk of perforation. We have employed this incision with almost no instances of perforation nor hematoma as it serves as a drainage pathway. This flap is elevated superiorly and cephalad for excellent exposure. It allows improved access to resect strips of cartilages in strategic places to effect midline placement. The quadrangular cartilage is dislocated from the ethmoid. Obstructive components of the bony septum are resected with Takahashi forceps. They can be morselized and replaced. Release of the ULC from the septum can also release deviating forces. Reconstituting their attachment to the septum should be completed prior to closure.

For inferior spurs, it must first be determined that they represent a functional problem. A Leptorhinne configuration has been observed to have airflow predominately adjacent to the middle meatus and middle turbinate and hence addressing obstructions in this area can most improve the airway for these nasal types. Platyrrhine noses have increasing flow along the nasal floor and may subsequently benefit more from treatment of septal spurs. If deemed necessary, we advocate direct excision of the spur with Takahashi forceps or drill. The use of the inferior, horizontal control incision should provide the superior mucosal reflection that should be adequate to cover the resulting defect created by the resection. This approach can ultimately save extra time and effort elevating the inferior mucosal reflection of the spur. Dr. Stucker's experience with almost no incidence of perforation or hematoma supports this technique.

The dorsum is next approached. If a dorsal hump is present, it is then removed with Kazanjian or osteotome. The open roof provides access for the medial osteotomies. If the roof is not resected, bilateral incisions between the ULCs and dorsal septum are made for access. We approach the depressed fragment initially with a medial osteotomy. Lateral pressure after just the medial osteotomy is oftentimes sufficient to elevate the nasal bones to preinjury position [46]. Animal studies have shown bony union in the membranous midfacial bones. Jenecke showed through cadaver dissections that the nasal bones predominately healed by bony reunion through histological examination, while the frontal process of the maxillary bone were more likely to undergo fibrous healing [70]. Many surgeons have noted the relative ease with which previous lateral osteotomies can be reopened. Other authors have made claims that fibrous healing is more likely to occur when soft tissue is interposed between fracture fragments. It is based on these observations and experiments that we approach depressed fragments with only a medial osteotomy initially. The lateralized nasal bone usually requires both medial and lateral osteotomies. It may be that the lateralized segment has more bone-to-bone contact and thus with more bony union than fibrous healing. Our medial osteotomies are performed with a 6-mm osteotome. We use a 2-mm osteotome endonasally pushed through mucosa immediately inferior to the inferior turbinate. The bone cut is begun 6 mm superior to the most inferior and lateral portion of the pyriform aperture [45]. No elevation of the periosteum is done. We advance superolaterally until the thicker bone of the nasomaxillary groove is encountered. Then our direction is aimed superomedially in this groove to meet with our medial osteotomy. The narrow width of the osteotome decreases soft tissue trauma and thus minimizes collapse. We preserve a triangular bony strut to maintain its attachment to the lateral nasalis muscle and ULCs. This decreases excessive narrowing which can compromise the airway at the INV (Fig. 72.8).

Based on the above protocol, we carried out a retrospective study, where the patients were asked to judge the success of their rhinoplasty on a cosmetic and functional standpoint. Our patients' subjective success rate was 93%, and the surgeon's success rate was 89%. Our approach belongs to the school that takes a more aggressive approach to the crooked nose and is not a strict camouflage method. Dr. Stucker's vast experience and sheer numbers support his approach given his high success rate. He has used this approach for crooked noses based on his experience of doing over 6,000 rhinoplasties during his career. It is done in a single stage and his revision rate for minor irregularities is less than 15%. His limited osteotomies, preserving periosteal support, produce a semi rigid reduction without destabilizing the bony structures allowing secondary healing to effect the results. The sole medial osteotomy is based on experimental evidence indicating that this is sufficient many times to mobilize the depressed fragment while offering more substantial stability to effect the intraop results. His septal whipstitch that he first introduced in 1978 aids in stabilizing fragments of the septum, along with unilateral elevation of the mucoperichondrial and mucoperiosteal layers. This "whipstitch" has been used by Dr. Stucker for over 26 years and has not been associated with sep-

72

tal hematoma nor perforation. Recently, a comparison between nasal packing and transseptal suturing was carried out in a rabbit model showing no significant difference in septal thickness or mucosal inflammation and damage between the two groups [47] further giving support to his septal stitch.

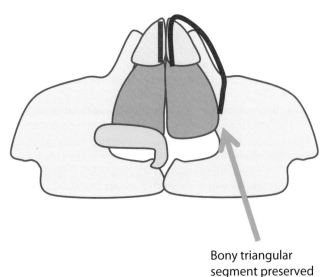

Bony triangular
segment preserved

Fig. 72.8 Medial and lateral osteotomies are used on the lateralized nasal bones (*red line*). On the side of the deviation with the medialized segment, only a medial osteotomy is essentially needed (*purple line*)

References

1. Sheen J (1987) Aesthetic rhinoplasty, 2nd edn. Mosby, St. Louis
2. Constantian M (1989) An algorithm for correcting the asymmetrical nose. Plast Reconstr Surg 83:801–811
3. Pirsig W, Kern E, Verse T (2004) Reconstruction of anterior nasal septum: Back-to-back autogenous ear cartilage graft. Laryngoscope 114:627–638
4. Menick F (1999) Anatomic reconstruction of the nasal tip cartilages in secondary and reconstructive rhinoplasty. Plast Reconstr Surg 104:2187–2198
5. Rees T (1986) Surgical correction of the severely deviated nose by extramucosal excision of osseocartilaginous septum and replacement as a free graft. Plast Reconstr Surg 78:320–330
6. Peer A (1933) Plastic surgery of the nose. J Med Soc 30:123
7. Malinac J (1948) Role of the septum in rhinoplasty. Am J Otolaryngol 48:189
8. Rohrich R, Gunter J, Deuber M, Adams W (2002) The deviated nose: Optimizing results using a simplified classification and algorithmic approach. Plast Reconstr Surg 110:1509–1523
9. Guyuron B, Uzzo C, Scull H (1999) A practical classification of septonasal deviation and an effective guide to septal surgery. Plast Reconstr Surg 104:2202–2209
10. Byrd S, Saloman J, Flood J (1998) Correction of the crooked nose. Plast Reconstr Surg 102:2148–2157
11. Pontius A, Leach J (2004) New techniques for management of the crooked nose. Arch Facial Plast Surg 6:263–266
12. Stucker F, Ansel D (1978) A case against nasal packing. Laryngoscope 88:1314–1317
13. Altreuter RW (1987) Nasal trauma. Emerg Med Clin North Am 5:293–300
14. Markowitz B, Manson P, Sargent L et al. (1991) Management of the medial canthal tendon and nasoethmoidal orbital fractures: The importance of the central fragment in classification and treatment. Plast Reconstr Surg 87:843–853
15. Dingman R, Natvig P (1969) The nose. Surgery of facial fractures. Saunders, Philadelphia, p 267
16. Colton J, Beekhius G (1986) Management of nasal fractures. Otolaryngol Clin North Am 19:73–85
17. Bailey B, Tan L (1998) Nasal and frontal sinus fractures. In: Baileys otolaryngology head and neck surgery 2nd edn, Chap 72. Lippincott-Raven, Philadelphia, p 1007
18. Rohrich R, Adams W (2000) Nasal fracture management: Minimizing secondary nasal deformities. Plast Reconstr Surg 106:266–273
19. Stucker F, Bryarly R, Shockley W (1984) Management of nasal trauma in children. Arch Otolaryngol 110:190–192
20. Goode R, Spooner T (1972) Management of nasal fractures in children: A review of current practices. Clin Pedia 11:526–529
21. Marks S, Loechel W (2000) Nasal and paranasal sinus surgery. Saunders, Philadelphia

22. Holt G (1989) Nasal septal fractures. In: English G (ed) Otolaryngology, vol 4. Lippincott, Philadelphia

23. Watson D, Parker A, Slack R, Griffiths M (1988) Local v general anesthetic in the management of the fractured nose. Clin Otolaryngol Allied Sci 13:491–494

24. Mayell M (1973) Nasal fractures: Their occurrence, management and some late results. J R Coll Surg Edinb 18:31–36

25. Crockett D, Mungo R, Thompson R (1989) Maxillofacial trauma. Pediatr Clin North Am 36:1471–1494

26. Waldron J, Mitchell D, Ford G (1989) Reduction of fractured nasal bones: Local vs. general anesthesia. Clin Otolaryngol Allied Sci 14:357–359

27. Courtney M, Rajapakse G, Duncan G, Morrisey G (2003) Nasal fracture manipulation: A comparative study of general and local anesthesia techniques. Clin Otolaryngol Allied Sci 28:472–475

28. Chaban R et al. (1988) Simulated septal deviations. Arch Otolaryngol Head Neck Surg 114:413–415

29. Cole P et al. (1988) The obstructive nasal septum. Effect of simulated deviations on nasal airflow resistance. Arch Otolaryngol Head Neck Surg 114:410–412

30. Howard B, Rohrich R (2002) Understanding the nasal airway: Principles and practice. Plast Reconstr Surg 109:1128–1144

31. Krouse J, Chadwick S, Gordon B, Derebery J (2002) Allergy and immunology, an otolaryngic approach. Lippincott, Philadelphia

32. Canady J (1994) Evaluation of nasal obstruction in rhinoplasty. Plast Reconstr Surg 94:555–559

33. Anand V, Isaacs R (1994) Nasal physiology and treatment of turbinate disorders. In: Rees T, LaTrenta S, Stilwell D (eds) Aesthetic plastic surgery. Saunders, Philadelphia

34. Kimmelman C (1989) The problem of nasal obstruction. Otolaryngol Clin North Am 22:253–264

35. Bridger G et al. (1970) Physiology of the nasal valve. Arch Otolaryngol Head Neck Surg 92:543–553

36. Grymer LF, Hilberg O, Elbrønd O, Pedersen OF (1989) Acoustic rhinometry: Evaluating the nasal cavity with septal deviation before and after septoplasty. Laryngoscope 99:1180–1187

37. Bridger G et al. (1981) Rib graft for nasal valve obstruction. Arch Otolaryngol Head Neck Surg 107:110–113

38. Constantian M (1993) Functional effects of alar malposition. Ann Plast Surg 30:487–493

39. Stucker F, Lian T, Sanders K A stepwise correction to the crooked nose. Am J Rhinol (in press)

40. Stucker F (1982) Management of the scoliotic nose. Laryngoscope 92:128–134

41. Sheen J (1984) Spreader grafts: A method of reconstructing the roof of the middle nasal vault following rhinoplasty. Plast Reconstr Surg 73:230–239

42. Boccieri A, Pacali M (2003) Septal crossbar graft for the correction of a crooked nose. Plast Reconstr Surg 111:629–638

43. Wexler M (1977) Surgical repair of the caudal end of the septum. Laryngoscope 87:304–309

44. Gunter J, Rohrich R, Adams W (2002) Dallas rhinoplasty: Nasal surgery by the masters, vols 1, 2. Quality Medical Publishing, St. Louis

45. Stucker F, Smith T (1976) The nasal bony dorsum and cartilaginous vault: Pitfalls in management. Arch Otolaryngol 102:695–698

46. Janeke J, Wright W (1973) A study of nasal fracture healing. Arch Otolaryngol 97:253–255

47. Genc E, Ergin T, Bilezikci B (2004) Comparison of suture and nasal packing in rabbit noses. Laryngoscope 114:639–645

Chapter 73

Nasal Valve Surgery

Richard L. Goode

Core Messages

- Valve collapse is an uncommon problem
- Needs careful preoperative evaluation
- Modified Cottle test helps diagnose
- High septal deflection may be a cause
- Cartilage battens placed in valve area best
- Banked costal cartilage is good source of cartilage

Contents

Introduction

A multitude of surgical procedures have been described to correct nasal valve insufficiency; all seem to be effective in the hands of their advocates but some appear more successful when performed by the average otolaryngologist. This chapter will describe my preferred surgical approach to this uncommon but important cause of nasal obstruction. Other chapters describe the anatomy and physiology of the valve in detail.

Weakness or collapse of the *internal* nasal valve is the most common location for obstruction. The *internal valve* is composed of the septum medially and the caudal end of the upper lateral cartilage laterally. The upper lateral cartilage is attached to the dorsal aspect of the septum forming an angle of 10–15° at the apex. The *external valve* lies caudal to the internal valve and consists of the alar margin with the lateral crus of the lower lateral cartilage laterally and the columella and medial crus of the lower lateral cartilage medially. A fibrous subcutaneous pad lies at the base of the nostril laterally and the nasal dilator muscles attach here. The apex is the inner aspect of the dome and the width and angulation here varies considerably between individuals. Obstruction due to weakness or collapse of the external valve is less common than at the internal valve; both are seen following an aggressive rhinoplasty, skin cancer surgery, nasal tip trauma, or paralysis of the dilator muscles.

There are no nasal constrictor muscles in the human, so narrowing of the nares occurs passively, secondary to increasing negative air pressure within the nose during inspiration and, to some extent, the Bernoulli effect of the airflow within the internal nasal valve area. In this effect, air passing through the narrow valve area has an increased velocity, which produces a localized decrease in air pressure, further contributing to collapse of the upper lateral cartilage against the septum. Rapid, short, inspiration, such as in a sniff, produces a very high negative air pressure, and invariably results in collapse of the valve. This collapse is normal and allows the individual to move excess mucus from the front to back of the nose.

The so called spring constant of the internal nasal valve cartilage defines how much the valve moves inward with increasing negative air pressure and is a measure of valve cartilage strength. No movement should occur during quiet nasal breathing with peak end inspiratory pressures of -5 to -10 cm of water. When increased airflow is desired, as during exercise, the inspiratory pressure becomes more negative and collapse begins in order to limit the nasal airflow so that the well known nasal functions of warming, cleansing, and humidifying the inhaled air can occur. This collapse is nonlinear, being minimal at lower pressures and increasing rapidly at higher negative air pressures. Some valve collapse is normal during rapid, deep breathing and varies between individuals as to amount based on valve anatomy and cartilage strength.

Diagnosis of Nasal Obstruction

A proper diagnosis of the cause(s) of nasal obstruction is, of course, essential in order to properly correct the obstruction. Many obstructions are transient or intermittent, due to allergic rhinitis, upper respiratory infections (URI), sinusitis, and vasomotor rhinitis. These are best treated medically and it is assumed that there has been failure of an adequate trial of medical management before proceeding to surgical treatment. Careful evaluation for nasal tumors, most commonly benign nasal polyps but including nasopharyngeal tumors of a more serious nature, should be a routine part of the evaluation. We consider nasal endoscopy as part of the initial evaluation.

The status of the inferior turbinates prior to vasoconstriction is important since they are often the sole or a major contributor to chronic nasal obstruction. The effect of a topical vasoconstrictor spray on symptoms of obstruction should be evaluated as part of the initial examination. Does it eliminate the obstruction completely on both sides? If not, what percent improvement?

Many individuals have nasal obstruction at night while in bed; some only have obstruction at this time. The inferior turbinates appear to swell more when the body is horizontal so an increase in obstruction would be expected. A short trial for 2–3 nights of a long-acting, over-the-counter nasal alpha adrenergic spray, such as oxymetazoline, will allow evaluation of the role of the turbinates in nocturnal nasal obstruction, similar to its effect on daytime obstruction.

The status of the septum is then carefully evaluated with emphasis on the caudal three centimeters, which is the most important area in the nose in regard to producing nasal obstruction. Since the dorsal septum in the area of the internal valve is the medial border of the valve, a deflection in this area will narrow or obliterate the superior valve opening, predisposing to abnormal valve collapse. A high septal deviation may be missed on routine anterior rhinoscopy, unless an effort is made to look superiorly into this important area. A high septal deflection may be misdiagnosed as a valve problem when it actually is a septal problem and best corrected by straightening the septum in this area.

Diagnosis of Valve Obstruction

Observation of the nasal valve area during resting, low-flow nasal breathing and then with more rapid, deeper breathing is the best single test. Normal valves do not obstruct during quiet breathing but may be seen to move slightly inward during deep breathing. Sniffing regularly collapses normal valves.

Some abnormal valves are collapsed even when mouth breathing and these are often easy to diagnose since the "pinched tip" stigmata of an overdone rhinoplasty or other nasal injury is apparent. More common are valves that appear normal at rest but collapse too easily during low- or moderate-flow nasal breathing. Many normal valves collapse to some extent during high-flow nasal breathing such as with strenuous exercise; as previously noted, this is normal and rarely requires surgical treatment.

The Cottle test or equivalent is an important test. We prefer to use a narrow probe to move various sites within the valve outwards, including the external valve. The amount of displacement needed and the exact location of maximal effect to eliminate obstruction is carefully noted and retested several times. We term this a modified Cottle test. The test is performed with and without a topical vasoconstrictor to assess the role of turbinate shrinkage in combination with opening the valve. A trial of a commercial over-the-counter valve dilator, such as Breathe Right nasal strips can also help assess valve collapse, both during the day and night [6].

Webs and scars in the superior valve area are looked for since these require different treatment than for a weak or missing valve cartilage. This is particularly a problem after rhinoplasty. In these cases, skin grafts or composite grafts from the concha may be required since the defect is not just cartilage but cartilage and skin. These reconstructions are beyond the scope of this chapter and are covered in other references [1].

As mentioned, damaged or weak valve cartilages may be collapsed at rest or collapse with normal or near normal inspiratory pressures. What is important is the individual's perception of the amount of "nasal dyspnea" produced by the collapse. This can vary considerably between patients so that minimal collapse in some is intolerable while the same amount or more in another produces no symptoms of obstruction.

Nasal "sniffers" who demonstrate how they cannot breathe through the nose by sniffing with resultant valve collapse must be educated that this is normal. They are not good surgical candidates!

Surgical Treatment

In the usual case of internal valve insufficiency I favor the approach of placing a stiff batten of appropriate size into a pocket made between the caudal edge of the upper lateral cartilage and the cephalic edge of the lateral crus of the lower lateral cartilage. (Fig. 73.1a) The pocket runs the same direction as the caudal border and extends to, but not above, the dorsal septum. Laterally, the end of the pocket lies just lateral to the bony pyriform process. The pocket is not angled but lies at right angles to the

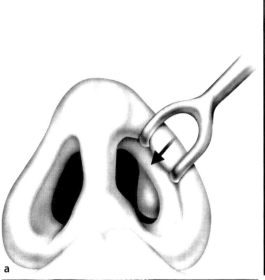
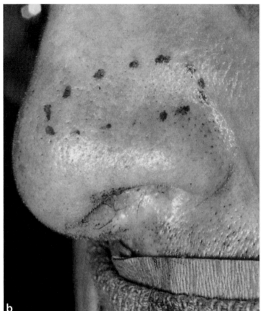
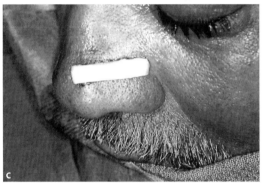

Fig. 73.1 **a** The *arrow* points to the caudal edge of the upper lateral cartilage comprising the lateral border of the internal nasal valve. Weak or absent cartilage in this area can allow valve collapse at rest or during normal nasal breathing producing obstruction. (With permission from Surgical Management of Sleep Apnea and Snoring. Taylor & Francis, New York, New York, 2005) **b** Outline of a typical pocket for a cartilage batten graft. The graft will lie at the junction of the upper and lower lateral nasal cartilages and stiffen the internal valve to prevent collapse. **c** Cartilage graft carved and ready for insertion and final size adjustment. It should extend from just below the dorsum of the septum to the naso-facial groove and be wide enough to correct the cartilage deficiency

plane of the nasal septum (Fig. 73.1b). The length of the batten is adjusted so as to meet the dorsal septum medially and lie just lateral to the bony pyriform process laterally, a distance of 2.5–3.5 cm in most cases (Fig. 73.1c).

The batten should be slightly convex to increase the distance between the septum and lateral valve area. It is inserted using a marginal or cartilage splitting incision and the pocket developed lateral to any remaining valve cartilages and made just slightly larger than the batten size required. Care is taken not to perforate the vestibular skin and the incision is made caudal to the pocket so it is not in contact with the batten (Fig. 73.2a).

The batten width depends on how wide an implant is required to eliminate valve collapse, usually about 5 mm, occasionally wider. The edges are beveled to minimize any later "edge lines." The thickness depends, in part, on the material used for the batten. It should be as thin as possible but be capable of providing the same support as normal valve cartilage. A millimeter or slightly less thickness is common. A normal angle of 15° at the medial contact point with the dorsal septum is another goal.

The greater the dorsal projection in the supratip area, the longer the batten must be. This requires a stronger batten material to support the longer span, similar to beams that support the roof of a house; the longer the span, the stronger the beam must be.

If no cartilage is present due to prior removal, the batten is placed where the cartilage was. If damaged or weak cartilage is present, that cartilage is removed. This decreases the thickness of the tissue in this area. Obviously, collapsed valves at rest, preoperatively, will be widened after implantation, which should not only correct the valve collapse but improve the cosmetic appearance of the lower nose. Valves that are weak but not collapsed preoperatively will be wider in the valve area following surgery.

Several choices are available for the batten material. *Septal cartilage*, if available, is good but may not be curved and care must be taken to get enough length for an adequate batten or battens, if two are needed. *Conchal cartilage* from the pinna is favored by many since it is an autograft, leaves a minimal cosmetic defect, and one side can usually provide adequate carti-

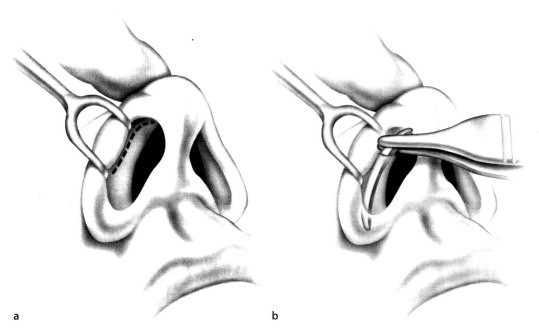

a   b

Fig. 73.2 **a** The *dotted line* shows the usual site of the marginal cartilage spitting incision used to develop the pocket for the implant. The incision should lie below the caudal border of the implant. The pocket is made with fine blunt tipped scissors and is only slightly larger than the implant. (With permission from Surgical Management of Sleep Apnea and Snoring. Taylor & Francis, New York, New York, 2005) **b** Insertion of the batten graft into the pocket is shown. Care must be taken to avoid breaking a cartilage implant during insertion. Residual damaged or weak cartilage in the area is removed to decrease width. The incision is closed with interrupted 4O chromic sutures (With permission from Surgical Management of Sleep Apnea and Snoring. Taylor & Francis, New York, New York, 2005)

73

lage for two implants. The incision may be made on the anterior or posterior surface of the pinna; I prefer the anterior approach. Again, obtaining adequate length of cartilage for battens in some ears can be a problem and excessive curvature may also be present.

Costal cartilage is the ideal material to use, in my opinion, but harvest of autograft costal cartilage has too many disadvantages for routine use. It makes a small operation into a big operation. Banked homograft costal cartilage is my preferred material. It is nonantigenic, has high tensile strength, carves well, has low long-term absorption, very low extrusion and infection problems, requires no donor site and is relatively cheap ($306.00 a bottle). This has been provided as irradiated cartilage in the past, but currently is provided frozen and sterile in an antibiotic solution. (Musculoskeletal Transplant Foundation, 125 May Street, Edison, NJ 08837-9948) A 3.0-cm long piece is usually needed to assure that adequate length is available. Multiple battens can be carved with a #10 Bard Parker scalpel changed frequently. It is easier if the cartilage is kept wet during carving. If a mistake is made or the batten fractures during carving or insertion, another can be carved. This is not usually possible with septum or conchal cartilage; errors may require another source of a batten. The major disadvantage of banked cartilage is the time required to carve the battens to the proper size and shape.

Alloplastic implants have been used as battens and, currently, Medpor, a perforated polyethylene material, is popular

[2]. These are provided preformed so that minimal trimming is required. I prefer the Romo type since they mimic the cartilage grafts that I carve. Extrusion may be a problem with these implants, more so, in my experience, than with homograft costal cartilage.

All battens are soaked in an antibiotic solution prior to implantation (80 mg of gentamicin used for IV injection in 250 cc of saline). Systemic prophylactic IV antibiotics are routinely used and started 30 min before the case begins. They are usually stopped after one dose.

The battens can be inserted though an endonasal or external approach; as previously stated, we prefer the endonasal approach for several reasons. It is faster and allows the surgery to be done in a procedure room under local anesthesia, if desired, which is more difficult with an open approach. There is no advantage to the additional incisions and exposure in the majority of the cases. Obviously, if a revision rhinoplasty is planned in addition to valve implants, an open approach may be preferred.

After placement of the batten into the pocket which has been carefully adjusted to allow minimal movement of the implant, the vestibular incision is closed with interrupted 4-O chromic sutures to provide a "waterproof" closure without tension. The immediate postimplant appearance is inspected, particularly in regard to right-left symmetry and width. Differences in symmetry need correction if present. In some noses a thicker or wider batten is needed on one side compared to the other. Unilateral implants are more difficult, since postoperative capsule formation around the implant may make it appear larger 1 year after surgery than in the operating room. Xeroform packing is placed in the anterior nares to support the implant and eliminate any dead space between the vestibular skin and the batten. This is removed in 3–4 days.

Troell et al. [5] described placing the batten in a pocket at the alar margin, similar to the effect produced by the nasal dilator muscles, and compared the results obtained in relieving nasal obstruction with a batten in the internal valve area such as described here. They found the external site produced slightly superior results but cosmetically was less appreciated. Stucker and Hoasjoe [4] and others have described another approach that appears to work well, placing a conchal cartilage graft horizontally over the septum in the valve area to widen the internal valve.

The postoperative cosmetic effect of an implant in a valve that does not appear pinched or collapsed preoperatively is a very important consideration. *It is not possible to widen the valve area on the inside without widening the valve area on the outside.* Beware the patient who states preoperatively: "Doctor, I don't care what my nose looks like, I just want to breathe." Excessive nasal widening postoperatively is not acceptable to patients, no matter what they say prior to surgery. "Excessive" may vary from patient to patient, so in order to make sure that the patient knows how much wider the nose will need to be to achieve an adequate airway, show them in a mirror the cosmetic result when the nasal valve is opened with the probe an adequate amount to relieve the obstruction; confirm that the appearance is acceptable.

The approach described here can be combined with spreader grafts [3] placed endonasally to further move the medial end of the batten laterally, if the batten does not appear to provide an adequate airway. I do not feel it is necessary to combine techniques in the usual case; the batten implants should be adequate.

High septal deflections in the valve area should be removed or straightened, if they contribute to valve collapse. The "one centimeter" of dorsal quadrilateral cartilage that is recommended to leave to avoid saddling is a rule of thumb. It may be necessary to remove more cartilage to relieve the obstruction, leaving only 5–6 mm. Each case must be individualized in order to produce a successful result. Obviously, as more septum in this area is removed, the nose is more susceptible to collapse following external trauma. In these cases, spreader grafts, sutured in place, may be needed on one or both sides to improve septal strength as well as relieve obstruction. We do not recommend removal of dorsal septum in this area to less than 5 mm; however, we try and do everything we can to improve obstruction at this site, the narrowest area of the airway.

Another important consideration is that individuals vary in the amount of nasal airway required to relieve symptoms of nasal obstruction. We term this the *nasal dyspnea threshold*. Some patients require so much nasal airway opening to relieve symptoms that the risk of a postoperative dry nose, *rhinitis sicca*, may become a problem, producing thicker mucus, and a higher propensity for nose bleeds. More commonly, they require excessive alar widening to produce the feeling of adequate airflow and, in my opinion, this is rarely a satisfactory postoperative solution.

Complications

Occasionally implants need to be removed or replaced. Homograft cartilage is relatively easy to remove. The usual reasons for removal are an inadequate airway or an unacceptable cosmetic result. If the nose appears too wide, the homograft cartilage graft can be sectioned near the base in the office using a scalpel after injection of a small amount of local anesthesia into the area. This decreases the curvature and resulting nasal width but also decreases the open area within the valve as well as the support.

Postoperative infection is rare, possibly in part due to soaking the implants in the antibiotic solution. Extrusion has not been a problem. I have had none in some 100 implants. Late absorption of homograft rib cartilage has been described but must be uncommon when used as a valve implant. I have not seen this in over 30 years time but many cases are lost to long-term follow-up.

Removal of implants has occurred in two cases due to an unhappy patient regarding the postoperative cosmetic result. The nose was thought too wide. This complication is about 2% of my total cases and occurred early in my series. Every operation has a learning curve.

Nasal valve insufficiency, its diagnosis and its correction, is an important part of nasal airway surgery and needs to be considered in the routine evaluation of nasal obstruction patients; it may not be the septum and/or turbinates.

Failure to achieve an "ideal" airway despite what appears to be a postoperative valve area of normal size and strength has occurred in 15–20% of cases. The airway was definitely better but the patients felt some obstruction was still present. The reasons are not clear in all cases. In one third, I thought the batten was too short, too narrow, or not curved enough to provide an adequate airway. Replacement of the batten produced success in most but not all of these cases. Lack of adequate reduction of the inferior turbinates was the cause in another one third, verified by the fact that a spray of a topical nasal vasoconstrictor following the valve surgery corrected the residual obstruction. In another one third, including the revision failure cases, I suspected a *nasal dyspnea syndrome* that I had missed in the preoperative evaluation. Opening the valve with the probe, making sure the septum was straight *and* spraying with a vasoconstrictor produced no significant improvement in the feeling of obstruction. While some resistance to nasal airflow is thought necessary in order to achieve "normal" nasal breathing, I am skeptical that a hyperpatent nasal airway is the reason for failure to achieve a feeling of adequate nasal breathing. All of our operations to correct obstructive symptoms are designed to open, not close, the nasal airway to produce the feeling of adequate nasal airflow.

Tips to Avoid Complications

- Precise size batten and pocket in optimal location
- Avoid "excessive" alar widening
- "Waterproof" pocket closure
- Topical and systemic antibiotics

Take-Home Pearls

- Careful preoperative evaluation
- Rhinoplasty is a common cause
- Select best implant material for batten
- Cartilage preferred: septum, concha, banked
- Endonasal approach
- Again, precise pocket in optimal location
- Replace absent or weak valve cartilage with batten
- Avoid excessively wide postop nares
- Strive to achieve nasal symmetry

References

1. Goode RL (1985) Surgery of the incompetent nasal valve. Laryngoscope 95:38–41
2. Romo T, Sclafani AP, Sabini P (1998) Use of a porous high-density polyethylene in revision rhinoplasty and in the platyrrhine nose. Aesthetic Plast Surg 22:211–221
3. Sheen JH (1984) Spreader graft: A method of reconstructing the roof of the middle nasal vault following rhinoplasty. Plast Reconstr Surg 73:230–239
4. Stucker FJ, Hoasjoe DK (1994) Nasal reconstruction with conchal cartilage: Correcting valve and lateral nasal collapse. Arch Otolaryngol Head Neck Surg 120:653–658
5. Troell RJ, Powell NB, Riley RW et al. (2000) Evaluation of a new procedure for nasal alar rim and valve collapse: Nasal alar rim reconstruction. Otolaryngol Head Neck Surg 122:204–211
6. Ulfberg J, Fenton G (1997) Effect of Breathe Right nasal strip on snoring. Rhinology 35:50–52

73

Chapter 74

Pediatric Septorhinoplasty

Gary Y. Shaw

Core Messages

- Significant pediatric nasal deformities should be corrected promptly to prevent long-term nasofacial deformities and psychological damage.
- Judicious repair will not adversely affect nasal growth.
- Nasal decortication (i.e., external open approach) is advantageous in pediatric nasal reconstruction.

Contents

Background

Classic teachings have long proposed that repair of pediatric nasal deformities should be delayed until maturation. With some notable exceptions (e.g., cleft lip/palate, choanal atresia, and nasal dermoid/encephalocoeles) this entailed waiting until approximately age 15–17 years in females and 16–18 years in males [1, 2]. This dictum was largely based upon poorly understood nasal growth center locations and animal studies that were not representative of realistic human surgical experience [3, 4]. This prevailing attitude unfortunately had condemned many children to endure significant functional and cosmetic deformities, which could have been avoided without risk to nasal and facial development.

As early as 1952, Goldman stated, "Early surgical correction of nasal and septal deformities is necessary to prevent the otherwise secondary severe nasal and facial deformities" [5]. These secondary deformities include retrognathic midface and unfavorable dental occlusion [6]. Jennes (1964) noted that clinical documentation of underdevelopment or deformity of the nasal dorsum resulting from uncomplicated surgical procedures on the septum is conspicuously sparse [7]. Furthermore, more recent, better-designed animal studies in cats [8], dogs [9], and guinea pigs [10] have shown conservative nasal surgery preserving mucoperichondrium cause little if any effect on nasal and midface growth. Several longitudinal human clinical studies have clearly shown judicious reconstructive nasal surgery in children from 1 to 14 years did not show any retardate effects on nasal or facial growth [7, 11, 12].

Nasal Embryology

The septum is felt to be integral in nasal growth and projection. In the third fetal month the septum is represented by two midline mesenchymal condensations, which gradually fuse. The sphenoid rostrum grows forward into the posterior septum. During the first post partum year ossification of the cephalic portion produces the perpendicular plate of the ethmoid [13]. The vomer develops bilaterally posterior and inferior to the septum with an ossification center in each side, which will eventually fuse. The suture line between the vomer and premaxilla is an area of growth and important in the management of bilateral cleft palate.

The nasal pyramid is derived from a single cartilaginous capsule. The nasal bones develop as membranous bone from a solitary ossification center of the capsule and eventually replace it. Additional contributions to the lateral vault of the nose come from the developing maxilla, which incorporates the adjacent cartilages of the nasal capsule. The developing maxilla also contributes the nasal spine and the maxillary crest both contribute to overall nasal projection. Chondrification of the nasal capsule begins at the third fetal month. Lateral in-growth will eventually develop into the upper and lower lateral cartilages and membranous septum [13].

Nasal Growth

Post partum nasal growth is generally felt to occur in three phases. There is rapid growth from birth to 2 years. Growth then slows considerably till approximately 10 years. Growth then increases reaching a crescendo at puberty. Extensive anthropomorphic measurements (in North American caucasians) by Farkas (1994) have determined nasal width, height, and bridge length have matured by age 14 years in the male and 12 years in the female. Nasal tip protrusion has reached maturation at age 16 in the male and 14 years in females [14].

While there are considerable individual anatomic variations, the external appearance of the infant nose has some common characteristics. The nose is broad with a low bridge and a round, elevated tip. The nostrils are almost circular and easily visible. As the infant ages the lower lateral cartilages extend down and the tip becomes more bulbous and the nostrils become less visible. Post puberty the lower lateral cartilages become firmer, the dorsum becomes higher, and most importantly, nasoseptal deformities which may have been imperceptible at an early age become more noticeable and potentially symptomatic.

Nasal deformities can be classified as: (1) Prenatal (familial), (2) Birth injury, (3) Preadolescent, (4) Postadolescent [15]. Prenatal abnormalities such as cleft lip nasal deformities are discussed elsewhere in the text (See Sec. 1, Chap. 15). While various theories exist for birth injury nasoseptal deformities, the most plausible theory appears to be intrauterine pressure during the first stage of labor. Supporting this contention, the most common presentation is left occiptoanterior while the most common septal deviation is to the right (approximately 80%) [16]. Cottle estimated that up to 7% of all births are complicated by irreversible nasal injury [17]. Often these injuries of preadolescent early childhood do not become clinically significant until after the nose is fully developed. Thus the decision for surgical correction must be made based not only on the acute injury but the predictive effect that it may have on nasal development. In many cases acute repair should be delayed for several weeks to allow adequate examination. Nevertheless, in those cases where functional abnormalities exist or significant deformities may be expected then corrective surgery is indicated. Several studies that have longitudinally examined the effect of judicious nasal septal surgery in prepubescent children have shown no significant growth retardation [11, 12, 14].

Acute Nasal Injury

When acute nasal injury occurs in a small child a thorough external and internal exam is necessary to determine if surgical repair is necessary. This often will entail restraining the child and assistance with a nurse and often a parent is necessary. Occasionally sedation is useful if head trauma is not present. Laceration of the nasal skin should be repaired in layered fashion if present. Palpation of the pyramid, presence of sharp edges, depressions, and crepitous should be noted. If there is active bleeding adequate hemostasis can often be achieved with cotton pledgets soaked with 9 parts 5% cocaine to 1 part 1/1000 epinephrine. There should be careful evaluation of the septum to determine septal hematoma, thickening with a blue or red discoloration, presence of mucosal tears or protruding cartilage and bone. The drainage of even a small septal hematoma is important to prevent septal necrosis and long-term deformity in the developing nose. Therefore, even if general anesthesia is needed, a complete exam is mandatory. Conversely, because the nasal framework in the child is proportionately more cartilaginous, nasal roentgenograms are generally not indicated.

If significant nasoseptal injury is detected, repair should be undertaken within a week. Once repaired, nasal packing is necessary to prevent recurrence of the hematoma. Antibiotics are necessary while packed. External splint and taping should be applied to prevent a dorsal hematoma. The parents should be instructed to look for any signs of increasing pain, fever, tenderness, or swelling. The child should be re-examined in 3 days. If possible, closed reduction would be preferable; however, if comminution exists or significant deformity, the rhinoplastic surgeon should perform open exploration. If cartilage is lost caudally or dorsally it should be replaced since subsequent deformity will occur. Ideally, implant material could be harvested from other nonsupportive nasal cartilage, perpendicular ethmoid plate, or vomer bone [18]. If suitable donor nasal tissue is not available then center cut rib cartilage, conchal cartilage, mastoid cortical bone, or outer table parietal calvarial graft could be utilized [19].

Chronic Nasal Deformity

Historically, many functional deformities in children have been left unrepaired. Concern for affecting midface growth has clouded the judgment of rhinoplastic surgeons. As stated earlier, many studies have demonstrated both in animals and humans that judicious nasal surgery is not only safe but can positively influence growth by avoiding late deformity through early correction.

Difficulty in nasal exposure in the pediatric patient has led many rhinoplastic surgeons to advocate the external approach [20–22]. This allows for direct exposure of the nasal skeleton with wide visualization of the nasal septum. Deformities in the caudal septum anterior to the nasal spine and/or the cartilaginous dorsum are best approached in this fashion. Repair of these severe septal defects often necessitate reconstruction. Unlike acute injury, often the entire cartilage septum must be exposed and removed. Once removed, a template can be drawn and if straight posterior septum is available it can be fashioned

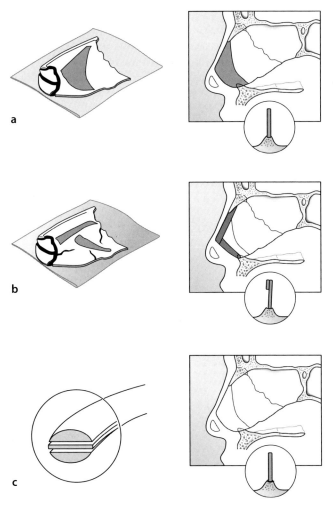

a

b

c

Fig. 74.1a–c Anterior nasoseptal reconstruction involves removal of cartilaginous septum and grafting in order of preference. (**a**) posterior central quadrilateral cartilage, (**b**) caudal and dorsal struts harvested from quadrilateral cartilage, (**c**) central cut rib cartilage (adapted from [19])

to place caudally (Fig. 74.1). As in acute injury, if adequate septal cartilage is not available then other donor material as previously outlined should be used. Abnormalities in the upper lateral cartilages affecting the nasal valve area causing nasal collapse can be reconstructed under direct vision. Defects in the lower lateral cartilages as seen in cleft lip nasal deformity (see Sec. 1, Chap. 15), can be precisely exposed and modified to make symmetric and directly sutured into place. If nasal bones are misaligned then careful osteotomy is performed.

Summary

While it has long been recognized that pediatric nasal deformities can cause severe long-term functional and cosmetic defor-

mities, there has been a reluctance to undertake surgical repair. This has been based on the misunderstood effect on midface growth centers. Often the very lack of surgical correction has allowed for significant midface deformities to occur. Good clinical judgment combined with judicious surgery can positively affect not only nasal function but otologic, sinus, and upper respiratory function, as well as the negative psychological effect that an uncorrected severe nasal cosmetic deformity can produce in the child.

Take-Home Pearls

- In acute nasal injuries a thorough internal and external nasal exam is necessary. Often sedation is necessary in the pediatric patient.
- Lost nasal support must be replaced.
- Donor site in order of preference includes: bony septum, center cut rib cartilage, conchal cartilage, mastoid cortical bone, or outer table calvarium.

References

1. Farkas LG, Posnick JC, Hreczko TM, Pron GE (1992) Growth patterns of the nasolabial region: A morphometric study. Cleft Palate Craniofac J 29:318–324
2. Beekhuis GJ, Wright WK (1965) Nasal Plastic Surgery. GP 32:136–140
3. Scott JH (1957) Studies in facial growth. Dent Pract 7:344–357
4. Sarnat BG, Wexler MR (1967) The snout growth after resection of nasal septum in the rabbits. Arch Otolaryngol 86:463–466
5. Goldman IB (1952) The maxillo-facial triad and its correction. J Int Coll Surg 17:167–180
6. Linder-Aronson S (1979) Respiratory function in relation to facial morphology and the dentition. Br J Orthod 6:59–71
7. Jennes ML (1964) Corrective nasal surgery in children. Arch Otolaryngol 79:145–151
8. Freng A, Haye R (1985) Experimental nasal septoplasty; Influence on nasomaxillary development in growing domestic cats. Acta Otolaryngol 100:309–315
9. Bernstein L (1973) Early submucus resection of nasal septal cartilage: A pilot study in canine pups. Arch Otolaryngol 97:273–278
10. Stenström SJ, Thilander BL (1970) Effect of nasal septal cartilage resections on young guinea pigs. Plast Reconstr Surg 45:160–170
11. Ortiz-Monasterio F, Olmedo A (1981) Corrective rhinoplasty before puberty: A long-term follow up. Plast Reconstr Surg 68:381–390
12. Walker PJ, Crysdale WS (1993) External septorhinoplasty in children: Outcome and effect on growth of septal excision and reimplantation. Arch Otolaryngol Head Neck Surg 119:984–989
13. Gilbert SG, Segal S (1958) Growth of the nose and septorhinoplastic problems in youth. Arch Otolaryngol 68:673–682
13. Farrior RT, Connolly ME (1970) Septorhinoplasty in children. Otolaryngol Clin North Am 3:345–364

14. Farkas LG, Hreczko TA (1994) Age-related changes in selected linear and angular measurements of the crainiofacial complex in healthy North American caucasians. In: Farkas L (ed) Anthropometry of the head and face, 2nd edn. Raven Press, New York, pp 89–102

15. Heinberg CJ (1956) Corrective surgery of the nasal framework. J Fla Med Assoc 45:276–289

16. Jazbi B (1977) Subluxation of the nasal septum in the newborn: Etiology, diagnosis, and treatment. Otolaryngol Clin North Am 10:125–138

17. Cottle MH (1951) Nasal surgery in children. Eye Ear Nose Throat Mon 30:32–45

18. Olsen N, Carpenter RJ, Kern EB (1980) Nasal septal injury in children. Arch Otolaryngol 106:317–320

19. Briant TDR, Middleton WC (1985) The management of severe nasal septal deformities. J Otolaryngol 14:120–124

20. Hugo SB (1987) Total septal reconstruction through decortication (external) approach in children. Arch Otolaryngol Head Neck Surg 113:173–178

21. Koltai PJ, Hoehn J, Bailey M (1991) The external rhinoplasty approach for rhinologic surgery in children. Arch Otolaryngol Head Neck Surg 118:402–405

22. Crysdale WS, Tatham B (1985) External septorhinoplasty in children. Laryngoscope 95:12–16

74

Facial Trauma

Chapter 75

Management of Trauma to the Nasal Bones and Septum

75

Fred G. Fedok, Michael P. Ondik, Todd W. Preston, and David Goldenberg

Core Messages

- A thorough history and physical should be part of any nasal fracture evaluation. Visual inspection, manual palpation and anterior rhinoscopy are essential. A thorough exam of the septum is also necessary to rule out septal hematoma and to properly access any septal deformity.
- Management of nasal injuries frequently requires individualization and an understanding of the patient's overall condition, associated injuries, age, and likelihood of reinjury.
- While traditional closed manipulation may be appropriately indicated in simple nasal fractures, it may frequently produce suboptimal results in more complex fractures or noses with pre-existing deformity. Practitioners should be prepared to perform reduction using either the described modified open or open technique.

Contents

Epidemiology

It has been reported that there are as many as 52,000 nasal fractures occur per year and that they account for more than 30% of all facial fractures [9, 12]. These numbers are most likely a low estimate since a large number of these injuries are not reported and may even go undiagnosed. As with most facial fractures, these injuries occur largely in the younger, physically active segments of the population and are usually males, although they do occur in patients from various walks of life and ages. While the most common mechanism is blunt trauma, these fractures also occur via penetrating and high-energy injuries. Finally, nasal fractures occur not only in isolation, but also frequently in conjunction with more extensive facial fractures.

Anatomy

Visually, the major aesthetic subunits of the external nose are typically described as: the nasal dorsum, the nasal tip and columella, the paired lateral nasal sidewalls, the alar lobules, and the alar facets laterally. Recreating these elemental subunits as distinct, individual anatomic entities during rhinoplasty or nasal reconstruction is essential if one is to provide an optimal nasal appearance. Maintaining and restoring the soft tissue and skeletal elements of the nose in physiologic relationship with each other is essential to restoring the function of the nose.

The External Soft Tissues of the Nose

The thickness and character of the skin of the nose varies from anatomic region to region. Beginning at the root of the nose, the nasal skin is rather thick. It thins considerably at the level of the nasofrontal suture and remains thin until reaching the lower third of the nose. At the lobule, the skin thickens considerably as it contains numerous sebaceous glands. The thickness of nasal skin along the caudal progression has many ramifications for the rhinoplasty surgeon. Very thin skin will reveal imperfections and inordinate detail of the osseocartilaginous skeleton whether native or surgical creations. In contrast, overly thickened skin may forestall efforts to impart definition and projection to a nose. In trauma situations, restorative rhinoplasty can be limited by the condition of the skin.

When one examines the skin moving from superficial to deep, the following are observed: the soft tissue elements are the epithelium; the subcutaneous tissue, which contains a variable amount of sebaceous glands; and the Subcutaneous Musculo-Aponeurotic System (SMAS), which contains all the nasal musculature. When possible, operations of the external nasal skeleton should take place within the plane deep to these tissues.

The Cartilaginous Framework

The upper lateral cartilages form the outer skeletal structure of the middle nasal compartment. The upper lateral cartilages underlay the nasal bones for a distance of 3–10 mm; disruption of this relationship traumatically can lead to nasal deformity or narrowing of the nasal airway at this point. These paired, triangular-shaped cartilages are joined in the midline to the cartilaginous septum for most of their length. The nasal tip is the mobile lower third of the nose, encompassing the lobule, columella, nostrils, and alae. Projecting laterally from the lobule are the paired alar sidewalls, forming the lateral walls of the nostrils, and joining the face at the alar–facial junction. The alar cartilages originate within the columella, just lateral to the septum at the nasolabial junction. They curve medially to meet the septum, and then quickly flare laterally and cephalically to form the cartilaginous structure of the nasal lobule. The alar cartilage is divided into three unequal segments, delineated by the two major inflection points in its curvature: the narrow medial crura, intermediate crura, and the upper lateral crura.

The Nasal Bones

The upper third and bony compartment of the nose is formed by the medially and posterior sloping ascending processes of the maxilla, articulating superiorly with the frontal bone and medially with the paired nasal bones, which continue medially to meet each other in the midline. The paired nasal bones contain a medial groove to receive the perpendicular plate of the ethmoid below. The sturdiest part of the bony compartment is the root of the nose, at which the ascending processes and nasal bones articulate with the frontal bone at a point labeled the nasion. The nasal bones are thickest at this point, becoming progressively thinner as they flare outward caudally, where they overlap with, then articulate with the upper lateral cartilages.

The Septum

The septum has both cartilaginous and bony components. The bony nasal septum is composed of the perpendicular plate of the ethmoid bone and the vomer. The perpendicular plate articulates with and bisects the tented up paired nasal bones and the frontal bone superiorly. Posterior and postero-superiorly the perpendicular plate extends to reach the sphenoid bone.

Inferiorly, it articulates with the vomer and quadrangular cartilage. The vomer, in turn, is set inferiorly in a groove provided by the maxillary crest of the maxilla and the superior aspect of the palatine bone. The perpendicular plate and vomer diverge anteriorly in the midsagittal plane, allowing the quadrangular cartilage to insinuate between the two via a network of fibrous attachments. The bony septum actually provides little support for the distal nasal dorsum; most of this support is derived from the anterior two thirds or the cartilaginous septum. The cartilaginous septum continues caudally past the upper lateral cartilages to intercalate with the alar cartilages, finally ending in attachment to the nasal spine of the maxilla.

Blood Supply of the Nose

The arterial supply of the nose comes from both the internal and external carotid arteries. This high flow system is important in the temperature regulation and pressure regulation of nasal airflow.

Innervation of the Nose

The trigeminal nerve provides sensation to the external nose via its ophthalmic and maxillary subdivisions. The facial nerve supplies motor innervation to the mimetic muscles of the nose.

Evaluation of the Patient with Nasal Injuries

The goal of the preoperative assessment is for the surgeon to aesthetically and anatomically diagnose what nasal components have been fractured or injured. The examination of this common injury can be performed expeditiously. A multitude of clinical questions, as detailed later, should be answered by a thorough examination. With this anatomic diagnosis at hand, the examiner should then be able to approach the patient within a framework that allows optimal management, reduction, and repair.

The examination of the patient is facilitated if the nose, when possible, is decongested. Visual inspection, manual palpation, and anterior rhinoscopy are essential. If possible, nasal endoscopy can be carried out to increase the acquisition of meaningful clinical data.

Visually, one can assess the overall appearance of the patient and their nose. The integrity of the nasal skin should be assessed. Is the skin intact, or are there lacerations or avulsions of soft tissue? If so, then an assessment should be made as to whether the lacerations involve deeper skeletal structures of the nose or the nasal lining.

Globally, the examiner should determine if the nose is straight, if there is a deviation, or if there is a C-shaped deformity. If these findings are present, the examiner should ascertain which components of the nose are crooked and why. In addition, the position of caudal septum should be assessed by manual palpation. Via visual inspection and palpation, the integrity

75

of dorsal support can be determined. Has the nose maintained normal midline support, or is there an acute saddle deformity and if so what anatomic disruption is contributing?

The nasal bones should be examined. Based on visualization and palpation, are there fractures of the nasal bones? If so, are the fractured nasal bones displaced; are the nasal bones dislocated or comminuted? Are there segments missing, and are the fractured segments mobile?

The tip and lower two thirds of the nose should be examined. Is there an injury to the cartilaginous framework? Has there been an avulsion of an upper lateral cartilage from its corresponding nasal bone (this injury is frequently under-diagnosed)? Is there an unusual mobility at the rhinion suggesting a fracture of the midline cartilaginous structures?

Determining the status of the septum is frequently underemphasized; however, appropriate appreciation and management of septal injuries is essential to the restoration of optimal nasal function and appearance. The following features should be assessed. The examiner should assess whether midline support has been disrupted, and if so, by what anatomic injury? Is the septum fractured? Is the septum dislocated? Are there mucosal lacerations? Is there cartilage missing? What is the condition of the mucoperichondrium and mucoperiostium; are there significantly sized areas of exposed cartilage? Is the entire septal cartilage present; has there been a loss of cartilage? And finally, the examiner should look for and document the presence or absence of a septal hematoma. If present it should be expeditiously and appropriately managed.

Photographs should be done similar to the views obtained for rhinoplasty evaluation. Planar radiographs and computerized tomography rarely add more valuable data than that obtained through the physical examination and medical history.

Injury Patterns and Classifications

A number of classification systems for nasal fractures have been published [7, 17]. None are universally accepted and applied, though; the surgeon should approach each nasal fracture patient within an anatomic diagnostic framework from which to consider management [11]. In a manner, the authors have found it helpful to categorize these injuries as depicted in Table 75.1, which is a modification of the classification system as proposed by Rohrich [17]. For example, the patient pictured in Fig. 75.1 suffered a nasal-septal injury. Based on the photograph alone, the patient's injury would be considered to represent a Type III injury.

Management

Although there are several general considerations in the management of patients with nasal injuries, some individualization is usually necessary. The individualization of care will be influenced by the overall condition of the patient, associated injuries, the age of the patient, and the likelihood of the patient's reinjuring the nose in a similar fashion, i.e., one might be hesitant to repair a minor fracture in a boxer, as well as a variety of other factors.

Timing of Repair

All soft tissue injuries should be addressed in a manner in accordance with the generally accepted principles of acute wound care. Acute management of nasal skeletal elements can be done

Table 75.1 Classification of nasal/septal fractures

I. Simple Straight (Unilateral or Bilateral)	
	Unilateral or Bilateral Nasal Fractures without causing deviation or disruption of nasal midline
II. Simple Deviated (Unilateral or Bilateral)	
	Unilateral or Bilateral Nasal Fractures with mild deviation or disruption of nasal midline either secondary to septal fracture or septal dislocation
III. Severe Nasal and Septal Fractures	
a. Unilateral	
b. Bilateral	
c. Comminuted	Unilateral or Bilateral Nasal Fractures with severe deviation or disruption of nasal midline either secondary to severe septal fracture or septal dislocation, may be associated with comminution of the nasal bones and septum which interfere with reduction of fractures
IV. Complex Nasal and Septal fractures	
	Severe injuries that may include comminution of nasal and septal structures, severe lacerations and soft tissue trauma, acute saddling of nose, open compound injuries, and avulsion of tissue

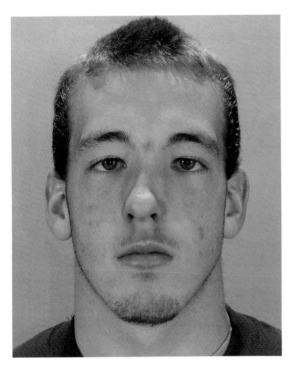

Fig. 75.1 Frontal photograph of patient who suffered nasal–septal frac-ture. Based on this photograph alone, the patient's injury would be con-sidered to represent a Type III injury

either before significant swelling has occurred or soon after it has subsided, but usually before 14 days. If repair is delayed lon-ger than that time period, the surgeon will encounter early bone malunion and remodeling.

All situations in which there is an immediate saddling of the nasal dorsum should be promptly managed surgically to estab-lish dorsal nasal support before significant scar contraction oc-curs. Type I, II, and III fractures can also be approached acutely in this time frame if there are no contraindications. It should be noted, that in IIIc situations the mobility afforded by comminu-tion will at times allow successful closed manipulation.

In Type IV fractures there should be a prompt repair of lacer-ations and coverage of exposed skeletal elements. Other aspects of treatment may have to be delayed until there is sufficient resolution of edema and softening of the skin so that proper contouring may take place. Delays of definitive treatment for up to 6 weeks and more may be necessary if there has been excessive tissue trauma. Even in these cases, however, early re-establishment of central dorsal support and acute wound repair is recommended.

Surgical Management Options

Observation

A suggested algorithm for management of nasal injuries and fractures is depicted in Fig. 75.2. When it has been determined that there is minimal displacement of the nasal bones, minimal soft tissue injury, and minimal compromise of the nasal airway, it is the opinion of these authors that it may be acceptable to recommend observation and to undertake no active surgical or manipulative intervention. Any definitive reparative rhino-plasty procedure that might be contemplated should be delayed for 6 weeks or more. This extended time frame will allow swell-ing and other healing to progress to the point that an accurate assessment of the nasal condition can be surmised.

Closed Manipulation

In this chapter closed manipulation refers to those methods of reduction that do not involve the use of incisions to expose anat-omy or to introduce instruments. Under local or general anes-thesia, the patient's fractures nasal bones and/or septum are mo-bilized and reduced digitally. At times this is aided with the used of blunt instruments such as the Boise elevator or Ash forceps. Traditional closed manipulation is best applied in those patients where there has been an actual subluxation or displacement of the nasal bones without a great deal of an actual fracture of the nasal bones themselves. This sometimes occurs in the younger patient with some elasticity to their nasal bones. These patients may present with an actual dislocation of the nasal bones, with-out comminution of the bones themselves. At times, the patient will present with bilateral subluxations, displaying an "open book" deformity. In some of these situations, there is a palpable "click" that occurs when the nasal bones snap into position. The limitations of this technique are seen in patients with unstable nasal fractures that do not remain in reduction after manipu-lation. This technique will also be unsuccessful in patients that have significant pre-existing or newly acquired septal deviation that impedes reduction and stabilization. In limited situations, a dislocated septum can be successfully replaced back into the midline using Ash forceps. Although this is the most commonly employed technique for the acute management of nasal frac-tures, suboptimal results have been reported in up to 30–50% of patients [13–16, 18].

Modified Open with Osteotomies

The Modified Open Technique is a limited version of an open technique in which intranasal incisions are made for the intro-duction of osteotomes. The senior author applies this technique to a significant number of young and older patients who pres-ent with asymmetric fractures, either unilateral or bilateral, of the nasal bones. There may be a "greensticked" or incompletely fractured segment that results in a "trapping" of one side of the nasal dorsum closed through impaction of the nasal bones or lack of successful reduction of the asymmetric or incomplete fractured bones. In many of these situations, when only closed manipulation of the nasal bones is attempted, there is failure of the nasal bones to reliably reduce and stabilize into a sym-metrical position. The end result is a persistence of asymmetry or deviation and malunion.

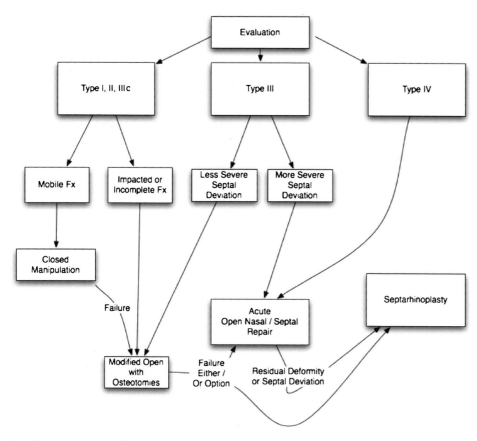

Fig. 75.2 Suggested nasal fracture management algorithm

Such patients frequently benefit from manipulation of the nasal bones into position after undergoing bilateral micro-osteotomies. Unilateral or bilateral osteotomies can convert asymmetric or impacted fractures into complete symmetric segments that can then be manipulated, reduced, and more reliably stabilized in position in a manner similar to that employed in the elective rhinoplasty situation. To avoid undo soft tissue trauma, 2 mm osteotomes are commonly used. Usually only lateral osteotomies are carried out [1, 2].

As with closed manipulation, the position of the septum may impede the success of this technique. It has been suggested that if the septum has a superior horizontal fracture, or if the dorsum is deviated more than 50% its width of the dorsum, then successful correction might only be achieved after open septoplasty [4, 10]. If these physical findings are noted, the patient should be informed that the modified open with osteotomies might prove to be unsuccessful. A secondary procedure may then be necessary or other treatment offered as described later in the text [19].

Modified Open with Osteotomies

The Open/Nasal Septal Repair refers to an aggressive approach to the acute management of complicated injuries using existing lacerations and/or external and intranasal incisions. With this approach the surgeon can reduce, graft, and fixate fractured anatomic components under direct visualization. In patients with comminuted fractures of the nasal bones and septum with loss of dorsal support or an acute saddle nose deformity, there is reason to carry out an acute open nasal or septal repair with reduction of the nasal bones and septum to normal positions with grafting of the septum if necessary. The acute open approach will also be necessary in most cases of compound injuries where there has been extensive soft tissue laceration and injury to the bony and cartilaginous skeleton. In trauma situations where there is severe septal deviation, or if a severe septal deviation is preventing adequate nasal bone reduction, open acute septoplasty may be warranted [3, 5]. These open approaches can frequently be carried out through pre-existing lacerations.

Formal Septorhinoplasty

Formal open septoplasty nasal fracture is employed in two general clinical situations. As noted earlier, this is sometimes the best approach to employ when there has been minimal displacement and treatment is delayed until swelling has resolved. This might be utilized when the patient's threshold for satisfaction is high, thus necessitating optimal symmetric results.

The other broad indication is as a secondary procedure after initial acute management [6]. Depending on the vast variability of clinical situations where soft tissue trauma may vary from minimal to massive, the delay may extend from 6 weeks to a year after the injury and previous acute management.

Special Situations

The Younger Patient

The younger patient with significant nasal trauma should be approached in a manner consistent with how one would prioritize any significant deforming or functionally impairing injury in the same child. To delay correction of a significantly displaced nasal or septal fracture is not warranted. So as to minimize possible impairment of nasal growth, repairs should be aimed at repositioning anatomic components and nasal dimensions. Structure should be restored and maintained, i.e., one should avoid removing segments of the cartilaginous or bony septum [12].

Nondisplaced Fracture

The minimally displaced fracture and septum may require no active intervention if there is no anticipated impact on form or function. However, it is important that such patients have at least a second assessment after swelling subsides.

"The Smashed Nose"

Severe crush, severe soft tissue injuries, acute saddle nose deformity and other high-energy injuries should be managed with a multiple-staged approach. In these cases the early priority is to re-establish central support, and repair lacerations of soft tissue and fractures of cartilaginous structures. Final definitive repair will have to be delayed until edema and swelling have subsided and adequate vascular coverage over septal components has been re-established.

Postoperative Care

Externally stabilizing dressings should be applied similarly to rhinoplasty care. Where there have been significant septal injuries, internal soft silastic splints may provide stabilization and aid in the prevention of synechia. Packing is only occasional necessary.

Complications and Limitations

Complications include scarring, infection, asymmetries, external deformity, saddling, septal deviation, septal perforation, airway obstruction, and need for additional procedures.

Tips to Avoid Complications

- Define the injury precisely and anatomically before planning any intervention.
- Manage the patient's expectations regarding the outcome of the repair. (Remember: what you tell the patient before the operation is informed consent; what you tell them after is an excuse.)
- Even if no surgical intervention is going to be planned, re-evaluate the patient after any traumatic swelling has resolved (usually 1–2 weeks).

Take-home pearls

- Nasal injuries frequently occur in the presence of other trauma. A thorough history must be taken in order to assess for concurrent injuries to other structures such as the eye, lacrimal system, teeth, and oral cavity.
- Always rule out the possibility of a septal hematoma and realize that these can easily be mistaken for a septal deviation; an undiagnosed and untreated septal hematoma can result in a septal perforation.
- Ask the patient to provide a premorbid photograph for an objective point of comparison.

References

1. Berman WE (1995) Nasal osteotomies-two parts. Ear Nose Throat J 74(5):318–319
2. Berman WE (1995) Nasal osteotomies-second and final part. Ear Nose Throat J 74(7):457–461
3. Burum JS, Oh SJ (1998) Indirect open reduction through intercartilaginous incision and intranasal Kirschner wire splinting of comminuted nasal fractures. Plast Reconstr Surg 102(2):342–349
4. Colton JJ, Beekhuis GJ (1986) Management of nasal fractures. Otolaryngol Clin North Am 19(1):73–85
5. Fernandes SV (2004) Nasal fractures: The taming of the shrewd. Laryngoscope 114:587–592
6. Goldman IB (1964) When is rhinoplasty indicated for correction of recent nasal fractures. Laryngoscope 14:689–700
7. Gollom J (1963) Problems in management of nasal fractures. Arch Otolaryngol 78:66–69
8. Gunter JP, Cochran CS (2006) Management of intraoperative fractures of the nasal septal "L-strut": Percutaneous Kirschner wire fixation. Plast Reconstr Surg 117(2):395–402
9. Illum P (1986) Long-term results after treatment of nasal fractures. J Laryngol Otol 100:273–277
10. Mondin V, Rinaldo A, Ferlito A (2005) Management of nasal bone fractures. Am J Otolaryngol 26:181–185

75

11. Murray JM, Maran AGD, Mackenzie IJ, et al (1984) Open v closed reduction of the fractured nose. Arch Otolaryngol 110:797–802

12. Perkins SW, Dayan SH (2002) Management of nasal trauma. Aesthetic Plast Surg 26 Suppl 1:3

13. Renner G (1991) Management of nasal fractures. Otolaryngol Clin North Am 24(1):195–213

14. Ridder GJ, Boedeker CC, Fradis M, et al (2002) Technique and timing for closed reduction of isolated nasal fractures: A retrospective study. Ear Nose Throat J 81(1):49–54

15. Roberts G (1950) The management of nasal fractures. Laryngoscope 60:557–563

16. Robinson JM (1984) The fractured nose: Late results of closed manipulation. N Z Med J 97:296–297

17. Rohrich RJ, Adams Jr. WP (1999) Nasal fracture management: Minimizing secondary nasal deformities. Plast Reconstr Surg 106(2):266–273

18. Rubinstein B, Strong B (2000) Management of nasal fractures. Arch Fam Med 9:738–742

19. Staffel JG (2002) Optimizing treatment of nasal fractures. Laryngoscope 112:1709–1719

Chapter 76

Fractures of the Zygomaticomaxillary Complex

Emre A. Vural and Mimi S. Kokoska

Core Messages

- Indications for treatment of ZMC fractures include lack of stability and displacement causing functional and/or cosmetic deficits.
- Ophthalmologic evaluation should be considered in ZMC injuries.
- Existing deficits, management options, and risks should be discussed with the patient and documented in the medical record.
- Adjacent nondisplaced bone and contralateral facial projection are useful references for adequate reduction.

Contents

Background and Anatomy

The malar eminence forms the most anterolateral projection on each side of the midface. It is comprised primarily from the zygomatic bone (Fig. 76.1). The zygomatic bone firmly abuts the frontal bone superolaterally at the zygomaticofrontal (ZF) suture. This attachment is in continuity with the zygomaticosphenoid suture in the lateral orbital wall. On its medial and inferior aspects, the zygomatic bone is attached to the maxilla at the zygomaticomaxillary (ZM) suture and alveolus forming the ZM buttress. ZM suture line extends to the inferior orbital rim. Laterally, the zygomatic bone attaches to the zygomatic process of the temporal bone to form the zygomatic arch. Various terms have been ascribed to malar eminence fractures including "tripod fracture" and "zygomatic fracture." There are four common distinct areas of injury that may require reduction and fixation in typical isolated fractures of the malar eminence. They include the inferior orbital rim, ZF suture, ZM buttress and zygomatic arch. The zygomaticosphenoid suture may also provide another helpful reference for reduction and realignment of fractured bone segments. Therefore, the term "tripod" is almost universally accepted as a misnomer, since it implies only three relevant anatomic regions. Similarly, the term "zygomatic fracture" does not fully represent fractures to the malar eminence, since separation of the ZM suture without maxillary involvement is quite rare and these fractures almost always involve maxilla to a various extent at the ZM buttress. Therefore we prefer the term "zygomaticomaxillary complex (ZMC) fractures" in defining the common pattern of multiple fractures involving the malar eminence. The malar eminence is akin to the apex, and the sutures or buttresses represent the legs of a pyramid or tetrapod. Traumatic injuries which cause a shortened leg will result in rotation of the malar eminence toward the shortened side. Forces which cause inferior displacement or lateralization of the zygomaticomaxillary complex will increase orbital volume, which can result in enophthalmos. Although most nondisplaced ZMC fractures can be managed conservatively without any surgical intervention, reduction and fixation is warranted for most displaced fractures of the ZMC, since the human eye can detect as little as one millimeter of dimensional difference. Important anatomic structures that can be directly or indirectly injured or

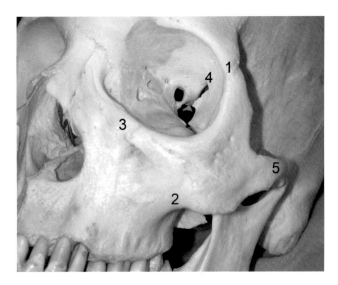

Fig. 76.1 The left zygoma bone and its abutting sutures or buttresses: (*1*) Frontozygomatic suture (*2*) Zygomaticomaxillary buttress (*3*) Inferior orbital rim (*4*) Zygomaticosphenoid suture (*5*) Zygomatic arch

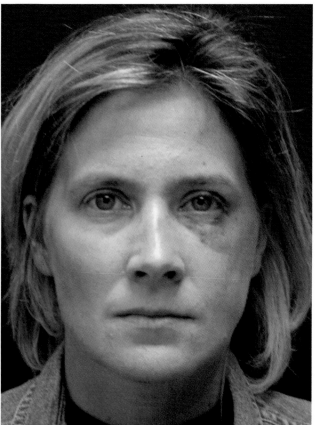

affected in a typical ZMC fracture include the eye, extraocular muscles, infraorbital nerve, lateral canthal tendon, masseteric and temporalis muscles, and mandibular coronoid process. The degree of involvement of any of these anatomic structures in a ZMC fracture defines the variety and severity of the symptoms and physical exam findings as discussed in the following section. The ZMC region is the third (after nasal and mandibular) most commonly fractured facial area. The majority of ZMC fractures occur in men, with a ratio of 4:1 in some series. These injuries are most commonly seen in the second to third decades of life and are most commonly associated with altercations. The infraorbital nerve and vessels (transmitted through the infraorbital foramen) are the main neurovascular structures contained in the ZMC region. The zygomaticofacial artery and vein and nerves (branches of cranial nerve V2) are relatively small and course out of the anterolateral zygoma.

Diagnosis

Clinical Presentation and Examination

The extent and direction of zygomaticomaxillary displacement and resultant facial deformity depends on the magnitude and direction of the inciting force, as well as the strength of the bone and its contacts. Patients who present with ZMC injury should be ruled out for multisystem injuries including cervical spine assessment and intracranial bleed when warranted by the circumstances of the inciting trauma. Patients presenting with acute zygomaticomaxillary complex fractures will frequently exhibit ecchymosis, edema, and tenderness in the overlying soft tissues. There may be evidence of malar flattening and/or depressed lateral cheek if there is a depressed arch fracture (Fig. 76.2).

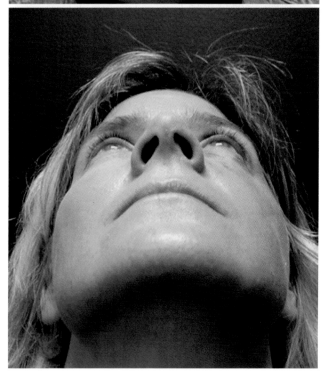

Fig. 76.2 Clinical evidence of left malar flattening with overlying ecchymosis, subconjunctival hemorrhage, and soft tissue swelling associated with a displaced zygomaticomaxillary complex fracture

76

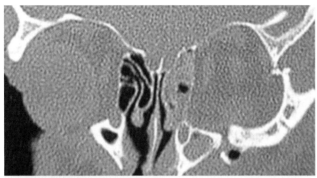

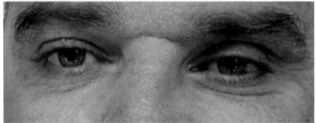

Fig. 76.3 Displaced left zygomaticomaxillary complex fracture with resultant increase in orbital volume and enophthalmos. Note the increased excursion from left upper eyelash margin and eyelid crease

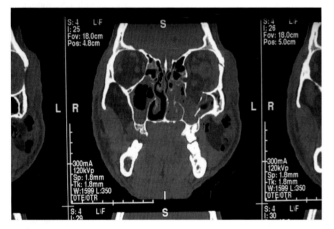

Fig. 76.4 Coronal CT scan demonstrating a left zygomaticomaxillary complex fracture with a displaced orbital floor fracture

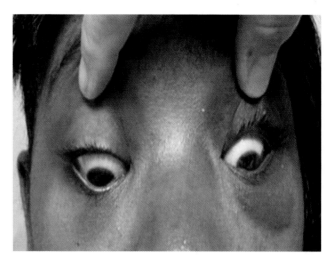

Fig. 76.5 Patient with inferior gaze restriction and diplopia due to entrapment of left inferior rectus muscle

Forces which cause inferior displacement or lateralization of the ZMC will increase orbital volume which will result in enophthalmos (Fig. 76.3). In contrast, medial displacement of the ZMC may cause exophthalmos by decreasing the volume of the orbital socket and these patients typically present with lateral subconjunctival hemorrhage due to the impact of medially displaced bone on the eye. It should be noted that enophthalmos may be due to a concurrent orbital floor fracture in a patient with ZMC fracture (Fig. 76.4). Diplopia suggests the presence of extraocular muscle entrapment, particularly the inferior rectus muscle (Fig. 76.5). Ophthalmologic consultation and forced duction test may be indicated in injuries to the ZMC. If there is direct globe injury or a fracture of the orbital wall, then it is prudent to have an ophthalmologist examine the eye, since there is a 10–60% incidence of significant intraocular sequelae with blunt orbital trauma with and without blow out fractures [1, 2].

In addition to orbital abnormalities, ZMC fractures can affect mastication through impingement by a depressed zygomatic arch on the temporalis muscle and coronoid process of the mandible. This can result in trismus and pain with mastication. Stepoffs are frequently detected on palpation along the frontolateral and inferior orbital rim and zygomatic arch. There may be hypoesthesia in the anterior cheek and upper lip from fracture and compression of the infraorbital foramen and nerve [3]. The mucosa in the upper gingivobuccal sulcus may be ecchymotic and swollen, with or without a palpable stepoff in the zygomaticomaxillary buttress. It is important to thoroughly document the clinical examination and review morbidity and possible outcomes with the patient, since there may be temporary or permanent functional and aesthetic deficits.

Imaging

Historically, plain films were used to confirm the presence of ZMC fractures (Fig. 76.6). However, in complex ZMC fractures, axial and coronal facial CT scans are presently the standard since they provide better resolution of the fractures and three-dimensional anatomy is better appreciated on CT scans. This is especially important for assessing facial projection and orbital volume, as well as for surgical planning (Fig. 76.7). In addition, CT scans provide useful information regarding the degree of orbital bone dehiscence, and the state of intraorbital contents and their relationship to the fracture site [4]. In most cases, the CT can delineate if there is muscle entrapment or only orbital fat within an orbital fracture (Fig. 76.4).

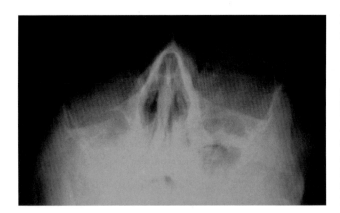

Fig. 76.6 Plain radiograph (Water's view) showing a displaced right inferior orbital rim fracture

Classification

Although ZMC fractures have been classified into types A, B, and C [5]. Type A injuries are isolated to one leg of the pyramid. Type B injuries fracture all legs of the tetrapod and type C involve comminuted fractures to the zygoma. This classification is not used commonly in the clinical setting, since defining and listing specific fractures provide more relevant information that the surgeon can act upon. For example, the degree of displacement is also important to cite when describing the fracture, since that is frequently an indication for surgical intervention in ZMC fractures.

Treatment

Indications

The indications for open reduction and fixation of ZMC fractures include lack of stability and displacement causing functional and/or cosmetic deficits. If fractures are nondisplaced or they are inherently stable, then the ZMC fractures will likely heal without sequelae. However, these patients should be kept on soft diet for 2–3 weeks to prevent displacement of the zygomatic arch from masseteric pull and to reduce the patient discomfort. To prevent subcutaneous emphysema or further risk of bacterial contamination, it is important to counsel patients to avoid blowing their nose or valsalva maneuvers in the acute setting of ZMC complex fractures which involve the maxillary sinus or medial orbital walls. The functional deficits which may be improved with reduction with or without fixation include hypoesthesia of the infraorbital nerve distribution, diplopia, pain, mandibular mobility, and trismus. The facial derangements which warrant surgical treatment include dystopia, enophthalmos or exophthalmos, malar or zygomatic displacement, and soft tissue deformities.

Approaches/Incisions

To access the superolateral orbit for repairing ZF fracturs, a lateral brow incision or an upper eyelid blepharoplasty incision can be used. A 1.5-cm incision following the curve of the superolateral orbital rim provides sufficient exposure to the fracture

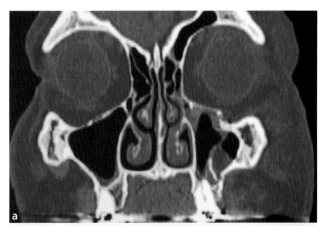
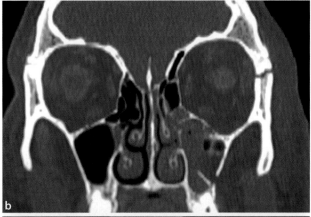
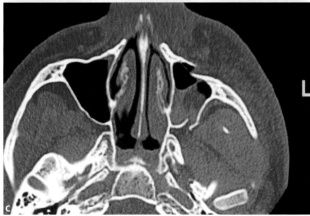

Fig. 76.7 **a**. Coronal CT scan showing inferior displacement of the left zygomaticomaxillary complex. **b**. Coronal CT scan with the left zygomaticomaxillary complex fractures specifically showing a fracture of the zygomaticofrontal suture with extension into the zygomaticosphenoid suture. **c**. Axial CT scan showing a posteromedial displacement of the zygomaticomaxillary complex

site (Fig. 76.8). If the lateral brow incision is extended into the eyebrow, then the incision should be beveled in the direction of the hair follicles to preserve the hairs and encourage coverage of the incisional scar. Although hemicoronal or bicoronal approaches are used by some surgeons, authors of this chapter find these approaches unnecessary in most cases. The risks of an unsightly scalp scar, temporal atrophy, and facial nerve injury should be weighed against the need for open exposure of the zygomatic arch for repair. Significant fragmentation and instability is an indication for exploration and reduction with fixation (Fig. 76.9). More recently, endoscopic guided repair of the zygomatic arch has been described. The inferior orbit can be accessed through a transconjunctival approach or a subciliary incision. Lateral canthotomy may be necessary in order to increase the exposure to the inferior orbital rim and orbital floor

in some cases. The subciliary approach can safely be performed by placing an incision about 2 mm below the eyelash-line in the lower eyelid and elevating the lower eyelid skin deep to the underlying pretarsal and preseptal orbicularis oculi muscle (Fig. 76.10). After obtaining sufficient skin-muscle flap elevation, the fracture can be exposed by incising the periosteum at the inferior orbital rim. Subciliary incisions do not always result in unsightly scars or cause eyelid malpositions, if these incisions are closed appropriately (Fig. 76.11). The incised periosteum at the inferior orbital rim should be reapproximated with absorbable sutures to cover the underlying hardware. After redraping the skin-muscle flap, subciliary incision should be closed in a "skin only" fashion with the material of surgeon's choice. If subciliary and lateral brow incisions are to be used together, special attention must be paid to leave at least a 4- to 5-mm distance

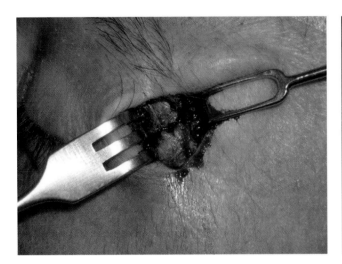

Fig. 76.8 Lateral brow incision for access to a fracture in the zygomaticofrontal suture

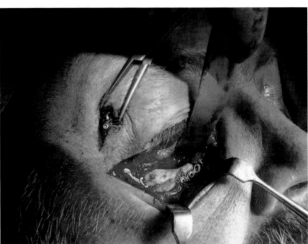

Fig. 76.10 Subciliary incision and approach to orbital region

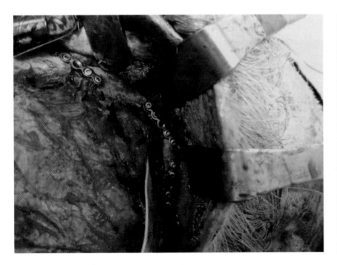

Fig. 76.9 Hemicoronal approach for zygomatic arch comminution and instability

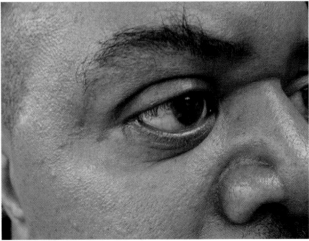

Fig. 76.11 Lateral brow and subciliary incisions that are healing well

between these two incisions at the lateral canthal region, to preserve a skin bridge between the incisions. A transconjunctival approach can be performed through the lower lid conjunctiva and the periosteum of the inferior orbital rim at the inferior conjunctival fornix. To reduce the risk of iatrogenic injury to the lacrimal system the incision should remain lateral to the lacrimal puncta in the medial extent of both transconjunctival and subciliary incisions. Both transconjunctival and subciliary approaches provide access to the orbital floor if necessary. A gingivobuccal incision provides adequate access to body, ZM buttress and inferior aspects of the ZMC complex, as well as the inferior orbital rim (Fig. 76.12). It is important to preserve an adequate cuff of gingiva to decrease the risk of wound dehiscence and plate exposure (Fig. 76.13). In addition, it is equally important to counsel patients to avoid traumatizing the incision with their tongue, digits, or toothbrush. In some cases, the or-

bital floor can also be accessed or visualized through an anterior maxillary wall defect. The surgeon should be careful about identifying and preserving the infraorbital nerve during exposure of fractures involving the inferior orbital rim and anterior maxilla. The zygomatic arch can be elevated through the posterosuperior part of gingivobuccal incision as described by Keen. The Gillies incision within the temporal hairline can be used to place an elevator directly under the zygomatic arch to reduce the fracture. The authors have found that when the incision is made deep to the deep temporal fascia, the elevator easily dissects naturally to a plane deep to the arch, which is optimal for elevating the fractures and essentially eliminates any risk to the facial nerve. In most cases where there is stable fixation at the other points of ZMC fractures, the zygomatic arch can be reduced without the need for rigid fixation. Although endoscopic approaches have been described for the orbital, zygomatic arch and midface fractures, it remains controversial as to whether there is clinical benefit to using the endoscope for the patient with ZMC fractures [6–8]. Of course, an existing open traumatic wound or laceration can be used if it is overlying or adjacent to the fracture sites (Fig. 76.14)

Reduction

Once adequate exposure of all the fracture sites is achieved, displacement and stability of the bone segments can be assessed. If there is fracture displacement, the fracture should be cleaned of debris and soft tissue to allow bone-to-bone contact of fractured segments. Reduction of displaced fractures can be accomplished by one or a combination of the following maneuvers: push, pull, or rotate. Since the entire ZMC region cannot usually be viewed in one frame, it is critical to have exact realignment of the fracture sites. In cases where there are impacted zygoma segments, bone hooks, heavy clamps, or elevators are frequently required to mobilize and reduce the bone fragments into the correct position. Multiple approaches or points of force may be needed to reduce a segment. The best reference for correct reduction

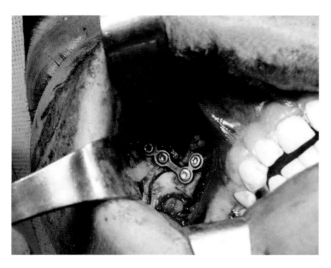

Fig. 76.12 Gingivolabial approach to the zygomaticomaxillary region

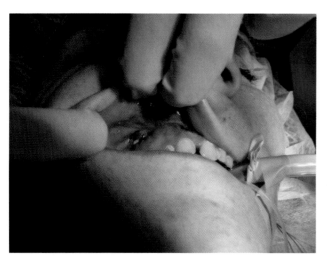

Fig. 76.13 Exposed hardware that was placed through a gingivolabial incision

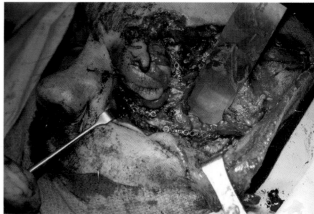

Fig. 76.14 Open reduction through existing traumatic lacerations

is normal nondisplaced bone, including the frontal orbital process, posterior zygomatic arch, maxillary alveolus, inferomedial orbital rim, edge of the posterior orbital floor, and nasomaxillary process. Another useful reference is the contralateral facial projection for comparing relative facial projection and symmetry during the reduction and fixation process. Visualization of all fractured sites or buttresses is helpful during the reduction and initial fixation process.

Fixation

Fracture fixation can be performed with resorbable or nonresorbable materials. Resorbable materials are perfect tools in pediatric practice, since they may affect facial skeletal growth less than titanium plating systems. One of the various commercially available titanium plating systems can safely be used for any ZMC fracture fixation. The surgeon should remember to use relatively small-size plates (1.2 or 1.3 mm) in the ZF region, infraorbital rim, or zygomatic arch in order to reduce visibility or palpation of these plates through the skin. ZM buttress should be repaired with a larger-size plate such as 1.5 mm. At least two screws should be placed on each side of the fracture lines. After three-dimensional reduction is obtained, the surgeon should start internal fixation at a fracture point which is approximated to a firm, normal nondisplaced bone.

Complications

A fracture traversing through the infraorbital foramen or canal can cause temporary or permanent infraorbital nerve hypoesthesia or anesthesia due to varying degrees of nerve damage. Insufficient evaluation or management of a concurrent orbital floor fracture may cause enophthalmus, dystopia, and/or diplopia on the affected side. Failure to address a ZMC fracture affecting mastication may cause permanent trismus and/or occlusal problems. Insufficiently reduced ZMC fractures may lead to permanent facial asymmetries, such as malar flattening. Globe injuries are possible following trauma to ZMC or during surgery for correction of ZMC fractures. Ectropion or scleral show can result from lower eyelid incisions. Corneal abrasion can result from the inciting trauma, iatrogenic injury, or corneal exposure.

References

1. Kreidl KO, Kim DY, Mansour SE (2003) Prevalence of significant intraocular sequelae in blunt orbital trauma. Am J Emerg Med 21:525–528

2. Petro J, Tooze FM, Bales CR, et al (1979) Ocular injuries associated with periorbital fractures. J Trauma19:730–733

3. Fogaca WC, Fereirra MC, Dellon AL (2004) Infraorbital nerve injury associated with zygoma fractures: Documentation with neurosensory testing. Plast Reconstr Surg 113:834–838

4. Ellis E 3rd, Reddy L (2004) Status of the internal orbit after reduction of zygomaticomaxillary complex fractures. J Oral Maxillofac Surg 62:275–283

5. Zingg M, Laedrach K, Chen J, et al (1992) Classification and treatment of zygomatic fractures: A review of 1,025 cases. J Oral Maxillofac Surg 50:778–790

6. Lee C, Jacobovicz J, Mueller RV (1997) Endoscopic repair of a complex midfacial fracture. J Craniofac Surg 8:170–175

7. Czerwinski M, Lee C (2006) The rationale and technique of endoscopic approach to the zygomatic arch in facial trauma. Facial Plast Surg Clin North Am 14:37–43

8. Strong EB (2004) Endoscopic repair of orbital blow-out fractures. Facial Plast Surg 20:223–230

Chapter 77

Treatment of Frontal Sinus and Nasoethmoid Orbital Fractures

77

Fred G. Fedok, David Goldenberg, and Sunny S. Park

Core Messages

- There is a significant risk of intracranial injury in patients with frontal sinus and nasoethmoid orbital fractures
- Goal of treatment is to restore form and function
- Understanding of anatomy is essential to providing appropriate management of injuries and physiology

Contents

Introduction

The treatment of fractures of the facial skeleton is dependent on the surgeon's grasp of principles of repair, knowledge of the local anatomy, and familiarity with current surgical technique. The proximity of the frontal area and the nasoethmoid orbital (NEO) areas allows a combined consideration of the management of injuries.

Frontal sinus fractures are one of the more common fractures in patients with craniofacial injuries. They are caused by high velocity impacts such as motor vehicle accidents and falls. Management continues to be controversial and thus there is no universally accepted algorithm.

In contrast, NEO fractures are among the least common craniofacial injuries. Typically, they are caused by high-energy impacts to the midface from motor vehicle accidents, penetrating injuries, falls, assaults, and industrial accidents [10]. Associated injuries to adjacent structures occur and involve the eye, anterior cranial fossa, and adjacent bony structures of the face.

Pertinent Anatomy

The paired frontal sinuses are located within the frontal bone. The borders for each frontal sinus include its anterior and posterior walls, the orbital roof inferiorly and the intersinus septum medially. The sinuses are in direct relation with the supraorbital rims inferior-laterally and the anterior cranium superiorly. The dimensions of each adult-sized sinus vary; the height ranges from 5–66 mm, the width 17–49 mm and the average volume is 6–7 cc [2, 6]. The anterior table is curved and composed of cortical bone that is twice as thick as the posterior table. Consequently, the anterior table of the frontal sinus is more resistant to fractures compared to other facial bones and resists up to 400–1,000 kg before breaking [18, 35].

In humans, the frontal sinus usually does not pneumatize until they have reached the age of 2 [25]. By the age of 6 years, the sinuses become radiographically identifiable. By the age of 15, the sinuses reach adult size and may continue to grow until the age of 20 [2, 22]. Although, the frontal sinuses are usually paired, unilateral sinus can be seen in 15% of skulls and complete aplasia is seen in 5% [2].

Normal functioning of the frontal sinuses requires patent nasofrontal ducts (NFD). The NFDs, which provide for drainage and aeration of the frontal sinuses, are located in the inferior-medial aspect of the frontal sinuses and communicate with their ipsilateral middle meati. At times, the NFDs are less well defined, however, communication from the sinuses to the nose then continues through the frontal recess, which is bounded by lamina papyracea laterally, middle turbinate medially, ethmoid bulla posteriorly, and agger nasi cells anteriorly [16]. The frontal sinuses and the NFDs are lined with mucous producing pseudostratified ciliated columnar epithelium. Occlusion of the NFDs results in mucous retention, mucocele, infection, and other complications.

The major vertical buttress or central fragment of the NEO region is made up of the frontal process of the maxilla, the nasal bones, the frontal bone, the lamina papyracea and the lacrimal bone. This vertically reinforced segment contains the point of insertion of the medial canthal ligaments. Thus, this central fragment must be reconstructed in the management of these injuries if normal medial canthal architecture is to be maintained [15]. In the midline, the perpendicular plate of the ethmoid and the cartilaginous septum provide support under the nasal bones [30]. The major horizontal buttress of this region includes the frontal bone and the infraorbital rims.

The most important soft tissue structure in the area is the medial canthal ligament [36]. The medial canthal ligament divides into three limbs prior to the insertion on the bony structures. An anterior limb inserts into the nasal bone anterior to the anterior lacrimal crest. The posterior limb attaches to the posterior portion of the lacrimal fossa and a superior limb attaches both here, as well as to the maxilla and to the lacrimal sac.

The lacrimal cannulicular system begins at the upper and lower puncta and runs within the medial portions of the upper and lower eyelids. Either as part of a common canaliculus or individually, these ducts join the lacrimal sac in the lacrimal fossa. In spite of the fact that in this location the lacrimal duct and sac are anatomically vulnerable to trauma, they usually do not require repair.

Evaluation and Classification of Injuries

The clinical presentation of frontal sinus fractures varies greatly depending on associated injuries to the adjacent structures such as the brain and the eye. The spectrum of initial symptoms ranges from a paucity of symptoms to changes in mental status. The most common finding is a laceration of the forehead [35]. Other signs and symptoms include periorbital ecchymosis, subconjunctival hemorrhage, bony irregularity, edema, tenderness, crepitus, superior orbital rim defects, sensory loss, and cerebrospinal fluid (CSF) leak [32].

Computerized tomography (CT) is the cornerstone of diagnostic imaging. Both axial and coronal views are preferred (Fig. 77.1). By studying these fractures in two planes, information about structures running perpendicular to these complimentary radiographic planes is optimally displayed. The axial

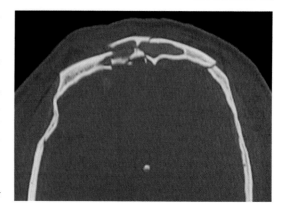

Fig. 77.1 Computerized tomogram (CT) of an adult patient with frontal sinus fracture involving anterior and posterior tables of frontal bone

views reveal the integrity of the ethmoid labyrinth and the degree of intrusion of the NEO complex in an anterior-to-posterior direction. The axial views will also contribute important information regarding the status of the NFDs. The coronal views help determine the status of the orbit. In addition, three-dimensional (3D) CT can be reconstructed from two-dimensional (2D) images without additional radiation exposure. This technique is superior in demonstrating the spatial relationships of fracture fragments in midfacial trauma [20, 24].

Pneumocephalus or displacement of a posterior table fracture by more than the thickness of the posterior table should raise the suspicion of a dural tear. Since up to 55% of all frontal sinus fractures involve some injury to the NFD, a careful evaluation of the NFD is necessary [35]. In addition to the clinical examination and CT, the NFDs should be evaluated in the operating room. Ethylene blue or fluorescein dye can be used to test the patency of NFD [35].

Classification of Fractures

Recently, Metzinger et al. have analyzed frontal fractures in terms of six characteristics [16] (Table 77.1).

The diagnosis of NEO injuries is made based on both physical examination and CT findings [11]. Traumatic telecanthus, or widening of the inner canthal distance, may be present. Typically, the normal range for the intercanthal distance ranges between 30 and 35 mm. The intercanthal distance should be 50% or less of the interpupillary distance. An eyelid traction test or palpation over the point of insertion of the medial canthal ligament may confirm the presence of an NEO injury. In more stable injuries, a bimanual examination may be necessary [12].

If there is comminution of the underlying perpendicular plate of the ethmoid, the nasal support may be destroyed and there may be retrodisplacement of the nasal dorsum with saddling and intrusion. Concomitant fractures and dislocation of the septal cartilage will result in a total loss of nasal support. Depending on the degree of injury, other findings such as vertical dystopia may be present. Finally, there may be other additional

77

Table 77.1 Metzinger classification of frontal sinus fractures [16]

Open vs. closed

Linear vs. comminuted

Displaced[a] vs. non-displaced

Anterior wall and/or posterior wall

With or without nasofrontal duct involvement

With or without CNS involvement

[a]Dislocated when >1 thickness of anterior/posterior table is involved

Table 77.2 Markowitz classification of NEO injuries

Type 1	Single-segment central fragment fracture
Type 2	Single-segment or comminuted central fragment fracture external to medical canthal tendon insertion
Type 3	Comminution within the central fragment with extension beneath the medial canthal tendon insertion

Table 77.3 Gruss classification of NEO injuries

Type 1		Isolated bony NEO injury
Type 2		Bony NEO and central maxilla
	2A	Central maxilla only
	2B	Central and one lateral maxilla
	2C	Central and bilateral lateral maxilla
Type 3		Extended NEO injury
	3A	With craniofacial injuries
	3B	With LeFort II and III fractures
Type 4		NEO with orbital displacement
	4A	With oculo-orbital displacement
	4B	With orbital dystopia
Type 5		NEO with bone loss

associated fractures causing instability of the maxilla, malocclusion, and forehead deformity.

Two recognized classifications that have been developed in the description of NEO fractures are that of Markowitz [15] and Gruss [10] (Tables 77.2, 3). While Markowitz focused on various fracture patterns of the NEO complex itself, Gruss characterized fractures of the NEO complex as either isolated or in combination with adjacent maxillofacial injuries.

Goals of Treatment and Priorities

Frontal Sinus Fractures

The main goal of treatment is to provide a sinus safe from the development of a mucocele and other infections. Appropriate treatment can include sinus preservation and observation, obliteration or cranialization. Secondary goals include cosmesis by re-establishing the frontal bony contour to its preinjury state.

NEO Fractures

The goals of treatment include re-establishing the bony and soft tissue architecture of the NEO region to its natural state. Surgical management of NEO injuries involves considerations of orbital volume and integrity, the integrity of the medial canthus, the status of nasal support, and the function of the frontal sinus and lacrimal drainage systems. Adequate acute management is necessary as late correction of abnormality is frequently only minimally rewarding.

Management of Frontal Sinus Fractures and Nasoethmoid Orbital Fractures

Surgical Approaches/Exposure

There are several generally accepted routes to the exposure of these fractures. The first of these is via existing lacerations. The existing lacerations that frequently occur with these injuries will provide limited access to the area that is adjacent to the laceration.

To some, the coronal incision is considered the gold standard for the repair of frontal sinus fractures [16]. The coronal approach provides exposure to the frontal sinus, the region of the glabella, the nasal bones, and the superior and medial orbits. With careful dissection, this approach also provides access to the medial canthal tendon insertions. In cases where there is only an anterior table fracture with an intact NFD, a minimally invasive endoscopic approach can be used. This approach requires two incisions, one at the midline of the scalp and the other over the fracture. It offers direct visualization, good aesthetic outcome and minimal tissue manipulation, avoids neurovascular injury, and shortens hospital stay [4].

Access to the orbital floor is provided by either a subciliary skin muscle flap-like approach to the inferior rim or a transconjunctival approach [8]. Buccal-gingival incisions allow the exploration of the medial and lateral maxillary buttresses. At times, horizontal or small curved medial canthal incisions have provided additional access without cosmetic compromise. A midfacial degloving approach can provide adequate exposure for the reduction of NEO and midface fractures without creating external incisions [5].

Specific Management Techniques

Frontal Sinus Fractures

There are a variety of treatment options for frontal sinus fractures. In general, there are four different management choices: observation, reconstruction of bony contour, obliteration, and cranialization. The decision for type of treatment depends on the bony contour, displacement of bone, and NFD involvement. However, specific techniques among surgeons may differ.

The management for the anterior table fractures is generally agreed upon among surgeons. Observation may be done when there is a nondisplaced fracture of the anterior table without NFD involvement [16, 27, 35]. Management involves the use of serial CT scans to evaluate sinus function [29]. A simple, linear, displaced fracture without NFD involvement may be adequately exposed, reduced appropriately, and rigidly fixed [21]. In addition, the aforementioned endoscopic approach can be used and has shown promising results [4, 26].

For the reduction and fixation of frontal fractures, permanent microplates have been used most commonly. Recently, bioresorbable plates have been developed and are made of biocompatible, nontoxic material that is resorbed within 1 to 2 years [3].

A comminuted depressed fracture (open or closed) without NFD involvement should be treated with reconstruction of the anterior table. If there is more than a 1.5-cm bony defect, grafting is advised. Choices for grafts include calvarial outer table, rib, iliac crest bone, or alloplasts.

In cases where there has been a disruption of the NFDs many surgeons propose obliteration or cranialization. These two methods are similar in that the frontal sinus is ablated by

sinusotomy, the mucosa is removed, and the NFD is occluded. Specifically, the mucosa can be removed with a sharp periosteal elevator. Then the sinus walls are drilled with a high-speed burr to completely clear the mucosal fragments from fracture lines and the foramen of Breschet. The duct can be plugged with a pericranial graft, bone graft, or fibrin glue. For obliteration, the sinus is filled with fat, cancellous bone, muscle, or alloplasts [17, 19, 23, 34, 37]. Autogenous fat and bone continue to be used and both are equally effective for obliteration. Some say fat grafts are relatively resistant to infections and thus these have been used most widely [35]. In addition to the grafts mentioned above, a pericranial flap can be used.

The management of posterior table fractures is much more controversial than that of anterior table fractures (Fig. 77.2). As a result, a wide range of treatment options exist, and management may differ significantly depending on the surgeon. Open exploration is recommended by some authors for almost all posterior table fractures while others use algorithms based on CSF leak and NFD involvement.

A closed, linear nondisplaced posterior table fracture without CSF leak or NFD injury may be observed but will need a repeat CT to rule out late CSF leak or meningoencephalocele at follow-up [16, 35]. Some authors report that open repair is not necessary even when there is minimal (less than one table width) displacement as long as there is no CSF leak [21]. On the other hand, others argue that open exploration is warranted for all posterior table fractures [6].

A closed, comminuted posterior table fracture should be considered for exploration as the risk of long-term complications is high. Either cranialization or obliteration can be done if the NFD is involved without a CSF leak [16]. Cranialization and dural repair is done if CSF leak is present. However, in cases

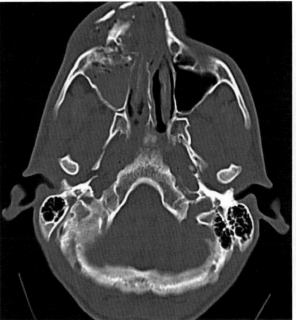 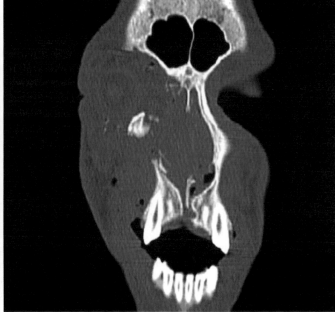

Fig. 77.2 Axial and coronal CT of a patient with severe Type III right nasoethmoid orbital fracture with marked displacement of the central fragment

where there is severe comminution of the posterior table, cranialization should be considered.

Cranialization involves ablating the frontal sinus by sinusotomy or craniotomy, removal of mucosa, occluding the NFD, reconstruction of the anterior wall and placing a pericranial flap between the bone and the brain [16]. Small tears of the dura can be repaired with absorbable sutures or fibrin glue while a patch graft of fascia lata or pericranium may be necessary for larger defects [27].

Fractures of the Nasoethmoid Orbital Region

The first step in the repair of these fractures is usually the repair and reduction of the buttresses of the surrounding bony architecture, or the management of the frontal sinus, if this is necessary [7]. These can be performed in either order. The management of an associated frontal sinus injury has been discussed previously.

The management of the medial canthal ligaments is most important. In blunt injuries to this area, the medial canthal tendon usually maintains its integrity and bony attachments. Instead of actual tears of the medial canthal ligament, the medial canthal ligaments usually remain attached to the fractured segments of the central fragment bones (Fig. 77.3). In the situation where

there is a large Type I or monoblock injury, re-establishment of normal inner canthal distance may be established through the use of rigid plating of the monoblock segment to the adjacent stable bone. When there has been comminution of the central fragment as in Type II injuries, precise reduction and fixation of these comminuted fragments may not be possible, except by the use of transnasal wiring.

In the placement of transnasal wires, the wires are passed at a point posterior and superior to the lacrimal fossa. Improper placement of the wire anterior to this point will result in a wide-appearing nose and an anteriorly displaced medial canthal tendon. Alternatively, a properly placed transnasal wire will reduce the central fragment and re-establish the inner canthal distance.

In the case of Type III injuries where the medial canthal attachment is disrupted, a separate transnasal wire may have to be placed so that a 5-0 Prolene suture that has been placed through the medial canthal ligament can be attached to the wire. The medial canthal ligaments are then directed to a point posterior and superior to the lacrimal fossa. Reduction and fixation of the fracture sites is performed using either microplates or wire osteosynthesis.

The orbital volume must be reconstructed in a similar fashion as performed in the cases of zygomatic complex fractures or orbital blowout fractures. Bone or porous polyethylene are usually the preferred graft materials to be used for reconstruction.

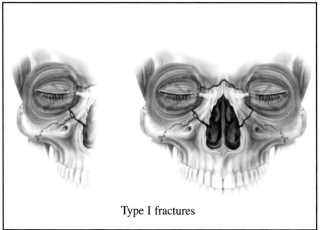

Type I fractures

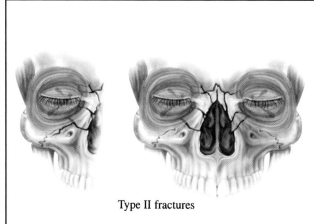

Type II fractures

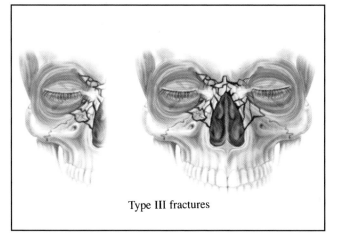

Type III fractures

Fig. 77.3 Illustration of the classification of nasoethmoid orbital fractures as proposed by Markowitz. In Type I injuries, the central fragment remains intact and maintains the insertion of the medial canthal ligament. In Type II injuries, the central fragment is comminuted, but maintains the insertion of the medial canthal ligament. In Type III injuries, the central fragment is comminuted, and does not maintain the insertion of the medial canthal ligament [7] (Copyright holder: The Montage Media Corporation. Permission pending)

The lacrimal system rarely has to be addressed at the time of the initial injury unless there has been a direct laceration. In these cases, the canaliculi should be cannulated and repaired with absorbable suture. Re-establishment of the major buttresses about the orbit and the maxilla is accomplished through the techniques performed with zygomatic complex-malar fractures or Lefort and other midface fractures. Immediate bone grafting may be necessary to reconstruct support and contour [1].

The establishment of nasal support is another key task to be performed during the management of NEO injuries. At times, the septum is only dislocated, and this can be replaced in the midline on the maxillary crest and supported in place with intranasal rigid or semi-rigid temporary splints. Very commonly, the perpendicular plate of the ethmoid is fractured along with septum and the nasal bones, causing complete loss of nasal support. Severe saddle nose deformity results unless the support of the nasal dorsum is re-established. This frequently must be accomplished through the use of a cantilevered bone graft that is secured at the glabella either with lag screw or miniplate technique. In the placement of these dorsal grafts, precise contouring is required.

The Pediatric Patient

Facial fractures are uncommon in children, accounting for only approximately 5% of all maxillofacial fractures [9, 32]. Only 10% of children with maxillofacial fractures were found to have a frontal sinus fracture [32].

While the management of the pediatric patient is controversial, strategies similar to those used for adults are recommended. The main goals remain the same: to prevent long-term complications such as meningitis, CSF leaks, frontal sinusitis, and mucocele and cosmetic deformity. Complications are similar to the adult population and include mucocele, delayed CSF leak, meningitis and cosmetic defects.

Complications and Management of Complications

Tips to Avoid Complications

- Provide complete evaluation of injuries using physical examination and imaging studies.
- In the case of frontal sinus fractures consider long-term follow-up.
- In the case of nasoethmoid orbital fractures, stabilization and reduction of the medial canthal ligament insertion is paramount.

While there is no standard length for follow-up, all patients with frontal sinus fractures should have long-term surveillance. Some authors suggest that patients should be followed for at least 5 years with yearly CT scans [35]. Because there are reports of mucocele development up to 35 years after initial trauma, others advocate follow-up for a lifetime [33].

The most common complication is mucocele or mucopyocele. Symptoms are related to the adjacent structures such as the eye and the brain, and can include headache, proptosis, diplopia, nasal congestion, edema of the forehead, and rhinorrhea. Treatment is cranialization and/or obliteration, and this may require multiple services including neurosurgery and ophthalmology depending on the extent of the mucocele. Other possible complications include cellulitis, nonunion, malunion, supraorbital anesthesia or dysesthesias, contour abnormalities, chronic sinusitis, and frontal headaches [16].

Brain abscess, encephalitis, cavernous sinus thrombosis, and meningitis can result when the intracranial contents are in communication with the nasal cavity. Meningitis occurs in 6% of cases as a complication of frontal sinus fractures [31]. Appropriate intravenous antibiotics should be initiated and an urgent neurosurgical consult is necessary.

Late enophthalmos can occur even when the orbital volume has been re-established at the time of the initial repair [13, 14, 32]. If this is recognized early within the first few weeks, the patient can be taken back to the operating room and additional grafting material can be placed in the orbital floor. However, when it occurs late or is discovered late, large changes in globe position are sometimes extremely difficult to repair. Similarly, the late correction of posttraumatic telecanthus and medial canthal abnormalities is at best very difficult, and at times impossible [28]. Therefore, it is crucial to perform the appropriate surgery as early as possible after the injury.

Of the secondary problems, airway obstruction and saddling of the dorsum appear most commonly.

Take-Home Pearls

- Evaluate Frontal Sinus and Nasoethmoid Orbital Fractures using axial and coronal computerized tomography
- Surgical management requires appropriate exposure, many times necessitating a coronal approach.
- Perform postoperative computerized tomography as soon as the patients condition permits, so inadequacies of management can be recognized early and corrected.

References

1. Antonyshyn O, Gruss JS, Galbraith DJ, et al. (1989) Complex orbital fractures: A critical analysis of immediate bone graft reconstruction. Ann Plast Surg 22(3):220–235
2. Bernstein L (1971) The Caldwell-Luc operation. Otolaryngol Clin North Am 4(1):69–77
3. Bhanot S, Alex JC, Lowlicht RA, et al. (2002) The efficacy of resorbable plates in head and neck reconstruction. Laryngoscope 112(5):890–898
4. Chen DJ, Chen CT, Chen Y, et al. (2003) Endoscopically assisted repair of frontal sinus fracture. J Trauma 55(2):378–382

5. Cultrara A, Turk JB, Har-El G (2004) Midfacial degloving approach for repair of naso-orbital-ethmoid and midfacial fractures. Arch Facial Plast Surg 6(2):133–135

6. Donald PJ (1995) Frontal sinus fractures. In: Donald P, Gluckman JL, Rice DH (eds) The sinuses. Rave Press, New York, pp 369–399

7. Fedok FG (1995) Comprehensive management of nasoethmoid-orbital injuries. J Craniomaxiollofac Trauma 1(4):36–48

8. Fedok FG (1996) The transconjunctival approach in the trauma setting: Avoidance of complications. Am J Otolaryngol 17(1):16–21

9. Ferreira P, Marques M, Pinho C, et al. (2004) Midfacial fractures in children and adolescents: A review of 492 cases. Br J Oral Maxillofac Surg 42(6):501–505

10. Gruss JS (1986) Complex nasoethmoid-orbital and midfacial fractures: Role of craniofacial surgical techniques and immediate bone grafting. Ann Plast Surg 17(5):377–390

11. Holt GR, Holt JE (1985) Nasoethmoid complex injuries. Otolaryngol Clin North Am 18(1):87–98

12. Leipziger LS, Manson PN (1992) Nasoethmoid orbital fractures. Current concepts and management principles. Clin Plast Surg 19(1):167–193

13. Manson PN, Clifford CM, Su CT, et al. (1986) Mechanisms of global support and posttraumatic enophthalmos: I. The anatomy of the ligament sling and its relation to intramuscular cone orbital fat. Plast Reconstr Surg 77(2):193–202

14. Manson PN, Ruas EJ, Iliff NT (1987) Deep orbital reconstruction for correction of post-traumatic enophthalmos. Clin Plast Surg 14(1):113–121

15. Markowitz BL, Manson PN, Sargent L, et al. (1991) Management of the medial canthal tendon in nasoethmoid orbital fractures: The importance of the central fragment in classification and treatment. Plast Reconstr Surg 87(5):843–853

16. Metzinger SE, Guerra AB, Garcia RE (2005) Frontal sinus fractures: Management guidelines. Facial Plast Surg 21(3):199–206

17. Mickel TJ, Rohrich RJ, Robinson JB Jr (1995) Frontal sinus obliteration: A comparison of fat, muscle, bone, and spontaneous osteoneogenesis in the cat model. Plast Reconstr Surg 95(3):586–592

18. Nahum AM (1975) The biomechanics of maxillofacial trauma. Clin Plast Surg 2(1):59–64

19. Owens M, Klotch DW (1993) Use of bone for obliteration of the nasofrontal duct with the osteoplastic flap: A cat model. Laryngoscope 103(8):883–889

20. Remmler D, Denny A, Gosain A, et al. (2000) Role of three-dimensional computed tomography in the assessment of nasoorbitoethmoidal fractures. Ann Plast Surg 44(5):553–563

21. Rice DH (2004) Management of frontal sinus fractures. Curr Opin Otolaryngol Head Neck Surg 12(1):46–48

22. Rohrich RJ, Hollier LH (1992) Management of frontal sinus fractures. Changing concepts. Clin Plast Surg 19(1):219–232

23. Rohrich RJ, Mickel TJ (1995) Frontal sinus obliteration: In search of the ideal autogenous material. Plast Reconstr Surg 95(3):580–585

24. Saigal K, Winokur RS, Finden S, et al. (2005) Use of three-dimensional computerized tomography reconstruction in complex facial trauma. Facial Plast Surg 21(3):214–220

25. Stammberger HR, Kennedy DW (1995) Paranasal sinuses: Anatomic terminology and nomenclature. Anatomic Terminology Group. Ann Otol Rhinol Laryngol Suppl 167:7–16

26. Strong EB, Kellman RM (2006) Endoscopic repair of anterior table—Frontal sinus fractures. Facial Plast Surg Clin North Am 14(1):25–29

27. Swinson BD, Jerjes W, Thompson G, et al. (2004) Current practice in the management of frontal sinus fractures. J Laryngol Otol 118(12):927–932

28. Tessier P (1986) Complications of facial trauma: Principles of late reconstruction. Ann Plast Surg 17(5):411–420

29. Tiwari P, Higuera S, Thornton J, et al. (2005) The management of frontal sinus fractures. J Oral Maxillofac Surg 63(9):1354–1360

30. Vora NM, Fedok FG (2000) Management of the central nasal support complex in naso-orbital ethmoid fractures. Facial Plast Surg 16(2):181–191

31. Wallis A, Donald PJ (1988) Frontal sinus fractures: A review of 72 cases. Laryngoscope 98(6 Pt 1):593–598

32. Whatley WS, Allison DW, Chandra RK, et al. (2005) Frontal sinus fractures in children. Laryngoscope 115(10):1741–1745

33. Wilson BC, Davidson B, Corey JP, et al. (1988) Comparison of complications following frontal sinus fractures managed with exploration with or without obliteration over 10 years. Laryngoscope 98(5):516–520

34. Xie C, Mehendale N, Barrett D, et al. (2000) 30-year retrospective review of frontal sinus fractures: The Charity Hospital experience. J Craniomaxillofac Trauma 6(1):7–18

35. Yavuzer R, Sari A, Kelly CP, et al. (2005) Management of frontal sinus fractures. Plast Reconstr Surg 115(6):79e–95e

36. Zide BM, McCarthy JG (1983) The medial canthus revisited--an anatomical basis for canthopexy. Ann Plast Surg 11(1):1–9

37. Zonis RD, Montgomery WW, Goodale RL (1966) Frontal sinus disease: 100 cases treated by osteoplastic operation. Laryngoscope 76(11):1816–1825

Aesthetic Facial Surgery

Chapter 78

Concepts of Facial Beauty

Philip Young

Core Messages

- Our current understanding of facial aesthetics has not shown the ability to discriminate between what we find exceptionally beautiful from what is thought to be average.
- Previous theories such as Leonardo Da Vinci's Neoclassical Canons and others have concentrated on external landmarks on the face which people place minimal importance on when assessing beauty.
- A new theory should concentrate on what people find important when they look at someone's face.
- The Circles of Prominence, a new theory on facial aesthetics, finds that the iris is the most important element within a face when people assess for beauty.
- Every shape or distance within the face has an ideal from zero and infinity. Because we spend so much time concentrating on the iris, it is logical that this ideal is the width of the iris. After establishing this, the rest of the elements of facial beauty become more easily to elucidate.
- A more accurate theory on facial beauty will allow us to improve our patients' lives for the better.

Contents

Introduction

There is no doubt that facial beauty has a tremendous impact in our lives [4, 11, 12, 15] and it begins very early. The beautiful are treated and evaluated better in grade school, which is not reflected on standardized exams. This preferential treatment continues in the work environment as they are found to be promoted faster. Socially, they are 10 times more likely to get married. People judge the beautiful to be more ethical, more honest, healthier, and to have better personalities. Amazingly, even our own mothers treat us differently as babies depending on how we look.

In terms of sexual selection, how is beauty propagated? We obviously choose for it when we select our mates. But, Darwinian theory has always stated that function precedes form. However, there are many studies which show that all species choose their mates based on some aesthetic elements. The reasoning is that these external features indicate the health and reproductive status of the bearer. In humans, there is lack of definitive evidence which points to beauty indicating a healthier person. It may be that there hasn't been the right study that isolates and negates confounding factors which prove this. There have been studies showing that we do have the ability to appreciate beauty preferentially in that it is wired into our neuroanatomy supporting that humans do select for beauty [10]. The question then becomes, "If we do select for beauty is there an ideal that we are selecting for?"

There are many studies which support that an ideal exists. Logically, because there are different grades of beauty there must be a face that is considered to be the best. Some have theorized that culture influences what particular people find attractive and that there is no universal ideal. Recently, cross-cultural studies, however, have begun to disprove this thought hinting at an innate ability that transcends ethnic variables in facial architecture to support a basic compilation of shapes that define facial beauty [3, 4, 12]. Studies showing that babies spend more time looking at more attractive people based on adult preferences also support this idea that an ideal arrangement exists [11].

Cultural differences and preferences can also fit into the universal ideal. For example, Asians and African-Americans have their own unique variations that distinguish them from different ethnicities. They are accepted as the norm in their cultures but the compilation of the different shapes of the face, their arrangement, balance, and proportion are essentially the same in adherence to an ideal. These minor differences may be what heightens a particular individual's beauty by showing the viewer a unique representation within the face adherent to the ideal while heightening a factor based on cultural familiarity.

Despite the numerous articles on facial aesthetics attempting to find the answer for facial beauty [1, 3–5, 10, 12, 13, 19–22], the ultimate qualitative and quantitative definition remains elusive. Farkas and colleagues showed in 1984 that the seminal neoclassical canons did not represent average facial proportions and are a poor theory to use when describing facial aesthetics [7]. Others agree [25, 27–29]. Some believe that there exists a divine proportion based on the number phi, 1.618, where the face is divided proportionately [4, 5, 8, 11]. However, faces that fit into that scheme are not necessarily beautiful [5].

Previous Theories and Thoughts

Perhaps the answer for facial aesthetics lies in the orientation of our analysis. Previous theories such as the canons have been traditionally based on horizontal and vertical planes of reference in two dimensions. The Canons are: Canon 1 states that the distance from the vertex (top of head) to endocanthion (level of medial canthi) is equal to the distance from the endocanthion to mentum. Canon 2 states that the distance from trichion to nasion equals nasion to subnasale equals subnasale to mentum. Canon 3 states that the distance from vertex to trichion equals the distance from trichion to glabella equals glabella to subnasale equals subnasale to mentum. Canon 4 states that the height of the nose equals the height of the ear (the distance from nasion to subnasale is equal to the distance from the top of the ear to the bottom.) Canon 5 states that the distance between lateral and medial canthi is equal to the distance between the medial canthi. Canon 6 states that the distance between the medial canthi is equal to the interalar distance. Canon 7 states that interalar distance (distance between the lateral edges of the alae) multiplied by one and one half is equal to the distance from commissure to commissure. Canon 8 states that interalar distance is one quarter the distance from zygoma to zygoma. Canon 9 states that nose inclination is equal to ear inclination. When you examine the canons you notice one important principle. They depend on external landmarks that may play little or no relevance to the observer who encounters a new face. When people interact with each other, they spend very little time incorporating the hairline or the subnasale into their assessment of beauty. Theories based on elements unimportant to the observer's visual attention will ultimately fail. In order to the find the answer to facial beauty we need to base a new theory on what the observer concentrates on when they analyze a face. If possible we also need to incorporate our analysis in three dimensions. With this seminal piece of knowledge, the specifics of the theory can then be deduced.

Unlocking the Answers

The failure of the canons in their attempts to define beauty supports the idea that the external landmarks that they employ are not central in humans' assessment of beauty. One basic idea in the development of the Circles of Prominence (COP) is that the eye and specifically the iris define all elements of facial beauty as we will explain. With this premise, the rest of the shapes and dimensions of the face are defined. On a more simple scale, the face is an oval with multiple shapes of which the eyes, nose, and mouth are predominant. All organisms, humans notwithstanding, have a strong desire for order. When one asks a population to determine their preference for the location of a circle within a square, the majority of that population will choose that the circle is more desirable in the center of the square [19, 22]. This arrangement promotes symmetry and satisfies the organisms desire for order. This same idea applies to the face. The shapes in the face must be arranged in such a way that order is emphasized. Finding the exact order, therefore, really answers the question of facial beauty.

Another idea that is central to facial beauty is that subtleties within the face are vital to this appreciation. The transition from one shape and structure to the next must be done almost imperceptibly. Not surprisingly, our visual system is arranged to exactly appreciate these subtleties. Specifically, our minds identify very subtle gradations of light that help us to subjectively interpret in three dimensions. Ganglion cells in the retina are arranged in concentric circles linked by inhibitory pathways increasing the sensitivity of these cells to appreciate borders between light and darkness. The brain is thus highly stimulated by contrast, exactly wiring our minds to appreciate these gradations of light. In addition, because of their geometric arrangement they possibly have a preference for appreciating circular elements as well. It is within these gradations of light where the answer to facial beauty hides, and these subtleties are also what make us beautiful [5]. We must see no lines, blemishes, or highlights that deviate from this collection of shapes within our face that determine our aesthetics. We must see only gradations of light that demarcate these specific shapes and these shapes must be in balance, must exude symmetry [14], and must be in equal proportions.

These gradations of light, ironically, may also be the underlying reason why beauty has remained such a mystery. In the past we have relied on the saying that "Beauty is in the eye of the beholder," but there existed all along some basic arrangement of shapes through which minor variations (in millimeters) endowed uniqueness to that particular face. These minor variations in combination with the subtleties of shading are the elements that have precluded us from identifying this beautiful arrangement. In addition to this hindrance supplied by gradations of light, beauty is appreciated preferentially in the right hemisphere, which is separated from the analytical left hemisphere [10]. Coupled with the findings that beauty incites a predominant emotional response in the limbic system and the subconscious realm along with the findings that beauty is appreciated at all levels of the brain, the conscious and analytical part of our mind was further kept from discovering the answers [5, 10, 11].

Circles of Prominence: A New Theory on Facial Aesthetics

The Key to Facial Beauty is Found in the Iris

Previous work has shown that there exists a hierarchy of interest for the observer when assessing a new face [22]. Studies based on recordings of eye movements show that a person fixates first on the eyes, nose, and mouth, then other external landmarks but returns again and again to the eyes, nose, and mouth. Specifically, the observer fixates the most attention on the iris. The Circles of Prominence (COP) is based on this vital finding. Importantly, this theory is based on the frontal view in three dimensions by incorporating subtle shading which brings the element of depth. All shapes, sizes, and dimensions in the face (which are delineated by subtle gradations of light) are defined by the iris and specifically the diameter of the iris. The width of the nasal dorsum, the diameter of the nasal tip highlight, the diameter of the partial circle formed by the alae, the width of lower philtrum, the distance from subnasale to upper lip, and the height of the lower lip (Fig. 78.1) all should equal 1 iris width

(IW). This is logical because every shape or distance on the face has its own existence and there must be an ideal size for each of them. Incorporating mathematics, the values zero and infinity help us to make sense of many things in nature. So it does in the face. Because we spend so much time focusing our attention on the iris, the brain prefers the size of the iris as the ideal median between zero and infinity through which these structures are defined. When the diameter is greater, the attention is drawn away from the iris and other structures that are ideally an iris width and towards the larger structure. The ultimate result is that the beauty of the iris and eyes are decreased. When the structure is smaller, less attention is brought to it. Hence, it is better for the structure to be smaller than an iris width. However, the smaller the shape is from the iris the less association with other structures. This inequality detracts from the harmony promoted by having all of the shapes equal in size. Hence, the more equal shapes are to 1 IW the more aesthetic (Fig. 78.1). For the palpebral aperture, the greater exposure of the iris the better, but it should not exceed superiorly past 1–2 mm inferior to the superior margin of the limbus and inferiorly below the lower limbus.

Crucially, the iris, nasal tip, and lower lip are the primary COP. They are the most prominent structures within the eye, nose, and mouth units. To bring more ideal balance and proportion to the rest of the face all of the subsequent, larger COP and shapes that emanate from these primary COP should be based on multiples of the IW. This is also logical because as these shapes increase in size, the distance that separates these larger COP from the smaller COP also has an ideal that exists between infinity and zero. Again, because we spend so much of our time focusing on the iris, it is logical that the iris width serves repeatedly as the width which the brain finds ideal.

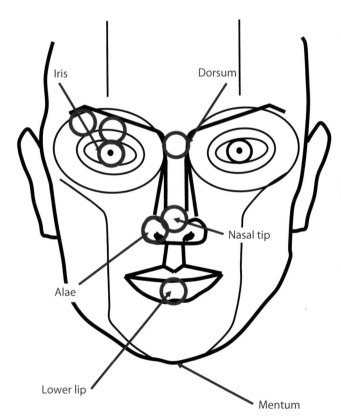

Fig. 78.1 All shapes, sizes and dimensions in the face (which are delineated by subtle gradations of light) are defined by the iris and specifically the diameter of the iris. The width of the nasal dorsum, the diameter of the nasal tip highlight, the diameter of the partial circle formed by the alae, the width of the lower philtrum, the distance from subnasale to upper lip, and the height of the lower lip all should equal 1 iris width (IW)

Balance Between the Eyes, Nose, and Mouth

Because progressively larger COP emanate from these structures, the distance between the primary COP should be equal to maintain balance. The most important distance is from the pupil to the midline. Specifically, from the center of the pupil to limbus, from limbus to caruncle, from lateral edge of caruncle to medial edge of canthus, from canthus to lateral edge of nasal sidewall, from sidewall to lateral dorsal edge, from dorsal edge to midline are all one half an IW length. Each of these distances have their own existence and thus must possess an ideal. Because they are not primary in their importance to the beauty of the face they are defined by one half the IW. The distance totals 3 IW. In turn, this defines the distances between other primary COP. From the pupil to midline, from the horizontal level of the pupil to the center of the nasal tip COP, from the nasal tip to the center of the lower lip COP, and from the lower lip to the mentum should all be equal to 3 IW (Fig. 78.2). The mentum serves as the lower boundary of the face. When these distances are unequal, they bring progressive tension to the circles that emanate from the first and primary COP in their relation with neighboring groups of COP (relate with Figs. 78.1–3). The result is that a decreased aesthetic value is placed on the observed by the observer. In other words, the main shapes within the larger oval shape of the face are the eyes, nose, and mouth and this description details the how this balance between these major units is achieved to satisfy the observers desire for order.

Relating the Eyes and Nose Through Three Oblique Lines

The next phase of the theory deals with three oblique lines that an observer visualizes. The first oblique (FO) line traverses from the central nasal tip COP through the pupil. The FO then centers a COP in the lateral upper lid (although not a definitive circle, its height from upper eyelid crease to brow is approximately 1 IW). The FO and the highlights of the nasal tip and lateral upper eyelid highlight bring attention to the eyes and iris. The arch of the eyebrow is really an evolutionary thinning of the lateral portion of the eyebrow to reveal the lateral eyelid highlight above the upper eyelid crease. The effect of the highlight is important to the beauty of the eye. The lateral upper eyelid highlight stands out because the middle and medial upper eyelid have a darker shade. It adds to the association dictated by the FO, and through the prominent highlight attracts significant at-

tention to the iris. The second oblique (SO) courses in a straight line beginning at the center of the lower lip and is parallel to the FO. It demarcates the upper limit of the cheek shadowing and the top of the superior helix of the ear (Fig. 78.4). The third oblique (TO) courses from the mentum and is also parallel to the first two and should demarcate the inferior border of the lobule (Fig. 78.4). These defining limits are a new thought on where the ear should be located as far as revealed in the literature and how it symmetrically harmonizes with other structures within the face. These obliques align the cheek shadowing, nasal tip, iris, lateral brow highlight, lower lip, and mentum. By doing so, a sense of harmony is achieved through the symmetrical alignment of these structures. The obliques, specifically the SO, also allow certain dynamics within the face to further accentuate this harmony. When we smile the commissures are pulled up by the zygomaticus major towards the top of the ear (this is inherent in the origin and insertion of this muscle). As the lower lip stays essentially at the same horizontal level, the commissures are pulled in line with the SO giving this part of the face dynamic symmetry further increasing the beauty of the face by accentuating the SO, and in turn the other obliques.

Further adding to these obliques are the vertical lines of shadowing that should bisect the pupil. As the flat portion of the central forehead takes a sloping posterior course, a vertical demarcation of shadowing is produced that lines up with the pupil. This effectively brings more attention to the iris (Fig. 78.4). The dental arches and their posterior course should also bring

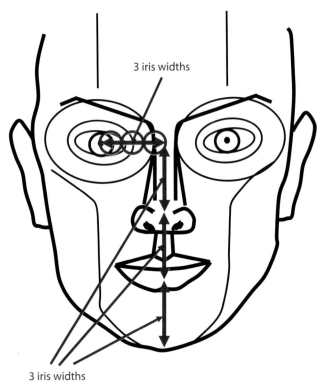

Fig. 78.2 Because progressively larger COP emanate from these structures, the distance between the primary COP should be equal to maintain balance. The most important distance is from the pupil to the midline. In turn, this defines the distances between other primary COP. From the pupil to midline, from the horizontal level of the pupil to the center of the nasal tip COP, from the nasal tip to the center of the lower lip COP, and from the lower lip to the mentum should all be equal to 3 IW

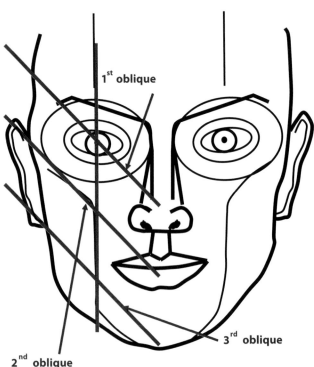

Fig. 78.3 The basic circles of prominence (iris, nasal tip, lower lip and mentum) are central in forming 3 obliques and 1 vertical that define the face and bring attention to the eyes

78

vertical shadowing within the cheek that is in line with the pupil, again bringing more attention to the iris. It may be that the development of the sinuses aid in forming these vertical lines of shadowing as part of the evolution of facial beauty. This vertical plane, SO and TO together, demarcates progressive shadowing of the cheek to further direct attention toward the central area of the face delineated by the COP of the eyes, nose, and mouth. These vertical lines are also tangential to the main lip unit at the nasolabial and melolabial folds (Fig. 78.4).

The Circles of Prominence Within the Eyes

The COP then takes on another more subtle level within the eye unit (Fig. 78.3). After the first COP, the iris, the second eye COP (Fig. 78.3) is delineated by the shadowing created by the upper eyelid crease, lower lid prominence produced by pretarsal muscular bunching, and the medial and lateral canthi (although the shape is more elliptical, we will refer to these ellipses as circles both in the eye and mouth). The upper lid crease and the shadowing below it extending to the lid margin should be one-half IW. The distance from the upper eyelid crease to the bottom of the brow should also be one-half IW, except in the lateral lid. As you approach the lateral portion of the eyelid the space between the upper eyelid crease to the bottom of the brow

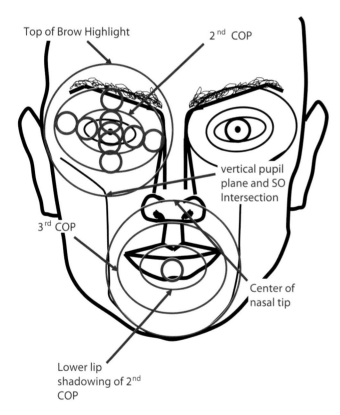

Fig. 78.4 The circles of prominence in the eye and mouth are equal in size and shape. All dimensions of the face are defined by the width of the iris; SO indicates second oblique

increases. The superior orbital rim adds to the highlight and should be about one IW above the lateral upper eyelid crease whereas the distance from crease to brow in the middle and medial third is one-half IW. The upper eyelid (ciliary margin to brow) above and medial to the pupil is thus one IW, in total, and this height is increased to 1 ½ IW as one approaches the lateral upper eyelid highlight. The crease should stay ½ IW from the upper lid ciliary margin from medial to lateral tapering towards the medial and lateral canthi. The lateral eyelid highlight is not necessarily at the lateral canthus, it is dictated more by the FO and the balance that this subtle line brings to the nose and eyes. Hence, this theory answers the age-old facial plastic question on where the arch of the eyebrow should lie. The arch should accentuate the lateral eyelid highlight in such a way that the highlight is in line with the FO. The result of this promotes harmony between these structures. The lower eyelid should have a shadowing one half IW extending below the margin. In short, the second eye COP is 2 IW high, 3 IW wide delineated by: the upper lid crease and shadowing extending below it to the lid margin, the lower lid shadowing, and the two canthi. Geometrically, the dimensions of the second eye COP is logical. The 2 IW high, 3 IW wide dimensions is an ellipse with radii 1 IW centered at the lateral edges of the iris. This same principle applies to the third eye COP (Fig. 78.3).

The third eye COP is delineated by the top of the eyebrows, lateral edge of the dorsum, center of the cheek highlight, and lateral orbital rim. The center of the cheek highlight is 1 IW below the inferior border of the lower lid's shadowing. The vertical dimension should extend from the top of the brow to the center of the cheek highlight, 4 IW. The medial limit of the horizontal dimension is dictated by the lateral edge of the dorsum (not the nasal sidewall) and the lateral limit by the lateral orbital rim, 5 IW wide. The third eye circle is 4 IW high, 5 IW wide. It is also an ellipse with a radii of 2 IW centered at the lateral edges of the iris. The height of the eyebrows should be, at most, ½ IW, any height greater than a ½ IW attracts attention to it and away from the eyes, ultimately, decreasing aesthetics. Notice how the brow hairs on the superior and inferior edge grow towards the center of the eyebrow axis. The purpose of this differential hair growth is to delineate a defined line that takes on a specific angle. As the hairs converge in the center, the angle and axis is accentuated, the importance of which will be discussed.

Although more prevalent in males with prominent brows, a fourth COP can be delineated by the following points: (1) The superior limit of a highlight, directly above the pupil, produced by the brow's prominence should be above the superior edge of the eyebrow by 1 IW. (2) Extending below the inferior edge of the third eye COP 1 IW is where the SO intersects the vertical shadowing in line with the pupil. This is the lower limit of the fourth COP. It demarcates where the cheek shadowing should markedly start to increase inferiolaterally from the SO and vertical papillary plane. The midline and lateral edge of the face at the horizontal pupillary plane are the (3) medial and (4) lateral limits. It is a circle 3 IW in radius centered at the pupil. In short there are four COP in the eye: (1) the iris; (2) the shadowing and bunching produced by the eyelids along with the canthi 2 IW high, 3 IW wide; (3) the lateral orbital rim, top of the eyebrow, lateral edge of the dorsum, and center of the cheek highlight

4 IW high, 5 IW wide; and (4) and a COP 3 IW in radius centered at the pupil (Figs. 78.3, 4).

Importantly, no COP should have any sharp delineation. All of the circles should be demarcated subtly by reflections of light. The transition of one unit or COP to the next is the point where there is a 50% difference from the shade of one unit to the next and this change should be imperceptible to promote beauty. Blemishes, wrinkles, and discoloration of any sort markedly detracts from the beauty of the face with all of its shapes in balance, proportion, and symmetry by violating the highlighting which leads to the circles we subjectively identify.

The Circles of Prominence Within the Mouth

The mouth is equivalent to the eye in terms of having subjectively recognizable COP (Fig. 78.3). The first mouth COP is the lower lip height, equal to one IW. Although not an overt, conspicuous circle, its height subconsciously connects with the other COP (iris, nasal tip, dorsum, philtrum, alae). This notion applies to the other structures, their shapes are subtle and their sizes should equal or be a proportion of the iris width while maintaining their own unique shape. The brain has a way of finishing shapes that are unfinished [19]. The second mouth COP begins with the shadowing produced by the downward and inward sloping of the upper lip, ½ IW high. The shadowing below the lower lip should be equivalent to the lower lid shadowing, ½ IW high, and completes the lower part of the second mouth COP. The vertical distance from top of upper lip to bottom of lower lip shadowing should be equal to 2 IW. The puckering of the lip should produce a subtle highlight that should be 3 IW wide, or the width of the second eye COP. Shadowing produced by the posterior course taken by the dental arch should help to produce gradual shadowing which, by doing so, emphasizes the highlight produced by the puckering. The height of the lower lip puckering markedly thins after the 3 IW as it approaches the commissures. The shadowing of the upper lip and the shade beneath the lower lip should be analogous to the second eye COP eyelid shadowing. All the associations are with the iris and eye COP to accentuate and associate with it. These associations continue with the mouth's third and fourth COP.

The aesthetics of the lips have not been elucidated to date. This is evident when one notices the awkward appearances of movie stars and their unattractive, recently augmented lips. The most famous surgeons have not reached an adequate understanding of lip aesthetics. Most surgeons mention that it is a gestalt or an artistic appreciation but cannot pinpoint the exact elements. Herein lies the inaccuracies and the resulting surgical manifestations. The lower lip is the center of attention within the mouth unit. This is based on a number of supporting pieces of information. Squamous cell cancer occurs 90% of the time on the lower lip, which supports the idea that most of the sunlight strikes the lower lip versus the upper lip. Practically speaking, when one observes the face in sunlight, you notice that the lower lip has the most light reflecting from it. This indicates that when one analyzes the face the highlight produced by the lower lip will attract more attention to it than the upper lip. To further support this thought, the lower lip is more ani-

mate than the upper lip. When a person speaks it is the lower lip that moves along with the jaw. All of these points suggest that the lower lip predominates as the anatomical center of attention within the mouth unit. With this premise, we theorize that the lower lip should serve as the primary COP from where we arrange the balance between the major units of the eye, nose,, and mouth (Fig. 78.2). Because of this importance it should be 1 IW in vertical dimension associating with the iris and other primary COP. The upper lip with its secondary role should be ½ IW. As mentioned before, shapes (or COP) should be related in size to strike associations and thus promote harmony. Hence, the iris equals the lower lip height and the second eye COP should equal the second mouth COP to support this order. The puckering of the lower lip should equal in exact dimension the palpebral fissure in an inverted fashion. This relation is further supported by the shadowing of the lids and of the lips delineated by the second COP. From a clinical standpoint, we should augment the lip mainly 3 IW in width and 1 IW in height within the lower lip. The upper lip should be no more than ½ IW in height and 1 IW in width gradually tapering laterally to promote this balance. When the upper lip exceeds these dimensions, it attracts more attention to it and upsets the balance between the eyes, nose, and mouth and the association between the lower lip puckering and the palpebral aperture (Fig. 78.3).

These associations continue in the third and fourth mouth COP. The third mouth COP begins from commissure to commissure, the distance is 5 IW and should be equal to the width of the third eye COP. The distance from subnasale to the center of the chin highlight should be 4 IW and equivalent with the distance from the top of the brow to the center of the cheek highlight. For the fourth mouth COP, the distance from tip to lower lip is the radius, 3 IW, by which one can draw a circle centered at the lower lip, equaling 6 IW in total height and width (Fig. 78.3). This circle is delineated by the nasal tip, melolabial folds, and the mentum. The width of the main lip unit is also the same distance from midline to the most lateral part of the face at the level of the pupil, 6 IW (Fig. 78.5, horizontal blue arrows). It is also equal to the interpupillary distance, further adding to the balance and harmony in the many dimensions within the face. The fourth COP is not the same shape as the first through third eye or mouth COP, it is nearly a perfect circle, but the fourth COP of the eye and mouth demarcate in the subjective mind's eye the limits in the eye unit and the limits of the mouth unit while associating with other distances (i.e., interpupillary and half-face width distances) connecting them all together. This adds to the subconscious association, with the other COP, between the two anatomic units of the eye and mouth. The fourth mouth COP also aids in the vertical shadowing that is limited by the vertical line bisecting the pupil, to help bring attention to the iris, further beautifying the eyes and, in turn, the face in general. The mentum, or lower limit of the fourth COP is 1 IW inferior to the third mouth COP; it is analogous to the point where the vertical plane of the pupil intersects with the SO (Fig. 78.5, green arrow). This is the same association found between the nasal tip and the brow prominence's upper limit 1 IW above the midpoint of the eyebrow (Fig. 78.5, pink arrow). In summary, the mouth has four COP: (1) the lower lip height that equals one IW; (2) the shadowing produced by the upper lip and area

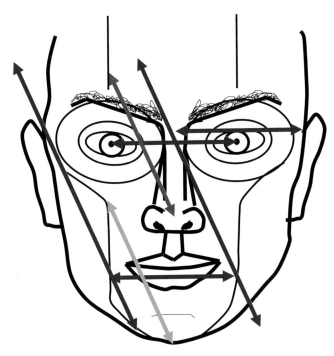

Fig. 78.5 Everything in the face is related. The largest circles of prominence (fourth COP) of the eye and mouth are equal to the interpupillary distance and half-face width (*blue arrows*)

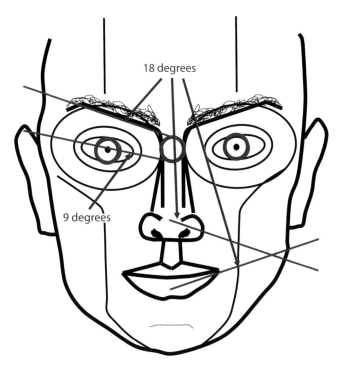

Fig. 78.6 The angles of the medial and lateral eyebrows, nasal tip to alae, and lower lip to commissures are 18°. The angle of the horizontal palpebral fissure is 9°. Everything in the face is related by shape, size and angles

inferior to the lower lip along with the lower lip pucker 2 IW high, 3 IW wide; (3) commissure to commissure and subnasale to the center of the chin highlighted area 4 IW high, 5 IW wide; and (4) the COP centered at the lower lip, with the radius = tip to lower lip, 3 IW, or 6IW in diameter (Fig. 78.3).

Harmonizing with Other Structures in the Face

Other structures are also delineated by the IW to continue the subtle association with the iris and eyes. The interbrow distance is 2 IWs delineated by the association between the mouth and eye fourth COP (Fig. 78.5, long diagonal blue arrow). The nasal base from ala to ala is 3 IW. The chin width is 3 IW. Bizygion distance is 12 IW, bigonion distance is 10 IW. The ear extends from the lateral part of the face by one IW. The nose at its root is 2 IW and is 3 IW at the base. The interpupillary distance is 6 IW (Fig. 78.5). Again, equal balance between shapes (equal distances between primary COP), proportion of all shapes (all shapes in multiples of IW), and symmetry between sides (right and left COP are equal) and within each COP (each COP is symmetric in its own dimension, i.e., elliptical or circular, and similar in shape between eye and mouth COP) contribute to a person's beauty. Again, when structures that are meant to be the same dimension as the IW are found to be larger than an iris width, it attracts unwanted attention. For example, if the ear protrudes more than an iris width away from the side of the head, it loses the association with the iris and attracts a greater amount of unwanted attention when it should be directed toward the eye and iris.

One question that has not been adequately answered by previous thinking is the angles of the eyebrows and horizontal eye fissures and how they fit into facial aesthetics (Fig. 78.6). There is also an ideal angle formed by the nasal tips and the centers of the alar prominences. Moreover, an angle must exist for the lips, from the center of the lower lip to the commissure shadow. Again, these angles have their own existence and must have an ideal, between zero and infinity. The eyebrow should produce an 18° angle from medial brow to the arch. This is the same angle (18) from the arch to the lateral extent of the brow. As stated above, the third eye COP is 4 IW high and 5 IW wide, the ratio of the main eye dimensions is 4/5 = 0.8. Twenty percent (reciprocal of 4/5) of 90° is 18°, this was a coincidental finding. The ideal angle of the eyebrow may be related to a center position between the eyes. If a phantom circle the size of the iris is drawn exactly in the midline on the horizontal plane of the iris, this serves as the focal point for this region of the face (Fig. 78.7). This phantom COP serves to help delineate the angles of the palpebral fissures and the eyebrows. A line tangential to the bottom of the circle intersecting the iris dictates the ideal angle for the palpebral fissure. Another line tangential to the top of this phantom COP intersecting a point 1 IW above the iris in the midline dictates the angle of the eyebrow. The phantom circle also serves as a focal point for the beginning of the nose as will be discussed. The importance of these relationships is that the structures of the eyes, eyebrows, and nose are tied in by this focal point (phantom circle) to serve as a way to transition these anatomical units subtlety from one to the other. Based on this,

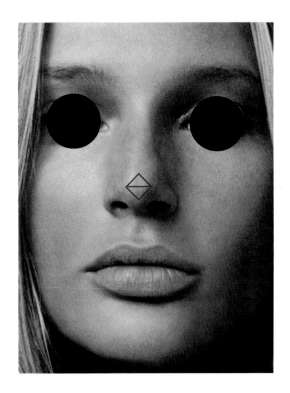

Circles of Prominence and Nasal Aesthetics

Within the nose, a theory must be quantifiable in order for surgeons to apply it in the operating venue. Most chapters on aesthetics use some form of the canons as the basis for understanding. On frontal view the tip should have four landmarks: two tip-defining points, a supra-tip break point, and the columellar-lobular angle. These points should demarcate two equilateral triangles. If they do not, it should be ascertained why and tip modification can be carried out to correct the discrepancies (Fig. 78.8). A vertical line drawn through the plane of the upper lip should then divide the nose equally from this plane to the alar base plane (distance B) and from the upper lip plane to the plane through the tip-defining point. This will indicate the projection of the tip and whether an increase or decrease is indicated (distance A should equal B, Fig. 78.9). Chin projection should be 3 mm posterior to the upper lip plane. Another way to determine the adequacy of tip projection is measuring the distance from the tip-defining point to the radix (nasal length) and tip projection from alar cheek junction to the tip-defining points. The ratio of nasal length to tip projection should be 1–0.67 (Fig. 78.10). The ideal nasal length from radix to tip defining point (RT) should equal stomion to mentum (SM) or 1.6 times TS, tip to stomion (Fig. 78.11). Tip rotation is determined by drawing a line through the upper lip plane. Another line drawn from the anterior and posterior points of the nostril forms an angle with the upper lip plane. This angle is

the ideal angle from endocanthion to exocanthion was discovered to be 9°. Other structures that should take on an angle are the relationship between the tip and alae and the center of the lower lip to the commissures, both 18°. Because some of the structures (alae, brows, commissures at rest, canthi) do not fit into the obliques, the angles just described allow them to associate with other structures to further create an association that promotes harmony and order. When the angles deviate from the others, tension is created with the shapes involved. Attention is brought to the deviation and less balance and harmony with the other shapes becomes the subjective result.

The forehead also should have an ideal height. As described above, the superior limit of the brow prominence and the highlight it produces should be 1 IW from the superior midpoint of the eyebrow. This is the upper limit of the fourth eye COP (Fig. 78.3). Above this point the trichion should not be more than 3 IWs high. In short, the distance from the pupil to the forehead should not exceed 6 IW, or the distance from pupil to lower lip. The more this distance from pupil to trichion is equal to the distance from pupil to lower lip the more ideal because the association produces harmony. When the forehead is taller, more attention is directed to this unit. When it is smaller, there is less association or harmony with the central face found between the pupil and lower lip. Both situations occur at the expense of aesthetics.

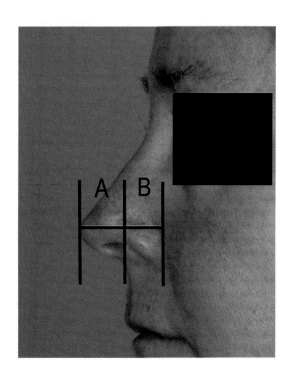

Fig. 78.8 A vertical line drawn through the plane of the upper lip which should divide the nose equally from this plane to the alar base plane (distance **B**) and from the upper lip plane to the plane through the tip defining point (distance **A**). This will indicate the projection of the tip and whether an increase or decrease is indicated (distance **A** should equal **B**)

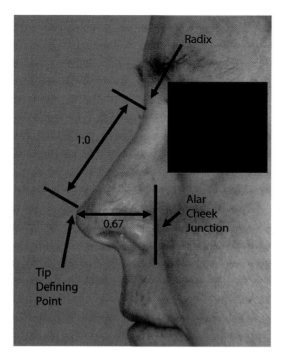

Fig. 78.9 Determining the adequacy of tip projection is done by measuring the distance from the tip defining point to the radix (nasal length) and tip projection from alar cheek junction to the tip defining points. The ratio of nasal length to tip projection should be 1 to 0.67

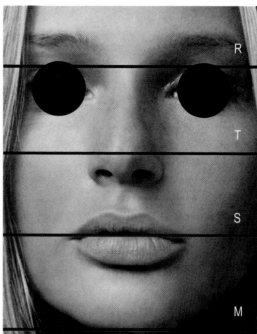

Fig. 78.10 The ideal nasal length from radix to tip defining point (**RT**) should equal stomion to mentum (**SM**) or 1.6 times **TS**, tip to stomion

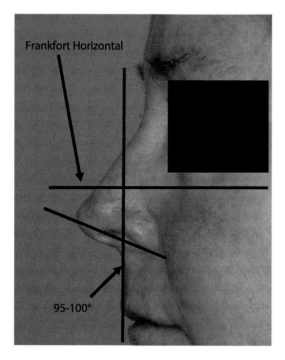

Fig. 78.11 Tip rotation is determined by drawing a line through the upper lip plane. Another line drawn from the anterior and posterior points of the nostril form an angle with the upper lip plane. This angle is ideally 95–100° in women and 90–95° in men

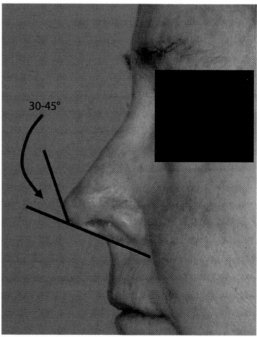

Fig. 78.12 Another angle exists called the columellar-lobular angle which is formed by the junction of the columella and the infratip lobule. This is ideally 30–45°

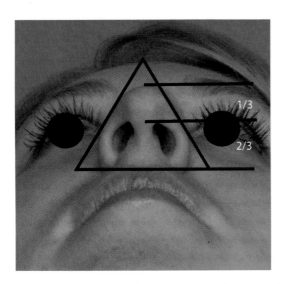

Fig. 78.13 From the worm's eye view, the nasal base should form an equilateral triangle. The ratio of the columella to the lobular portion of the nose should be 2:1

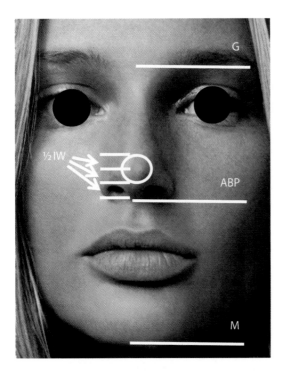

Fig. 78.14 An important term for nasal analysis is midface height (**MFH**) which is the distance from glabellar plane (**G**) to Alar Base Plane (**ABP**). Lower face height (**LFH**) is the distance from **ABP** to Mentum plane (**M**). MFH equals 3 mm less than **LFH**. The ideal nasal length (**RT**, Radix to Tip defining point) should be 0.67 x **MFH**. Nasal tip projection should be 0.67 **RT**. Ideal radix projection should be 0.28RT, the distance from corneal plane to the radix plane. From the center of the nasal tip to the bottom of the nasal tip COP, the distance is one half IW. The supertip breakpoint is really a depression that emphasizes the tip and is one half IW superior to the center of the nasal tip COP. It is a one half IW from lower edge of the nasal tip COP to the subnasale. From the subnasale to the top of the upper lip, the distance is 1 IW

ideally 95–100° in women and 90–95° in men (Fig. 78.12). Another angle exists called the columellar-lobular angle, which is formed by the junction of the columella and the infratip lobule. This is ideally 30–45° (Fig. 78.13). From the worm's eye view, the nasal base should form an equilateral triangle. The ratio of the columella to the lobular portion of the nose should be 2:1 (Fig. 78.14). An important term for nasal analysis is midface height (MFH) which is the distance from glabellar plane (G) to Alar Base Plane (ABP). Lower face height (LFH) is the distance from ABP to Mentum plane (M). MFH equals 3 mm less than LFH. The ideal nasal length (RT, Radix to Tip defining point) should be 0.67 × MFH. Nasal tip projection should be 0.67 RT. Ideal radix projection should be 0.28 RT, the distance from corneal plane to the radix plane (Fig. 78.15) [26].

Although, much of their ideals are based on the canons, which have been shown to be incorrect, these aesthetic values are adequate for determining surgical maneuvers based on years of ad hoc experience. However, these ideals again are based on external landmarks which observers find less important. The ideals for the width of the dorsum and tip have been loosely determined to date. Our only real approach to this is that the dorsum should be outlined by two slightly curved divergent lines extending from the superciliary ridges to the tip-defining points.

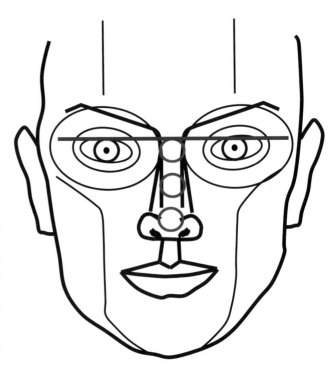

Fig. 78.15 The start of the nasal length should be where the irises horizontally line up at the top of the nose

As stated above, because we concentrate so much of our time looking at the iris it logically serves as the ideal for these values (dorsal width and tip width). The alae and their shape and size have not received adequate attention as well. This theory states that the alae are ideally circular in appearance from a frontal view and that they should subtlety emulate the iris. Instead of following dogmatic values to determine the nasal length, the balance between the horizontal pupillary plane and the center of the nasal tip should ideally be 3 IW. The start of the nasal length should be where the irises horizontally line up at the top of the nose (Fig. 78.15). This ideal location for the radix, at the horizontal plane through the top of the irises, is logical because it connects the nose perceptually with the iris along with the angles of the eyebrows and palpebral fissure, as stated above. This connection allows the viewer to naturally proceed from the eyes to the nose and then the mouth. In terms of tip aesthetics, from the center of the nasal tip to the bottom of the nasal tip COP, the distance is ½ IW. The supertip breakpoint is really a depression that emphasizes the tip and is ½ IW superior to the center of the nasal tip COP. It is a ½ IW from lower edge of the nasal tip COP to the subnasale. From the subnasale to the upper lip the distance is 1 IW. From the root of the nose to the base (top to bottom), it should widen from 2 IW to 3 IW. It is ½ IW from the lateral edge of sidewall to the lateral edge of the dorsum. The dorsum is 1 IW. The alae are 1 IW and the tip is 1 IW, which in horizontal dimension adds up to the sum of 3 IW.

Conclusion

The theory is subtle because it is based on shades of light. It is based on the most important structure on the face, the iris. Simply put, there are multiple shapes on the face and an evolutionary force must have determined the specific size of each of those shapes. Extremes in dimensions are unaesthetic. Between the extremes an ideal must exist which the mind settles on and prefers. The iris is the center of attention in the face and should, therefore, be the structure on which every dimension on the face is based. The formulation of this theory began with the understanding that symmetry, proportion, and balance are important aspects when dealing with any structure that is a compilation of different shapes [19]. The shapes that attract the most attention on the face are the irises followed by the nasal tip and lips [22]. From there an observer's eyes shift to examine other shapes then returns again to the iris and then repeats this cycle to continue analyzing. In regards to the neoclassical canons, it would not seem likely that an observer would concentrate on the trichion, glabella, or other insignificant external landmarks which occupy prominent points in those theories. These structures are not important to the observer. Rather, a new theory should focus on what a person actually concentrates on, namely the iris. Because every shape and size on the face has its own existence, the ideal distance logically is dictated by the width of the iris. With this known, the quantitative and qualitative elements become more clarified.

Because the iris, tip of the nose, and lower lip are the most prominent features, they need to be equal in size (Fig. 78.1) and the distances between them should be equal. Since each of the smallest COP represent the base for larger COP, any deviation of this balance between them will bring tension to the larger COP (which emanate from the primary COP) arrangement with other COP within the face [19, 22]. All of the structures of the face emphasize the iris including the vertical forehead and cheek shadowing which should line up with the pupil in a vertical plane as well as the obliques, and other primary COP. As indicated above, the shapes in the mouth are related to the shapes in the eye. All of the COP in each of these anatomic parts should be equal in shape and size. Notice how the dimensions of the first through fourth COP are the same shape in the eye and mouth units. The subconscious result is that when a person speaks, smiles, or sings the mouth brings to life the eye and subsequently the face as a whole.

The angles formed by the brows, nasal tip and alae, lower lip and commissures, and canthi are defined as being either 18° or 9° (Fig. 78.6). When looking at Figure 78.4, the obliques are 45° from the horizontal. The angle formed by the mentum to the point where the SO intersects the vertical plane through the pupil should be 67.5° or midway between 90° and 45°. This is also true with the angle formed by the line connecting the nasal tip and the superior edge of the brow prominence that is in line with the vertical plane through the pupil (Fig. 78.5, pink arrow). In short, the angle 67.5 is essentially the angle associating the mouth with the eye. The alignment of the other structures within the face to specific angles (i.e., nasal tip/alae, lower lip/commissure, endocanthion to exocanthion) at 18° and 9° brings balance to these structures that do not fit within the confines of the obliques and eye/mouth angles. In total, all of the structures and shapes of the face are adherent to either 90°, 67.5°, 45°, 18°, 9° or 0°. The phantom circle between the eyes also serves as a regional focal point for the viewer to follow a smooth transition from the eye, brows, and eye unit into the nose. Although the values for the angles need further refinement and scientific evidence (along with other minor elements of this theory), the principle that all of the structures of the face need some association with the other neighboring structures remains sound. When all of the shapes associate with each other; symmetry, balance, and harmony is achieved and the ultimate result is beauty.

The problem with theories in the past are the external landmarks that they were based on, which people did not find important. However, these external landmarks were easier to base a theory on compared with subtleties of light that change with the orientation of the face. This theory concentrates on the forms that attract a person's attention and theorizes how the mind puts together the shapes of the face, and how a person decides why a face is beautiful or not. From there the quantitative elements become better defined. Because the COP is based on mathematics, simple geometry, and what a viewer finds important, these elements together with the adherence to existing anatomy make this theory an original thought that could stand the test of time. The difficulty with this theory is that it is dependent on shades of light. Although the very elements viewers' use to judge beauty, these elements are not conspicuous to identify, nor easily adjusted through surgery. The use of computers to quantitate these grades of shading or differential light projection in photography could aid our appreciation of how these subtleties impact our perception of the face. If we could translate these studies to quantify variances that may be adjustable through surgical means, our ability to improve our patients' lives for the better will be changed forever.

References

1. Crumley RL, Lanser M (1988) Quantitative analysis of nasal tip rhinoplasty. Laryngoscope 98:202–208

2. Ferrario VF, Sforza C, Poggio C, Tartaglia G (1995) Facial morphometry of television actresses compared with normal women. J Oral Maxillofac Surg 53:1008–1014

3. Perrett DI, May KA, Yoshikawa S (1994) Facial shape and judgements of female attractiveness. Nature 368:239–242

4. Alam, M, Dover J (2001) On beauty: Evolution, psychosocial considerations, and surgical enhancement. Arch Dermatol 137:795–807

5. Jefferson Y (1996) Skeletal types: Key to unraveling the mystery of facial beauty and its biological significance. J Gen Orthod 7:7–25

6. Farkas LG, Kolar JC (1987) Anthropometric guidelines in cranioorbital surgery. Clin Plast Surg 14:1–15

7. Farkas LG, Hreczko TA, Kolar JC, Munro IR (1985) Vertical and horizontal proportions of the face in young adult North American caucasians: Revision of neoclassical canons. Plast Reconstr Surg 75:328–337

8. Seghers MJ, Longacre JJ, deStefano GA (1964) The golden proportion and beauty. Plast Reconstr Surg 34:382–386

9. Gonzalez-Ulloa M (1962) Quantitative principles in cosmetic surgery of the face (Profileplasty). Plast Reconstr Surg 29:186–197

10. Chen AC, German C, Zaidel DW (1997) Brain asymmetry and facial attractiveness: Facial beauty is not simply in the eye of the beholder. Neuropsychologia 35:471–476

11. Drury NE (2000) Beauty is only skin deep. J R Soc Med 93:89–92

12. Larrabee WF (1997) Facial beauty: Myth or reality? Arch Otolaryngol Head Neck Surg 123:571–572

13. Vioarsdottir US, O'Higgins P, Stringer C (2002) A geometric morphometric study of regional differences in the ontogeny of the modern human facial skeleton. J Anat 201:211–229

14. Enquist M, Stefano G (1998) Evolutionary biology: The secret of faces. Nature 394:826–827

15. Etcoff NL (1994) Beauty and the beholder. Nature 368:186–187

16. Enquist M, Arak A (1994) Symmetry, beauty, and evolution. Nature 372:169–172

17. Skiles MS, Randall P (1983) The aesthetics of ear placement: An experimental study. Plast Reconstr Surg 72:133–140

18. O'Higgins P, Johnson DR, Moore WJ, Flinn RM (1990) The variability of patterns of sexual dimorphism in the hominid skull. Experientia 46:670–672

19. Tolleth H (1987) Concepts for the plastic surgeon from art and sculpture. Clin Plast Surg 14:585–597

20. Farkas LG, Kolar JC (1987) Anthropometrics and art in the aesthetics of women's faces. Clin Plast Surg 14:599–615

21. Flowers RS (1987) The art of eyelid and orbital aesthetics: Multiracial surgical considerations. Clin Plast Surg 14:703–721

22. Menick FJ (1987) Artistry in aesthetic surgery. Clin Plast Surg 14:723–735

23. Farkas LG, Eiben OG, Sivkov S, Tompson B, Katic MJ, Forrest CR (2004) Anthropometric measurements of the facial framework in adulthood: Age-related changes in eight age categories in 600 healthy white North Americans of European ancestry from 16–90 years of age. J Craniofac Surg 15:288–298

24. Ruff CB (1980) Age differences in craniofacial dimensions among adults from Indian Knoll, Kentucky. Am J Phys Anthropol 53:101–108

25. Borman H, Ozgur F, Gursu G (1999) Evaluation of soft-tissue morphology of the face in 1050 young adults. Ann Plast Surg 42:280–288

26. Gunter JP, Rohrich RJ, Adams WP (2002) Dallas rhinoplasty. Quality Medical Publishing Chaps. 4–10

27. Porter JP (2004) The average African American male face: An anthropometric analysis. Arch Facial Plast Surg 6:78–81

28. Porter JP, Olson KL (2001) Anthropometric facial analysis of the African American woman. Arch Facial Plast Surg 3:191–197

29. Choe KS, Sclafani AP, Litner JA, Yu GP, Romo T (2004) The Korean American woman's face: Anthropometric measurements and quantitative analysis of facial aesthetics. Arch Facial Plast Surg 6:244–252

Chapter 79

Implants and Fillers for Facial Plastic Surgery

79

William E. Silver, Mathew J. Dickson, and Louis M. DeJoseph

Core Messages

■ Structural augmentation and soft tissue volumization are critical components to complete facial rejuvenation. The modern facial plastic surgeon must balance surgical resuspension with volumization to achieve the desired results. Therefore, implants and fillers will forever play a crucial role in the treatment of the aging face.

Contents

Introduction

As reconstructive and cosmetic surgical techniques have advanced, so too has the need for suitable grafting materials for augmentation of soft tissue, cartilage, and bone of the face. Consequently, a large number of potential grafting materials, both synthetic and biological, have been developed and are available to the facial plastic surgeon. When choosing a graft, the surgeon must consider many factors including its inherent mechanical properties, biocompatibility, potential for reabsorption, resistance to infection, and cost. The purpose of this chapter is to review the properties of various implant materials and fillers available to the facial plastic surgeon, and to consider their clinical strengths and weaknesses.

Implant Materials

Bone

Bone is composed of both organic and inorganic materials. The inorganic component, calcium hydroxyapatite ($Ca_{10}(PO_4)_6$ (OH_2)), gives bone its hardness and strength. The organic component, known as osteoid, is composed of various cell types including osteoblasts and osteoclasts, type I collagen, and other noncollagenous proteins.

When considering bone as a grafting material, it is important to recognize its two forms; cancellous and cortical. Cortical bone is dense, lined by periosteum, and relatively poorly vascularized. The use of cortical bone is osseoconductive, thus without bony contact, a cortical bone graft will resorb over time. Cancellous bone is trabeculated, more highly vascularized. With its abundant supply of osteoblasts, cancellous bone may have some osseoinducitve potential, thus the graft is less likely to resorb. Ideally, bone grafts should contain both cancellous and cortical bone.

Bone grafts are incorporated into the recipient site in several steps. First, the graft is revascularized through its haversian system. Next, the graft is demineralized to varying degrees over the next several months. Once established, the graft remineralizes and reverts to its original structure. It has been noted that bone derived from membranous sources are revascularized significantly faster than endochondral bone, and are resorbed to a lesser extent [1, 2].

Free autologous grafts can be harvested from the parietal skull, iliac crest, and occasionally rib, and thus its use carries the morbidity of an additional incision. Heterologous bone treated by freeze drying or exposure to gamma radiation is available for use. Numerous vascularized free flaps can be harvested with bone, most notably the fibular, scapular, and iliac crest.

Bone is more often used in reconstruction rather than cosmetic surgery. Both free bone grafts and vascularized free flaps are used in mandibular reconstruction following trauma or neoplastic extirpation. Other uses include orbital, zygomatic, malar, and nasal reconstruction [3]. In the nose, calvarial bone grafts have been used for dorsal augmentation, insertion of columella struts for nasal tip ptosis, and insertion of nasal battens for nasal valve collapse [4].

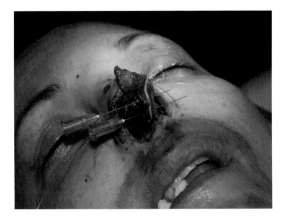

Fig. 79.3 Intraoperative picture of auricular cartilage seen in **Fig. 79.2** being placed as a medial crural strut

Cartilage

Autologous cartilage is perhaps the most widely used grafting material in facial plastic surgery. It is harvested from the nasal septum, the auricle, or rib cage. In the past, preserved heterologous cartilage was used with great success, and with a very limited host immune response. Some evidence points to a greater

rate of resorption of preserved cartilage when compared to fresh autologous cartilage. The use of heterologous cartilage has ceased over concerns regarding the transmission of infectious diseases.

While the precise composition of cartilage may vary at each anatomic site, essentially cartilage is composed of chondrocytes, type II collagen, proteoglycans, and water. Cartilage itself is avascular. Chondrocytes obtain their nutrition from simple diffusion of molecules through the aqueous component. This allows the graft to survive in its implantation site without the need for neovascularization. Thus, cartilage can be implanted in superficial sites such as the nasal dorsum.

Autologous cartilage offers many advantages as a grafting material. It incites no host response, and does not act to harbor infection. It is strong, flexible, and easily shaped via carving. It is readily available, and often easily obtained especially when harvested from the nasal septum or ear (Figs. 79.1–79.3). Fresh autologous cartilage grafts have long-term survival. Resorption is estimated at 12–50% [5].

There are few disadvantages associated with the use of autologous cartilage. Depending on the harvest site, there may be the need for a second incision, thereby increasing the morbidity of the operation. This is much more likely in revision rhinoplastic surgery. Also, there is some evidence that costal cartilage has a propensity to warp [6, 7].

Because of its excellent characteristics, cartilage has found wide use in facial plastic surgery, especially in the areas of rhi-

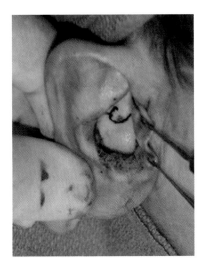

Fig. 79.1 Intraoperative picture of conchal cartilage being harvested from the patient's right ear

79

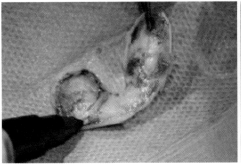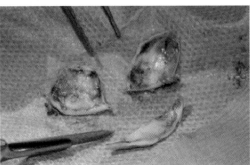

Fig. 79.2 Intact conchal cartilage (*left*). Divided conchal cartilage (*right*)

noplasty and auricular reconstruction. In the nose, cartilage can be used for direct augmentation such as onlay grafts on the tip, columella, or dorsum. It can be used for structural support for existing tissues, such as when used as a medial crural strut. It can be fashioned into a spreader graft for use in internal nasal valve reconstruction. Onlay cartilage grafts can also be used to substitute for lost alar cartilage and can even be morselized to "paper thin" and used as a camouflage over new structured nasal domes or to just cover little irregularities at the conclusion of the rhinoplastic procedure.

For the ear, costal cartilage can be used to recreate the contours of the helix and the defective cartilaginous framework of the ear.

Fat and Dermis

Reports of using autologous fat date back over a century [8]. Its use has increased in recent years with the advances of tumescent liposuction [9].

Autologous fat has the advantage of abundant supply, and with proper technique, harvesting carries a relatively low morbidity. Its texture is inconspicuous in the soft tissues of the face. It can be used both as a free graft and as an injectable filler. As with all autologous materials, there is no host immune response, and very low risk of infection. Lastly, compared with synthetic materials, the associated cost is low. The major disadvantage associated with fat is resorption, which has been estimated by some authors at 20–90% [10].

Fat can be used in the treatment of acquired facial defects, HIV-associated lipodystrophy, filling of rhytids and folds such as the ML folds and tear troughs, and cosmetic augmentation of the lips [11–13].

Dermal grafts are prepared by removing the epithelium from a portion of skin as in a split thickness skin graft, and then removing the subcutaneous fat. Dermal grafts have the disadvantages of increased morbidity from the donor site, and the post-surgical risk of epithelial cyst formation if not all the epithelium is removed.

Davis et al. have reported on the use of free dermal fat grafts in facial reconstruction. Sixty-six percent of patients were treated successfully. They state that resorption can be minimized by keeping the fat less than 1.5 cm thick [14].

Acellular heterologous dermis (AlloDerm LifeCell, Branchburg, New Jersey) is banked human dermis that is treated to maintain the dermal matrix, but remove any antigenic components. It is strong and pliable, and supports revascularization [15, 16]. It has been used to smooth out irregularities of the nasal dorsum, or rolled to fill in the melolabial folds or augment the lips. Its longevity varies with each situation and has been shown to be resorbed as much as 100%. Therefore, it should not be used for permanent augmentation.

Expanded Polytetrafluoroethylene

Expanded Polytetrafluoroethylene (e-PTFE) is a synthetic fluorocarbon polymer which can be fashioned into an inert, micro porous material suitable for use in the body. It has an extensive history of use as vascular grafts and patches, as well as a mesh in hernia repair. It is chemically similar to polytetrafluoroethylene (Teflon), but has been stretched under special conditions to create a specific micro architecture. Electron microscopy reveals nodes of solid PTFE connected by fine PTFE fibers, with the resulting pores measuring 10–30 μ. This has clinical significance in that such a pore size allows for minimal tissue ingrowth. E-PTFE has been shown to be highly biocompatible, with minimal inflammation and capsule formation [17]. These factors allow for straightforward removal of the implant at a later time if necessary. Furthermore, e-PTFE maintains its structural integrity and pliability after implantation.

Manufactured in many forms, Gore-Tex (WL Gore, Flagstaff, AZ), Soft Form (Collagen Corporation, Palo Alto, CA), and Advantage (Atrium Medical Corporation, Hudson, NH), are available as thin sheets or as cylindrical strands.

With its natural feel, and ease of use, e-PTFE has gained a prominent role in soft tissue augmentation of the face. In its tubular forms, e-PTFE can be used for lip augmentation or effacement of deep furrows such as the melolabial folds (Fig. 79.5) or mental crease. Alternatively, sheets of e-PTFE can be cut and used for dorsal nasal augmentation. Godin et al. have reported on the use of Gore-Tex implants in rhinoplasty, both secondary and revision. They found no cases of implant displacement or extrusion, and an infection rate of only 2.2% [18]. Lohuis et al. studied 66 patients after nasal dorsal augmentation using e-PTFE and found no incidence of infection or complication related to the implant [19]. The senior author recommends pressure loading the porous implant with Clindamycin (300 mg. in 15 cc of saline) before insertion (Figs. 79.6, 79.4).

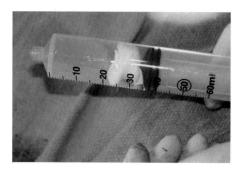

Fig. 79.4 Strips of e-PTFE being impregnated with Clindamycin solution prior to implantation

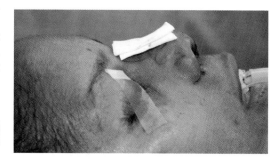

Fig. 79.5 Intraoperative photograph of e-PTFE cut sheeting being measured for dorsal nasal augmentation

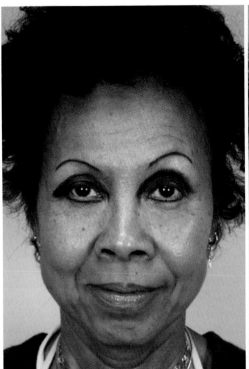
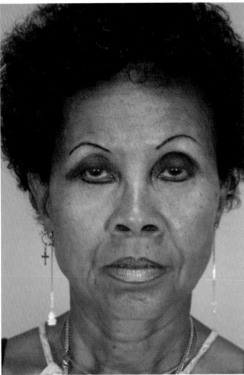

Fig. 79.6 Preoperative (*left*) and postoperative (*right*) photographs of a patient having undergone implantation of e-PTFE to the ML folds

A major difference in the micro-pour implants compared to the solid implants is that if the porous implant becomes infected it must be removed and replaced at a later date; whereas if a solid implant becomes infected there may be a chance to be successful in treating this with antibiotics. The same is true if exposure of a porous implant occurs, it must be removed, whereas with local treatment a solid implant may heal if careful local treatment is given in time. A porous implant should not be placed in the nose if there is exposure to the nasal cavity for the reasons mentioned above. A corollary to this is that the implant should be placed far away from the introducing incision. Thus, if using a porous dorsal nasal implant it should be introduced via an external incision rather than and intercartilaginous one.

79

Silicone Elastomer

Silicone elastomer, often referred to as Silastic (Dow Corning, Midland, MI), is based on the monomeric unit dimethylsiloxane. It is unique in that it is based on a silicone rather than carbon chain, as many other polymers are. At shorter polymer lengths, the silicone assumes a liquid form. As the polymer chain increases in length, the resulting material becomes more viscous. Silastic is produced by a process of vulcanization, whereby very long strands of polydimethylsiloxane are cross linked, resulting in a nonporous, solid material. Silastic can be made in varying degrees of firmness, and can be carved by the surgeon at the time of surgery, and is autoclavable.

Despite public fears in the past over silicone breast implants, Silastic is nontoxic and essentially inert. Several studies have demonstrated a mild tissue reaction to silastic, characterized by a thin fibrous capsule formation with little or no surrounding inflammation [20, 21]. Silastic maintains its structural integrity over time. Custom made shapes and sizes can be designed and produced for a specific defect using CT scan defect reproductions to mold the implant to fit the exact defect. This can be ordered though Implantech (Implantech associates inc., Ventura, CA).

Difficulties associated with using silastic can include capsule formation and dislocation. Being nonporous, silastic does not allow tissue ingrowth, nor does it adhere to the surrounding fibrous capsule. This may result in poor anchoring of the implant, with resulting mobility and migration. Additionally, there have been reports of extrusion, especially with thin soft tissue coverage.

Silastic has found wide use as an implant in facial plastic. It can be used successfully to augment the chin, nasal dorsum, and malar region. Its use in mentoplasty is well established. Preformed implants in various sizes and configurations are available (Figs. 79.7, 79.8). Being stiff and incompressible, some surgeons feel that silastic is ideal for augmenting bony tissue. Some authors have noted mandibular bone erosion following implantation. Saleh et al. studied 20 patients with radiographs after augmentation mentoplasty with silastic implants [22]. They found up to 2 mm of bony absorption in 19% of patients. However, two thirds of the patients had absorption limited to 0.5 mm. The senior author has not seen any dental complications from the mild radiological bone absorption in literally hundreds of cases in over 35 years of their use for chin augmentation.

Several studies have show silastic to be a suitable implant for malar augmentation [23, 24]. Metzinger et al. reviewed 60

Porous High Density Polyethylene

Polyethylene is another synthetic polymer which is composed of repeating ethylene subunits. When first fabricated, these polymers were highly branched, which created a low-density polyethylene. This material was, in fact, used for soft tissue augmentation of the face, but was limited due to low tensile strength and high extrusion rate. Later, chemical processes were developed which created polyethylene molecules with very little branching, thus creating high-density polyethylene (HDPE).

HDPE can be fabricated as a porous material, with pore sizes of 100–150 μm (Medpor, Porex Corporation, Fairburn, GA). It can be contoured at the time of surgery with a scalpel, scissors, or heated and molded manually, all while maintaining the porous structure. It is supplied in sterile packaging, and cannot be resterilized.

Porous High Density polyethylene (PHDP) has sufficient pore size to allow for tissue and osseous ingrowth. This leads to greater stability in the tissues, and can even result in stability against bone [20].

PHDP has had extensive use in bony reconstruction of the face. It has been used with varying success for orbital reconstruction, nasal dorsal, microtia and auricular repair, malar augmentation, and mandible contouring [27]. In its thin form (.85 mm) it can be used as the senior author has used it as a lateral nasal valve reinforcement implant and has been used to replace the lower lateral cartilage in nasal reconstruction [28] (Fig. 79.9).

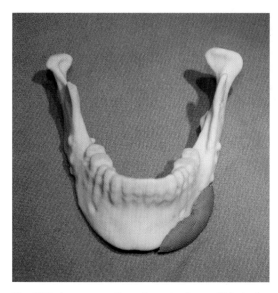

Fig. 79.7 An exact replica of a patient's mandible is shown with the sculpted model for a custom Silastic implant. Careful planning insures proper fit against the bone, proper postoperative mandibular contour, and avoidance of impingement of the mental nerve

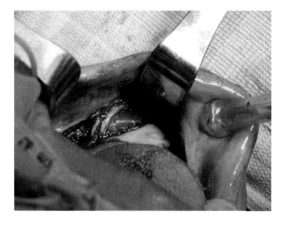

Fig. 79.8 Intraoperative photograph of the custom Silastic implant seen in **Fig. 79.5** being implanted. The mental nerve is clearly seen

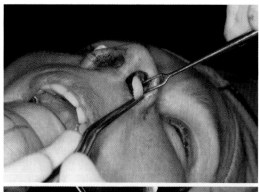
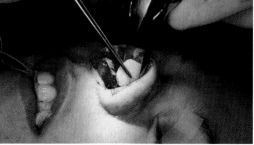

Fig. 79.9 Intraoperative photographs of a Porex implant being used for correction of lateral nasal valve collapse. Insertion can be accomplished via an endonasal (*above*) or external (*below*) approach

patients undergoing silastic malar augmentation. They found a 16.4% incidence of adverse sequelae, which included misalignment, displacement, and infraorbital hypesthesia. Only 3.4% required revision surgery [23].

Silastic's role in nasal augmentation is more limited. The thin soft tissue covering of the nasal dorsum may lead to higher complication rates. These can include mobility of the implant, visible implant edges under the skin, abnormal skin color or sensation, and extrusion [25, 26].

Liquid silicone will be discussed below under "Fillers."

Polyester Mesh

Mersilene (Ethicon, Somerville, NJ) is a synthetic polyester fiber, similar to Dacron (Dupont), composed from polyethylene terephthalate. Mersilene is used as a nonabsorbable suture material and can be woven into a mesh for use in soft tissue augmentation. As a mesh it has excellent tensile strength, which is maintained after implantation. It is soft and pliable, allowing for good conformation to underlying bone, and is difficult to palpate beneath the skin. Furthermore, its structure allows for tissue ingrowth, contributing to stability within the host tissues. No fibrous capsule is formed around the implant. Mersilene mesh is autoclavable, and can be cut at the time of surgery without fraying.

Mersilene mesh is most widely used in chin augmentation. Rolled Mersilene mesh has been successfully used by several authors [29, 30]. Gross et al. [28] reported on 264 patients over 14 years who underwent chin augmentation with Mersilene mesh. They found a 0.8% rate of infection, a 1.5% displacement rate, with no incidence of extrusion, or bony absorption.

Mersilene mesh has also been used in nasal augmentation. Colton and Beekhuis [31] used Mersilene mesh primarily for nasal dorsal augmentation, but also in the tip and lobule with success. They reported a 3.5% infection rate. Soaking the implant in Clindamycin (300 mg in 15 cc of saline) is also preferred when using Mersilene mesh for a rolled or layered implant. In special situations the mesh can be "buried" in a soft tissue pocket to be later removed after tissue ingrowth has taken place. It then can be carved and reinserted. This will reduce the chance of extrusion under thin skin such as in the nasal dorsum since tissue ingrowths are already present.

Titanium

Titanium is a metallic element well known for its strength, light weight, and resistance to corrosion. When used for medical implantation, Titanium is alloyed. Titanium implants are biocompatible and allow for osseous integration. Titanium is nonmagnetic, and thus does not interfere with magnetic resonance imaging.

Titanium's use in the head and neck are generally limited to bony reconstruction, plating, dental implants, or floor of the orbit support after a blow out fracture. Its hardness precludes its use in soft tissue augmentation. However, the senior author has used thin titanium mesh for stenting the external nasal valve in cases of dynamic valve collapse. This is a process of shaping a small circular titanium screen mesh and putting radial cuts around the sides and overlapping sequentially the slits, forming a slight concave shape. This slightly concave "disc" can then be inserted at the time of a rhinoplastic procedure or as an isolated procedure through a rim incision over the predetermined lateral nasal valve area (Fig. 79.10). It is thin, nonreactive, stays in place, and can rarely be felt by the patient after the healing is complete. On occasion the implant has been removed and repositioned because of misplacement. No extrusions or infections have occurred in over 100 cases.

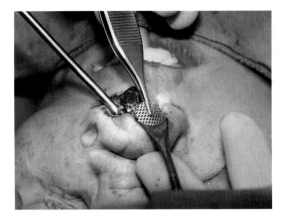

Fig. 79.10 A titanium mesh is shown being inserted for correction of lateral nasal valve collapse

Facial Fillers

The choices of facial filler material available to the cosmetic surgeon have drastically changed over the last several years. The materials are as varied as the patients we encounter during daily practice. One filler material will not suffice in all patients. This portion of the chapter will describe different fillers where they are utilized in specific clinical situations.

Collagen

The original facial filler substance, bovine collagen, was introduced over 30 years ago as Zyderm and its counterpart Zyplast. This was the mainstay of facial fillers until recent times. Both of these products require a skin test prior to placement, but have a long and excellent safety record. In an effort to reduce allergic reaction and skin test requirements, the Inamed Corporation introduced a human collagen formulation called CosmoPlast and CosmoDerm. These products are mainly used to fill fine facial lines and contour deficiencies. They are also useful for accentuating an attenuated lip white roll, as this filler provides excellent definition for this area. The only drawback is longevity, which ranges from 2 to 4 months. Its usage has been limited by the increased longevity of the newer fillers, but it still maintains a role in our facial filler practice.

Hyaluronic Acid

Hyaluronic acid (HA) fillers comprise the next generation of facial fillers and volume enhancement. Marketed under the names Restylane, Hylaform, and Juvederm, they have become a gold standard of facial injectables. HA poses a reduced risk of allergic reaction because all HAs are chemically identical across all species and do not require a skin test prior to injection. Another advantage is longevity of 4–6 months. These products are useful for volumization of the lips and lip borders (Fig. 79.11),

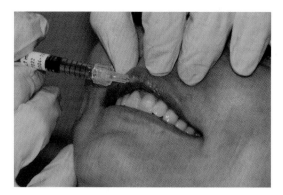

Fig. 79.11 A photograph of a patient having lip augmentation with injectable hyaluronic acid

nasolabial folds, cheek and chin augmentation, and recently the nasojugal groove or "tear trough" (Fig. 79.12). Overcorrection is not necessary with these fillers, as was the case with collagen. Future formulations and varied particle size HAs will further expand the usefulness of this class of fillers.

Calcium Hydroxlapatite

Radiesse (formerly Radiance, BioForm Medical Inc.) is a biocompatible implant composed of calcium hydroxlapatite (CaHa) microspheres varying in size from 25 to 40 μ in diameter. These microspheres are suspended in a carboxymethylcellulose gel carrier. This product has been used in other applications in medicine including oral and maxillofacial defects, vocal cord augmentation, and radiographic tissue marking. As a component of bone, the material does not elicit an immune response and as such does not require a skin test prior to injection. The mechanism of action for this filler is one of initial volume application and augmentation at the desired site. It is now known that the fillers' longevity can be attributed to the microspheres acting as a soft tissue ingrowth framework as the carrier gel dissolves over several months. The longevity of these fillers ranges

from 9 to 18 months. It is well suited for deep facial folds, nasolabial folds, and wrinkles, facial contouring such as malar and chin augmentation, and nasal contouring for nasal deformities. The filler is not well suited for lip augmentation because it has been shown to develop nodule formation over time when used in lip volumization. Injections of both calcium hydroxlapatite and hyaluronic acid, whether in the mid and lower part of the face, are typically performed after local anesthetic blocks.

Poly-L-lactic Acid

Poly-L-lactic acid (PLA) is a substance that has been used for years in surgery for absorbable suture material, tissue anchoring systems, surgical sealant meshes, and solid implants (absorbable screws and plates). The injectable facial filler form sold under the name Sculptra (Dermik Laboratories) is unique among facial fillers in that the material doesn't provide the augmentation, but rather it stimulates production of dermal collagen which augments the site. No skin testing is required with this product. It has FDA approval for HIV-induced facial lipoatrophy and is very useful in this application. Education of patients with the application and expectations with this product are paramount to satisfaction. The augmentation is not immediate since it relies on the patients' tissue growth for volume. Also Sculptra is injected every 4–6 weeks for 3–6 treatments depending on the amount of correction required. The filler is used as a general facial volumizer, not a specific wrinkle or fold correction material. It works well for cheek augmentation, temporal wasting, and perioral and jaw line volumization. Patient participation is also required with facial massage to evenly distribute and stimulate the product for several days after injection.

Liquid Silicone

From an historical perspective liquid silicone (3,000–5,000 centistokes) has been used in "micro-droplet" technique to fill in very small defects for years. However, it was discontinued in the late twentieth century when the FDA placed a moratorium on

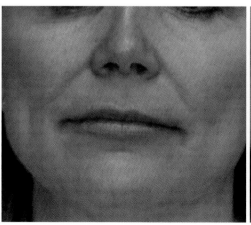
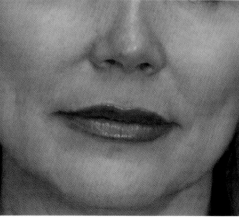

Fig. 79.12 Pre- and postprocedural photographs of the same patient in **Fig. 79.8** having had lip augmentation and filling of the ML folds with hyaluronic acid

its use as an injectable filler. Recently the FDA allowed its use in ophthalmology to treat retinal detachments. This product, AdatoSil 5000 is manufactured by Bausch and Lomb Surgical (Claremont, CA), and is 5,000 centistokes. Some clinicians are beginning to use this material as an off label use. Close follow-up will be necessary before the authors can recommend its use as a filler.

This section of the chapter is not meant to be an in-depth guide to facial fillers or the technique of application. Rather it is to serve as a general guideline for common usage applications for facial fillers available to the facial plastic surgeon.

References

1. Kusiak JF, Zins JE, Whitaker LA (1985) Early revascularization of membranous bone. Plast Reconstr Surg 76:510–514

2. Zins JE, Whitaker LA (1983) Membranous versus endochondral bone: Implications for craniofacial reconstruction. Plast Reconstr Surg 72(6):778–785

3. Dingman RO (1950) Use of iliac bone in the repair of facial and cranial defects. Plast Reconstr Surg 6:170–175

4. Romo T 3rd, Jablonski RD (1992) Nasal reconstruction using split calvarial grafts. Otolaryngol Head Neck Surg 107(5):622–630

5. Ortiz-Monasterio F, Olmedo A, Oscoy LO (1981) The use of cartilage grafts in primary aesthetic rhinoplasty. Plast Reconstr Surg 67(5):597–605

6. Gibson T, Davis WB (1958) The distortion of autogenous cartilage grafts: Its cause and prevention. Br J Plast Surg 10:257–274

7. Kridel RW, Konior RJ (1993) Irradiated cartilage grafts in the nose. A preliminary report. Arch Otolaryngol Head Neck Surg 119(1):24–31

8. Neuber F (1893) Fettransplantation. Chir Kongr Verhandl Deutsch Gesellsch Chir 22:66

9. Newman J, Burgmeister H, Shahar Y (1992) Facial lipotransplant surgery. Facial Plast Surg 8(3):140–148

10. Ersek RA (1991) Transplantation of purified autologous fat: A 3-year follow-up is disappointing. Plast Reconstr Surg 87(2):219–227

11. Glashofer M, Lawrence N (2006) Fat transplantation for treatment of the senescent face. Dermatol Ther 19(3):169–176

12. Strauch B, Baum T, Robbins N (2004) Treatment of human immunodeficiency virus-associated lipodystrophy with dermafat graft transfer to the malar area. Plast Reconstr Surg 113(1):363–370; discussion 371–372

13. Colic MM (1999) Lip and perioral enhancement by direct intramuscular fat autografting. Aesthetic Plast Surg 23(1):36–40

14. Davis RE, Guida RA, Cook TA (1995) Autologous free dermal fat graft. Reconstruction of facial contour defects. Arch Otolaryngol Head Neck Surg 121(1):95–100

15. Choe JM et al. (2001) Autologous, cadaveric and synthetic materials used in sling surgery: Comparative biomechanical analysis. Urology 58(3):482–486

16. Menon NG et al. (2003) Revascularization of human acellular dermis in full-thickness abdominal wall reconstruction in the rabbit model. Ann Plast Surg 50:523–527

17. Mass CS, Gnepp DR, Bumpous J (1993) Expanded polytetrafluoroethylene (Gor-Tex soft-tissue patch) in facial augmentation. Arch Otolaryngol Head Neck Surg 119:1008–1014

18. Godin MS, Waldman R, Johnson CM (1995) The use of expanded polytetrafluoroethylene (Gore-Tex) in rhinoplasty. A 6-year experience. Arch Otolaryngol Head Neck Surg 121:1131–1136

19. Lohuis PJ, Watts SJ, Vuyk HD (2001) Augmentation of the nasal dorsum using Gore-Tex: Intermediate results of a retrospective analysis of experience in 66 patients. Clin Otolaryngol Allied Sci 26(3):214–217

20. Mass CS, Merwin GE, Wilson J, Frey MD, Maves MD (1990) Comparison of biomaterials for facial bone augmentation. Arch Otolaryngol Head Neck Surg 116:551–556

21. Tang L, Eaton J (1995) Inflammatory responses to biomaterials. Am J Clin Pathol 103:466–471

22. Saleh HA, Lohuis PJ, Vuyk HD (2002) Bone resorption after alloplastic augmentation of the mandible. Clin Otolaryngol Allied Sci 27(2):129–132

23. Metzinger SE, McCollough EG, Campbell JP, Rousso DE (1999) Malar augmentation: A 5-year retrospective review of the silastic midfacial malar implant. Arch Otolaryngol Head Neck Surg 125(9):980–987

24. Silver WE (1992) Malar augmentation. Facial Plast Surg 8(3):133–139

25. Zeng Y, Wu W, Yu H, Yang J, Chen G (2002) Silicone implant in augmentation rhinoplasty. Ann Plast Surg 49:495–499

26. Beekhuis GJ (1967) Use of silicone-rubber in nasal reconstructive surgery. Arch Otolaryngol 86:88–91

27. Menderes A, Baytekin C, Topcu A, Yilmaz M, Barutcu A (2004) Craniofacial reconstruction with high-density porous polyethylene implants. J Craniofac Surg 15(5):719–724

28. Romo T 3rd, Sclafani AP, Jacono AA (2000) Nasal reconstruction using porous polyethylene implants. Facial Plastic Surg 16(1):55–61

29. Gross EJ, Hamilton MM, Ackermann K, Perkins SW (1999) Mersilene mesh chin augmentation: A 14-year experience. Arch Facial Plast Surg 1:183–189

30. McCollough EG, Horn DB, Weigel MT, Anderson JA (1990) Augmentation mentoplasty using Mersilene mesh. Arch Otolaryngol Head Neck Surg 116:1154–1158

31. Colton J, Beekhuis GJ (1992) Use of Mersilene mesh in nasal augmentation. Facial Plast Surg 8(3):149–156

32. Stucker F, Wong F, Shaw G (1992) Facial augmentation with rolled mesh material. Facial Plast Surg 8(3):183–187

Chapter 80

Botox: Its Use in Facial Lines and Wrinkles

Jerome S. Schwartz, Phillip C. Song, Andrew Blitzer, and William Binder

Core Messages

- Botulinum toxin injections of the facial muscles has been found over the past 2 decades to be safe and effective means of minimizing or eliminating facial lines and wrinkles.

Contents

Introduction

The recent interest in the use of botulinum neurotoxin (BoNT) for the treatment of hyperfunctional muscular disorders, dysautonomia, and headache is astonishing. Initial fears concerning the injection of a potentially lethal paralytic agent into a human being for therapeutic purposes have gradually been replaced by an optimistic eagerness to explore additional uses for this incredible toxin. Our current level of comfort with botulinum toxin therapy is demonstrated by the hundreds of new physicians who incorporate its use within the scope of their medical practices each year. Among the American public, Botox, the only FDA-approved type-A botulinum toxin available in the USA, has essentially become a common household name. While the 21st century may well mark the Golden Age for therapeutic botulinum toxin administration, physicians must strive to utilize sound technique and judicious practices when handling one of nature's most potent toxins.

This chapter will describe the historical perspectives, pharmacology, and clinical indications for botulinum toxin administration. The reader will gain insight into current practices, including diagnostic evaluation, toxin preparation, and techniques of administration based upon our experiences with over 1,000 patients within the past 20 years. A discussion of the common adverse effects and complications of BoNT as well as future considerations will be addressed.

Historical Perspective of Botulinum Toxin

The effects of botulinum toxin on the human nervous system were first described during the 18th and 19th centuries in Bavaria, where outbreaks of a specific disease pattern characterized by skeletal muscle and enteric tract paralysis, dry skin, lack of tear fluid and saliva, pupillary dilatation, and respiratory failure were recognized. Justinus Kerner, a medical officer and romantic poet, published two complete monographs in 1820 and 1822 detailing the symptomotology, time course, and clinical presentation in 280 patients who suffered from what was later termed *botulism* [1]. The term *botulism* was derived from the sausage *botulus (*meaning blood sausage in Greek*),* which was a common food product consumed in both Eastern and Western Europe. Kerner hypothesized that a substance, or toxin, that formed within spoiled *botulus* sausage must have been responsible for the outbreak of disease. Kerner later suggested the potential therapeutic use of botulinum toxin to treat hyperfunctional motor movements, such as chorea, and speculated on its use in disorders with hypersecretion [2].

In 1895, the Belgian scientist Emile Pierre van Ermengem, a professor of bacteriology and disciple of Koch, had correctly postulated the bacterial origin of the BoNT. He reported on 23 individuals who had become paralyzed following the consumption of spoiled ham. Extracts of the ham were fed to laboratory animals which resulted in a botulism-like paralysis, with only minute quantities required to cause mortality. From the infected ham, van Ermengem isolated the anaerobic bacterium, grew the organism in culture, and named it *Bacillus botulinus* [2]. The organism was later renamed *Clostridium botulinum.*

During the 1920s and 1930s, a rise in botulism correlated with the advent of the canning industry in the USA. Efforts by Drs. Herman Somner at the University of California, San Francisco and K.F. Meyer at the Hooper Foundation in San Francisco resulted in the isolation of novel strains of the organism and crude forms of BoNT. Techniques for reliably killing canned clostridial spores, including food salting, acidification, and heating were defined, and the California canning industry was saved.

Over the next few decades, the potential for botulinum toxin as a biological warfare agent was realized. Large quantities of crude toxin were easy to produce within a few days' time, and fear that foreign nations were capable of producing toxin in quantities sufficient to cause widespread casualties led to the development of the Army's Chemical Corps botulinum research laboratory at Fort Detrick. Concentration and crystallization techniques headed by Lammana, Duff, and Schantz in the mid-1940s resulted in the characterization of several of the toxin's seven known serotypes.

Clinical applications for BoNT were pioneered by Drachman [3] and Scott [4] in the 1970s. Following Drachman's successes using the toxin to paralyze the hind limb of chicks, Dr. Scott, in 1977, injected the extraocular muscles in human with BoNT to correct strabismus [2]. Botulinum toxin serotype A (BoNT-A) subsequently received its initial FDA approval in 1989 for the treatment of blepharospasm and strabismus. Recognizing its potential therapeutic benefits, researchers expanded the utility of BoNT to include a variety of hyperfunctional muscle disorders such as the dystonias (torticollis, spasmodic dysphonia, hemifacial spasm, oromandibular dystonia, and writer's cramp), spastic paresis following stroke, demyelinating disease, tremor and sphincteric hyperfunction of the enteric and urogenital tracts. In 1994, Drobic and Laskawi [5] extrapolated from Kerner's original observations that patients with botulism presented with decreased salivary and sweat gland function. Recognizing the toxin's effects at autonomic nerve terminals, they initiated the use of BoNT for the treatment of Frey syndrome (gustatory sweating), which paved the way toward treating palmar and axillary hyperhidrosis. Jean and Alistair Carruthers [6], and Blitzer, Brin et al. [7] are credited with recognizing the cosmetic use of BoNT in patients who noted decreased facial wrinkling following treatment for blepharospasm. Their initial studies focused upon re-establishing facial symmetry by targeting selective agonist-antagonist muscle groups of the face, adjusting brow height and flattening folds. Today, botulinum toxin is administered for a variety of functional and cosmetic facial disorders. Binder noted that botulinum toxin demonstrated benefit in treating migraine and tension-type headaches [7–10]. Anecdotal reports from patients receiving BoNT for glabellar lines with coexistent migraine or tension type headaches suggested an improvement in overall headache severity, duration, and frequency [11]. Several studies have confirmed these initial reports [12–14], and headache is currently an off-label indication for BoNT injection.

There are currently five formulations of BoNT-A (Botox, Dysport, Linurase, Xeomin, and Neuronox) approved for clinical use. Botox (Allergan, Inc., Irvine, CA) is the only BoNT-A toxin currently available in the USA and has been approved for the treatment of strabismus and blepharospasm (1989), cervical dystonia (torticollis) (2000), hyperfunctional glabellar lines (2002), and hyperhidrosis (2004). Myobloc (Solstice Neurosciences, Inc., South San Francisco, CA) was approved in 2000 for the treatment of cervical dystonia and remains the only BoNT-B toxin available in the USA.

Pharmacologic Basis

The bacterium *Clostridium botulinum* produces seven serologically distinct toxins that are potent neuroparalytic agents. These are designated A, B, C, D, E, F, and G [15, 16]. Although the various neurotoxins are antigenically distinct, they possess similar molecular weights and share a common subunit structure [16]. BoNT exerts its effect at the neuromuscular junction through the inhibition of acetylcholine release, resulting in paralysis. BoNT has no known effect on either the synthesis or storage of acetylcholine [17–19]. Nerve endings that are poisoned with the toxin can still be induced to release normal quanta of acetylcholine, although nonphysiologic techniques must be used.

The currently accepted mechanism of action of BoNT involves the toxin's enzymatic role as a zinc (Zn^{2+}) endopeptidase [17]. Das Gupta and Tepp [20] reported that proteolysis of one or more neuronal proteins most likely results in the intracellular lesion that inhibits neurotransmitter release. Located on the toxin's light chain is a *VAMP/synaptobrevin-2(VAMP/SYB-2)*-specific protease. It appears that presynaptic neurotransmitter release is significantly impaired following an ATP-dependent enzymatic cleavage of the neuronal docking protein, known as the VAMP/SYB-2 complex. Cleavage of the protein moieties interferes with the binding and fusion of a neurotransmitter-containing vesicle to the plasma membrane and therefore impedes exocytosis-mediated neurotransmitter release [21–23].

Measuring variations in muscle fiber diameter and using acetylcholinesterase staining as indices of denervation, Borodic and colleagues [24] showed that BoNT may diffuse up to 4.5 cm from the site of a single injection (i.e.,10 Botox U injected into rabbit longissimus dorsi). Because the size of the denervation field is largely determined by the dose of toxin and volume of injection, multiple point injections along the affected muscle rather than a single point injection might, therefore, contain the biologic effects of the toxin within the boundaries of the target muscle and reduce complications.

Using glycogen depletion, estimated by periodic acid-Schiff staining, of the anterior tibialis muscle of rat in response to repetitive, prolonged stimulation (3 mAmp at 20 HZ for 10 min) of the common peroneal, Sharri and Sanders [25] studied the effects of dose, volume, and site of injection. In normal controls, after 10 min of stimulation, glycogen depletion was most evident closest to the midbelly, which naturally contained the highest concentration of motor endplates. The area of glycogen-retained muscle fibers increased as the injection was given closer to the motor end plate band region. No quantifiable paralysis was measured when the same dose (0.2 Botox U) was given 1 cm inferior to the band. The area of paralysis increased with the dose and dilution (larger volume) up to 50 mm^2, the total cross-sectional area of the tibialis anterior muscle. Filippi and coworkers [26] found in a rat model that BoNT decreased the afferent discharge of muscle spindles. Therefore, the relief in dystonic muscle spasm could be, in part, due not only to a partial motor paralysis, but also to a decrease of the reflex muscular tone.

Studies to assess the long-term effects of exposure to toxin are still emerging. In experimental models, long-term exposure results in denervation atrophy. In one human study, long-term exposure reportedly resulted in fibrosis and atrophy in the orbicularis oculi muscles [27]. In another study, however, necrosis or inflammation were not observed [28]. Weakness or altered electromyographic changes in muscles distal to the site of injection have not been reported. There are detectable abnormalities, however, on single-fiber electromyography (EMG) [29–32]. It is not yet known how long these abnormalities persist or whether they have any clinical significance [33].

There is a paucity of data regarding use during pregnancy. In one report, of nine patients treated during the course of pregnancy (dose unspecified), one gave birth prematurely; "this was thought not to be related to the drug" [34]. Currently, the authors recommend not injecting patients who are pregnant or lactating.

Although the authors have treated certain patients with preexisting neuromuscular junction disorders, they recommend proceeding with caution when treating patients with myasthenia gravis, Eaton-Lambert syndrome, and motor neuron disease, particularly when large doses are required, such as in the treatment of cervical dystonia. The actual amount of toxin entering the systemic circulation after injection is thought to be minute; however, and this theoretic concern should be balanced against the severity of the hyperkinetic symptoms. Antibody formation has occasionally been found in some patients receiving large doses for the management of torticollis. These antibodies appear to destroy the toxin, preventing adequate responses despite large doses. Most antibody tests involve a biologic assay; however, there has been a report of an enzyme-linked immunosorbent assay, which should yield quantifiable data regarding antibody production to toxin [35].

Storage and Reconstitution of Botulinum Toxin

There are currently five formulations of BoNT-A (Botox, Dysport, Linurase, Xeomin, and Neuronox) and one type B complex (Myobloc) approved for clinical use. Only Botox and Myobloc are currently available in the USA for injection. These products have different dosing, safety, and efficacy characteristics and familiarity with each complex is essential prior to administration. There are no well-established methodologies to calculate equivalent doses [36].

Lyophilized BoNT-A (Botox, Allergan, Inc., Irvine, CA) is the only type A toxin currently available in the USA. Unreconstituted Botox may be stored in a refrigerator at 2–8ºC for up to 24 months. Each vial contains 100 U of vacuum-dried, purified BoNT-A. While the package insert recommends reconstitution with preservative free saline, we have found an equal efficacy and increased patient comfort when the toxin is reconstituted with 0.9% benzyl alcohol preserved saline. Recommendations for reconstitution and storage of Botox are shown in Table 80.1. The authors typically dilute each vial with either, 2 or 4 ml of saline to prepare a 50 U/mL or 25 U/mL (5.0 or 2.5 U per 0.1 mL) stock, respectively. Further dilutions are performed by adding additional saline, keeping a uniform volume of 0.1 mL.

BoNT-B (Myobloc, Solstice Neurosciences, Inc., South San Francisco, CA) is available in 2,500 U and 5,000 U/mL vials prediluted with 0.05% human serum albumin. Although less commonly used for cosmetic therapy, it serves an important role in the treatment of patients who may have developed resistance to Botox. In a study comparing the effects of BoNT-B vs. BoNT-A injections for patients with adductor SD, Blitzer [37] reported a conversion ratio of 52:1 U of BoNT-B: BoNT-A. This dose adjustment has been used for cosmetic and other hyperfunctional muscle disorders of the head and neck with good overall results.

Table 80.1 Recommendations for storage and reconstitution of Botox *

Parameter	Recommendation
Diluent	Preserved 0.9% saline
	Nonpreserved 0.9% saline*
Concentration	2.5 or 5 U/0.1 ml or similar concentration to deliver required dose
Storage	
Before reconstitution	Between 2–8ºC for up to 24 months
After reconstitution	4 h at 2–8ºC
	Up to 6 weeks at 4ºC

Preprocedural Evaluation

The evaluation begins with a careful medical history, paying particular attention to prior cosmetic surgery, trauma, medications, allergies and propensity to bleeding, and scarring. The patient's face is closely observed for areas of maximal muscle pull. Photographs are useful for documentation and postprocedural comparison, and should be taken with the face at rest and with activity demonstrating the undesirable lines. The patient is asked to perform tasks such as frowning, squinting, and raising the eyebrows, which will produce the action-induced hyperkinetic facial lines of the forehead, glabella, and periorbital region. In addition, having the patient smile, grimace, and pucker may reveal mid- and lower facial wrinkling in the perioral, mental, and platysmal regions. With careful analysis of the facial lines, the physician should distinguish those which are functional (dynamic wrinkles amenable to BoNT therapy) from those which are sequelae of actinic damage or aging (static wrinkles). Deep lines within the forehead or midface may require a combination of BoNT and a dermal filler agent for an optimal cosmetic outcome.

The patient's face is then marked in the regions which demonstrate maximal muscle pull. It should be realized that locations of hyperfunctional lines do not necessarily correlate with the locations of the muscle bellies, rather, they demonstrate the pleating effect of the muscles on the overlying skin. Injecting toxin into the hyperfunctional lines without addressing the adjacent muscle will result in a suboptimal effect. The area to be injected may be iced or treated with EMLA or compounded "BLT" (Benzocine, Lidocaine, & Tetracaine) cream to minimize the discomfort associated with the injections.

Despite the paucity of data, patients who are pregnant or lactating should not be injected as the effects on the fetus or newborn remain unknown. Although we have treated selected patients with neuromuscular disorders, caution is advised when injecting patients with diseases such as myasthenia gravis, Eaton-Lambert myasthenia, or motor-neuron disorders. Amin-

oglycoside antibiotics may potentiate the effect of a given dose of BoNT; therefore, we do not recommend injections in patients receiving aminoglycoside therapy [44].

Treatment of the Upper Face

Glabellar Rhytids

The primary muscles responsible for creating vertical glabellar wrinkling are the corrugator supercilii, the procerus, and the depressor supercilii. Fibers from the medial orbicularis oculi and frontalis muscles may interdigitate in this region and contribute as well. The corrugator muscles act to depress and medialize the medial brow, and in doing so, they create vertical skin pleats in the interbrow region. The physician must recognize that the lines do not correlate anatomically to the corrugator muscle belly, and that toxin injections directly into the lines may result in suboptimal denervation and effect. This is particularly evident when injecting the procerus muscle. We usually use a higher location to inject the muscle belly than where the transverse wrinkle is present over the upper portion of the nose. Taking into account the complexity of muscular activity in this region as well as the effect of muscle pull on the medial

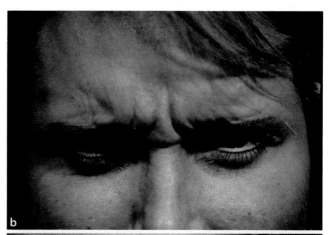

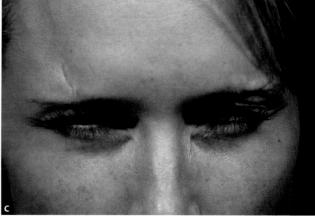

Fig. 80.1 a Injection sites for glabellar lines. Typically between 10–25 units of BTX-A are injected over 5 injection sites over the glabella region. **b** Patient with glabellar lines caused by significant corrugator muscle contraction. **c** The same patient after BTX-A injection

brow is of paramount significance when injecting BoNT into the glabella.

The glabellar injections primarily manage the hyperactivity of the corrugator and procerus muscles. Among members of the Botox Consensus group [41], most recommended the injection of between 5 and 7 points, with men often requiring more sites than women. Some members advocated dividing the total required dose by region: 20% procerus, each corrugator 15%, each superomedial orbicularis 15%, and each of two orbicularis sites above the midpupillary line10%. We typically inject each corrugator with 2.5U/0.1 ml at two distinct sites and the procerus with 2.5–5 U/0.1 ml at one site. We add additional toxin to the superomedial orbicularis depending upon the desired effect upon the medial brow (Fig. 80.1).

The muscle bellies lie deep to the subcutaneous tissue, and hence the injections should be placed deep to the hypodermis. After the patient is asked to wrinkle the glabella, the corrugator muscles may be pinched between the thumb and index finger. The needle is directed away from the supraorbital rim and the muscle belly is impaled (Fig. 80.2). Injections should remain at least 1 cm above the supraorbital rim, and the lateral injection should not lie further laterally than the midpupillary line to avoid lateral brow ptosis.

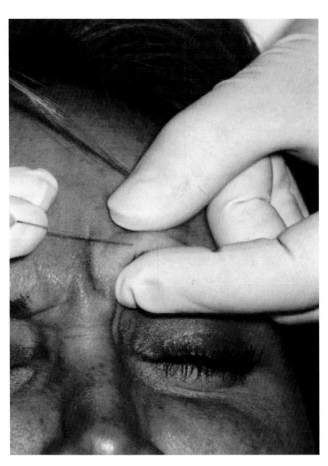

Fig. 80.2 The corrugator muscle may be pinched between the thumb and index finger. The needle is directed away from the supraorbital rim and the muscle belly is impaled

Horizontal Forehead Lines

The broad, fan-shaped frontalis muscles contract vertically, resulting in brow elevation as well as horizontal forehead pleating. BoNT-A injections across the forehead help to alleviate horizontal forehead lines, and when properly executed should preserve some element of facial animation. The goal of injection is to weaken, not paralyze the frontalis muscle completely. We have found that most patients will have significant reduction in the number and degree of horizontal lines following BoNT-A injections to the frontalis muscle belly. Treatments are individualized according to the location and extent of rhytid formation, as individual variability is common, precluding a cookbook approach to injection.

We have found that forehead injections of the glabellar and frontalis regions should span an area demarcated by V-shape, with its apex located at the nasal root (Fig. 80.3). Injections are generally kept at least 1 cm above the supraorbital rim to avoid brow ptosis, lid levator ptosis, and lack of expressivity. It is also important to realize that only the lower 2 cm of frontalis muscle is primarily responsible for brow elevation. If injections are applied lateral to the midpupillary line, they should be placed superiorly to avoid lateral brow ptosis and allow for residual lateral forehead expression (Fig. 80.4). We have found that between 6 and 12 injection sites substantially reduces forehead lines, with male patients often requiring more sites than female patients. Each site should lie at least 1 to 1.5 cm from an adjacent injection site. We generally inject 2.5 units per 0.1 ml per injection site with overall doses ranging from 10 to 30 units (Fig. 80.3). Should the patient present with a particularly hyperactive re-

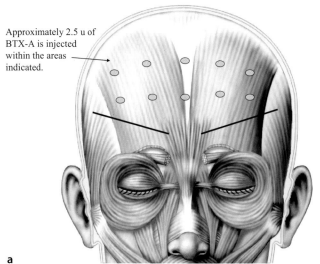

Approximately 2.5 u of BTX-A is injected within the areas indicated.

a

Fig. 80.3 a The area of the forehead generally treated to reduce the hyperfunctional lines caused by frontalis muscular contraction. The dosage and number of injections vary depending on the number of forehead lines. This can range between 12.5 and 40 units and 6 to 12 or more injection sites. BTX-A is usually not injected below an oblique line drawn from the medial brow to a point at least 1 cm. above the lateral aspect of the brow. **b,c** *see next page*

gion just above the lateral brow, the region may be injected with caution, and should brow ptosis occur, a small injection to the superolateral orbicularis oculi (brow depressor) may help stabilize the brow's position.

Brow Adjustment

In order to appreciate the effects of BoNT-A on brow position, one must understand the dynamic muscular forces acting upon the brow. Final brow position is determined by an interaction between the primary brow elevator (frontalis muscle), brow depressors [medial orbicularis oculi (depressor supercilii), procerus, and superolateral orbicularis oculi], and brow medializer (corrugator supercilii). Treating vertical glabellar lines through injections to the corrugator and procerus muscles results in medial brow elevation—known as "the Botox brow lift." This effect results from unopposed medial frontalis activity with an upward pull on the brow. Similarly, medial forehead injections to the frontalis may result in lateral brow elevation, especially if Crow's feet (lateral orbicularis oculi) injections are performed. These "Spock eyes" result from unopposed lateral frontalis upward pull on the brow. Huang and coworkers [37] found that BoNT-A injections to both the lateral infrabrow region and corrugator supercilii resulted in mean brow elevations at rest of 1.9 mm (right) and 3.1 mm (left). In some cases, brow elevation is a wanted result, as in the female patient who desires a high-arched brow appearance. Among most male patients brow elevation is an undesired outcome and the clinician should be aware of techniques to minimize or alter these effects.

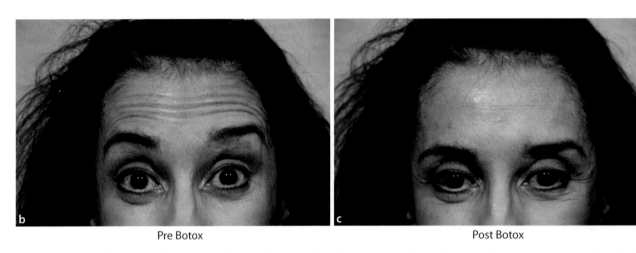

Pre Botox   Post Botox

Fig. 80.3 (*continued*) **b** Patient with horizontal forehead lines caused by significant frontalis muscle contraction, **c** the same patient 3 weeks after BTX-A

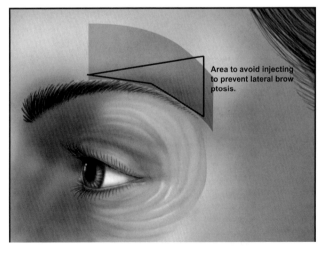

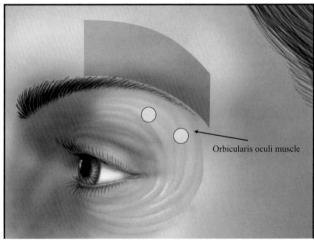

Fig. 80.4 The *shaded area* above the eyebrow represents an area from the mid-pupillary line extending laterally to a point approximately 1–1.5 cm in vertical height over the lateral most portion of the eyebrow. This area should avoid injection to prevent lateral brow ptosis. However, in patients with no tendency or redundancy of suprabrow skin this are may be injected to prevent excess elevation of the brow ("Spock Look")

Fig. 80.5 Injecting the superior lateral aspect of the orbicularis oculi muscle with BTX-A (2.5–5 U) weakens the depressor effect of the orbicularis oculi muscle in this area and reduces the amount of brow ptosis if it is necessary to inject the infero-lateral portion of the frontalis muscle

80

The medial brow can often be elevated by injecting the depressor supercilii (medial orbicularis oculi/procerus overlap) or medial corrugator with a small amount (1–2.5 U/0.1 ml injection) of toxin. The lateral brow can be raised with a similar dose applied to the superolateral orbicularis oculi muscle at the junction of the orbital rim and temporal line (Fig. 80.5). The medial brow may be depressed by injecting the frontalis muscle medial to the midpupillary line and superior to the corrugator muscle belly. Laterally, the brow may be depressed by injecting the lateral frontalis muscle with a small dose of BoNT-A; however, this may result in complete loss of forehead expression if the forehead is overweakened laterally and medially (Fig. 80.4). The techniques for brow positioning may also be applied to eyebrow asymmetries arising from facial nerve trauma, congenital anomaly, or habitual, maladaptive behavior.

Treatment of the Midface

Crow's Feet

Muscle contraction of the lateral orbicularis oculi muscle results in a radial pattern of lateral periorbital lines, most notable upon forceful smiling. This muscle functions in eye closure, blinking, and squinting. In this region of the face, the musculature lies just deep to the dermis, which accounts for the significant degree of skin pleating. The lateral periorbital region often demonstrates wrinkling of various etiologies. The clinician should recognize the fine rhytids associated with either aging or photodamage that remain and are present at rest, and differentiate those from hyperfunctional muscle lines. The former may be better treated with fillers, chemical peeling, or laser resurfacing and not BoNT-A whereas the latter will naturally respond well to muscle weakening.

Crow's feet region injections are typically performed at a subdermal or intradermal depth. The first injection site is placed lateral to the lateral canthus at a distance of at least 1 cm. The patient is asked to squint, and the regions of hyperactivity are noted. We generally mark additional sites superiorly and inferiorly along a vertical line through the lateral canthus. When injecting the lateral orbicularis oculi muscle the needle should be directed away from the globe to prevent inadvertent intraorbital diffusion with a resultant lateral rectus palsy, diplopia, epiphora, or mild ectropion. Each injection should result in a small bleb, which may be massaged away from the globe radially. We typically inject 3 sites on each side with doses of 2.5–5 U per 0.1 ml

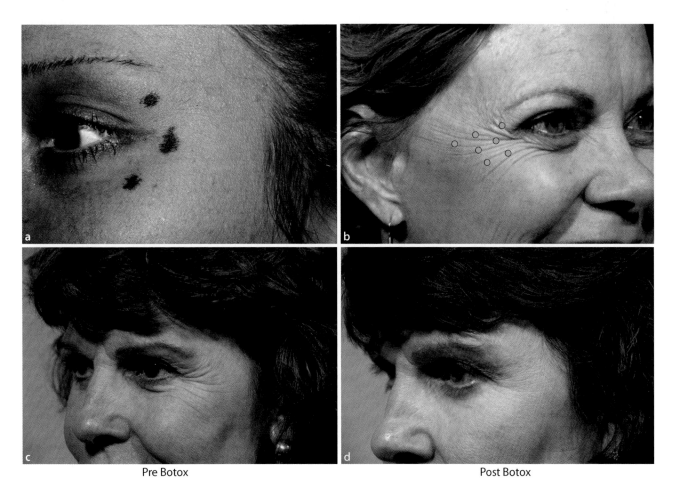

Pre Botox   Post Botox

Fig. 80.6 **a** Typical sites of injection for the lateral orbital lines or crow's feet. Between 5 and 10 units of BTX-A are injected over 3 injection sites per side for the crow's feet. **b** Additional sites are added if the lines extend laterally. **c** Patient with visible crow's feet prior to BTX-A injection. **d** The same patient 2 weeks after BTX-A injection. **e,f** *see next page*

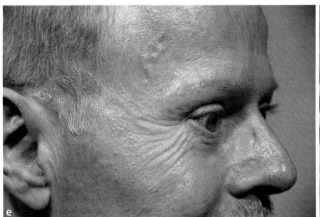 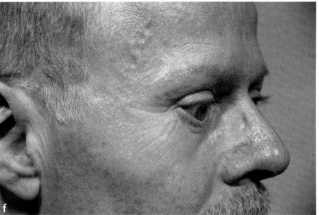

Fig. 80.6 (*continued*) **e** Patient with noticeable lateral orbital lines or crow's feet. **f** The same patient 3 weeks after BTX-A treatment

injection or 7.5–15 U per side. If the lines continue out laterally we will add injection sites to the primary treatment regimen and inject the lateral crow's feet lines as far as they continue to extend into the temporal area (Fig. 80.6a–f).

Nasal Scrunch and Nasal Flare

Nasal scrunch or "bunny lines" originate at the lateral nasal dorsum and radiate laterally toward the nasofacial groove (Fig. 80.7c). They result from contraction of the transverse portion of the nasalis muscle. The muscle originates from the maxilla and inserts upon the nasal dorsum, often interdigitating with the inferior fibers of the procerus muscle. In addition, a transverse nasal line may be evident, which results from procerus muscle contraction. Chemodenervation of the nasalis and procerus will often soften nasal scrunch and transverse nasal lines, respectively.

The midface should be observed at rest while the patient performs a facial scrunch maneuver. Nasal scrunch lines are treated with a single injection at the nasofacial groove or lateral nasal wall at least 1 cm inferior to the medial canthus (Figs. 80.7a, b) A small, superficial dose of 1–2.5 U per 0.1 ml on each side is usually adequate. A single 2.5 U per 0.1 ml midline injection at the nasal dorsum will address any transverse nasal line (Figs. 80.7c, d).

Occasionally, patients will complain of undesirable nasal alar flaring. Flaring results from contraction of the alar portion of the nasalis muscle. The Carruthers have described a technique to weaken the nasal flare using BoNT-A. A single 5-U injection is directed to the nasal alar rim bilaterally. Smaller injection volumes allow for an excellent result with minimal risk of toxin diffusion to the levator muscles of the upper lip.

Narrowed Palpebral Fissure

The orbicularis oculi muscle surrounds both the bony orbit and tarsal plates conferring sphincteric closure and palpebral aper-

ture narrowing during contraction. Hypertrophy of the pretarsal division of the orbicularis oculi may give the appearance of a narrowed palpebral fissure as well as fine pretarsal rhytids during squinting. Asian patients sometimes desire a more round-eyed or "Western" appearance yet may be hesitant to proceed with surgical correction. BoNT-A can be used to improve eyelid contouring and sculpting by widening the palpebral aperture nonsurgically.

The pretarsal muscle may be infiltrated beneath the ciliary lash line bilaterally. Injections should be performed either intra- or subdermally as the muscle lies superficially in this region. Patients to be considered for this treatment should have normal lid laxity judged by snap test, and patients who have undergone prior subciliary blepharoplasty or lid surface peeling should be approached with extreme caution. In a study of 15 female patients, Flynn and coworkers [39] injected 2 U of Botox, 3 mm inferior to the pretarsal orbicularis within each lower lid. They noted that 86% of patients demonstrated a 1.9-mm increase in palpebral fissure height at rest, and a 2.9-mm increase with smiling. We have found that a single pretarsal injection of 1.25–2.5 U per side also helps to smoothen the appearance of pretarsal rhytids.

Treatment of the Lower Face and Neck

Perioral Lip Rhytids

"Smoker's" or "lipstick" lines are circumoral lines which radiate outward from the lips and are most obvious during puckering maneuvers. They result from skin pleating secondary to orbicularis oris contraction. The orbicularis oris is a sphincteric muscle which encircles the mouth and allows for lip closure and puckering. It extends from the inferior nasofacial groove superiorly to the supramental crease, lying between the skin and mucous membrane of the oral cavity. Perioral rhytids have also been associated with heredity, photodamage, whistling, and playing musical instruments which require embouchure [40]. Although

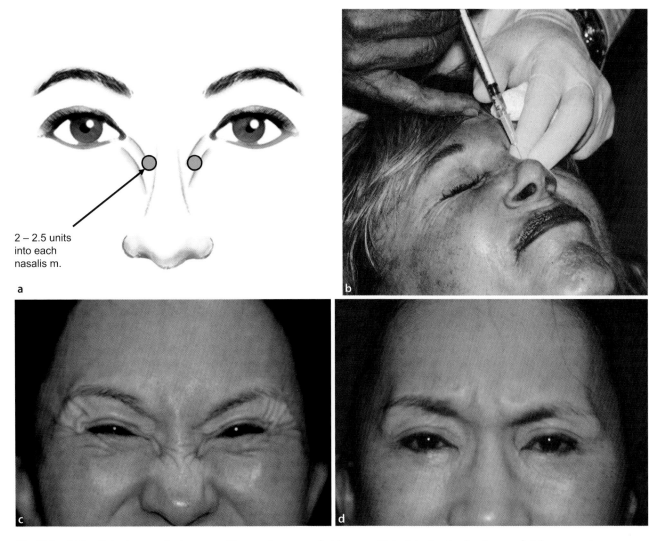

2 – 2.5 units
into each
nasalis m.

Fig. 80.7 **a,b** Nasalis best approached over nasal bones, above naso-facial groove. Note: Injection too low in naso-facial groove can cause upper lip ptosis; or too lateral can cause lower eyelid weakness. **c** Patient with bunny lines caused by significant nasalis muscle contraction. **d** The same patient 3 weeks after BTX-A injection

primarily a disorder of muscle contractility, perioral rhytids are difficult to treat with chemodenervation alone. Unlike many of the aesthetic facial muscles, the orbicularis oris muscle plays a crucial functional role in maintaining oral competency. Over-weakening of the orbicularis with BoNT-A may result in deficits in lip proprioception, dysarthria, dysphagia, and drooling. As such, we have found that a combination regimen of small, superficial doses of BoNT-A and injectable dermal filler materials, with or without laser resurfacing, gives the best cosmetic and functional outcome in this area.

Treatment of the perioral area remains highly individualized. Among members of the Botox Consensus Group, the number of perioral injection sites varied from 2 to 11, included either upper lip alone or both lips, and target either the orbicularis oris, depressor anguli oris (DAO), or mentalis muscles [41]. Our injection technique utilizes microdoses to produce a microparesis

of the superficial fibers of the orbicularis oris. The Carruthers [40] describe an injection regimen using a total of 6 U of toxin diluted into 0.24 ml (2.5 U/0.1 ml), distributed among 8 injection sites. Each site receives 0.75 U (0.03 ml) per injection. Our experience has shown that 4–6 injection sites using 1 U BoNT-A per injection is effective (Fig. 80.8). Patients are educated that chemodenervation alone will not get rid of these lines and are offered concomitant filler injections (i.e., hyaluronic acid gel or collagen) to optimize the aesthetic effect.

Mouth Frowning

The depressor anguli oris (DAO) originates from the inferior border of the mandibular body and inserts upon the subcutaneous aponeurosis of the oral commissure region. Contraction of

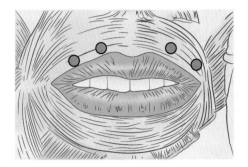

Fig. 80.8 Perioral lip lines. Inject 1–2 units of Botox per site up to 4 sites, symmetrically at the vermillion border. Do not inject into the philtrum or cupid's bow and avoid the lateral quarter and corners of the mouth

the DAO tends to pull the oral commissure inferiorly, imparting an expression of dissatisfaction or bitterness. In addition, DAO contraction may contribute to the production of melolabial "Marionette" lines. These lines extend from the oral commissure inferiorly to the lateral mentum. Superomedially the DAO overlaps with the depressor labii inferioris, and injections in this region may impair lower lip mobility. The DAO may be safely injected 1 cm above its mandibular origin to reduce the mouth frown. This corresponds to a location 7 mm lateral to the commissure and 7–10 mm inferior [42]. A single dose of 2.5–5 U per side usually suffices to weaken, not paralyze the muscle and improve the cosmetic appearance of the commissure and reduce prominent melolabial lines.

Chin Wrinkling and Mental Crease

Excessive chin wrinkling may be caused by a loss of subcutaneous fat and dermal connective tissue. The appearance may resemble the texture of an orange peel, "peau d' orange," due to the visibility of the underlying mentalis and depressor labii inferioris musculature (Fig. 80.9). Weakening, not paralyzing, the mentalis muscle near its mandibular attachment with BoNT-A helps to soften the coarse wrinkling. We inject the right and left divisions of the mentalis muscle with 2.5–5 U BoNT-A per 0.1 ml injection. The needle should target the lower one-half of the mentalis muscle, just lateral to the chin prominence (Fig. 80.10). The patient should be asked to wrinkle the chin, and audible motor unit potentials should confirm the proper location. Injecting too far superiorly should be avoided, as accidental chemodenervation of the depressor labii inferioris and orbicularis oris may result in oral incompetence and drooling. The toxin may be massaged by the physician in a side-to-side direction to augment the regional distribution. The use of soft tissue augmentation, such as collagen or hyaluronic acid-based filler materials, significantly adds to the contouring effect of chemodenervation. In most cases, BTX-A is all that is required for the effects of the hyperfunctioning mentalis muscle

(Fig. 80.11). Added effects of skin breakdown may require a combined modality regimen of augmentation and botulinum toxin to afford the best aesthetic result.

A prominent mental crease or furrow lying just superior to the mentum may be improved with BoNT-A chemodenervation. Often, a hypertrophic mentalis muscle pad is present along the midline of the chin. By denervating some of the muscle and inducing a moderate atrophy, the clinician may nonsurgically reduce the prominence of the mental crease and establish a more pleasing lower facial contour. Either a single midline dose of 10 U (5 U per 0.1 ml) or bilateral paramedian 5 U injections to the mentalis muscle, as described above, generally suffices. Injections must be kept below the half-way point from the inferior mentum to the vermillion border to avoid oral incompetence.

Platysmal Bands

Prominent platysmal bands may be softened with BoNT chemodenervation. These bands typically are arranged in vertical ridges from the mentum inferiorly to the clavicles. As part of rhytidectomy, platysmal plication or imbrication procedures are often necessary to eliminate the redundant anterior neck bands and turkey gobbler deformity. Chemodenervation may provide an alternative to surgery in younger and more selective patients with sufficient elasticity to the neck muscles.

The platysmal bands may be marked in both horizontal and vertical directions to facilitate the injections. Usually 3–4 injection sites along the platysmal band is sufficient to produce the desired outcome. Injection is performed with a hollow-bore, 1.5-inch, 27-gauge, Teflon-coated monopolar EMG needle. The

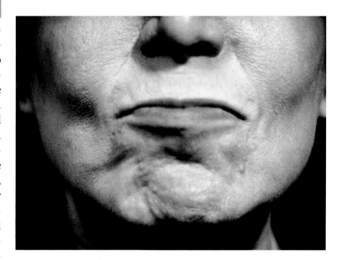

Fig. 80.9 The "Popply chin" is due to a hyperfunctional mentalis muscle causing excessive chin wrinkling. This is often secondary to labial incompetence with malocclusion or microgenia, often seen after mentoplasty and also caused by dermal atrophy at site of origin of mentalis muscle

80

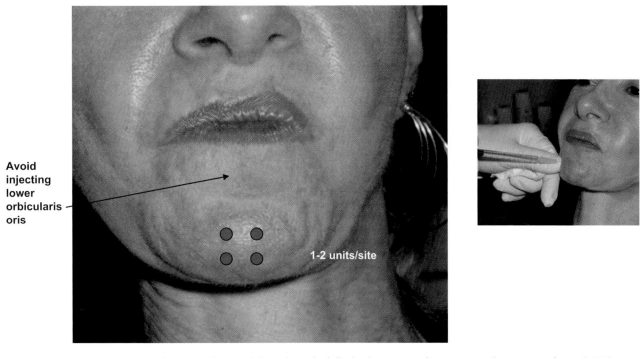

Avoid
injecting
lower
orbicularis
oris

1-2 units/site

Fig. 80.10 Inject 1–2 units into each site, evenly spaced throughout the hillocks. (maximum of 5–10 units and maximum of 6 sites). Make sure injection sites are medial

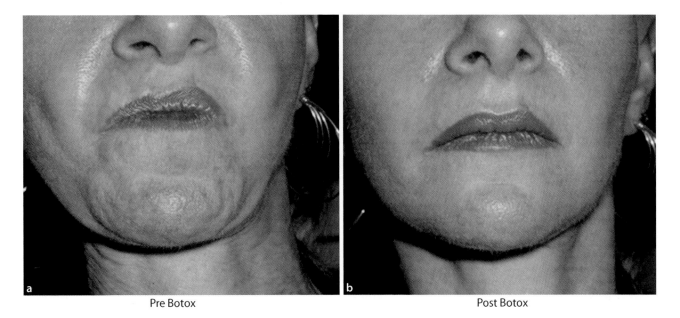

Pre Botox   Post Botox

Fig. 80.11 **a** Patient with hypermentalis muscle function causing the "peau d'orange" appearance to the chin area. **b** The same patient after BTX-A injection to the mentalis muscle

patient can activate the platysma by lowering the lower lip. The needle is inserted through the skin at the anterior edge of the band and advanced along the length of the band (Figs. 80.12, 13). Once the muscle belly has been identified (via EMG motor unit signal), the toxin may be delivered as the needle is withdrawn. We injected each site with 2.5–5 U/0.1 ml or approximately 7.5–20 U per side [43].

Postprocedural Care

The postprocedural period is characterized by a gradual onset of muscle weakness with maximal response at approximately 2 weeks. For the first 48 hr, the patients are instructed not to massage the facial muscles, which could inadvertently spread the free toxin to adjacent muscles. Intradermal blebs, itching, small ecchymoses, and mild erythema may be noted during the first few days, and generally resolve without further sequelae. Patients are instructed to return to the office after 2–3 weeks to re-evaluate the effect of the toxin. Additional photographs

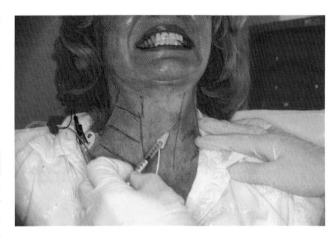

Fig. 80.12 Neck bands develop perpendicular to the pull of the platysma muscle. Edges become accentuated with age-related loss of subcutaneous fat A Teflon-coated monopolar EMG needle is used to guide the needle through the width of the muscle. The toxin is injected on withdrawal of the needle

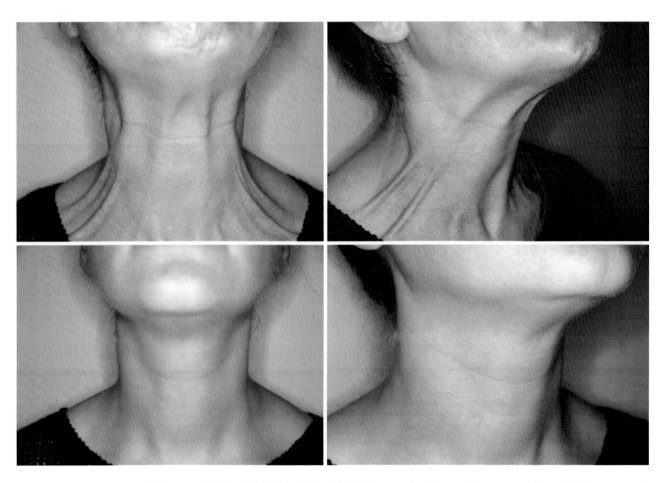

Fig. 80.13 BTX-A injection of platysma. The *above* "Before" and *below* "After" photographs illustrate the treatment effect of BTX on a patient's platysma bands 2 weeks after injection

80

may be taken at this time, and both the patient and physician may rate the degree of muscle hyperfunction on a 0- to 3-point scale [44].

Should the hyperfunctional lines remain bothersome to the patient, additional toxin may be administered. The dosage and location of the injections are determined by the region and degree of persistent hyperactivity present. An appropriate effect is considered when the hyperfunctional lines have disappeared, and a smooth, symmetric contour has been achieved. The patients are instructed to return when the facial lines have once again become prominent, usually between 3 to 6 months. Interestingly, in some patients who have been treated multiple times, the BoNT effect appears to last for longer periods with successive injections. We believe these patients may have become conditioned to the muscular disuse, whereby the patient's behavioral modification allows them to avoid wrinkling of the skin.

Adverse Effects of Botulinum Toxin

Adverse effects are often mild or transient, and can usually be minimized through proper injection technique. The most significant adverse effects involve sequelae of weakening or paralyzing muscles at or near the injection site. Most local complications are cosmetic in nature; however, inactivation of periorbital muscles when treating the glabella and forehead may result in visual disturbances. Adverse effects reported during the treatment of the upper and midface include: blepharoptosis, brow ptosis, diplopia, and muscle weakness at the site of injection [45]. Various minor sequelae associated with needle injections are also discussed.

Eyelid Ptosis (Blepharoptosis)

Although relatively few occurrences of eyelid ptosis have been reported the physician should be aware of this potential complication when injecting the corrugator muscles. Eyelid ptosis may occur when BoNT extravasates through the superior aspect of the orbital septum, causing paralysis of the levator palpebrae superioris muscle. The risk increases if injections are placed at or under the middle of the eyebrows in the vicinity of the mid-pupillary line [46]. Caution is advised in elderly patients where the orbital septal thickness may be reduced. The onset of ptosis may occur between 2 and 10 days following injection and persist for up to 2–4 weeks. Proper injection technique, including the use of small injection volumes, maintaining digital pressure at the superior orbital rim during injection, and placing injections at least 1 cm above the supraorbital rim at the mid-pupillary line significantly reduce the risk of ptosis [47]. Treatment involves the use of mydriatic eye drops (i.e., 2.5% phenylephrine hydrochloride) three times daily until symptoms resolve [48].

Brow Ptosis

Transient brow ptosis has been reported following treatment of forehead wrinkles with BoNT-A. This complication may arise secondary to inferolateral frontalis muscle weakness (lateral brow ptosis) or supraorbital frontalis weakness (middle brow ptosis). As the frontalis muscle contributes to brow elevation, weakening of this muscle can result in brow droop. Proper injection technique is essential to avoiding brow ptosis. BoNT-A injections should be performed at least 2 cm above the supraorbital rim, and up to 4 cm in patients with low set brows. Not rendering the frontalis muscle completely immobile but weakened can achieve a comparable goal while preserving some forehead movement. Ptosis correction involves injecting BoNT to either the ipsilateral superolateral orbicularis oculi muscle (lateral depressor) or corrugator and superomedial orbicularis oculi muscles (medial depressors) depending upon the presentation.

Diplopia

Diplopia is a disabling but fortunately rare complication which can be avoided through cautious BONT-A infiltration. Double vision may occur from inadvertent extravasation of toxin beyond the orbital septum to the lateral rectus muscle within the orbit. Most cases have occurred during treatment of the orbicularis oculi muscle with BoNT-A. The orbicularis oculi muscle surrounds the palpebral fissure circumferentially, and extends beyond the orbital rim just deep to the subcutaneous tissue. Diplopia may be prevented by injecting just below the epidermis, 1 cm outside the orbital rim or 1.5 cm lateral to the lateral canthus. The needle should be directed away from the orbit to prevent extravasation of the toxin toward the globe. Should diplopia arise, immediate referral to an ophthalmologist is recommended.

Minor Sequelae

Minor sequelae that can occur secondary to BONT-A injection at any site include: pain, edema, erythema, ecchymosis, and short-term hypoesthesia. The pain, edema, and erythema associated with an intramuscular injection may be reduced by applying ice to the face following injections. Ecchymosis can be minimized by having the patient avoid aspirin, nonsteroidal anti-inflammatory agents, and vitamin E for 7 days prior to injection. Careful attention to small subcutaneous vessels or palpation of larger vessels can help avoid ecchymosis and inadvertent intravascular injection. Pain associated with injections can be minimized by infusing slowly with a 30- or 32-gauge needle directly into the muscle belly avoiding the periosteum.

Conclusions

Botulinum toxin chemodenervation provides the cosmetic surgeon with an alternative technique with which to treat a variety of hyperfunctional muscle disorders of the face and neck. BoNT therapy may be initiated as monotherapy, or utilized in conjunction with alternative cosmetic procedures such as chemical peels, laser resurfacing, or facial cosmetic surgical procedures. Once feared for the devastating harm it inflicted on many unfortunate individuals, botulinum toxin has once again surfaced into the public's eye. Through careful technique and judicial use of the toxin, many patients are enjoying an improvement their facial cosmesis without the risks associated with more complicated surgical procedures. Botulinum toxin therapy remains an important adjunct in the field of facial aesthetics.

References

1. Erbguth FJ, Naumann M (1999) Historical aspects of botulinum toxin: Justinus Kerner (1786–1862) and the "sausage poison". Neurology 53:1850–1853

2. Scott AB (2004) Development of botulinum toxin therapy. Dermatol Clin 22:131–133

3. Drachman DB (1971) Neuropoisons. In: Simpson LL (ed) Plenum Press, New York, pp 315–339

4. Scott AB (1981) Botulinum toxin injection of eye muscles to correct strabismus. Trans Am Opthalmol Soc 79:734–770

5. Drobik C, Laskawi R (1994) Frey-Syndrom: Behandlung mit botulinum-toxin. HNO Aktuell 2:142–144

6. Carruthers JD, Carruthers A (1992) Treatment of glabellar frown lines with C. botulinum-A exotoxin. J Dermatol Surg Oncol 18:17–21

7. Blitzer A, Brin MF, Keen MS, Aviv JS (1993) Botulinum toxin for the treatment of hyperfunctional lines of the face. Arch Otolaryngol Head Neck Surg 119:1018–1023

8. Binder W (1994) Method for reduction of migraine headache pain. US Patent 5,714,468, 3 Feb 1998

9. Binder W, Brin M, Blitzer A, Schoenrock L (2000) Botulinum toxin type A (BOTOX) for treatment of migraine headaches: An open-label study. Otolaryngol Head Neck Surg 123:669–676

10. Binder W, Brin M, Blitzer A, Pogoda J (2001) Botulinum toxin type A (BOTOX) for treatment of migraine headaches. Semin Cutan Med Surg 20:93–100

11. Carruthers A (1999) Improvement of tension-type headache when treating wrinkles with botulinum toxin A injections. Headache 39:662–665

12. Blumenfeld A (2003) Botulinum toxin type A as an effective prophylactic treatment in primary headache disorders. Headache 43:853–860

13. Blumenfeld A (2002) Botulinum toxin type A (BOTOX) as an effective prophylactic treatment in headache. Cephalalgia 22(Suppl 1):20

14. Binder WJ, Brin MF, Blitzer A, et al. (2000) Botulinum toxin type A (BOTOX) for treatment of migraine headaches: An open label study. Otolaryngol Head Neck Surg 123:669–676

15. Simpson LL (1984) The binding fragment from tetanus toxin antagonizes the neuromuscular blocking actions of botulinum toxin. J Pharmacol Exp Ther 229:182–187

16. Simpson LL, DasGupta BR (1983) Botulinum neurotoxin type E: Studies on mechanism of action and on structure-activity relationships. J Pharmacol Exp Ther 224:135–140

17. Shaari CM, Sanders I (1994) Assessment of the biological activity of botulinum toxin. In: Jankovic J, Hallet M (eds) Therapy with botulinum toxin. Marcel Dekker, New York, pp 159–170

18. Gundersen CB (1980) The effects of botulinum toxin on the synthesis, storage, and release of acetylcholine. Prog Neurobiol 14:99–119

19. Simpson LL (1989) Peripheral actions of the botulinum toxins. In: Simpson LL (ed) Botulinum neurotoxin and tetanus toxin. Academic Press, New York, pp 153–178

20. DasGupta BR, Tepp W (1993) Protease activity of botulinum neurotoxin type E and its light chain: Cleavage of actin. Biochem Biophys Res Commun 190:470–474

21. Barinaga M (1993) Secrets of secretion revealed. Science 260:487–489

22. Biasi J, Chapman ER, Link E, et al. (1993) Botulinum neurotoxin A selectively cleaves the synaptic protein SNAP-25. Nature 365:160–163

23. Binz T, Blasi J, Yamasaki S, et al. (1994) Proteolysis of SNAP-25 by types E and A botulinal neurotoxins. J Biol Chem 269:1617–1620

24. Borodic GE, Pearce LB, Smith K, Joseph M (1992) Botulinum A toxin for spasmodic torticollis: Multiple vs. single injection points per muscle. Head Neck 14:33–37

25. Shaari CM, Sanders I (1993) Quantifying how location and dose of botulinum toxin injections affect muscle paralysis. Muscle Nerve 16:964–969

26. Filippi GM, Errico P, Santarelli R, Bagolini B, Manni E (1993) Botulinum A toxin effects on rat jaw muscle spindles. Acta Otolaryngol 113:400–404

27. Borodic GE, Cozzolino D (1989) Blepharospasm and its treatment, with emphasis on the use of botulinum toxin. Plast Reconstr Surg 83:546–554

28. Harris CP, Alderson K, Nebeker J, Holds JB, Anderson RL (1991) Histologic features of human orbicularis oculi treated with botulinum A toxin. Arch Ophthalmol 109:393–395

29. Poewe W, Schelosky L, Kleedorfer B, Heinen F, Wagner M, Deuschl G (1992) Treatment of spasmodic torticollis with local injections of botulinum toxin. One-year follow-up in 37 patients. J Neurol 239:21–25

30. Quinn N, Hallett M (1989) Dose standardization of botulinum toxin. Lancet 1:964

31. First ER, Pearce LB, Borodic GE (1989) Dose standardization of botulinum toxin. Lancet 1:1035

32. Sanders DB, Massey EW, Buckley EG (1985) EMG monitoring of botulinum toxin in blepharospasm. Neurology 35:272

33. Habermann E (1974) 125I-labeled neurotoxin from Clostridium botulinum A: Preparation, binding to synaptosomes and ascent to the spinal cord. Naunyn Schmiedebergs Arch Pharmacol 281:47–56

34. Scott AB (1989) Clostridial toxins as therapeutic agents. In: Simpson LL (ed) Botulinum neurotoxin and tetanus toxin. Academic Press, New York, pp 399–412

35. Doellgast GJ, Triscott MX, Beard GA (1993) Sensitive enzyme-linked immunosorbent assay for detection of Clostridium botulinum neurotoxins A, B, and E using signal amplification via enzyme-linked coagulation assay. J Clin Microbiol 31:2402–2409

36. Jankovic J, Brin MF (1997) Botulinum toxin: Historical perspective and potential new indications. Muscle Nerve Suppl 6:S129–S145

37. Blitzer A (2005) Botulinum toxin A and B: A comparative dosing study for spasmodic dysphonia. Otolaryngol Head Neck Surg 133:836–838

38. Huang W, Rogachevsky AS, Foster JA (2000) Brow lift with botulinum toxin. Dermatol Surg 26;55–60

39. Flynn TC, Carruthers JA, Carruthers A (2001) Botulinum-A toxin treatment of the lower eyelid improves infraorbital rhytids and widens the eye. Dermatol Surg 27:703–708

40. Carruthers J, Carruthers A (2004) Aesthtic uses of botulinum toxin A in the periocular region and mid and lower face. Op Tech Otolaryngol Head Neck Surg15:134–138

41. Carruthers J, Fagien S, Matarasso SL (2004) Consensus recommendations on the use of botulinum toxin type A in facial aesthetics. Plast Reconstr Surg 114:1S–22S

42. Wynn R, Bentsianov BL, Blitzer A (2004) Botulinum toxin injection for the lower face and neck. Op Tech Otolaryngol Head Neck Surg 15:139–142

43. Blitzer A (2002) Botulinum neurotoxin A for the management of lower facial lines and platysmal bands. In: Lowe NJ (ed) Textbook of facial rejuvenation. Martin Dunitz, London, pp 171–176

44. Blitzer A, Binder WJ, Brin MF (1999) Botulinum toxin injections for facial lines and wrinkles. In: Blitzer A, Binder WJ, Boyd JB, Carruthers A (eds) Management of facial lines and wrinkles. Lippincott Williams & Wilkins, Philadelphia, pp 303–313

45. Silberstein S, Mathew N, Saper J, et al. (2000) Botulinum toxin type A as a migraine preventative treatment. For the BOTOX Migraine Clinical Research Group. Headache 40:445–450

46. Klein AW (2004) Complications with the use of botulinum toxin. Dermatol Clin 22:197–205

47. Klein A (1996) Cosmetic therapy with botulinum toxin: Anecdotal memoirs. Dermatol Surg 22:757–759

48. Burns RL (1998) Complications of botulinum exotoxin. Presented at the 25th annual clinical and scientific meeting of the ASDS, Portland, 13–17 May 1998

Chapter 81

Chemical Facial Resurfacing: The Modified Phenol-Crotinoil Peel

81

James R. Shire and Edwin A. Cortez

Contents

Background

The principle of skin resurfacing is the process of controlled re-epithelization. These procedures are used to improve surface irregularities that include pigmentation disorders and the treatment of wrinkles, acne scars, and other texture disorders. Techniques of resurfacing have been available for decades if not centuries, and consist mainly of dermabrasion, lasers, and chemical peels. The techniques may very but the mechanism and guidelines of replacing damaged epithelium with new skin remain constant. Yes we want to provide smooth skin with even texture, tone, and color, but not at the expense of a natural skin appearance. Therefore, one must understand and avoid the major complications of resurfacing, which are loss of pigmentation and scarring. The evolution of skin resurfacing has been motivated by "secret formulas" with mysterious ingredients, technologic advancements, and economic and market pressures.

The use of dermabrasion has fallen out of favor due to the difficulty to obtain consistent results and the additional risk to medical personnel due the aerosolized epithelium and blood with the increased incidents of HIV and hepatitis in the population.

The utilization of CO_2 lasers road the wave of the high tech revolution and was propagated by the media as much as by science. The advantage of laser resurfacing is that it is easy to perform with minimal training and it gave relatively consistent results. The problem with the laser is the high rate of hypopigmentation, scarring, and texture change, not to mention the high cost of the machine itself. In the early to mid 1990s we saw a remarkable increase in resurfacing procedures followed by a fear and reluctance of the patient towards resurfacing due to the large number of poor results created by the laser.

The use of chemical peels can be divided into three categories: light, intermediate, and deep, depending on the depth of penetration. In addition, there is a plethora of chemical agents available that are useful in resurfacing.

Phenol and phenol-croton oil have been the bases for many peels throughout history [5]. Lay peelers were the providers of this service until 1962 when the Baker formula was published (Table 81.1). This became the formula that was used by plastic surgeons and dermatologists and was the "gold standard" by

Table 81.1 Classic Baker formula (1962)

Phenol USP 88%: 3 cc
Distilled water: 2cc
Crotin oil: 3 drops
Septisol: 8 drops

which all other resurfacing modalities were compared. During this period no one questioned this classic formula or the role of the croton oil [1]. In addition there was a set of absolute dogma taught:

- Phenol was the active ingredient, and there is an "all-or-none" effect;
- Phenol peels deeper in lower concentrations. Highly concentrated phenol prevents deeper penetration of the dermis by denaturing keratin while lower concentrations would penetrate deeper;
- The loss of pigmentation or the porcelain mask is the result of phenol;
- Uncontrollable toxicity of phenol;
- Addition of a soap lowers surface tension thus increases penetration of the phenol;
- Croton oil was thought to be only an irritant.

For years the Baker-Gordon Peel has been used with varied results, some good and some poor. This is due in large part to the steep learning curve in the "art" of peeling. Controlling the variables in the technique takes experience. These variables include skin type and patient selection, skin preparation and degreasing, preparing or mixing the formula, application technique and the number of passes, use of occlusive dressing or not, and post-peel after care, wet verses dry wound, etc.

These ideas persisted for over 30 years. In the mid to late 1990s Stone [3, 4] and Hetter [1, 2] both published communications and articles on the use of modified phenol peels and the roles of croton oil and phenol concentration in chemical peeling. In doing so the old ideas and beliefs have changed, dispelling the myths of the past. Hetter showed that [1]:

- Phenol greater than 50% peels deeper with increasing concentrations to a maximum with 88% USP phenol.
- Unoccluded phenol less than 35% does not peel the skin.
- Unoccluded 88% USP phenol without croton oil produces only a light peel.
- Phenol does not have an "all-or-none" effect.
- Croton oil contains a powerful cytotoxic resin.
- Minute amounts of croton resin will cause skin burns.
- Small amounts of croton oil added to phenol will cause peeling or skin burns.
- Peel depth increases with increasing concentrations of croton oil.
- The depth of the peel is increased by tape occlusion, petroleum-based ointments, and multiple applications of croton oil in phenol.

Technique

Using the updated evidence and studies on modified phenol peels and phenol-croton oil peels provided in a series of articles by Stone [3, 4] and Hetter [1, 2] in recent years, the following chemical peel technique has been developed. It has been used by both authors here with superior results and lack of complications. The peeling process involves the pre-peel and post-peel care as well as the actual peeling itself.

Pre-peel Considerations

Patient selection is crucial in obtaining the optimum results. In general patients with fair or lighter complexions are the best candidates. Those patients with olive complexion and/ or marked solar damage, and those with freckled skin require full-face peeling and are not good candidates for regional, periorbital, or perioral peels. Regional peels in these patients will leave obvious demarcation lines and create a color disparity that will require the patient to wear makeup. Blacks and Asian are not good candidates due to the increased risk of splotchy complexion with areas of hyperpigmentation and hypopigmentation.

Preoperative evaluation and a complete, thorough history and physical examination are crucial. Evaluation of cardiac, hepatic, and renal function as well as any disorder that affects healing such as diabetes, collagen-vascular disease, history of radiation treatments, medications like Accutane, and a history of herpes outbreaks are documented. We require a current EKG, CBC, and basic chemistry profile (including electrolytes, BUN, and liver function test). Standard photos are taken.

The preoperative consultation includes a frank discussion of the principles of resurfacing and the procedure itself. Before and after photos including documented pictures of the healing process are reviewed with the patient. The healing process is explained in detail to all patients and their families including the swelling, discomfort, weeping of the skin, and keeping the skin moist, and the postpeel erythema. Consent forms are signed and risk and complications are reviewed and questions are answered. Prescriptions are given at the preop visit for Duricef (cefadroxil monohydrate) 500 mg (every 12 h for 7–10 days post peel), Medrol (methylprednisolone) Dose Pack (as directed over 6 days post peel), Lortab (hydrocodone bitartrate and acetaminophen) 7.5/500 or Toradol (ketorolac tromethamine) as needed for discomfort, and Valtrex (valacyclovir HCL GlaxoSmithKline) 500 mg every 12 h beginning 2 days prior to the procedure and ending 10 days post peel. The patient is instructed to purchase Eucerin cream (Beiersdorf, Inc) and Aquaphor (Beiersdorf, Inc). A complete written post-peel manual of care, restrictions, dos and don'ts, is reviewed and given to the patient. The authors do not use or recommend the use of any exfoliating agents, retinoids, or hydroquinones for 1 month prior to the peel. Patient-applied pretreatments can vary individually and we do not want to change the epidermal kinetics.

The Phenol-croton oil peel should be limited to the face, and not extended down to the neck. Peeling the neck results in hypertrophic scarring.

81

Formula Preparation

In any one patient the skin thickness, epidermal damage, depth, and amount of rhytides vary, therefore the strength and depth of the peel should correspond. The formula used by the authors is based on the classic Baker-Gordon formula with varying amounts of croton oil used. This modified formulation is supported by the work of Hetter [1, 3] who has shown that 33% phenol can produce a medium light, medium heavy, or heavy peel if the concentration of croton oil is changed from 0.35% to 0.7% to 1.1%, respectively. The depth of peel from 88% phenol has been shown to be less than that produced by 62.5% phenol, which was less than that produced by 48.5% phenol (Baker-Gordon formula).

The phenol comes as a liquid solution in a concentration of approximately 88% USP. Distilled water is used as a diluent. Septisol, a liquid soap, is used as a saponifying agent. Croton oil is a powerful cytotoxic resin that increases the depth of peel with increased concentrations.

We use four different mixtures or formulas to vary the depth of peels (Table 81.2).

We prepare a fresh batch of each mixture prior to each case. The authors strongly recommend that each surgeon mixes his own formulas and does not entrust this job to a pharmacist, nurse, or other personnel. The formulas are compounded in individual 30-ml amber glass bottles that are labeled with the concentration, date, and patient (Fig. 81.1). These ingredients do not mix homogenously, and must be continuously stirred during the application.

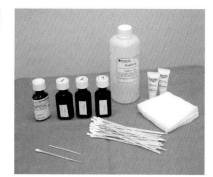

Fig. 81.1 Set up tray for peel procedure including the different peel formulas, acetone, applicators, and Eucerin cream

The face is divided into treatment zones by marking a topographic map (Fig. 81.2). These areas represent the differences in skin thickness, level of skin appendages, and will determine which peel mixture is to be used. The facial zones are:
- Zone 1: perioral, chin, and lower nose
- Zone 2: cheeks and upper nose
- Zone 3: forehead
- Zone 4: eyelids, periorbital extending to the temples, and preauricular area

Zone 1 is peeled usually with the strongest concentration. Zones 2 and 3 are peeled with the next strongest concentration. Zone

The Peel Procedure

All patients are peeled under conscience sedation anesthesia, and monitored with EKG and pulse oximeter. The patient's face is cleansed with Septisol to make sure all makeup is off and the skin is clean. Then the face is degreased with acetone on a 2×2 gaze sponge to remove any surface oils. This is an extremely important step to allow a more even peel.

Nerve blocks are used to reduce the post-peel discomfort. Marcaine (bupivacaine) 0.75% plain is used to block the infraorbital, supraorbital, and mental nerves.

Table 81.2 Four different mixtures or formulas to vary the depth of peels

Baker-Gordon 3 Drop	Modified 2 Drop	Modified 1 Drop	Straight Phenol 88% USP
3 ml phenol	3 ml phenol	3 ml phenol	3 ml phenol
2 ml water distilled	2 ml water	2 ml water	
8 drops Septisol	8 drops Septisol	8 drops Septisol	
3 drops croton oil	2 drops croton oil	1 drop croton oil	

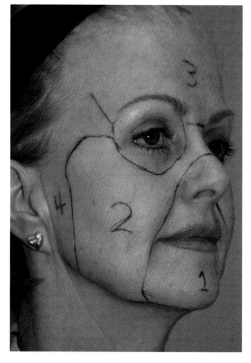

Fig. 81.2 The face is sectioned into five treatment zones

4 is peeled using the straight phenol solution. As to which formula is used where, it is determined by each individual patient. The peel solution is chosen and stirred continually to keep it in suspension. Six-inch cotton tip applicators are used to apply the solutions. The deep rhytides are treated first by applying the solution on a pointed applicator stick to the base of the rhytides or wrinkle lines. The area is covered by rolling a saturated cotton tip applicator to the area. The entire zone is painted to provide an even and complete coverage. With this application an immediate grayish white frost is observed. We usually begin at Zone 1 and then proceed to Zones 2, 3, and 4 allowing about 15–20 min between zones. The depth of peel is determined by how the skin is prepped, the formula used, the amount of solution applied, the number of application layers, and the amount of rubbing that is done with the swab. This is the reason experience, technique, and the "art" of peeling are critical in obtaining superior results. In general terms the 3 Drop or 2 Drop solutions are used in Zone 1. The 1 Drop or occasionally the 2 Drop or straight phenol is used in Zones 2 and 3 . It should be noted that the use of the 3 Drop or Baker-Gordon peel is rarely used anymore in our practices. When an even frost is obtained, a moist dressing of Eucerin cream is heavily applied. The patient is monitored for a minimum of 1 h post op and usually has only mild to moderate discomfort due to the nerve blocks. Toradol or Lortab is used for supplemental relief.

Post-peel Care

What must be stressed is the importance of the post-peel healing phase to the final result (Fig. 81.3).The following instructions are given to the patient in writing and are verbally reviewed. The instructions are based on hundreds of chemical peels and designed to answer the patient's questions and result in the most favorable healing.

Moderate to severe swelling will occur especially around the eyes and mouth. Swelling peaks by the second or third day and should subside by the fifth or sixth day. The patient should remain head elevated as much as possible. Within 24 to 36 h the peeled area resembles a deep sunburn with the skin darkening and serum oozing from the skin. Approximately 24 h after the procedure the patient is instructed to wash their face by standing in a shower with a fine wide spray and letting the tepid water flow over the face. The purpose of the shower is to give moisture to the skin, not remove the cream. After the shower, the face is left to air dry, and then Eucerin cream is applied. The Euc-

erin cream should be applied like frosting a cake. This process is done five to six times per day. The Eucerin is reapplied between showers as needed. Initially the patient is seen daily to monitor the progress of the healing and the compliance of the patient, and to reassure the patient about the process. The peeling is usually complete between the ninth and fourteenth day. On the seventh to eighth day Eucerin is replaced with Aquaphor. When the peeling is complete, about the tenth to fourteenth day, the new epidermis is an intense pink, which will begin to fade after the second week. The pink color will remain for 6–12 weeks, continually decreasing in intensity. As mentioned, all patients are treated with Valtrex preoperatively and postoperatively to prevent outbreaks of herpes or "fever blisters."

Complications

In our experience serious complications are rare and mostly avoidable. However, complications and undesirable result are discussed with the patients.

Hypopigmentation to some degree is the most commonly reported post-phenol-peel reaction. But the surgeon must understand and be able to explain to the patient that although the removal of sun-damaged skin, solar dyschromias, and freckles is a lightening of the current skin condition, it is in fact a return to the patient's original skin coloring. (The patient is directed to compare the new skin to an area that has not had sun exposure.) The severe pigmentation loss and porcelain complexion is due to the use of waterproof tape or Vaseline occlusive dressing and is the reason phenol has received an unfair poor reputation in the past. Pigmentation demarcations are noted in areas of transition between the peeled and unpeeled. Therefore patient selection, peeling technique formula choice, and the practice of regional peeling are critical.

Scarring has not been a problem with the modified phenol-croton oil peels. In the past scarring has been related to older techniques. These were usually minor and could be treated with watchful waiting and interlesional steroid injections. It has been noted that patients who have undergone lower lid blepharoplasty can get ectropion. This can occur in any lid that is tightened and special care must be taken even with the lighter peeling solutions such as the straight phenol.

Post-peel hyperpigmentation can be a problem and the patient needs to be well educated on sun sensitivity and exposure. It appears more commonly in patients with type III skin and those who do not protection their skin from the sun during

81

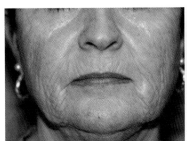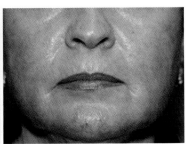

Fig. 81.3 Before and after example of modified phenol-croton oil peel

the erythematous period. The use of sun blocks that protect against UVA and UVB both is essential. This sensitivity to the sun may last for several months. Patients are advised on the use of sunscreens and that future tanning should be avoided. The prolonged erythema may be treated with mild topical steroids for a limited period [2 weeks of Hytone (hydrocortisone) 2.5% cream every 12 h].

Though infections can occur in an open peel, it is very rare and has not been encountered by the authors. Patients are given prophylactic post-peel antibiotics Duricef 500 mg/BID for 7 days. The more common infection is perioral herpes simplex. It is estimated that over 50% of the population has been exposed to the herpes virus, therefore all patients are treated with Valtrex 500 mg /BID beginning 2 days preoperative and 10 days post peel. With this protocol, there have been no herpetic breakthroughs. Herpetic infections are usually superficial but can result in scarring.

Milia may occur post peel as a consequence of the healing process. These are small inclusion cysts that appear in the first 2–4 weeks after the peel and are temporary. Patients are informed of this and are reassured and instructed to leave them be and let the milia resolve. Also patients that have fair skin with a red, flushing complexion can have increase in telangiectasia. If telangiectasia persists beyond the erythema stage, it can be treated with a Diolite 532 nm (Iridex Corp.) laser or a similar device.

Persistent rhytides cause patient disappointment. This can be avoided with proper patient selection and the use of the proper peel solution. Repeat focal touch-up [4] peels can be performed after 9 months or so and can be done as an office procedure.

Conclusion

Some of our happiest and most grateful patients are the resurfaced patients. For years the gold standard in resurfacing has been the Baker-Gordon peel. However, the theories of action appear to have been based on fallacies. The idea that phenol was the only active ingredient and that croton oil was only a slight irritant that could be omitted has been dispelled in recent decades. With the studies of both Stone and Hetter, we modified the classic Baker-Gordon peel into a resurfacing spectrum by varying the amount of croton oil in each formula. Then selecting the correct formula for the appropriate skin type, skin damage, and facial zone provides the ability to maximize the results and minimize the complications. The strict adherence to detailed preoperative preparation, formula preparation and selection, and postoperative care and follow up have shown consistent superior results.

Tips to Avoid Complications

- Avoid dark skinned individuals and Asians
- Avoid patients who will have marked areas of demarcation
- Avoid regional peels (do the entire face)
- Make the peel solution yourself immediately prior to the procedure
- Discourage using any stratum corneum thinners 1 month preop (i.e., retinoids)
- Treat prophylactically with Valtrex and antibiotics
- See patients daily for 1 week after the peel
- Treat hyperpigmentation early
- Don't peel lax lower lids
- Patient should be 1 year off Accutane

Take-Home Pearls

- Patient selection is critical
- Patient education is extremely important; i.e., show prospective patients photos of patients during peel procedure and process
- Pay attention to details; i.e., preparation of solution, stirring solution, proper application, postop care
- Hit a triple—don't go for a home run!

References

1. Hetter GP (2000) An examination of the phenol-croton oil peel: Part: i. dissecting the formula. Plast Reconstr Surg 105(1):227–239
2. Hetter GP (2000) An examination of the phenol-croton oil peel: Part iv. face peel results with different concentrations of phenol and croton oil. Plast Reconstr Surg 105(3):1061–1083
3. Stone PA (1998) The use of modified phenol for chemical face peeling. Clin Plast Surg 25(1):21–44
4. Stone PA, Lefer LG (2001) Modified phenol chemical face peels. Facial Plast Surg Clin North Am 9(3):351–376
5. Stuzin JM (1998) Phenol peeling and the history of phenol peeling. Clin Plast Surg 25(1):1–19

Chapter 82

Laser Facial Resurfacing

Edmund A. Pribitkin

82

Core Messages

- The laser does not resurface skin. It ablates skin.
- The upper reticular dermis heals by reorganization, but the lower reticular dermis heals by scar formation.
- Vary treatment parameters according to detailed facial analysis.
- Fully involve the patient in the recovery process.

Contents

Basic Principles

Successful laser facial resurfacing presupposes a thorough knowledge of the skin's structure and the physiology of wound healing. Achievement of a youthful postoperative appearance following laser treatment relies upon dermal regeneration from deeper, less photo-aged cells. The laser, itself, does not resurface the skin. It is simply a tool employed to ablate aged skin layers while minimizing the injury to healthier surrounding skin structures. The surgeon and patient working in tandem create the conditions necessary for successful wound healing following laser tissue ablation.

Basic principles of laser-tissue interaction apply to all types of lasers. Laser energy may be transmitted, absorbed, scattered, or reflected by varying tissue types. The majority of skin resurfacing lasers (carbon dioxide, Er:YAG) vaporize the skin while minimizing the surrounding zones of coagulative necrosis and thermal conductivity. The volume of tissue ablated varies directly with laser power density, whereas the thermal damage to adjacent tissue varies directly with the intensity and duration of laser exposure. For example, a carbon dioxide laser with a wavelength of 10,600 nm will be primarily absorbed by the water content of the skin resulting in a typical single pass penetration depth of 120–200 μ and a collateral thermal effect of 40–60 μ. Increases in power density will result in deeper penetrations but will also increase the risk of thermal injury unless dwell times are minimized. Typically, the depth of skin penetration will determine the degree and nature of skin regeneration in a patient with normal skin adenexae. Lasers may freshen the appearance by ablating just the epidermis or may achieve more significant corrections of superficial blemishes and wrinkles by penetrating into the papillary dermis. Correction of deeper wrinkles by more aggressive ablation into the reticular dermis involves greater risks and requires more healing time. Histologically, the upper reticular dermis heals by reorganization and the lower reticular dermis heals by scar formation.

Initial Consultation and Pretreatment Regimen

The initial encounter with the patient explores the patient's concerns and determines whether the patient exhibits proper motivation and has realistic expectations regarding the outcome of the resurfacing. More importantly, the initial encounter should explore whether a patient can be an active participant in the healing process following laser resurfacing. Patients who cannot follow postoperative instructions make poor resurfacing candidates (Fig. 82.1) and may wish to seek nonablative skin treatments which affect dermal collagen without exfoliation. Such nonablative techniques (Nd:YAG, broad-band high intensity pulsed light and flashlamp dye) cannot achieve the degree of skin rejuvenation seen with ablative laser resurfacing techniques, but offer a marked reduction in recuperative time.

A detailed medical and dermatological history should screen for relative contraindications to the procedure (Table 82.1). Individuals with pigmented skin lesions should be evaluated by a dermatologist for biopsy prior to resurfacing. Individuals with a history of keloid or hypertrophic scar formation should avoid the dermal injury induced by laser resurfacing. Atrophic (Acne) scars respond poorly to resurfacing; however, the skin surrounding these scars may be treated. Atrophic scars may also be excised or punch grafted and these sites subsequently resurfaced Individuals with a history of hyperpigmentation or hypopigmentation following inflammatory skin conditions may expect these difficulties to occur following resurfacing (Fig. 82.2). Pregnant ladies, those who are breastfeeding, or individuals undergoing estrogen-based fertility or gender changing

Table 82.1 Relative contraindications to laser skin resurfacing

Hypertrophic or keloid scar formation
Atrophic scar formation
Hyperpigmentation
Hypopigmentation
Uncontrolled herpetic ulcers
Isotretinoin therapy
Collagen vascular disorders
Elevated estrogen levels
Prolonged oral corticosteroid therapy
Poorly motivated or non-compliant patient

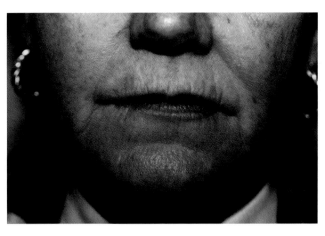

Fig. 82.2 Patient with hypopigmentation following chemical peel may expect similar results following laser resurfacing

therapies should also avoid laser resurfacing due to the risk of hormonally induced hyperpigmentation. Fever blisters may also be triggered to occur following surgery (Fig. 82.3). Individuals with collagen vascular diseases or immunological deficiencies may experience delayed wound healing following resurfacing. Similarly, numerous medications including systemic corticosteroids and topical fluorinated corticosteroids retard skin healing and can result in areas of atrophic scar formation (Fig. 82.4). Other medications and herbal therapies [e.g., fluoroquinolones, tetracyclines, sulfonamides, thiazide diuretics, tricyclic antidepressants, Saint John's Wort (*Hypericum perforatum),* kava kava (*Piper methysiticum*)] can increase skin sensitivity to thermal injury and should be avoided perioperatively. Patients with a previous history of external beam skin irradiation should avoid laser skin resurfacing due to the destruction of skin adenexae, which aid in reepithelialization. Similarly, individuals undergoing therapy with Accutane (isotretinoin) should not undergo resurfacing for 12 months following cessation of therapy due to the delays in skin re-epithelialization seen following the reduc-

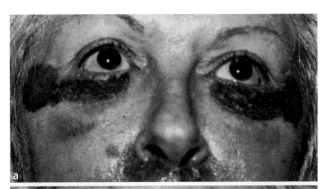

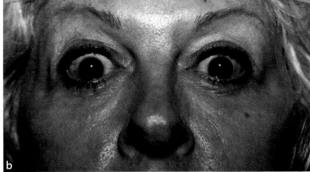

Fig. 82.1 **a,b** Patient with initial poor postoperative hygiene and eventual results following intensive counseling and postoperative therapy

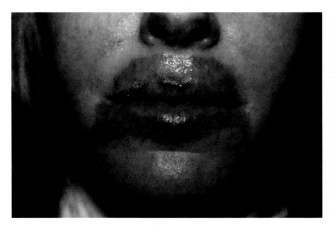

Fig. 82.3 Perioral postoperative Herpes Simplex outbreak

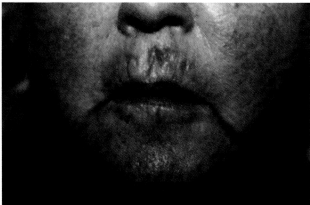

Fig. 82.4 Delayed wound healing seen in patient on chronic high dose oral corticosteroid therapy for collagen vascular disease

Table 82.2 Fitzpatrick skin types

1	Very white	Freckled always burns
2	White	Usually burns
3	White to olive	Sometimes burns
4	Brown	Rarely burns
5	Dark brown	Very rarely burns
6	Black	Never burns

Table 82.3 Glogau's photo-aging groups

	Age	Wrinkles	Keratoses	Make-up use
1	20s	Histologically present	None	Minimal
2	30s	In motion	Early	Little
3	40s	At rest	Actinic changes	Always
4	>50s	Severe	Possible carcinoma	Poor cover

tion of skin appendages by this medication. Those patients who have undergone previous deep chemical peels, dermabrasion, or laser resurfacing may undergo further resurfacing following a healing period of 6–12 months.

The surgeon should perform a facial analysis to determine the patient's skin type, epidermal and dermal thickness, and degree of chronological and photo-aging. We generally characterize patients according to their Fitzpatrick skin type [1] (Table 82.2) and Glogau's photo-aging group (Table 82.3) [2]. Individuals with darker skin types are a greater risk of postinflammatory pigmentary changes, whereas individuals with lighter skin types may experience prolonged postoperative erythema. In addition to noting the depth and character (static vs. dynamic) of wrinkles, we note the presence of posttraumatic, herpetic, and acne type scarring and counsel patients regarding limited improvements in these areas. The majority of patients will also exhibit interzonal variations in epidermal and dermal thickness [3], which must be considered when applying laser energy to the different parts of the face. Generally speaking, these interzonal variations will decrease in proportion to the degree of photo-aging (Fig. 82.5).

Dr. Michael Stevens has delineated the goals of pretreatment skin conditioning to include inducing a uniform, well-hydrated stratum corneum, increasing mitotic activity in the basal layers, epidermis, and adenexae of the skin, increasing epidermal growth factors, increasing dermal hydration, regulating melanocyte function, and reducing acne, comedones, and folliculitis [4]. For 1 month prior to surgery, our patients apply topical retinoic acid 0.0125–0.05% bid. In those patients with severe photo-aging requiring increased penetration, retinoic acid is applied after washing the face with a 10% alpha-hydroxy acid preparation. All patients also apply a gel consisting of 4% hydroquinone and kogic acid to decrease the risk of postinflammatory hyperpigmentation. In patients with acne difficulties, topical Clindamycin 1% is employed. Botulinum toxin injections administered 2 weeks prior to laser resurfacing can improve re-epithelialization by decreasing facial movement across the treatment zone. On the day of surgery, patients are instructed to wash with phisohex and apply no makeup. Both antistaphylococcal antibiotics and antiviral medications are prescribed for 10 days.

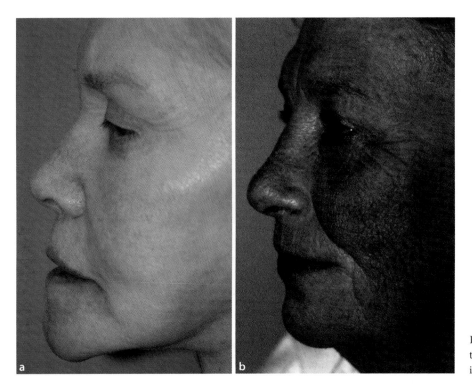

Fig. 82.5a,b Normal interzonal variations in skin thickness (**a**) diminish with increased photo-aging (**b**)

Operative Technique

All centers performing laser resurfacing must adhere to laser safety precautions including the use of protective eyewear and laser masks, evacuation of the laser plume, appointment of a laser safety officer, and posting of clearly marked procedure room signs indicating that a laser is in use. Procedures may be performed under general anesthesia, sedation, regional blocks, or local infiltration. When using local infiltration we employ hyaluronidase to minimize distortion of tissues and to aid in the spread of the anesthetic. On the day of surgery, the procedural consent form is reviewed with the patient and all questions answered. The consent should include specific language regarding the potential for permanent darkening, lightening, or blotchiness of the skin, persistence of wrinkling, formation of atrophic or hypertrophic scars as well as unforeseen difficulties that are acknowledged to be beyond the practitioner's control. We also include a clause whereby the patient agrees to assume responsibility for the postoperative care of the resurfacing procedure. On the day of surgery, the patient's face is prepared again with a phisohex wash and degreased with acetone.

The surgeon must be familiar with all aspects of a given laser operating system, because each laser comes with specific operating instructions that are unique to that particular piece of equipment. Nonetheless, certain broad recommendations apply across the spectrum of laser systems. Laser resurfacing should not be performed simultaneously with any surgery involving subcutaneous dissection—injuries to the subdermal plexus increase the risk of skin loss with consequent atrophic or hypertrophic scarring. Dynamic lines (e.g., Crow's feet) and lower lid laxity cannot be corrected with laser resurfacing. Botulinum toxin treatments may be used for the former, whereas the latter respond better to directed lid tightening procedures. Similarly, deep nasolabial folds and marionette lines often require treatment with fillers rather than laser resurfacing.

Entire regional subunits rather than individual trouble spots should be treated. The surgeon should resurface the entire treatment zone with steady, linear passes and minimal overlap. Interzonal variations in skin thickness demand alterations in laser power density. Accordingly, power density should be decreased in areas of thin skin (eyelids) or fair skin. The power density should also be decreased along the hairline and as treated skin transitions to untreated skin. The depth of skin ablation may be judged by the appearance of the wiped skin: penetration through the epidermis appears pink, into the papillary dermis gray, and into the reticular dermis a chamois color (Fig. 82.6). The skin should be wiped clean of any laser char before a second pass is performed—char will not vaporize but will heat and cause surrounding thermal injury. The medial canthi, lateral canthi, and the oral commissures should not be treated for fear of inducing ulcerations, delayed healing, and hypertrophic scarring. Great care should be exercised as the facial skin transitions into the neck skin at the angle of the mandible. Here, fewer skin adenexae exist from which to regenerate injured epithelium.

Following treatment, the skin is cleansed of any char with gentle iced saline sponges and icepacks are applied. Postoperatively, an occlusive skin dressing will reduce crust formation, pruritus, erythema, and pain [5]. Numerous authors have advocated commercial bio-occlusive dressings, but petroleum jelly applied frequently in thin coatings will work effectively for most

82

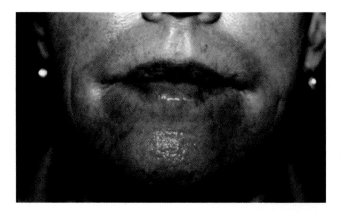

Fig. 82.6 The depth of skin ablation may be judged by the appearance of the wiped skin penetration through the epidermis appears pink, into the papillary dermis gray, and into the reticular dermis a chamois color

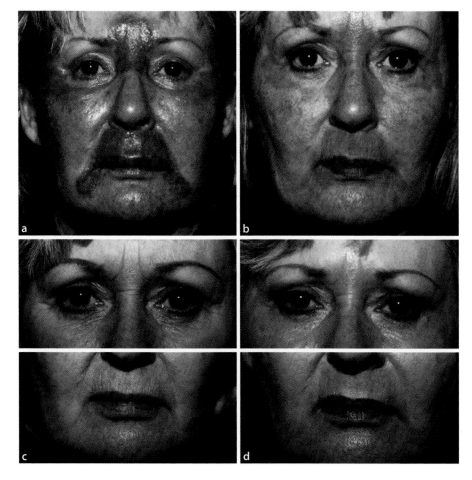

Fig. 82.7a–d Good candidate with fair skin with moderate wrinkling (c) but with postoperative inflammation due to topical triple antibiotic ointment (a) with resultant postinflammatory hyperpigmentation (b) requiring 6 months to resolve (d)

patients. Patients must expect mild burning, erythema, edema, and a weeping exudate for up to 1 week postoperatively. This will lessen with frequent washings of 1 tablespoon of vinegar mixed in 1 cup of tap water. Commercial antibiotic ointments, steroid creams, and moisturizers can potentially incite inflammation and should be avoided (Fig. 82.7). Patients may apply cosmetics only after the skin is fully re-epithelialized (7–10 days following a deep laser resurfacing). Patients will note gradual improvement in their appearance over the course of 6 weeks to 12 months. Laser resurfacing of the perioral subunit (Fig. 82.8), periorbital subunit (Fig. 82.9), and of the full face (Fig. 82.10) can yield dramatic improvements in patient appearance.

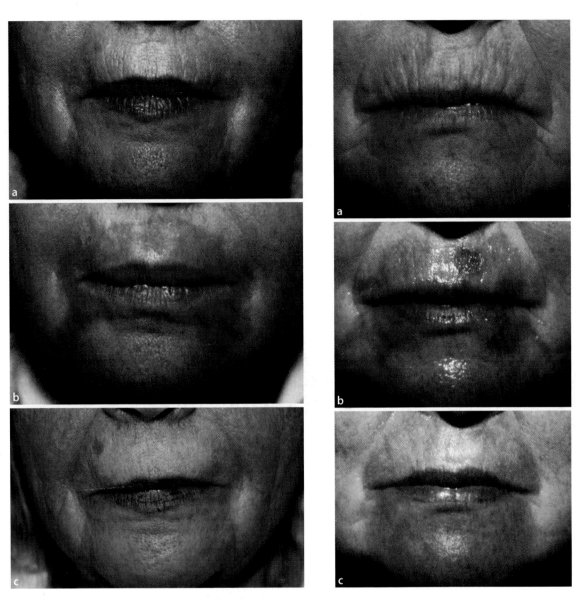

Fig. 82.11a–c Even individuals with lighter skin (a) can develop hyperpigmentation (b) 6 months postop), but this will respond to bleaching agents, although occasionally with eventual hypopigmentation (c) 10 years postop)

Fig. 82.12a–c Preoperative oral rhytids (a) treated with carbon dioxide laser resurfacing with perioperative herpetic ulceration (b) resulting in atrophic scarring, which largely resolves over 6 months (c)

Complications

Frequent and detailed follow-up serves to prevent the majority of complications. Early complications treated with appropriate antimicrobial agents include Herpes Simplex virus and staphylococcus aureus infections (Fig. 82.3). Candidal infections often respond to oral fluconazole or to Lotrisone cream. Inflammatory or hypersensitivity reactions may lead to postinflammatory hyperpigmentation (Fig. 82.7) and must be treated with immediate removal of the offending agent, topical hydrocortisone cream, and occasionally oral corticosteroids.

Late complications include persistent erythema, hyperpigmentation, hypopigmentation, scarring, and persistent wrinkles. Again, topical hydrocortisone cream, limited sun exposure and time will generally reduce inflammation and erythema. Hyperpigmentation must be treated aggressively with limited sun exposure and bleaching agents such as 4% hydroquinone and kogic acid (Fig. 82.11). Hypopigmentation is generally more accepted by patients and can usually be effectively camouflaged with make-up. Scarring typically results from either overly aggressive laser resurfacing, poor skin regeneration, or as the result of a posttreatment herpetic outbreak. Hypertrophic scars may be treated with commercial silicone-based preparations and judicious injection of intralesional steroids. Although they will often thicken over months, atrophic healing areas may require skin grafting or serial excision (Fig. 82.12). Persistent rhytids will respond to repeated resurfacing (Fig. 82.13).

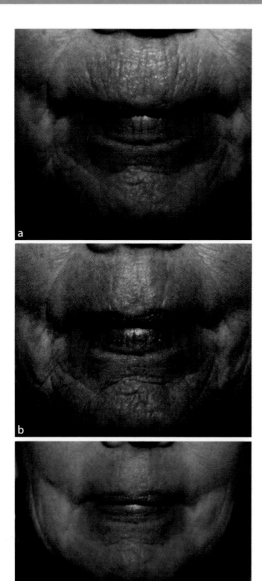

Fig. 82.13a–c Preoperative (**a**), 6 months following initial carbon dioxide perioral laser resurfacing (**b**) and 6 months following repeat procedure (**c**)

Conclusion

A thorough understanding of wound healing and the capabilities/limitations of modern laser delivery systems are a prerequisite to successful laser facial skin resurfacing. Proper patient selection, preoperative skin preparation and support throughout the healing period will enable patients to achieve a marked improvement in the appearance of photo-aged skin while minimizing complications.

Tips to Avoid Complications

- Optimize conditions for skin regeneration perioperatively.
- Observe laser safety guidelines.
- Observe interzonal variations in skin thickness.
- Do not try to fully ablate dynamic rhytids.

Take-Home Pearls

- Decrease power density in areas of thin or fair skin.
- Avoid medial canthi, lateral canthi, and oral commissures.
- Avoid areas with few skin adenexae.
- Continually check clinical endpoints-wipe char.

References

1. Fitzpatrick TB (1988) The validity and practicality of sun-reactive skin types I through VI. Arch Dermatol Jun; 124(6):869–871
2. Glogau RG (1996) Aesthetic and anatomic analysis of aging skin. Semin Cutan Med Surg 15:134–138
3. Pellacani G, Seidenari S. (1999) Variations in facial skin thickness and echogenicity with site and age. Acta Derm Venereol 79(5):366–369
4. Stevens M (1996) Optimizing the results of your resurfacing by pre-procedure and post-procedure skin conditioning, Int J Aesthetic Restor Surg 4(2):133–136
5. Newman J (1998) Closed dressings after laser skin resurfacing. Arch Otolaryngol Head Neck Surg 124:751–757

Chapter 83

Soft Tissue Augmentation with Injectable Fillers

83

David A. F. Ellis and Evelyn Linda Maxwell

Core Messages

- There is a wide variety of injectable fillers available to to-day's facial plastic surgeon. Each individual filler has its own unique set of indications, advantages, and disadvantages. It is the responsibility of the facial plastic surgeon to fully understand the patient's aesthetic goals as well as the mechanism of action of each particular filling agent. Careful injection technique is of paramount importance in obtaining a safe and pleasing aesthetic result.

Contents

Introduction

Injectable soft tissue fillers have begun to play an increasingly important role in facial rejuvenation, soft tissue augmentation, and treatment of acne and other scarring. Injectable fillers may be used exclusively or in conjunction with facial cosmetic surgical and nonsurgical procedures [1]. Over the past 20 years, there has been remarkable innovation and improvement in the types of injectable fillers available to facial plastic surgeons. This chapter will focus specifically on the fillers we use or have used in our practice and will cover the evolution of injectable fillers from the early and controversial liquid silicone introduced in the 1960s to new and innovative products of the 21st century such as Bio-Alcamid.

Indications

There are numerous indications for injectable fillers; however, specific fillers are better suited to specific indications. In general, the indications for injectable fillers include the correction of grooves and wrinkles of the face. Facial regions particularly suitable to injectables include the lip-cheek groove, the horizontal forehead lines, the glabellar frown lines, and down-turned corners of the mouth. A second indication for injectables includes filling of subcutaneous skin defects such as irregularities of the nose or chin. In fact, an expanding area of facial cosmetic surgery includes the nonsurgical rhinoplasty, in which injectable fillers, rather than surgery, are used to reshape and recontour the nose. Injectable fillers are particularly useful in correcting cosmetic deformities in cases where previous rhinoplasty has been performed. The third indication for injectable fillers is the improvement of acne scars. The use of injectable fillers for acne scars that are wide, shallow, and depressed yields the most satisfactory and most predictable results. Narrow, deep acne scars and ice pick acne scars are less likely to improve significantly with the use of injectable fillers. Finally, the fourth and most common indication for injectable filler is lip augmentation. There is a wide variety of techniques that may be used to improve various aspects of the upper and lower lips. A simplified way of thinking about lip augmentation is to decide whether

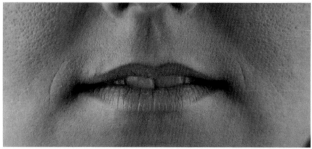

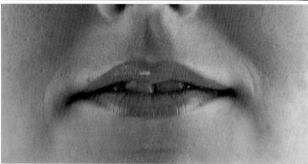

Fig. 83.1 Upper lip augmentation with a temporary injectable filler. Note the improvement in the central upper one-third of the lip (pout)

lip augmentation or lip definition is the desired goal. Improving lip definition involves enhancing the junction of the red and white lip and filling the vermilion border. On the other hand, lip augmentation traditionally implies increasing the volume of the red lip. In this case, the injectable filler is placed in the red lip substance. Injectable fillers may also be used to enhance specific areas of the lips such as the philtrum of the lip and the middle third (pout) (Fig. 83.1).

This chapter will focus on reviewing our experience with different types of injectable fillers, injection technique and site-specific injection.

The Ideal Injectable Filler

Presently, a single ideal injectable filler does not exist. The selection of a particular injectable filler is influenced by a number of factors including patient and clinical factors. Clinical factors include the availability of the filler, the anatomical region to be treated, the type of correction or improvement desired, and physician comfort and expertise with the product. Patient factors include the degree of correction or improvement and desired longevity of the result. As well, the patient's age, general health, and underlying medical conditions may influence the choice of filler. For example, a young patient with no previous exposure to facial plastic procedures who desires lip augmentation may be best served with a temporary injectable filler. This will allow both the patient and physician to evaluate the patient's clinical response to and satisfaction with the filling agent. In general, an ideal filler is long lasting or permanent and potentially remov-

able. It is nontoxic and nonallergenic. It is easy to store and to administer. There should be minimal if any side effects and the material should be noncarcinogenic. Virtually all injected fillers will incite a mild degree of host reaction and, in the case of permanent fillers, a fibrous capsule may develop. However, it is important that injectable fillers do not elicit chronic inflammation and that the body is able to stimulate neo-collagen growth in order to improve augmentation and prevent particle migration. In other words, it is of utmost importance that these materials demonstrate optimal biocompatibility [2].

Adverse Events

Complications and adverse reactions to most injectable fillers may be organized according to the time-frame in which they develop. Short-term reactions are fairly common and may be considered to be a natural consequence of injection. Some patients may experience some degree of discomfort or pain, mild swelling, redness, and/or bruising. Much of these side effects may be attributed to the skill and level of expertise of the injector as well as the caliber needle used, and use of topical anesthetics and/or ice. Serious and fortunately rare short-term complications such as embolism have been reported [3]. For the most part, this is an entirely avoidable situation if the area of injection is gently aspirated to assess entry into the vascular system prior to injecting. Intermediate reactions, which are rare, may occur from 2 to 12 months after injection and may be seen after injection of any permanent filler. Some intermediate-level adverse reactions include nodules, swelling, fistulas, ulcers, exudates, and scarring [4]. Finally, delayed or long-term adverse reactions may present as tender areas of induration or nodularity. If these lesions do not resolve spontaneously, they will often respond to local steroid injection if no infection is present [4].

Xenogenic Fillers

One of the first injectable fillers, Zyderm, was composed of highly purified bovine collagen mixed with local anesthetic. It was used as a dermal filler. However, skin testing was required and there was a 3% allergy rate to bovine collagen. Seventy percent of positive reactions occur within the first 72 h and those reactions consist of redness, firmness, tenderness, and swelling with or without pruritus at the test site (undersurface of right forearm). Delayed reactions may occur up to 4 weeks after the test. In patients with a negative skin test after 4 weeks, collagen injection may proceed; however, most clinicians will repeat the skin test and not proceed until two negative skin tests have been achieved. Fillers have evolved to include temporary materials such as hyaluronic acid gel and calcium hydroxyapatite and permanent materials such as acrylic beads coupled to collagen or hyaluronic acid. Injectable fillers can be further subdivided into classes based on the source of the product. Fillers are derived from a variety of sources that include xenogenic (from other species), allogeneic (from other humans), autogeneic (from one's own tissue) and synthetic or alloplastic. Amongst the xenogenic

83

fillers, Zyderm as discussed previously was the first. Artecoll is probably the most commonly used xenogenic injectable filler at present. It is a permanent filler derived from bovine collagen and polymethacrylate beads. Other xenogenic fillers include Zyplast, Fibrel (derived from porcine collagen), and Hyalform (hyaluronic acid gel derived from rooster comb). Zyplast (The Collagen Corp., Palo Alto, CA), which was introduced in 1985, is a similar formulation as rapidly-degraded Zyderm I and Zyderm II. However, Zyplast contains collagen that is conjugated to glutaraldehyde. This cross-linkage makes Zyplast more stable and longer lasting than its Zyderm predecessors. Zyplast is injected into the deeper soft tissues at the mid-recticular dermis level [5]. Zyplast fell somewhat out of favor following rare (9 in 10,000) incidences of skin necrosis, particularly in the glabellar region, due to the vascular occlusion in the deeper dermis [6, 7].

Allogeneic and Autogeneic Fillers

Allogeneic fillers are used less commonly in facial plastic surgery but include Dermalogen, which is derived from pooled cadaveric dermis. There are numerous other types of pooled cadaveric dermal fillers including micronized AlloDerm and Fascian. CosmoDerm and CosmoPlast (INAMED Corporation) are human-based collagen treatments and offer a similar aesthetic profile as Zyderm and Zyplast, with the exception of not requiring a skin test. Autogeneic injectable fillers are materials derived from the patient's own tissue and include materials such as harvested dermis, cartilage, and bone. The main problem with these materials is the strong tendency for resorption of the agent. We have had significant success with autologous fat harvest and transfer. Fat transfer provides a significant amount of filler for large defect areas. For example, the hollow of the cheeks and deep nasolabial folds may be filled with fat. Although it is a more invasive surgical procedure compared to other injectable fillers, fat transfer has several advantages. Firstly, fat transfer yields greater volume and is suited to large defect areas. Secondly, once the fat graft takes, the results are truly permanent. And thirdly, in carefully selected patients, fat grafting is more cost effective than other injectable fillers. However, there are disadvantages to the procedure as well. As mentioned previously, it is a surgical procedure that requires local anesthetic. There is donor site morbidity, albeit minimal. Successful fat transfer requires two procedures since there is about a 60% take-rate after a single procedure. Finally, the procedure is time consuming and requires experience and technical expertise.

Fat transfer is performed under local anesthesia in the operating room. The mid-trunk area of the patient is injected with diluted xylocaine. Careful dilution (1 mL of 1% xylocaine per 9 mL of normal saline) of the anesthetic is important since larger volumes of anesthetic are required to anesthetize the trunk than are required to numb smaller regions of the head and neck. Other donor sites include the inner thigh and buttocks; however, most individuals usually have enough adipose tissue in the trunk. Once the area is anesthetized, the entire abdomen and trunk is prepped and draped in a sterile fashion. Retrieval of autolo-

gous fat is performed with a 13- or 14-gauge needle attached to a 10-mL syringe using a modified Coleman technique [8]. This method provides gentle fat harvest in contrast to the liposuction cannula and closed suction, which have a tendency to fracture and damage fat cells. The fat is then placed in a centrifuge in a balanced fashion and spun for 10 min. The supernatant is then poured off and a dry gauze sponge is twisted and placed into the syringe to touch the top layer of fat and absorb the dead and fractured fat cells. Approximately 20 mL of fat need to be harvested to yield viable graft material. An 18-gauge needle is then attached to the syringe and the fat is injected in the desired area. The fat is injected in small parcels as the syringe is withdrawn from the tissue and is deposited in a grid-like pattern to ensure uniform distribution of the material. The donor site is closed in one layer with an absorbable suture in a horizontal mattress fashion. The recipient puncture site is closed with a drop of histoacryl glue or a small piece of sterile adhesive tape. The patient is warned before the procedure to expect bruising and swelling of both the donor and recipient site and that at least a second session will be required to achieve maximum results.

Other autologous and allogenic filling substances, with which we have less familiarity, include Isolagen (autologous fibroblasts harvested from 3 mm skin punch biopsy: Isolagen Laboratories, Paramus, NJ), Autologen (autologous dermal collagen obtained from intraoperative skin resection: Collagenesis, Inc., Beverly, MA), Dermalogen (pooled cadveric tissue composed of collagen, elastin, and glycosaminoglycans: Collagenesis, Inc., Beverly, MA), and Alloderm (acellular dermis obtained from banked homogenic skin: The Woodlands, TX).

Permanent Injectable Fillers: Artecoll, Dermalive, Silicone, Bio-Alcamid

Permanent injectable fillers have found significant demand in facial plastic surgery. One of the earliest permanent injectable fillers was liquid silicone which has since fallen out of favor due to the possible link between silicone breast implant leakage, siliconomas [9], and collagen vascular and other autoimmune diseases. In many communities, liquid injectable silicone is not available and is off the market. Liquid silicone is available in a variety of viscosities ranging from 300 to 10,000 centistokes with the latter being the most viscous. A rule of thumb: the higher the viscosity of the liquid silicone, the less migration of the product in the soft tissues. Using a 25-gauge needle, the silicone is injected in a linear pulse technique. Small aliquots of 0.1 mL are injected in a linear pattern, resembling a string of closely spaced pearls. A fibroblastic inflammatory reaction occurs around each silicone droplet, preventing product migration and resulting in a permanent effect.

Artecoll is one of the most commonly used injectable fillers in facial plastic surgery and was pioneered in Germany in the early 1990s [10]. It is U.S. Food and Drug Administration (FDA) approved for medical use under the name Artefill. Artecoll is composed of 0.3% lidocaine; 3.5% bovine collagen coupled to tiny beads of polymethacrylate (PMMA), each bead measuring 32–40 microns in diameter; buffers; and water. One milliliter of Artecoll contains roughly six million PMMA microspheres, with each PMMA microsphere being about 4–5 times the size of a human red blood cell. The mechanism of action of Artecoll takes advantage of the body's ability to encapsulate a foreign body with connective tissue. In essence, the bovine collagen acts as a transport medium for the PMMA beads. The collagen transport medium dissolves after it is introduced into the host. The PMMA microspheres remain separated in vivo and stimulate the host to deposit new native collagen around each microsphere. Encapsulation of the PMMA beads by the body's own collagen is usually complete in 2–3 months. Hence, there is a loss of volume between injection sessions as the bovine collagen dissipates and usually three to four injection sessions, 2–3 months apart, are required to achieve full correction.

The indications for Artecoll are similar to those of most injectable fillers with one exception. Indications for Artecoll include lip augmentation, correction of well-defined wrinkles and grooves, improvement of acne scars, and correction of contour defects. The fifth indication for Artecoll is the desire for permanent results. In fact, patient desire for a temporary correction or enhancement is a contraindication to Artecoll injection. Other contraindications to Artecoll include allergy to lidocaine or collagen, use of systemic steroids, immunosuppression, and known collagen vascular and/or autoimmune disease.

Injection technique is of paramount importance for successful use of Artecoll. Artecoll must be stored in a refrigerated environment and be slightly warmed to body temperature before use. To warm the Artecoll, the syringe of product may be gently rolled between the palms for several seconds. Traditionally, a 25-gauge needle is used to inject the product into the deep reticular dermis. Perhaps the most important technical point in Artecoll injection is ensuring the product is placed in the proper skin layer. Artecoll is best suited for injection in the deeper skin layers; in the case of the tear-trough deformity, Artecoll should be judiciously injected in the immediate supraperiosteal layer of the infraorbital soft tissue. Injecting Artecoll too superficially, for example in the papillary dermis, can result in unsightly blanching of the overlying skin and undesirable palpable nodules. A linear threading injection technique yields the most uniform results (Fig. 83.2).

Once the syringe of Artecoll has pierced the skin and is in the correct tissue plane, the syringe is slowly withdrawn while simultaneously injecting the Artecoll under constant pressure. Multiple passes are performed through the same puncture site in a fanning pattern to ensure even distribution of the product. The nondominant fingers are used to control the placement of the needle and product. Finally, once the injection is complete, the product is gently massaged within the tissue to ensure as smooth a contour as possible. The patient is warned that there will be slight redness and possibly swelling for the following 48 h in addition to the fact that 3–4 injections will be required in the future.

Artecoll has many advantages over other injectable fillers, particularly the long-lasting aesthetic effect it has on tissues. However, the use of Artecoll does carry some risks and potential complications. Firstly, success with Artecoll is extremely operator-dependent and, technically, Artecoll injection is unforgiving. For this reason, we usually do not recommend Arte-

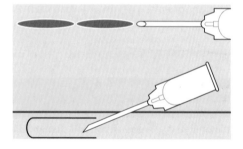

Fig. 83.2 The linear threading technique (*the lower cartoon*) is the preferred method injection as opposed to the microdroplet technique (*the upper cartoon*)

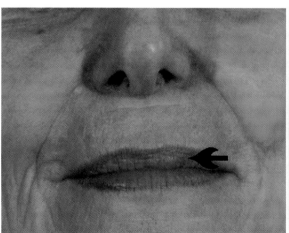
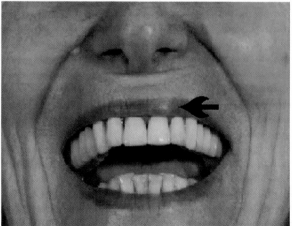

Fig. 83.3 An example of an Artecoll granuloma in the upper lip

83

coll to patients who are naïve about injectable fillers. We also do not recommend Artecoll to inexperienced injectors. Other risks associated with Artecoll include overcorrection, which is, fortunately, not common. Overcorrection and excessive injection of Artecoll is a difficult problem to fix; however, when required, needle aspiration and/or surgical excision may be performed. Patients may experience prolonged inflammation and in some cases, formation of telangiectasia which usually resolves in 6–9 months with watchful waiting. There have been incidences of hypertrophic and/or keloid scarring of the skin overlying the injected Artecoll and late-forming granulomas and nodules [11]. In these cases, local steroids and surgical excision and/or scar revision may be required. Improvement in the preparation technique of Artecoll, including washing the PMMA beads to remove electrostatically charged contaminants, has resulted in a decrease in granuloma formation. Nevertheless, there exists a 0.01% risk of granuloma formation (Fig. 83.3).

And finally, there is a risk of allergy and even anaphylaxis to one or several components of Artecoll. Indeed, one of the controversies surrounding Artecoll is whether or not skin testing must be performed prior to injection. If skin testing is chosen, intradermal skin testing must be performed at least 4 weeks prior to planned injection. Other areas of controversy concerning Artecoll include potential risk of transmission of bovine spongiform encephalitis (BSE) and other prion disease.

DermaLive and DermaDeep, products that are conceptually similar to Artecoll, are permanent injectable fillers that combine hyaluronic acid and 45–65-μm fragments of hydroxyethyl methacrylate and ethyl methacrylate, respectively. Dermalive is composed of acrylic microbeads coupled to hyaluronic acid gel in a buffered solution. The technique and indications for Dermalive are similar to those for Artecoll. However, because Dermalive does not contain a xenogenic component, no skin testing is required and thus is favored by many facial plastic surgeons. The side effect profile of this material includes palpable nodules, erythema and fibrosis, all of which can usually be treated by local steroid injection.

One of the newest permanent injectable fillers is Bio-Alcamid (Polymekon Research, Italy). Originally designed for soft tissue augmentation in HIV patients suffering from severe facial lipodystrophy, a side effect of the antiretroviral medications used to treat the disease [12], Bio-Alcamid is a nontoxic, nonabsorbable gel polymer composed of 4% alkyl-imide groups and 96% water [13]. Bio-Alcamid is a cohesive, radiolucent, elastic material that is non-water soluble. It does not contain any xenogenic components or proteins and as such it is nonallergenic. Bio-Alcamid is a large volume injectable filler and as such is indicated in the head and neck in areas such as the cheek hollows. In our practice, we have successfully injected the product into deep nasolabial groves, deep marionette lines and along the zygomatic arch. It is injected subcutaneously with a 14-, 16- or 18-gauge needle in a macro droplet technique; the product is injected in 0.5-mL aliquots before the needle is withdrawn from the tissues. Moreover, a larger aliquot size is preferred since smaller aliquots are less predictable. The product then becomes encapsulated by a thin (0.02 mm) collagen capsule [14], which prevents product migration and allows the injected filler to be identified and removed if necessary at a later date. In addition to the increased predictability of larger aliquots, aliquots greater than 0.5 milliliters are easier to identify and potentially alter or explant at a later date. In fact, once the filler is injected, it essentially acts as an endoprosthesis due to the nature of the collagen encapsulation. Bio-Alcamid is easily modified even after significant time has elapsed by simply evacuating excess product with a large-bore syringe once the implant has been identified (by palpation and chart consultation). Once encapsulated, the product feels soft and of the same consistency as normal adipose tissue.

Patients are empirically given prophylactic broad-spectrum antibiotics and postprocedure antibiotics for the following 5–7 days. In our practice, we have had no infections. An infection rate of 0.6% has been reported in the literature and has been attributed to staphylococcal infection [14]. The infections were treated with antibiotics; however, removal of the implant was required in each case. Other potential complications include asymmetry, overcorrection, prolonged swelling, and bruising (Figs. 83.4, 5).

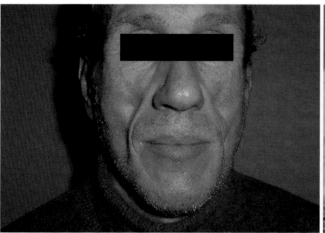
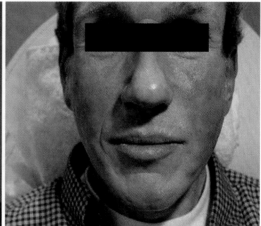

Fig. 83.4 Midface lipoatrophy improved by Bio-Alcamid injection

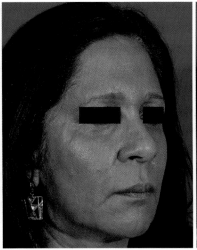
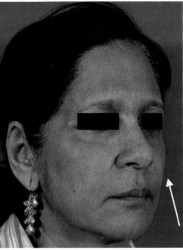

Fig. 83.5 Midface sag, a natural occurrence in the aging process is improved with Bio- Alcamid injection

Temporary Injectable Fillers: Perlane, Restylane, Restylane Fine Lines, Restylane Sub Q, Juvederm, Hyalform

Non-animal stabilized hyaluronic acid gel (Q-Med AB, Uppsala, Sweden) has proved to be an advantageous soft tissue injectable filler currently used worldwide, although not approved by the U.S. Food and Drug Administration (FDA). Hyaluronic acid (HA) is a glycosaminoglycan compound composed of alternating D-glucuronic acid and N-acetyl-D-glycosamine monosaccharide units. HA occurs naturally in the body in the extracellular dermal matrix of the skin, in the synovial fluid of joints, etc. It is avidly binds water (hygroscopic) to become very viscous and is highly biologically compatible. As it is a naturally occurring substance, no allergy testing is required and there is no risk of animal-protein disease transmission. Like collagen, HA is metabolized by the liver to carbon dioxide and water over a 3- to 6-month period, making HA an excellent but temporary injectable filling material.

All injections are done during routine office visits and require about 10–15 min. Patients can usually return to normal activity after the procedure. Immediately after injection, there is usually slight redness and swelling which resolves within several hours. Rarely is there bruising.

A variety of temporary injectable fillers based on stabilized HA gel have been in use for many years with good success. HA products are obtained through bacterial fermentation of a ubiquitous streptococcus line. The key to successful soft tissue augmentation and contour correction is understanding the dynamic interaction of different dermal tissue densities and the HA concentration within the specific filling material. Each dermal layer has a specific tissue density and each HA gel product has a specific particle size. For example, Perlane contains 8,000 particles per milliliter, Restylane contains 100,000 particles per milliliter, and Restylane Fine Lines contains 200,000 HA particles per milliliter. All three products contain the same concentration of HA (20 mg/mL) but contain different HA particle sizes. It is important to match the HA particle size with the density of the dermal layer. Larger particle HA, such as Perlane, must be injected in the deep dermis. Restylane Fine Lines, containing the smallest HA particle size, must be injected into the superficial papillary dermis, and Restylane, containing intermediate size HA particles, should be injected in a plane between the papillary and reticular dermis. All HA products are injected using the same technique. The linear threading technique is used with the nondominant fingers ascertaining and maintaining the correct needle position and injection plane. Injection of Restylane Fine Lines with a 30-gauge needle should result in mild blanching of the overlying epidermis as the product is injected into the superficial dermis. Injection of this small-particle HA in a deep plane will result in rapid dissipation and migration of the particles; in other words, in a deeper dermal layer, the small particles will just float away. Restylane Fine Lines is useful for filling fine rhytids of the lips and oral commissure and for crow's feet. On the other hand, injection of larger particle HA products should be at a deeper level and should not result in any blanching at all. Injecting these products in a superficial plane may result in scarring, nodularity, and a poor aesthetic result.

Restylane Sub Q is a newer version of non-animal stabilized hyaluronic acid with a concentration of 20 mg/mL. However, the Restylane Sub Q bead size is larger (2,000 µm) and the product offers increased volume and longevity with a safety profile similar to that of its shorter-acting relatives.

In our practice, we use extensively stabilized HA gels for soft tissue augmentation with rare complications and unwanted side effects. The most common complication we experience is undercorrection and/or asymmetry. On rare occasions, patients may experience prolonged redness and/or swelling, but these issues are self-limited and usually resolve over the course of days. There have been reports in the literature of cutaneous hypersensitivity to an impurity during the bacterial fermentation process [15]. There has also been a report of a sterile cyst

83

that developed after multiple injections [16]. The overall rate of adverse events, which is comprised mainly of hypersensitivity reactions, is 0.06% [17].

Juvederm 15 and Juvederm 30 (both INAMED Corporation) are HA gels with a concentration of 24 mg/mL. Juvederm 15 has a normal viscosity but has a smaller particle size and is appropriate for superficial injection. Juvederm 30 has a higher viscosity, larger particle size, and more stable cross-linking, causing it to have a longer half-life. It is injected in the deeper dermis.

Conclusion

In conclusion, the types and availability of different injectable fillers have increased dramatically over the past decades with newer and better fillers being developed constantly. It is imperative for a facial plastic surgeon to not only know what is available but also to understand the mechanism, indications, and contraindications for each product to ensure optimal aesthetic results and patient safety and satisfaction.

Tips to Avoid Complications

- Always aspirate prior to injecting any filler to avoid embolism.
- Skin test susceptible patients as indicated.
- Inject the appropriate filling agent into the appropriate skin layer.
- Understand fully the patient's desires and expectations.
- A thorough knowledge of skin anatomy and physiology is a prerequisite.

Take-Home Pearls

- For best results, use the nondominant hand to guide needle and product placement.
- For lip definition, inject into the red lip-white lip junction, just superior to the vermilion border.
- For lip augmentation, inject into the red-lip substance.

References

1. Haneke E (2004) Polymethyl methacrylate microspheres in collagen. Semin Cutan Med Surg 23:227–232
2. Laeschke K. (2004) Biocompatibility of microparticles into soft tissue fillers. Semin Cutan Med Surg 23:214–217
3. Lemperle G, Hazan-Gauthier N, Lemperle M. (1995) PMMA microspheres (Artecoll) for skin and soft tissue augmentation: Part II. Clinical investigations. Plast Reconstr Surg 96:627–634
4. Christensen L, Breiting V, Janssen M, Vuust J, Hogdall E (2005) Adverse reactions to injectable soft tissue permanent fillers. Aesthetic Plast Surg 29:34–48
5. Cheng JT, Perkins SW, Hamilton MM. (2002) Collagen and injectable fillers. Otolaryngol Clin North Am 35:73–85
6. Zimmerman US, Clerici TJ (2004) The histological aspects of fillers complications. Semin Cutan Med Surg 23:241–250
7. Hanke CW, Higley HR, Jolivette DM (1991) Abscess formation and local necrosis after treatment with Zyderm or Zyplast collagen implant. J Am Acad Dermatol 25:319–326
8. Coleman WP, Lawrence N, Sherman RN, Reed RJ, Pinski KS (1993) Autologous collagen? Lipocytic dermal augmentation: A histopathological study. J Dermatol Surg Oncol 19:1032
9. Austad ED (2002) Breast implant-related silicone granulomas: the literature and the litigation. Plast Reconstr Surg 109:1724–1730
10. Lemperle G, Ott H, Charrier U, Hecker J, Lemperle M (1991) PMMA microspheres for intradermal implantation: Part I. Animal research. Ann Plast Surg 26:57–63
11. Reisberger EM, Landthaler M, Wiest L, Schroder J, Stolz W (2003) Foreign body granulomas caused by polymethylmethacrylate microspheres. Arch Dermatol 139:17–20
12. Protopapa C, Sito G, Caporale D, Cammarota N (2003) Bio-Alcamid in drug-induced lipodystrophy. J Cosmet & Laser Ther 5:1–5
13. Pacini S, Ruggiero M, Cammarota N, Protopapa C, Gulisano M (2003) Bio-Alcamid, a novel prosthetic polymer, does not interfere with morphological and functional characteristics of human skin fibroblasts. Plast Reconstr Surg 111:489–491
14. Pacini S, Ruggiero M, Morucci G, Cammarota N, Protopapa C, Gulisano M (2002) Bio-Alcamid: A novelty for reconstructive and cosmetic surgery. Ital J Anat Embryol 107:209–214
15. Lupton JR, Alster TS (2000) Cutaneous hypersensitivity reaction to injectable hyaluronic acid gel. Dermatol Surg 26:135–137
16. Shafir R, Amir A, Gur E (2000) Long-term complications of facial injection with Restylane. Plast Reconstr Surg 106:1215–1216
17. Friedman PM, Mafong EA, Kauvar AN, Geronemus RG (2002) Safety data of injectable non-animal stabilized hyaluronic acid gel for soft tissue augmentation. Dermatol Surg 28:491–494

Chapter 84

Blepharoplasty

Stephen W. Perkins and Rami K. Batniji

84

Core Messages

- A thorough understanding of the eyelid anatomy is essential to both proper diagnosis and surgical planning.
- During the evaluation of the patient considering upper lid blepharoplasty, the forehead should be assessed for ptosis. The surgeon should also evaluate the upper lid to rule out blepharoptosis.
- Evaluation of both lower eyelid position and laxity is an essential component of the preoperative examination of the patient considering lower lid blepharoplasty.
- During lower lid blepharoplasty, conservative resection of skin and muscle as well as suspension of the orbicularis oculi muscle to the periosteum of the lateral orbital rim will maintain proper lower lid position.
- Dry eyes should be managed aggressively.

Contents

Introduction

Blepharoplasty remains one of the most common surgical procedures performed in facial plastic surgery for both men and women. Indeed, according to a survey of members of the American Academy of Facial Plastic and Reconstructive Surgery, blepharoplasty was the third most common cosmetic surgical procedure performed on the male patient in 2004, following hair restoration and rhinoplasty [1]. Whereas the initial motivation for the patient seeking surgery of the upper lids may be a functional defect, an interest in aesthetic improvement, or a combination of the two factors, it is an interest in aesthetic improvement that is the primary motivating factor for the patient considering lower lid surgery. In fact, it is not uncommon for a patient to present earlier in life wishing to address the "tired" look associated with age-related changes to the upper and/or lower lids. Upper and lower lid blepharoplasty will be reviewed in this chapter.

Relevant Surgical Anatomy of the Upper and Lower Lids

A thorough understanding of the eyelid anatomy is essential to both proper diagnosis and surgical planning. The upper and lower lids consist of three lamellae [1]. The anterior lamella consists of skin and pretarsal orbicularis oculi muscle. The middle lamella contains the orbital septum, which is an extension of the periosteum of the orbital rim. The posterior lamella consists of the tarsus and conjunctiva; the inferior retractor muscles are also found within the posterior lamella of the lower lid. Orbital fat is located posterior to the orbital septum and is compartmentalized: the upper lid consists of a medial (nasal) fat pocket and a middle fat pocket while the lower lid consists of lateral, central, and medial pockets with the inferior oblique muscle dividing the middle fat pocket from the medial fat pocket. In the upper lid, the lacrimal gland is a grayish structure and is found laterally.

The Aging Eyelid Complex

Progressive loss of organization of elastic fibers and collagen lead to dermatochalasis (loss of skin elasticity and subsequent excess laxity of lower eyelid skin) [1]. Additionally, the orbital septum weakens with age leading to steatoblepharon (pseudoherniation of orbital fat) [1]. Orbicularis oculi muscle hypertrophy is also associated with age-related changes of both the upper and lower eyelid complex [1]. In the lower lid, festoons may form as a manifestation of aging. Festoons are folds of orbicularis oculi muscle in the lower lid that hang in a hammock-like fashion from the medial to lateral canthi; festoons may contain protruding orbital fat. Malar mounds refer to skin and fat that bulge from the malar prominence. Age-related changes of the midface, such as ptosis and volume loss of the midfacial soft tissue, may contribute to the formation of malar mounds [1]. When ptosis and volume loss of the midfacial soft tissue occur in conjunction with pseudoherniation of orbital fat, a double convexity contour is noticeable and the nasojugal groove, or tear trough deformity, deepens [1].

Preoperative Assessment

History

During the consultation, one must assess the motivating factors that lead the patient to consider blepharoplasty. Typically, the patient is bothered by hooding of the upper lid and fullness of the lower lid, which make the patient appear tired and older; the patient seeking upper and/or lower lid blepharoplasty desires to achieve a younger and refreshed look about the eyes.

The preoperative assessment of the patient seeking rejuvenation of the upper and/or lower eyelid complex includes a history to evaluate for systemic disease processes, such as collagen vascular diseases and Grave's disease, dry eye symptoms,, and visual acuity changes. It is important to delineate whether the changes to the upper and/or lower lids are related to the age-related changes to the lids (dermatochalasis and steatoblepharon) or a manifestation of a systemic process, such as allergy or an endocrine disorder. For example, while a patient with Grave's disease may have upper lid retraction and exophthalmos, the myxedematous state of hypothyroidism may mimic dermatochalasis. Therefore, a screening thyroid stimulating hormone (TSH) level should be obtained if one suspects a thyroid disorder. As well, if any unusual history is gleaned from the preoperative assessment, it may be prudent to obtain an ophthalmologic evaluation prior to endeavoring upon blepharoplasty. Finally, it is important to discuss the limitations of blepharoplasty with the patient and the role of adjuvant procedures. For example, the patient seeking periorbital rejuvenation with significant crow's feet may benefit from botulinum toxin treatment while the patient demonstrating fine wrinkling, "crepe" paper skin may find significant improvement with skin resurfacing.

Physical Examination

The physical examination should include evaluation of the patient's skin, paying particular attention to the Fitzpatrick skin type and areas of previous scars to assess the patient's tendency for wound healing, pigment issues, hypertrophic scar, and keloid formation. Consider adjunctive treatments in patients demonstrating crow's feet and/or fine wrinkling of the skin.

Assess visual acuity and extraocular movements on all patients. A visual field test may be necessary for the individual with significant upper lid dermatochalasis resulting in a visual field defect; this individual would benefit from functional upper lid blepharoplasty. During the evaluation of the patient considering upper lid blepharoplasty, the forehead should be assessed for ptosis as this may confound the dermatochalasis seen in the upper lid. The surgeon should evaluate the upper lid to rule out blepharoptosis. The ideal position of the upper lid is at the level of the superior limbus. If unilateral blepharoptosis is identified, it behooves the surgeon to rule out blepharoptosis in the contralateral eye as Herring's Law may apply in this situation.

Pseudoherniation of orbital fat can be demonstrated on the direction of the patient's gaze. Gaze in the superior direction will accentuate the lower central and medial fat pockets, whereas superior gaze in the contralateral direction will accentuate the lateral pocket.

Evaluation of both lower eyelid position and laxity is an essential component to the preoperative examination. The ideal position of the lower eyelid margin is at the inferior limbus [1]. A snap test and lid distraction test are key components to the evaluation of lower eyelid laxity. A snap test is performed by grasping the lower eyelid and pulling it away from the globe. When the eyelid is released, the eyelid returns to its normal position quickly. However, in a patient with decreased lower eyelid tone, the eyelid returns back to its position more slowly. The lid distraction test is performed by grasping the lower eyelid with the thumb and index finger; movement of the lid margin greater than 10 mm demonstrates poor lid tone and a lid tightening procedure would be indicated. Finally, a Schirmer's test is indicated if there is concern for dry eye syndrome.

Upper Lid Blepharoplasty

It behooves the surgeon to be meticulous in the surgical markings for upper lid blepharoplasty prior to surgery as a difference of 1 to 3 millimeters (mm) from one lid to the next may create noticeable asymmetries. Therefore, the surgical markings for both upper lids are made using a fine tip marker and small calipers. With the patient looking up, the supratarsal crease is identified and measured from the lid margin using small calipers; this denotes the location of the inferior limb of the surgical marking. This measurement ranges from 8–12 mm (10–11 mm in females; 8–9 mm in males) (Fig. 84.1). The inferior limb of the marking is curved gently and parallels the lid margin; the inferior limb of the marking is carried medially to within 1–2 mm of the punctum and laterally to the lateral canthus. If the marking is carried along the curve of the lid crease lateral to the lateral canthus, the final closure scar line will bring the

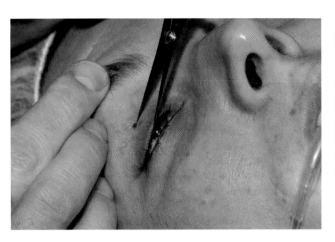

Fig. 84.1 The supratarsal crease is identified with the patient looking upward; the supratarsal crease is then measured from the lid margin using small calipers. This denotes the location of the inferior limb of the surgical marking and ranges between 8–12 mm

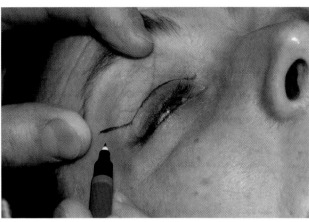

Fig. 84.2 The marking sweeps diagonally upward from the lateral canthus to the lateral eyebrow margin

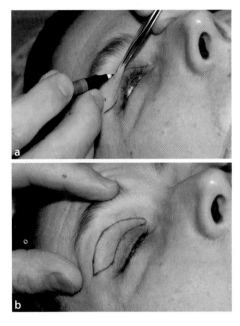

Fig. 84.3a,b The superior limb of the surgical marking is made. Smooth forceps are used to pinch the excess amount of upper eyelid skin so as to roll the lashes upward (a). The superior limb is connected with the inferior limb medially and laterally (b)

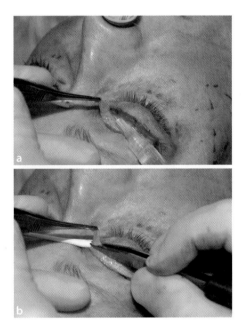

Fig. 84.4a,b A small opening is made in the orbital septum to access the middle and medial fat compartments. Gentle pressure on the globe demonstrates redundant fat from each compartment; forceps are used to grasp the herniated fat. Local anesthesia is infiltrated at the base of the herniated fat (a) and then the base is cauterized (b). Excision of the fat is then performed at the cauterized base

upper lid tissue downward, thus resulting in a hooded appearance. In an effort to avoid this unsightly result, the marking sweeps diagonally upward from the lateral canthus to the lateral eyebrow margin (Fig. 84.2). This modification of the lateral incision makes it easy for women to camouflage with makeup. Medially, the nasal-orbital depression should not be violated as an incision in this area may result in a webbed scar; ending the

incision medially within 1–2 mm of the punctum avoids this result. Next, the superior limb of the surgical marking is made. This is facilitated by a smooth forceps which is used to pinch the excess amount of upper eyelid skin so as to roll the lashes upward (Fig. 84.3). The surgeon's contralateral hand is used to reposition the eyebrow superiorly so as to isolate the perceived contribution of brow ptosis from upper lid dermatochalasis.

Alternatively, if the patient is planned for a forehead lift at the same time as the upper lid blepharoplasty, the surgeon may elect to perform the forehead lift first and then measure the appropriate amount of upper lid skin excision necessary to provide rejuvenation of the upper lid complex while minimizing the risk of lagopthalmos.

Typically, isolated upper lid blepharoplasty can be performed under local anesthesia with intravenous sedation. Two percent lidocaine with epinephrine (1:50,000) is infiltrated deep to skin but superficial to the orbicularis oculi muscle, thus minimizing the risk of ecchymosis caused by the injection of local anesthesia. Stabilization of the skin in the eyelid is paramount to making the "skin-only" incision of the upper eyelid; therefore, the help of an assistant is required to place tension on the skin. A round handled scalpel with a #15 Bard Parker blade is ideal for following the curves of the upper lid surgical markings. Once the skin incision is made, the skin is then sharply dissected from the underlying orbicularis oculi muscle with the blade or dissecting beveled scissors. The preseptal orbicularis oculi muscle is then evaluated. If it is atrophic or very thin, then the muscle need not be excised. However, most often, a thin strip of preseptal orbicularis oculi muscle is excised medially, thus exposing the fat compartments. If the muscle is robust, then the excision is performed along the entire length of the lid.

Attention is then directed to the pseudoherniation of orbital fat. A small opening is made in the orbital septum overlying the middle and medial fat compartments. Gentle pressure on the globe demonstrates redundant fat from each compartment. Using a Griffiths-Brown forceps, the herniated fat is grasped from its respective compartment and, unless the patient is under general anesthesia, the fat is infiltrated with local anesthesia to minimize discomfort associated with subsequent cautery and excision of the redundant fat (Fig. 84.4). Meticulous hemostasis is of utmost importance to not only maintain a clear operative field, but also minimize the risk of postoperative bleeding. Indeed, once fat removal is completed from both compartments, bipolar cautery is used to ensure hemostasis prior to closure.

The preferred technique for skin closure is as follows (Fig. 84.5): 7-0 blue polypropylene suture is used in an interrupted fashion to reapproximate the skin edges. While a 6-0 mild chromic or fast absorbing gut suture may create an inflammatory response and subsequent milia, a 7-0 size suture rarely produces milia. The upper lid blepharoplasty incision closure is then completed with a running 6-0 blue polypropylene in a subcuticular fashion with knots tied at the medial and lateral aspects of the incision (Fig. 84.6).

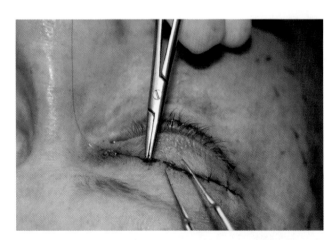

Fig. 84.5 Skin closure is performed with blue polypropylene sutures used in an interrupted fashion to reapproximate the skin edges; the remainder of the skin closure is performed with 6-0 blue polypropylene suture in a subcuticular fashion with knots tied at the medial and lateral ends

84

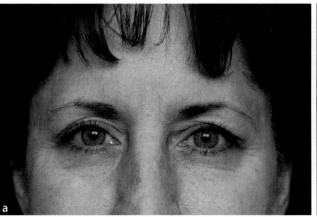
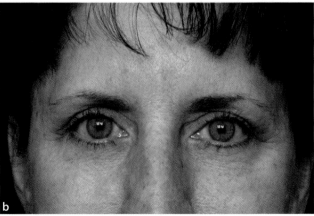

Fig. 84.6a,b An example of a patient before (a) and after (b) upper lid blepharoplasty

Lower Lid Blepharoplasty

Lower lid blepharoplasty may be performed via a transconjunctival or transcutaneous approach. Among the transcutaneous approaches, the skin-muscle flap is the most commonly used technique by the senior author (SWP). The indications for this technique include true vertical excess of lower eyelid skin, orbicularis oculi muscle hypertrophy, and presence of pseudoherniation of orbital fat. The incision is 2 mm inferior to the lower lid margin and extends from the lower punctum medially to a position 6 mm lateral to the lateral canthus; lateral extension of the incision to this position minimizes rounding of the canthal angle. Following the skin incision, fine curved scissors are used to dissect through the orbicularis muscle at the lateral aspect of the incision (Fig. 84.7a). Then, blunt scissors are positioned posterior to the muscle at the lateral aspect of the incision and,

with spreading motions of the blunt scissors, the skin-muscle flap is elevated off the orbital septum along an avascular plane (Fig. 84.7b). The subciliary incision is then completed using the scissors in a beveled manner to ensure the preservation of the pretarsal portion of the orbicularis oculi muscle, thus minimizing the risk of postoperative lower lid malposition. Small openings are made in the orbital septum to obtain access to the orbital fat compartments. Gentle palpation of the globe results in herniation of orbital fat through the aforementioned openings of the orbital septum. Bipolar cautery is used to cauterize the fat pad prior to excision; prior to cauterization, local anesthesia is infiltrated in the fat pocket to minimize pain. This procedure is performed for the lateral, middle, and medial fat pockets. Gentle palpation of the globe following resection of orbital fat allows for reassessment of orbital fat. A conservative approach to fat resection is maintained to avoid the creation of a sunken

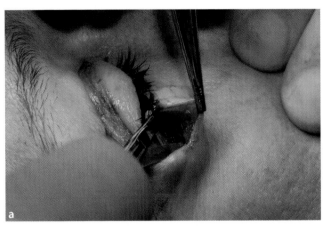
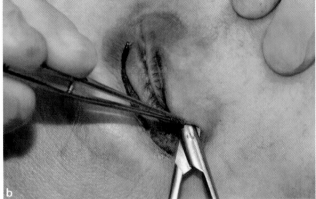

Fig. 84.7 **a** The incision is 2 mm inferior to the lower lid margin and extends from the lower punctum medially to a position 6 mm lateral to the lateral canthus. Following the skin incision, fine curved scissors are used to dissect through the orbicularis muscle at the lateral aspect of the incision, thus exposing the orbital septum. **b** Outwardly-beveled blunt scissors are introduced posterior to the muscle at the lateral aspect of the incision and, with spreading motions of the blunt scissors, the skin-muscle flap is effectively elevated off the orbital septum along an avascular plane to the level of the inferior orbital rim inferiorly and the incision superiorly

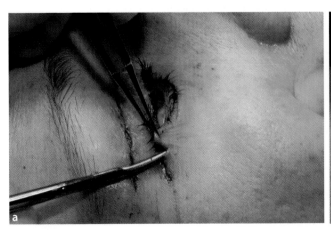
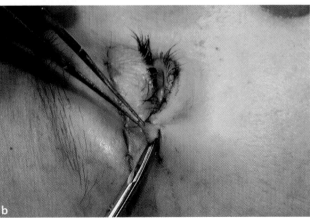

Fig. 84.8 **a** Maximal stretch effect is achieved by single-finger pressure at the inferomedial portion of the melolabial mound. Then, an inferiorly-directed segmental cut is made at the lateral canthus to determine the amount of excess skin and muscle to excise. A tacking suture is placed to maintain the position of the skin-muscle flap. **b** The overlapping skin and muscle are excised. Conservative resection will decrease the incidence of postoperative lower eyelid malposition **c** *see next page*

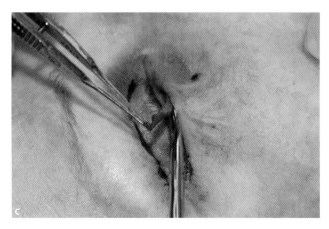

Fig. 84.8 (*continued*) **c** If orbicularis oculi muscle hypertrophy is evident, an additional 1- to 2-mm strip of muscle is resected to prevent overlapping of muscle and ridge formation with closure of the subciliary incision

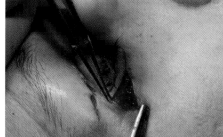
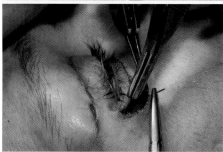
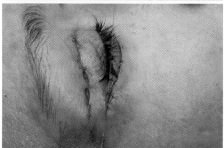
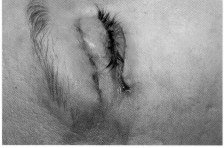

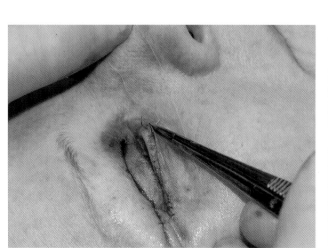

Fig. 84.10 The subciliary incision is closed with 7-0 blue polypropylene suture at the lateral canthus in a simple, interrupted fashion; the remainder of the incision is closed with 6-0 mild chromic suture in a running fashion

Fig. 84.9 Suspension of the orbicularis oculi muscle to the periosteum of the lateral orbital rim at the tubercle with 5-0 polyplyconate (Maxon) maintains proper lid position

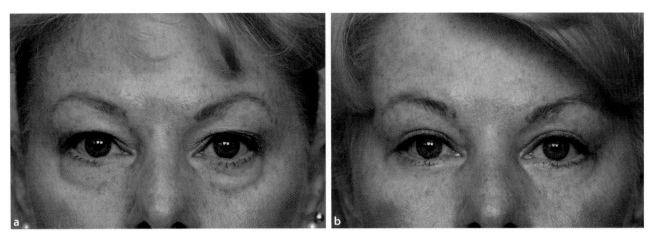

Fig. 84.11a,b Preoperative (**a**) and postoperative (**b**) photographs following transcutaneous lower blepharoplasty

appearance. Then, the skin-muscle flap is repositioned. If mildly sedated, the patient is asked to open their mouth and look up; this maneuver allows for maximal separation of wound edges and subsequent conservative resection of skin and muscle. On the other hand, if the patient is completely sedated, single-finger pressure at the inferomedial portion of the melolabial mound will create the same maximal stretch effect. Following this, an inferiorly directed segmental cut is made at the lateral canthus to determine the amount of excess skin to excise (Fig. 84.8a). A tacking suture is placed to maintain the position of the skin-muscle flap; eyelid scissors are then used to excise the overlapping skin (Fig. 84.8b). If orbicularis oculi muscle hypertrophy is evident, a 1- to 2-mm strip of muscle is resected to prevent overlapping of muscle and ridge formation with closure of the subciliary incision (Fig. 84.8c). Conservative resection of both

skin and muscle will decrease the incidence of postoperative lower eyelid malposition. Additionally, suspension of the orbicularis oculi muscle to the periosteum of the lateral orbital rim will assist in maintaining proper lid position (Fig. 84.9). If there is evidence of festoons or malar mounds, an extended lower lid blepharoplasty is performed inferior to the infraorbital rim; the redundant orbicularis oculi muscle and/or malar mounds are addressed by advancing the entire skin-muscle flap and suborbicularis oculi fat (SOOF) unit superior-laterally [1]. Following muscle suspension, the subciliary incision is closed (Fig. 84.10) with 7-0 blue polypropylene suture at the lateral canthus in a simple, interrupted fashion; the remainder of the incision is closed with 6-0 mild chromic suture in a running fashion (Fig. 84.11).

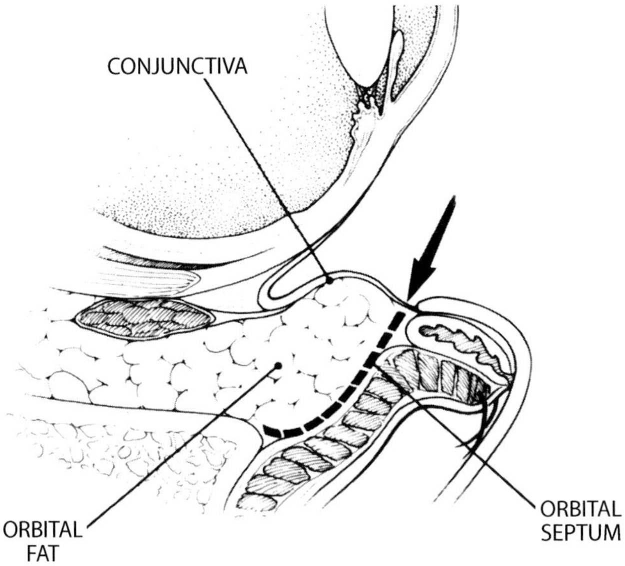

Compared to the transconjunctival approach, the transcutaneous approach affords the ability to correct true vertical excess of lower lid skin and orbicularis oculi hypertrophy. However, there are specific indications for the transconjunctival approach [1]. For example, young patients with excellent elasticity, presence of hereditary pseudoherniation of orbital fat, and no evidence of skin excess are ideally suited for the transconjunctival approach. Additionally, patients with Fitzpatrick skin types V–VI may benefit from the transconjunctival approach as the transcutaneous lower lid blepharoplasty scar may depigment in these patients. Finally, the transconjunctival approach results in transection and release of the inferior retractor muscles, thus allowing for a temporary rise in the lower lid position. This fact makes the transconjunctival approach an ideal procedure for secondary lower lid blepharoplasty [1]. During transconjunctival blepharoplasty, a preseptal approach via an incision located

CONJUNCTIVA

ORBITAL
FAT

ORBITAL
SEPTUM

Fig. 84.12 The preseptal approach to the transconjunctival blepharoplasty utilizes an incision located inferior to the tarsus and not deep to the inferior fornix, thus allowing for a more anterior to posterior approach to the fat pockets [1]

inferior to the tarsus and not deep in the inferior fornix; this allows for a more anterior to posterior approach to the fat pockets (Fig. 84.12) [2].

Postoperative Course

Immediately following surgery, ointment (antibiotic/steroid ophthalmic) is applied to the eye and the suture lines. Cold compresses are applied in the recovery room and the patient is instructed to apply the cold compresses until the second postoperative day as swelling occurs during this time. To that end, head of bed elevation is important as this also minimizes postoperative swelling.

Postoperative swelling may interfere with normal tear production and flow. Indeed, epiphora may result. In order to minimize the risk of dry eye, it is imperative to instruct the patient of the importance of the routine use of artificial tears throughout the day and an ointment in the evenings. The ointment is applied to the suture lines on a regular basis throughout the day as well.

The patient is instructed to restrain from physical activity for the first 48 h and is encouraged to avoid any form of heavy lifting, bending, or straining for 2 weeks postoperatively to minimize the risk of hematoma formation.

The medial knot of the upper lid subcuticular suture is removed on the first postoperative day. However, the subcuticular suture remains in place until 1 week postoperatively, when all sutures are removed. At that time, the patient is provided with a makeup consultation by the esthetician to allow for cosmetic camouflage and makeup application.

Complications of Blepharoplasty

Dry Eyes

As previously mentioned, postoperative edema interferes with normal tear flow. The astute surgeon should identify the signs and symptoms of dry eye; these include a dry or scratchy sensation to the eye, epiphora, and presence of conjunctival bleb. If identified early and managed aggressively, one will avoid the problem of exposure keratitis. First, the patient is educated with respect to the issue at hand as some patients may find it difficult to comprehend that the eye is dry when they are experiencing copious amounts of epiphora. Second, the generous and frequent use of artificial tears throughout the day and ointment in the evenings is re-emphasized. One may consider transitioning to a more viscous artificial tear product in those individuals demonstrating a conjunctival bleb. If the conjunctival bleb is persistent and/or quite prominent, other maneuvers such as placement of a Frost suture or taping of the lower eyelid may be of benefit.

Hematoma

Hematomas after blepharoplasty may range from a small collection under the suture line that is self-limiting to an expanding hematoma that may extend into the retrobulbar space. The incidence of hematomas is lowered by a thorough history prior to surgery. A review of medications is essential; one must not only inquire about such medications as aspirin and ibuprofen, but also herbal medications which may increase the risk of postoperative hematoma. Meticulous hemostasis intraoperatively with bipolar cautery also minimizes the risk of hematoma. Additional maneuvers that will minimize the risk of hematoma include control of the blood pressure both intraoperatively and perioperatively, head of bed elevation, application of cold compresses, and aggressive treatment of postoperative nausea with antiemetic medication.

Most hematomas are self-limiting. However, organization of the hematoma beneath the skin may present as an indurated mass beneath the skin and subsequently form into a thickened scar. Therefore, treatment with steroid injection may be required. Although rare, a retrobulbar hemorrhage is an emergency as there is an undeniable risk of blindness associated

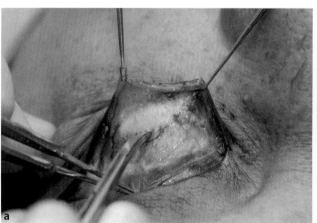
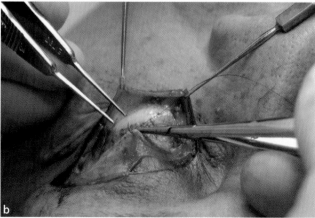

Fig. 84.13a–c Blepharoptosis repair. Intraoperative evaluation demonstrates intraoperative dehiscence of the levator muscle (**a**). Subsequently, 7-0 silk sutures are used in a mattress fashion to reapproximate the levator aponeurosis to the upper tarsal border (**b, c**) **c** *see next page*

with the increased pressures that result in either retinal artery occlusion or ischemic optic neuropathy. A lateral canthotomy with inferior cantholysis performed immediately will alleviate the pressure. As well, an ophthalmologic consultation should be requested.

Adjunctive Procedures

Repair of Upper Lid Blepharoptosis

Repair of upper lid blepharoptosis is possible during upper lid blepharoplasty; the upper lid blepharoplasty is performed first in the standard manner with excision of redundant skin and prolapsed fat.

Following this, the orbital septum is opened in a horizontal fashion and then retracted inferiorly with single hook retractors. This exposes the preaponeurotic fat, which is then resected or retracted to expose the entire levator aponeurosis up to Whitnall's ligament and down to the anterior face of the tarsus. Intraoperative evaluation confirms the etiology of blepharoptosis, which is typically levator dehiscence or separation (Fig. 84.13a). Preoperative photographs are reviewed to confirm the location and extent of the blepharoptosis. Subsequently, 7-0 silk is used to suture the levator aponeurosis to the upper tarsal border in a mattress fashion (Fig. 84.13b, c). Care is taken to make sure the suture is not exposed through the conjunctiva. The suture is tightened to achieve the appropriate position of the upper lid. If needed, multiple mattress sutures are placed.

The incision is then closed as in a standard upper lid blepharoplasty.

Fat Transposition

Many methods have been utilized to efface the tear trough deformity including fat grafts, injections with fat or injectable fillers [1], alloplastic implants [1], and transposition of pedicled orbital fat over the orbital rim [1]. Fat transposition via a transcutaneous approach in conjunction with lower lid blepharoplasty is the preferred method of addressing a tear trough deformity. Preoperatively, the tear trough deformity is marked out with a pen. Lower lid blepharoplasty with extension below the infraorbital rim is performed. Once the orbital fat from the medial pocket is isolated from the orbital septum, it is transposed

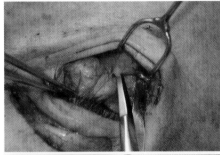
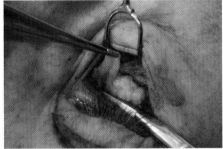
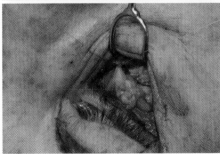

Fig. 84.14 Fat transposition. A pocket is created posterior to the orbicularis oculi muscle but anterior to the periosteum. The medial fat pocket is released from the surrounding orbital septum and subsequently sutured over the infraorbital rim into the previously made pocket with 6-0 polyglycolic acid (Dexon)

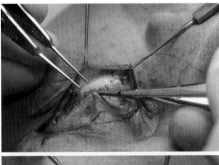
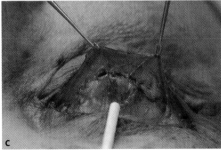

Fig. 84.13a–c (*continued*) Blepharoptosis repair.. Subsequently, 7-0 silk sutures are used in a mattress fashion to reapproximate the levator aponeurosis to the upper tarsal border (**b, c**)

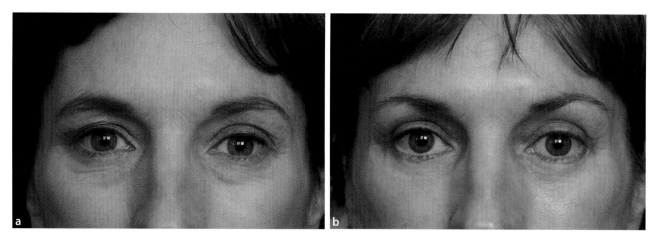

Fig. 84.15a,b Preoperative (**a**) and postoperative (**b**) photographs demonstrating effacement of the tear trough deformity following transcutaneous lower lid blepharoplasty with fat transposition

over the orbital rim and positioned into a pocket posterior to the orbicularis oculi muscle and anterior to the periosteum to efface the tear trough deformity. The transposed orbital fat is then secured to the periosteum using interrupted 6-0 polyglycolic acid (Dexon) sutures (Fig. 84.14). The contour of the orbital fat is then softened with the use of bipolar cautery. Subsequently, the lower lid blepharoplasty is completed as previously described (Fig. 84.15).

Lateral Canthoplasty

Several intraoperative maneuvers will minimize postoperative lower lid malposition during lower lid blepharoplasty, such as preservation of the pretarsal orbicularis oculi muscle, conservative resection of skin and muscle, and suspension of the orbicularis oculi muscle to the periosteum of the lateral orbital rim. If the lower lid demonstrates malposition or poor tone preoperatively, then a lateral canthoplasty is performed in conjunc-

tion with lower lid blepharoplasty. Following lateral canthotomy and inferior cantholysis, the tarsus is dissected from the skin, muscle, and conjunctiva. The tarsal strip is then attached using permanent suture to the medial aspect of the lateral orbital rim

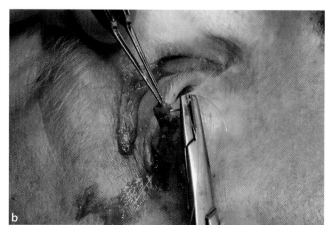

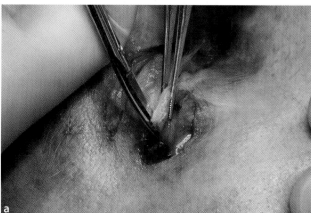
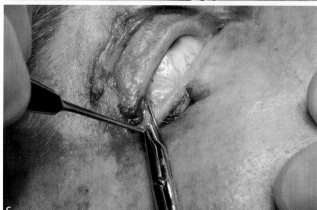

Fig. 84.16 a–c Lateral canthoplasty. Following lateral canthotomy and lateral cantholysis, the tarsus is separated anteriorly from the skin and orbicularis oculi muscle and posteriorly from the conjunctiva. 5-0 polypropylene (Prolene, usually clear) is passed through the periosteum of the medial aspect of the lateral orbital rim in a postero-superior position (**a**) and the tarsus (**b**) to improve lid position and support (**c**)

periosteum in a postero-superior position. Then, the appropriate amount of lower lid is excised (Fig. 84.16a–c).

Skin Resurfacing

Lower lid blepharoplasty cannot effectively efface periorbital fine wrinkling of skin. Therefore, skin resurfacing can be performed in conjunction with lower lid blepharoplasty. However, vertical contracture of the lower eyelid may occur following blepharoplasty and result in lower lid malposition. Additionally, skin resurfacing may result in skin tightening of the lower eyelid and subsequent ectropion. Therefore, it is essential to evaluate both lid position and lid support prior to performing skin resurfacing in conjunction with lower lid blepharoplasty and consider canthoplasty if the lower eyelid demonstrates malposition and/or poor support.

Ideal candidates for skin resurfacing of the lower eyelid include patients with Fitzpatrick skin types I–III. An 88% phenol peel or CO_2 laser resurfacing for the lower lid skin is the preferred method of skin resurfacing and are safely performed in conjunction with the transcutaneous blepharoplasty. However, as previously discussed, one should consider performing a lateral canthoplasty if the lower eyelid demonstrates malposition and/or poor support.

Conclusions

Rejuvenation of the lower eyelid complex in the male patient requires proper preoperative evaluation. In doing so, the facial plastic surgeon can select the proper treatment modality. Blepharoplasty performed in conjunction with fat transposition, canthoplasty, and/or skin resurfacing can result in a less tired, more youthful appearance of the lower eyelid complex.

Acknowledgment

The authors would like to acknowledge Nancy A. Rothrock for her assistance in the preparation of digital images used in this manuscript.

References

1. American Academy of Facial Plastic and Reconstructive Surgery (2004) Membership Survey
2. Verity DH, Collin JR (2004) Eyelid reconstruction: State of the art. Curr Opin Otolaryngol Head Neck Surg 12:344–348
3. Friedman O (2005) Changes associated with the aging face. Facial Plast Surg Clin North Am 13:371–380
4. Rankin BS, Arden RC, Crumley AL (2002) Lower eyelid blepharoplasty. In: Papel ID (ed) Facial plastic and reconstructive surgery, 2nd edn. Thieme, New York, pp 196–207
5. Bernardi C, Dura S, Amata PL (1998) Treatment of orbicularis oculi muscle hypertrophy in lower lid blepharoplasty. Aesthetic Plast Surg 5:349–351
6. Mendelson BC, Muzaffar AR, Adams WP (2002) Surgical anatomy of the midcheek and malar mounds. Plast Reconstr Surg 110:885–896
7. Kawamoto HK, Bradley JP (2003) The tear trough procedure: Transconjunctival repositioning of orbital unipedicled fat. Plast Reconstr Surg 112:1903–1907
8. Moses JL (1995) Blepharoplasty: Cosmetic and functional. In: McCord CD, Tantenbaum M, Nunery W (eds) Oculoplastic surgery, 3rd edn. Raven Press, New York, pp 285–318
9. Becker FF, Deutsch BD (1995) Extended lower lid blepharoplasty. Facial Plast Surg Clin North Am 3:189–194
10. Perkins SW (1995) Transconjunctival lower lid blepharoplasty. Facial Plast Surg Clin North Am 3:175–187
11. Fedok FG, Perkins SW (1996) Transconjunctival blepharoplasty. Facial Plast Surg 12:185–195
12. Perkins SW, Dyer WK, Simo F (1994) Transconjunctival approach to lower eyelid blepharoplasty: Experience, indications, and techniques in 300 patients. Arch Otolaryngol 120:172–177
13. Kane MA (2005) Treatment of tear trough deformity and lower lid bowing with injectable hyaluronic acid. Aesthetic Plast Surg 29:363–367
14. Flowers RS (1993) Tear trough implants for correction of tear trough deformity. Clin Plast Surg 20:403–415
15. Goldberg RA (2000) Transconjunctival orbital fat repositioning: Transposition of orbital fat pedicles into a subperiosteal pocket. Plast Reconstr Surg 105:743–748
16. Perkins SW, Latorre RC (2000) Blepharoplasty. In: Romo T, Millman AL (eds) Aesthetic facial plastic surgery. Thieme, New York, pp 262–287

Chapter 85

Rhytidectomy

Jon B. Chadwell and Devinder S. Mangat

Core Messages

- Realistic goals and appropriate patient selection are paramount to the success of facelift surgery.
- Detailed preoperative evaluation of the patient's past medical history, medication list, and psychosocial history will go a long way to avoiding postoperative complications and achieving the patient's goals.

Contents

Introduction

Rhytidectomy is one of the most common cosmetic procedures performed. With advances in technique and training, rhytidectomy is no longer viewed as a radical operation as it was at the turn of the century. As evidenced by the "baby boomer" generation, people no longer want to look their age; rather they want to look as young as they feel. There used to be a "secretive" and negative connotation attached to cosmetic surgery and something considered only by the wealthy elite. As a result of media coverage and television shows in this youth-oriented society, cosmetic surgery has become much more mainstream and available to people from all walks of life. People that have careers where appearance is a priority will benefit from facial rejuvenation surgery and sometimes use it as an advantage in a competitive work environment.

Cosmetic surgery, however, is not a panacea for the aging process. Rhytidectomy is performed to rejuvenate the sagging face, but aging still continues regardless. The keys to successful cosmetic surgery are careful selection of patients, a thorough facial analysis, and appropriate selection of an operative procedure. It is important for prospective patients to realize that even though significant improvements can be achieved there are always certain risks and limitations associated with the face-lift procedure.

This chapter will discuss one approach to face-lift surgery beginning with the preoperative evaluation through the complete postoperative period. Clearly, this is not a comprehensive review of rhytidectomy, but it is one approach that has worked well for the senior author for over 26 years.

History

European surgeons are credited with pioneering the rhytidectomy in the early 20th century. Eugene Hollander from Berlin published the first description of the face-lift operation in 1912. He wrote about a procedure that eliminated sagging cheeks by doing fusiform excisions in pre- and postauricular areas. However, Eric Lexar may have actually performed the first operation to remove wrinkles in 1906. Cosmetic surgery at this time was

85

practiced in secrecy, and the practitioners were not interested in sharing ideas. As a result, the procedure remained nothing more than a subcutaneous dissection with skin excision for another half of a century. Prior to the early 1970s, the face-lift procedure consisted of raising a skin flap and performing a skin tightening only which did not produce long-term results and was frequently associated with wide unsightly scars.

It was not until 1975 that Skoog wrote about subfascial dissection [10]. Metz and Peyronnie are credited with describing this fascial layer as the superficial musculoaponeurotic system (SMAS) [6]. This served as one of the biggest developments in face-lift surgery since the early descriptions of the procedure itself. By understanding the SMAS, rhytidectomy outcomes were improved and long-lasting results were achieved.

It was not until the 1960s and 1970s that the blanket of secrecy and shame that was associated with cosmetic surgery was lifted, allowing communication and education about the procedure to occur more freely. As a result, techniques improved, as did the results. In the past 20 years the procedure has become mainstream, and it continues to evolve with some that are technically complex and others that are less invasive.

Patient Evaluation

Consultation

Contact with a prospective cosmetic surgical patient begins long before consultation with the physician. Initial interaction often begins with a phone inquiry about a consultation with the facial plastic surgeon. At this time, it is imperative that the individual taking the call be pleasant and informative. Although this is not a substitute for consultation with the physician, he or she should be capable of detailing what the practice has to offer, describe procedures and postoperative expectations in general terms, and quote approximate fees that are in a comparable range for the community. This is information that is often requested during the initial contact. Being able to provide it not only educates the patient but also empowers the patient to have the confidence to schedule the consultation.

Upon scheduling a consultation a packet of information should be sent to the patient. The packet should include a physician background brochure, a preconsultation medical questionnaire, brochures describing the procedures for which the patient scheduled the consultation, and a letter detailing the process and thanking them for scheduling a consultation. By including this information the consultation will be more efficient and informative for both parties, and a well-informed patient usually results in a happy patient.

The consultation is an opportunity for a prospective surgical patient to interact with key members of the staff, visit the facility, and meet the surgeon. This time should be unhurried, personal, and private. During the consultation the surgeon should develop a rapport with the patient and determine the patient's motivation for seeking improvement in their appearance. A detailed history should be obtained in addition to a head, neck, and facial examination. Following this, reasonable recommendations can be made and realistic expectations can be described to the patient.

Facial photography is an integral part of the consultation. Standard views for face-lift surgery include frontal, right and left oblique, and right and left lateral. Close ups can also be taken of the platysmal banding, the ears, and perioral rhytids. With the use of digital photography and modern imaging software, expected changes in the patient's appearance can be visually demonstrated to the patient. These photos can also be used to illustrate any facial asymmetries that are present preoperatively and will probably be present postoperatively. Incision placement can also be shown on these photos.

General Health

Given that this is purely elective surgery, all organ systems should be functioning satisfactorily. Preoperatively, the patient should have a physical examination by the surgeon or the primary care physician. In patients over the age of 50, a routine EKG is obtained and a chest x-ray is requested when the patient has a history of smoking or lung disease. Laboratory studies are ordered only as indicated following history and physical examination.

Review of Systems

The preconsultation medical questionnaire is a valuable tool to identify the presence of medical conditions that may preclude the patient from undergoing rhytidectomy. Cardiovascular disease is not a contraindication to surgery; however, the patient will need to be evaluated by their cardiologist and cleared for surgery. The single most important variable in the preoperative medical evaluation of potential rhytidectomy patient is the status of their blood pressure. Uncontrolled hypertension, in our opinion, is an absolute contraindication to performing face-lift surgery. Hypertension significantly increases the dreaded risk of hematoma formation and a less than ideal result. Diabetes and autoimmune disease are not absolute contraindications to surgery, unless they are advanced or uncontrolled. Patients with a history of easy bleeding or bruising, especially with previous surgery, should undergo coagulation studies. Renal and kidney disease are also important to recognize preoperatively. How well a person healed following any previous surgery is usually a good measure of the patient's ability to heal. It is obviously important to know if the patient has had previous cosmetic surgery. An individual who has had multiple prior cosmetic procedures especially by multiple physicians may not be a good surgical candidate. Obesity is not a contraindication to surgery, but the results may be disappointing. Encouraging a patient to lose weight prior to surgery will ultimately lead to a happier patient. If the patient is actively dieting or planning significant weight loss, then surgery should be delayed until this is complete.

Social History

Smoking is not an absolute contraindication to surgery but will definitely influence the planned procedure. An individual who smokes more than one pack per day is a poor candidate for face-lift surgery. Up to a one pack per day smoker should be encouraged to cut down or stop smoking for 1 month prior to surgery and should have a more conservative procedure with a "shorter" flap and no tension on the skin flap.

Medications

A history of aspirin, nonsteroidal anti-inflammatory, or other anticoagulant use should be elicited, because these medications need to be discontinued 2 weeks prior to rhytidectomy. We prohibit the use of antidepressants or any herbal supplements for 2 weeks prior to surgery because these agents cause excessive intraoperative bleeding. Use of isotretinoin, chronic steroids, and other immune suppressing agents is a relative contraindication to face-lift. Allergies to medications used for surgery and postoperatively should be noted and addressed preoperatively.

Emotional Health

Prospective surgical patients should be emotionally stable prior to surgery. If the patient is currently under significant emotional stress, surgery should be delayed until their situation stabilizes. If the patient has a history of mental illness, clearance from the managing therapist should be sought prior to surgery. It is important to very carefully evaluate patients during the consultation and identify the uncommon but very real individual with "Body Dysmorphic Disorder" [9]. These patients should not be candidates for surgery until they have undergone psychiatric evaluation and treatment.

Facial Analysis and Patient Selection

The aging process brings about very specific changes in the skin and soft tissues of the face and it is important to identify these in order to render the correct treatment. With aging the face loses volume, the skin thins, and the tissues begin to sag. Rejuvenative facial surgery is directed at reversing these changes. Rhytidectomy removes excess skin in addition to repositioning and tightening the soft tissues of the cheeks and neck. Understanding the limitations of the procedure and selecting appropriate patients is the key to successful rhytidectomy, and this is accomplished with accurate facial analysis.

Ideal anatomic candidates demonstrate good skin tone, minimal photodamage, few fine wrinkles, a strong chin, shallow melolabial folds, good facial bony structure, and a high cervicomental angle. Patients that are poor candidates for rhytidectomy exhibit heavy, inelastic skin, significant actinic damage, fine wrinkling, deep melolabial folds, a low hyoid position, receded mandible, and low submandibular glands. During the consultation, facial analysis must be undertaken to adequately address the above-mentioned areas. The results should be shared with the patient to provide the best insight into what the expected outcomes will be and what limitations their anatomical factors present.

Facial analysis for rhytidectomy should be systematic and detailed including all aspects of the face.

1) Skin – Fitzpatrick type, actinic damage, rhytids, the presence and amount of adipose, elasticity and texture of the skin
2) Hair – hairlines, quantity, texture, style
3) Soft Tissue – depth of melolabial folds, presence jowling, amount of submental fat (subplatysmal and subcutaneous), malar mounds, submandibular gland position
4) Muscle – platysmal banding
5) Bone – position of chin, hyoid, and malar eminences

Following thorough facial analysis, recommendations can be made to the patient whether there may be alternative procedures to rhytidectomy, additional procedures to rhytidectomy, or no procedures at all. Any recommendations need to be tempered with the patient's goals and expectations. Computer imaging often can be used to demonstrate expected results, or the changes can simply be demonstrated in front of a three-way mirror by manipulating the tissues into the anticipated postoperative position. At this time the location of incisions can be shown to the patient, and the typical postoperative course and potential risks of the procedure can be explained to the patient.

Realistic goals are paramount to the success of cosmetic surgery. Helping the patient understand that the procedure simply serves to remove excess skin, reposition jowling, recreate the neckline, and to a lesser degree efface deep creases like the melolabial fold, will go a long way to achieving patient satisfaction. Patients with unreasonable expectations or misguided motivations need to be identified during consultation. These patients may simply need to be redirected and educated about what reasonable expectations are. However, if this cannot be accomplished, they should not be considered to be good surgical candidates. On the other hand, patients seeking surgery to achieve a natural rejuvenated appearance, improve self esteem, and ones that are not motivated by others are likely to be happy with the outcomes. Beware of the patient that brings photographs of models and is striving for perfection.

If there are factors that may affect the result but don't preclude the procedure from being done, then the patient should be made aware of these. For example, patients with diabetes or a history of smoking may require shorter flaps. Obese patients may not achieve as sculpted a resulted because of excessive facial adipose tissue and inelastic tissues.

Anatomic Considerations

A detailed understanding of the anatomy of the face and neck are prerequisites for performing safe and effective rejuvenative surgery of the face and neck. The skin, muscles of facial expression, SMAS, and nerves are the key anatomic components of the face and neck.

Skin

Rhytidosis, adiposity, elasticity, and quantity of skin all factor into the evaluation for rhytidectomy. The development of rhtyids is multifactorial. Rhytids differ in character ranging from etched lines, like "crow's feet" or "smoker's lines," to deep folds, like the melolabial folds or infracommisural folds (drool lines),

85

and their treatment may varies from skin resurfacing to soft tissue augmentation. Excessive facial adiposity contributes to facial fullness and roundness which can be difficult to remedy. With respect to rhytidectomy significant amounts of adipose tissue can cause less than optimal results. Elasticity of the skin correlates with the amount of lift that can be obtained; therefore, rhytidectomy performed in very inelastic skin achieves an overall poorer result. Rhytidectomy addresses excess skin very effectively when combined with SMAS suspension.

Muscles of Facial Expression

There are twenty-four paired muscles in the face that contract to produce facial expression. These muscles, in conjunction with the loss of skin elasticity, subcutaneous fat atrophy, and sun exposure lead to formation of rhytids. The lines of facial expression run perpendicular to the orientation of the facial muscles. Chemodenervation (Botox) is one way to alleviate the contribution of muscle contraction to rhytid formation. The forehead muscles and platysma are really the only facial muscles which can be altered surgically. Approaching other facial muscles and altering them is not something that is recommended or safe.

The platysma is a thin, paired muscle that extends from the lower face to the upper chest and over the lateral aspect of the neck. It is typically deficient in the anterior 3–5 cm of the central neck. Because of this deficiency, platysmal banding and the "turkey gobbler" deformity can develop. However, the "turkey gobbler" can result from excessive skin, fat, and is usually caused by a low hyoid. A thorough physical examination should be used to determine the cause of this deformity. A "turkey gobbler" deformity is frequently present in combination with a weak, receding chin. The use of a chin implant, in this case, will dramatically improve the result of the rhytidectomy. The need for a chin implant during a rhytidectomy usually has to be recommended by the physician since the patients are not aware of this deficiency.

SMAS

The superficial muscular aponeurotic system (SMAS) is a fibrous tissue layer of tissue contiguous with the galea in the scalp and the platysma in the neck. It envelops the facial musculature and extends anteriorly to attach to the dermis in the cheek area via firm fibrous connections. Superiorly, the SMAS is firmly adherent to the zygomatic arch and continuous with the superficial temporal fascia, also known as the temporoparietal fascia. In the preauricular area it can be recognized as the shiny layer overlying the parotidomasseteric fascia, which is the superficial layer of the deep cervical fascia.

Mitz and Peyronnie first described the SMAS in 1976 as a dynamic fibromuscular web, and although procedures had been performed on the SMAS prior to this, repositioning and suspension of the SMAS has been one of the most significant advancements in face-lift surgery over the last three decades. One-layer rhytidectomies were skin only operations and have been abandoned by most surgeons. Over time, skin tends to re-

stretch; however, because the SMAS is attached to the skin in the cheek, SMAS tightening has led to a much improved and long-term result.

Nerves

By virtue of elevating a skin flap, rhytidectomy disrupts many cutaneous sensory nerves causing loss of sensation which is an unavoidable consequence of face-lift surgery. Loss of sensation in the periauricular typically returns in 6–8 weeks, but in some cases can take 6–12 months.

Larger nerves at risk during face-lift surgery include the greater auricular nerve and branches of the facial nerve. The great auricular nerve is encountered as it crosses over the sternocleidomastoid muscle when elevating the flap over the superficial layer of the deep cervical fascia. Damage to this nerve results in numbness of the auricle and periauricular skin. Injury to motor branches of the facial nerve can be a devastating complication of face-lift surgery. During deep plane techniques the facial nerve branches are at greater risk.

The frontal branch of the facial nerve is at risk as it becomes more superficial over the zygomatic arch. In this area the nerve is just beneath the superficial temporal fascia and crosses the zygomatic arch halfway between the lateral canthus and the root of the helix. The marginal mandibular division of the facial nerve can also be at risk as it drops below the margin of the mandible under the platysma. The buccal branch can also be injured anterior to the parotid gland as the nerve becomes more superficial which requires that the dissection in this area be subdermal.

Adjunctive Procedures

A patient often comes in for a consultation to have just a face-lift. In the process of analyzing their face it may become apparent that their result would be enhanced by one of several additional procedures.

The patient may have significant actinic damage and fine rhytids, dermatochalasis of the upper eyelids, brow ptosis, deep melolabial folds, or microgenia. These changes may require skin resurfacing, blepharoplasty, forehead lift, autologous fat transfer to the melolabial folds, or chin implant respectively, to achieve maximal results. This is something that the surgeon is obligated to discuss with the patient and recommend that it be performed at the same time if feasible.

The Face-lift Procedure

A multitude of rhytidectomy techniques exist. Within this chapter one method will be described which has been employed effectively for more than 25 years. Deep plane rhytidectomy and composite subperiosteal face-lifts will not be discussed but can easily be reviewed in other publications. The time-proven SMAS face-lift will be detailed below.

Preparation

All patients are instructed to wash their face and hair the night before surgery with a surgical soap like pHisoHex or Hibiclens which disinfects the skin and hair. By lowering the bacterial count, the need to perform a preoperative prep is eliminated. Oral antibiotics, such as cephalosporins, are initiated one day prior to surgery and continued 7 days after surgery. No hair needs to be trimmed or shaved.

The patient is positioned on a "dental-type chair" or operating table equipped with a headrest which enables the surgeon to be seated and place the patient's head in the most optimal position, "in the lap." Incisions are carefully marked with a marking pen. The hair is then parted along these markings. Hair above the markings is retracted with 1-inch tape placed circumferentially around the head. A surgical towel is then stapled to the tape as a head drape. Hair below the marking is taped in small bunches. This prevents having to trim or cut hair while keeping it out of the operative field (Fig. 85.1).

Anesthesia

The type of anesthesia administered for rhytidectomy is determined by many variables including the patient's preference, patient's health, and surgeon's preference. In our practice local anesthesia with sedation has been the most effective and reliable technique for rhytidectomy. Local anesthesia with sedation provides adequate anesthesia, analgesia, and amnesia in a safe, monitored fashion. General endotracheal anesthesia is also a perfectly acceptable option. It does not obviate the need for injection of local anesthetic, because its vasoconstrictive properties are still necessary. General endotracheal anesthesia may introduce additional risks to the procedure. There are pros and cons to each technique. The type of anesthesia used is usually determined by the surgeon's preference and comfort level.

One hour preoperatively Valium 10–20 mg and Dramamine 100–200 mg are given orally with a sip of water. If the patient's blood pressure is greater than 130/80, 0.1 mg of clonidine (Catapres) is administered at this time. The oral preoperative medications not only relax the patient and induce some amnesia, but they avoid the need for excessive intravenous sedation during the procedure.

This type of "Twilight" anesthesia is produced using a combination of propofol and midazolam, and fentanyl is used for analgesia as well as to supplement the effects of midazolam. A bolus of propofol is usually administered just prior to injecting the local anesthetic. Local anesthesia is accomplished with 2% lidocaine containing 1:100,000 epinephrine for the incisions, 1% lidocaine containing 1:100,000 epinephrine for the flaps to be elevated, and 0.5% lidocaine containing 1:200,000 epinephrine for the submental area. A crucial component of the injection is the epinephrine, because it provides hemostasis. Both sides of the face are not injected at the same time to reduce the risk of lidocaine toxicity and decrease the side effects from the epinephrine. The time from injection to making incision is at least 15 min, in order to provide adequate time for vasoconstriction to occur.

Incisions

The incisions selected for rhytidectomy should accomplish two primary goals: (1) create imperceptible scars, (2) avoid unattractive changes in the hairline. The face-lift incisions used by the authors accomplish these two goals.

In the preauricular area, the sideburn hair should be preserved for the most part and this is accomplished by placing the incision at the inferior border of the sideburn hair or in the case of a very low sideburn placing the horizontal limb at about 15° to the horizontal and no higher than at the level of the superior insertion of the helix (Fig. 85.2). Temporal incisions should be avoided, because they provide little or no additional lift in the lateral brow or temporal region. The vector of lifting is primarily superior and slightly posterior in the preauricular area; therefore, a temporal incision will only provide lift at the ex-

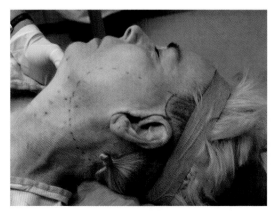

Fig. 85.1 Hair preparation and draping

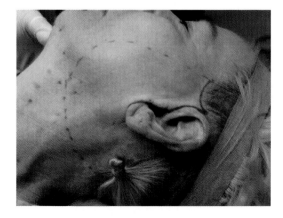

Fig. 85.2 Close-up view of the markings for the preauricular incision and intended flap length

pense of displacing the temporal hairline. Incisions that follow the anterior border of the temporal hairline should be avoided because they are difficult to camouflage. The preauricular incision then follows the natural curvature of the auricle, into the insura, along the posterior margin of the tragus, and then along the junction of the lobule and the face.

The postauricular incision should be placed onto the conchal bowl and above the postauricular sulcus (Fig. 85.3). As the incision heals and contracts the scar will end up in the postauricular sulcus. If the postauricular incision is placed in the sulcus, the resulting scar will be visible on the mastoid skin. At approximately the level where the antihelix touches the mastoid bone when it is pressed against the scalp, the postauricular incision should transition gently into the occipital area; a notch is placed where the incision crosses the postauricular sulcus to prevent horizontal scar band from formation. This will allow the postauricular hairline to not be notched and camouflage the scar. After the excess postauricular skin is removed, the flap is advanced superior and slightly posterior thus realigning the hairlines. However, when the postauricular hairline is very posterior or there is a significant amount of skin that will need to be removed from the postauricular flap, then the incision should be placed along the postauricular hairline or a few millimeters behind and parallel to the hairline. At no point should the incision be directed along the hairline toward the anterior neck skin.

Management of the Submental Area

The submental area is handled in one of two ways, and this is determined by a few different variables. These include the amount of excess skin in the neck, amount of submental fat, and presence of platysmal banding. If there is no platysmal banding, minimal submental fat, and only a minimal-to-moderate amount of excess skin, then only submental liposuction is used. If there is platysmal banding, significant submental fat, or large amount of excess skin, then a submental platysmaplasty is performed.

Submental liposuction is carried out through a small, 0.5- to 1-cm, incision (Fig. 85.4). Initially, a 1-cm flap is elevated inferiorly in the middle of the subcutaneous plane. A 3-mm blunt liposuction cannula is then passed in a radial fashion from mandibular body to mandibular body between the sternocleidomastoid muscles and down to the superior margin of the thyroid cartilage. At first pass no suction is applied and tunnels are created in the subcutaneous plane approximately 5 mm apart leaving most of the fat away from the skin. While passing the cannula, the opposite hand tents the skin up and guides the cannula through the neck. After tunnels have been created the fat to be suctioned has been separated from the skin. Suction is then applied, and the fat is removed while the cervicomental angle can be contoured. Judicious removal of fat should be exercised and a layer of fat should be preserved to allow subtle redraping of the skin. Aggressive liposuction and using the cannula with openings directed at the skin should be avoided to prevent dermal injury and possible subdermal scarring down the road. Submental liposuction will not only remove fat but also serves to elevate a large submental flap so that the excess skin can be addressed with the posterior dissection during the face-lift. The incision is closed with 5.0 fast absorbing chromic suture.

Submental platysmaplasty involves first performing submental liposuction as described above, but through a slightly larger incision, approximately 2–3 cm. The tunnels created during liposuction are then connected using Metzenbaum scissors to create a submental flap in the subcutaneous plane. Excess tissue in the midline, including subplatysmal fat and medial borders of the platysma, are clamped with a Kelly and excised. The cut edges of the platysma are then reapproximated with a running, locking 5.0 Maxon suture starting just above the thyroid cartilage and continuing to the mentum. The incision is closed with 5.0 fast absorbing chromic suture. By creating this submental corset, a sharper cervicomental angle is achieved, platysmal banding is eliminated, and excess submental tissue is removed.

Flap Elevation and Management of the SMAS

Flap length is determined by a number of factors including the amount of jowling, excess skin, elasticity of the skin, depth of melolabial folds, tobacco use, and pre-existing medical condi-

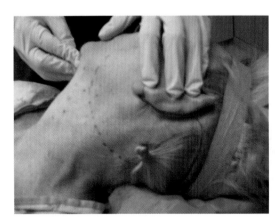

Fig. 85.3 Markings for the occipital and postauricular incisions

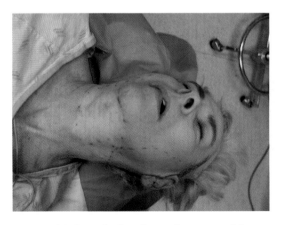

Fig. 85.4 Markings for the submental incision and flap

tions. Historically, "long" flap techniques were employed where the two cheek-neck flaps were connected in the submental area. With the advent of SMAS suspension techniques, "long" flap techniques generally have been abandoned. This decreases the following risks of using "long" flap techniques:
1) Higher incidence of postoperative hematomas
2) Potential for flap necrosis

3) Longer operative time
4) More postoperative edema and ecchymosis

"Short" flap techniques involve elevating only a limited skin flap of 4–6 cm to expose the SMAS. Then the SMAS is suspended and the excess skin is trimmed. After excision of the skin, the skin flap may only be 1–2 cm in some areas.

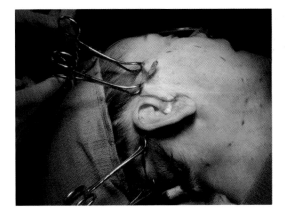

Fig. 85.5 Incisions with nonpenetrating towel clamps in place to retract the flap during elevation

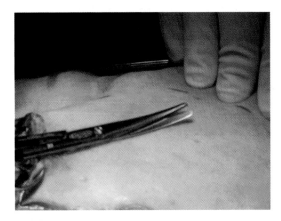

Fig. 85.6 Curved blunt-ended facelift scissors used to elevate the skin flaps

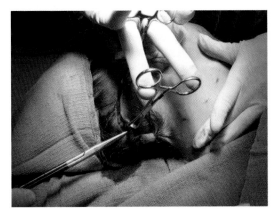

Fig. 85.7 Elevation of the flap in the subcutaneous plane

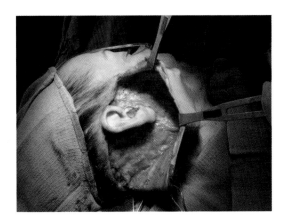

Fig. 85.8 The elevated flap

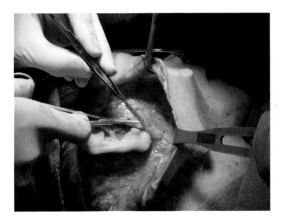

Fig. 85.9 Excising a strip of SMAS

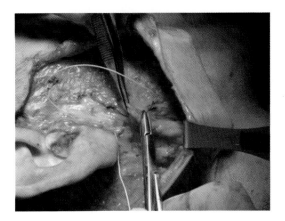

Fig. 85.10 Imbricating the SMAS with a 2.0 Dexon

Currently, the technique we most commonly use involves more of "medium" length flap with SMAS suspension. Margins of the skin flap are just lateral to the lateral canthal region and melolabial fold, to the jowl and mid-body of the mandible, connect the submental tunnels, and then extend over the mastoid to meet the inferior aspect of the occipital incision. The plane of dissection is the subcutaneous layer for the entire skin flap making sure to leave some fat down on the SMAS and some up on the dermis. Flap elevation is accomplished by placing two non-penetrating towel clamps on the sideburn incision and two on the occipital incision, then using curved blunt-ended face-lift scissors to tunnel and divide the intervening tissue (Figs. 85.5–8). In hair-bearing areas care should be taken to stay deep to the hair follicles. Optimal management of the submental area involves making a submental incision and approaching it directly in addition to the cheek-neck flap.

Multiple methods are available for SMAS management; the most common techniques are plication, imbrication, and SMAS flap maneuvers. Our preferred approach is SMAS imbrication. A strip of SMAS is excised and two ends are imbricated with a 2.0 Dexon suture (Figs. 85.9, 10). This not only advances the SMAS but suspends it in a posteriosuperior direction. This avoids potential damage to the buccal and marginal mandibular branches of the facial nerve that can occur using deep plane maneuvers while achieving the same results.

Plication of the SMAS is similar to imbrication, but does not involve excising any SMAS. The SMAS is simply suspended in a posterosuperior direction. However, this may result in bunching of tissue in the preauricular area. Plication is most applicable in the slender face that has little or no supra-SMAS fat.

Various SMAS flap techniques exist. In some cases an incision is made in the SMAS in the preauricular area extending from the zygomatic arch, around the lobule to the anterior border of the sternocleidomastoid muscle. A SMAS flap is elevated to the anterior border of the parotid. The excess SMAS is excised and the flap is secured to the tragal perichondrium and mastoid periosteum. Deep plane maneuvers are another technique that involves elevating a SMAS flap to the anterior border of the masseter and connecting this with the tissue superficial to

the platysma. However, this technique carries additional risk of injury to the buccal and marginal mandibular branches of the facial nerve.

By utilizing a SMAS technique a two-layer suspension is achieved. This offers the following advantages over the skin only techniques:

1) By suspending the SMAS a more significant and lasting improvement can be obtained.
2) SMAS suspension decreases tension on the skin closure; therefore, minimizing the risks of widened scars, skin necrosis, and overall poor wound healing.
3) SMAS techniques obviate the need for "long" flap procedures and all of the risks associated with them.

Flap Insetting and Closure

The goal of rhytidectomy is to obtain a rejuvenated appearance without creating an operated or "swept" look. To achieve this goal and avoid unsightly scars and earlobe deformities meticulous repositioning and insetting of the flaps is crucial. Tension should be placed primarily on the SMAS suspension, allowing the skin flaps to be under minimal or no tension. Around the earlobe the closure should be tension free.

In order to determine the appropriate amount of skin to excise the flap should be redraped in a posterosuperior direction over the auricle and secured at the pre- and postauricular incision lines with surgical staples (Fig. 85.11). A Pitanguy flap demarcator can be used with methylene blue to accurately and incrementally mark where the flaps will be inset (Fig. 85.12). The sideburn is marked first followed by the posterior hairline, and the excess skin is then removed (Figs. 85.13, 14). The postauricular area is then cut with Metzenbaum scissors to free the lobule, and then the preauricular flap is demarcated (Figs. 85.15, 16). It is crucial to avoid extending the incision in the postauricular skin too far in order to avoid a "pixie" ear deformity by allowing the lobule to remain "bunched" up during insetting and closure around the earlobe. The occipital area is then demarcated and excess skin is excised (Fig. 85.17). The two staples are

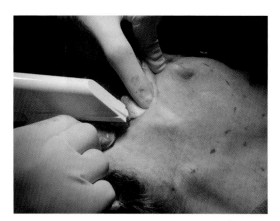

Fig. 85.11 Placing the initial postauricular staple in the redraped flap

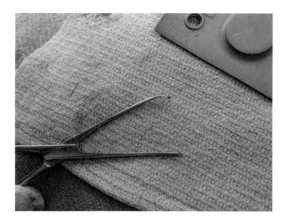

Fig. 85.12 The Pitanguy flap demarcator

then removed and the flaps and surgical bed are irrigated with saline and absolute hemostasis is obtained with bipolar cautery. At this point the opposite flap is injected. Following this the excess preauricular skin is removed leaving plenty of skin to recreate the tragus (Fig. 85.18). The tragal flap should be defatted to allow it to accurately reseat. Tisseal fibrin glue is sprayed under the flaps, and the flaps are restapled and pressure applied over them for 2 min to allow the glue to set (Figs. 85.19, 20). Closure is performed with surgical staples in the posterior hairline and sideburn; a few mattress sutures are placed around the earlobe with 5.0 plain gut, and the pre- and postauricular incisions are closed with running locking 5.0 plain gut (Fig. 85.21).

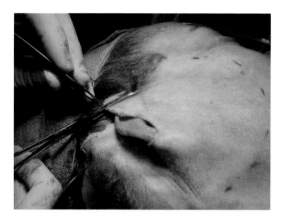

Fig. 85.13 Demarcating the sideburn

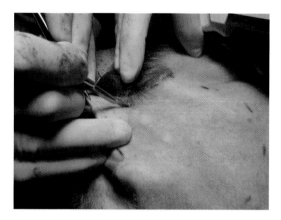

Fig. 85.14 Excising the excess sideburn skin

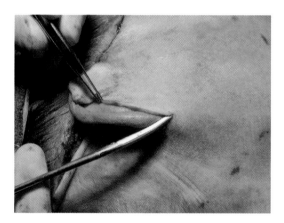

Fig. 85.15 Releasing the lobule

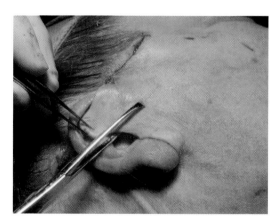

Fig. 85.16 Demarcating the preauricular flap

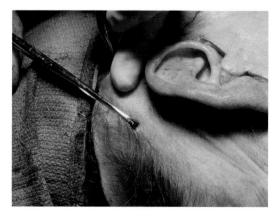

Fig. 85.17 Demarcating the occipital flap

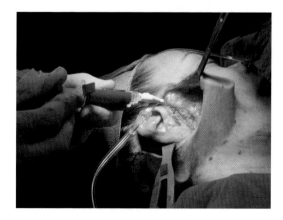

Fig. 85.18 Excising the excess preauricular skin

Postoperative Management

After surgery the patient's face and hair is cleaned, and a circumferential compressive dressing is placed for 24 h. Antibiotic ointment is applied over the pre- and postauricular incisions. Strips of cotton are then layered over the flaps; Kerlix is then wrapped around the head followed by a Coban elastic dressing (Figs. 85.22–24). The dressing should be snug but not too tight. The area over the neck should be cut to free the thyroid cartilage so the patient does not suffer dysphagia or feel suffocated. Overnight the patient is observed with nursing supervision.

On postoperative day one, the dressing is removed, and an elastic sling is placed to be worn for 1 week. Any serous fluid should be evacuated with an 18-gauge needle. The pre- and postauricular incisions are cleaned with peroxide and antibiotic ointment is applied. This routine should be carried out three times daily for the next week. All patients are given a booklet

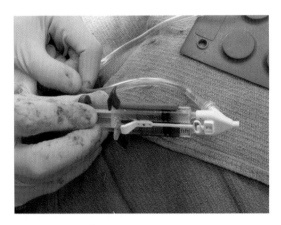

Fig. 85.19 Tisseal sprayer

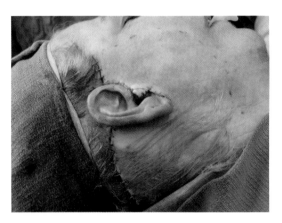

Fig. 85.20 Tisseal fibrin glue being sprayed under the flap

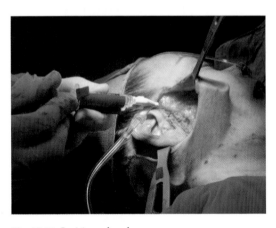

Fig. 85.21 Incisions closed

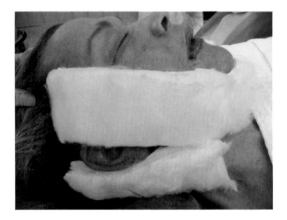

Fig. 85.22 Cotton strips in place

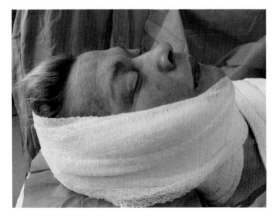

Fig. 85.23 Kerlix in place

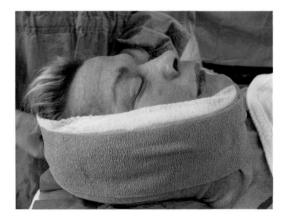

Fig. 85.24 Coban in place

that details their postoperative course including activity, medications, diet, wound care, expectations, and restrictions. This will serve as reference for the patient and family to help provide them with some reassurance.

At 7 days the patient is seen in follow-up for suture and staple removal. Sometimes only half of the staples are removed if the wound is not well healed, and in this case the patient is seen back in 2–3 days to have the rest of the staples removed. Follow-up visits are then planned for 3, 6, and 12 months. Often the patient will experience some emotional ups and downs, possibly some regrets, and probably some insecurity during the immediate postoperative period. It is very reassuring for patients to receive a call from the surgeon or the nurse on the second day after surgery to answer questions and provide reassurance. Patients should know that you are available all the time to answer questions and provide reassurance. They should feel comfortable calling or returning to the office whenever they need to. This is crucial to their long-term satisfaction.

Evaluation by an esthetician 1–2 weeks after face-lift for makeup coverage and skin care is an invaluable tool during the postoperative period. Patients should be educated about the sensations they will experience as the cutaneous neural regeneration occurs like hypersensitivity and hypesthesias. If hypertrophic scarring begins to develop, intralesional steroids should be utilized at 4–6 weeks after surgery.

Complications

Even though we know an ounce of prevention is worth a pound of cure, not all complications in surgery are preventable. However, careful patient selection, tempering perfection with conservatism, and meticulous surgical technique will all go a long way to achieving optimal results and avoiding complications. Preoperative discussions with the patient about postoperative expectations lead to more satisfied patients after surgery. If a complication does occur, it is best to discuss this with the patient and family and outline a management plan. At this point frequent office visits should be encouraged to avoid the patient feeling abandoned.

Hematoma

By virtue of elevating large flaps with significant undermining, hematomas are a potential complication in face-lift surgery. It is the most serious complication associated with rhytidectomy, and occurs between 1 and 15% of patients [2, 8]. The wide range exists because of the definition of hematomas. Expanding hematomas usually develop acutely within the first 12 h. Symptoms and signs of acute hematoma are pain more significant than usual or out of proportion to the opposite side, firmness of the flap, facial edema, and buccal ecchymosis. These types of hematomas require immediate operative intervention with evacuation, irrigation, and control of bleeding. Keeping the patient overnight with nursing observation helps to detect and treat a hematoma early, which will prevent a prolonged healing period. Following this, consideration should be given to placing a drain and a compressive dressing should be reapplied. Delay in treatment of acute hematomas may predispose the patient to flap necrosis as a result of compromised blood supply and may result in a wound infection as this material serves as an ideal culture medium.

Predisposing factors for hematoma include hypertension, nausea and vomiting, a rocky postanesthesia period, being a male, and medications that affect coagulation. Hypertension increases the incidence of hematoma by 2.6 times [11]. Careful blood pressure control is crucial to avoiding hematoma. Our patients are given 0.1–0.2 mg of clonidine preoperatively if their blood pressure is above 130/80, and postoperatively hypertension and nausea is closely monitored and controlled. A list of medications that increase the risk of bleeding is distributed to the patient preoperatively. All nonsteroidal anti-inflammatory drugs, aspirin-containing products, and vitamin E need to be stopped 2 weeks in advance of surgery and for 1 week postoperatively. It has been our experience that most antidepressants predispose patients to easy bleeding, and we advise our patients to work with their treating physician to get weaned off these drugs 2 weeks in advance of surgery. Patients on anticoagulants, like Coumadin and Plavix, need to consult with the managing physician to stop these medications before surgery, and laboratory evidence of corrected clotting capability needs to be obtained. Males are more likely to develop hematoma because of the increased blood supply to the hair follicles of the beard.

Small hematomas and seromas can be recognized during the first 24 h after surgery and such fluid collections should aspirated with an 18-gauge needle. Clots detected under the flap may be evacuated if they are still soft by making a small opening in the incision and using a liposuction cannula to retrieve the clot. Following this, pressure is applied and a compression dressing may need to be reapplied. If the hematoma has become hard, then intralesional steroids may need to be used in order to prevent potential fibrosis and skin puckering and this may take months to resolve.

Flap Necrosis

Skin flap necrosis results from compromised circulation at the distal ends of the flap where the blood supply is in a random pattern. Factors that contribute to flap necrosis are as follows:
1) Overly thin flap causing damage to the subdermal plexus
2) Too long of a flap
3) Excessive tension on the skin closure
4) History of smoking
5) Systemic medical conditions that cause vascular disease like diabetes and autoimmune disorders
6) Unrecognized hematoma
7) Excessive pressure from dressings

The most common site for skin loss is over the mastoid and the preauricular area.

Cyanosis caused by venous congestion and loss of capillary refill may lead to a poor chance of skin survival. Prevention is the best treatment for flap loss. Preoperatively, smokers should abstain from smoking for at least 4 weeks prior to and after surgery, as their risk for flap necrosis is significantly increased. Smokers should be made aware of this risk, and their flaps should be shorter, slightly thicker, and closed under absolutely no tension. If skin necrosis does occur, limited debridement of only the eschar should be undertaken, and the wound should be kept covered with antibiotic ointment to keep it moist and cleaned 2–3 times daily with peroxide solution. The patient should also be kept on antibiotics while this heals by secondary intention and have frequent office visits for observation, debridement, and reassurance. Often the resultant scar is acceptable and revision is rarely necessary.

Nerve Injury

Facial nerve injury is a very uncommon occurrence in rhytidectomy; it has been reported in 0.5–2.6% of patients undergoing face-lift surgery [3, 8]. Branches of the facial nerve at risk during face-lift are the frontal, marginal, buccal, and zygomatic in that order. Detailed understanding of facial nerve anatomy is imperative to preventing facial nerve injury. Damage to the frontal branch can be avoided with careful dissection between the sideburn and lateral canthus. The course of the frontal branch of the facial nerve can be approximated by drawing a diagonal line that starts over the parotid just under the lobule and intersect with a point halfway between the root of the helix and the lateral canthus. The branch becomes more superficial as it crosses the zygomatic arch. Marginal branch injury is sustained when subplatysmal dissection is undertaken. The buccal and zygomatic branches are at risk at the anterior border of the parotid where they become more superficial.

The greater auricular nerve is the most commonly injured nerve in face-lift surgery, occurring in 1–7% of cases [5]. Damage to this nerve will result in numbness of the lower ear and surrounding, and neuroma formation is also a possibility. This nerve is located on the anterior border of the sternocleidomastoid muscle and dissection in this area should remain superficial and should avoid violating the muscle or its investing fascia. This precaution should protect the nerve. If damage to the nerve is noted intraoperatively, then the perineural sutures should be placed to reanastomose the cut ends of the nerve.

Scarring

Scars are an unavoidable consequence of rhytidectomy; however, the ideal scars should be imperceptible. Hypertrophic scars, on the other hand, are very prominent and over time can widen and become more noticeable. They may be related to excessive tension on the closure and typically develop between 2 weeks and 3 months. Some patients with Fitzpatrick skin types IV–VI may be more susceptible to developing hypertrophic or even keloid scars. As soon as they are recognized intralesional steroids should be used and may have to be repeated two or three times. Scar revision should be avoided for 6–12 months.

Alopecia

Loss of hair can occur in the area of the sideburn and the occipital hairline. Often this is the result of traumatic alopecia caused by follicular shock, which is temporary and resolves in 3–6 months. However, permanent hair loss can result from damage to the hair follicles during flap elevation or excessive tension on the flap at closure. When alopecia does not resolve after waiting a period of 6–9 months, then hair transplants or direct excision can be performed depending on the circumstances.

Infection

Infection is a rare complication of rhytidectomy, probably because of the exceptional vascularity in the head and neck region. Unrecognized hematomas will predispose patients to wound infections. If infection occurs, it is usually a cellulitis that will respond to an extended course of oral antibiotics with good antistaphylococcal and antistreptococcal coverage. In the unusual event that an abscess develops, then incision and drainage should be performed immediately. Cultures should be taken, and consideration may need to be given to packing the wound open, and systemic antibiotics may also be necessary.

Earlobe Deformity

Satyr's ear, or Pixie ear deformity, is the result of excess traction on the lobule during closure and the healing period. The lobule develops a "pulled down" appearance, and there is no demarcation between the lobule and the facial skin. When the flaps are trimmed and inset, they should essentially create a sling around the lobule, and it should simply flip out from under the flap and rest there under absolutely no tension and appear "bunched" up.

Parotid Injury

Damage to the parotid gland is very rare; however, it can result in development of a sialocele or fistula. If a sialocele develops, then it should treated with aspiration and pressure dressings. Damage to the parotid gland recognized intraoperatively should be oversewn.

Surface Irregularities

Lumps and bumps under the flap may persist for months. These irregularities are not permanent and are usually the result of fat necrosis or localized hematomas. Intralesional steroids and massage may hasten their resolution.

A submental concavity can result if excessive submental tissue is removed and/or the platysmal bands are not brought together in the midline. This is referred to as the "cobra" deformity. This is avoided by not performing excess direct removal of fat in the midline but resorting to conservative liposuction technique.

Pain

Postoperative pain is usually minimal and very easily controlled with oral analgesics. Persistent localized pain may be caused by neuritis or neuroma, which resolves spontaneously or the neuritis is treated with nerve block, and neuromas may be excised.

Dyschromia in Flaps or Scars

Hyperpigmented scars are more likely to occur in Fitzpatrick skin types III–VI and may require intralesional steroid injections or treatment with a tunable dye laser. Hyperpigmentation or "bruising" of the flap is sometimes a concern which resolves spontaneously.

Secondary Rhytidectomy

Generally patients can expect the results of a primary rhytidectomy to last 8–10 years. This length of time is variable and is determined by many factors including not only surgical technique but also patient factors like skin quality and their overall ability to heal. Aging, however, continues after surgery despite all the best efforts, and in the first 6–12 months some relaxation of the skin may occur. Patients should be reassured that the surgery was performed in a manner to rejuvenate their appearance while retaining a natural appearance. Overtightening of tissues can result in a "pulled look" and potentially lead to complications. Even when some relaxation of the tissues occurs the individual will still look younger than their chronological age. Rejuvenation surgery should be viewed as an ongoing process, and occasional touch ups being necessary. Residual subplatysmal banding and fullness can be addressed with a platysmaplasty. Recurrence of jowls can be remedied with a cheek lift. Deepening of the melolabial folds, a situation not addressed well in rhytidectomy anyway, can be treated with autologous fat transfer or other filler materials.

In primary rhytidectomy one of the benefits of the surgery is the development of a thin fibrous layer of scar tissue between the skin and fascial layer that resists some of the relaxation of tissues and prevents some further signs of aging. During secondary rhytidectomy this fibrous layer may allow a decent plane of dissection and serve as a strong layer to resuspend the SMAS. This may be the reason why the results of secondary rhytidectomy last longer than in primary rhytidectomy. Otherwise techniques used in secondary rhytidectomy are similar to those used in primary rhytidectomy, except that scars may be removed and repositioned favorably and care needs to be taken to maintain the hairlines. During primary or secondary rhytidectomy it is essential to preserve a natural pre- and postauricular hairline and camouflage all scars appropriately.

Tips to Avoid Complications

- The risk of postoperative hematoma can be reduced with management of hypertension throughout the perioperative period and having patients discontinue all medications that have anticoagulative properties preoperatively.
- Excessively thin or long flaps, history of smoking, systemic diseases like diabetes and autoimmune disorders, excessive tension on the skin closure, steroids and other immunosuppressive therapies, excessive pressure from dressings, and unrecognized hematomas all can contribute to flap necrosis.
- Avoid excess traction on the lobule during closure to help prevent Pixie ear deformity.

Take-Home Pearls

- The cheek-neck rhytidectomy serves to remove excess skin, reposition jowling, and recreate the neckline.
- Facelift incisions should be chosen so that they result in imperceptible scars and avoid unattractive changes in the hairline.
- The strength of a facelift and longevity of the result comes from appropriate management of the SMAS.

References

1. Berman W (1991) Rhytidectomy. Aesthetic facial surgery. Lippincott, Williams and Wilkins, Philadelphia, pp 513–531
2. Lawson N (1993) The male face-lift: An analysis of 115 cases. Arch Otolaryngol Head Neck Surg 119:535–539
3. Liebman E, Webster R, Gaul J, Griffin T (1988) The marginal mandibular nerve in rhytidectomy and liposuction surgery. Arch Otolaryngol Head Neck Surg 114:179–181
4. Mangat D, McCollough E, Maack R (1986) Rhytidectomy. In: Cummings CE et al. (eds) Otolaryngology—Head and neck surgery, 2nd edn. Mosby, St. Louis, pp 532–550
5. McKinney P, Katrana D (1980) Prevention of injury to the great auricular nerve during rhytidectomy. Plast Reconstr Surg 66:675–679
6. Mitz V, Peyronnie M (1976) The superficial musculoaponeurotic system (SMAS) in the parotid and cheek area. Plast Reconstr Surg 58:80–88
7. Perkins S, Dayan S (2002) Rhytidectomy. Facial plastic and reconstructive surgery. Thieme, New York, pp 153–170
8. Rees A, Aston S (1978) Complications of rhytidectomy. Clin Plast Surg 5:109–119

85

9. Sarwer D, Crerand C, Didie E (2003) Body dysmorphic disorder in cosmetic surgery patients. Facial Plast Surg 19:7–17

10. Skoog T (1974) Plastic surgery: The aging face. Plastic Surgery: New methods and refinements. WB Saunders, Philadelphia, pp 300–330

11. Straith R, Raju D, Hipps C (1977) The study of hematomas in 500 consecutive face lifts. Plast Reconstr Surg 59:694–698

Otoplasty

Alan R. Burningham and Fred J. Stucker

86

Core Messages

- The lateral conchal resection combined with Mustarde's mattress sutures corrects most pediatric and adult osteoplasty candidates.
- A sterile orthopedic stockinet rolled down over the head and endotracheal tube after prepping allows bilateral access and complete sterile mobility of the head.
- Wet Cottonoid dressing after liberal coating with A&D ointment is a propitious dressing and serves as a cast once dry. It is routinely removed on the fifth or sixth postoperative day.
- Removal of the dressing and examination of the surgical site is done immediately with any bleeding, pain, or fever.

Contents

Introduction

The primary goal of otoplasty surgery for the protruding ear or lop ear deformity is to create a normal-appearing ear with acceptable protrusion, symmetry, and form. The most common defects that prompt surgical consultation are a poorly developed or absent antihelical fold and an abnormally large concha.

Various techniques have been employed to correct the primary defects in the protruding ear. The first published technique by Ely in 1881 consisted of a full thickness excision of skin and cartilage [1]. Many other techniques have been developed and reported over the years. In 1910, Luckett developed the concept of managing the existing cartilage to create a normal appearing ear. The most well-known technique was introduced by Mustarde in 1963 [2]. This technique, which has almost become synonymous with otoplasty, involves placement of multiple mattress sutures on the posterior surface of the pinna to create the antihelix. Furnas described a technique to address the contribution of the conchal bowl to protrusion with concha to mastoid sutures [3]. These and other techniques have produced very good results and have withstood the test of time with various modifications.

The conchal excess may be addressed in a variety of ways. The most commonly described is the conchal-mastoid suture described by Furnas [3]. In this technique the conchal cartilage is repositioned posteriorly against the mastoid periosteum with a permanent suture. This technique, however, may cause narrowing of the external auditory meatus, even if the sutures are placed properly. A modification of this technique involves splitting the conchal bowl at its base and suturing the flap to the periosteum [4]. We favor resection of the excessive cartilage from the lateral portion of the conchal bowl, as will be described below.

Surface Anatomy of External Ear

The external ear is composed of a complex cartilaginous structure covered by skin and the lobule, which does not contain cartilage. The skin over the anterior surface is densely adherent to the underlying perichondrium, while the skin on the posterior

86

surface has a loose connective tissue layer that allows for some mobility of the skin. The cartilaginous framework of the ear has a distinct shape and surface morphology (Fig. 86.1). From a structural standpoint, the primary goal in otoplasty is to create a natural-appearing antihelical fold, superior crus, fossa triangularis, and scapha.

In addition to creating a natural and normal-appearing external ear structure, the surgeon must also address the excessive protrusion of the external ear seen in the primary deformity. The normal parameters are well described [4]. Protrusion from the mastoid of greater than two centimeters is noticeable to the patient and family as a protruding ear.

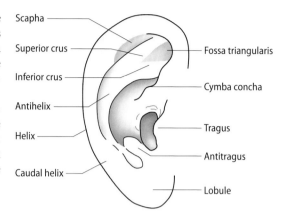

Fig. 86.1 Surface anatomy of external ear

Preoperative Evaluation

A careful preoperative inspection of the ears is necessary for achieving the optimal result from surgery. The patient's ears should be evaluated relative to each other and individually for position, size, relationship to mastoid, and each component of the ear including the helix, antihelix, concha, tragus-antitragus, and lobule. We typically perform otoplasty on patients at age 4 or 5 since the ear has developed to almost adult size, but the cartilage is still relatively thin and pliable. In addition, this is before most patients begin school, and therefore avoids the potential for ridicule by his or her peers. Preoperative full face and close-up photo-documentation is always performed. The protrusion of the ear is measured at three locations: the superior helix, mid-helix at the external canal meatus, and at the lobule. This may be done at either the preoperative evaluation or on the day of surgery.

Surgical Technique—Lateral Conchal Resection with Mattress Suture Placement

Since most patients undergoing otoplasty are children age 4–6 years old, the procedure is typically done in the operating room under general anesthesia. For adults, the procedure can easily be done under local anesthesia, usually with sedation. Intra- and postoperative antibiotics are typically administered.

When performing the case under general anesthesia in children, the patient is placed in the supine position. After induction and intubation with an oral RAE endotracheal tube, the ears are carefully examined. The amount of skin that will need to be excised is estimated by rolling the pinna posteriorly over a finger to create the desired antihelical fold. The skin excision is then marked based on the estimation, and the ends are tapered to create a fusiform shape. The posterior auricular skin is injected subcutaneously with 1% lidocaine with epinephrine 1:100,000 solution before skin preparation. The patient is then draped in the standard fashion. A sterile stockinet is placed over the head and endotracheal tube, and holes are cut in the stockinet over the ears. This permits access to both ears for comparison during the procedure while maintaining a sterile surgical field.

The posterior auricular skin is then incised with a #15 blade, and the skin and subcutaneous tissue marked for excision are dissected in a subdermal plane and removed. Next, the junction

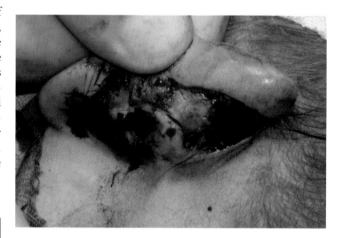

Fig. 86.2 Exposure of the cauda helix from posterior auricular incision, left ear

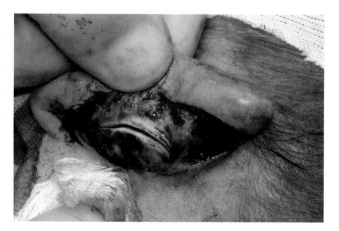

Fig. 86.3 Incision in cauda helix

of the cauda helix and the lateral conchal cartilage are exposed by sharp dissection and separated (Fig. 86.2). There is often a cleft present in this area and the spreading action of the scissors will often result in separation of the cartilage. If not, the cartilage is sharply divided at this cleft. Separation in this location insures that the natural roll of the cauda helix is preserved in the reconstructed ear.

Most patients have some degree of conchal excess preoperatively, so most of our patients undergo lateral conchal resection. The amount of cartilage removed is determined by returning the ear to the normal, anatomical position and creating the desired antihelical fold over the surgeon's finger. This maneuver allows one to see how much conchal cartilage needs to be excised to allow the midportion of the helix to set back once the antihelical fold is created. The typical width of excised cartilage varies; we typically err on a conservative resection and remove additional cartilage as necessary to produce the desired result. The incision in the cartilage extends longitudinally and parallel to the inci-

sion at the junction of the lateral conchal cartilage and the cauda helix (Fig. 86.3). The excised cartilage is crescent shaped, and the anterior perichondrium is not resected (Fig. 86.4).

The antihelix is then created using mattress sutures as described by Mustarde [2]. Three to four permanent sutures of 4-0 nylon are usually necessary to create the desired contour (Fig. 86.5). Braided sutures are avoided because of their tendency to saw through the cartilage. A Keath needle may be dipped in methylene blue to mark the desired location of the mattress sutures prior to placement. When some experience has been gained with the procedure, this step is easily eliminated. After all sutures have been placed, they are sequentially tied. A final inspection for hemostasis is performed and, the postauricular skin incision is closed with a running 4-0 chromic suture.

The same procedure is performed on the opposite side. It is useful to measure the protrusion of the first side prior to operating on the opposite side. Measurements from the mastoid to the

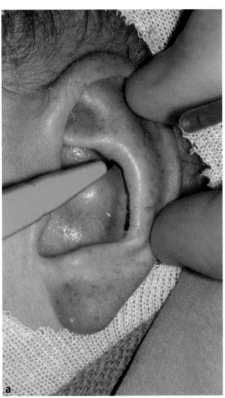
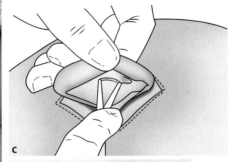
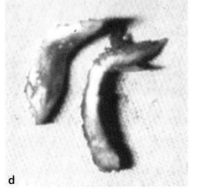

Fig. 86.4a–d Crescent-shaped conchal cartilage resection. (a) Location of conchal cartilage to be resected marked on lateral surface of left ear. (b) Intraoperative view. (c) Schematic representation. (d) Resected cartilage

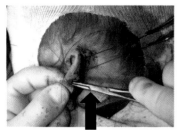

3 mattress sutures strategically placed, and tested but not tied (tagged)

once all mattress sutures are placed and tested, they are tied from top to bottom

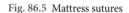

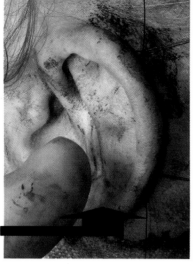

Fig. 86.5 Mattress sutures

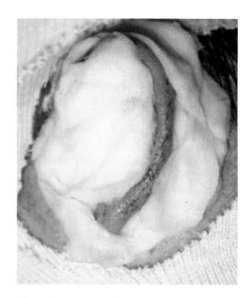

Fig. 86.6 Wet cotton dressing

lateral surface of the pinna are taken at three locations: the superior helix, superior rim of the conchal bowl, and inferior rim of the conchal bowl. All measurements should be 2 cm or less. Although it is not necessary to produce exactly the same measurements on the opposite side, the numbers serve as a useful aide when trying to create a symmetric final result. In addition, protrusion of the lobule may be addressed by simple excision of skin from the posterior lobule.

The appropriate dressing for the ear is a critical aspect of the procedure. The incision on the posterior auricle is coated with ointment, and a cotton ball coated with ointment is placed in the canal. Cotton balls soaked in warm saline are then placed into the folds and interstices of the ear and in the postauricular sulcus (Fig. 86.6). The cotton is covered with fluffed gauze and a mastoid dressing is applied. As the cotton dries and the moisture is wicked into the fluffed gauze, it creates a cast of the ear. The dressing is removed on the fifth postoperative day. The dressing is removed early and promptly if there is excessive pain or bleeding. Once the dressing is removed, the patient is instructed to wear a headband over the ears while sleeping to prevent inadvertent nocturnal trauma which can disrupt the sutures.

Summary

There are many techniques for managing the protruding ear. We believe that our remarkably simple and easily reproduced technique is both versatile and safe. In over 35 years of practice, this has been the senior author's preference for correcting the protruding ear (Fig. 86.7). A telephone survey conducted by our institution revealed that most patients were very to completely satisfied with the perception, appearance, and symmetry of their ears after the operation (unpublished data).

There are numerous advantages to the combined conchal cartilage resection and mattress suture technique. First, removing strips of cartilage along the lateral portion of the concha provides a smooth transition from the helix to the antihelix when the mattress sutures are placed. Second, cartilage removal prevents excessive projection of the newly created antihelix; therefore preventing a telephone ear deformity. Finally, cartilage resection avoids the need for concha-mastoid sutures, which have been associated with meatal stenosis.

Complications from the procedure occur in less than 3% of cases [6]. Suture failures requiring reoperation typically occur within the first 6 months after the procedure. It is important to make patients aware of this risk so that they may take the necessary precautions such as avoiding contact sports or at least wearing a headband for protection. We have not seen failures after 6 months.

Postoperative hematomas may be treated by needle drainage in the office and bolster placement (Fig. 86.8). Mild wound infections respond well to oral antibiotic therapy. Conchal skin bunching or redundancy may be treated with direct skin excision. In African-American populations caution is advised because of the possibility of keloid formation (Fig. 86.9). These may be treated with carbon dioxide laser resection followed by steroid injections if large, or steroid injections alone if small.

In summary, the combined conchal cartilage resection and mattress suture technique is a reproducible, versatile, and safe approach to the protruding ear. The technique improves the protrusion, symmetry, and form of the ear by addressing the poorly developed or absent antihelical fold and the abnormally large concha. It has been used for many years and has produced consistently good long-term results in both children and adults.

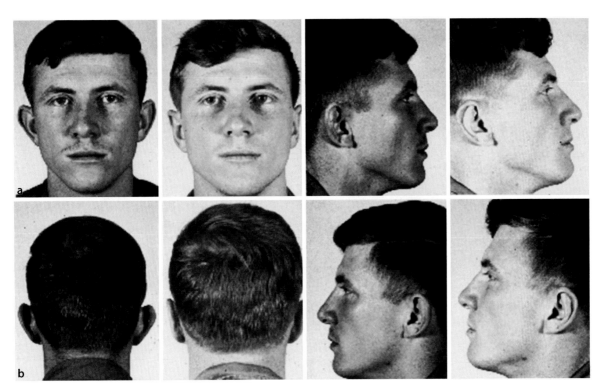

Fig. 86.7a,b Adult preoperative (*left*) and postoperative (*right*) photos. (**a**) Front view. (**b**) Side view

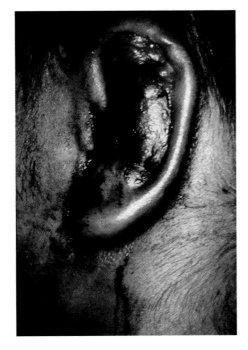

Fig. 86.8 Auricular hematoma following otoplasty

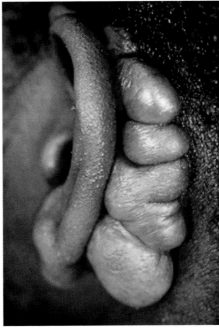

Fig. 86.9 Posterior auricular keloid following otoplasty

86

References

1. Ely ET (1881) An operation for prominence of the auricles. Arch Otolaryngol 10:97
2. Mustarde JC (1968) The correction of prominent ears using simple mattress sutures. Br J Plast Surg 16:170–176
3. Furnas DW (1968) Correction of prominent ears by concha-mastoid sutures. Plast Reconst Surg 42:189–192
4. Spira M, Stal S (1983) The conchal flap: An adjunct in otoplasty. Ann Plast Surg 11:291
5. Nachlas NE (2002) Otoplasty. In: Papel ID (ed) Facial plastic and reconstructive surgery. Thieme, New York, pp 309–321
6. Stucker FJ, Christiansen TA (1977) The lateral conchal resection otoplasty. Laryngoscope 87:58–62
7. Stucker FJ, Vora NM, Lian TS (2003) Otoplasty: An analysis of technique over a 33-year period. Laryngoscope 113:952–956

Chapter 87

Cleft Lip and Palate

Samson Lee and Jonathan Sykes

87

Core Messages

- Multidisciplinary care is necessary in the care of the cleft lip/palate patient.
- Knowledge of the embryology and anatomy aids in surgical planning and comprehension of cleft lip/palate surgical techniques for repair.
- Assessment of the cleft lip/palate patient includes ability to feed, audiologic, otologic, genetic, and speech assessment in addition to assessment of the anatomic defect.
- The Millard approach is the basis for our cleft unilateral lip and bilateral cleft lip repair.

Contents

Introduction

Cleft lip with or without cleft palate is a common congenital disorder affecting children. Patients with cleft deformities experience a multitude of problems including problems with speech, swallowing, hearing, and cosmetic appearance. The care of the cleft lip and palate patient requires a multidisciplinary approach spanning multiple specialties including speech pathology, otolaryngology, genetics, facial plastic surgery, pediatrics, orthodontics, oral maxillofacial surgery, and audiology. This chapter aims to provide the reader with the ability to understand the genetics, incidence, anatomy, embryology, and classification of these disorders. Surgical techniques to repair cleft lip and palate will be outlined.

Embryology and Anatomy

Embryology of cleft lip and palate can be divided into two important time correlates. The first stage occurs at 4–7 weeks gestation and involves the development of the structures of the upper lip, nose, and primary palate. The second stage occurs at age 8–12 weeks gestation and involves the development of the secondary palate [1] (Table 87.1).

At the end of the fourth embryonic week, the neural crest-derived facial prominences appear from the first pair of pharyngeal arches. The primary palate that forms at 4–7 weeks is formed by fusion of the median nasal prominences. The median nasal prominences fuse in the midline to form the philtrum, premaxilla, lateral and central incisors, columella, nasal tip, and hard palate anterior to the incisive foramen. The maxillary prominences form each lateral half of the upper lip, cheek, zygoma, maxilla, and the secondary palate [2].

During formation of the secondary palate, the developing tongue initially separates the palatal shelves. In normal development, palatal closure proceeds from anterior to posterior from the incisive foramen to the uvula from weeks 8–12. This development is closely intertwined with the development of the mandible. With mandibular growth, the tongue moves anteriorly and away from the palatal shelves allowing them to fuse in the midline. If there is relative micrognathia with posterior tongue malposition, cleft palate can result. Thus, a common malforma-

87

tion, which exhibits palatal clefting, is Pierre-Robin sequence (micrognathia, glossoptosis, and a U-shaped cleft palate). The severity of the cleft of the palate can be correlated to the severity of micrognathia in most cases ranging in severity from a complete cleft of the secondary palate to bifid uvula to submucous soft palate cleft [3].

Study of the normal lip is useful in dictating the ideal repair for the cleft lip deformity. The upper lip can be divided into four anatomical subunits: philtrum, upper lip, and two lateral subunits. The goal of any reconstruction of the upper lip is to utilize these subunits and to try to minimize incision lines outside of these subunits and to place scars on the borders of these subunits. The upper lip is bordered by the nasal columella and ala, which are useful adjuncts in terms of hiding incision lines to achieve the best cosmetic result possible.

The lip can be further subdivided into the round roll of epithelium (the white skin roll) just above the vermilion-cutaneous junction. The red portion of the lip can also be further divided into the wet and dry portion of the lip. The orbicularis oris muscle lies underneath the cutaneous layer in two circumferential bands of muscle within the vermilion portion of the lip and within the cutaneous portion of the lip. Recreation of these circumferential muscles from their abnormal insertions is critical in maximizing lip appearance and in achieving oral competence and the best functional result possible [4].

In the unilateral cleft lip deformity, the muscle fibers are directed superiorly along the margins of the cleft. In an incomplete cleft lip, the fibers are hypoplastic across the width of the cleft or are absent all together. There is increased muscle bulk in the lateral segment comparatively to the medial segment. The vermilion also tends to be thinner on the medial side. The pull from the abnormal insertions of the orbicularis oris muscle in combination with the relative hypoplasia of the maxilla on the cleft side results in a significant and characteristic nasal deformity as outlined in Table 87.2 [5, 6].

In the bilateral cleft, the orbicularis oris fibers are absent in the prolabium segment. Again, the abnormal insertion of the orbicularis fibers in combination with a protracted and misplaced premaxillary segment results in a characteristic nasal deformity as outlined in Table 87.3 [6, 7].

The cleft palate demonstrates abnormal insertion of the muscle fibers of the levator veli palatini and tensor veli palatini. These fibers insert into the posterior edge of the hard palate and medial cleft edges. A unilateral complete cleft palate defect has continuation of the oral and one side of the nasal cavity. A bilateral complete cleft palate defect has continuation of both sides of the nasal cavity and the oral cavity with visualization of the vomer. Secondary cleft palate defects and submucous cleft palate defects have similar patterns of abnormal muscle insertion without involvement of the bony hard palate [5].

Incidence and Genetics

The incidence varies according to ethnic background. Whites have an incidence of 1/1000, blacks 0.41/1000, Asian 2.1/1000, and Native Americans 3.6/1000. Forty-five percent of these congenital malformations occur as complete clefts of the lip, alveolus, and palate while 25% involve the cleft lip and/or alveolus only, and isolated cleft palate is about 30%. There is sex differentiation of 2:1 (M:F) for cleft lip with or without palate and 1:2 (M:F) for isolated cleft palate [8–10].

Table 87.1 Development of the secondary palate

Embryologic correlate	Anatomical structure
Median nasal process	Central upper lip (philtrum)
	Columella and Nasal Tip
	Premaxilla and Primary Palate
	Lateral and Central Incisors
Maxillary process	Lateral upper lip
	Maxilla and zygoma
	Cheek
	Secondary palate

Table 87.2 Characteristics of unilateral cleft nasal deformity

Anatomical site	Characteristic
Nasal tip	Deflects toward noncleft side with columella
	Long lateral and short medial crus of lower cartilage on cleft side
	Cleft side alar base posterior, lateral, and inferiorly displaced
	Absent nasal floor and sill (variable) on cleft side
	Nostril on cleft side horizontally oriented and widened
Septum	Caudal septum toward noncleft side
	Cartilaginous and bony septum toward cleft side
External valve	Compromised by webbing of nasal vestibule and displacement of lower lateral crus
Upper cartilages	Weakened support leads to collapse on inspiration
	Abnormal scroll
Internal valve	Compromised by weakened support of upper cartilage and septal deviation.
Upper third nose	Wide dorsum
	Bony deficiency on cleft side

Cleft lip, with or without cleft palate, can be further divided into syndromic versus nonsyndromic. Nonsyndromic is defined as an inherited disorder without other recognizable anomalies. Nonsyndromic cleft lip, with or without palate, is not associated with other head and neck anomalies, no organ system problems, no teratogens, no environmental exposure history, and otherwise normal physical and mental well-being. These nonsyndromic cases are thought to be a result of multiple factors with no known Mendelian inheritance pattern. Recently, a group of investigators has further classified nonsyndromic clefts into further subcategorization based on expressive phenotypes associated with the cleft lip with or without cleft palate [11]. Clefting has been associated with environmental factors as well such as smoking, phenytoin, retinoids, alcohol use, folate deficiency, corticosteroid use, and valproic acid [12]. Syndromic clefting is a recognized pattern of human malformation or syndrome associated with clefting. The etiology of syndromic clefts may be single gene transmission, chromosomal aberrations, teratogenic effects, or environment. Over 200 syndromes have shown to include facial clefting as recognized syndromes [3].

Classification

Cleft lip can be classified into several categories with or without an associated cleft palate. Cleft lip can be unilateral or bilateral. A complete unilateral or bilateral cleft lip deformity extends all the way into the nasal sill. This deformity is always associated with an alveolar cleft. An incomplete cleft lip does not extend all the way into the sill. Incomplete cleft lips usually do not have orbicularis oris muscle fibers in the incomplete cleft segment. A microform cleft lip is characterized by notched mucosal margin, thin medial vermilion, elevated medial peak of Cupid's bow, furrowed philtral column, hypoplastic orbicularis oris, and possibly a minor nasal deformity. These categories apply to both unilateral and bilateral cleft lip. The palate is divided into primary (anterior to the incisive foramen) and secondary (posterior to the incisive foramen). These clefts of the palate can also be complete or incomplete. A submucous cleft palate is similar to a microform cleft lip in that there is minimal distortion of visible cutaneous structures but there is abnormal insertion of palatal musculature resulting in potential speech problems. A submucous cleft palate may or may not have a bifid uvula.

Preoperative Assessment

The most important factor on initial evaluation is the infant's ability to feed. This is a greater issue with children with cleft palate, as most children with cleft lip are able to feed normally. There is a lack of efficiency of the suck secondary to the continuity of the nasal and oral cavities. This can be addressed by specially designed nipples, such as the McGovern nipple. Babies may benefit from a palatal prosthesis. These patients should be followed weekly to ensure that they are gaining weight. In the first week of life, it is normal to lose 10% of the birth weight [13]. Most surgeons consider the rule of 10s in determining if the child is ready for surgery (Hgb 10, Wgt 10lbs, age 10 weeks). Additional anomalies or suspected syndromic background require full evaluation by a pediatric geneticist. The pinch test should be performed to assess whether the cleft will be able to be closed primarily without too much undue tension. Preoperative orthopedics can be extremely helpful in reducing the width of a cleft lip and can ultimately improve surgical results [14–16]. Lip adhesion has grown out of favor as an adjunct to repairing the wide cleft with the advent of presurgical orthopedics. If lip adhesion is performed, it usually is done at 6–8 weeks in preparation for definitive lip repair at 4–6 months. Otologic and audiologic assessment is important in cleft palate patients to ensure proper speech development. This usually requires placement of PE tubes by age 3 months. When considering multiple procedures in cleft lip and palate patients, the timeline shown in Table 87.4 is a useful guide [4].

Table 87.3 Characteristics of bilateral cleft nasal deformity

Anatomical site	Characteristic
Nasal tip	Short columella with deviation towards less involved side. Long lateral crus and shortened medial crus. Splaying of medial crura resulting in bifid tip. Alar bases are posterior, inferior, and laterally displaced. Nostrils are wide and horizontally oriented.
Septum	Deviated towards less involved side.
External valve	Compromised by displacement of lower cartilage and webbing of nasal vestibule.
Upper cartilages	Weakened support leads to collapse on inspiration. Abnormal scroll.
Internal valve	Compromised by weakened support of upper cartilage and septal deviation.
Upper third nose	Wide dorsum. Bony deficiency on both sides.

Table 87.4 Timetable for surgical management of cleft lip and palate

Age	Procedure
3 months	Repair of cleft lip, initial tip rhinoplasty, and placement PE tubes if required (Grommet)
10–15 months	Repair of cleft palate and replacement of PE tubes (T-tubes)
4–6 years	Correction of velopharyngeal insufficiency if present
9–11 years	Alveolar bone grafting
16–18 years	Formal cleft rhinoplasty and orthognathic surgery

Procedure Unilateral Cleft Lip Repair and Rhinoplasty (Millard Rotation and Advancement Flap)

In 1952, Tennison described a technique based on Z-plasty to lengthen the lip and close the cleft lip defect [17]. Randall refined this technique based on the Z-plasty termed the triangular repair [18]. The most commonly used technique for repair of the unilateral cleft lip is the Millard rotation advancement flap introduced in the mid-1950s [19]. The initial procedure is usually preceded by placement of tympanostomy tubes in cases associated with a cleft palate. Prior to placement of the tubes, local anesthetic injection of 1% lidocaine with 1:100,000 epinephrine is used sparingly to aid in vasoconstriction of the surgical field. The patient is marked at the key points as originally described by Millard (Table 87.5, Fig. 87.1a). This allows the delineation of the various flaps (Fig. 87.1b) which will be utilized for repair (Table 87.6) [19].

The distance between points 1 and 2 is measured, should normally be between 2 and 4 mm, and is used to establish the location of point 3, which represents the high point of Cupid's bow on the cleft side of the upper lip. Thus, the distance from point 1 to 2 is equal to the distance from point 1 to 3. Point 3 marks the starting point of the incision for the "A" or rotation flap.

The "A" flap is generated by an incision from point 3 to point 5. Point "x," the back cut point, is made at a variable distance from point 5 and is determined by estimating the amount of tissue needed to create symmetric philtral ridges and to make up for the discrepancy in vertical height of the lip at the philtral ridge. Point "x" should never cross the philtral ridge on the

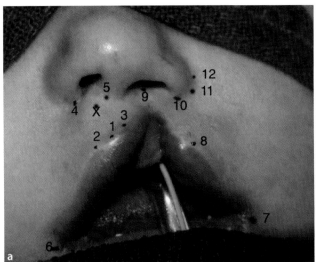

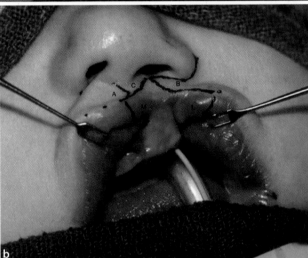

Fig. 87.1 **a** Intraoperative photograph of patient with left incomplete unilateral cleft lip. The standard skin markings *1–12* plus *X* are denoted on this patient. **b** Intraoperative photograph of the same patient with a left unilateral cleft lip and palate. The incision lines have been drawn out and the major flaps *A* and *B* and the minor flaps *C*, *M*, and *L* are shown

Table 87.5 Reference points for Millard rotation advancement cleft lip repair

Point	Definition
1	Low point of Cupid's bow
2	Peak of Cupid's bow, noncleft side (NCS)
3	Medial peak of Cupid's bow, cleft side (CS)
4	Alar base (NCS)
5	Columellar base
X	Backcut point
6	Commissure (NCS)
7	Commissure (CS)
8	Lateral peak of Cupid's bow (CS)
9	Medial tip of advancement flap
10	Midpoint of alar base
11	Lateral alar base
12	Maximum extent of alar incision

Table 87.6 Reference points for Millard rotation advancement cleft lip repair

Point	Flap
A	Downward medial rotational flap
B	Lateral advancement flap
C	Columellar base soft tissue (noncleft side)
M	Medial mucosal flap
L	Lateral mucosal flap

noncleft side but should lie medial to it, so that the back cut of the rotation flap runs parallel and medial to the normal philtral ridge on the noncleft side. This helps to maintain a scar-free philtral ridge on the noncleft side and improves the ultimate cosmetic result of cleft lip repair.

Point 8 marks the starting point for the incision for the "B" or advancement flap. Point 9 is the medial-most point of the advancement flap and is placed at a distance from point 8 that is equivalent to the distance between point 3 and point 5 + "x." Thus, the philtral ridge is formed by the union of the cleft edge on the side of the advancement flap (line 8 to 9) and the cut edges of the rotation flap on the noncleft side (line 3 to x). It is helpful to measure the distance from point 4 to 5 in order to create symmetry of the alar bases by measuring point 5 to 10. It is also helpful to measure the vertical distance from points 2 to 4 which should equal points 8 to 10. This will help ensure equal vertical heights on both sides of the cleft.

Undermining is also performed along the mucosal portion of the lip to separate the orbicularis fibers from the mucosal surface to help prevent a whistle deformity. Undermining is performed on the face of the maxilla to provide release of both the medial rotational and lateral advancement sides. This also allows release of the misaligned orbicularis fibers into a more correct horizontal orientation. A complete alotomy should be performed with a cut adjacent to the inferior turbinate along the pyriform aperture to allow full mobility of the advancement flap. Care should be taken to avoid injury to the infraorbital nerve.

The ala is then actively repositioned by suturing it to the nasal septum with a long-acting monofilament suture. Additional undermining of the nasal tip can be performed through the alar base incision or along the medial advancement side to help release the lower cartilages from the overlying skin to help provide nasal tip symmetry. The mucosal incisions are then closed with advancement of the "m" and "l" flaps into both gingivolabial sulci to help provide fullness to the lip. Next the cutaneous vermilion border is precisely realigned. The "C" flap can be set into the nasal sill if necessary. The superior aspect of the lateral advancement flap is advanced into the superior junction of the border between the medial rotational flap and the "C" flap. Attention is then turned to the optional placement of bolster sutures through the nasal tip to help provide symmetry of the nasal domes. This is described in detail in other references [20, 21].

Bilateral Cleft Lip Repair

Lip adhesion or presurgical orthopedics can be used to help reposition the premaxilla in patients with bilateral cleft lip deformities. Occasionally, osteotomies are required in order to reset the premaxilla posteriorly into its native position [22, 23]. The Millard technique is our most common approach to bilateral cleft lip deformities (Fig. 87.2) [7].

Point 1 is the midpoint of the vermilion-cutaneous junction of the prolabium. Both high points of Cupid's bow (points 2 and 3) are measured 2–3 mm on each side of point 1. Two slightly curvilinear lines connect points 2 and 3 to points 4 and 5, respectively. These planned incision lines represent the new phil-

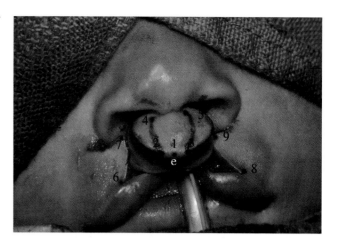

Fig. 87.2 Intraoperative photograph of a patient with a bilateral cleft lip and palate. In this patient, the lateral lip flaps have been cut and the markings for the height of the lateral lip flaps are denoted. The central prolabium and premaxilla have been marked but not yet incised. The markings on the central segment are also shown

tral edges. The two flaps lateral to these flaps will be used to reconstruct the medial and inferior aspects of the nasal sill. Points 6 and 8 are marked at the vermilion cutaneous junction on the lateral lip. The distance from points 6 to 7 should be the same as the distance from points 2 to 4. The distance from points 8 to 9 should equal the distance from points 3 to 5. A vermilion flap is created on each side to recreate the vermilion portion of the flap. These edges will join the "e" flap centrally (Fig. 87.2).

After markings are made, the area is infiltrated with 1% lidocaine with 1:100,000 epinephrine. Incisions are made along the mid-prolabial flap, which are based superiorly along with the "e" flap. The remaining vermilion of the prolabial segment is pedicled inferiorly and dissected free. The lateral lip incision and flaps are created and extended along the alar crease. Alotomies are performed bilaterally similar to a unilateral repair dissecting on the face of the maxilla with care to protect the infraorbital nerve. Lateral gingivobuccal sulcus incisions are created for further relaxation. This allows mobilization of the orbicularis oris muscle to the midline. The vermilion flap is sutured superiorly to mucosally line the anterior premaxilla. The lateral lip mucosal flaps are sutured in the midline with care taken to resuture the orbicularis muscle in the midline. The central prolabial skin flap is placed into position between the lateral lip segments creating the philtrum. The small "e" flap is tucked behind the lateral vermilion flaps to recreate the central tubercle. The two lateral prolabial flaps are sutured to recreate the medial and inferior nasal sill.

Unilateral Cleft Palate Repair by Two-Flap Palatoplasty [24]

Local anesthetic injection of 1% lidocaine with 1:100,000 epinephrine is used to inject the palate area first, followed by place-

---

ment of tympanostomy tubes, which allows the epinephrine to have time to take effect. Initially, the uvula is trimmed medially slightly. The incisions along the medial border of the cleft are performed just slightly favoring the oral side in order to avoid short changing the nasal layer in terms of closure (Fig. 87.3a). The incisions are carried from the tip of the uvula to the primary palatal defect anteriorly. Lateral incisions are made around the curvature of the maxillary tuberosity along the alveolar ridge toward the first medial cut. Care must be taken to avoid entry into a tooth bud. Dissection is carried all the way medially and then carried posteriorly towards the anterior extent of the secondary palate with care taken to protect the greater palatine neurovascular foramen (Fig. 87.3b). Additional mobility is now gained by dissecting behind posteriorly to the greater palatine neurovascular foramen to gain more mobility in the flap medially. Additional dissection can be performed with a right-angled scissors in the space of Ernst to separate the nasal layer from the muscular layer and provide medial mobility. The hamulus can be fractured if necessary to provide improved medial movement of the flap.

Additional nasal layer can be obtained from the nasal septum or vomer if necessary. Once adequate mobility is ensured, the flaps are closed sequentially starting with the nasal layer. 4-0 PDS suture is used to reapproximate the muscular layer of the palate (Fig. 87.3c). Additional 4-0 Vicryl sutures are used to close the mucosal oral layer with several deep-tacking sutures

performed grabbing all three layers to eliminate dead space. Additional tacking sutures can be performed anteriorly and laterally to the alveolar ridge oral mucosa (Fig. 87.3d). There is frequently quite a bit of empty space between the tacking sutures. This does not present a problem as this area granulates within several weeks. Bilateral cleft palate repair is similar to two-flap palatoplasty with the exception of bilateral vomer flaps, which are used to help close the nasal layer. Postoperative care consists of arm restraints and syringe feeding for 2-3 weeks.

Secondary Cleft Plate Repair with Furlow Palatoplasty [25]

The double opposing Z-plasty is drawn with methylene blue. The incision takes place with care taken not too close the edge of the hard palate. If the defect is an isolated soft palate defect the incision is along the medial surface of the oral mucosal side. If the procedure is being performed for a submucous cleft, the palate is incised through and through initially. In general there is a thicker fibrofatty layer between the oral mucosal surface and the muscle layer, while there is minimal tissue between the muscle of the soft palate and the nasal mucosa making the dissection more difficult (Fig. 87.4a). The abnormal insertion of the levator veli palatini muscle fibers are released from their attachments to the bony hard palate so that they will be reoriented in the

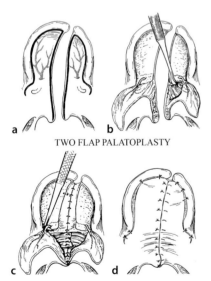

TWO FLAP PALATOPLASTY

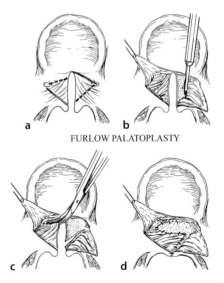

FURLOW PALATOPLASTY

Fig. 87.3a–d Two-flap palatoplasty. **a** The incisions for two-flap palatoplasty. Note that the lateral incision goes around the hamular process, extents on to anterior hard palate just behind the incisal ridge and extents on to the medial cleft edge down through the uvula. **b** Flaps are elevated with care being taken to identify and preserve the greater palatine neurovascular structures. **c** After elevation of all flaps the nasal layer is closed from the anterior palate to the uvula and the soft palate musculature is realigned into an optimal position. **d** Two-flap palatoplasty after closure of the oral layer of the palate. Note that the two palatal flaps are positioned with lateral coapting suture to the alveolus ridge

Fig. 87.4a–d Furlow palatoplasty. **a** Incisions for furlow palatoplasty are shown. The oral incisions are noted by a *straight line* and the nasal incisions for the double reversing z-plasty are shown with a *dotted line*. **b** Elevation of the oral and nasal flaps is accomplished. Note that the soft palatial musculature is elevated with the oral flap on the patients *left* side and the soft palatial musculature is allowed to remain with the nasal mucosa on the patients *right* side. **c** Realigning of soft palate musculature in posterior sling in a z-plasty fashion. d Closure of all oral mucosal layers in a z-plasty so as to lengthen the palate

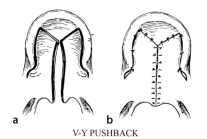

V-Y PUSHBACK

Fig. 87.5a,b V-to-Y Pushback. **a** Incisions noted in *dark black lines* for three-flap palatoplasty V-to-Y pushback. **b** Lengthening of the palate achieved after elevation of all flaps and closure of these flaps creating additional length to the soft palate

correct direction when reconstructing the palate (Fig. 87.4b). Once the flaps have been raised, the double opposing Z-plasty is performed with tenotomy scissors with care taken not to get to close to the posterior margin of the hard palate which makes closure of the nasal layer difficult. The nasal layer is closed first with the apex of the Z-plasty recreated first to redistribute the tension evenly along the length of the incision. The muscle layer is closed separately followed by the oral mucosal layer; care is taken to recreate the uvula (Fig. 87.4c, d). Postoperative instructions are similar for two-flap palatoplasty. Complications are similar as well.

A V-Y pushback technique is useful for wider secondary clefts and for those that extend partially into the hard palate. The oral mucoperiosteal flaps in this closure lie opposite the primary canine teeth. Dissection of the oral and nasal flaps is similar to the two-flap palatoplasty (Fig. 87.5a). Use of mucosa overlying the vomer is advocated if extension of the cleft goes into the hard palate. The velar musculature should be dissected free from the posterior aspect of the hard palate and closure is performed as described in the two-flap palatoplasty procedure (Fig. 87.5b).

Tips to Avoid Complications for Cleft Lip Repair

- Measure preoperatively to ensure symmetric vertical height between marked points.
- Wide undermining improves mobility of the flap and reduces tension on the wound repair.
- Remove sutures early to avoid suture marks.
- Use arm restraints and syringe feeding to avoid stress on the wound.
- Place several muscle approximation sutures to provide strength to the closure.

Tips to Avoid Complications in Cleft Palate Repair

- Avoid injury to the greater palatine neurovascular bundle.
- The oral layer is much thicker than the nasal layer with a thick layer of fibrofatty tissue making the nasal layer dissection more difficult.
- Avoid undue tension by wide but careful undermining.
- Use arm restraints and syringe feeding to avoid trauma to the wound.
- Pre- and postoperative steroids help reduce swelling and greatly improve patient recovery time.

Take-Home Pearls

- Surgical success relies on knowledge of the anatomy and ability to deviate from standard technique when necessary.
- Multidisciplinary care is in the patient's best interests including other medical specialty evaluations.

References

1. McCarthy J (1990) Cleft lip and palate and craniofacial anomalies. In: McCarthy JG (ed) Plastic surgery, vol 4. WB Saunders, Philadelphia, pp 2515–2552
2. Gaare JD, Langman J (1977) Fusion of nasal swellings in the mouse embryo: Surface coat and initial contact. Am J Anat 150:461–475
3. Gorlin R, Cohen M, Levin L (1990) Syndromes of the head and neck, 3rd edn. Oxford University Press, New York
4. Sykes J (2002) Diagnosis and treatment of cleft lip and palate deformities. In: Papel I (ed) Facial plastic and reconstructive surgery, 2nd edn. Thieme, New York, pp 813–829
5. Sykes J, Senders C (1993) Anatomy of the cleft lip, palate, and nasal deformities. In: Myers A (ed) Biological basis of facial plastic surgery. Thieme, New York, pp 57–71
6. Coleman J, Sykes J (2002) Cleft lip rhinoplasty. In: Papel I (ed) Facial plastic and reconstructive surgery. Thieme, New York, pp 830–843
7. Millard D (1977) Cleft craft: The evolution of its surgery, vol 2. Bilateral and rare deformities. Little Brown, Boston
8. Gorlin RJ CM, Levin LS (1990) Syndromes of the head and neck, 3rd edn. Oxford University Press, New York
9. Dionsisopoulos T, Williams H (1997) Congenital anomalies of the mouth, palate, and pharynx. In: Tewfik T (ed) Congenital anomalies of the ear, nose, and throat. Oxford University Press, New York, pp 229–242
10. Forrester MB, Merz RD (2004) Descriptive epidemiology of oral clefts in a multiethnic population, Hawaii, 1986–2000. Cleft Palate Craniofac J 41:622–628

87

11. Weinberg SM, Neiswanger K, Martin RA, et al. (2006) The Pittsburgh oral-facial cleft study: Expanding the cleft phenotype. Background and justification. Cleft Palate Craniofac J 43:7–20

12. Eppley BL, van Aalst JA, Robey A, Havlik RJ, Sadove AM (2005) The spectrum of orofacial clefting. Plast Reconstr Surg 115:101e–114e

13. Senders C, Sykes J (1999) Unilateral cleft lip. In: Cotton RT Myer C (eds) Practical pediatric otolaryngology, 1st edn. Lippincott-Raven, Philadelphia, pp 789–807

14. Reisberg DJ (2004) Prosthetic habilitation of patients with clefts. Clin Plast Surg 31:353–360

15. Evans CA (2004) Orthodontic treatment for patients with clefts. Clin Plast Surg 31:271–290

16. Grayson BH, Maull D (2004) Nasoalveolar molding for infants born with clefts of the lip, alveolus, and palate. Clin Plast Surg 31:149–158, vii

17. Tennison C (1952) The repair of the unilateral cleft lip by the stencil method. Plast Reconstr Surg 9:115–119

18. Randall P (1959) A triangular flap operation for the primary repair of unilateral clefts of the lip. Plast Reconstr Surg 23:331–336

19. Millard D (1976) Cleft craft: The evolution of its surgery. Vol. I. The unilateral deformity. Little Brown, Boston, pp 79–88

20. Sykes J, Senders C (1990) Surgery of the cleft lip nasal deformity. Op Tech Otolaryngol Head Neck Surg 1:219–224

21. Senders C, Sykes J (1995) Surgical treatment of the unilateral cleft nasal deformity at the time of lip repair. Facial Plast Surg Clin North Am 3:69–77

22. Aburezq H, Daskalogiannakis J, Forrest C (2006) Management of the prominent premaxilla in bilateral cleft lip and palate. Cleft Palate Craniofac J 43:92–95

23. Mulliken JB, Wu JK, Padwa BL (2003) Repair of bilateral cleft lip: Review, revisions, and reflections. J Craniofac Surg 14:609–620

24. Bardach J, Salyer K (1987) Surgical techniques in cleft lip and palate. DC Decker, Philadelphia

25. Furlow L (1986) Cleft Palate repair by double opposing Z-plasty. Plast Reconstr Surg 78:724–736

Subject Index